Haematology and Blood Transfusion
Hämatologie und Bluttransfusion 40

Springer
Berlin
Heidelberg
New York
Barcelona
Budapest
Hong Kong
London
Milan
Paris
Santa Clara
Singapore
Tokyo

T. Büchner W. Hiddemann B. Wörmann
G. Schellong J. Ritter U. Creutzig (Eds.)

Acute Leukemias VI

Prognostic Factors and Treatment Strategies

With 298 Figures and 288 Tables

Springer

Prof. Dr. T. BÜCHNER
Department of Internal Medicine

Prof. Dr. G. SCHELLONG
Prof. Dr. J. RITTER
Priv. Doz. Dr. U. CREUTZIG
Department of Pediatrics
University of Münster
Albert-Schweitzer-Strasse 33
48145 Münster
Germany

Prof. Dr. W. HIDDEMANN
Priv. Doz. Dr. B. WÖRMANN
Department of Internal Medicine
University of Göttingen
Robert-Koch-Strasse 40
37075 Göttingen
Germany

ISSN 0949-7021
ISBN-13: 978-3-642-64379-8 e-ISBN-13: 978-3-642-60377-8
DOI: 10.1007/978-3-642-60377-8

Softcover reprint of the hardcover 1st edition 1997

Cover design: Design & Production GmbH, Heidelberg

Typesetting: Thomson Press (India) Ltd., Madras

SPIN: 10528377 23/3134/SPS – 5 4 3 2 1 0 – Printed on acid-free paper

Preface

Under the old and new subtitle "Prognostic Factors and Treatment Strategies" this 6th volume of ACUTE LEUKEMIAS, again, provides new updates from major multicenter clinical trials under the aspect of both, the effects of different treatments tested and different biologic characteristics of the individual diseases. Thus, intensified chemotherapy, the use of growth factors, the induction of differentiation, and the transplantation of stem cells are addressed. Among biologic characteristics, cytomorphology, cytogenetics, molecular genetics, immunophenotypes and minimal residual disease are evaluated according to their prognostic relevance as well as potential therapeutic consequences. Beyond the anti-leukemic treatment strategies, prevention and treatment of opportunistic infections representing an important part of the management for acute leukemias is updated in an own section. In addition, new data from laboratory work on leukemia cell biology and pharmacology contribute to the basis of further clinical research and progress against acute leukemias.

The high quality of inputs by scientists from around the world together with the special concept of the series ACUTE LEUKEMIAS, again, helped to make this book a useful state of the art report for both, clinical oncologists and basic scientists.

The editors wish to thank Beate Kosel for her excellent contribution as a coordinator of the editorial work.

September, 1996

T. Büchner · W. Hiddemann · B. Wörmann
J. Ritter · U. Creutzig

Table of Contents

Leukemia Cell Biology: Cytokines

Leukemia Cell Biology

Residual Leukemia

New Strategies: Antifungal Treatment

Pharmacology

ALL in Children

ALL in Adults

AML in Children

Secondary Leukemia, Myelodysplastic Syndrome

Authors and Institutions

AMADORI, S.
Department of Human Biopathology, Division of Hematology, University of Rome, University 'La Sapienza', Via Benevento 6, 00161 Rome, Italy

ANDREEVA, S.
Kiev Research Institute of Hematology and Blood Transfusion, Kiev, Ukraine

ANNINO, L.
Department of Human Biopathology, Division of Hematology, University of Rome, Via Benevento 6, 00161 Rome, Italy

ARCHIMBAUD, E.
Hematology Service, Hospital Edouard Herriot, 69437 Lyon Cedex 03, France

AUL, C.
Department of Internal Medicine, Division of Hematology and Oncology, Heinrich-Heine-University, Moorenstraße 5, 40225 Düsseldorf, Germany

BARTRAM, C.R.
Section of Molecular Biology, Department of Pediatrics II, University of Ulm, Helmholtzstraße 10, 89081 Ulm, Germany

BEHRE, G.
Department of Hematology/Oncology, University of Göttingen, Robert-Koch-Straße 40, 37075 Göttingen, Germany

BELOGUROWA, M.
Department of Pediatric Oncology and Hematology, Center of Advance Medical Technologies, Hospital Nr. 31, Pr. Dinamo 3, St. Petersburg, Russia

BERGMANN, L.
Department of Internal Medicine, Division of Hematology and Oncology, J.W. Goethe University, Theodor-Stern-Kai 7, 60590 Frankfurt/M., Germany

BEYER, J.
University Hospital Rudolf Virchow, Division Hematology/Oncology, Free University of Berlin, Spandauer Damm 130, 14050 Berlin, Germany

BIONDI, A.
Department of Pediatrics, University of Milano, 'Fondazione M. Tettamanti, Ospedale Nuovo San Gerardo, Via Donizetti, 106, 20052 Monza, MI, Italy

BISHOP, J.
Division of Haematology and Medical Oncology, Peter MacCallum Cancer Institute, St. Andrews Place, East Melbourne, Victoria 3002, Australia

BOOS, J.
Department of Pediatrics, Pediatric Hematology and Oncology, University of Münster, Albert-Schweitzer-Straße 33, 48149 Münster, Germany

BORKHARDT, A.
Children's University Hospital, Hematology/Oncology, Feulgenstraße 12, 35392 Giessen, Germany

BRETTREICH, S.
Children's University Hospital, Hematology/Oncology, Feulgenstraße 12, 35385 Giessen, Germany

BÜCHNER, T.
Department of Internal Medicine, University of Münster, Albert-Scheitzer-Straße 33, 48149 Münster, Germany

BURNETT, A.
Department of Haematology, University of Wales College of Medicine, Health Park, Cardiff CF4 4XN, UK

BUSKE, C.
Department Internal Medicine, Hematology and Oncology, University of Göttingen, Robert Koch-Straße 40, 37075 Göttingen, Germany

CAMITTA, B.
Pediatric Hematology/Oncology, Midwest Children's Cancer Center, Medical College of Wisconsin, 8701 Watertown Plank Road, Milwaukee, WI 53226, USA

CHUDOBA, I.
Institute of Human Genetics and Anthropology, University of Jena, Kollegiengasse 10, 07747 Jena, Germany

CHYBICKA, A.
Department of Children Hematology and Oncology, Wroclaw University of Medicine, Bujwida 44, 50-345 Wroclaw, Poland

CREUTZIG, U.
Department of Pediatrics, Hematology/Oncology, University of Münster, Albert-Schweitzer-Straße 33, 48149 Münster, Germany

DEERBERG. J.
Department of Human Genetics, University of Kiel, Schwanenweg 24, 24105 Kiel, Germany

DEGOS, L.
University Hospital of Hematology, Hospital Saint-Louis, 1, Avenue Claude Vellefaux, 75010 Paris, France

DEMIDOVA, L.A.
National Research Center for Hematology, Novozykowsky 40, 125167 Moscow, Russia

DENGLER, R.
Medical Clinic, Division Hematology/Oncology, University of Munich, Ziemssenstraße 1, 80336 Munich, Germany

DE WITTE, Th.
Department of Internal Medicine, Division of Hematology, University Hospital Nijmegen, Geert Grooteplein 8, P.O. Box 9101, 6500 HB Nijmegen, The Netherlands

DIGHIERO, G.
Blood Transfusion Center, Institute Pasteur, 28, Rue du Dr. Roux, 75724 Paris, France

DONSKAYA, S.
Kiev Institute of Medical Training, Regional Hospital, Pediatric Hematology/Oncology, ul. Baggowutowskaja 1, 252022 Kiev, Russia

DREYLING, M.
University of Chicago, Department of Hematology, 5841 South Maryland Avenue, MC 2115, Chicago, IL 60637, USA

DUBROVINA, E.
Research Institute for Pediatric Hematology, 117, Leninsky Avenue, Moscow 117513, Russia

ECKHOF-DONOVAN, S.
Children's Hospital, Division of Pediatric Hematology and Oncology, Heinrich-Heine-University, Moorenstraße 5, 40225 Düsseldorf, Germany

EINSELE, H.
Medical Hospital, Department II and Section of Transplantimmunology, Otfried-Müller-Straße 10, 72076 Tübingen, Germany

ELSTNER, E.
UCLA School of Medicine, Division of Hematology/Oncology, Cedars-Sinai Medical Center, 8700 Beverly Blvd., Los Angeles, CA 90048-1865, USA

ESTEY, E.
Department of Hematology, The University of Texas M.D. Anderson Cancer Center, 1515 Holcombe Blvd., Box 47, Houston, TX 77030, USA

FENAUX, P.
University Hospital of Lille, Department of Internal Medicine, Division of Hematology, Place de Verdun, 59037 Lille, France

Fiere, D.
Hematology Service, Hospital Edouard Herriot, Pav. E bis, Place d'Arsonval, 69437 Lyon Cedex 03, France

Fink, F.M.
Department of Pediatrics, University of Innsbruck, Anichstraße 35, 6020 Innsbruck, Austria

Gaynon, P.
UW Children's Hospital, University of Wisconsin, 600 Highland Avenue, K4/430, Madison, WI 53792-4672, USA

Gieseler, F.
Department of Internal Medicine, University of Würzburg, Klinikstraße 8, 97070 Würzburg, Germany

Gluzman, D.F.
Institute of Experimental Pathology, Oncology and Radiobiology, Vasilkovskaya Str. 45, 252022 Kiev, Ukraine

Goldstone, A.H.
The University College London Hospitals, Dept. of Clinical Haematology, University College Hospital, Grafton Way, London WC1E 6 AU, UK

Griesinger, F.
Department of Internal Medicine, Hematology/Oncology, University of Göttingen, Robert-Koch-Straße 40, 37075 Göttingen, Germany

Griffin, J.
Division of Hematologic Malignancies, Dana-Farber Cancer Institute Division of Tumor Immunology, 44 Binney Street, Boston, MA 02115, USA

Haase, D.
Department of Hematology and Oncology, University of Göttingen, Robert-Koch-Straße 40, 37075 Göttingen, Germany

Haferlach, T.
Second Medical Department, Christian-Albrechts-University, Chemnitzstraße 33, 24116 Kiel, Germany

Harbott, J.
Oncocytogenetic Laboratory, University of Gießen, Children's Hospital, Feulgenstraße 12, 35385 Gießen, Germany

Harousseau, J.L.
University Hospital, Department of Hematology, University of Nantes, Place Alexis Ricordeau, B.P. 1005, 44035 Nantes Cedex 01, France

Hasle, H.
Department of Pediatrics, Odense University Hospital, 5000 Odense C, Denmark

Heil, G.
Department of Internal Medicine III, Medical Hospital, University of Ulm, Robert-Koch-Straße 8, 89081 Ulm, Germany

Heinecke, A.
Department of Medical Biostatistics, University of Münster, Domagkstraße 9, 48149 Münster, Germany

Heinemann, V.
Department of Internal Medicine III, Hematology, University Hospital Großhadern, University of Munich, Marchioninistraße 15, 81377 München, Germany

Heußner, P.
Department of Internal Medicine, Division of Hematology/Oncology, Universtiy of Rostock, Ernst-Heydemann-Straße 6, 18055 Rostock, Germany

Hiddemann, W.
Department of Hematology and Oncology, University of Göttingen, Robert-Koch-Straße 40, 37075 Göttingen, Germany

Hoelzer, D.
Department of Internal Medicine, Division of Hematology, J.-W. Goethe-University, Theodor-Stern-Kai 7, 60596 Frankfurt, Germany

Holowiecki, J.
University Department of Hematology, Reymonta Straße 8, 40029 Katowice, Poland

Horowitz, M.
International Bone Marrow Transplant Registry, Statistical Center, Medical College of Wisconsin, 8701 Watertown Plank Road, P.O. Box 26509, Milwaukee, WI 53226, USA

Jahns-Streubel, G.
Department of Hematology and Oncology, University of Göttingen, Robert-Koch-Straße 40, 37075 Göttingen, Germany

Kaczorowski, S.
Department of Immunology, Maria Sklodowska-Curie Memorial Cancer Center and Institute of Oncology, Wawelska 15, 02–781 Warsaw, Poland

Kaleita, Th.
Childrens Cancer Group, 440 E. Huntington Dr., P.O. Box 60012, Arcadia, CA 91066–6012, USA

Kaspers, G.J.L.
Department of Pediatrics, Free University Hospital, De Boelelaan 1117, 1081 HV Amsterdam, The Netherlands

Keating, M.J.
M.D. Anderson Cancer Center, Texas Medical Center, 1515 Holcombe Boulevard, Houston, TX 77030, USA

Kienast, J.
Department of Internal Medicine A, University of Münster, Albert-Schweitzer-Straße 33, 48149 Münster, Germany

KOENIGSMANN, M.
Division of Hematology and Oncology, Benjamin Franklin Hospital of the Free University of Berlin, Hindenburgdamm 30, 12200 Berlin, Germany

KOLLER, E.
Ludwig Boltzmann Institute for Leukemia Research and Hematology, Hanusch Hospital, Pav. 4/4, Heinrich-Collinstraße 30, 1140 Vienna, Austria

KRAUTER, J.
Department of Internal Medicine III, University of Ulm, Robert-Koch-Straße 8, 89081 Ulm, Germany

KRAUZE, A.
Warsaw University Medical School, Department of Pediatric Hematology-Oncology, Dzialkowska 1, 01-184 Warsaw, Poland

KULICZKOWSKY, K.
Department of Haematology, University of Wroclaw, ul. Pasteura 4, 50-307 Wroclaw, Poland

LAMPERT, F.
Department of Pediatrics, University of Gießen, Feulgenstraße 12, 35385 Giessen, Germany

LANGE, B.
The Children's Hospital of Philadelphia, Division of Oncology, 324 South 34th Street, Philadelphia, PA 19104-9786, USA

LARSON, R.
Section of Hematology/Oncology, University of Chicago Medical Center, 5841 S. Maryland Avenue, MC-2115, Chicago, IL 60637-1470, USA

LINK, H.
Department of Hematology and Oncology, Medical College of Hannover, Konstanty-Gutschow-Straße 8, 30623 Hanover, Germany

MAHLMANN, S.
Howard Hughes Medical Institute, University of California, Los Angeles, 5-748 Mac Donald Building, 10833 Le Conte Avenue, Los Angeles, CA 90024-1662, USA

MASCHAN, A.A.
Institute of Children Hematology, 117, Leninski Avenue, 117513 Moscow, Russia

MAYER, R.
Division of Medical Oncology, Dana-Farber Cancer Institute and the Department of Medicine, Harvard Medical School, 44 Binney Street, Boston, MA 02115-6084, USA

MCCULLOCH, E.A.
Ontario Cancer Institute, Princess Margaret Hospital, 610 University Ave., Toronto, Ontario M5G 2M9, Canada

MEIERHOFF, G.
German Collection of Microorganisms and Cell Cultures, D S M, Mascheroder Weg 1b, 38124 Braunschweig, Germany

MESSNER, J.A.
Department of Medicine, The Princess Margaret Hospital, University of Toronto, 500 Sherbourne Street, Toronto, Canada M4X IK9

MESTICE, A.
Hematology Service, University of Bari, Viale Luigi Eimadi 111/0, 70124 Bari, Italy

METZKE, S.
Institute of Human Genetics and Anthropology, University of Jena, Kollegiengasse 10, 07740 Jena, Germany

MINNING, H.
Department of Internal Medicine, Division of Hematology/Oncology, Heinrich-Heine-University, Moorenstraße 5, 40225 Düsseldorf, Germany

MONTSERRAT, E.
Postgraduate School of Hematology "Farreras Valenti", Department of Medicine, University of Barcelona, Villarroel 170, 08036 Barcelona, Spain

NOWAK, R.
Medical Clinic of the Technical University of Dresden, Department of Hematology/Oncology, Fetscherstraße 74, 01307 Dresden, Germany

NOWAK-GÖTTL, U.
Department of Pediatrics, Pediatric Hematology and Oncology, University of Münster, Albert-Schweitzer-Straße 33, 48149 Münster, Germany

NÜSSLER, V.
Department of Internal Medicine III, University Hospital Großhadern, University of Munich, Marchioninistraße 15, 80377 Munich, Germany

OELSCHLÄGEL, U.
I. Medical Clinic Carl Gustav Carus of the TU Dresden, Department of Hematology, Fetscherstraße 74, 01307 Dresden, Germany

ORFAO, A.
Unit of Cytometry, University of Salamanca, Paseo de San Vicente s/n, 37007 Salamanca, Spain

PACHMANN, K.
Brandenburgerstraβe 30, 95448 Bayreuth, Germany

PANZER-GRÜMAYER, E.R.
Children's Cancer Research Institute, St. Anna Kinderspital, Department of Blood Group Serology, Kinderspitalgasse 6, 1090 Vienna, Austria

PAROVICHNIKOVA, H.
National Research Center for Hematology, Novozykovski pr. 4a, 125167 Moscow, Russia

Pavlovsky, S.
Centor de Internacion e Investigacion Clinica, Angelica Ocampo, Jose E. Uribura, 1450 Buenos Aires-1114 Capital Federal, Argentina

Petti, M.C.
Department of Human Biopathology, Division of Hematology, University "La Sapienza", Via Benevento 6, 00161 Rome, Italy

Pförtner, J.
Department of Hematology and Oncology, University of Göttingen, Robert-Koch-Straße 40, 37075 Göttingen, Germany

Pott-Hoeck, C.
Department of Hematology and Oncology, University of Göttingen, Robert-Koch-Straße 40, 37075 Göttingen, Germany

Pui, C.H.
Department of Hematology-Oncology, St. Jude Children's Research Hospital, University of Tennessee, 332 North Lauderdale, P.O. Box 318, Memphis, TN 38101-0318, USA

Ravindranath, Y.
Children's Hospital of Michigan, Division of Hematology/Oncology, Wayne State University, 3901 Beaubien Boulevard, Detroit, MI 48201–2196, USA

Reiffers, J.
Department of Internal Medicine Paul Broca, University of Bordeaux, 146 rue Léo-Saignat, 33076 Bordeaux, France

Reuss-Borst, M.
Second Department of Internal Medicine, University of Tübingen, Otfried-Müller-Straße 10, 72076 Tübingen, Germany

Ritter, J.
Children's Hospital, University of Münster, Albert-Schweitzer-Straße 33, 48149 Münster, Germany

Rohatiner, A.Z.S.
Medical Oncology Unit, St. Bartholomew's Hospital, 45, Little Britain, London, West Smithfield, EC1A 7BE, UK

Rowley, J.D.
Section Hematology/Oncology, University of Chicago, Medical Center, 5841 S. Maryland Avenue, MC 2115, Chicago, IL 60637–1470, USA

Runde, V.
Department of Internal Medicine, Heinrich-Heine-University, Moorenstraße 5, 40225 Düsseldorf, Germany

San Miguel, J.F.
Department of Hematology, University Hospital, University of Salamanca, Salamanca 37007, Spain

SAVCHENKO, V.
National Research Center for Hematology, Novozykovski pr. 4a, 125167 Moscow, Russia

SCHAISON, G.
Department of Pediatric Hematology, Hospital Saint Louis, 1 Avenue Claude Vellefaux, 75010 Paris, France

SCHELLONG, G.
Department of Pediatrics, Division of Hematology/Oncology, University of Münster, Albert-Schweitzer-Straße 33, 48149 Münster, Germany

SCHIFFER, C.A.
Division of Hematologic Malignancies, University of Maryland Cancer Center, 22 South Greene Street, Baltimore, MD 21201, USA

SCHLIEBEN, S.
Oncogenetic Laboratory, Children's University Hospital, Feulgenstraße 12, 35392 Giessen, Germany

SCHOCH, C.
Department of Internal Medicine II, University of Lübeck, Ratzeburger Allee 160, 23538 Lübeck, Germany

SCHRAPPE, M.
Department of Pediatrics, Center of Pediatrics and Cytogenetics Hanover, Konstanty-Gutschow-Straße 8, 30625 Hannover, Germany

SCHULZ, A.
Department of Internal Medicine I, University Hospital Cologne, University of Cologne, Josef-Stelzmann-Straße 9, 50924 Cologne, Germany

SCHUMACHER, A.
Department of Internal Medicine A, University of Münster, Albert-Schweitzer-Straße 33, 48149 Münster, Germany

SERIU, T.
Section of Molecular Biology, Department of Pediatrics II, University of Ulm, Helmholtzstraße 10, 89081 Ulm, Germany

SILIES, H.
Department of Pediatrics, Pediatric Hematology and Oncology, University of Münster, Albert-Schweitzer-Straße 33, 48149 Münster, Germany

SILLING, G.
Anemonenweg 25, 50858 Cologne, Germany

SPECCHIA, G.
Hematology Service, University of Bari, Piazzale G. Cesare 11, 70124 Bari, Italy

STARK, B.
The Center for Pediatric Hematology Oncology and Cancer Cytogenetic Laboratory, The Schneider Children's Medical Center of Israel, Petah-Tiqva 49202, Israel

STAUCH, M.
Department of Internal Medicine II, Division Oncology-Hematology, University of Jena, 07740 Jena, Germany

STEINMETZ, H.T.
First Department of Internal Medicine, University Hospital, University of Cologne, Josef-Stelzmann-Straße 9, 50924 Cologne, Germany

STOCKSCHLÄDER, M.
Center for Bone Marrow Transplantation, Department of Hematology-Oncology, University Hospital Eppendorf, Martinistraße 52, 20246 Hamburg, Germany

TAFURI, A.
Hematology, Cell Kinetics Laboratory, Universita "La Sapienza" of Rome, Via Benevento 6, 00161 Rome, Italy

THOMAS, X.
Hematology Service, Hopital Edouard Herriot, Place d'Arsonval, 69437 Lyon Cedex 03, France

TOSI, S.
MRC Molecular Haematology Unit, Institute of Molecular Medicine, John Radcliffe Hospital, Headington, Oxford OX3 9DU, UK

TOUW, I.
Erasmus University Rotterdam, Department of Hematology, P.O. Box 1738, 3000 Rotterdam, The Netherlands

URASINSKI, T.
Ist Pediatric Department, Pomeranian Medical Academy, U1. Unii Lubelskiej, 1, 71-344 Szczecin, Poland

VORWERK, P.
Children's Hospital, Department of Hematology and Oncology, Otto-von-Guericke University, Halberstädter Straße 13, 39112 Magdeburg, Germany

VOSE, J.M.
Department of Internal Medicine, University of Nebraska Medical Center, 600 South 42nd, Box 983330, Omaha, NE 68198-3330, USA

WAGNER, H.M.
Department of Internal Medicine I, Division Hematology and Oncology, University of Regensburg, 93042 Regensburg, Germany

WANDT, H.
Medical Hospital 5, Department of Internal Medicine, Institute of Medical Oncology and Hematology, Flurstraße 17, 90419 Nuremberg, Germany

WERBER, G.
Department of Pediatrics, Pediatric Hematology and Oncology, University of Münster, Albert-Schweitzer-Straße 33, 48149 Münster, Germany

WIELENGA, J.J.
Department of Hematology, University Hospital Dijkzigt Rotterdam, Department of Hematology, Room L 407, Dr. Molewaterplein 40, 3015 GD Rotterdam, The Netherlands

WIERNIK, P.
Albert-Einstein Cancer Center and Montefiore Medical Center, 111 E. 210th St., Bronx, NY 10467, USA

WITZ, F.
University Hospital, Department of Internal Medicine A, Hematology, 54511 Vandouevre Les Nancy, France

WÖRMANN, B.
Department of Hematology and Oncology, University of Göttingen, Robert-Koch-Straße 40, 37075 Göttingen, Germany

WOLFROM, Ch.
Children's Hospital, University of Berlin, UKRV, Reineckendorfer Straße 61, 13347 Berlin, Germany

ZANDER, A.R.
University Hospital Eppendorf, Bone Marrow Transplantation Center, Martinistraße 52, 20246 Hamburg, Germany

ZARITSKEY, A.
The Centre for Advanced Medical Technology, Pavlov Medical University, pr. Dinamo 3, 197042 St. Petersburg, Russia

ZEIS, M.
Department of Internal Medicine II, University of Kiel, Chemnitzstraße 33, 24116 Kiel, Germany

ZÜHLSDORF, M.
Department of Internal Medicine, Division of Haematology and Oncology, University of Münster, Albert-Schweitzer-Straße 33, 48149 Münster, Germany

Leukemia Cell Biology: Cytogenetics

Acute Leukemias VI
Prognostic Factors
and Treatment Strategies
Büchner et al. (eds)

Chromosome Translocations Play a Key Role in Leukemogenesis

J.D. Rowley

Introduction of Janet Rowley F. Lampert

Dear organizers, colleagues, ladies and gentlemen, it is an honor, a pleasure and a privilege to introduce to you Janet Davison Rowley, physician and scientist, oncocytogeneticist and professor, author of many superb research articles and book chapters, coeditor of over 10 prestigious journals, many times honorary doctor and adviser to famous institutions, 1993 president of the American Society of Human Genetics, recipient of over 15 awards, including the first Kuwait Cancer Prize in 1984 and the General Motors Foundation's Charles Mott Prize in 1989 - and also a wife and mother of 4 sons. What a remarkable personality!

Although she was born in New York City, and had a year's training in radiobiology (1961-1962) and a year's sabbatical (1970-1971) in Oxford Janet Rowley lived, studied and worked most of her life in the city of Chicago. At the University of Chicago, her alma mater, she has moved from research assistant to professor in the Department of Medicine.

Like many physicians looking through the microscope, Dr. Rowley was fascinated by the little worm-like bundles you see in cell divisions - the chromosomes. By applying chromosome banding techniques, which were first developed by Lore Zech in Sweden, she examined the different cell populations of human leukemia and found and defined many clinically important non-random chromosome rearrangements. She opened our eyes to leukemia aetiology at the cellular and, now, at the molecular level.

Dr. Janet Rowley's most popular publication, a "citation classic" with over 1000 citations, appeared in 1973 (*Nature* 243: 290–293: "A new consistent chromosomal abnormality in chronic myelogenous leukemia identified by quinacrine fluorescence and Giemsa staining"). Even in 1993, with 61 citations, this 4-page letter including 5 illustrations and 1 table was cited more often than any other of her many publications in that year. This famous *Nature* paper shared the fate of many other important publications: it was first rejected. It was finally accepted in a revised and improved version including the results of 9 (instead of 5) patients with chronic myelocytic leukemia, clearly demonstrating the translocation (not deletion) of material from chromosome 22 to chromosome 9.

That chromosome alterations cause the transformation of a normal cell into a malignant cell, and thus generate cancer, was postulated over 80 years ago by the Würzburg zoologist Theodor Boveri in his famous 64-page booklet *zur Frage der Entstehung maligner Tumoren*, which was published in 1914, shortly before his untimely death at the age of 53. Boveri foresaw many facts now familiar to the oncologist: the cellular nature and the unicellular origin of cancer, risk factors such as age and chronic irritation, the two-step triggering, and even growthrepressing versus growth-stimulating chromosomal elements. But his book ended with a question: Is there a way, are there means, to prove the validity of this hypothesis?

I think the time has come now to firmly underline the chromosome theory of cancer ori-

Departments of Medicine and of Molecular Genetics and Cell Biology, University of Chicago, Chicago, IL 60637-1470, USA

gin, and there is no one more capable of providing the convincing answers than Janet Rowley!

Abstract. The recurring cytogenetic abnormalities seen in the leukemias, lymphomas, and sarcomas are frequently translocations or, less often, inversions which are closely associated with particular morphologic subtypes of these tumors. Rearrangements involving chromosome band 11q23 are common in acute leukemia, both lymphoblastic and myeloid (monoblastic), and are less common in lymphoma. Although several different genes have been cloned from 11q23 translocation breakpoints, the great majority involve the *MLL* (*ALL1, Htrx, HRX*) gene. The central part of the gene codes for multiple zinc fingers which show homology to the *Drosophila trithorax* gene. About 70% of infants with acute leukemia will have *MLL* rearrangements. *MLL* is involved in five common translocations as well as in at least 25 uncommon or rare translocations, insertions and deletions. The translocation breakpoints occur within an 8.3 kb region which can be detected with a 0.74 kb cDNA probe which is useful for diagnosis and for monitoring patients during the course of their disease. Patients who have previously received drugs that inhibit topoisomerase II often develop acute leukemia with translocations involving 11q23 which break *MLL* in the same 8.3 kb region. The translocation leads to a fusion gene on the derivative 11 chromosome with a chimeric transcript, consisting of 5′ *MLL* and the 3′ segment of the other gene. The molecular dissection of these rearrangements will provide insights into the biology of *MLL* and into the interaction of *MLL* with topoisomerase II inhibitors.

Introduction

The molecular analysis of recurring structural chromosome abnormalities in human neoplasia has led to the identification of a number of genes involved in these rearrangements [1, 2]. Translocations and other rearrangements involving chromosome band 11q23 are of particular scientific interest because they occur frequently in a variety of hematologic neoplasms, including acute lymphoblastic (ALL) and acute myeloid leukemias (AML), as well as in mixed lineage leukemias and in lymphomas [1–4]. In addition to leukemias that occur de novo, balanced 11q23 translocations are also observed in therapy related leukemias, most commonly of the myeloid lineage [5].

11q23 translocations occur in about 7% of ALL and in up to 80% of ALL in children under the age of 1 year. 11q23 translocations are also seen in 6–8% of AML and in about 60% of infants with AML [6]. The t(4;11) is most common in ALL and the t(9;11) and t(11;19) are the most common in AML [4,7]. The t(11;19) is complicated because two translocations have been identified involving different breakpoints in 19p with different phenotypic features. About 65% of patients have a t(11;19)(q23;p13.3) and ALL; it is most common in infants and young children. One-third have a t(11;19)(q23;p13.1) and they are generally older children or adults with AML-M4 and M5 [8]. Patients with both ALL and AML often present with high leukemic blast cell counts and have a poor prognosis. This involvement of 11q23 in both the lymphoid and myeloid leukemias as well as in biphenotypic leukemias has led to the hypothesis that rearrangements of the involved gene may affect a pluripotential progenitor cell capable of either myeloid or lymphoid differentiation. However, before the gene at the translocation breakpoint was cloned, it was unclear whether several genes might be involved in the different translocations.

Mapping and Cloning the *MLL* Gene

Pulsed field gel electrophoresis (PFGE) and fluorescence in situ hybridization (FISH) have both been used to map the region containing the 11q23 breakpoints in leukemias [7]. Using FISH, we showed that a yeast artificial chromosome that contained a 330 kb insert of human DNA with the *CD3* gene cluster at the centromeric end of the YAC, spanned the breakpoint region in leukemias with the t(4;11), t(6;11), t(9;11), and t(11;19) [7] (Fig. 1A, B). Subsequently, we identified a gene named *MLL* for myeloid-lymphoid leukemia or mixed lineage leukemia that spans the breakpoint in these translocations [9]. The gene is transcribed from centromere to telomere (Fig. 1B). It is also called *ALL-1*,[10] *Htrx1* [11], or *HRX* [12] because of homology of some regions to the *trithorax* gene of *Drosophila melanogaster*. The designation *MLL* is currently accepted by the Human Genome Nomenclature Committee and it will be used here. The gene is

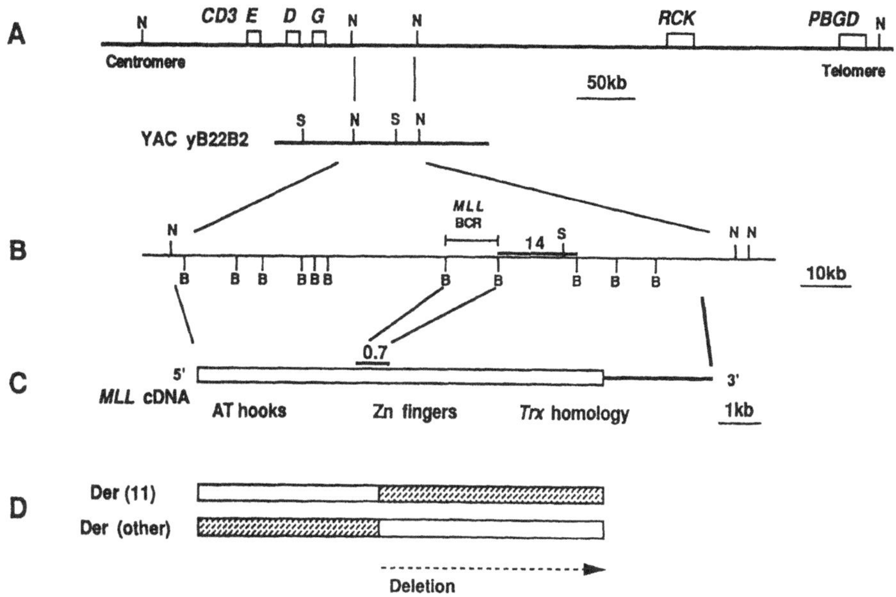

Fig. 1. **A** A partial map of 11q23 showing the location of nearby genes. Below, partial restriction map of YAC showing alignment to larger genomic map above and to the *MLL* gene in B. **B** A partial map of *MLL* showing the location of the 8.3 kb breakpoint cluster region (*BCR*) and the clone 14 probe used in FISH studies. **C** Diagram of the cDNA with the position of the 0.7 kb probe and the general location of important motifs. **D** Representation of the two derivative chromosomes formed as a result of the translocation. The zinc fingers are translocated to the der(other) chromosome and part or all of *MLL* telomeric to the breakpoint is deleted in about 25% of de novo acute leukemia patients. *N NotI*; *S SFiI*; *B BamHI*; *trx trithorax*, *der(11)*, derivative 11 chromosome; *Der(other)*, other derivative chromosome

estimated to be over 100 kb in size. There are multiple sized cDNAs, some of which are seen only in specific tissues; the largest of these is a 15 kb cDNA which should code for just over 3900 amino acids and a protein of about 430 kDa [10,12]. The *MLL* gene is expressed in a wide variety of human tissues, including spleen, liver, brain, and in both T and B cell lines.

Although the function of the normal *MLL* is unknown at present, it has several motifs suggesting that it is a transcription factor. There are DNA binding motifs called AT hooks which are at the amino-terminal portion and are related to high mobility group (HMG) proteins. We have recently shown that the AT hook region of the *MLL* protein binds to cruciform DNA [13]. The DNA sequence also encodes a series of zinc fingers which could also bind DNA. This region is homologous to the *trithorax* gene; however, the *trithorax* gene does not contain the AT hook domain. We have also identified a repression domain and a separate activation domain on functional studies.

We have identified a 0.7 kb *Bam*HI cDNA fragment which detects rearrangements in *Bam*HI digested DNA in all 21 cases of the t(4;11), all 7 t(6;11), all 11 t(9;11), and in 7 cases with both types of t(11;19) (involving breaks in 19p13.1 and 19p13.3) that we have examined [6] (Fig. 1C). We also detected rearrangements in 16 rare 11q23 translocations with the other breakpoint at bands 1p32, 10p11, 10p13, 10q22, 15q15, 17q21, 17q25, and 22q12 in patients with AML, 1q21 and 2p21 in patients with ALL and in three patients with lymphoma [6]. We have thus delineated an 8.3 kb breakpoint cluster region in all of the common and most of the rare translocations, insertions and inversions involving 11q23. These observations have been confirmed by others [17, 14].

This 0.74 kb cDNA probe that spans the breakpoint region should have broad application in clinical diagnosis because it detects all of the rearrangements in DNA digested with a single enzyme. This should allow the rapid detection of leukemia in children and will be especially important in leukemic infants under 1 year of age in whom the single most common chromosomal abnormality is a translocation involving 11q23. The importance of identifying leukemic infants with an 11q23 translocation is emphasized by a number of recent studies of these patients. Chen et al. showed that 70% of infants with ALL had an *MLL* rearrangement and they had a 15% projected event-free survival at a median follow-up of 46 months compared with 80% in infants with normal *MLL* [15]. Pui et al. found that 68% of infants with ALL had MLL rearrangements, especially those under 6 months of age; the leukemic cells expressed myeloid antigens, and the patients had an almost fivefold increased risk of an adverse event [16]. In addition, this cDNA probe should be effective for monitoring response to chemotherapy and for evaluation of minimal residual disease following treatment. It has been shown by a number of studies that the use of reverse transcriptase PCR (RT-PCR) is an effective means for detecting cells with the translocation, even when it is not found by cytogenetic analysis [17].

We have also used this same probe to study the location of 11q23 translocations in patients with t-AML [18]. We studied patients with t-AML, 12 of whom had detectable 11q23 rearrangements. Ten of the 12 had received prior treatment with topoisomerase II (topo II) inhibitors, usually the epipodophyllotoxins, and nine had *MLL* rearrangements. All of the patients who had *MLL* rearrangements had received prior treatment with topo II inhibitors. The use of FISH showed that the one patient with topo II exposure who had no *MLL* rearrangement had a break in 11q23 centromeric to *MLL*.

In our series of 58 de novo acute leukemia patients with *MLL* rearrangements we found that 16 had only a single rearranged band using the 0.74 kb cDNA probe [6]. To determine which derivative chromosome was represented by each of the rearranged bands on Southern blot analysis, we developed probes that could distinguish the centromeric and telomeric portions of the 0.74 kb cDNA fragment [19]. On Southern blot analysis, the centromeric probe detected the germline band and one of the rearranged bands which corresponded to the derivative 11 [der(11)] chromosome containing the 5′ portion of the *MLL* gene. The telomeric probe identified the germline band as well as the derivative chromosome of the other translocation partner. In cases with two rearranged bands, both derivative chromosomes were present, whereas in those with only one rearranged band, it was identified only by the centromeric probe [19] (Fig. lD).

Although about 95% of 11q23 translocations involve *MLL*, breakpoints in other translocations may involve other genes on 11q23 and the antigen receptor loci on chromosome 14 (both 14q11 and 14q32) or a new gene, *PLZF*, at the breakpoint in a t(11;17)(q23;q12) seen in a few patients with atypical acute promyelocytic leukemia [20]. Therefore, band 11q23 contains breakpoints for at least four different cancer-related translocations [7].

Mapping of Breakpoints Within the 8.3 kb BamHI Breakpoint Cluster Region

In an effort to understand the mechanism associated with these translocations, we have mapped the location of the *MLL* breakpoints in DNA from 31 patients with de novo leukemia (including one cell line and one non-Hodgkin lymphoma patient), and 8 t-AML patients [21]. We divided the 8.3 kb *Bam*HI fragment that contained all of our breakpoints into two regions defined by the restriction enzyme *Xba*I; the centromeric half is 4.57 kb (53%) and is region I, and the telomeric half of 3.87 kb (47%) is region II. DNA from all patients demonstrated the expected germline bands as well as one or two rearranged bands with the various *MLL* probes. In region I, 23 (74%) de novo patient breakpoints mapped uniformly throughout the region, whereas the breakpoints in eight patients (26%) mapped to region II ($p = 0.02$) (Fig. 2). In our 8 t-AML patients, one breakpoint mapped within the 1.6 kb *Eco*RI/*Bgl*II fragment between exons 6 and 7, near the centromeric portion of the breakpoint cluster region, and one mapped near the middle of the breakpoint cluster region; breakpoints in six t-AML patients mapped to region II ($p = 0.1$). These patients were all treated with topo II inhibitors for a prior neoplasm and most of them received one of the epipodophyllotoxins, e.g. etoposide or teniposide [18]. We found no association between region I or II breakpoints and leukemia phenotype, translocation partner or telomeric *MLL* deletions.

A total of 107 de novo patient breakpoints, which map either within or just outside the breakpoint cluster region, have been reported in

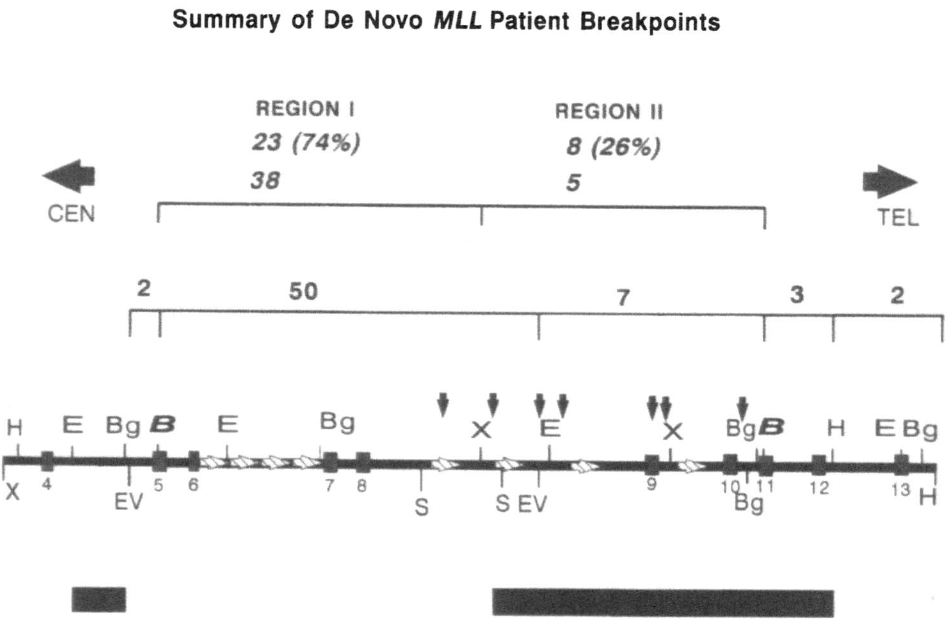

Fig. 2. Relationship of *MLL* breakpoints to regions I and II in de novo leukemia patients. The upper two sets of numbers represent our patient breakpoints (*top*) and patient breakpoints in the literature defined by *Xba*I restriction enzyme analysis. The bottom row represents breakpoints recorded in the literature as defined by *Eco*RI/*Bgl*II restriction enzyme analysis. *Grey boxes*, exons; *white striped arrows*, *Alu* repeats; *black arrows*, topoisomerase II consensus sites; *solid black bars below map*, scaffold attachment sites; *X*, *Xba*I; *H*, *Hind* III; *Bg*, *Bgl* II; *EV*, *Eco*RV; *B*, *Bam*HI; *S*, *Sac*I

the literature [21] (Fig. 2). Including our patients, a total of 138 patient breakpoints have now been studied. Forty-three patients reported on by others were studied using the *Xba*I restriction enzyme, and we can thus compare the breakpoint distribution directly with our results. For 57 patients only *Eco*RI or *Eco*RV were used and thus region I contained an additional 822 bp or 1196 bp telomeric of the *Xba*I restriction site respectively. Comparison of our data with this second group of patients is therefore general rather than exact. For those 43 patients whose DNA was digested with *Xba*I, 38 breakpoints (36%) mapped in region I and 5 in region II. Pooling these data with our XBa results, we find 61 patient breakpoints mapping in region I and 13 mapping in region II ($p \leqslant 0.005$). Of the 57 patients whose DNA was digested with *Eco*RI, 50 breakpoints (47%) mapped in region I, whereas 20 mapped in region II. In addition, 2 breakpoints (1.8%) mapped centromeric to region I, and 5 (4.6%) mapped telomeric to region II. In all of the studies, region I appears to be a genomic hotspot for breakage associated with translocations in de novo leukemia.

This distribution of breakpoints is very different from that seen in the t-AML patients. In our 8 t-AML patients, we observed 2 breakpoints in region I and 6 in region II ($p = 0.1$). Domer et al. (personal communication) mapped 8 t-AML patient breakpoints in the 8.3 kb *Bam*HI fragment and also observed that 2 mapped to region I and 6 to region II. At present, too few t-AML patient breakpoints have been mapped to assess the significance of the difference in the distribution of their breakpoints between region I and II compared with de novo patients. Thus, the critical question of whether the mechanism of translocation is similar in t-AML patients and de novo patients is still unanswered. But even with this small sample size we observe a potentially important trend showing 3 times as many t-AML patient breakpoints in region II as in region I. Clearly these AML patients, both de novo and therapy related, provide an important resource for resolving this issue.

Chromatin Structure Model of the Breakpoint Cluster Region

We and others had assumed, because of the very close association of *MLL* rearrangements in t-AML patients with prior exposure to drugs targeting topo II, that the breakpoints in all of the *MLL* translocations would occur in topo II consensus cleavage sites. Because no genomic breakpoints in t-AML patients have been sequenced, we cannot relate the breakpoints to topo II sites. It is clear from the data obtained from mapping the breakpoints in the de novo AML patients that the great majority map in a region that is largely devoid of topo II consensus cutting sites [21]. This analysis is complicated by the correct definition of a topo II consensus binding and cleavage site. Using high stringency criteria, only one breakpoint maps to a topo II site. On the other hand, eight of 13 breakpoints map to *Alu* domains. Our present information suggests that *Alu* sequences play a more important role than topo II sites, at least in the rearrangements in de novo patients. However, at present, it is unclear how these elements contribute to *MLL* rearrangements.

Molecular Consequences of the *MLL* Translocation

In reciprocal translocations, the identification of the derivative chromosome containing the critical junction is essential. Based on data from Southern blot analysis, FISH, and cytogenetic analysis of complex translocations, we proposed that the der(11) contains the critical junction [6,7]. Based on all of the data, we propose the following model. As a result of the translocation, 5′ *MLL* sequences on the der(11) are joined to the 3′ sequences from a large number of other chromosomal breakpoint regions - 22 detected in our laboratory alone [6] and seven additional breakpoints detected by others in patient samples or cell lines for a total of 29 different breakpoints presumably representing different genes.

Analysis of the cDNA from cell lines and patient samples has revealed that at least for 11 different 11q23 translocations cloned at present, the rearrangement results in a fusion gene with an in-frame fusion mRNA on the der(11) chromosome [7,10,12]. Thus it seems likely that there will be at least 29 (and probably more) different fusion genes all with essentially the same region of *MLL* at the 5′ end.

The genes on the other translocation partners have variable motifs, although some of them share some sequence homology, especially 3′ serine and proline rich regions, suggesting that they may have similar biological functions [10,12]. Adding to the complexity is the fact that some partner genes are localized to the nucleus, whereas a few are present in the cytoplasm. At present, we have relatively little functional information about *MLL* or the other fusion partners. Finally, several patients have been identified whose cells do not have a translocation but rather have trisomy 11 or, in one case, a normal karyotype. In these patients, molecular analysis has revealed a tandem duplication of exons 2 through 6 or 2 through 8, leading to an in-frame fusion *MLL* protein [22, 23]. All of our interpretation is based on motifs identified from analysis of the DNA sequences of these genes. *MLL* has two different DNA binding motifs. We have recently shown that the 5′ AT hook region binds cruciform DNA similar to the HMG proteins [13]. The contribution of the gene on the partner chromosome is unknown. It should be emphasized that essentially the same segment of *MLL* is present in the 5′ part of the fusion gene and that the t(4;11) patients have primarily ALL with some myeloid features, whereas the t(9;11) patients generally have myeloid leukemia with some lymphoid features. This indicates that the predominant phenotype of the leukemic cell is closely associated with the genes contributed by the partner chromosome, emphasizing that in chromosome translocations, especially those leading to fusion genes, both partners are essential components of the resulting phenotype.

Biological Consequences of Consistent Chromosome Abnormalities

The cloning of many of the chromosome translocation breakpoints and the identification of the involved genes has had a major impact on our understanding of at least one critical event in the transformation of a normal cell to a leukemic cell. The translocations in the lymphoid leukemias and lymphomas that involve the immunoglobulin genes in B lineage tumors and the T cell receptor genes in T lineage tumors result in inappropriate expression of the other gene in the translocation with no alteration in its protein structure. In contrast, all of the translocations cloned to date in the myeloid leukemias result in a fusion mRNA and a chimeric protein. Fusion genes are also formed in the 9;22, 1;19, 4;11 and 11;19 translocations in ALL [7].

Cloning of the translocation breakpoints has led to the identification of a number of new genes. It has been pointed out repeatedly that all of the genes cloned from the breakpoints in acute leukemia have been transcription factors [24]. In fact, one could argue that cloning these junctions is a very effective method for identifying new transcription factors.

Our new sophistication regarding the genetic changes in hematologic malignant diseases provides us with some very critical new diagnostic tools. Standard Southern blot analysis of tumor DNA can reveal clonal rearrangements of genes using the appropriate probes. PCR can increase the sensitivity of detection of these aberrations; sometimes the sensitivity is too great to be clinically applicable. The fusion genes are especially suited for RT-PCR, a technique in which the fusion mRNA is copied into cDNA and then, with appropriate primers from each gene, the fusion gene is amplified by PCR. Based on the position of the primers, the size(s) of the expected fusion product is known and can be compared with that actually obtained. Our increasing precision in identifying the genetic changes in the malignant cells comes at a most opportune time, because physicians will soon be in a position to use targeted therapy aimed at the specific genetic defect in the malignant cells. To use this targeted therapy effectively requires a precise genotype of the malignant cells. Although a number of genes will be involved and they will undergo various types of genetic changes, those reflected in chromosomal changes may be amongst the easiest to monitor clinically. Thus the leukemias with chromosomal translocations provide an attractive model system for beginning specific gene therapy in tumors.

Acknowledgments. This research has been carried out with the help of many of my colleagues: Dr S. Manuel Diaz, Michelle LeBeau, Norah McCabe, Robert Burnett, Michael Thirman, Nancy Zeleznik-Le, Sheryl Zieman-Vander Poel, Heidi Gill Super, and Pamela Broeker. It has been supported by funds from The National Cancer Institute, CA42557, and the Department of Energy, DE-FG02-86ER60408.

References

1. Rowley J.D. Recurring chromosome abnormalities in leukemia and lymphoma. Semin Hemat 1990: 27: 122–36.
2. Sandberg A.A. The chromosomes in human cancer and leukemia, 2nd Edition. Elsevier, New York, 1990.
3. Kaneko Y., Shikano T., Maseki N., Sakurai M., Sakurai M., Takeda T., Hiyoshi Y., Mimaya J., Fujimoto T. Clinical characteristics of infant acute leukemia with or without 11q23 translocations. Leukemia 1988: 2: 672–76.
4. Mitelman F., Kaneko Y., Berger R. Committee on chromosome changes in neoplasia; Chromosome Coordinating Meeting. (Cuticchia AJ., Pearson PL., Klinger HP., eds) pp 1992: 700–726. Genome Priority Reports Vol. 1, Basel, Karger, 1993.
5. Pedersen-Bjergaard J., Rowley J.D. The balanced and the unbalanced chromosome aberrations of acute myeloid leukemia may develop in different ways and may contribute differently to malignant transformation. Blood 1994: 83: 2780–2786.
6. Thirman M.J., Gill H.J., Burnett R.C., Mbangkollo D., McCabe N.R., Kobayashi H., Ziemin-van der Poel S., Kaneko Y., Morgan R., Sandberg A.A., Chaganti R.S.K., Larson R.A., Le Beau M.M., Diaz M.O., Rowley J.D. Rearrangement of the *MLL* gene in acute lymphoblastic and acute myeloid leukemias with 11q23 chromosomal translocations. New Engl J Med 1993: 329: 909–914.
7. Rowley J.D. Rearrangements involving chromosome band 11q23 in acute leukemia. In: Seminars in Cancer Biology, 4: 377–385, 1994. Editor: Rabbitts, T.H., Academic Press, London.
8. Huret J.L., Brizard A., Slater R., Charrin C., Bertheas M.F., Guilhot F., Hahlen K., Kroes W., van Leeuwen E., Schoot E.V.D., Beishvizen A., Tanzer J., Hagemeijer A. Cytogenetic heterogeneity in t(11;19) acute leukemia: Clinical, hematological and cytogenetic analyses of 48 patients: Updated published cases and 16 new observations. Leukemia 1993: 7: 152–60.
9. Ziemin-van der Poel S., McCabe N.R., Gill H.J., Espinosa III R., Patel Y.D., Harden A.M., Le Beau M.M., Smith S.B., Rowley J.D., Diaz M.O. Identification of a gene (*MLL*) which spans the breakpoint in 11q23 translocations associated with human leukemias. Proc Natl Acad Sci USA 1991: 88: 10735–39.
10. Gu Y., Nakamura T., Alder H., Prasad R., Canaani O., Cimino G., Croce C.M., Canaani E. The t(4;11) chromosome translocation of human acute leukemias fuses the ALL-1 gene, related to Drosophila Trithorax, to the AF-4 gene. Cell 1992: 71: 701–08.
11. Djabali M., Selleri L., Parry P., Bower M., Young B.D., Evans G.A. A trithorax-like gene is interrupted by chromosome 11q23 translocations in acute leukemias. Nature Genetics 1992: 2: 113–18.
12. Tkachuk D.C., Kohler S., Cleary M.L. Involvement of a homolog of Drosophila Trithorax by 11q23 chromosomal translocations in acute leukemias. Cell 1992: 71: 691–700.

13. Zeleznik-Le N.J., Harden A.M., Rowley J.D. 11q23 translocations split the AT-hook cruciform DNA binding region and the transcriptional repression domain from the activation domain of the mixed lineage leukemia (*MLL*) gene. Proc Natl Acad Sci USA in press.
14. Hunger S.P., Tkachuk D.C., Amylon M.D., Link M.P., Carroll A.J., Welborn J.L., Willman C.L., Cleary M.L. *HRX* involvement in de novo and secondary leukemias with diverse chromosome 11q23 abnormalities. Blood 1993: 81: 3197–3203.
15. Chen C-S., Sorensen P.H.B., Domer P.H., Reaman G.H., Korsmeyer S.J., Heerema N.A., Hammond G.D., Kersey J.H. Molecular rearrangements on chromosome 11q23 predominant in infant acute lymphoblastic leukemia are associated with specific biologic variables and poor outcome. *Blood* 1993: 9: 2386–93.
16. Pui C-H., Behm F.G., Downing J.R., Hancock M.L., Shurtleff S.A., Ribeiro R.C., Head D.R., Mahmoud H.H., Sandlund J.T., Furman W.L., Roberts W. M., Crist W.M., Raimondi S.C. 11q23/*MLL* rearrangement confers a poor prognosis in infants with acute lymphoblastic leukemia. Journal of Clin. Onc. 1994: 12: 909–915.
17. Borkhardt A., Repp R., Haupt E., Brettreich S., Buchen U., Gossen R., Lampert F. Molecular analysis of *MLL*-1/AF4 recombination in infant acute lymphoblastic leukemia. Leukemia 1994: 8: 549–553.
18. Super H.G., McCabe N.R., Thirman M.J., Larson R.A., Le Beau M.M., Pedersen-Bjergaard J., Preben P., Diaz M.O., Rowley J.D. Rearrangements of the *MLL* gene in therapy-related acute myeloid leukemia-in patients previously treated with agents targeting DNA-topoisomerase II. Blood 1993: 82: 3705–3711.
19. Thirman M.J., Mbangkollo D., Kobayashi H., McCabe N.R., Gill H.J., Rowley J.D., Diaz M.O. Molecular analysis of 3' deletions of the *MLL* gene in 11q23 translocations reveals that the zinc finger domains of *MLL* are often deleted. Proc Amer Asso Cancer Res (Abstract) 1993: 34: 495.
20. Licht J.D., Chomienne C., Goy A., Chen A., Scott A.A., Head D.R., Michaux J.L., Yu W., DeBlasio A., Miller Jr. W.H., Zelenetz A.D., Willman C.L., Chen Z., Cen S-J., Zelent A., Macintyre E., Veil A., Cortes J., Kantarjian H., Waxman S. Clinical and molecular characterization of a rare syndrome of acute promyelocytic/leukemia associated with translocation (11;17). Blood 1995: 85: 1083–1094.
21. Broeker P., Super H.G., Thirman M.J., Tanabe S., Zeleznik-Le N.J., Rowley J.D. Mapping breakpoints in the *MLL* gene relative to LJ topoisomerase II cleavage sites, Alu sequences and scaffold attachment regions. Submitted.
22. Schichman S.A., Caligiuri M.A., Yansong G., Strout M.P., Canaani E., Bloomfield C.D., Croce C.M. All-1 partial duplication in acute leukemia. Proc. Natl. Acad. Sci. 1994: 91: 6236–6239.
23. Schichman S.A., Caligiuri M.A., Strout M.P., Carter S.L., Yansong G., Canaani E., Bloomfield C.D., Croce C.M. *ALL*-1 tandem duplication in acute myeloid leukemia with a normal karyotype involves homologous recombination between *Alu* elements. Cancer Research 1994: 54: 4277–4280.
24. Rabbitts T.H. Chromosomal translocations in human cancer. Nature 1994: 372: 143–149.

Acute Leukemias VI
Prognostic Factors
and Treatment Strategies
Büchner et al. (eds)

Fifty-nine Cases of Acute Myeloid Leukemia with Inversion inv(16) (p13q22): Do Additional Chromosomal Aberrations Influence Prognosis?

C. Schoch[1], T. Büchner[2], M. Freund[3], H. Link[4], H. Bartels[5], T. Haferlach[6], H. Löffler[6], C. Sauerland[7], and C. Fonatsch[7]

Abstract. The influence of additional chromosome aberrations on the clinical outcome of patients with inv(16) is unclear. We analyzed 59 cases of acute myeloid leukemia carrying a pericentric inversion 16; 56 were de novo AML and 3 were secondary AML after treatment with cytotoxic drugs for a primary tumor. Additional chromosome aberrations were observed in 17 patients (29%). Eight of them showed an additional chromosome 8, 3 an additional chromosome 22. Different structural rearrangements in addition to inv(16) were found in 6 patients. In all three patients suffering from secondary AML, additional chromosome anomalies were observed. Clinical follow-up data were available for 51 patients. Seven patients (14%) died within 1 month after diagnosis of AML due to infection or bleeding; 20 (39%) are alive 3–109 months after diagnosis (median follow-up 36 months). Secondary clonal chromosome abnormalities in patients with a pericentric inversion 16 had no negative influence on prognosis.

Introduction

The pericentric inversion inv(16)(p13q22) represents one of the most common structural rearrangements in acute myeloid leukemia (AML). It occurs in 2%–7% of patients with AML [1–5]. Nearly all cases show a morphology consistent with AML FAB group M4 with bone marrow eosinophilla [6–8]. A related chromosomal abnormality is a translocation between the two homologous chromosomes 16, t(16;16)(p13;q22). While morphological and clinical characterisitics are identical in patients with inv(16)(p13q22) and with t(16;16)(p13;q22), cases with rearrangements involving only the breakpoint in 16q22 seem to belong to a different entity [9,10]. Therefore, rearrangements of chromosome 16 with breakpoints at both 16p13 and 16q22 seem to be specific aberrations most closely associated with AML M4eo. Recently Claxton et al. showed that the molecular consequences of t(16;16) are similar to those of inv(16), both resulting in the generation of a chimeric messenger RNA transcript by fusing the CBFB (core binding factor B gene encoded at 16q22) to MYH11 (smooth muscle myosin heavy chain gene encoded at 16p13) [11].

Patients with a inv(16) in their leukemic blasts show a high complete remission rate and are thought to have the longest survival of all AML entities [2, 3, 12–14].

Usually inv(16) is the sole cytogenetic abnormality. The reported incidence of clonal chromosome aberrations in addition to inv(16) varies between 24% and 57% [1, 3, 9, 10, 15–18]. The influence of additional chromosome aberrations on the clinical outcome of patients with inv(16) remains unclear.

[1]AG Tumorcytogenetik, Medizinische Universität zu Lübeck, Ratzeburger Allee 160, 23538 Lübeck, Germany
[2]Medizinische Universitätsklinik A, Münster, Germany
[3]Abt. Hämatologie/Onkologie der Universität Rostock, Germany
[4]Abt. Hämatologie/Onkologie, Medizinische Hochschule Hannover, Germany
[5]Städtisches Krankehaus Süd, Lübeck, Germany
[6]2. Medizinische Klinik, Universität Kiel, Germany
[7]Institut für Medizinische Informatik und Biomathematik, Münster, Germany

Materials and Methods

Chromosome analyses were performed on short term (4 h, 24 h, 48 h, 72 h) cultures of blood and/or bone marrow cells. For methods of cell cultivation, chromosome preparation and staining see Stollmann et al. 1985 [19]. A modified GAG banding [20] was used to classify the chromosomes according to the ISCN [21].

Patients were treated according to the protocols of two German cooperative AML study groups (AMLCG, using 6-thioguanine, cytosine arabinoside, daunorubicin and mitoxantrone, and the AML study of the Süddeutsche Hämoblastose-Gruppe, treating with cytosine arabinoside, daunorubicin, etoposide, amsacrine and mitoxantrone), except patients 46, 56 and 59, who suffered from secondary AML and received only palliative treatment. Patient 48 was treated with idarubicin, cytosine arabinoside and amsacrine.

Six patients received allogeneic bone marrow transplantation (BMT) (4 in 1st CR, 2 in 2nd CR); 2 patients underwent autologous BMT (1 in 1st and 1 in 2nd CR).

For 49 patients appropriate cytomorphological data were available, all were classified as AML M4eo according to FAB criteria.

Results

Of fifty-nine cases of AML carrying a pericentric inversion 16 were studied cytogenetically; 56 occurred de novo, 3 were observed secondarily after treatment with cytotoxic drugs for a primary tumor. Patient 46 was treated for a high-grade B-cell non-Hodgkin's lymphoma, patient 56 for breast cancer and patient 59 for a low-grade non-Hodgkin's lymphoma.

Clinical and cytogenetic data are summarized in Tables 1 and 2. Thirty-four patients were female, 25 were male. The mean age was 40 with a range of 20–72 years at initial diagnosis. The mean leukocyte count was 42 900/μl, with a range of 1000–272 000/μl.

Additional chromosome aberrations were observed in 17 patients (29%) (Table 2). Eight of them showed an additional chromosome 8, while in 3 patients an additional chromosome 22 was observed. Different structural rearrangements in addition to inv(16) were found in 6 patients. In all three patients suffering from secondary AML, additional chromosome anomalies were observed.

Figure 1 shows the G-banded karyotype of patient 49 with an inv(16)(p13q22) and gain of chromosomes 8 and 21 in addition.

In Fig. 2 the G-banded karyotype of patient 54 with an inv(16)(p13q22) and a balanced translocation between the short arm of chromosome 2 and the long arm of chromosome 13 is presented.

Clinical follow-up data were available for 51 patients. CR was achieved in 80.4%. The median survival time was 22 months after initial diagnosis. Seven patients (14%) died within 1 month after diagnosis of AML due to infection (4), intracerebral bleeding (2) or cardiac arrest (1); 3 additional patients died within 3 months because of spesis (2) or pulmonary insufficiency (1). Death occurred in 3 patients due to persitence of leukemia and in 17 patients due to relapse 5–46 months after initial diagnosis. One patient died in first complete remission of unknown cause. Twenty patients (39%) are alive 3–109 months after diagnosis (median follow-up 36 months).

Patients with secondary clonal chromosome abnormalities showed no worse outcome than patients with only a pericentric inversion 16. Seven out of 12 patients with additional chromosome aberrations for whom clinical follow-up data are available are alive 9–79 months after initial diagnosis. All 3 patients suffering from secondary AML and showing additional chromosome anomalies died shortly after diagnosis.

Figure 3 shows the survival of patients with and without clonal chromosome aberrations in addition to inv(16).

Discussion

Patients with an inv(16) in their leukemic blasts show a high CR rate but only sparse data are available on long term outcome. The second follow-up of the Fourth International Workshop on Chromosomes in Leukemia [13] reported on 13 patients with inv(16), 4 of them surviving longer than 9 years. Plantier et al. [14] followed 19 patients with inv(16), 14 remaining in first remission, 11 of them with a follow-up greater than 44 months.

The main objective of our study was to investigate the long term outcome in a larger group of patients with AML and inv(16)(p13q22) and to examine whether the occurrence of additional chromosomal aberrations has an influence on prognosis.

Table 1. Clinical data of 42 patients with inv(16)(p13q22) without additional chromosomal aberrations

Patient	Sex	Age	Leukocyte count (µl)	Bone marrow transplanatation	Cause of death	Outcome, months
1	f	20	65 900	–	Pneumonia	Dead < 1
2	f	20	32 600	Allogeneic in 1st CR	–	Alive 36+
3	f	21	77 000	–	Relapse	Dead 12
4	f	21	132 900	–	–	Alive 3+
5	m	22	120 000	–	Relapse	Dead 15
6	f	23	187 600	–	Pneumonia	Dead < 1
7	f	25	164 800	Autologous in 1st CR	Relapse	Dead 22
8	m	27	–	Allogeneic in 1st CR	–	Alive 82+
9	f	27	51 200	–	Relapse	Dead 5
10	f	27	85 700	–	Sepsis	Dead 3
11	f	29	77 600	–	Sepsis	Dead 3
12	m	30	–	–	Relapse	Dead 25
13	m	30	32 900	Allogeneic in 1st CR	–	Alive 20+
14	f	31	22 000	–	Relapse	Dead 35
15	f	31	29 000	Allogeneic in 2nd CR	Relapse	Dead 17
16	f	31	35 000	Allogeneic in 2nd CR	–	Alive 37+
17	f	31	96 000	–	–	Alive 32+
18	f	34	72 000	–	–	Alive 7+
19	f	36	123 000	Autologous in 2nd CR	Relapse	Dead 22
20	m	37	57 000	–	–	Alive 28+
21	f	38	42 900	–	Relapse	Dead 12
22	f	40	49 800	–	Intracerebral bleeding	Dead 1
23	f	43	–	–	Relapse	Dead 13
24	f	44	7 800	–	Pneumonia	Dead 1
25	m	46	157 000	–	Relapse	Dead 19
26	m	47	50 200	–	Relapse	Dead 29
27	m	48	272 000	–	Intracerebral bleeding	Dead < 1
28	f	48	40 000	–	–	Alive 26+
29	f	49	100 000	–	Relapse	Dead 19
30	m	52	38 500	–	Pneumonia	Dead 1
31	f	53	87 000	–	–	Alive 70+
32	f	55	40 000	–	–	Alive 61+
33	f	56	12 000	–	Relapse	Dead 17
34	f	57	19 800	–	Relapse	Dead 43
35	m	58	21 400	–	Relapse	Dead 37
36	f	60	28 000	–	Relapse	Dead 46
37	m	60	26 500	–	–	Alive 109+
38	m	64	15 900	–	Cardiac arrest	Dead 1
39	f	64	93 400	–	–	Alive 88+
40	m	31	197 000	Allogeneic in 1st CR	–	–
41	m	34	–			–
42	m	41	50 000			–

We could confirm a high CR rate in patients with inv(16), but the long term outcome in our collective is dissatisfying. Compared to patients with t(8;21)(q22;q22) studied at our institution, patients with inv(16)(p13q22) show a worse outcome, mostly due to a higher early death rate but also to a higher relapse rate.

Seventeen of 59 patients (29%) showed additional clonal chromosome aberrations, a low rate compared the to 57.2% stated by Johansson et al. [18], who compiled 229 cases of AML with inv(16)(p13q22) reported in the literature. As in our collective, gain of chromosomes 8 and 22 occurred most frequently.

We did not observe a negative influence on prognosis of additional chromosome anomalies. This is in line with data from Holmes et al. [16] and Campbell et al. [17], who each studied 25 patients with inv(16) and found no effect of additional chromosome aberrations on prognosis. However, if a higher rate of long term remission can be reached, certain secondary

Table 2. Clinical data of 17 patients with clonal chromosomal aberrations in addition to inv(16)(p13q22)

Patient	Sex	Age	Leukocyte count (μl)	Additional clonal aberrations	Cause of death	Outcome, months
43	m	34	37.000	-/+8	-	Alive 20+
44	f	51	15.000	+8	-	Alive 35+
45	f	37	3.900	+8	-	Alive 38+
46	m	50	25.900	+8	Pulmonary insufficiency	Dead 3
47	f	51	115.000	+8	Persistence of leukemia	Dead 5
48	f	72	1.000	+8, +21	-	Alive 9+
49	m	23	10.700	+8/+8, +21		
50	m	20	100.000	-/+9		
51	f	50	2.990	+22/+13, +22		
52	m	31	68.700	-/+22	-	Alive 74+
53	m	33	2.000	-/+22	Unknown in 1st CR	Dead 7
54	m	57	125.800	-/t(2;13)(p24;q14)		
55	f			t(3;17)(p23;q21-23), +8		
56	f	48	2.000	r(7)(p15q11.2-21)	Persistence of leukemia	Dead 7
57	m	25	7.000	del(9)(q22)	-	Alive 19+
58	m	27		-/t(13;18)(q21;q21)	-	Alive 79+
59	m	67	26.000	del(20)(q11)	Persistence of leukemia	Dead 3

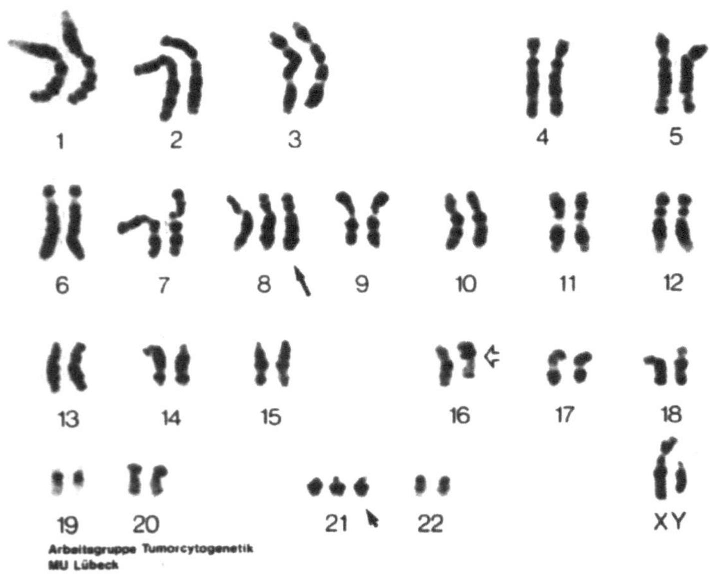

Fig. 1. G-banded karyotype of patient 49: 48,XY, +8,inv(16)(p13q22),+21

chromosome aberrations might turn out to be of prognostic value.

Acknowledgments. We thank PD Dr. Wandt, Klinikum der Stadt Nürnberg, Dr. Lengfelder, Klinikum der Stadt Mannheim, Dr. Grüneisen, Städtisches Krankenhaus Berlin-Neukölln, Prof. Dr. Hiddemann, PD. Dr. Wörmann, Universität Göttingen, Prof. Dr. Diehl, Universität Köln, Prof. Dr. Wagner, Dr. Schwieder, Medizinische Universität zu Lübeck, Prof. Dr. Andreesen, Dr. Hollerbach, Universität Regensburg, Prof. Dr. Thiel, Universitätsklinikum Benjamin Franklin Berlin, Prof. Dr. Schneider, Medizinische Einrichtungen der Universität Düsseldorf for providing tumor material and clinical data. The

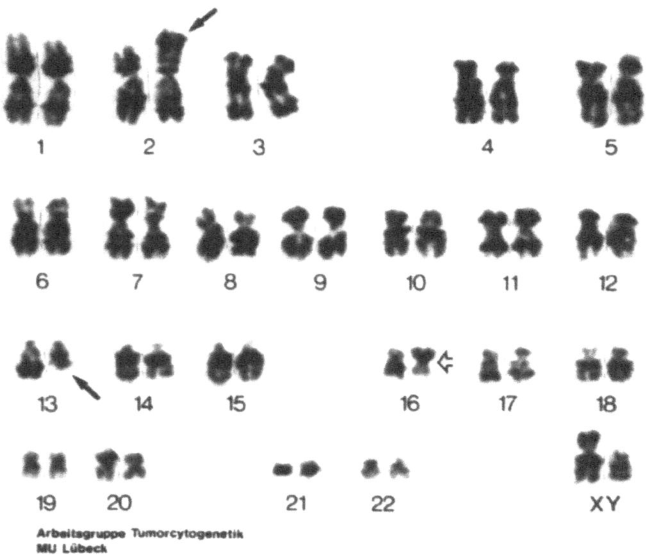

Fig. 2. G-banded karyotype of patient 54:46, XY, t(2;13)(p24;q14),inv(16)(p13q22)

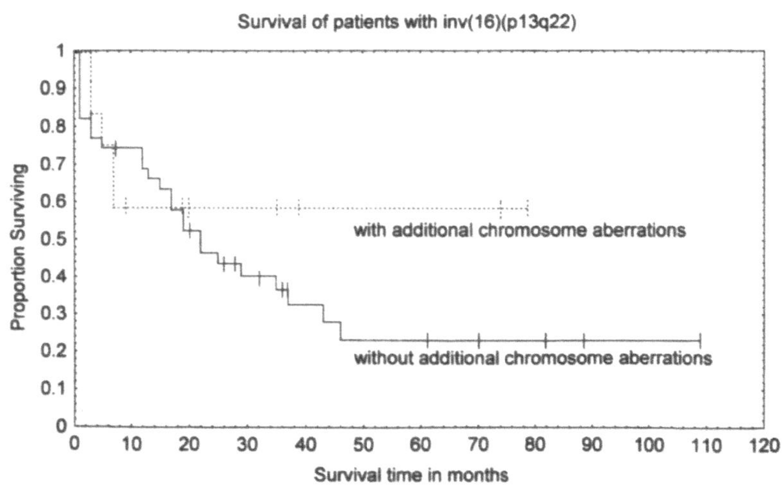

Fig. 3. Outcome of 51 patients with inv(16). The *continuous line* represents the survival of 39 patients with inv(16) as the sole anomaly at initial diagnosis; the *dashed line* marks the survival of 12 patients who showed clonal chromosome aberrations in addition to inv(16)

technical assistance of N. Erbe, U. Kolbus, U. Koop, B. Höschler and P. Müller is gratefully acknowledged.

References

1. Berger R, Flandrin G, Bernheim A, Le Coniat M, Vecchione D, Pacot A, Derré J, Daniel M-T, Valensi F, Sigaux F, Ochoa-Noguera ME: Cytogenetic stud-

ies on 519 consecutive nonlymphocytic leukemias. Cancer Genet Cytogenet 29, 9–21, 1987
2. Fenaux P, Preudhomme C, Lay JL, Morel P, Beuscart R, Bauters F: Cytogenetics and their prognostic value in de novo acute myeloid leukemia: a report on 283 cases. Br J Haematol 73, 61–67, 1989
3. Keating MJ, Cork A, Broch Y, Smith T, Waltes RS, McCredie KB, Trujillo J, Freireich EJ: Toward a clinically relevant cytogenetic classification of acute myelogenous leukemia. Leukemia Res 11(2), 119–133, 1987
4. Arthur DC, Berger R, Golomb HM, Swansbury GJ, Reeves BR, Alimena G, Van Den Berghe H, Bloomfield CD, De la Chappella A, Dewald G, Garson OM, Hagemeijer A, Kaneko Y, Mitelman F, Pierre RV, Ruutu T, Sakurai M, Lawler, SD, Rowley JD: The clinical significance of karyotype in acute myelogenous leukemia. Sixth International Workshop on Chromosomes in Leukemia, London 1987. Cancer Genet Cytogenet 40, 203–216, 1989
5. Morasi C, Köller U, Koller-Weber E, Schwarzinger I, Schneider B, Jäger U, Vahls P, Nowotny H, Pirc-Danoewinata H, Steger G, Kreiner G, Wagner B, Lechner K, Lutz D, Bettelheim P, Haas OA: Prognostic impact of karyotype and immunologic phenotype in 125 adult patients with de novo AML. Cancer Genet Cytogenet 61, 14–25, 1992
6. Bennett JM, Catovsky D, Daniel MT, Flandrin G, Galton DAG, Gralnick HR, Sultan C: Proposal for the classification of the acute leukemias. Br J Haematol 33, 451–458, 1976
7. Bennett JM, Catovsky D, Daniel MT, Flandrin G, Galton DAG, Gralnick HR, Sultan C: Proposed revised criteria for the classification of acute myeloid leukemia: a report of the French-American-British Cooperative Group. Ann Intern Med 103, 626–629, 1985
8. Second MIC Cooperative Study Group. Morphologic, immunologic, and cytogenetic (MIC) Working Classification of the acute myeloid leukemias. Cancer Genet Cytogenet 30, 1–15, 1988
9. Larson RA, Williams SF, Le Beau MM, Bitter MA, Vardiman JW, Rowley JD: Acute myelomonocytic leukemia with abnormal eosinophils and inv(16) or t(16;16) has a favourable prognosis. Blood 68, 1242, 1986
10. Betts DR, Rohatiner AZS, Evans ML, Rassam SMB, Lister TA, Gibbson B: Abnormalities of chromosome 16q in myeloid malignancy: 14 new cases and a review of the literature. Leukemia 6, 1250–1256, 1992
11. Claxton DF, Liu P, Hsu HB, Marlton P, Hester J, Collins F, Deisseroth AB, Rowley JD, Siciliano MJ: Detection of fusion transcripts generated by the inversion 16 chromosome in acute myelogenous leukemia. Blood 83, 1750–1756, 1994
12. Berger R, Bernheim A, Ochoba-Noguera ME, Daniel M-T, Valensi F, Siguax F, Flandrin G, Boiron M: Prognostic significance of the chromosomal abnormalities in acute nonlymphocytic leukemia: A study of 343 patients. Cancer Genet Cytogenet 28, 293–299, 1987
13. Swansbury GJ, Lawler SD, Alimena G, Arthur D, Berger R, Van Den Berghe H, Bloomfield CD, De la Chappelle A, Dewald G, Garson OM, Hagemeijer A, Mitelman F, Rowley JD, Sakurai M: Long-term survival in acute myelogenous leukemia. A second follow-up of the Fourth International Workshop on Chromosomes in Leukemia. Cancer Genet Cytogenet 73(1), 1–7, 1994
14. Plantier I, Lai JL, Wattel E, Bauters F, Fenaux P: inv(16) may be one of the only 'favaourable' factors in acute myeloid leukemia: A report on 19 cases with prolonged follow-up Leuk Res 18(12), 885–888, 1994
15. Le Beau MM, Larson RA, Bitter MA, Vardiman JW, Golomb HM, Rowley JD: Association of an inversion of chromosome 16 with abnormal marrow eosinophils in acure myelomonocytic leukemia: A unique cytogeneticclinicopathological association. N Engl J Med 309, 630–636, 1983
16. Holmes RI, Keating MJ, Cork A, Broach Y, Trujillo, Dalton WT, McCredie KB, Freireich EJ: A unique pattern of central nervous system leukemia in acute myelomonocytic leukemia associated with inv(16)(p13q22). Blood 65, 1071–1078, 1985
17. Campbell LJ, Challis J, Fok T, Garson OM: Chromosome 16 abnormalities associated with myeloid malignancies. Genes, Chromosomes & Cancer 3, 55–61, 1991
18. Johansson B, Mertens F, Mitelman F: Secondary chromosomal abnormalities in acute leukemias. Leukemia 8(6), 953-962, 1994
19. Stollmann B, Fonatsch Ch, Havers W: Persistent Epstein-Barr virus infection associated with monosomy 7 or chromosome 3 abnormality in childhood myeloproliferative disorders. Br J Haematol 60, 183–196, 1985
20. Fonatsch Ch, Schaadt M, Kirchner H, Diehl V: A possible correlation between the degree of karyotype aberrations and the rate of sister chromatid exchanges in lymphoma lines. Int J Cancer 26, 749-756, 1980
21. ISCN 1991, Guidelines for Cancer Cytogenetics, Supplement to: An International System for Human Cytogenetic Nomenclature, Publisher: S. Karger, 1991

Acute Leukemias VI
Prognostic Factors
and Treatment Strategies
Büchner et al. (eds)

Chromosome Abnormalities and Karyotype Evolution in the Stem Cell Compartments of AML and MDS

D. Haase[1], M. Feuring-Buske[1], S. Könemann[1], W. Verbeek[1], C. Troff[1], C. Fonatsch[2], W. Hiddemann[1], and B. Wörmann[1]

Abstract. The phenotype of the (pre)leukemic stem cell in AML and MDS has not been identified as yet. We have investigated whether cells with a stem cell-like immunophenotype (CD34+/CD38−) are involved in the leukemogenic process. In 12 patients with AML and in one patient with MDS the identification of (pre)leukemic cells was performed by classical cytogenetics. Highly purified (96–98% purity) cellular subpopulations were generated by fluoresence activated cell sorting according to the expression of CD34 and CD38. Following brief incubation with a cytokine cocktail (EPO, G-CSF, GM-CSF, IL-3, SCF) the sorted subpopulations were processed for chromosome analysis. In 9/12 AML patients clonal karyotype abnormalities were observed in the unsorted material. In 7/9 cases the chromosomal changes found in unsorted specimens were also detected in the immature stem cell-like population (CD34+/CD38−). In 9/9 cases the karyotype abnormalities were diagnosed in the population of committed progenitors (CD34+/CD38+). Additional secondary abnormalities were also demonstrable in both subpopulations in a case of M4Eo with inv(16). In a patient with secondary MDS RA, 2 subpopulations, CD34+/CD38− and CD34+/CD38+, were sorted together (CD34+/ 38+ −) because of the rarity of available cells. Cytogenetic analysis revealed a mosaic of normal and abnormal cells with 5 different dependent cell clones. All abnormal cell clones were demonstrable in the CD34+, sorted cell population. The relevance of our findings for pathogenesis, autologous stem cell transplantation and targeted gene therapy are discussed.

Introduction

In MDS and secondary AML the hematopoietic stem cell supposed to be the cellular target for leukemia initiating genetic defects [1]. However, as yet, no direct proof of genetic defects in leukemic stem cells is available. In de novo AML with a differentiated phenotype, the leukemic transformation is thought to occur in cells at the maturational stage of the bulk leukemic population. The phenotype of the (pre)leukemic stem cell in AML and MDS has not been identified as yet. However, in normal human bone marrow immature hematopoietic precursors can be identified by the expressional pattern of the cell surface marker molecules CD34 and CD38 [2]. The antigenic profile of the early hematopoietic maturational pathway is well conserved in myeloid blasts [3]. We have investigated whether cells with a stem cell-like immunophenotype (CD34+/CD38−) are involved in malignant transformation in de novo AML, secondary AML and MDS.

Materials and Methods

Patients

Bone marrow aspirates from 12 patients with AML and one patient with MDS were analyzed. According to the FAB classification [4,5], diag-

[1]Dept. of Hematology and Oncology, University of Göttingen, Robert-Koch-Str. 40, 37075 Göttingen, Germany
[2]Tumor Cytogenetics Working Group, Medical University of Lübeck, Ratzeburger Alle 160, 23538 Lübeck, Germany

noses were M0 (1 case), M1 (1 case), M2 (1 case), M2 following MDS (1 case), M4 (3 cases), M4 following PNH (1 case) and M4Eo (4 cases). The patient with MDS had RA without excess of blasts secondary to an ovarian cancer 3 years before MDS, treated surgically with subsequent chemotherapy (carboplatin/cyclophosphamide and treosulfan).

Immunophenotyping and Cell Sorting

Immunological characterization was carried out at diagnosis by multiparameter flow cytometry [2] (Fig. 1). The maturational profile was analyzed by a set of monoclonal antibodies directed against CD34, CD38 and HLA-DR. Subpopulations of cells with the antigenic profile of early (CD34+/CD38−) and committed (CD34+/CD38+) hematopoietic progenitor cells were isolated with a fluorescence-activated cell sorter (FACS Vantage, BDIS) equipped with a 488 nm laser. In the case of secondary MDS, due to the small number of positively stained cells, CD34+/CD38− and CD34+/CD38+ cells were sorted together.

In Vitro Culturing and Cytogenetics

The FACS-isolated cells as well as an unsorted bone marrow specimen were incubated for 24–72 h in RPMI 1640 supplemented with a cytokine cocktail (100 U/ml G-CSF, 100 U/ml GM-CSF, 100 U/ml IL-3, 1 U/ml Epo, 50 ng/ml SCF). Chromosome preparation and modified GAG-SSC staining was performed as described [6]. The karyotypes were classified according to the International System of Chromosome Nomenclature, ISCN [7]. FISH of one aspirate with trisomy 8 was performed as recommended (Imagenetics, manual). Mitotic indices were determined in 7 patients with AML by counting the mitotic figures within 1000 cells.

Results

Cellular Yield

In AML the frequency of cells with the immunophenotype of early progenitors (CD34+/CD38−) ranged from 0.05% to 12.1% (see Table 1). In the case of MDS-RA it was 0.03%. The frequency of committed progenitors (CD34+/CD38+) ranged between 0.13% and 66.7% in AML (Table 1) and was 0.28% in the patient with MDS. The absolute number of CD34+/CD38− cells available after cell sort ranged between 4.5×10^3 to 6×10^5. The number of CD34+/CD38+ cells ranged from 4.5×10^3 to

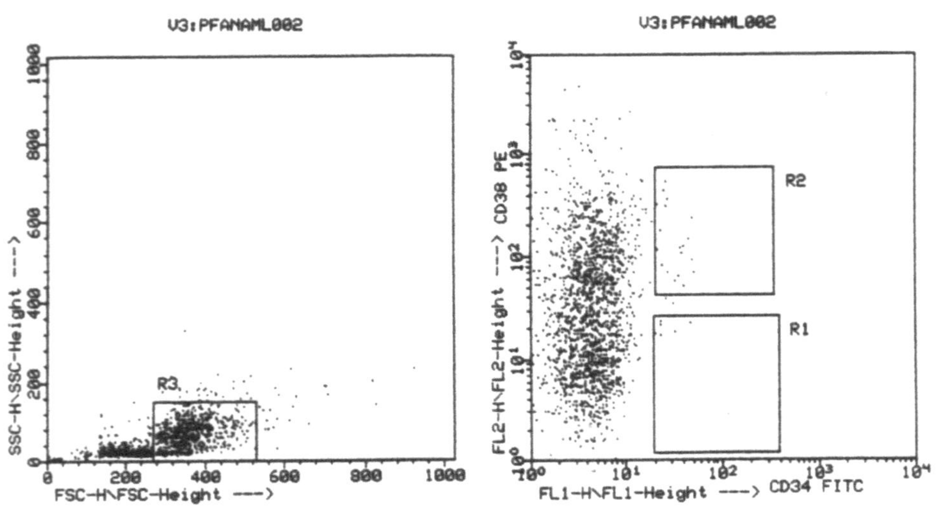

Fig. 1. Four-dimensional flow cytometric analysis of the bone marrow from a patient (Pf) with AML M4Eo. 10^4cells were acquired in list mode on a FACScan with four gates (R1–R4) showing the four different maturational subpopulations (R1, CD34+/CD38−; R2, CD34 +/CD38+; R3; CD34−/CD38+; R4; CD34−/CD38−) that were sorted in accordance with their light scatter characteristics (R5, R6)

Table 1. Yield of cellular subpopulations after sorting procedure

Patient age/sex	FAB type	Number of cells after the sort(× 10^3)		Relative frequency	
		CD34+/38–	CD34+/38+	CD34+/38– (%)	CD34+/38+(%)
Wi/32/m	M0	4.5	4.5	0.18	0.42
No/46/m	M1	55	60	12.14	6.02
Ko/8/m	M2	12	50	0.15	1.12
Mo/60/m	M2	30	70	0.60	1.42
Re/71/f	M4	100	1000	1.21	17.72
Wo/73/m	M4	5	100	0.05	6.76
TE/60/f	M4	45	52	0.14	0.13
Mu/58/f	M4	50	500	1.01	15.97
Ha/51/m	M4Eo	20	200	3.88	53.91
Mi/34/f	M4Eo	30	100	5.80	66.70
Gr/30/f	M4Eo	600	2000	6.86	56.58
Pf/81/m	M4Eo	70	390	1.13	35.56

2×10^6. In the case of MDS, 2.5×10^4 and 2×10^5 sorted CD34+/CD38– and CD34+/CD38+ cells, respectively, were available. The mean mitotic index in AML was <1 in the unsorted control population, 17 in the CD34+/CD38– populations and 33 in the CD34+/CD38+ populations (Table 2).

Table 2. Cytogenetic findings and mitotic activity in sorted cellular subpopulations

Patient	FAB type/ prephase	Karyotype	Number of analyzed metaphases			Mitotic index (related to 1000 cells)		
			Un-sorted	CD34+/ CD38–	CD34/ CD38+	Un-sorted	CD34+/ CD38–	CD34+/ CD38+
Wi	M0	Normal	2	5	2	< 1	50	1
No	M1	Normal/	16	0	3	2	2	6
		2q+	18	2	8			
Ko	M2	Normal/	n.d.	-	2	n.d.	n.d.	n.d.
		–7	n.d.	-	18			
Mo	M2/	Normal/	7	-	0	n.d.	n.d.	n.d.
	MDS	+8	17	-	3			
	normal (FISH)		n.d.	10	2			
	+8 (FISH)		n.d.	32	14			
Re	M4	Normal	21	9	17	< 1	8	73
Wo	M4/	Normal/	16	19	11	1	224	58
	PNH	del(6)(p12p23)	11	10	5			
Te	M4	Normal/	13	2	13	< 1	14	24
	+4	10	11	1				
Mu	M4	Normal	25	24*	4	n.d.	n.d.	n.d.
Ha	M4Eo	Normal/	4	-	-	n.d.	n.d.	n.d.
		inv(16)(p13q22)	10	-	1			
Mi	M4Eo	Normal/	2	2	0	< 1	40	33
		inv(16)		5	4	5		
Gr	M4Eo	Normal/	2	2	0	< 1	40	33
		inv(16)	4	34	36			
Pf	M4Eo	Normal/	0	0	0	< 1	17	35
		+8,inv(16)/	18	22	19			
		+8, – 12,inv(16)	3			1		

* = after colony assay; n.d., not done; -, no metaphases available; 0, metaphases available, but not in this cell population with the respective karyotype

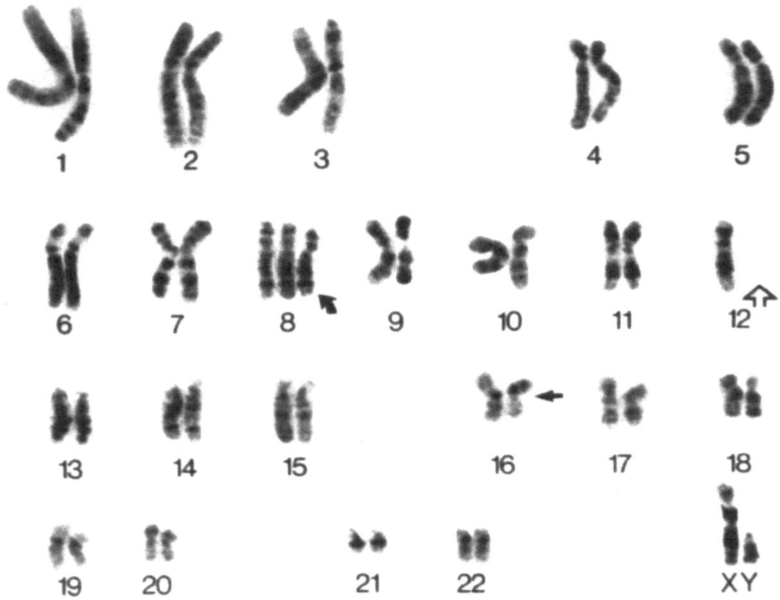

Fig. 2. Giemsa-banded karyogram of a flow-sorted CD34+/CD38− bone marrow cell from a patient (Pf) with AML M4Eo

Cytogenetics

Nine of 12 patients with AML and one patient with MDS had clonal karyotype abnormalities (2q+ in AML M1; −7 in M2; +8 in M2; 6p− in M4; +4 in M4; inv(16) in 3 cases of M4Eo; inv(16), +8,+12 in a further case with M4Eo (Fig. 2, Table 2) and 5q− and complex abnormalities in MDS-RA) (Table 3, Figs. 3–5). In AML, in 7/9 cases the chromosomal changes diagnosed in the unsorted bone marrow were also found in the immature stem cell-like population (CD34+/CD38−). In MDS, likewise all 5 abnormal cell clones initially characterized in the unsorted material were detectable in the CD34+ population. In 9/9 cases of AML the karyotype abnormalities occurred in the subpopulation of committed progenitors (CD34+/CD38+). Additional, secondary karyotypic abnormalities were found in the CD34+/CD38− population in a case of M4Eo. In the MDS specimen karyotype evolution was observed in the unsorted control population as well as in the CD34+ population. A mosaic of normal and abnormal metaphases was found in the immature cell populations in 5 cases with AML and in the committed progenitors in 4 patients with

Table 3. Cytogenetic findings in a case of secondary MDS and RA

Karyotype	*n*=47 unsorted	*n*=36 CD34+
46, XX	21.3%	0
Clone A:46, XX,del (5)(q15q33)	6.4%	5.6%
Clone B:46, XX,5q−,del(17)(p12)	4.3%	11.1%
Clone C:46, XX,5q−,17p− der(17)(?)	6.4%	2.8%
Clone D:46, XX,5q−, 17p− der 17,−20	53.2%	58.2%
Clone E:46, XX, 5q−,−7,17p− der17	8.5%	22.2%

n, Number of completely analyzed metaphases

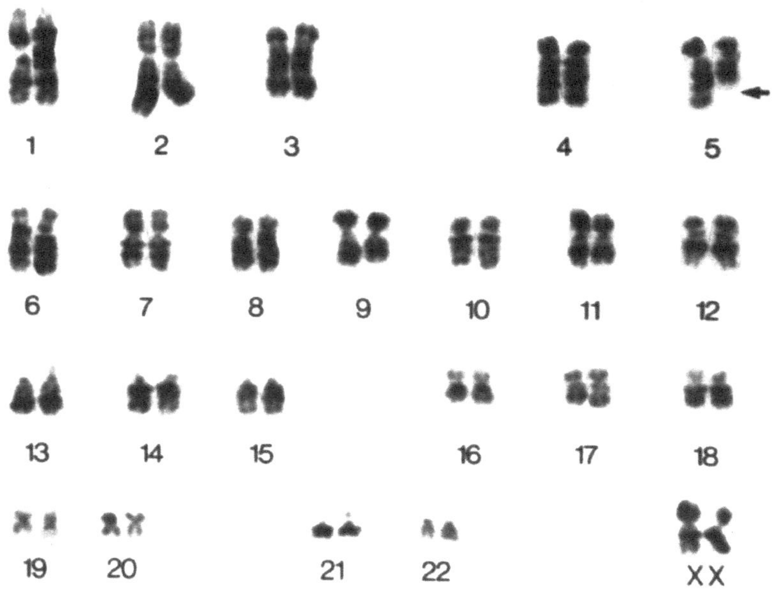

Fig. 3. Giemsa-banded karyogram of a flow-sorted CD34+ bone marrow cell from a patient with secondary MDS RA from clone A

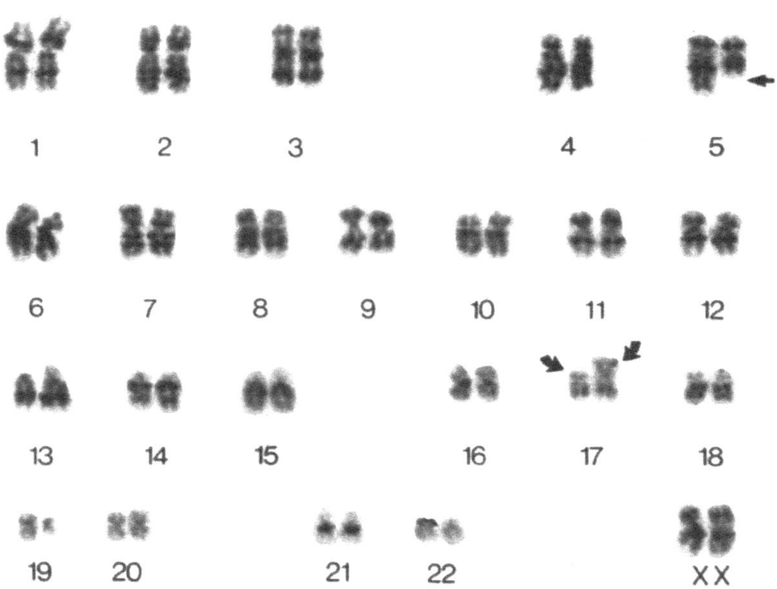

Fig. 4. Giemsa-banded karyogram of a flow-sorted CD34+bone marrow cell from a patient with secondary MDS RA from clone C

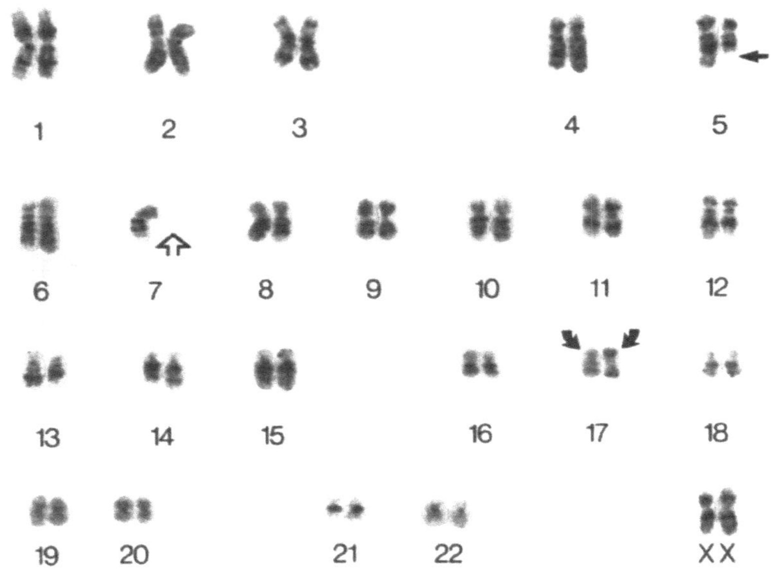

Fig. 5. Giemsa-banded karyogram of a flow-sorted CD34+ bone marrow cell from a patient with secondary MDS RA from clone E

AML. In the patient with MDS, normal cells were found only in the unsorted specimen.

Discussion

While MDS [1] and secondary AML are considered as stem cell diseases, de novo AML are not. Our cytogenetic analyses of highly purified progenitor and stem cell-like cells, obtained by FACS, revealed an abnormal karyotype in 10 of 13 patients examined. In all 9 informative AML cases with metaphases in the CD34+/CD38- population and in the patient with MDS (CD34+/CD38+ –), the abnormalities characterized in the unsorted controls were likewise demonstrable in the stem cell-like population. Secondary abnormalities and karyotype evolution in MDS were also found in the stem cell compartments. It is noteworthy that in some patients there was a mosaic of normal and abnormal cells within the immature progenitor population. The observation that not only disease initiation but also disease progression occur at the level of immature progenitors is of pathogenetic relevance. The presence of both normal CD34+/CD38– cells and abnormal CD34+/CD38– cells in the same patient might translate into future therapeutic autologous transplantation strategies if a discrimation of both CD34+/CD38– subpopulations can be achieved.

While our findings strongly support the concept of the pluripotent origin of the leukemic clone in MDS and secondary AML, they are surprising in the patients with de novo AML, especially in M4Eo with inv(16). It can be derived from our data that in AML, independent of the phenotype of the bulk leukemic population, the leukemogenic event occurs on the immature progenitor level (M3 may be an exception). This would imply that the maturational level of the leukemic cell population is not a reflection of the phenotype of the initial leukemic mother cell but is determined by the genetic abnormality itself, regularly occurring at the level of the immature stem cell.

References

1. Janssen JWG, Buschle M, Layton M et al. (1989). Clonal analysis of myelodysplastic syndromes: Evidence of multipotent stem cell origin. Blood 73: 248–254
2. Terstappen LWMM, Loken M (1990) Myeloid cell differentiation in normal bone marrow and acute

myeloid leukemia assessed by multi-dimensional flow cytometry. Analyt Cell Pathol 2: 229–240.
3. Terstappen LWMM, Safford M, Unterhalt M et al. (1992). Flow cytometric characterization of acute myeloid leukemia. IV. Comparision to the differentiation pathway of normal hematopoietic progenitor cells. Leukemia 6: 993–1000
4. Bennet J, Catovsky D, Daniel M-T et al. (1976) Proposals for the classification of acute leukemias. A report of the French-American-British Cooperative Group. Br J Haematol 33: 451–458
5. Bennett JM, Catovsky D, Daniehl M-T et al. (1982) Proposals for the classification of the myelodysplastic syndromes. Br J Haematol 51: 189–199
6 Fonatsch C, Schaadt M, Kirchner H et al. (1980) A possible correlation between the degree of karyotype aberrations and the rate of sister chromatid exchanges in lymphoma lines. Int J Cancer 26: 749–756
7. ISCN (1991) Guidelines for Cancer Cytogenetics, Supplement to an International System for Human Cytogenetic Nomenclature. F. Mitelman (ed.). S. Karger, Basel

Acute Leukemias VI
Prognostic Factors
and Treatment Strategies
Büchner et al. (eds)

Karyotypic Abnormalities in Secondary Leukemia of Children

J. Harbott[1], I. Reinisch[1], J. Ritterbach[1], U. Creutzig[2], W.-D. Ludwig[3], P. Gutjahr[4], A. Borkhardt[1], and F. Lampert[1]

Abstract. Over a period of 10 years the bone marrow of 38 children with secondary leukemia was cytogenetically analyzed. After comparison of all karyotypes, chromosomes 5, 7, and 11 were found to be most frequently involved in numerical or structural aberrations. Whereas in ANLL chromosomes 5 and 7 predominated, chromosome 11 was found in all groups, but mainly in ALL. The breakpoints of different rearrangements were always located in band 11q23.

In 4 of 6 children with secondary ALL the chromosomal abberrations were one of the immunophenotype-specific abnormalities. In ANLL, however, a FAB-type-specific anomaly was found only once. In 5 of 6 patients with ANLL after a prephase of MDS the original karyotype of MDS appeared also in ANLL. In 3 of these 5 additional abnormalities appeared, confirming the progress of the disease.

Introduction

With the improvement in survival, which has been achieved for many childhood neoplasms by the use of multiple agent chemotherapy combined with radiation, the appearance of secondary hematological malignancies has increased. Chromosomal analyses may give more information about the origin of this disease through the evaluation of specific breakpoints and the localization of specific genes. Cytogenetics will also help to distinguish (late) relapses and secondary leukemias by the comparison of the karyotypes with that of initial diagnosis.

Therefore, we analyzed the leukemic karyotypes of 29 children with secondary leukemia and MDS whose bone marrow was sent to our laboratory over a period of 10 years. In addition, the cytogenetic results of 6 children with AML after a prephase of MDS were compared.

Materials and Methods

Bone marrow and blood samples which were mailed to our laboratory were prepared directly and/or incubated in RPMI 1640 + 20% FCS (10^6 cells/ml) for 24 and 48 h. The cell suspension was then brought to hypotonic solution (KCl, 15 min) and fixed in methanol-acetic acid (3:1). After washing several times, the cells were dropped on to a cold wet slide to spread the metaphases. G-banding was performed after a trypsin pretreatment (10–15) 3–5 days later. Karyotyping was done according to the Third International Workshop on Leukemia 1980 [1] and the ISCN 1985 and 1991 [2,3].

Results

Of 29 children with secondary hematological malignanacies, 19 had AML (Table 1). The latency period between primary and secondary malignancy ranged from 11 months to 11 years, with a

[1]University Children's Hospital, Feulgenstrasse 12, 35385 Giessen, Germany
[2]University Children's Hospital, 48129 Münster, Germany
[3]Robert-Rössle-Klinik, Dept. Oncology/Molecular Biology, 13122 Berlin, Germany
[4]University Children's Hospital, 55101 Mainz, Germany

Table 1. Karyotype of 19 children with secondary AML. LOF, Lost to follow-up. The karyotype of primary malignancy was only analyzed in patient 8, 15, and 17 (see text). The latency period is years; months

Patient no.	Primary malignancy Diagnosis	Secondary malignancy			
		Latency	Diagnosis	Cytogenetics	Outcome
1	NBL	3;4	AML-M2	45,XX,del(5)(q31),add(17)(p11),–19	Alive 12/94
2	PNET	4;5	AML-M2	45,XX,add(2)(q35),inv(3)(p21p27), – 5, add(12)(p13),mar	Alive 1/95
3	ALL	4;3	AML	45,XX,–7	LOF
4	ALL	11;1	AML	46,XY,t(4;11)(q21;p23)inc	Died 7/93
5	NHL	1;8	AML-M0	46,XY,t,(10;12)(p13;q21)	Died 6/86
6	Hepatoblastoma	2;3	AML-M5	46,XY	Died 7/92
7	c-ALL	8;7	AML-M4	46,XY	Died 4/92
8	c-ALL4	4;10	AML-M2	46,XY	Died 4/91
9	Hodgkin IIB	2;7	AML-M4	46,XX,del(5)(q13q31)	Died 5/87
10	ALL	1;8	AML-M1	46,XX,t(9;11)(p22;q23)	Died 1/90
11	Hodgkin	4;3	AML-M1	47,XY,t(10;21)(p12;q22),+19	CR
12	Hodgkin	2;3	AML-M5	47,XY,t(1;11)(p32;q23),+8	LOF
13	ALL	6;3	AML-M1	46,XY,r(7)(p22q22)	Prelapsed
			AML-M1	46,XY,–7	LOF
14	NHL (B-cell)	0;11	AML-M5	46,XX	Died 9/84
15	c-ALL	4;6	AML-M4	near tetraploid	Died 11/91
16	Synovial Sarcoma	4;4	AML-M4	47,XY,+11	Died 4/89
17	c-ALL	1;3	AML-M4	no result	Died 9/91
18	Wilms tumor	0;0	AML-M2	46,der(1p),add(5)(p15.1),del(5)(q22), del(7)(q22)	Died 8/87
19	Rhabdomyosarcoma	5;0	AML-M4	1mar	Died 1/85

median of 3 years, 4 months. One child with Wilms tumor was diagnosed as having AML in the same month. The child died 1 month later. To date, only 3 of these children are known to be alive, while 3 others are lost to follow-up. The survival time, after the diagnosis of secondary AML, ranged from 0 to 32 months with a median of 6 months. The FAB type of 17 children was known: 6 of them had M4, while M1 (n=3), M2 (n=4), and M5 (n=3) were found less often. M3, M6 and M7 were not detected as a secondary malignancy, and only one patient had M0.

Unfortunately, the karyotype of the primary disease was only known from 3 patients, where c-ALL was diagnosed. Two had no sub-type-specific abnormalities, while the third had a hyperdiploid karyotype with more than 50 chromosomes.

Chromosomal abnormalities of the secondary AML were detected in 14 children; 4 had a normal karyotype, and one had no result. Only 2 patients showed numerical changes exclusively, e.g., –7, +11, whereas in the majority structural abnormalities were found, at times accompanied by the loss or gain of a whole chromosome.

Chromosomes 5, 7 and 11 were most frequently involved in the aberrations. In chromosomes 5 and 7 the breakpoints were located in various bands of the long arms, while in chromosome 11 the breaks always occurred in the band 11q23.

Secondary ALL was less frequent (n=6) (Table 2). The median latency period was 5 years, 11 months, ranging from 1 year, 3 months to 20 years, 7 months. Four children had c-ALL, one had pre-pre-B-ALL, and the immunophenotype of the last one remained unclear. Two children died 3 and 15 months, respectively, after being diagnosed with secondary ALL, and 4 are in complete remission between 4 and 8.5 years. The karyotype of these patients showed aberrations of chromosome 11q23 in 3 of 5 cases.

Three of 4 patients with secondary MDS had an abnormal karyotype (Table 3). All showed abnormalities involving chromosome 7: twice a –7 and once a partial monosomy of the long arm (7q22). Three of the 4 children are alive; the outcome of one is unknown.

The karyotype of 6 children with AML after a prephase of MDS was analyzed successfully during MDS as well as during leukemia (Table 4). Two patients had a normal karyotype of MDS with additional chromosomal abnormalities.

Table 2. Karyotypes of 6 children with secondary ALL

Patient no.	Primary malignancy Diagnosis	Secondary malignancy			
		Latency	Diagnosis	Cytogenetics	Outcome
1	c-ALL	5;11	ALL	46,XX	Unknown
2	Nephroma	9;7	c-ALL	46,XY,t(2;16)(p13;q24),t(9;22)(q34;q11)	Died 1/89
3	ALL	8;5	c-ALL	51,XY,T(1;19)(q23;P13),t(2;11)(q13;q23),+6,+7,+13,+der(19)t(1;19),tder(19)t(1:19)	Died 5/88
4	Medulloblastoma	3;6	c-ALL	Hyperdiploid > 50	2nd CCR
5	NBL	20;7	c-ALL	46,XX,del(11)(q23)	CCR
6	NBL	1;3	pre-pre-B-ALL	46,XY,t(4;11)(q21;q23)	CCR

Table 3. Karyotypes of 4 children with secondary MDS

Patient no.	Primary malignancy Diagnosis	Secondary malignancy			
		Latency	Diagnosis	Cytogenetics	Outcome
1	Lymphoma (T-cell)	8;8	MDS	44,XY,-4, del(5)(q13q22), − 7, − 12, der(17)t(12;17)(p11;p11), +mar	LOF
2	T-ALL	2;5	CMML	46,XX,add(7)(q22)[3]/idem, add(3)(q26?[8], add(5)(q35)[6], − 10[3], +2mar[3][cp21]	CCR
3	NBL	4;3	AML-M1	46,XY	Alive 11/94
4	Germ cell tumor	2;5	MDS	45,XX,t(4;11)(q21;q23), − 7	Alive 2/95

Table 4. Karyotypes of 6 children with AML and a prephase of MDS

Patient no.	Diagnosis	Cytogenetics	Latency	Outcome
1	MDS-RA	45,XY, − 7	2;6	Died 4/94
	AML-M4	45,XY,r(6)(p23;q21), − 7		
2	MDS	47,der(11)t(1;11)(q21;q23), +mar	2;1	Died 2/94
	AML	47,der(11)t(1;11)(q21;q23), +mar/48,XY,idem, +2mar		
3	CMML	46,XY	0;5	Died
	AML-M1	48,XY, +8, +21		10/90
4	MDS	46,XY,der(10)(q26),der(15)t(1;15)(q21;p11),inv(16)(p13q22)	0;1	LOF
	AML-M4	47,XY,der(10)(q26),der(15)t(1;15)(q21;p11),inv(16)(p13q22), +mar		
5	CMML	46,XY	0;2	Died
	AML-M5	46,XY		10/92
6	MDS-RAEB-T	46,XY	0;10	LOF
	AML-M2	46,XY		

Discussion

During a period of 10 years the bone marrow karyotype of 25 children with secondary hematological malignancies were analyzed (Fig. 1). By comparing the results it could be shown that the band 11q23 was most frequently involved. A rearrangement of this band was found in ALL as well as AML and MDS. In patients with AML and MDS, however chromosomes 5 and 7 were far more often involved in aberrations. Abnormalities of the latter were never found in

Fig. 1. Chromosomal breakpoints of secondary malignancies

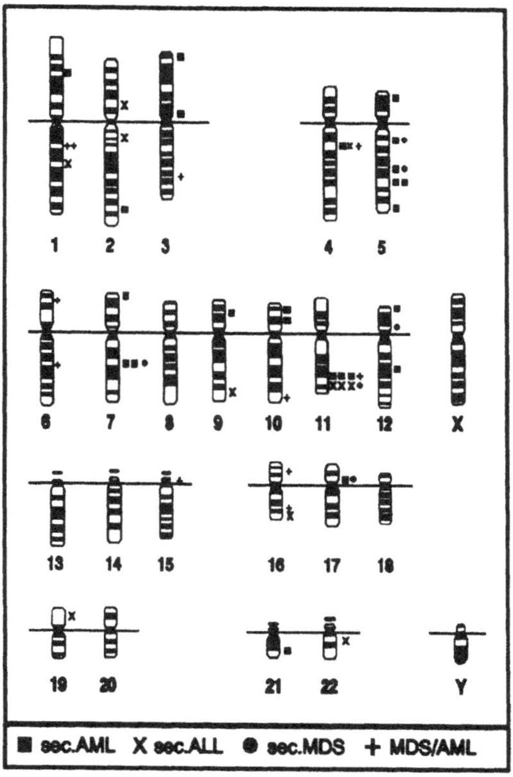

children with ALL. It is interesting to note that 4 of 5 ALL patients with an abnormal karyotype showed one of the subtype-specific abnormalities: t(9;22), t(1;19), t(4;11), and hyperdiploidy >50. On the other hand 3 of 5 had an aberration involving 11q23, which seems to be typical for this type of disease [4-6].

In children with AML, only one had a t(9;11); not, as expected, in M5, but in M1. Other FAB-type-specific aberrations like t(8;21) or inv(16) were not detected. These results are in accordance with other authors who describe a frequency of chromosome 5 and 7 abnormalities of 60%-70% in secondary AML, while specific aberrations are found in only 10% of cases [7-10]. Partial or complete monosomies of the chromosomes 5 and 7 are normally rare in childhood AML and more frequent in adults [11,12].

For comparsion with the cytogenetic results of secondary malignancies, 6 children with AML after a prephase of MDS were analyzed. In 4 of them a karyotypic evolution could be detected: three times the original aberrations of MDS were found in AML, as well as the appearance of additional abnormalities as described by others [13,14]. Three patients had a normal karyotype in the MDS marrow and one of them switched to abnormal. The remaining two showed no evolution. Only one child had an 11q23 aberration and another one a monosomy of chromosome 7(-7). Both abnormalities, however, were detected in MDS and AML as well. These findings confirm that AML is a progression of the same disease and not a secondary malignancy.

Acknowledgment. For excellent technical assistance we thank Mrs Christina Böth, Doris Erb, Sabine Gräf-Höchst, Astrid Jaeckel, and Susanne Kühn. This study was supported by the Parents' Leukemia Research Fund, Gießen and by Forschungshilfe Station Peiper.

References

1. Third International Workshop on Chromosomes in Leukemia 1980 (1981) Clinical significance of chromosomal abnormalities in acute lymphoblastic leukemia. Cancer Genet Cytogenet 4: 111–137

2. ISCN (1985) An International system for human cytogenetic nomenclature. Karger, Basel
3. ISCN (1991) Guidelines for cancer cytogenetics, supplement to an international system for human cytogenetic nomenclature. S. Karger, Basel
4. Pedersen-Bjergaard J (1992) Acute lymphoid leukemia with t(4;11) (q21;q23) following chemotheraphy with cytolastic agents targeting at DNA-topoisomerase II. Leuk Res 16: 733–735
5. Zaccaria A, Alimena G, Baccarani M, Billströrm R, Carbonell F, Castoldi GL, Fuscaldo K, Hecht F, Hossfeld DK, Mitelman F, Rosti G, Sandberg AA, Tassinari A, Testoni N, Tura S (1987) Cytogenetic analyses in 89 patients with secondary hematologic disorders - results of a cooperative study. Cancer Genet Cytogenet 26: 65–74
6. Lennard A, Jackson GH, Carey PJ, Bown N, Middleton P, Proctor SJ (1991). Secondary acute lymphoblastic leukemia with 4:11 translocation following treatment for Hodgkin's disease: case report and review of the literature. Leukemia 5: 624–627
7. Heim S (1992) Cytogenetic findings in primary and secondary MDS. Leuk Res 16: 43–46
8. Rubin CM, Arthur DC, Woods WG, Lange BJ, Nowell PC, Rowley JD, Nachman J, Bostrom B, Baum ES, Suarez CR, Shah NR, Morgan E, Maurer HS, McKenzie SE, Larson RA, Le Beau MM (1991) Therapy-related myelodysplastic syndrome and acute myeloid leukemia in children: correlation between chromosomal abnormalities and prior therapy. Blood 78: 2982–2988
9. Fenaux P, Laï JL, Quiquandon I, Preudhomme C, Dupreiz B, Facon T, Lorthois C, Lucidarme D, Bauters F (1991) Therapy related myelodysplastic syndrome and leukemia with no "unfavourable" cytogenetic findings have a good response to intensive chemotherapy: a report on 15 cases. Leuk Lymphoma 5: 117–125
10. Pedersen-Bjergaard J, Philip P, Larsen SO, Jensen G, Byrsting K (1990) Chromosome aberrations and prognostic factors in therapy-related myelodysplasia and acute nonlymphocytic leukemia. Blood 76: 1083–1091
11. Creutzig U, Ritter J, Ludwig WD, Harbott J, Löffler H, Schellong G (1993) AML classification by morphologic, immunologic, and cytogenetic parameters - occurrence of subtypes in study AML-BFM-87. Klin Pädiatr 205: 272–280
12. Ritterbach J, Harbott J, Creutzig U, Ritter J, Lampert F (1992) Oncocytogenetic investigations in children with acute non-lymphocytic leukemia (ANLL) chronic myeloid leukemia (CML), and myelodysblastic syndromes (MDS). Ann Hematol 64: 86
13. Rosenbloom B, Schreck R, Koeffler HP (1992) Therapy-related myelodysplastic syndromes. Hematol Oncol Clin North Am 6: 707–722
14. Pedersen-Bjergaard J, Philip P, Pedersen NT, Hou-Jensen K, Sverjgaard A, Jensen G, Nissen NI (1984) Acute nonlymphocytic leukemia, preleukemia, and acute myeloproliterative syndrome secondary to treatment of other malignant diseases II. Cancer 54: 452–462

Acute Leukemias VI
Prognostic Factors
and Treatment Strategies
Büchner et al. (eds)

Deletion of Chromosome 6p as Primary Karyotypic Anomaly in Secondary Acute Nonlymphocytic Leukemia

S. Metzke[1], M. Herold[2], G. Anger[2], and U. Claussen[1]

Abstract. Various structural rearrangements on the short arm of chromosome 6 have been repeatedly reported in therapy-related hematological malignancies, but very rarely as solitary anomaly. Here we report a case of acute nonlymphocytic leukemia (ANLL) after radiochemotherapy for Hodgkin's disease, with a deletion of chromosome 6 (p21pter). This is the first case of deletion 6p as a solitary chromosomal anormaly reported in therapy-related ANLL. This case strongly supports the nonrandom involvement of chromosome 6p in induced leukemias.

Introduction

Structural rearrangements on the short arm of chromosome 6 with involvement of p21pter have been repeatedly reported in therapy-related acute nonlymphocytic leukemias (ANLL), myelodysplastic and myeloproliferative syndrome (MDS, MPS) and malignant lymphomas (ML) [1-8]. Most often 6p rearrangements have been observed in complex karyotypes including aberrations of chromosomes 5 or 7, or both. Only occasionally have 6p rearrangements been described as a single anormaly [2,7]; no isolated deletion of 6p has been described in therapy-related ANLL. The associations of 6p rearrangements with both clinical history of exposure to mutagens and complex aberrations with abnormalities of chromosomes 5 or 7 have suggested that the 6p region may contain a chromosomal region that is preferentially rearranged in induced hematologic malignancies [7].

Here we report a case of ANLL after treatment for Hodgkin's disease (HD) with combination radiochemotherapy, associated with an isolated deletion of the short arm of chromosome 6 which occurred as the only cytogenetic event.

Materials and Methods

Cytogenetic study was performed at the time of diagnosis of leukemia on bone marrow (BM) cells, using short term (24-48 h) cultures, without addition of mutagens. Chromosomes were identified using conventional Giemsa staining and GTG-banding method and were designated according to the International System for Human Cytogenetic Nomenclature [11]. FISH was performed with a directly labeled painting probe specific for chromosome 6 (VYSIS, Framingham, no. 30-608314).

Case Report

A 41-year-old man referred to us in Febraury 1987 with a 6-week history of fever, weight loss and fatigue. Physical examination showed enlargement of supraclavar lymph nodes, histologically diagnosed as Hodgkin's disease (HD), nodular sclerosis, stage IIb. Radiological examination showed a mediastinal tumor mass. Liver and spleen were not palpable.

[1]Institute of Human Genetics and Anthropology, 07740 Jena, Germany
[2]Department of Internal Medicine, Klinikum Erfurt, 99012 Erfurt, Germany

From February to October 1987, the patient received polychemotherapy, including six cycles of CMT [total dose (TD) vinblastine 10 mg, CTX 1.2 g, procarbazine 100 mg, prednisolone 60 mg, daunorubicin 40 mg, vincristine 2 mg, Cytostasan 50 mg, bleomycin 15 mg i.m]. Supraclavar and cervical as well as mediastinal radiotherapy (25 Gy total, involved fields) was administered from May to June 1987. Despite these treatments only partial remission (PR) was achieved. Therefore, from October 1987 to July 1988, the patient received six cycles of CLMP (TD CCNU 100 mg, chlorambucil 20 mg, MTX 7.5 mg, prednisolone 50 mg). A complete remission (CR) was achieved but the patient relapsed (cervical nodes) 9 months later. From April to November 1989 he was treated with six cycles CLMP (TD CCNU 120 mg, chlorambucil 20 mg, MTX 7.5 mg, prednisolone 50 mg) and from October to November 1989 cervical radiotherapy was also administered (20 Gy total, involved field). CR was achieved.

In May 1992, owing to the patient's fever and podagra, a complete blood count was performed, but showed no abnormalities. In August 1992, 33 months after final treatment, the blood count showed anemia, thrombopenia and a white blood cell (WBC) count of $5.9 \times 10^9/l$ with 30% blasts. BM analysis showed 80% blasts, and ANLL-M2 was diagnosed according to the French-American-British (FAB) criteria. The patient was treated thereafter with Ina-Ara-C and Ham and remained in PR until the time of writing.

Results

Of 38 analyzed BM cells, 27 showed a 46, XY,del(6)(p21pter) karyotype (Fig. 1). The partial deletion of 6p was confirmed by fluorescence in situ hybridization (FISH) using a chromosome 6 specific painting probe (Fig. 2)

Discussion

Involvement of the short arm of chromosome 6 in structural rearrangements, other than t(6;9), have been observed in ANLL, MDS, MPS, and ML [1–8]. The almost constant involvement of segment p21pter appears to be particularly frequent among iatrogenically induced ANLL or MDS. More than 80% of the cases with 6p rearrangements described in the literature had

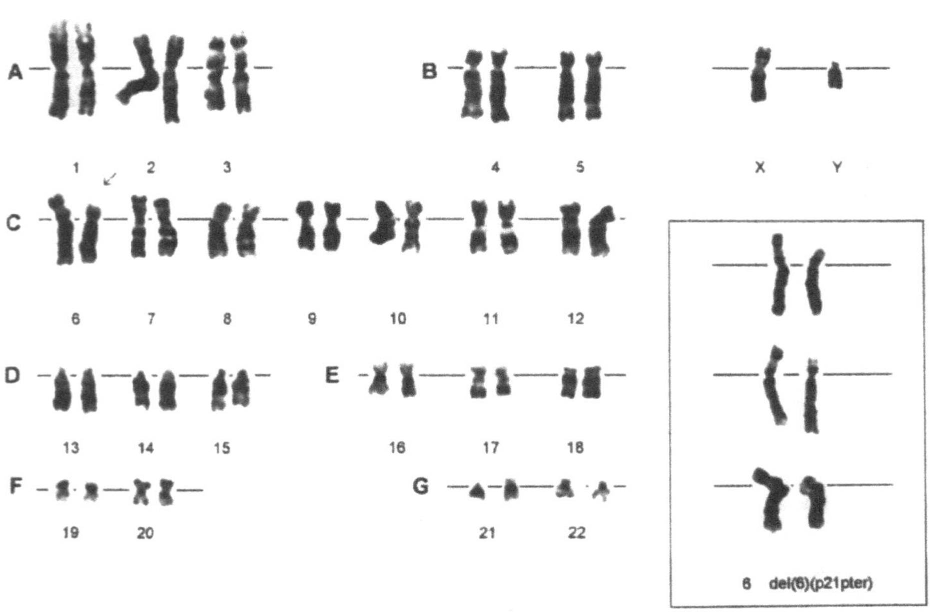

Fig. 1. Karyotype of patient 1 at time of diagnosis of therapy-related ANLL. 46,XY,del(6)(p21pter)

an antecedent history of therapeutic or environmental exposure to carcinogens. In nearly all cases, these rearrangements of 6p were observed in complex karyotypes, mostly associated with aberrations of chromosomes 5 and 7, which typically occur in secondary leukemias [1–8].

Only very rarely have rearrangements of chromosome 6p been reported as a single anormaly. Mancini et al.[7] reported a case of therapy-related ANLL after treatment for HD with an unbalanced t(6;?11) (6qter→ 6p23::?11q13→?11-qter). The deletion 6p (p21pter) described here was confirmed by FISH and seems to be the only cytogenetic event. The association of 6p involvement with both a clinical history of exposure to mutagens and/or abnormalities of chromosomes 5 and 7 has been interpreted as a hint that the region 6p21pter may contain critical sites that are preferentially rearranged in induced hematologic malignancies [7]. The exclusive involvement of 6p in our patient fits well with this hypothesis and strongly supports the idea that a rearrangement of 6p is the initial specific karyotypic anomaly. Rearrangements of this region may play a role in early steps of mutagen-related disorders. Consequently, 6p21 may contain a gene responsible for repair of damage by ionizing radiation and/or DNA-damaging agents. A comparable situation has been described by Thacker et al. [9] for the human XRCC2 gene at 7q36.1. Loss of heterozygosity of this gene by deletion of this region may cause higher sensitivity to mutagens and may lead to secondary hematologic malignancies.

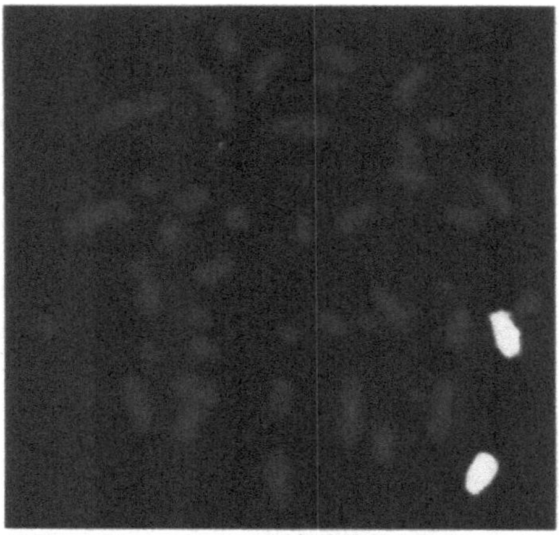
(a)

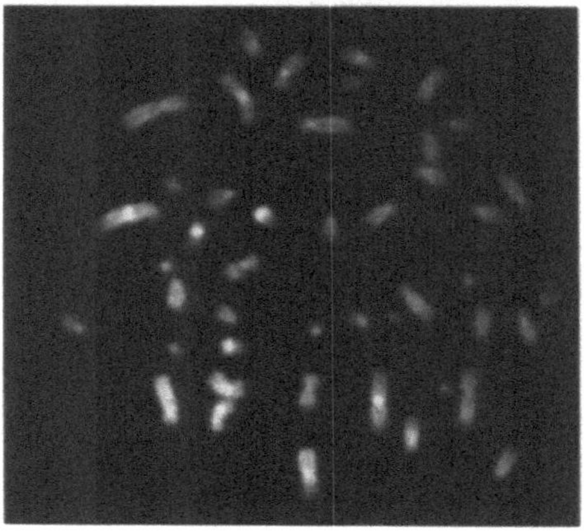
(b)

Fig. 2a,b. Flourescence in situ hybridization showing that no material of chromosome 6 is rearranged to other chromosomes. **a** Chromosomes 6-specific painting probe; **b** DAPI counterstain

Acknowledgment. This work was supported by Dr. Rainald Stromeyer Stiftung, TS 194/01/95.

References

1. Mecucci C, Michaux JL, Louwagie A, Boogaerts M, Van Den Berghe H: The short arm of chromosome 6 is nonrandomly rearranged in secondary myelodysplastic syndromes. Cancer Genet Cytogenet 31, 1988, 147–155.
2. Huret JL, Schoenwald M, Brizard A, Guilhot F, Vilmer E, Tanzer J: Chromosome 6p rearrangements appear to be secondary charges in various haematological malignancies. Leuk Res 13, 1989, 819–824.
3. Philip P, and Pedersen-Bjergaard J: Cytogenetic, clinical and cytologic characteristics of radiotherapy-related leukemias. Cancer Genet Cytogenet 31, 1988, 227–236.
4. Jotterand-Bellomo M, Parlier V, Petite J, Beris P: A new case of myelodysplastic syndrome with 6p rearrangement. Cancer Genet Cytogenet 44, 1990, 271–274.
5. Le Beau MM, Albain KS, Larson RA, Vardiman JW, Davis EM, Blough RR, Golomb HM, Rowley JD: Clinical and cytogenetic correlations in 63 patients with therapy-related myelodysplastic syndromes and acute nonlymphocytic leukemia: further evidence for characteristic abnormalities of chromosomes no.5 and 7-J Clin Oncol 4, 1986, 325–345.
6. Pedersen-Bjergaard J, Philip P, Larsen SO, Jensen G, Brysting K: Chromosome aberrations and prognostic factors in therapy-related myelodysplasia and acute nonlymphocytic leukemia. Blood 76, 1990, 1083–1091.
7. Mancini M, Mecucci C, Cedrone M, Rondinelli MB, Aloe-Spiriti MA, Alimena G: Unbalanced 6p trans-

location as primary karyotypic anomaly in secondary acute nonlymphocytic leukemia. Cancer Genet Cytogenet 60, 1992, 93–95.
8. Shekhter-Levin S, Mirro J, Penchansky L, Sherer ME, Wlad N, Gollin SM: Acute myeloblastic leukemia with a pericentric inversion of chromosome 6 in a child with Down syndrome. Cancer Genet Cytogenet 73, 1994, 157–160.
9. Thacker J, Tambini CE, Simpson PJ, Tsui LC, Scherer SW: Localization to chromosome 7q36.1 of the human XRCC2 gene, determining sensitivity to DNA-damaging agents. Hum Mol Genet 4, 1995, 113–120.
10. Nagarajan L, Louie E, Tsujimoto Y, Ar-Rushdi A, Huebner K, Croce LM: Localization of the human pim oncogene (PIM) to a region of chromosome 6 involved in translocations in acute leukemias. Proc Natl Acad Sci USA 83, 1986, 2556–2560.
11. ISCN 1991. Guidelines for Cancer Cytogenetics, Supplement to An international system for human cytogenetic nomenclature, Mittelman F., Karger S., Basel 1991.

Acute Leukemias VI
Prognostic Factors
and Treatment Strategies
Büchner et al. (eds)

Molecular Cytogenetic Analysis of 7q Abnormalities in Acute Leukemia

S. Tosi[1,5], J. Harbott[2], M. Fitchett[3], F. Ross[4], A. Biondi[5], and L. Kearney[1]

Abstract. Abnormalities of the long arm of chromosome 7 are commonly observed in acute myeloid leukemia (AML) and myelodysplastic syndromes (MDS). These often involve deletions of 7q. We applied fluorescent in situ hybridization (FISH) using a chromosome 7 paint and a 7q telomere-specific probe for a better characterization of 7q abnormalities in a series of patients with acute leukemia. Of the six patients studied, five had structural abnormalities of 7q involving band q22: four of these were deletions and one had additional material on 7q. Only one patient had a breakpoint of 7q31. Four patients had a complex-karyotype: only two had chromosome 7 aberrations as the sole abnormality. The use of FISH revealed the presence of an interstitial deletion in only two patients analysed so far. A further two patients with reported 7q deletions were shown to have unbalanced translocations, with additional material present on 7q. The remaining two patients with other abnormalities of 7q were also identified as having unbalanced translocations. We are continuing these studies in conjunction with FISH using locus-specific probes from 7q to define the critical deleted region involved in abnormalities of 7q in acute leukemia.

Introduction

The application of conventional cytogenetic techniques such as chromosomal banding and, more recently, molecular methods has allowed the identification of recurrent chromosomal aberrations in approximately 80% of patients with de novo AML [1]. Among the unbalanced chromosomal aberrations in AML and MDS, the complete or partial loss of chromosome 5 or 7 is very common [2]. The loss or deletion of chromosome 7 has been associated with a variety of myeloid disorders of both adults and children and is a frequent finding in therapy related MDS and AML [1, 3, 4, 6]. Monosomy 7 and deletions of the long arm of chromosome 7 are not restricted to any FAB subtype and they generally confer a very poor prognosis, with poor response to the therapy and low survival times [5,6]. Chromosome 7 abnormalities have also been reported in acute lymphoblastic leukemia (ALL), although translocations are more commonly observed than deletions [7]. The reported cytogenetic breakpoints in 7q deletions are variable; however, there appear to be two distinct critical regions: 7q22 and 7q32–34 [8]. Both terminal and interstitial deletions have been described [7].

The aim of the present study was to obtain an improved interpretation of the karyotype in a series of patients with acute leukemia carrying abnormalities of 7q using FISH. The reported abnormalities included interstitial and terminal deletions, as well as uncharacterised add(7q) chromosomes present both as part of a complex karyotype and as the sole cytogenetic abnormality.

[1]MRC Molecular Haematology Unit, Institute of Molecular Medicine, John Radcliffe Hospital, Oxford, UK
[2]Oncocytogenetic Laboratory, Children's Hospital, Giessen, Germany
[3]Department of Medical Genetics, Churchill Hospital, Oxford, UK
[4]Wessex Regional Genetics Laboratory, Salisbury, UK
[5]Clinica Pediatrica dell'Universita' di Milano, Ospedale S. Gerardo, Monza, Italy

Materials and Methods

Patient Material

Archival methanol-acetic acid-fixed chromosome preparations from bone marrow cells of 6 patients with acute leukemia and abnormalities of the long arm of chromosome 7 were selected for our study. The patient material was collected from three different centres where the cytogenetic analysis was previously performed (patients 1 and 2: Children's University Hospital, Giessen, Germany; patient 3: Churchill Hospital, Oxford, UK; patients 4, 5 and 6: Wessex Regional Laboratory, Salisbury, UK). All the patients considered in our study were suffering from acute leukemia: 5 out of 6 had AML and 1 had ALL. Two of the 6 patients analysed were children and 4 were adult (Table 1).

Probes

The probes utilized were (1) a commercially available biotinylated chromosome 7 α satellite/7q telomere probe (Oncor, Gaithersburg, Md), and (2) a chromosome 7 paint which was obtained by degenerate oligonucleotide primer-polymerase chain reaction (DOP PCR) amplification of flow sorted chromosomes [9].

Fluorescence In Situ Hybridization

The chromosome 7 centromere-7q telomere probes were used following the manufacturers' instructions. The chromosome 7 paint was applied by competitive in situ suppression hybridization as previously described [10]. In both cases the detection was performed using avidin-fluorescein in isothiocyanate (FITC) and biotinylated anti-avidin antibody (Vector Laboratories). Slides were mounted in antifade medium (Vectashield, Vector Laboratories) containing propidium iodide and 4, 6-diamidinophenylindole (DAPI) as counterstain. Cells were examined under epifluorescence, and images were captured and stored using a Bio-Rad MRC600 confocal laser scanning microscope.

Results

The clinical and cytogenetic features of the 6 patients analysed in our study, together with the FISH results, are summarized in Table 1.

Cases 1 and 3

Previous conventional cytogenetic analysis of these two patients revealed the presence of one chromosome 7 carrying a terminal deletion with breakpoint at band q22. In the first patient the karyotype was complex, with the presence of structural abnormalities involving other chromosomes, whereas in patient 3 the del(7) was present as the sole abnormality. In both cases chromosome painting revealed that the chromosome described as del(7) was only partially painted and, in patient 1, hybridization signals specific for 7q telomere were present only on the normal chromosome 7. These results suggest the presence of an unbalanced translocation with loss of 7q telomeric sequences, rather than the reported terminal deletion.

Cases 2 and 4

A complex karyotype was reported in both of these cases. In patient 2 the presence of an undefined der(7)(q22) was described, and in

Table 1. Clinical and cytogenetic features of the six patients analyzed

Patient no.	Age (years)/sex	Diagnosis	Reported abnormalities	7paint	7q telomere
1	10 /F	c-ALL	del(7)(q22)[a]	Partially painted	Deleted
2	13 /F	AML-M0	der(7)(q22)[a]	Fully painted	ND
3	44 /F	t-AML	del(7)(q22)[b]	Partially painted	ND
4	76 /F	AML	del(7)(q22q36)[a]	Fully painted	Retained
5	74 /F	AML	add(7)(q22)[b]	Partially painted	Deleted
6	24 /M	AML	add(7)(q31)[a]	Partially painted	Deleted

c-ALL, acute lymphoblastic leukemia, common type; t-AML, therapy related acute myeloblastic leukemia; ND not determined
[a]Part of a complex karyotype
[b]Present as sole abnormality

patient 4 an interstitial deletion, del(7)(q22q36), was observed. In these two cases both chromosomes 7 appeared fully painted by FISH, and, in case 4, it was possible to demonstrate that the 7q telomere was retained on the del(7) (Fig. 1 A). These results suggest the presence of an interstitial deletion in this case.

Cases 5 and 6

In these two cases the cytogenetic analysis revealed the presence of add(7) with breakpoints at band q22 (patient 5) and band q31 (patient 6). In both cases the chromosome 7 paint revealed one chromosome fully painted and one partially painted, with additional material present on 7q. The chromosome 7 telomere probe identified, in each case, two chromosomes with a chromosome 7 centromere, only one of which had 7q telomere present: the telomeric sequences did not appear to be present on any other chromosome (Fig. 1C, D). These results confirmed the cytogenetic findings and suggested the presence of an unbalanced translocation with loss of material from chromosome 7.

Discussion

In the present study we applied FISH with a chromosome 7 paint and 7q telomere probe in a small series of patients in whom prior cytogenetic analysis identified structural abnormalities of 7q. These were interpreted by banding analysis as terminal deletions (cases 1 and 3), interstitial deletions (case 4), or der(7) and add(7) (cases 2, 5 and 6). The present study has allowed more precise definition of the karyotype: in 4 of 6 cases (cases 1, 3, 5 and 6), structural abnormalities defined as del(7q), der(7) or add(7)

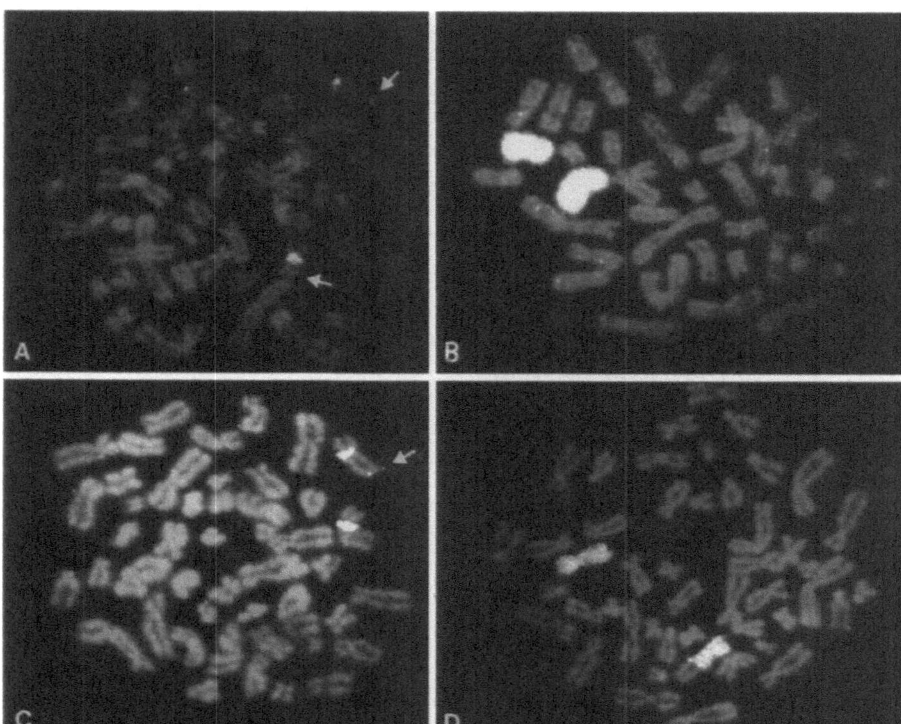

Fig. 1. FISH results using **A,C** chromosome 7 α satellite/7q telomere probe and **B,D** chromosome 7 paint on patients 4 and 6. **A,B** In patient 4 both chromosomes 7 are fully painted and hybridization signals are seen on both 7q telomeres. **C,D** In patient 6 the abnormal chromosome 7 is only partially painted and lacks 7q telomere signals. *Arrows* indicate hybridization spots on 7q telomeres

were reinterpreted as unbalanced translocations with deletion of the telomeric sequences, while the remaining 2 patients (cases 2 and 4) had "true" deletions, at least one of which (case 4) was interstitial since the telomeric sequences were retained on the del(7). In all the cases loss of material from chromosome 7q was confirmed.

Abnormalities of 7q are often observed as part of complex karyotype. However, in the present series, correct cytogenetic interpretation did not appear to be dependent on whether the del(7) was present as part of a complex karyotype or as the sole abnormality. In fact in the only case (no. 3) in which the del(7) was apparently the sole chromosomal aberration, FISH revealed the presence of an unbalanced translocation. This study demonstrates the importance of using FISH for a better characterization of chromosomal abnormalities: the use of paints may enable the detection not only of translocations or insertions, but also of evident loss or gain of chromosomal material. The application of probes specific for telomeres is essential in order to define whether a deletion is terminal or interstitial. The technique of FISH with whole chromosome paints is now being applied not only for the study of hematological malignancies [11, 12] but also for the analysis of solid tumors [13], and it seems that, in both fields, this relatively simple technique may lead to a general revision of the chromosomal assessment even in those cases with apparently simple rearrangements.

The region of interest in 7q deletions has not been defined in size, nor have the breakpoints been accurately characterized, although it has been reported that one of the most common breakpoints is at band 7q22 and that the critical deleted region always comprises band 7q32 to 7qter [6, 8]. It is not yet established whether true terminal deletions exist, or whether all deletions are interstitial. In the present series, at least one of the reported del(7q) cases was an interstitial deletion. However, all of the unbalanced translocations identified also had deletions of 7q which included the telomere.

This preliminary characterization obtained using chromosome paint and probes specific for chromosome 7 centromere and 7q telomere, in combination with probes for specific loci in the long arm of chromosome 7, will help in future studies to narrow down the deleted region in those patients with unbalanced chromosome aberrations. Such a molecular cytogenetic definition of chromosomal rearrangement involving 7q may allow a better correlation between clinical groups and karyotype. A precise definition of deletion breakpoints and the minimum size for deletions may eventually lead to a better definition of prognostic groups and to the development of more appropriate treatment strategies.

Acknowledgments. S.T. is supported by a fellowship from the *Associazione Italiana Ricerca sul Cancro* (AIRC).

References

1. Pedersen-Bjergaard J, and Rowley J (1994) The balanced and the unbalanced chromosome aberrations of acute myeloid leukemia may develop in different ways and may contribute differently to malignant transformation. Blood 83: 2780–2786
2. Le Beau MM, Albain KS, Larson RA, Vardiman JW, Davis EM, Blough RR, Golomb HM, Rowley JD (1986) Clinical and cytogenetic correlations in 63 patients with therapy related myelodysplastic syndrome and acute nonlymphocytic leukemia: further evidence for characteristic abnormalities of chromosome no. 5 and 7. J Clin Oncol 3: 3: 325–345
3. Mufti GJ (1992) Chromosomal deletions in the myelodysplastic syndrome. Leuk Res 16: 35–41
4. Gadner H, and Haas OA (1992) Experience in pediatric myelodysplastic syndromes. Hematology/Oncology Clinics of North America 6: 655–672
5. Yunis JJ, Lobell M, Anersen MA, Oken MM, Mayer MG, Rydell RE, Brunning RD (1988) Refined chromosome study helps define prognostic subgroups in most patients with primary myelodysplastic syndrome and acute myelogenous leukemia. Br J Haematol 68: 189–194
6. Pedersen-Bjergaard J, Philip P, Larsen SO, Jensen G, Byrsting K (1990) Chromosome aberrations and prognostic factors in therapy-related myelodysplasia and acute nonlymphocytic leukemia. Blood 76: 1083–1091
7. Mitelman F (1991) The catalog of chromosome aberrations in cancer. Fourth Ed. Wiley-Liss. New York
8. Neuman WL, Rubin CM, Rios RB, Larson RA, Le Beau MM, Rowley JD, Vardiman JW, Schwartz JL, Farber RA (1992) Chromosomal loss and deletion are the most common mechanisms for loss of heterozygosity from chromosome 5 and 7 in malignant myeloid disorders. Blood 79: 1501–1510
9. Telenius H, Pelmear AH, Tunnacliffe A, Carter NP, Behmel A, Ferguson-Smith MA, Nordenskjold M, Pfragner R, Ponder BA (1992) Cytogenetic analysis by chromosome painting using DOP-PCR amplified for sorted chromosomes. Genes Chromosom Cancer 4: 257–263

10. Kearney L, Watkins PC, Young BD, Sacchi N (1991) DNA sequences of chromosome 21-specific YAC detect the t(8;21) breakpoint of acute myelogenous leukemia. Cancer Genet Cytogenet 57: 109–119
11. Gibbons B, Lillington DM, Monard S, Young BD, Cheung KL, Lister TA, Kearney L (1994) Fluorescence in situ hybridization studies to characterize complete and partial monosomy 7 in myeloid disorders. Genes Chromosom Cancer 10: 244–249
12. Kobayashi H, and Rowley J (1995) Identification of cytogenetically undetected 12p13 translocations and associated deletions with fluorescence in situ hybridization. Genes Chromosom Cancer 12: 66–69
13. Sahlin P, Mark J, Stenman G. (1995) Detection of hidden structural rearrangements by FISH in pleomorphic adenomas. Genes Chromosom Cancer 12: 81–8

Acute Leukemias VI
Prognostic Factors
and Treatment Strategies
Büchner et al. (eds)

Unusual Karyotype 46,XX,inv(8)(p21q24),del(20)(q11q13) in a Case of Acute Leukemia M6 in a Child

S. Donskaya[1], S. Andreeva[2], A. Galántha[2], L. Sclysarenko[3], and N. Derbenyova[1]

Introduction

Specific structural chromosome abnormalities are connected with different types of acute myeloid leukemia and have proved to be helpful in establishing the precise diagnosis and the prognosis of disease. For FAB M6 subtype, many karyotype changes have been described and classified as minor and major karyotype abnormalities (MIKA and MAKA) [1]. Here we report the combination of two clonal chromosome changes in a child with M6 AML.

Patient and Cytogenetic Study

The patient, a 5-year-old girl, was admitted to the hospital in June 1994 because of hepatosplenomegaly. She had lost weight and had suffered weakness in the previous two months. Physical examination showed liver and spleen enlargement (6.0 cm and 5.0 cm below the costal margin, respectively) and general lymphadenopathy (0.5–1.0 cm in diameter). Initial hematologic data were: Hb 10.6 g/dl; RBC $3.4 \times 10^{12}/l$; WBC $12.8 \times 10^9/l$ with 10% of blast cells; platelets $74.0 \times 10^9/l$. Bone marrow aspiration showed 52.6% of erythroblasts among all nucleated cells and 32.8% myeloblasts for all nucleated cells (69.2% for all nonerythroid cells), and FAB M6-AML was diagnosed.

Chromosome analysis was carried out on unstimulated bone marrow cells which were incubated in RPMI 1640 and 20% FCS for 24 h. The cell suspension was brought to hypotonicity with KCl (20 min) and fixed in methanol–acetic acid (3:1). Then the suspension was washed four or five times. The cells were pipetted onto cold wet slides to spread metaphases. G-banding was done, after trypsin pretreatment (1–3 s), 7 days later. The subsequent karyotyping followed the recommendations of the ISCN [2].

At diagnosis 100 metaphases were counted and 10 were karyotyped. Chromosome analysis showed the existence of three clones: 46,XX, del (20)(q11q13); 46,XX,inv(8)(p21p24), del(20) (q11q13) (Fig. 1). The existence of the third clone was revealed by the presence of 8.0% of tetraploid metaphases (Fig. 2).

The patient was treated according to protocol BFM-AML-78 but did not achieve remission after the induction course: control bone marrow showed 76.4% of erythroid cells and 44.4% of erythroblasts with atypical features and 14.8% myeloblasts; liver and spleen were still enlarged (4.0 and 5.0 cm below the costal margin respectively).

After prolongation of treatment only short episodes of leukopenia with stable persistence of blasts in peripheral blood were registered, and after 2 months palliative treatment with low-dose Ara-C was begun. The child died of disease progression 5.5 months after diagnosis.

[1]Kiev Institute of Medical Training, Kiev, Ukraine
[2]Kiev Institute of Hematology and Blood Transfusion, Kiev, Ukraine
[3]R.E. Kavetsky Institute of Experimental Pathology, Oncology and Radiobiology, Academy of Sciences, Ukraine

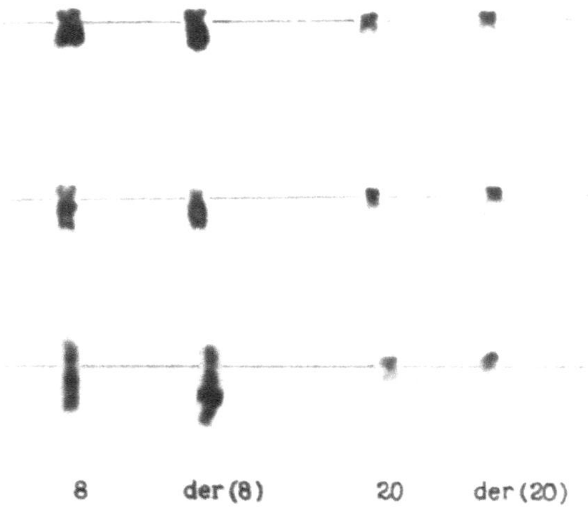

Fig. 1. Karyotype of G-banded bone marrow cells from a 5-year-old girl with M6 AML with inv(8) (p21q24), del(20)(q11q13)

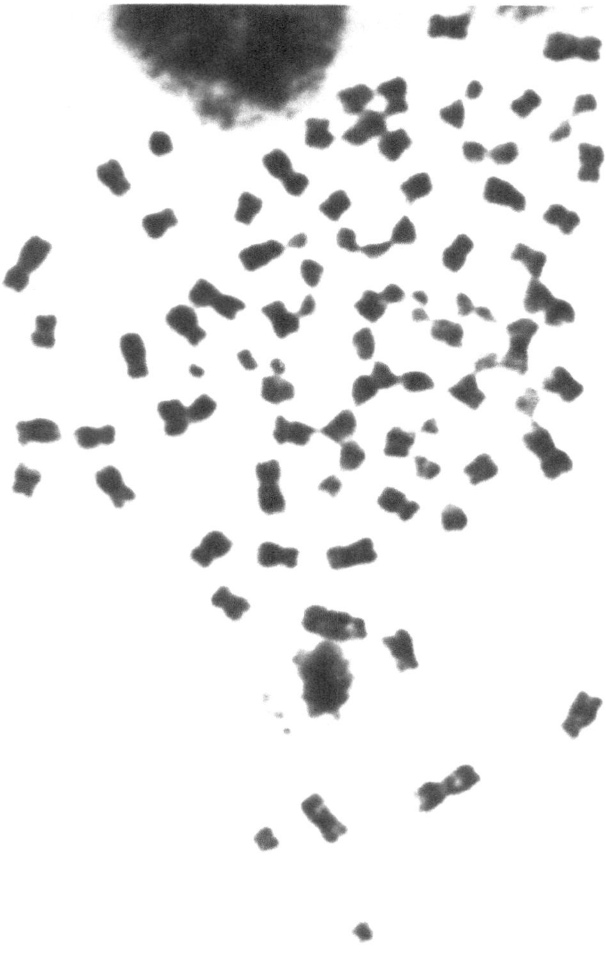

Fig. 2. Hypotetraploid metaphase from bone marrow of a 5-year-old girl with M6 AML

Discussion

The cytogenetic characteristics in M6 AML are very heterogeneous. One anomaly registered in our case, inv(8)(p21q24), was described earlier [3] as connected with the M6 variant of AML. In the literature, involvement of the short arm of chromosome 8 is very rare among different types of chromosome 8 aberrations in AML variants [4].

The other karyotyping abnormality, del(20)(q11q13), has not been previously described in AML but has been seen as a karyotype marker of polycythemia vera [5].

It is interesting that one clone presented del(20)(q11q13) and another two abnormalities connected with pathologic erythroblasts. This could be connected with a specific clinical picture at presentation, because our patient had no initial anemia syndrome, which is known as one of the typical features for such variant AML. We propose that such a combination of cytogenetic anomalies could be responsible for the initial chemoresistance of the leukemic clone.

Acknowledgments. We gratefully acknowledge Professor F. Lampert, Dr. J. Harbott, and Dr. R. Engel of the Children's Hospital, University of Giessen, for their teaching, consultation and continous support of our research and practical work. We are also very grateful to Professor G. Schellong from the University Children's Hospital, Münster, for his regular consultation and constant help in our treatment policy.

References

1. Sakuari M, Sandberg AA (1976). Chromosomes and causation of human cancer and leukemia. XIII. An evaluation of karyotypic findings in erythroleukemic. Cancer 37: 790–804
2. ISCN (1991). Guidelines for Cancer Cytogenetics. Supplement to an International System for Human Cytogenetic Nomenclature. S. Karger, Basel, 54p.
3. Santoro A, Carbone P, Caradonna F, Fabbiano F, Mitro S, Caronia F (1993) A New Pericentric inv (8) in Acute Nonlymphocytic Leukemia. Cancer Genet Cytogenet 65: 77–78.
4. Bertheas MF, Jaubert J, Vasselon C, Reunaud J, Promier G, Le Petit JC, Hagenieijer A, Brizard CP (1989) A complex t(3;8;17) Involving Breakpoint 8p11 in a Case of M5 Acute Nonlymphocytic Leukemia with Erythrophagocytosis. Cancer Genet Cytogenet 42: 67–73.
5. Human Cytogenetics. A Practical Approach. Volume II. Malignancy and Acquired Abnormalities. Second Edition. (Ed. Rooney DE, Czepulkowski BH). Oxford New York Tokyo. Oxford University Press. 293 p

Acute Leukemias VI
Prognostic Factors
and Treatment Strategies
Büchner et al. (eds)

Acute Myeloblastic Leukemia M2 with the 8;21 Translocation Associated with Granulocytic Sarcoma

E. Dubrovina, O. Kryzhanovsky, A. Maschan, E. Samochatova, L. Baydun, and O. Bartseva

Abstract. A 13-year-old girl presented with 2 compact painless subcutaneous tumors of 3 cm on the scalp in June 1993. Peripheral blood count was Hb 95g/l, Er 3.2 time $\times 10^{12}$/leukocytes- 21×10^9/l: blasts 74%, neutrophils 9%, lymphocytes 14%, monocytes 3%. After bone marrow puncture, AML FAB M2 was diagnosed. Cytogenetic analysis of bone marrow showed two clones: 1, 46 XX (20%) and clone 2, 46 XX t(8;21) (q22;q22) and t(1;17) (q21;p13) (80%). CSF examination revealed 9 cells/ml WBC with blasts on the cytocentrifuged specimen. A tumor mass in the spinal canal (L2-L3) compressing the spinal cord was also revealed by CT scan. A complete remission was achieved after induction chemotherapy acccording to the BFM-AML-87 protocol. The patient received the 6 week consolidation phase, but intensification of treatment with high-dose Ara-c and VP-16 was omitted due to the 10-fold increase in hepatic enzymes. Then the patient received maintenance therapy. Two months after completion of consolidation the patient was admitted with urine retention. Three separate large masses were palpable in the abdomen. Laparoscopy disclosed tumor masses in the uterus and both ovaries. Bone marrow examination revealed more than 50% of blasts. Relapse treatment consisted of: one course of Ara-C 1000mg/m^2 every 12 h for 4 days, VP-16 100mg/m^2 per day for 4 days and mitoxantrone 8 mg/m^2 per day for 3 days; one course of the same doses of Ara-C for 4 days plus amsacrine 100 mg/m^2 per day for 3 days and L-asparaginase 6000 IU/m^2 6 h after the last dose of Ara-C. After the treatment the second remission was achieved in January 1994. Autologous BMT without ex vivo purging was performed in July 1994 after conditioning with melphalan 190 mg/m^2. After bone marrow reconstitution, immunotherapy with IL-2 (5 MU/m^2 s.c. for 5 days every 2 weeks) was begun and is being continued. The second remission has lasted for 12 months.

Conclusion

Patients with AML M2 with t(8;21) who have granulocytic sarcoma may be at high risk of early relapse. A thorough search for GS must be recommended in patients with AML M2 with t(8.21). Those who have such an association can not be included in the low risk prognostic group and require intensive systemic chemotherapy.

Introduction

The incidence of acute myeloid leukemia (AML) meeting the morphological criteria of M2 type according to the French-American-British (FAB) classification is reported as 28% [1]. Cytogenetically, approximately 40% of patients with M2 t(8;21) while over 90% of patients with t(8;21) have a diagnosis of M2 [2]. Over 50% of patients with t(8;21) have additional changes [3]. A critical event in the pathogenesis may be the formation of a novel chimeric gene and message as the result of the two genes' fusion – *eto* from chromosome 8 and AML1 from chromo-

Russian Institute of Pediatric Hematology, Moscow, Russia

some 21 [4,5]. It is generally believed that characteristic features of the M2 with t(8;21) include a high complete remission rate and the longest relapse-free survival durations with conventional chemotherapy [6]. Other favorable prognostic features that emerged from the AML-BFM-83 study and are currently in use in the AML-BFM-93 protocol are a WBC count less than 20,000/μl [7] and the presence of Auer rods.

Granulocytic sarcoma (GS) or chloroma is observed in 3–7% cases of AML both as a primary manifestation and in relapse [8]. These tumors are discrete extramedullary collections of immature leukemic cells that may occur anywhere but most often arise adjacent to cranial, facial and spinal bones [9]. Evidence is accumulating that GS is frequently associated with t(8;21) - up to 38% in some series of adult patients with AML [9]. To date, only 18 such cases in children have been reported and little is known about the prognostic significance of the association. We describe here the disease course of a pediatric patient with AML and t(8;21) who developed GS.

Case Report

A 13-year-old girl presented in June 1993 with high-grade fever, nausea, dizziness, weakness in the lower extremities and urine retention. At admission, the clinical examination revealed a painless subcutaneous mass in the right temporal region. Liver, spleen, and lymph nodes were not enlarged. The bladder was distended to the umbilicus. A tumor mass in the spinal canal (L2-L3) compressing the spinal cord was revealed by computed tomography. Examination of the CSF showed leukemia cells. Needle aspiration of the subcutaneous mass demonstrated a granulocytic sarcoma. The peripheral blood count was Hb 95g/l, Er 3.2×10^{12}/l leukocytes 21×10^9/l: blasts 74%, neutrophils 9%, lymphocytes 14%, monocytes 3%. The bone marrow showed AML FAB M2 with Auer rods. Karyotype analysis showed 2 clones: abnormal clone 46, XX t(8;21)(q22;q22), t(1;17)(q21;p13) (80%) and normal 46 XX (20%). A complete remission was achieved after induction chemotherapy according to the BFM-AML-87 protocol. The patient received the 6-week consolidation phase, but intensification of treatment with high-dose Ara-C and VP-16 was omitted due to acute hepatitis C development. Then the patient received maintenance therapy. Two months after completion of consolidation the patient was admitted with complaints of urine retention. Three separate large masses were palpable in the abdomen. Laparoscopy disclosed tumor masses in the uterus and both ovaries. Bone marrow examination revealed more than 50% of blasts. Relapse treatment consisted of one course of Ara-C 1000 mg/m^2 every 12 h for 4 days, VP-16 100 mg/m^2/day for 4 days and mitoxantrone 8 mg/m^2/day for 3 days; one course of the same doses of Ara-C for 4 days plus amsacrine 100 mg/m^2/day for 3 days and L-asparaginase 6000 IU/m^2 6 h after the last dose of Ara-C. After the treatment the second remission was achieved in January 1994. Autologous BMT without purging was performed in July 1994 after conditioning with melphalan 190 mg/m^2. After bone marrow reconstitution, immunotherapy with IL-2 (5 MU/m^2 s.c. for 5 days every 2 weeks) was begun. The second remission has lasted for 12 months.

Discussion

This case demonstrates that the prognostic significance of the translocation t(8;21) is debatable. As patients are usually easily brought into remission with conventional treatment, those who have GS in association with this cytogenetic abnormality may be at high risk of early relapse. As long as GS may not be widely recognized a thorough search for such lesions in patients with t(8;21) is recommended. The subgroup of patients with GS probably requires more intensive systemic therapy, such as allogeneic or autologous stem cell transplantation. Besides, local radiotherapy may be of no use as the disease may recur at any other site.

Acknowledgments. The technical assistance of T. Churkina is gratefully acknowledged.

References

1. Blood Textbook of hematology. JH Jandl, ed. Boston: Little Brown & Co, 1987.
2. Sandrerg AA. 1990. The chromosomes in human cancers and leukemia. 2nd ed. New York: Elsevier, 1990.
3. Walker H, Smith FJ, Betts DR. Cytogenetics in acute myeloid leukemia. Blood Reviews; 1994, 8: 30–36.
4. Downing JR, Head DR, Curcio-Brint AM. An AML1/ETO fusion transcript is consistently detect-

ed by RNA-based polymerase chain reaction in acute myelogenous leukemia containing the t(8;21) (q22;q22) translocation. Blood 1993; 81: 2860–2865.
5. Maseki N, Miyoshi H, Shimizu K, et al. The 8;21 chromosome translocation in acute myeloid leukemia is always detectable by molecular analysis using AML1. Blood 1993; 81: 1573–1579.
6. Arthur DC, Berger R, Golomb HM, et al: The clinical significance of karyotype in acute myelogenous leukemia. Cancer Genet. Cytogenet, 1989; 40: 203–216.
7. Creutzig U, Ritter J, Schellong G: Identification of two risk groups in childhood acute myelogenous leukemia after therapy intensification in study AML-BFM-83 as compared with study AML-BFM-78. Blood, 1990, 75: 1932–1940.
8. Muss HB, Moloney WC: Chloroma and other myeloblastic tumors. Blood. 1973, 42: 721–728.
9. Tallman MS, Hakimian D, Shaw JM, et al.: Granulocytic sarcoma is associated with the 8;21 translocation in acute myeloid leukemia. Journal of Clinical Oncology, 1993, 4: 690–697.

Acute Leukemias VI
Prognostic Factors
and Treatment Strategies
Büchner et al. (eds)

Cytogenetic Subgroups in Childhood Acute Myeloblastic Leukemia at the Schneider Children's Medical Center of Israel

B. Stark[1,2], M. Jeison[2], R. Gobuzov[2], I. Kadyshevitch[2], D. Luria[3], S. Ash[1], I. Cohen[1], Y. Goshen[1], S. Fischer[1], J. Stein[1], H. Tamary[1], I. Yaniv[1], and R. Zaizov[1,2,3]

Abstract. Specific cytogenetic aberrations in acute myeloblastic leukemia (AML) have been found to have important, independent prognostic significance. Consistent incidence of variations of the cytogenetic subtypes have been related to age, ethnic origin, geographical area, and exposure to environmental factors. In our pediatric AML population treated from 1988 to 1994, of the 40 patients (4 with t-AML) with successful karyotypes, 85% had clonal aberrations. Incidence of chromosomal abnormalities in decreasing order was t(8;21) in 20%, t/del (11q23) in 15%, t/inv(3q) in 7.5%, and t(15;17), t(3;5), del(9q) and t(6;9) in 5% (patients) each. Isolated trisomy 8, monosomy 7, t(8;19) variant of t(8;16), t(10;11;12) were also found in one patient each. No inv/del(16q) was detected in this cohort. Outcome with a short follow-up did not differ in general to that previously reported. To confirm this unique cytogenetic profile of a relatively high incidence of the favorable t(8;21) together with a high incidence of relatively rare, nonrandom, unfavorable aberrations, the study should be extended to a larger group of children.

Introduction

Nonrandom cytogenetic abnormalities have repeatedly been specifically associated with the type and specific lineage subtype of leukemia [1-5]. The frequency of some of the aberrations has also been nonrandomly correlated with age; for example, a higher frequency of t/del(11q23), t(8;21), inv(16q), and −7/7q−or−5/5q− in acute myeloblastic leukemia (AML) is observed in infancy, childhood, adulthood, and old age, respectively [2,4,6]. A consistent difference in the cytogenetic profile of AML has been noted among various ethnic groups, such as a higher proportion of t(8;21) and t(15;17) in blacks and Orientals than in whites [2,7]. These consistent variations may reflect genetic factors, although they do not preclude exogenous environmental factors. Specific chromosomal abnormalities have been reported to be related to specific types of carcinogens, such as balanced translocation of 11q23, or 21q22 with topoisomerase II inhibitors, and −7/7q− and −5/5q− with alkylating agents and pesticides in secondary or therapy-related AML (t-AML) [8-11].

The specific chromosomal aberrations in AML have a significant prognostic value [5,12-19]. Their different response to chemotherapeutic agents has recently been introduced in the planning of treatment stratification [19]. When comparing results from different geographic areas and planning a new treatment design, these epidemiological differences should be taken into consideration.

We present the cytogenetic profile of the pediatric AML population treated from 1988 to 1994 by the AML BFM-87 protocol at the Schneider Children's Medical Center of Israel (SCMCI).

[1]Department of Pediatric Hematology and Oncology
[2]Cancer Cytogenetic Laboratory
[3]Flow-Cytometry Laboratory, The Schneider Children's Medical Center of Israel, Beilinson Medical Campus, Petah Tiqva 49202, and Sackler Faculty of Medicine, Tel Aviv University, Tel Aviv, Israel

Materials and Methods

Between July 1988 and December 1994, 47 children less than 20 years of age with AML (de novo and therapy-related) were admitted to the Pediatric Hematology-Oncology Department of the SCMCI. The diagnosis of AML was based on standard FAB morphologic and cytochemical criteria [20], including staining with periodic acid-Schiff reagent, acid phosphatase, myeloperoxidase, Sudan black, chloroacetate esterase, and alpha-naphthyl acetate esterase.

Cytogenetic studies were performed on bone marrow samples obtained at diagnosis. Direct or 24- to 48-h unstimulated cultures, with or without methotrexate synchronization, were processed according to standard methods; briefly, colcemid (final concentration 0.05 μg/ml) incubation for 25–40 min, exposure to hypotonic solution (KCl 0.075 mol/l) for 30 min, and then G banding of slide metaphase preparation with trypsin and Giemsa staining. Chromosome abnormalities were identified and classified according to the ISCN [21].

Adequate cytogenetic analysis was achieved in 40 children (in five children analysis was not done, and in two others metaphases could not be obtained). Thirty-six children had de novo AML, one of whom (referred from abroad) was in first relapse; four others had t-AML. All children, except for one, were treated with the AML modified BFM-87 protocol [22], with the addition of IT triple injections, but without cranial irradiation. In higher risk patients, allogeneic bone marrow transplantation (BMT) was performed in patients with matched donor, and in the last year autologous BMT was also performed.

Results

Cytogenetics

Of the 40 adequately banded patients, six (15%) had an apparently normal karyotype (Table 1). In the remaining 34 patients (85%), clonal chromosomal abnormalities could be identified. The majority (22/34) of the cases were pseudodiploid; among the others, one had 51 chromosomes, two had 47 chromosomes (+19 and isolated +8), and eight had 45 chromosomes. Hypodiploidy was due to loss of sex chromosome in four patients [in three it accompanied t(8;21)], loss of chromosome 7 in three patients (in one as the sole aberration and in two accompanying 3q aberrations), and loss of 9 or 22 in one patient (no. 25). Complex karyotype was found in two patients (nos. 13, 15), and in five patients (nos. 7, 9, 12, 16, 24) additional clones evolving from the original one could be identified already at diagnosis. Most of the chromosomal abnormalities were of the known consistent nonrandom aberrations, although a few of them are known to occur very rarely. Results of chromosome analysis and clinical findings on patients 17, 33 [23] and 30 [24] have been published previously.

Of the major karyotypic subgroups detected in our series, t(8;21) was the most common, occurring in eight patients (20%); t/del (11q23) was found in six patients (15%), and rearrangement involving 3q21 of q26 in three (7.5%). Translocation t(15;17) was found in only two patients. Trisomy 8 and monosomy 7, both as sole aberrations, could be identified in one patient each. The rare aberrations t(3;5), del (9q) (as the sole aberration), and t(6;9) or its variant were found in two patients each. The t(8;19) variant of t(8;16) and t(10;11;12), the variant of t(10;11)(p13;13), were found in one patient each. No inv/del(16q) and t(9;22) were observed.

Clinical Presentation and Outcome

Of the 40 patients successfully analyzed, 30 were of Jewish origin and 10 of Moslem origin; 24 were male and 16 were female (Table 2).

In the t(8;21) subgroup, three out of the eight patients were Moslem; median age was 6 years, (range 3.8–16.8), and median WBC was 24×10^9/l. All were uniquely characterized by blast cell morphology of FAB-M2, most of them with Auer rods. However, one child (no. 6) had preceding myelodysplastic syndrome (MDS) and presented with refractory anemia with excess of blast in transformation (RAEB-T). By immunophenotype (results not shown), all eight patients were strongly positive for HLA-DR and CD34 and frequently mildly positive for CD13 and/or CD33; three patients were weakly positive for T-cell marker CD7, two for NK-cell marker CD56, and only two for the B-cell marker CD19. All achieved remission after one induction course of the AML BFM-87 protocol, including the girl who presented in relapse after 24 months (no. 3). Two children have relapsed

Table 1. Chromosomal findings in childhood AML (40 patients)

Chromosome group	Patient no.	Karyotypes
t(8;21)	1	46,XX,t(8;21)(q22;q22)[3]
	2	46,XX,t(8;21)(q22;q22)[6]
	3[a]	46,XX,t(8;21)(q22;q22)[11]/46,XX[3]
	4	46,XX,t(8;21)(q22;q22)[5]
	5	45,X,-Y,t(8;21)(22;q22)[14]
	6	45,X,-Y,t(8;21)(q22;q22)[15]/46,XY[2]
	7	46,XX,t(8;21)(q22;q22)[22]/46,idem,add(2)(q35)[17]/ 46,idem,del(9)(q22),del(11)(p13)[7]
	8	45,X-Y,t(8;21)(q22);q22)[19]
t/del(11)(q23)	9	51,XY,+4,+8,+13,+16,+19,t(9;11)(p22;q23)[12]/ 52,idem,+del(1)(p2)[2]
	10[b]	46,XY,t(9;11)(p21;q23)[21]/46,XY[1]
	11[b]	46,XY,t(9;11)(p22;q23)[17]
	12	46,XY,t(1;11)(q21;q23)[17]/46,idem,add(19)(p13?)[7]
	13	46,XX,del(6)(q21q24),add(11)(q23or24),der(18?)[15]
	14	46,XY,del(11)(q23)[16]/46,XY[1]
t/inv(3q)	15	45,XY,-1,der(1)t(1;7)(p11;q11),add (3)(q26?),-7,-11, der(11)t(1;11)(p?;p11?),-13,+mar1,+mar2,+mar3
	16	46,XX,t(3;21)(q21;q22)[9]/46,idem,add(2)(q?),add(4)(q23?)[7]/ 46,idem,add(1)(p36),add(4)(q23)[3]
	17[b]	45,XX,inv(3)(q21;q26),-7[3]/46,XX[2]
t(3;5)	18	46,XY,t(3;5)(q25;q35)[9]/46.XY[1]
	19	46,XX,t(3;5)(q25;q34)[20]
t(15;17)	20	46,XX,t(15;17)(q22;q21)[16]/46,XX[3]
	21	46,XY,t(15;17)(q22;q21),inv(12q12q?)[17]/46,XY[2]
del(9q)	22	46,XY,del(9)(q13q22)[5]
	23	46,XY,del(9)(q13q22)[18]/46,XY[2]
t(6;9)	24	46,XY,t(6;9)(p23;q34)[6]/46,idem,del(16)(q21)[3]/46,XY,[3]
	25	45,XX,del(6)(p23),-9,-22,+mar[17]
Miscellaneous	26	46,XY,del(6)(q?)[5]/46,XY[3]
	27	46,XY,t(2;X)(q13or14;q26or25)[7]/46,XX[1]
	28	47,XY,add(7)(p11or15),+19[14]/46,XY[6]
	29	45,XY,-7[11]/46,XY[9]
	30	46,XX,t(8;19)(p11;q13)[6]/46,XX[15]
	31	47,XY,+8[2]
	32	46,XY,t(10;11;12)(p12or13;q13or14;q12)[10]
	33[b]	46,XY add(11)(p15)[11]
	34	45,X,-X,add(14)(q32)[2]
Normal	35–40	

[a]Presented at relapse
[b]Therapy-related leukemia (t-AML)

8 and 9 months after diagnosis, including the child with preceding MDS. Two patients underwent bone marrow transplantation (BMT) in first remission, and one of them (no. 1) died of infection. Four of the eight patients are alive in first continuous complete remission (CCR) at 10–31 months since diagnosis.

Among the t/del(11q23) subgroup, all were of Jewish origin. Three patients had t(9;11), one de novo AML, and two were young adults with t-AML appearing 1.9 and 3.3 years after the diagnosis of Ewing's tumor and Hodgkin's lymphoma treated with ifosfamide, VP-16, vincristine, actinomycin D, cyclophosphamide and doxorubicin (IV-VACA) and with four courses of cyclophosphamide, vincristine, procarbazine, prednisone – adriamycin, bleomycin, vinblastine, decarbazine (COPP-ABVD), respectively.

Table 2. Clinical and blast cell characteristics and outcome of the 40 childhood AML patients with adequate cytogenetic analysis

Patient no.	Age/sex (years)	L/S (cm)	Extra medullary	Peripheral blood				Bone marrow			Outcome			BMT Rm/Rl
				WBC (× 10⁹/l)	Blst (%)	Hb (g/dl)	Plat (10⁹/l)	FAB (M)	Auer	Blst (%)	CR (*n*)	CCR (months)	Status	(*n*)/(*n*)
1	7.5/F	2/1	LN	10	38	9.7	49	2		60	+1	13	Dd, Inf	All 1
2	4.5/F	1/0		19	26	6.5	61	2Eo	+	30	+1	31+	Al, 1st Rm	
3[a]	10.0/F	1/0	LN	4	12	5.6	110	2Eo	+	40	+1	24	Al, 2nd Rm	All 2
4	5.2/M	6/3	LN	23	45	8.8	1400	2Eo	+	50	+1	8	Dd, Rl	Au /2
5	8.5/M	2/0		124	84	6.7	18	2	+	80	+1	22+	Al, 1st Rm	Au 1
6	4.1M	0/0	Facialis	28	26	7.0	147	2	+	10	+1	9	Al, Rl	
7	3.8/F	4/0		34	89	5.9	17	2Eo	+	90	+1	11+	Al, 1st Rm	
8	16.8/M	3/3		19	78	8.5	15	2	+	90	+1	10+	Al, 1st Rm	
9	11.0/M	6/0	Orbit, gums	12	70	7.0	65	5		95	+1	6	Dd, Rl	All 2
10[b]	16.5/M	0/0		2	47	9.3	15	5		95	None	0	Dd, Rl	All /2
11[b]	16.6/M	0/0	CNS	183	99	9.9	9	5		95	+2	10+	Al, 1st Rm	All 1
12	2.0/M	3/0	Bone, FSP	6	17	7.2	140	2		80	+1	25+	Al, 1st Rm	Au 1
13	0.2/F	3/1		270	95	8.7	308	4		99	+1	12	Al, 2nd Rm	All /1
14	8.0M	0/0	Gums	22	60	11.1	224	5		95	+1	1+	Al, 1st Rm	
15	4.5/M	2/0	Myelobl	12	0	10.6	400	2Eo		30	+1	3	Dd, Rl	
16	0.7/F	7/8		13	73	7.9	16	1		95	+1	17	Dd, Rl	
17	6.2/F	0/0		5	14	6.7	10	1	+	60	None	0	Dd, Rl	
18	4.8/M	2/0		10	10	3.8	9	6	+	30	+1	56+	Al, 1st Rm	
19	9.5/F	2/0		7	5	9.2	20	2		25	+1	5+	Al, 1st Rm	
20	20.0/F	0/0		5	67	9.5	24	3V	±	90	None	0	Dd, Bld	
21	14.9/M	0/0	DIC	140	95	7.4	31	3	+	90	None	0	Dd, Bld	
22	6.4/M	0/4	LN	8	16	7.6	113	2	+	30	+1	9	Dd, Rl	
23	2.5/M	2/1		85	93	7.8	46	4	+	100	+2	1+	Al, 1st Rm	
24	13.5/M	1/0	Bone	18	31	6.9	77	4		90	+2	1+	Al, 1st Rm	
25	6.4/F	5/8		31	41	4.4	43	4		80	+3	7+	Al, 1st Rm	All 1
26	1.2/M	0/0	Gums	52	7	9.0	104	5		95	+1	3+	Al, 1st Rm	
27	1.2/F	7/4		280	98	9.5	90	4		99	+2	12+	Al, 1st Rm	Au 1
28	1.5/M	6/9		25	57	4.2	10	7		85	None	0	Dd, Ind	
29	2.8/M	0/0		25	22	9.0	25	2		90	+1	10	Al, 2nd Rm	All /1
30	15.5/F	1/0		5	7	10.9	61	4		98	+1	18+	Al, 1st Rm	Au 1
31	15.0/M	0/0	Gums	1	1	6.2	88	5		95	+1	7+	Al, 1st Rm	Au 1
32	0.4/M	4/0	CNS, skin	4	0	8.5	234	5		70	+2	11	Dd, Rl	Au 1

Table 2. (*contd.*)

Patient no.	Age/Sex (years)	L/S (cm)	Extra medulary	Peripheral blood				Bone marrow			Outcome			BMT Rm/Rl
				WBC ($\times 10^9/l$)	Blst (%)	Hb (g/dl)	Plat ($10^9/l$)	FAB (M)	Auer	Blst (%)	CR (*n*)	CCR (months)	Status	(*n*)/(*n*)
33[b]	9.0/M	0/0		100	10	10.0	39	2		15	None	0	Dd, Rl	All /1
34	12.0/F	3/0	LN	10	90	7.0	16			99	+1	32+	Al, 1st Rm	
35	16.5/F	0/0		10	90	7.0	16	1		99	+1	24+	Al, 1st Rm	
36	12.5/M	4/5	Gums	37	1	9.4	70	4		45	+1	6	Dd, Rl	
37	7.5/M	1/0	LN	73		9.5	124	2		90	+1	9	Dd, Rl	
38	11.0/F	0/0		5	36	10.0	96	4Eo		90	+1	34+	Rl, 1st Rm	
39	6.3/M	4/4	FSP	62	61	10.0	84	4		90	+2	11	Dd, Rl	
40	6.0/F	5/0		1	0	4.3	24	7			+1	48+	Al, 1st Rm	

Abbrevations: L/S, liver/spleen; LN, lymph node; FSP, fibrinogen split product; DIC, disseminated intravascular coagulopathy; Myelobl, myeloblastoma; Blst, blasts; Plat, Platelets; CR, complete remission; *n*, following number of induction courses; CCR, first continuous complete remission; Dd, died; Al, alive; Inf, infection; Rm, remission; Rl, relapse; Bld, Bleeding; Ind, induction; BMT, bone marrow transplantation; Au, autologous BMT; All, allogeneic BMT.

[a]Presented at relapse

[b]Therapy-related leukemia (t-AML)

One boy presented with pancytopenia, and the other with hyperleukocytosis and CNS involvement. All had FAB M5 morphology. Other abnormalities of 11q23 occurred in three patients, including two infants with M2 and M4 blasts. Immunophenotype in two patients was positive for myelomonocytic CD33, CD15, and CD11B antigens, and for the NK CD56 and T cell CD7 or CD4 antigens. Response to treatment was poor in the two t-AML patients, with slow or no remission. One of them underwent BMT and is alive in CCR more than 10 months later. Another two de novo patients relapsed 6 and 12 months after diagnosis, and another two are alive in first CCR 1 and 24 months after diagnosis.

The aberrations t/inv(3q) were observed in three children. In one with inv(3)(q21q26) and monosomy 7, t-AML developed 5 years after high doses of alkylating agents were administered for neuroblastoma; this patient has been described elsewhere [23]. The other two children were an infant with t(3;21) and few evolving clones, with de novo M1 leukemia, and a young boy with complex karyotype including add(3q), unbalanced t(1;7), −7 and presence of markers. The latter patient presented with supraclavicular myeloblastoma, high thrombocyte count and dysmegakaryopoiesis in bone marrow. Blast cell morphology of the t/inv(3q) was M1, M2, and immunophenotype was positive in addition to the myeloid CD13, CD33 to the T-cell marker CD7. Response to treatment was poor, and all patients relapsed and died of leukemia.

The t(15;17) aberration occurred in two adolescents presenting with or subsequently developing severe disseminated intravascular coagulopathy (DIC) and fatal bleeding. One of them had the microgranular variant, and both had low expression of HLA-DR antigen and positive reaction to CD2. Both died within a few weeks of bleeding, during induction; one was treated with retinoic acid, and the other received low dose cytarabine. In two children with prominent myelodysplastic features in bone marrow, one with erythroleukemia, t(3;5) was detected, and responded to the AML-BFM-87 protocol. In two young boys del(9q) was found; one of them had presented with preceding MDS which progressed to AML, M2 blasts with Auer rods. One child responded slowly to induction, the other relapsed within a few months. In two children, t(6;9) or its suspected variant was associated with M4 leukemia without basophilia; one had myelodysplastic features. Response to treatment and remission achievement was slow in one patient, and the other responded only to allogeneic BMT.

In one girl t(8;19) variant of the t(8;16) was associated with M4 leukemia and autophagocytic vacuoles [24]. She is alive in first CCR following autologous BMT 19 months after diagnosis. In one 4-month-old infant t(10; 11;12) was associated with M5 leukemia with extensive extramedullary involvement of the eyes, CNS, testicles, and skin, which preceded BM infiltration. He responded poorly and relapsed after a few months following autologous BMT.

Discussion

The incidence of clonal chromosomal abnormalities in childhood AML is relatively high in comparison to adults (Table 3) [25–36]. In our series, a successful yield was achieved in 95% of the analyzed karyotypes, and of these, 85% abnormal clones were detected. The most frequent nonrandom aberration in pediatric patients is t(8:21) which, in our series, occurred in 20%, comparable to the pediatric BFM and Johannesburg series [29,36], and lower than Chicago and Moscow series [26,31]. This translocation was found in a higher proportion of the black and Oriental patients than in the white ones, both in adults and children [2,7,29]. Although t(8;21) is very specific to AML M2 type with Auer rods, one child in our series had preceding MDS, which is rarely reported [37]. We could not confirm the high incidence of CD19 expression in this type of leukemia, as claimed by others [38]. Favorable prognoses have been observed for patients with t(8;21) on previous and more recent AML protocols [1,5,12–17,34], and they seem to benefit from very high dose cytarabine [18,19]. In our series all children achieved remission after one course of induction, and only two of the seven newly diagnosed children have relapsed; however, follow-up, as yet, is too short to draw conclusions.

The second most frequent aberration in our series was t/del(11q23), similar to other pediatric series, where it rates second or third, occurring much more often in children than in adults (Table 3). Rearrangement of 11q23 is the most common aberration in infants with mixed and myeloid leukemias, and in childhood t-AML fol-

Table 3. Incidence of major cytogenetic subgroups in pediatric and adult AML

Study period	Pediatric									Adult		
	CMCI	BFM [36]	SJCRH [33]	St-Ls [32]	CCSG [30]	WMSJ [29]	Chcg [26]	RCHP [35]	4IWCL [2]	4IWCL [2]	CALGB/MN [5]	BFM [36]
	88–94	87–92	80–87	77–86	79	78–82	77–81	–	80–82	80–82	80–86	85–91
Total patients (no.)	47	307	155		266	31					387	704
Successful karyotypes (no.)	40	147	121	130	195	26	26	30	102	613	307	342
Cytogenetic subgroups[a]												
Normal	15	20	20	31	51	27	20	20	43	45	38	48
t(8;21)	20	17	11.6	13	6	15	43	10	12	5.7	5.5	8
t/del(11)(q23)	15	17	13	11	4	4	8	15	12	3.4		2
inv/del(16q)	0	8	12.4	3	3	8		22		1.4	5.2	8
t(15;17)	5	3	7.4	8	4	8	12	10	8	6	6.5	4
+8	2.5	13	5.8	1	9				3	5.5	10	8
−7/7q−	2.5	4	5	2	4	8		3	3	5.7	5.5	4
−5/5q−	0	1							2	6.1		3

lowing topisomerase II inhibitors [34,39,40]. Most have M5 or M4 leukemia, with a relatively high incidence of CNS involvement and high blast count. Prognosis in infants and in t-AML is very grave, much poorer than in adults and in de novo leukemia [34,40–42]. Lately, different molecular breakpoints of the MLL or HRX gene on 11q23 have characterized de novo AML versus t-AML, and childhood and adults versus infant de novo AML [41,42], which may explain the different biological course.

In our series, the two children with t-AML had a grave prognosis, with one responding only to allogeneic BMT. Among the de novo patients, two, including the infant, relapsed within a year, and the other two are alive in first CCR, one of them following BMT, with short follow-up.

The second or third most frequent aberration in pediatric series in inv/del(16q), associated with M4 leukemia, usually with eosinophilia, and a favorable prognosis. This was the most prevalent aberration in the St. Jude series and the Australian series [33–35]. In our series it was not detected, and more cases have to be studied to eliminate technical artifacts. The promyelocytic M3-specific t(15;17) was detected only in two young adults (5%), a rate comparable to that of the BFM series and lower than in other pediatric and adult series. It occurs more frequently among black and Oriental pediatric AML patients [29], and clusters of M3, including the variant form, have been reported in northern Italy [43] and in South America [43]. Although considered to have a favorable prognosis, the two patients in our series died on induction from bleeding.

It is noteworthy that a group of rare, nonrandom aberrations, t/inv(3q), t(3;5), del(9q), t(6;9) [44–49], which were reported only anecdotally in other pediatric series, were found in a relatively high proportion of our series – in two patients each, altogether eight (15%) of the 36 de novo patients. These aberrations have been associated either with MDS or myelodysplastic features, and bear a very poor prognosis [19,44–49]. The children in our series had a grave outcome; three responded slowly to induction, and four relapsed. Only two are alive in first CCR after more than a few months.

It would be a challenge to explore the genetic and/or environmental factors which may predispose individuals to these specific rare cytogenetic subtypes of myeloid leukemia in our pediatric population. Moreover, effective chemotherapeutic agents should be tailored to this relatively large group of children with poor prognosis.

Acknowledgment. This work is supported by the Israel Cancer Association.

Addendum. In a recent childhood AML de novo study from Chicago by Rowley's group [50], different AML subtype incidences from the previous study [26] were noted. Out of 120 patients 115 had adequate samples for analysis. Normal karyotype was found in 15%, t(8;21) in 8%, t(11)(q23) in 18%, inv(16) in 8%, t(15;17) in 10% and -7/del(7q) in 5%.

References

1. The Fourth International Workshop on Chromosomes in Leukemia, 1982. Introduction. Cancer Genetic Cytogenet 1984;11: 251–360.
2. The Fourth International Workshop on Chromosomes in Leukemia, 1982. Overview of association between chromosome pattern and cell morphology, age, sex, and race. Cancer Genet Cytogenet 1984; 11: 265–274.
3. Mitelman F, Heim S. Quantitative acute leukemia cytogenetics. Genes Chromosome Cancer 1992; 5: 57–66.
4. Rowley JD, Alimena G, Garson M, Hagemeijer A, Mitelman F, Progogina EL. Collaborative study of the relationship of the morphological type of acute nonlymphocytic leukemia with patient age and karyotype. Blood 1982; 59: 1013–1022.
5. Bloomfield CD, de la Chapelle A. Chromosome abnormalities in acute nonlymphocytic leukemia: Clinical and biologic significance. Semin Oncol 1987; 14: 372–383.
6. Mertens F, Johansson B, Mitelman F. Age- and gender-related heterogeneity of cancer chromosome aberrations. Cancer Genet Cytogenet 1993; 70: 6–11.
7. Johansson B, Mertens F, Mitelman F. Geographic heterogeneity of neoplasia-associated chromosome aberrations. Genes Chromosomes Cancer 1991; 3: 1–7
8. Larson RA, le Beau MM, Ratain MJ, Rowley JD. Balanced translocations involving chromosome bands 11q23 and 21q22 in therapy-related leukemia. (Letter) Blood 1992; 79: 1892–1893.
9. Pedersen-Bjergaard J, Philip P, Larsen SO, et al. Therapy-related myelodysplasia and acute myeloid leukemia. Cytogenetic characteristics of 115 consecutive cases and risk in seven cohorts of patients treated intensively for malignant diseases in the Copenhagen series. Leukemia 1993; 7: 1975–1986.
10. Cuneo A, Fagioli F, Pazzi I, et al. Morphologic, immunologic and cytogenetic studies in acute myeloid leukemia following occupational exposure

to pesticides and organic solvents. Leukemia Res 1992; 16: 789-796.
11. Buckley JD, Robison LL, Swotinsky R, et al. Occupational exposures of parents of children with acute nonlymphocytic leukemia: A report from the Children's Cancer Study Group. Cancer Res 1989; 49: 4030-4037.
12. Keating IJ, Smith TL, Kantarjian H, et al. Cytogenetic pattern in acute myelogenous leukemia: A major reproducible determinant of outcome. Leukemia 1988; 2: 403-412.
13. Yunis JJ, Lobell M, Arnesen MA, et al. Refined chromosome study helps define prognostic subgroups in most patients with primary myelodysplastic syndrome and acute myelogenous leukaemia. Br J Haematol 1988; 68: 189-194.
14. Samuels BL, Larson RA, Le Beau MM, et al. Specific chromosomal abnormalities in acute nonlymphocytic leukemia correlate with drug susceptibility in vivo. Leukemia 1988; 2: 79-83.
15. Schiffer CA, Lee EJ, Tmiyasu T, Wiernik PH, Testa JR, Prognostic impact of cytogenetic abnormalities in patients with de novo acute nonlymphocytic leukemia. Blood 1989; 1: 263-270.
16. Fenaux P, Preudhomme C, Lai JL, Morel P, Beuscart R, Bauters F. Cytogenetics and their prognostic value in de novo acute myeloid leukemia: A report on 283 cases. Br J Haematol 1989; 73: 61-67.
17. Marosi C, Köller U, Koller-Weber E, et al. Prognostic impact of karyotype and immunologic phenotype in 125 adult patients with de novo AML. Cancer Genet Cytogenet 1992; 61: 14-25.
18. Bloomfield CD, Lawrence D, Arthur DC, Berg DT, Schiffer CA, Mayer RJ. Curative impact of intensification with high-dose cytarabine (HiDAC) in acute myeloid leukemia (AML) varies by cytogenetic group. (Abstract) Blood 1994; 84(Suppl 1): 111a.
19. Bloomfield CD. Prognostic factors for selecting curative therapy for adult acute myeloid leukemia. Leukemia 1992; 6(suppl 4): 65-67.
20. Bennett JM, Catovsky D, Daniel MT, et al. Proposed revised criteria for the classificaiton of acute myeloid leukemia. Ann Intern Med 1985; 103: 626-629.
21. Mitelman F. ISCN 1991 - Guidelines for Cancer Cytogenetics. Supplement to an International System for Human Cytogenetic Nomenclature. Recommendations of the International Standing Committee on Human Cytogenetic Nomenclature. Karger, Basel, 1991.
22. Creutzig U, Ritter J, Zimmermann M, Schellong G. Does cranial irradiation reduce the risk for bone marrow relapse in acute myelogenous leukemia? Unexpected results of the Childhood Acute Myelogenous Leukemia Study BFM-87 J Clin Oncol 1993; 11: 279-286.
23. Stark B, Jeison M, Shohat M, et al. Involvement of 11p15 and 3q21q26 in therapy-related myeloid leukemia (t-ML) in children. Cancer Genet Cytogenet 1994; 75: 11-22.
24. Stark B, Resnitzky P, Jeison M, et al. A distinct subtype of M4/M5 acute meyloblastic leukemia (AML) associated with t(8:16)(p11:p13) in a patient with the variant t(8:19)(p11:q13) (Case report and review of the literature). Leukemia Res 1995; in press.
25. Hagemeijer A, Hahlen K, Abels J. Cytogenetic follow-up of patients with nonlymphocytic leukemia. II. Acute nonlymphocytic leukemia. Cancer Genet Cytogenet 1981; 3: 109-124.
26. Kaneko Y, Rowley JD, Maurer HS, Variakojis D, Moohr JW. Chromosome pattern in childhood acute nonlymphocytic leukemia. Blood 1982; 60: 389-399.
27. Slater RM, Behrendt H, de Waal FC. Chromosome studies on acute nonlymphocytic leukemia in children. Pediatr Res 1983; 17: 398-405.
28. Brodeur GM, Williams DL, Kalwinsky DK, Williams KJ, Dahl GV. Cytogenetic features of acute nonlymphoblastic leukemia in 73 children and adolescents. Cancer Genet Cytogenet 1983; 8: 93-105.
29. Bernstein R, Macdougall LG, Pinto MR. Chromosome patterns in 26 South African children with acute nonlymphocytic leukemia (ANLL). Cancer Genet Cytogenet 1984; 11: 199-214.
30. Woods WG, Nesbit ME, Buckley J, et al. Correlation of chromosome abnormalities with patient characteristics, histologic subtype, and induction success in children with acute nonlymphocytic leukemia. J Clin Oncol 1985; 3: 3-11.
31. Prigogina EL, Fleischman EW, Puchkova GP, et al. Chromosomes in acute nonlymphocytic leukemia. Hum Genet 1986; 73: 137-146.
32. Leverger G, Bernheim A, Daniel M-T, Flandrin G, Schaison G, Berger R. Cytogenetic study of 130 childhood acute nonlymphocytic leukemias. Med Pediatr Oncol 1988; 16: 227-232.
33. Raimondi SC, Kalwinsky DK, Hayashi Y, Behm FG, Mirro J Jr, Williams DL. Cytogenetics of childhood acute nonlymphocytic leukemia. Cancer Genet cytogenet 1989; 40: 13-27.
34. Kalwinsky DK, Raimondi SC, Schell MJ, et al. Prognostic importance of cytogenetic subgroups in de novo pediatric acute nonlymphocytic leukemia. J Clin Oncol 1990; 8: 75-83.
35. Tiedemann K, Waters KD, Tauro GP, Tucker D, Ekert H. Results of intensive therapy in childhood acute myeloid leukemia incorporating high-dose melphalan and autologous bone marrow transplantation in first complete remission. Blood 1993; 82: 3730-3738.
36, Creutzig U, Buchner T, Ritter J, et al. Comparison of biological data and prognosis in childhood and adult AML. (Abstract) Ann Hematol 1995; 70(suppl II): A108.
37. Mitelman F, Kaneko Y, Trent J. Report of the committee on chromosome changes in neoplasia. Cytogenet Cell Genet 1991; 58: 1053-1079.
38. Hurwitz CA, Raimondi SC, Head D, et al. Distinctive immunophenotypic features of t(8;21)q22;q22) acute myeloblastic leukemia in children. Blood 1992; 80: 3182-3188.
39. Rowley JD. 1993 Robert R deVillier Lecture. Chromosome translocatoins: Dangerous liaisons.

40. Sandoval C, Head DR, Mirro J Jr, Behm FG, Ayers GD, Raimondi SC. Translocation t(9;11)(p21;q23) in pediatric de novo and secondary acute myeloblastic leukemia. Leukemia 1992; 6: 513–519.
41. Rowley JD. Chromosomal translocations play a key role in leukemogenesis. Ann Hematol 1995; 70(suppl II): A102.
42. Griesinger F. Biology and detection of t(4;11). Ann Hematol 1995; 70(suppl II): A103.
43. Caniu-Rajnoldi A, Biondi A, Jankovic M, et al. Diagnosis and incidence of acute promyelocytic leukemia (FAB M3 and M3 variant) in childhood. (Letter) Blood 1993; 81: 2209–2211.
44. Fonatsch C, Gudat H, Lengfelder E, et al. Correlation of cytogenetic findings with clinical features in 18 patients with inv(3)(q21q26) or t(3;3)(q21; q26). Leukemia 1994; 3: 1318–1326.
45. Rubin CM, Larson RA, Anastasi J, et al. t(3;21)-(q26;q22): A recurring chromosomal abnormality in therapy-related myelodysplastic syndrome and acute myeloid leukemia. Blood 1990; 76: 2594–2598.
46. Horiike S, Taniwaki M, Misawa S, et al. The unbalanced 1;7 translocation in de novo myelodysplastic syndrome and its clinical implications. Cancer 1990; 65: 1350–1354.
47. Raimondi SC, Dube ID, Valentine MB, et al. Clinicopathologic manifestations and breakpoints of the t(3;5) in patients with acute nonlymphocytic leukemia. Leukemia 1989; 3: 42–47.
48. Kwong YL, Chan TK, Chan LC. Interstitial deletion of the long arm of chromosome 9 as the sole anomaly in acute myeloid leukemia is associated with dyserythropoiesis. (Letter) Leukemia 1992; 6: 64–65.
49. Lillington DM, Mac Cullum PK, Lister TA, Gibbons B. Translocation t(6;9)(p23;q34) in acute myeloid leukemia without myelodysplasia or basophilia: Two cases and a review of the literature. Leukemia 1993; 7: 527–531.
50. Martinez-Climent JA, Lane NJ, Rubin CM, et al. Clinical and prognostic significance of chromosomal abnormalities in childhood acute myeloid leukemia de novo. Leukemia 1995; 9: 95–101.

Acute Leukemias VI
Prognostic Factors
and Treatment Strategies
Büchner et al. (eds)

FISH Analysis in Acute Leukemia with Initially Abnormal Karyotypes and Normal Karyotypes in Relapse

I. Chudoba[1], S. Metzkel[1], K. Blumenstengel[2], H.-J. Fricke[2], K. Junker[1], C. Bleck[1], K. Höffken[2], and U.Claussen[1]

Abstract. In acute leukemias the finding of cytogenetically completely different results at different phases of the disease is a recurrent phenomenon. The question arising from these findings is whether cytogenetic investigations may not be sensitive enough to detect the malignant cell clone at certain stages of the disease.

We present three cases with aberrant karyotypes at initial diagnosis prior to therapy and with normal cytogenetic results in hematological relapse. Bone marrow (BM) samples with numerical aberrations intitially and normal karyotypes in relapse were analyzed by fluorescence in situ hybridization (FISH). This method provides higher sensitivity, and the examined cell population is enlarged by cells with no mitotic activity. In case 1, at the initial phase of AML-M1 a trisomy 21 was diagnosed. In FISH analysis on interphase nuclei in remission as well as in relapse the trisomic cell line was not detectable any more. The chromosomal analysis in remission revealed a minor constitutional mosaicism 46, XY/47, XYY, confirmed by FISH. In case 2, ac-ALL with the abnormal karyotype of 47,XX,4p-,der (9)t(1;9)(q11;p12), i(17q), −20,+21,+mar[6]/46,XX[5] was diagnosed. Again the chromosome 21-specific probe was chosen in order to characterize the malignant cell clone. Whereas an abnormal finding with an additional chromosome 21 was confirmed in the first BM sample by FISH, all subsequent investigations of BM samples (in remission and in relapse) revealed no cells with trisomy 21 any more. In case 3, a trisomy 8 was found at the initial chromosome analysis in a BM sample from a patient with AML-M2. FISH analysis confirmed the trisomy 8 in the first BM sample. In remission and a subsequent relapse no cells with trisomy 8 were found any more.

In all three cases the FISH investigations yield results consistent with the cytogenetic findings of a normal karyotype in the later stage of the disease.

Introduction

Different approaches have been made to reveal that acute myeloid leukemia (AML) is a clonial disorder. The monoclonality of the leukemic cell population was demonstrated by conventional cytogenetic [1] as well as biochemical [2] and molecular [3] studies. Therefore, it is generally assumed that at a certain stage of hematopoiesis one single normal cell has been transformed and serves as the ancestral cell from which leukemia arises.

The detection of the same chromosomal abnormality in at least two cells in conventional cytogenetic preparations of a bone marrow sample is regarded as proof of the malignancy of the examined cells. But not in all cases are chromosomal changes detectable. In AML, however, about 45%–55% of cases reveal no cytogenetic aberrations [4] and in acute lymphoblastic leukemia (ALL) the range is 20%–30% [5]. Nevertheless, once clonal chromosomal aberrations are identified, patients who achieve complete remission (CR) generally lose their karyotypic anomalies [6]. A patient entering a subsequent acute leu-

[1]Institute of Human Genetics and Anthropolgy, Jena, Germany
[2]Hospital of Internal Medicine II, Jena, Germany

kemic phase after CR is referred to as having a relapse. A relapse would imply that the malignant clone from the initial disease was not eradicated by the therapy and again dominates the bone marrow (blasts > 30%). Hence, a chromosomal aberration diagnosed initially should be identifiable at relapse. We present three cases of acute leukemias with chromosomal anomalies found at the initial cytogenetic examination carried out prior to therapy and with normal karyotypes at relapse.

Materials and Methods

Conventional cytogenetic examinations as well as fluorescence in situ hybridization (FISH) were carried out on bone marrow (BM) samples from patients diagnosed as having acute leukemias. The bone marrow was processed according to standard procedures, and at least 20 metaphases were analyzed, preferably from two different cell cultures. In 5 of 13 examinations a low mitotic index did not allow the evaluation of 20 cells. FISH was carried out according to the producer's recommendations (Oncor) using a chromosome 21-specific DNA probe (D21S65) hybridizing on 21q22 (Oncor), Y chromosome-specific alpha satellite DNA cocktail (DYZ1 and DYZ3; Oncor) and an alpha satellite chromosome 8-specific DNA probe (D8Z2; Oncor).

Results

Case 1

BM of a 42-year-old male with an AML-M1 has been investigated with conventional cytogenetic methods. The initial chromosome analysis revealed the abnormal karyotype of 47,XY,-+21[20]. Two months later, at a second cytogenetic examination and after chemotherapy, only normal metaphases ($n = 21$) were observed. A third cytogenetic examination was processed 17 months after the initial investigation (still in remission) and revealed an additional Y chromosome in 5 of 74 metaphases. The additional chromosome was confirmed by FISH to be the Y chromosome. After these findings the first chromosome preparation was reexamined; the additional chromosome again was clearly identified as a chromosome 21. In addition FISH was carried out with the Y chromosome-specific DNA probe, showing only 1 signal in 73 scored metaphases.

Three months later (20 months after initial diagnosis) the patient relapsed. The chromosomal analysis of the BM displayed only normal metaphases ($n = 20$). In order to enlarge the examined cell population and to check cells which did not enter mitosis, FISH examinations with a chromosome 21 cosmid probe and a Y chromosome-specific centromer probe were carried out. The data are shown in Table 1 and Fig. 1. Unfortunately, FISH examination with the chromosome 21 probe was not possible on the first BM due to the lack of cells. Nevertheless, for comparison the results of the conventional cytogenetic investigation and the FISH results are shown in Fig. 1. The data demonstrate that the initially diagnosed trisomy 21 could not be refound in later BM preparations, or even in relapse, by conventional cytogenetics or by FISH. FISH analysis with the Y chromosome-specific probe of the first and the third examination were processed on metaphases only. A detection rate of 2.7% (series 3) means

Table 1. Results of the conventional cytogenetic investigations and FISH analysis of case 1

Clinical diagnosis	Time (months)	Karyotype	Probe	Nuclei scored	Frequency [signals/nuclei in %]			
					1	2	3	4
AML-M1	0	47, XY,+21[20]	DYZ1/3	73(M)	100	0	0	0
Remission	2	46, XY[24]	21	200	2.5	93.5	3.5	0.5
			DYZ1/3	374	87.2	12.2	0.6	0
Remission	17	46, XY[72]/ 47,XYY[4]	21	368	2.7	94.3	3.0	0
			DYZ1/3	75(M)	97.3	2.7	0	0
Relapse	20	46,XY[20]	21	313	2.6	93.0	4.5	0
			DYZ1/3	300	97.4	2.6	0	0

M, Metaphases scored only

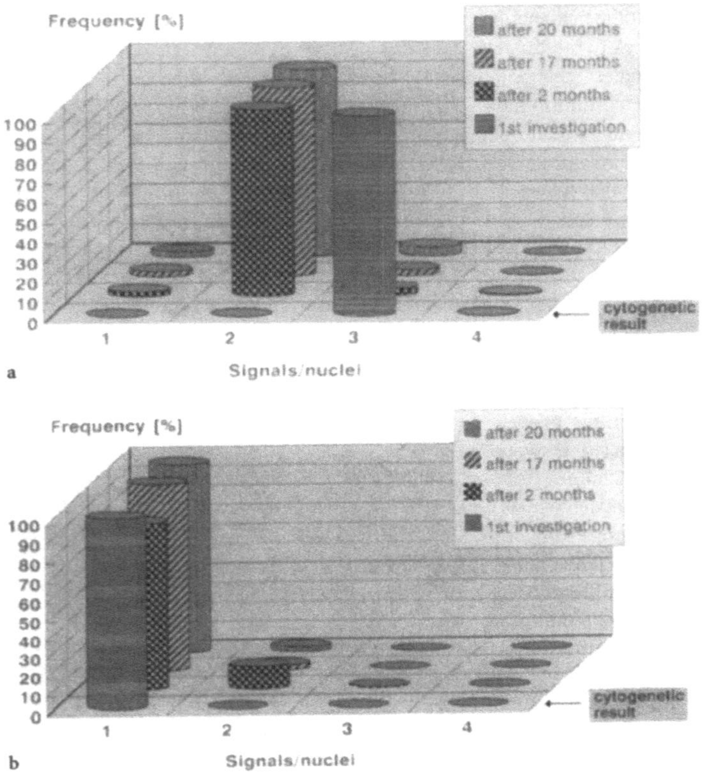

Fig. 1. **a** Results of cytogenetic and FISH analysis applied to chromosome 21 of patient 1 at different stages of the disease. **b** Results of cytogenetic and FISH analysis applied to the Y chromosome of patient 1 at different stages of the disease

that in 2 of 75 metaphases analyzed a second Y chromosome was clearly identified. Together with the results of the conventional cytogenetic investigation (5 of 74 metaphases with "+Y") the existence of a second cell line with an additional Y chromosome besides the normal cell line is evident in the BM sample in remission. The FISH investigation on interphase nuclei of the second BM sample also indicates the existence of a cell line with "+Y" (12.2% nuclei with two signals). Cells with "+Y" were detected only in remission. We interpret these findings as a minor constitutional mosaicism 46, XY/47XYY. Furthermore, the data clearly show that in later BM samples a cell line with an additional chromosome 21 could not be detected. The 3.0%–4.5% of nuclei showing three signals would be interpreted as method-related artifacts.

Case 2

Conventional cytogenetic investigation of the BM of a 19-year-old female with a c-ALL revealed an abnormal karyotype in about 55% of the cells (47,XX,4p-, der(9)t(1;9)(q11;p12), i(17q),−20,+21,+mar[6]/46,XX[5]). After complete hematological and cytogenetic remission the patient relapsed twice. Finally, only partial hematological remission was achieved and bone marrow transplantation was carried out. The patient died 30.5 months after the initial diagnosis because of severe GvH disease. Other conventional cytogenetic investigations performed later on in remission as well as in relapse revealed only normal metaphases. In FISH analysis trisomy 21 was chosen to characterize the karyotypic abnormal cell clone. The results are shown in Table 2 and Fig. 2. The preponder-

Table 2. Results of the conventional cytogenetic investigations and FISH analysis of patients

Clinical diagnosis	Time (months)	Karyotype	Probe	Nuclei scored	Frequency (signals/nuclei in %)			
					1	2	3	4
c-ALL	0	47, XX,4p-,der (9) t(1;9)(q11;p12), i(17q), – 20,+21, +mar[6]/46,XX[5]	21	235	n.s.	39.1	59.6	1.3
Remission	18.5	46,XX[24]	21	260	77	83.1	9.2	0
1st relapse	21	46,XX[5]	21	214	7.9	83.7	5.6	2.8
Remission	22	46,XX[13]	21	229	3.5	92.1	4.4	0
2nd relapse	25	46,XX[20]	21	224	2.2	94.6	2.7	0.5
Relapse	28	46,XX[21]	21	219	5.0	91.8	3.3	0
Death	30.5							

n.s., Not scored

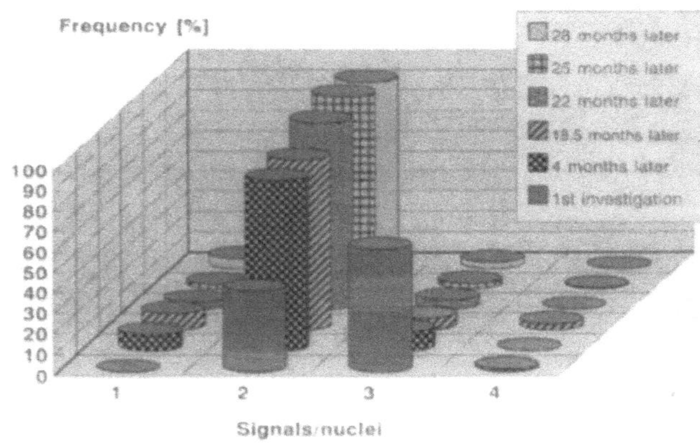

Fig. 2. Results of FISH analysis applied to chromosome 21 of patient 2 at different stages of the disease

ance of the abnormal cell line in the first BM sample was confirmed by FISH. Furthermore, FISH analysis confirmed all conventional cytogenetic results.

Case 3

At the age of 74 a woman was diagnosed as having AML-M2. Chromosomal analaysis of the BM revealed an abnormal karyotype trisomic for chromosome 8 in 81% of the cells examined. Twenty months later conventional cytogenetic investigation in remission showed only cells with a normal karyotype. The patient relapsed 4 months later (24 months after initial diagnosis), and again only normal metaphases could be detected in the BM. Retrospective FISH analysis of the cell preparation of the BM from the initial acute phase confirmed the trisomy 8, but the additional chromosome 8 was detected in only 46.8% of instances. Furthermore, the normal karyotypes obtained with conventional cytogenetic methods were confirmed as well. In remission and in relapse the trisomic cell line was no longer detectable (Table 3, Fig. 3).

Discussion

We applied FISH investigations to BM samples processed for conventional cytogenetic examinations. The patients revealed clonal abnormal chromosome findings in their BM examined in the first phase of acute leukemia, whereas in relapse only normal karyotypes were detected. The advantage of FISH over conventional cyto-

Table 3. Results of the conventional cytogenetic investigations and FISH analyses of patient[3]

Clinical diagnosis	Time (months)	Karyotype	Probe	Nuclei scored	Frequency (signals/nuclei in %)			
					1	2	3	4
AML	0	47,XX,+8[17]/46,XX[4]	D8Z2	1159	9.7	42.7	46.8	0.8
Remission	20	46,XX[20]	D8Z2	797	9.8	89.0	1.2	0
Relapse	24	46,XX[20]	D8Z2	419	9.1	90.2	0.2	0.5

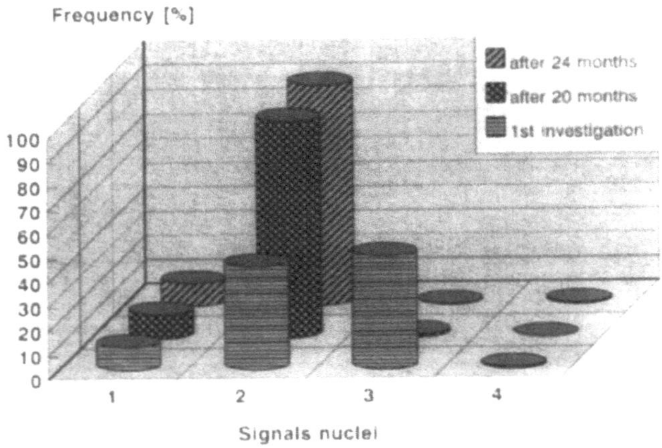

Fig. 3. Results of FISH analysis applied to chromosome 8 of patient 3 at differnt stages of the disease

genetics is that known chromosomal aberrations can be checked on interphase nuclei. In this manner a large number of cells can be evaluated, even if the chromosome morphology and spreading do not allow chromosomal analysis. Also, cells which have not entered mitosis and possibly represent a distinct biological entity can be included in the examination. In our cases FISH analysis confirmed the results obtained with conventional cytogenetic methods and revealed their reliability. Still, FISH analysis is undoubtedly more sensitive than conventional cytogenetics [7]. However, the results presented here raise more questions than they give answers. We found that the primarily detected chromosomally abnormal cell clones were no longer present, or at least were not part of the malignant cell clone in relapse. A possible explanation is that the chromosomally abnormal cell clones represent derivative cell clones. They might have emerged from the primarily transformed cell or cell clone and show karyotypic evolution. In this case, they are thought to have a stronger proliferation potential but are probably more sensitive to chemotherapy. After therapy the cytogenetically abnormal clones were eradicated, whereas the primarily transformed clones resided.

Another possibility is that the acute phase referred to as relapse actually represents therapy-related leukemia. This is unlikely, however, because clonal chromosomal aberrations are observed in 95% cases of therapy-related AML [8] and we found only metaphases in relapse in all three cases.

A further explanation might be the recurrence of leukemia. The therapy could have successfully eradicated the malignant cell clone and independent transformation of another cell could have taken place. In this case an intraindividual predisposition might exist, which could explain why a rather rare event should occur twice in the same patient. Alternatively, a possibly external leukemogenetic effect is able to transform more than one cell. In a primary phase the cell clone with the higher proliferation rate overgrows all other cells. This cell line chraracterized by the abnormal karyotype could be destroyed by the first chemotherapy while a second cell clone resists the therapy and emerges at a later time.

References

1. Bloomfield CD, de la Chapell A: Chromosome abnormalities in acute nonlymphocytic leukemia: clinical and biological significance. Semin Oncol (1987) 14: 372
2. Fialkow ER, Singer JW, Raskind WH et al: Clonal development, stem cell differentiation and clinical remission in acute nonlymphocytic leukemia. N Engl J Med (1987) 317: 468
3. Bartram CR, Ludwig WD, Hiddemann et al: Acute myeloid leukemia: analysis of ras gene mutations and clonality by defined, X-linked loci. Leukemia (1989) 3: 247
4. Poter A, Watmore AM: Cytogenetics in myeloid leukemia. In: Human cytogenetics, a practical approach, Volume II. Edited by; Rooney DE and Czepulkowski BH, 1992. IRL Press
5. Gibbons B, Czepulkowski BH: Cytogenetics in acute lymphoblastic leukemia. In: Human cytogenetics, a practical approach, Volume II.Edited by: Rooney DE and Czepulkowski BH, 1992. IRL Press
6. Bain BJ, The role of cytogenetics in the assessment of hematological disorders. In:Human cytogenetics, a practical approach, Volume II. Edited by; Rooney DE and Czepulkowski BH, 1922. IRL Press
7. Flactif M, Lai JL, Preudhomme C, Fenaux P: Flourescence in situ hybridization improves the detection of monosomy 7 in myelodysplastic syndromes. Blood (1994) 8: 1012–1018
8. Arthur DC, Bloomfield CD: Banded chromosome analysis in patients with treatment-associated acute nonlymphoblastic leukemias. Cancer Genetics and Cytogenetics (1984) 13: 189–198

Acute Leukemias VI
Prognostic Factors
and Treatment Strategies
Büchner et al. (eds)

Cytogenetic Findings of Acute Leukemias in the Ukraine

S. Andreeva[1], S. Donskaya[2], A. Galantha[1], O. Ryzak[2], and A. Nadgornaya[3]

Introduction

The role of specific structural abnormalities in the definition of subvariants in acute leukemias and estimation of prognosis for individual patients is well known [1, 2]. The value of numerical karyotypic characteristics, especially hypo- and hyperdiploidies as important criteria for prognosis in All and AML is also known [3].

There are some data about the incidence of near-tetraploidy in patients with different forms of acute leukemias. Our aim was to estimate the frequency of such phenomena among our patients with ALL and AML.

Materials and Methods

Bone marrow and peripheral blood specimens of 26 children and 9 adult patients with acute leukemias from the Kiev region were examined cytogenetically at diagnosis and, for 3 children, in relapse. Pediatric patients' ages ranged between 0.3 and 13 years (mean, 7.3), and the male: female ratio of 18:11. Adult patients' ages ranged between 23 and 73 years (mean, 48.8). Different ALL subvariants were identified by cytochemical investigation and immunophenotyping. FAB variants of AML were established using mainly morpho-cytochemical procedures.

Chromosome analysis was carried out on unstimulated bone marrow and peripheral blood cells, which were incubated in RPMI 1640 and 20% FCS for 24 h culture. The cell suspension was brought to hypotonicity with KCl (20 min) and fixed in methanol-acetic acid (3:1). Then the suspension was washed four or five times. The cells were pipetted onto cold wet slides to spread metaphases. G-banding was done after trypsin pretreatment (1–3 s) 7 days later.

The investigation was based on the analysis of at least five metaphases. The subsequent karyotyping followed the recommendations of the ISCN [4]. To be accepted as clonal, a chromosomal rearrangement or gain had to be detected in two cells, and monosomies had to be present in three cells. The percentage of hypotetraploidy was determined by scanning at least 50 metaphases with calculation of mean range.

Results

Five of the pediatric patients with newly diagnosed ALL (nos. 3, 5, 6, 7, 14) showed a normal karotype. In three patients with common ALL mosaic chromosomal patterns were found: a hyperdiploid and a normal clone (nos. 4, 8, 19) (Table 1). The technical quality did not allow identification of all of the supernumerary chromosomes. In two patients with B-ALL (nos. 2, 16) t(8;14)(q24;q32) were detected (Fig. 1). One of them (no. 16), had an additional abnormality – deletion of the long arm of chromosome 6, which was found as a sole change in one case of pre-B-ALL (no. 9). A patient with 0-ALL (no. 10) showed t(4;11)(q21;q23).

[1]Kiev Research Institute of Hematology and Blood Transfusion, Kiev, Ukraine
[2]Kiev Institute of Medical Training, Kiev, Ukraine
[3]R.E. Kavetsky Institute of Experimental Patology, Oncology and Radiobiology, Academy of Sciences, Ukraine

Table 1. Results of chromosomal analysis and clinical outcome of children with ALL and AML at diagnosis and relapse

Patient no.	Code	Sex	Age (years)	Karyotype	Percentage of near-tetraploidy	Remission	Overall survival (months)	Variant of disease
1	201	f	2.5	53,XXX,+6,+10,+12,+14, +18,+18/46,XX	0	+	33,0	C-ALL
2	203	m	5.5	46,XY,t(8;14)(q24;q32)	0	+	LFU	B-ALL
3	204	m	10.5	46,XY	0	+	31,0	0-ALL
4	206	f	11.0	46,XX/>51	14,3	+	26,0	pre-B-ALL
5	207	m	4.0	46,XY	0	+	31,0	pre-T-ALL
6	208	m	6.0	46,XY	0	+	29,0	pre-B-ALL
7	211	f	8.0	46,XX	0	+	27,0	C-ALL
8	217	f	4.5	>51/46,XX	0	+	27,0	pre-B-ALL
9	219	m	8.0	46,XY,del(6)(q23)	0	+	26,0	pre-B-ALL
1993								
10	301	m	0.3	46,XY,t(4;11)(q21;q23)/ 46,XY	0	–	0	0-ALL
11	302	m	12.0	45,XY,–20	21,4	+	LFU	M2 AML
12	305	m	7.0	46,XY	21,4	+	15,0	C-ALL
13	309	f	8.0	46,XY,t(15;17)(q22;q11)	0	+	15,0	M3 AML
14	310	m	3.0	46,XY	0	+	LFU	pre-B-ALL
15	312	m	7.5	38,–X,Y,–1,–3,–4 [cp3]	0	+	12,0	pre-T-ALL
16	316	m	7.0	46,XY,del(6)(q24) t(8;14)(q24;q32)	0	+	LFU	B-ALL
17	320	m		46,XY	47,1	+	12,0	T-ALL
1994								
18	402	m	13.0	46,XY	19,5	+	11,0	M4 AML
19	403	f	5.0	46,XY/>51	0	+	11,0	C-ALL
20	405	f	8.0	46,XX,t(15;17((q22;q11)/ 47,XX,t(15;17)(q22;q11),+8	0	+	4,0	M3 AML
21	406	m	12.0	46,XY	10,4	+	6,5	T-ALL
22	409	f	6.0	46,XX,inv(8)(p21q24), del(20)(q11q13)	8,0	–	1,0	M6 AML
23	413	m	3.0	46,XY	14,3	+	5,0	pre-T-ALL
24	413	m	4.0	45,X,–Y,t(8;21)(q22;q22)	8,1	+	2,5	M2 AML
25	417	f	11.0	45,XX,del(16)(q22)	0	+	2,0	M4 AML
26	421	m	6.5	32–45	0	+/–	1,0	M2 AML
Relapse								
27	422	m	8.0	46,XY/>51	0			pre-B-ALL
28	426	f	12.5	46,XX,t(9;22)(q34;q11)	0			pre-B-ALL
29	428	f	12.0	46,XX,del(1)(q23), i(17),der(13,21)(q10;q10)	15,0			C-ALL

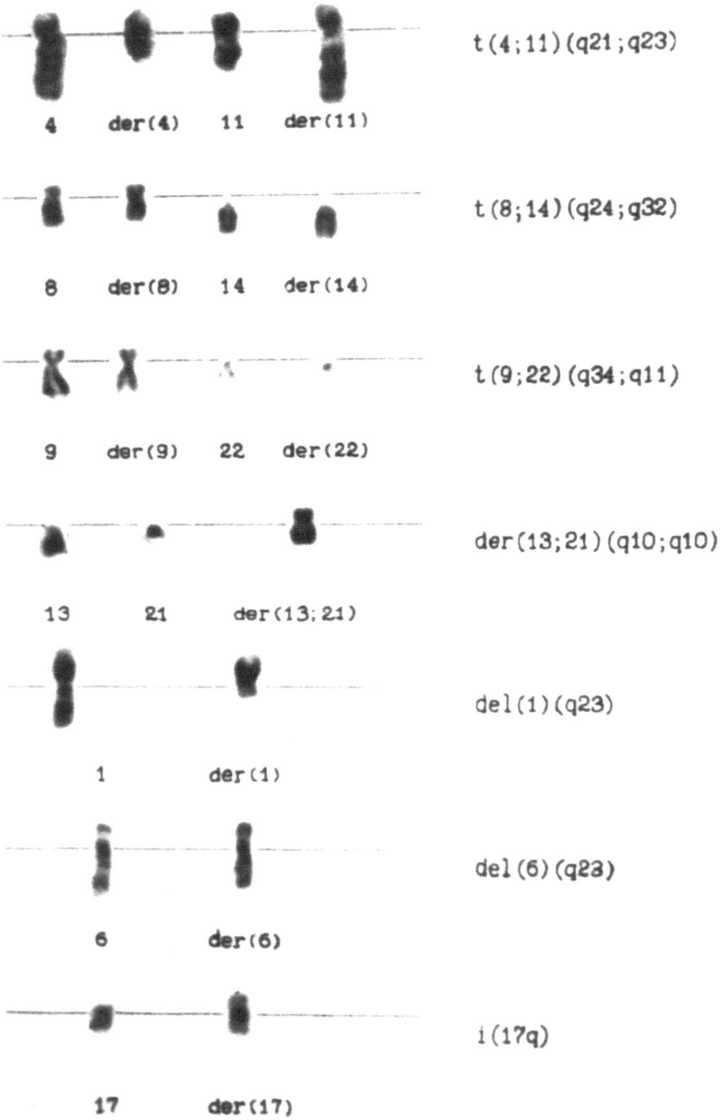

Fig. 1. Partial G-banded karyotypes from patients with ALL

In five cases of the total ALL group (27.0%) (nos. 4, 12, 17, 21, 23) we found a hypotetraploid clone and the fluctuation was from 10.4% to 47.1% (mean: 21.5%)(Fig. 2; Table 1). Eight patients with AML in the pediatric group had M2, M3, M4 and M6 FAB variants (Table 1).

In one case of M2 AML (no. 24) a specific structural abnormality, t(8;21)(q22;q22) (Fig. 3), was shown. Both patients with M3 (nos. 13, 20); showed t(15;17)(q22;q11), one of them (no. 20) had an additional clone with trisomy 8. One patient with M4 (no. 25) had del(16)(q22) and

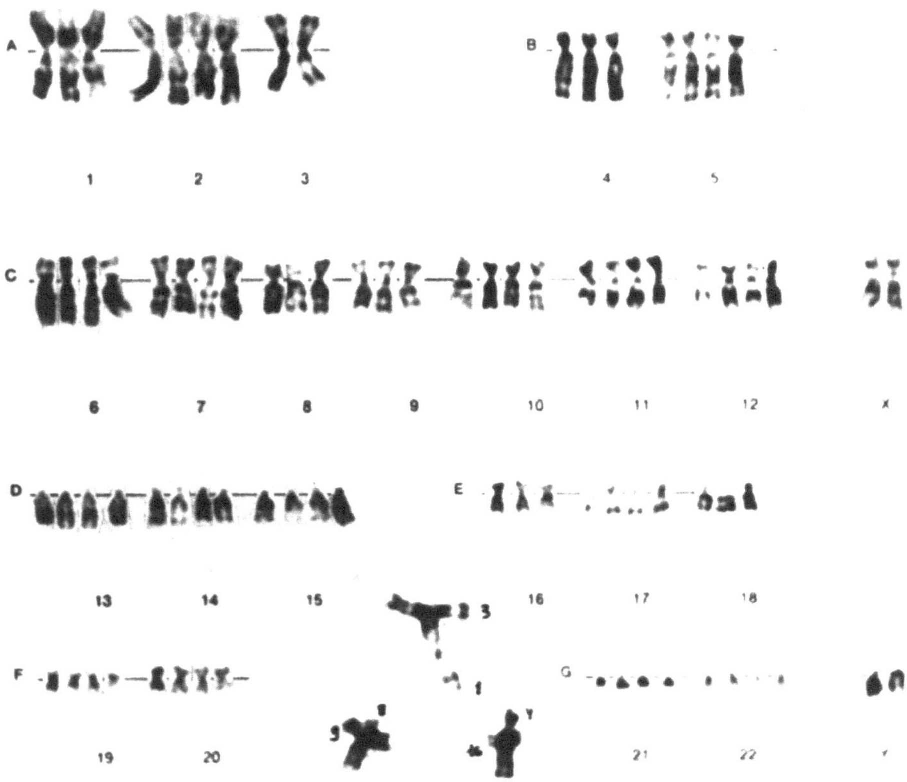

Fig. 2. Hypotetraploid G-banded karyotype of bone marrow cell from an AML patient with 90, XXYY, −3, −18

was classified as M4eo. A patient with M6 (no. 22) showed a combination of two structural abnormalities which was discussed separately.

In four cases of AML (50.0%) (nos. 11, 18, 22, 24) a hypotetraploid clone was found. The fluctuation was from 8.0% to 21.4% (mean: 4.2%).

The adult AML group consisted of three patients with M2, one with M3 and five with M4 disease (Table 2).

One case of M2 (no. 4) showed two clones with hypodiploidy and hypotetraploidy; in the other (no. 7), del(5)(q31q33) was registered. The patient with M3 had typical t(15;17) (q22;q11), and among the M4 cases two showed anomalies of chromosome 16:del(16) (q22) (no. 5) and inv (16)(p13q22) (no. 2); one displayed t(6;9) (p23; q34), ?17 (no. 6), and one had normal karyotype (no. 8).

In four of all nine cases (nos. 1, 3, 4, 9) (44.4%) a hypotetraploid clone was found with fluctuation from 6.7% to 14.0%(mean:9.4%).

Relapse

We also investigated three cases of ALL in relapse (Table 1). The first one (late bone marrow relapse; no. 28) showed t(9;22)(q34;q11). In the second (early bone marrow relapse; no. 27) the mosaic karyotype was detected: normal and hyperdiploid clones. The third one (early bone marrow relapse; no. 29) had a complex rearrangement: del(1)(q23), i(17q), robertsonian translocation-der(13;21)(q10;q10) and an additional hypotetraploid clone.

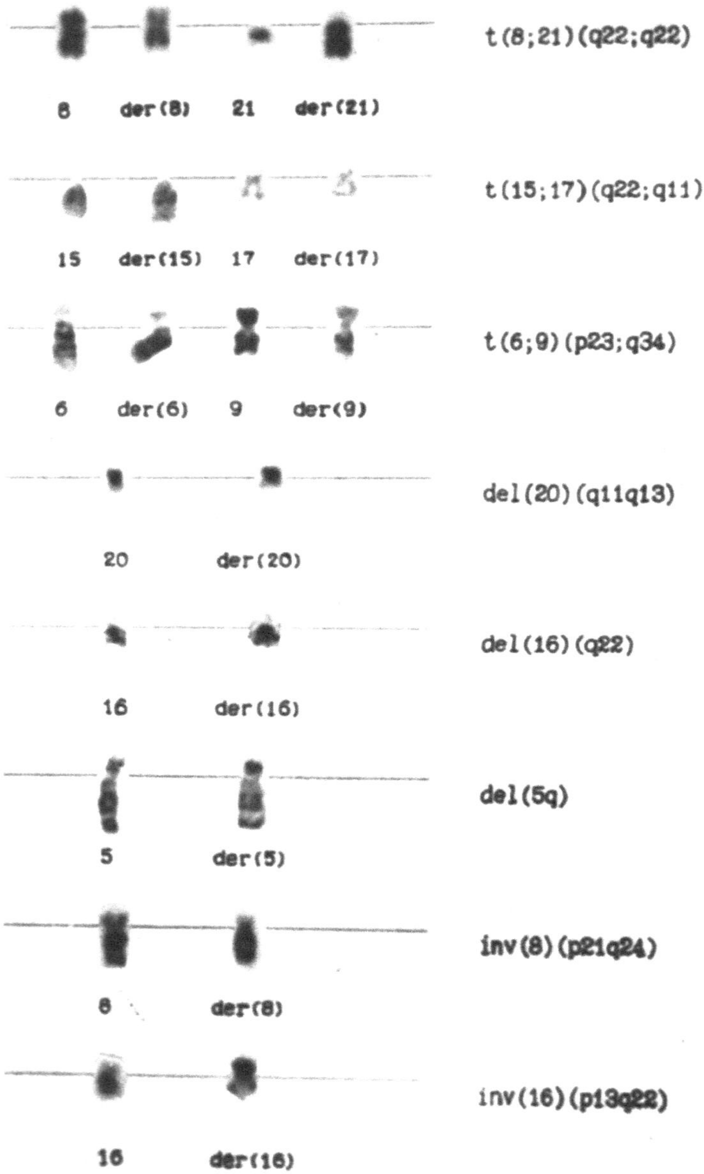

Fig. 3. Partial G-banded karyotypes from patients with AML

Treatment

Children with non-B-ALL were treated according to a modified BFM-ALL-90 protocol, except one infant with 0-ALL, who received no cytostatic therapy. All those treated achieved complete remission, and only one child (no. 4) had late bone marrow relapse and died during treatment according to the BFM-ALL-Rel. protocol.

B-ALL was treated using the B-NHL-BFM-90 protocol, and all patients achieved remission.

Table 2. Results of chromosomal analysis and clinical outcome of adult patients with AML at diagnosis

Patient no.	Code	Sex	Age (years)	Karyotype	Percentage of near-tetraploidy	Remission	Overall survival (months)	Variant of disease
1993								
1	318	f	23	46,XXt(15;17)(q22;q11)	11,0	–	0	M3 AML
2	322	f	70	46,XX,inv(16)(p13q22)	0	+	14,0	M4 AML
1994								
3	408	f	73	46,XX	6,7	–	2,0	M4 AML
4	410	f	33	33–38	14,0	–	1,0	M2 AML
5	411	m	27	46,XY,del(16)(q22)	0	–	1,5	M4 AML
6	418	m	66	46,XY,t(6;9)(p23;q34),?17	0	–	1,0	M4 AML
7	420	f	38	46,XX,del(5)(q31;q33)	0	–	0,1	M2 AML
8	423	f	55	46,XX	0	–	1,0	M4 AML
9	425	f	54	46,XX,del(11)(q21q23)	6,0	–	0	M2 AML

The pediatric group of AML received a standard scheme of cytostatic therapy following the BFM-AML-78 protocol. Complete remission was achieved in six patients: one girl (no. 22) with M6 was completely resistant to chemotherapy and died of leukemia progression. One patient with M3 (no. 20) died after achievement of complete remission of hemorrhagic complications, and in one case of M2 (no. 26) only partial bone marrow remission was achieved after the induction course.

All adult patients were treated by combinations of Ara-C anthracyclines (in medium doses): ("7+3" scheme), but remission was achieved only in one case (no. 2).

Discussion

Robertsonian translocation t(13;21)(q10;q10) in a child with common ALL is a very rare abnormality in hematopoietic malignancy [5]. This investigation revealed a very high incidence of hypotetraploidy among newly diagnosed cases of acute leukemia. It was connected with ALL of children and AML of both children and adults. In some cases the hypotetraploidy was registered in the clone with specific structural abnormalities, but in the others it was seen as an additional clone.

We could not conclude that this type of cytogenetic abnormality had a prominent influence on remission rate and overall survival because of the small numbers of patients in each group; but we intend to prolong observation and to add additional patients.

In the literature, the usual frequency of near-tetraploidy among patients with acute leukemias < 1.0% in pediatric ALL patients [6] and 2.0% in adults [7]. Near-tetraploidy in children has been associated with a reduction in therapy success[8]. Our investigation has shown very high incidences of such karyotype abnormality in both groups of patients. Additonally, near-tetraploidy is tending to increase in frequency from year to year (1992–1994).

Published data on chromosomal analysis in blast-transformed peripheral blood lymphocytes show that the frequency of near-tetraploidy in people living near Tchernobyl is higher than that in people living further from Tchernobyl [9]. All our patients lived near the Tchernobyl catastrophe zone.

Acknowledgments. We gratefully acknowledge Professor F. Lampert, Dr. J. Harbott, and Dr. R. Engel of the Children's Hospital, University of Giessen, for their teaching, consultation and continuous support of our research and practical work.

We are also very grateful to Professor G. Schellong of the University Children's Hospital, Münster, for regular consultation and help in our treatment practices.

References

1. Human Cytogenetics. A Practical Approach. V. II. Malignancy and Acquired Abnormalities. Second Edition. (Ed.Rooney DE, Czepulkowski BH), Oxford University Press, Oxford, NewYork, Tokyo

2. Harbott J, Ritterbach J, Ludwig W-D, Bartram CR, Borkhardt A, Jomka-Schaub G, Lampert F. Clinical Relevance of Chromosomal Aberrations in Childhood ALL: Cytogenetic Data of the German Therapy Studies. Acute Leukemias IV. Prognostic Factors, pp 317–321
3. Secker-Walker LM, Chessells JM, Stewart EL, Swansbury GJ, Richards S, Lawler SD (1989) Chromosomes and other prognostic factors in acute lymphoblastic leukemia: A long term follow-up. Brit. J. Haematol. 72: 336–342
4. ISCN (1991). Guidelines for Cancer Cytogenetics. Supplement to an International System for Human Cytogenetic Nomenclature. S. Karger, Basel. 54 p.
5. Horsman DE, Kalouusek DK (1990) Acquired Robertsonian Translocation in Hematologic Malignancy. A Rare Mechanism of Clonal Evolution. Cancer Genet Cytogenet 45: 193–196
6. Pui C-H, Crist WM, Look AT (1990) Biology and clinical significance of cytogenetic abnormalities in childhood acute leukemia. Blood 76: 1449–1463
7. Rieder H, Fonatsch C. Cytogenetic Findings in Acute Lymphoblastic Leukemia. Acute Leukemias IV. Prognostic Factors 413–419
8. Pui C-H, Carrol AJ, Head D, Raimondi SC, Shuster FG, Crist WM, Link MP, Borowitz MJ, Lomd VJ, Nash MB, Pullen DJ, Look AT (1990) Neartriploid and neartetraploid acute lymphoblastic leukemia of childhood. Blood 76: 590–596
9. Влияние низких доз ионизирующей радиации и других факторов окружающей среды на организм (1994) Киев, Наукова думка (ред М И Руднев) 216 с.

Acute Leukemias VI
Prognostic Factors
and Treatment Strategies
Büchner et al. (eds)

Detection of Minimal Tumor Cell Populations by FICTION

J. Deerberg, A. Rosenwald, K. Weber-Matthiesen, and B. Schlegelberger

Abstract. Sensitive techniques for the detection of minimal tumor cell populations are gaining in importance. In hematological disorders they are required for monitoring residual disease after therapy, detection of minimal bone marrow infiltration by malignant lymphoma cells and exclusion of tumor cell contamination after leukapheresis. The applicability of the combination of immunophenotyping and interphase cytogenetics, the FICTION technique, to detection of minimal tumor cell populations is demonstrated in a case of Hodgkin's disease.

Introduction

Sensitive techniques for the detection of minimal tumor cell populations are gaining in importance. In hematological disorders they are required for monitoring residual disease after therapy, detection of minimal bone marrow infiltration by malignant lymphoma cells and exclusion of tumor cell contamination after leukapheresis.

The use of the sensitive PCR technique is restricted to tumors with defined structural chromosome aberrations. Its application depends on the availability of DNA primers specific for the chromosome aberration to be analyzed. Since only primers for some common structural chromosome aberrations are available to date, this technique is restricted to a limited number of cases.

Fluorescence in situ hybridization (FISH) [1] appears suitable for tracing tumor cells with numerical chromosome aberrations. However, the sensitivity of FISH is limited: its detection limit ranges from 1-2% for cells with chromosome gains to 10-20% for cells with chromosome losses. The reason is that also a considerable portion of normal control cells contain irregular hybridization signal numbers due to artificial hybridization. Therefore, reliable results cannot be obtained using the FISH technique in cases with a low number of malignant cells, as found in minimal residual disease.

A solution to this problem could be to selectively analyze cells with tumor cell-associated immunophenotype by FISH. Physical enrichment of tumor cells with a certain immunophenotype, e.g., by FACS sorting, and subsequent FISH analysis is possible but too time consuming in routine diagnostics.

We suggest our new technique of combined immunophenotyping and interphase cytogenetics analysis (FICTION) [2-5] as a reasonable and less intricate alternative. By FICTION, cells with a tumor cell-associated immunophenotype are recognized by fluorescent immunostaining and, at the same time, studied for certain chromosome aberrations by FISH. If the immunophenotype of the tumor cells differs considerably from that of the normal cell population, tumor cells can be analyzed exclusively. In this way the detection limit of FISH may be overcome.

The applicability of FICTION was demonstrated in a case of Hodgkin's disease. Similar to minimal residual disease, the portion of tumor cells was very low (< 0.5% of total cells).

Department of Human Genetics, University of Kiel, Germany

Materials and Methods

Cytospin slides were prepared from a lymph node biopsy of a 23-year-old woman with Hodgkin's disease, lymphocyte predominant subtype, and stored at −70 °C. After thawing, cytospin slide preparations were fixed in acetone for 10 min at room temperature and incubated with monoclonal anti-CD30 antibody (Dakopatts, Hamburg). CD30 was visualized by a three step sequential incubation with Cy3-conjugated secondary antibodies (Jackson, West Grove, Pa.). All incubations were followed by three 2 min washes in phosphate buffer (0.1 M NaH_2PO_4, 0.1 M Na_2HPO_4, pH 8). Polyclonal antibodies were diluted 1:200 in PNM buffer (5% non-fat dry milk, 0.02% Na azide in phosphate buffer). For preserving the immunostaining, slides were fixed for 1 min in 1% paraformaldehyde and 10 min in ice-cold Carnoy's fixative (methanol:glacial acetic acid, 1:3). After a brief wash in phosphate buffer, the slides were dehydrated in a 70%, 85% and 100% ethanol series. For in situ hybridization, 1 µl hybridization mixture (1 ng of biotinylated chromosome 12 probe D12Z1, 50 ng sonicated salmon sperm DNA and 10% dextran sulfate in 60% formamide, 1 × SSC) was placed on the cell-containing area of the slide and covered with a round coverslip (8 mm diameter). After sealing with rubber cement, the slides were denatured at 73 °C for 5 min and hybridized at 37 °C for 2 h. Hybridization was followed by three 5 min washes in 50% formamide, 2 × SSC, pH 7.4 at 45 °C. After equilibration in phosphate buffer, the detection of the biotinylated probe was performed with FITC-conjugated avidin (Jackson). Detection can be amplified with a biotinylated goat anti-avidin antibody (Jackson) in the first step and FITC-conjugated avidin in the second step, and further by repetitive employment of steps one and two. Each step was followed by a brief wash in phosphate buffer. The antibodies were diluted 1:200 in PNM buffer. Finally, the slides were mounted in antifade solution (90% glycerol in phosphate buffer containing 23 mg/ml DABCO, Sigma, Deisenhofen, Germany). Microscopic evaluation was carried out with a Zeiss Axiophot microscope with appropriate filter sets for the fluorescence dyes (00 for Cy3, 09 for FITC).

Results

We performed FICTION analysis in a case of Hodgkin's disease to demonstrate that tumor cell populations of less than 0.5% can be detected by this method. Results are shown in Figs. 1 and 2. The CD30-positive Hodgkin and Reed-Sternberg (HRS) cells are clearly marked by the (red) Cy3 fluorescence. Thus, single CD30-positive cells against a background of bystander lymphocytic cells are easily detected. CD30-positive and -negative cells can clearly be distinguished. The (green) hybridization signals corresponding to the centromeric region of chromosome 12 are visible within the nuclei. The CD30-positive cells contain four copies of chromosome 12. All hybridization signals could be detected at microscopic analysis by focussing. Since some hybridization signals are at different focus levels, not all signals could be photographically documented. Background staining was minimal in our preparations.

Discussion

By means of FISH with centromeric DNA probes, numerically aberrant tumor cells can be identified by the number of hybridization signals. This holds particularly true in cases of Hodgkin's disease, since the malignant HRS cells often contain complex aberrations with irregular chromosome numbers [6]. On the other hand, the number of HRS cells is often far below 1% of total cells. Even if single cells with irregular hybridization signal numbers can be identified by the FISH technique within an overwhelming mass of reactive or normal cells they need not necessarily be malignant: even in normal tissue, cells with irregular hybridization signals (up to 2%) due to artificial hybridization can be found by FISH.

In Hodgkin's disease this problem can easily be overcome, since the malignant HRS cells strongly express the CD30 antigen, which is only rarely expressed on lymphocytic bystander cells. With the simultaneous demonstration of immunophenotypical and cytogenetic features (FICTION), even very low numbers of malignant cells ($<0.1\%$) can selectively be studied.

We presented the application of our FICTION technique in a case of Hodgkin's disease to clearly demonstrate that FICTION is a powerful tool for detecting minimal tumor cell populations with a certain tumor-associated antigen.

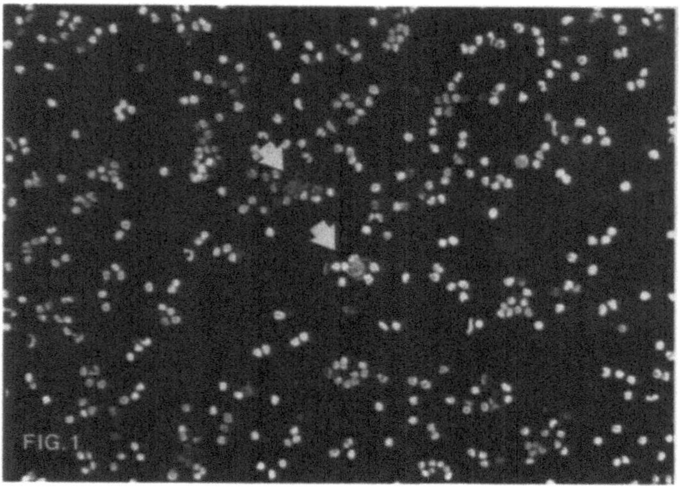

Fig. 1. FICTION technique in a case of Hodgkin's disease, lymphocyte predominant subtype. Cytocentrifuge slides were prepared from a lymph node suspension. Immunostaining against CD30, interphase cytogenetic analysis with centromeric chromosome 12 probe. In Hodgkin's disease, the malignant Hodgkin and Reed-Sternberg (HRS) cells strongly express the CD30 antigen. They usually make up much less than 1% of the lymph node cells. The microphotograph shows two HRS cells (*arrows*), positively immunostained for CD30, which are surrounded by more than 500 CD30-negative lymphocytes (DAPI-stained nuclei). At this low magnification the hybridization signals for chromosome 12 within the nuclei are not visible. The upper HRS cell is shown at higher magnification in Fig. 2

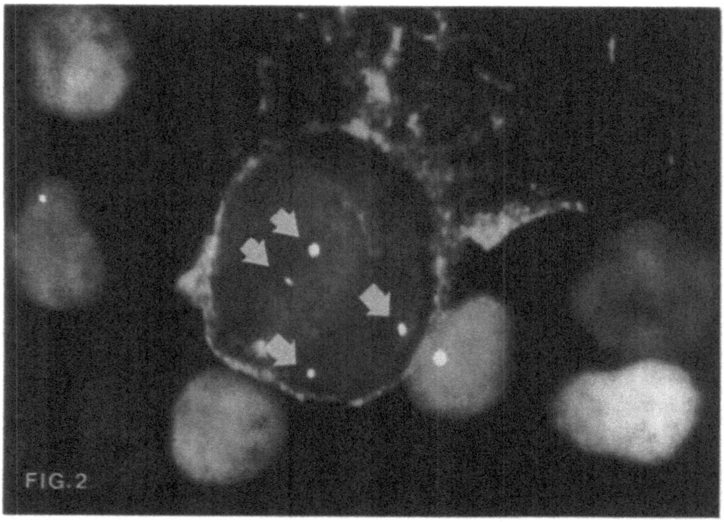

Fig. 2. CD30-positive HRS cell from Fig. 1 at higher magnification. Both immunophenotype and hybridization signals for chromosome 12 (*arrows*) are clearly visible. The HRS cell contains four chromosomes 12, whereas the bystander lymphocytes show exclusively regular signal numbers. Note that some signals are out of focus

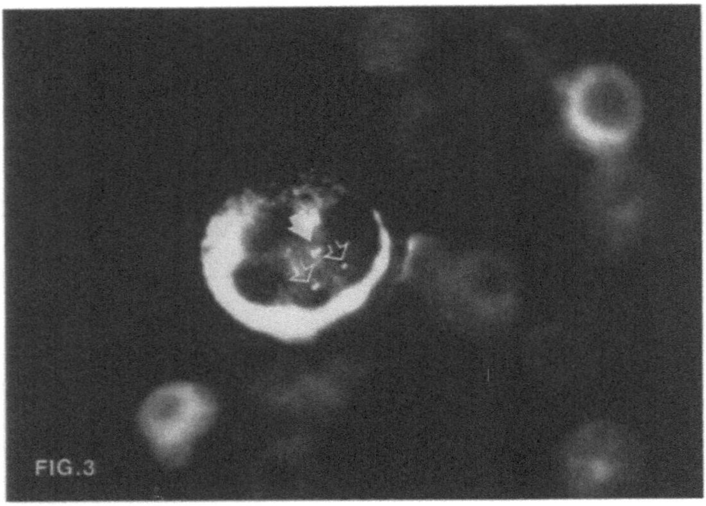

Fig. 3. CD19-positive lymphocyte from a case of ALL with the Philadelphia translocation t(9;22). The strong immunostaining of the cell for CD19 is clearly visible. Surrounding lymphocytes stained negative. Hybridization was performed with cosmid DNA probes for chromosomes 9 and 22. The cell contains one copy of chromosome 9 and one copy of chromosome 22 (*open arrows*). The *filled arrow* points at the Philadelphia chromosome t(9;22) composed of parts from chromosomes 9 and 22

This situation mostly pertains in some cases of minimal residual disease: tumor cells in common acute lymphatic leukemia (c-ALL), for example, which typically have a hyperdiploid karyotype with gain of different chromosomes, are usually CD10-positive. This antigen is not expressed on peripheral blood cells. Thus, employing FICTION with an antibody against CD10 and a DNA probe for a numerically aberrant chromosome, minimal fractions of malignant cells can be detected within smears or cytospin slides prepared from peripheral blood.

New developments in the field of interphase cytogenetics have extended the applicability of FISH to the detection of structural chromosome aberrations. This is true for the highly specific DNA probes, e.g., cosmids or YAC (yeast artificial chromosome)-generated DNA probes that enable the identification of structural chromosome aberrations like t(9;22) in chronic myeloid leukemia and some cases of acute lymphatic leukemia (ALL) (Fig. 3), or t(14;18) in cb-cc lymphoma within interphase cells. Using these DNA probes suitable for the detection of structural chromosome aberrations, FICTION can also be applied in cases of CML or cb-cc lymphoma to detect small tumor cell populations after therapy.

References

1. Cremer T, Landegent J, Bruckner A, Scholl H, Schardin M, Devilee P, Pearson P, Van der Ploog M (1986) Detection of chromosome aberrations in the human interphase nucleus by visualization of specific target DNAs. Hum Genet 74: 346–352
2. Weber-Matthiesen K, Winkemann M, Muller Hermelink A, Schlegelberger B, Grote W (1992) Simultaneous fluorescence immunophenotyping and interphase cytogenetics: a contribution to the characterization of tumor cells. J Histochem Cytochem 40: 171–175
3. Weber-Matthiesen K, Deerberg J, Muller-Hermelink A, Schlegelberger B, Grote W (1993) Rapid immunophenotypic characterization of chromosomally aberrant cells by the new FICTION method. Cytogenet Cell Genet 63: 123–125
4. Weber-Matthiesen K, Muller-Hermelink A, Deerberg J, Scherthan H, Schlegelberger B, Grote W (1993) Discrimination of distinct subpopulations within a tumor with double immunophenotyping and interphase cytogenetics. J Histochem Cytochem 41: 1641–1644
5. Weber-Matthiesen K, Pressl S, Schlegelberger B, Grote W (1993) Combined immunophenotyping and interphase cytogenetics on cryostat sections by the new FICTION method. Leukemia 7: 646–649
6. Tilly H, Bastard C, Delastre T, Duval C, Bizet M, Lenormand B, Dauce J-P, Monconduit M, Piquet H (1991) Cytogenetic studies in untreated Hodgkin's disease. Blood 77: 1298–1304

Leukemia Cell Biology: Molecular Biology

Acute Leukemias VI
Prognostic Factors
and Treatment Strategies
Büchner et al. (eds)

A Cloning Strategy to Identify Genes that Functionally Interact with Bcr-Abl for Transformation

S. Mahlmann[1], D.E.H. Afar[1], J. McLaughlin[3], A. Goga[2], and O.N. Witte[1,2,3]

Abstract. We have developed an expression cloning system to identify genes which functionally interact with Bcr-Abl for transformation. This system is based on a complementation strategy we used recently to define the signaling pathways activated by the Bcr-Abl tyrosine kinase. Point mutations were generated in domains of Bcr-Abl that may play a role in connecting its tyrosine kinase signal to downstream effector molecules. Hyperexpression of c-Myc, a gene known to act downsteam of a Bcr-Abl signal, was able to rescue one of these mutants. Based on this complementation, we developed an expression cloning strategy to identify unknown downstream genes in the complex signaling network of Brc-Abl. A lymphoid progenitor cDNA expression library was constructed in a retroviral vector and introduced into fibroblasts stably expressing a Brc-Abl point mutant. cDNA clones capable of complementing a mutant for transformation should result in colony formation in soft agar. We have obtained numerous colonies in several assays. PCR analysis of the genomic DNA from transformed fibroblasts revealed different cDNA inserts varying in size between 0.5 and 3 kb.

Introduction

Since the discovery of oncogenes as mutated forms of normal cellular counterparts, it has been suggested that cancer is the result of an alteration of a normal signal. A key to understanding cancer is to elucidate how signaling molecules functionally relate to each other within the cell to cause oncogenesis. For instance, signal pathways induced by the Bcr-Abl tyrosine kinase oncogene are involved in the pathogenesis of Philadelphia chromosome-positive leukemias [1]. Bcr-Abl is the result of a reciprocal translocation of chromosomes 9 and 22, which results in the fusion of two cellular genes encoding Bcr and Abl [2–4]. The resulting fusion gene encodes an activated protein tyrosine kinase. Two fusion proteins are detected in nature, P210 Bcr-Abl and P185 Bcr-Abl. In general, P210 is associated with chronic myelogenous leukemia (CML) and P185, which exhibits higher tyrosine kinase activity than P210, is associated with the more aggressive acute lymphocytic leukemia [5].

We describe here an expression cloning system to identify genes which functionally interact with Bcr-Abl for transformation. This sytem is based on a complementation strategy we used recently[6] to define the signaling pathways activated by the Bcr-Abl tyrosine kinase. Point mutations were generated in domains of Bcr-Abl that may play a role in connecting its tyrosine kinase signal to downstream effector molecules. The mutants were introduced into rat-1 cells by retroviral infection [7]. Single point mutations in the Src-homology (SH2) domain, the major tyrosine autophosphorylation site of the kinase domain, and the Grb-2 binding site in the Bcr region impaired the

[1] Department of Microbiology and Molecular Genetics, University of California–Los Angeles, Los Angeles, CA 90095-1662, USA
[2] Molecular Biology Institute, University of California–Los Angeles, Los Angeles, CA 90095-1662, USA
[3] Howard Hughes Medical Institute, University of California–Los Angeles, Los Angeles, CA 90095-1662, USA

transformation of fibroblasts by Bcr-Abl. Hyperexpression of c-Myc, a gene known to act downstream of a Bcr-Abl signal [8], was able to rescue only the SH2 mutant for transformation. Transformation resulted in colony formation in a soft agar assay [5].

The ability of c-Myc to differentially complement the Bcr-Abl point mutants signified that at least two different signaling pathways are generated by Bcr-Abl. In principle, every downstream gene in the complex signaling network of Bcr-Abl should complement at least one Bcr-Abl mutant for transformation. Colony formation in soft agar can therefore be used as a functional assay in an expression cloning approach to screen for novel genes complementing a Bcr-Abl mutant for transformation. This approach involves cDNA library transfer into fibroblasts and phenotypic selection of these cells over a period of several weeks. Traditionally, expression cloning techniques rely on cDNA transfection methods [9-11]. The most significant limitation in the use of stable transfection methods in fibroblasts [12-16] are the low efficiencies of cDNA tranfer and expression. To circumvent these problems, we adopted a retroviral cloning strategy orginally described by Rayner and Gonda [17]. Retroviral vectors have been shown to transfer and express cDNAs in mammalian cells with high efficiences [17, 18]. This includes gene transfer into fibroblasts [19]. We therefore constructed a retroviral lymphoid progenitor cDNA library. Retroviral stocks were generated and used to infect rat-1 cells, which express a transformation-defective mutant of Bcr-Abl. The infected cells were plated in soft agar and screened for colony formation. We obtained numerous colonies in several assays, indicating a panel of complementing cDNAs. This retroviral cloning system should also be useful for identifying downstream genes in signal pathways initiated by other oncogenes.

Material and Methods

cDNA Synthesis and Cloning

Poly $(A)^+$ RNA was prepared from lymphoid progenitor cells using guanidium thiocyanate, cesium chloride centrifugation, and oligo (dt) cellulose chromatography [20]. cDNA was synthesized [21] from 5 µg poly $(A)^+$ RNA using oligo (dt) primers. The blunt-ended cDNA was ligated to Eco RI adaptor (Promega) using the RiboClone Eco RI Adapter Ligation System (Promega) and following the recommendations of the suppliers. The cDNA was passed through a Sephary S-400 spin column (Pharmacia) to select for cDNA fragments greater than 500 bp. The size-selected cDNAwas ligated into the Eco RI side of the retroviral vector pSRaMSVtk. Construction of pSRaMSVtkneo has been described elsewhere [8]. The neofragment was removed by Xbal digestion and vector religation. After ligation, the reaction mixture was phenol-extracted and ethanol-precipitated in the presence of 20 µg glycogen (Boehringer). After washing the pellet was resuspended in 10 µl 10 m*M* $MgCl_2$ in preparation for electroporation.

Amplification of the Library

Aliquots of 1 µl (ca. 5 ng) of the resuspended ligation mixture were electroporated in to *E. coli* DA5α using a Gene Pulser apparatus (Bio Rad). The electroporated cells were grown for 1 h at 37°C in 1 ml SOC medium [20], plated out on 150-mm LB-ampicillin plates (100 µg ampicillin per milliliter), and grown overnight at 37°C. The cell density was 5000 per dish and 200 dishes were plated. Every ten dishes were pooled, and the cells were pelletized. supercoiled plasmid DNA was prepared from the pellet by alkaline lysis followed by purification on a CsCl Buchstabe gradient [20].

Preparation of Virus Stocks

Retrovirus stocks were prepared by transient transfection of 293T cells as described (22). Supernatant of 293T cells was collected at a rate of 5 ml every 8 h from 36 h after transfection until 60 h after transfection.

Generation of Indicator Lines and Soft Agar Colony Assay

Rat-1 cells expressing a Bcr-Abl mutant were generated as described [6]. Briefly, rat-1 cells were infected with helper-free retrovirus containing a Bcr-Abl cDNA mutant. The cells were selected in G418 (0.5 mg/ml) for 3-4 weeks. All indicator lines were maintained continuously in G418 to prevent the growth of cells that might have deleted the retroviral construct. The indicator lines were plated at a density of 2×10^5 cells per 15-cm^2 dish overnight. The cells were then infected with the retroviral cDNA stocks. Infection was performed for 3 h at 37°C, using 3 ml virus stock with 8 ug/ml polybrene. Forty-eight hours later, infected cells were plated in agar [23] at a density of 10^6 per 10-cm^2 dish in triplicate, dishes were refed at 1 week and screened for colonies at 4 weeks.

Recovery of Complementing Retrovirus

Transformed colonies were expanded in liquid culture and superinfected with replication-compotent Molony murine leukemia virus as described [24]. The rescued retrovirus was used to reinfect the indicator cell lines, which are subsequently plated in agar as described above.

Genomic DNA Isolation

Genomic DNA was isolated from cells using a proteinase K-sodium dodecyl sulfate procedure essentially as described by Hughes et al. [25].

Polymerase Chain Reaction of Genomic DNA Polymerase Chain Reactions

(PCRs) with 1 µg genomic DNA were performed essentially as described by Saiki [26]. The primers used for amplification were CTC TGA GTG ATT GAC TAC CCA C, which corresponds to vector 5' LTR (position 549–570), and CCC CGA CTG CAT CTG CGT GTT C, which corresponds to the thymidine kinase promoter region (position 153–164). The reactions were performed in a Perkin Elmer Thermocycler for 30 cycles, and the cycling parameters were denaturation at 94°C for 1 min, annealing at 58°C for 1 min, and extension at 72°C for 3 min. The reaction mixtures were denatured at 94°C for 5 min before cycling commenced, and a final 10 min extension was added after cycle 30.

Protein Analysis

Expression of Bcr-Abl proteins was measured by Western analysis using the monoclonal antibody pex5. Cell pellets were lysed in 10 m*M* Tris (ph 7.4) and 1% SDS at 100°C and analyzed as described [7].

Results and Discussion

Outline of the Protocol

An outline of the cloning strategy is shown in Fig. 1. It begins with the cDNA synthesis from a tissue that is appropriate for the isolation of the gene in question. The cDNA is cloned into a retroviral vector and amplified in *E. coli*. The

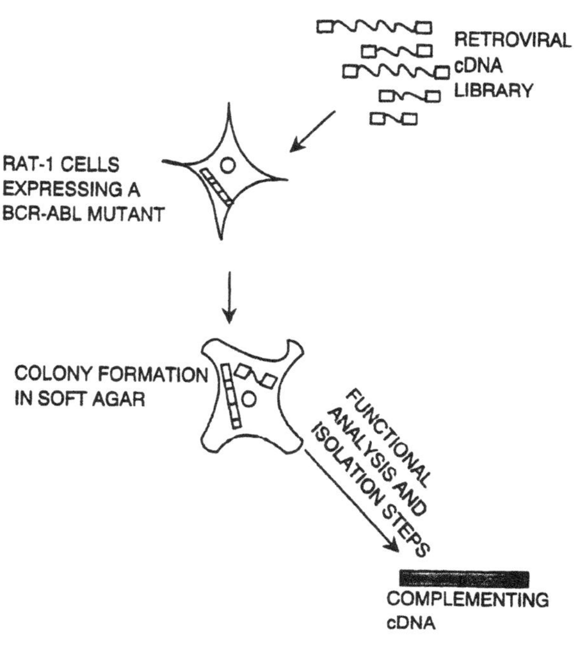

Fig. 1. Outline of the strategy for identifying cDNA clones that complement Bcr-Abl mutants for transformation (see text for details)

retroviral vector encoding the cDNA library is cotransfected with Psi(-) ecotropic packaging vector into 293T cells to generate helper-free retrovirus. Viral stocks are used to infect rat-1 cells, which express a transformation-defective mutant of Bcr-Abl. The infected cells are plated in soft agar and screened for colony formation. Colonies are expanded in culture and superinfected with a helper virus to rescue the complementing retrovirus. The rescued retrovirus is used to reinfect native rat-1 cells and rat-1 cells expressing a transformation-defective mutant of Bcr-Abl. In this way a complementing gene can be distinguished from an activated oncogene or just background colonies. The complementing genes are recovered by PCR from the retroviral DNA integrated in the original cell population.

Generation of a Lymphoid Progenitor cDNA Library

The cDNA was synthesized from a lymphoid progenitor cell line. This cell line can be transformed by Bcr-Abl [27]. The cDNA was cloned into the Eco RI side of the pSRaMSVtk vector (for details see Materials and Methods). We electroporated the retroviral vector containing the cDNA into *E. coli.* Electroporated cells were grown for 1 h at 37°C in LB medium and plated out on LB-ampicillin plates. With this method we were able to generate a library of 2×10^6 recombirants (1.5×10^7 clones/μg DNA). Insert analysis revealed an insert frequency of 86%, the insert size varied between 500 bp and 6 kb. To amplify the library the transformed cells were plated on 15 cm LB-ampicillin plates and grown overnight at 37°C. The bacteria had a density of 5000/plate. The library was not further amplified in liquid culture, because these conditions would favor the growth of cells harboring plasmids with small or no inserts. Colonies from every ten dishes were scraped into LB medium, pooled, and plasmid DNA was prepared. In this way, we pooled the plasmid DNA of 50 000 independent colonies. Twenty different pools were generated.

Generation of Retrovirus in 293T Cells

The human embryonic kidney cell line 293T [28] is a retroviral packaging cell line analogous to COS cells. This cell line expresses the SV 40 large T antigen, which allows the amplification of plasmids containing the SV 40 origin of replication. The retroviral cDNA was cotransfected with Psi(-) ecotropic packaging vector into 293T cells to generate helper-free retrovirus. We did independent transfections with retroviral cDNA from each pool to generate independent viral stocks. Each cDNA pool was used at least four times and we generated 80 different viral stocks. We used 293T cells for several reasons: (i) 293T cells are highly transfectable [22]; we routinely observe 80%–90% transfection efficiencies, compared to 10%–15% efficiencies for COS cells [7]. (ii) Viral titers generated in 293T cells after transient transfection are very high (10^6–10^7 infectious units per milliliter of cell supernatant). By Western bolt analysis we have determined that the highest viral titers for these cells are generated during the period from 36 h after transfection to 60 h after transfection (Fig. 2). Therefore, for 36 h after transfection, supernatant from 293T cells was collected at a rate of 5 ml every 8 h. The supernatants from each collection were pooled and frozen. The viral titers were assessed by slot hybridization [20]. Viral RNA was prepared and deposited at different dilutions onto a nitrocellulose membrane in a filtration manifold. The blot was probed with an LTR probe and the autoradiographic signals were compared to a signal generated by v-Abl RNA of a viral stock with a titer of 10^6 infections per milliliter. As shown in Fig. 3, the cDNA-containing retroviral stocks have nearly the same titer as the v-Abl viral stock.

The Bioassay

Previously we have shown that hyperexpression of c-Myc efficiently restores transformation activity to the Bcr-Abl SH2 mutant [6]. The complementation of signaling-defective point mutations by downstream genes is the basis of our bioassay. Theoretically, every retroviral cDNA that codes for a downstream protein in the signaling network of Bcr-Abl should complement at least one Bcr-Abl mutant for transformation and should lead to colony formation in soft agar. However, in the original complementation experiment, rat-1 cells which express a transformation-defective mutant of Bcr-Abl were infected with a viral stock containing only the c-Myc cDNA. Therefore c-Myc is orders of magnitude more highly represented than any clone of interest in a retroviral sublibrary. Our initial concern was therefore whether the agar assay is sensitive enough to screen for single genes in a complex library. To test this, we start-

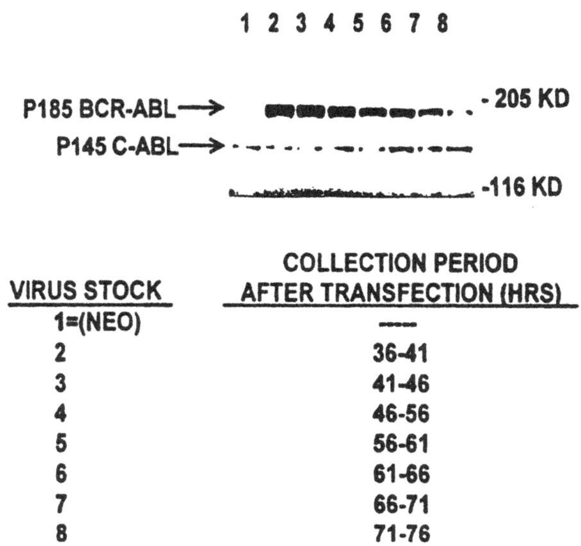

Fig. 2. Time course of virus production from 293T cells as determined by retroviral expression of Bcr-Abl in infected rat-1 cells. 293T cells were cotransfected with P185 Bcr-Abl plasmid DNA and a Psi(-)ecotropic packaging vector. Supernatant was collected at different time points after transfection as indicated. Supernatant from each collection period was independently used to infect rat-1 cells. Rat-1 cells were harvested 48 h after infection and analyzed by immunoblotting with monoclonal antibody to Abl (anti-Abl, pex5). Molecular size markers are indicated in kilodaltons. The positions of P185 Bcr-Abl and P145 C-Abl are indicated

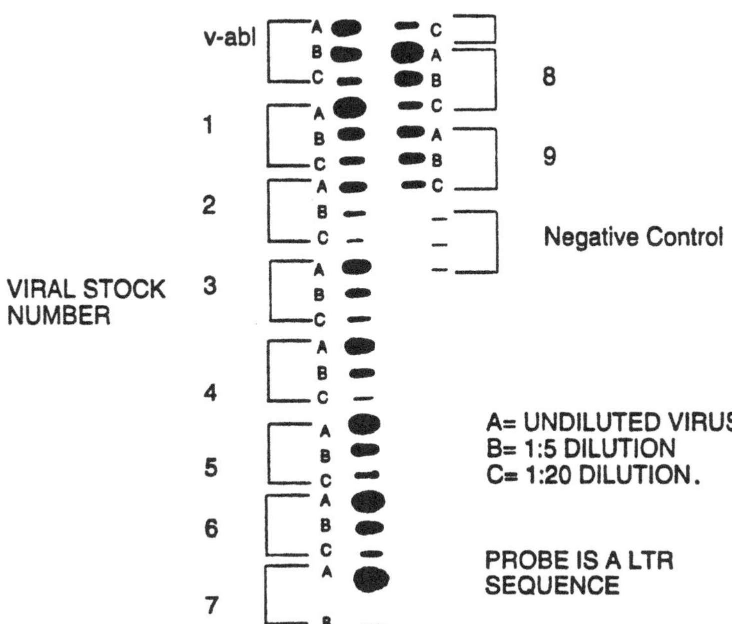

Fig. 3. Slot blot analysis of viral mRNA concentrations of independent stocks. The blot was probed with an LTR probe. The v-Abl stock that was used as a positive control had a titer of 10^6 infections/per milliliter. Each viral RNA was blotted in different concentrations as indicated

ed with a pilot experiment. As an indicator cell line we used rat-1 cells which express P 185 with a deletion in the SH2 domain. This mutation behaves in an identical fashion to P 185 with a point mutation in the phosphotyrosine binding site of the SH2 domain, but is less likely to revert back to wild-type Bcr-Abl than a point mutant. After G418 selection, rat-1 cells expressing ΔSH2 were infected with a c-Myc-containing retrovirus at different dilutions. An infection with the c-Myc virus stock diluted 1:1000 resulted in 7 ± 3 colonies in soft agar after 4 weeks. In contrast, infection with undiluted c-Myc virus resulted in more than 300 colonies after 3 weeks and led to acidification of the culture medium. Rat-1 cells expressing P 185 ΔSH2 which were superinfected with a retrovirus containing neo-cDNA did not form colonies in soft agar even after a cultivation period of 2 months. These data indicate that low representation of a complementing gene is still sufficient to lead to colony formation in soft agar. However, there is no final proof that complementation induced by rare messages can be detected in this way. On the other hand, the data show that expression of the Bcr-Abl mutant alone did not result in background colonies.

After this pilot experiment we tested the 80 viral stocks in independent agar assays. Each assay was done in triplicate. As shown in Fig. 4, in most of the assays no colony growth was observed. However, in some assays between one and four colonies were detected. In these cases colonies grew at least in two of the three plated assays.

We obtained a total of 50 colonies. They were isolated from the agar plates, grown in liquid culture, and some of them analyzed for the presence of a cDNA insert. To rescue the cDNA inserts we used a PCR approach, as outlined in Fig. 5. The primers used were complementary to sequences in the 5′ LTR and the TK promoter of the retroviral vector. PCR fragments between 3 kb and 500 bp were amplified. These data strongly indicate the utility of this retroviral cloning approach to identify genes that functionally interact with Bcr-Abl for transformation.

Functional Identification of Complementing Genes

To recover complementing retrovirus from transformed colonies and to determine the function of the cDNA insert, transformed cells expanded in liquid culture will be superinfected with replication competent Moloney murine leukemia virus [24]. Since only cDNAs from the library are contained within the retroviral genome, only library-derived cDNA will be rescued by the helper virus. The rescued retrovirus will be used to re-infect rat-1 cells expressing the SH2 mutant of Bcr-Abl, rat-1 cells expressing the other P 185 point mutants and native rat-1 cells. The strategy is outlined in Fig. 6. The advantage of this approach is that it provides a functional test for the genes of interest. In theory, if the retrovirus encodes only a complementing gene for the SH2 mutant, the rescued virus should only transform cells in conjuction with the SH2 mutant. If the rescued virus can also transform cells expressing the other point mutants, then the retrovirus may encode a gene that is downstream of several signaling pathways. If, however, the rescued virus is also capable of transforming native rat-1 cells, then the retrovirus most likely encodes an activated oncogene.

Alternatively, the function of the cDNA clones can be determined after subcloning and sequencing of the PCR fragments. Every clone with an open reading frame can be reintroduced in the retroviral vector and probed for complementation with a Bcr-Abl mutant.

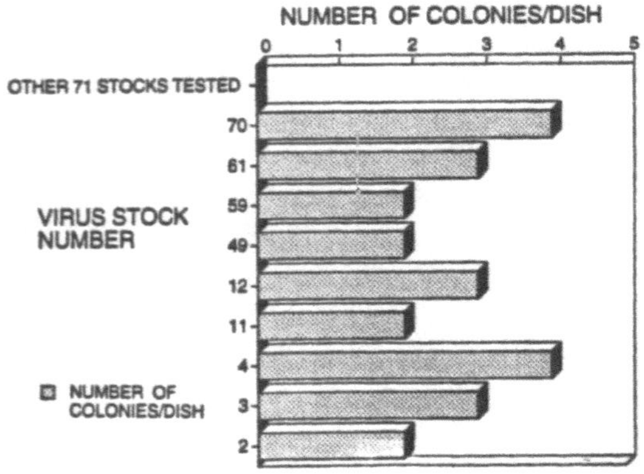

Fig. 4. Colony formation induced by different virus stocks. Rat-1 cells stably expressing P185 ΔSH2 were superinfected with retroviral stocks, each of them containing fractions of the cDNA library Eighty virus stocks were tested. The rat-1 cells were plated in soft agar 48 h after infection and screened for colony formation after 4 weeks

With the identification of downstream genes involved in Bcr-Abl signaling, we hope to gain an understanding of oncogenic signaling that is crucial to the development of therapeutic intervention. Furthermore, the described method should be useful for delineating signaling pathways generated by other oncogenes and signal transduction molecules.

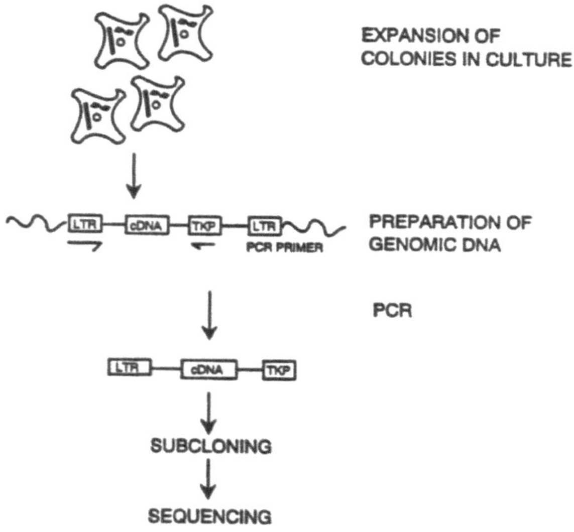

Fig. 5. Outline of the strategy for recovering complementing cDNA clones (see text for details)

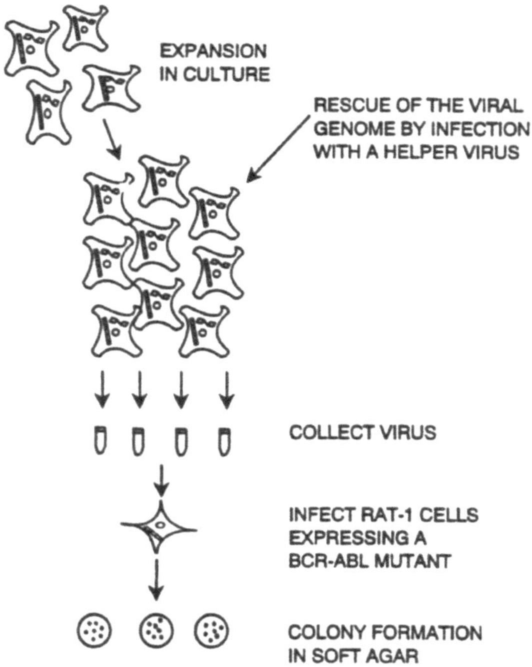

Fig. 6. Outline of the strategy for recovering complementing retrovirus (see text for details)

Acknowledgments. This work was supported by grant CA-53867 from the National Institutes of Health (O.N.W.), by the Howard Hughes Medical Institute, and fellowship support from the Deutsche Forschungsgemeinschaft (S. M.), the Medical Research Council of Canada (D. E. H. A.), and the UCLA Medical Scientist Training Program (A. G). O. N. Witte is an Investigator with the Howard Hughes Medical Institute.

References

1. Afar, D.E.H., A. Goga, L. Cohen, C. Sawyers, Jami McLaughlin, R. Mohr, and O.N. Witte, 1994 Genetic approaches to defining signaling by the CML-assoiciated tyrosine kinase BCR-ABL: in press.
2. Clark, S.C., J. McLaughlin, M. Timmons, A.M. Pendergast, Y. Ben-Neriah, L.W. Dow, W. Crist, G. Rovera, S.D. Smith, and O.N. Witte, 1988. Expression of a distinctive BCR-ABL oncogene in Ph1-positive acute lymphocytic leukemia (ALL). Science 239: 775–777.
3. Kurzroch, R., J. Gutterman, and M. Talpaz, 1988. The molecular genetics of Philadelphia chromosome-positive leukemias. N. Engl. J. Med. 319: 990–998.
4. Shtivelman, E., B. Lifshitz, R.P. Gale, and E. Canaai, 1985. Fused transcript of *abl* and *bcr* genes in chronic myelogenous leukaemia. Nature 315: 550–554.
5. Lugo, T.G., A. Pendergast, A.J. Muller, and O. Witte, 1990. Tyrosine kinase activity and transformation potency of bcr-abl oncogene products. Science 247: 1079–1082.
6. Afar, D.E.H., A. Goga, J. McLaughlin, O. Witte, and C.L. Sawyers, 1994. Differential rescue of BCR-ABL point mutants with c-MYC. Science 264: 424–426.
7. Muller, A.J., J.C. Young, A.-M. Pendergast, M. Pondel, N.R. Landau, D.R. Littman, and O.N. Witte, 1991. BCR first exon sequences specifically activate Bcr/Abl tyrosine kinase oncogene of Philadelphia chromosome positive human leukemias. Mol. Cell. Biol. 11: 1785–1792.
8. Sawyers, C.L., W. Callahan, and O.N. Witte, 1992. Dominant negative myc blocks transformation by ABL oncogenes. Cell 70: 901-910.
9. Aruffo, A. and B. Seed, 1987. Molecular cloning of a CD28 cDNA by a high-efficiency COS cell exp system. Proc. Natl. Acad. Sci. USA 84: 85773-8577.
10. Gearing, D.P., J.A. King, N.M. Gough, and N.A. Nicola, 1989. Expression cloning of a receptor for human granulocyte-macrophage colony-stimulating factor. EMBO J. 8: 3667–3676.
11. Mathews, L.S. and W.W. Vale, 1991. Expression cloning of an activin receptor, a predicted transmembrane serine kinase. Cell 65: 973–982.
12. Chan, A.M.-L., M. Chedid, E.S. McGovern, Popescu, N.C. , T. Miki, and S.A. Aaronson, 1993. Expression cDNA cloning of serine kinase transforming gene. Oncogene 8: 1320–1333.
13. Chan, A.M.-L., T.P. Fleming, E.S. McGovern, M. Chedid, T. Miki, and S. Aaronson, 1993. Expression cDNA cloning of a transforming gene encoding the wild-type G_12 gene product. Mol. Cell. Biol. 13: 762–768.
14. Miki, T., T.P. Fleming, D.P. Bottaro, J.S. Rubin, D. Ron, and S.A. Aaronson 1991. Expression cDNA cloning of the KGF receptor by creation of a transforming actocrine loop. Science 251: 72–75.
15. Miki, T., T.P. Fleming, M. Crescenzi, C. Molloy, S.B. Blam, S.H. Reynolds, and S.A. Aaronson, 1991. Development of a highly efficient expression cDNA cloning system: Application to oncogene isolation. Proc. Natl.Acad. Sci. USA 88: 5167–5171.
16. Miki, T., C.L. Smith, J.E. Long, A. Eva, and T.P. Fleming, 1993. Oncogene *ect2* is related to regulators of small GTP-binding proteins. Nature 362: 462–465.
17. Rayner, J.R. and T.J. Gonda, 1994. A simple and efficient procedure for generating stable expression libraries by cDNA cloning in a retroviral vector. Mol. Cell. Biol. 14: 880–887.
18. Wong, B.Y., H. Chen, W. Siu-Chung and P.M.C. Wong, 1994. High-efficiency identification of genes by functional analysis from a retroviral cDNA expression library. J. Virol. 68: 5523–5531.
19. Whitehead, I., H. Kirk, and R. Kay, 1995. Expression cloning of oncogenes by retroviral transfore of cDNA libraries. Mol. Cell. Biol. 15: 704–710.
20. Sambrook, J., E.F. Fritsch, and T. Maniatis, 1989. Molecular cloning. A laboratory manual. Cold Spring Harbor Laboratory Press, Cold Spring Harbor Laboratory.
21. Gubler, U. and B.J. Hoffman, 1983. A simple and very efficient method for generating cDNA libraries. Gene 25: 263–269.
22. Pear, W.S., G.P. Nolan, Scott, G.P. M.L. and D. Baltimore, 1993. Production of high titer helper-free retroviruses by transient transfection. Proc. Natl. Acad. Sci. USA 90: 8392–8396.
23. Lugo, T. and O.N. Witte, 1989. The BCR/ABL oncogene transforms Rat-1 cells and cooperates with v-myc. Mol. Cell. Biol. 9: 1263–1270.
24. Goga, A., J. McLaughlin, A.M. Pendergast, K. Parmar, A. Muller, N. Rosenberg, and O.N. Witte, 1993. Oncogenic activation of c-ABL by mutation within its last exon. Mol. Cell. Biol. 13: 4967–4975.
25. Hughes, S.H., F. Payvar, D. Spector, R.T. Schimke, H.L. Robinson, G.S. Payne, J.M. Bishop, and H.E. Varmus, 1979. Heterogeneity of genetic loci in chickens: analysis of endogenous viral and normal genes by cleavage of DNA with restriction endonucleases. Cell 18: 347–359.
26. Saiki, R.K. 1990. Amplification of genomic DNA, p. 13–20. In M.A. Innis, D.H. Gelfand, J.J. Sninsky, and T.J. White (eds.), PCR protocols: a guide to methods and applications, Academic Press, Inc., San Diego.

27. Young, J.C., M.L. Gishizky, and O.N. Witte, 1991. Hyperexpression of interleukin-7 is not necessary or sufficient for transformation of a pre-B lymphoid cell line. Mol. Cell. Biol. 11: 854–863.

28. DuBridge, R.B., P. Tang, H.C. Hsai, P.M. Leong, J.H. Miller, and M.P. Calos, 1987. Analysis of mutation in human cells by using an Epstein-Barr virus shuttle system. Mol. Cell. Biol. 7: 379–387.

Acute Leukemias VI
Prognostic Factors
and Treatment Strategies
Büchner et al. (eds)

Biology and Detection of t(4;11) Leukemias

F. Griesinger

Abstract. The elucidation of the genetic basis of various entities of acute leukemias has provided insight into the physiologic function in lymphohematopoiesis and the transforming potential of genes involved in malignant transformation. Furthermore, specific genetic alterations/chromosomal translocations are associated with distinct biologic and prognostic characteristics and serve as criteria for stratification to risk adapted therapy in acute lymphoblastic leukemia (ALL). The t(4;11) leukemias are characterized by a unique epidemiology and specific biologic features. t(4;11) Pre-pre-B-ALL has an incidence of 50%–60% in infant ALL with a preponderance in females, and an incidence of 5%–10% in pediatric and adult ALL. Immunophenotypically, this translocation is almost exclusively associated with a pre-pre-B-ALL phenotype and coexpression of the myeloid lineage-associated antigens CD15 and CDw65. Induction of differentiation into the myeloid lineage has been described, and it has been hypothesized that a common lymphoid and myeloid progenitor is transformed in t(4;11) pre-pre-B-ALL. Prognosis in infants has been dismal with chemotherapy alone. With intensification of postremission chemotherapy, prognosis may be more favorable in adults. MLL (ALL-1, Htrx, HRX) on 11q23, a potential DNA-binding protein with homology to *Drosophila trithorax*, and AF4 (FEL) on 4q21, a gene encoding a serine/-proline-rich protein of unknown function, are fused by the 4;11 translocation. MLL has been found to form fusion transcripts with at least 30 other translocation partners in both ALL and AML and it has been termed the most promiscuous potential oncogene in leukemia. 11q23 rearrangements occur in both de novo and secondary acute leukemias, the latter especially upon exposition to topoisomerase II inhibitor treatment. The common feature of all MLL fusion transcripts in the disruption of 5′ protein domains out of the physiological configuration and deletion of all or most of the zinc finger domains, which most likely transfers transforming potential to the fusion gene product. Genomic breakpoints within the MLL gene cluster within a small region of 8.3 kb. Various mechanisms may be involved in inducing MLL breaks such as recombinase, Alu-rich sequences, and inhibition of topoisomerase II. The latter mechanism mey be relevant in secondary acute leukemias upon topoisomerase II inhibitor treatment, as MLL breakpoints have been found to be localized preferentially in the vicinity of topoisomerase II binding sites in secondary leukemias. In the present overview, data will be presented regarding immunophenotyping of t(4;11) leukemias, the detection of the MLL-AF4 transcript by RT-pcr. An analysis of MLL-AF4 fusion transcripts in our series as well as in the literature shows that fusion transcripts are heterogeneous due to various exon usage and differential splicing. MLL exon usage may differ between adult and infant t(4;11) ALL, with infants fusing 3′ MLL exons rather than 5′ exons to AF4. Whether these differences are associated with a different biology and prognosis in different age groups has to be investigated in a homogeneously treated patient population.

Division of Hematology, Department of Internal Medicine, University of Göttingen, Robert Koch Str. 40, 37075 Göttingen, Germany

Introduction

Acute lymphoblastic leukemias (ALL) represent a variety of heterogeneous biologic disease entities which can be subdivided by the expression pattern of characteristic stage-associated differentiation antigens and by specific genetic aberrations detected by cytogenetic and molecular biology methods [1, 2]. Pre-pre-B-ALL carrying a t(4;11) (q21;q23) is a biologically well-defined subset of ALL [3]. Epidemiologically this type of leukemia makes up about 50% of all ALL cases in infants under the age of 1 year, the incidence in children over the age of 1 year is estimated to be 5%–6% and the incidence in adults about 10%. There is a preponderance of female patients in t(4;11) ALL [4–7]. Biologically t(4;11) leukemias are characterized by the coexpression of B-lymphoid differentiation antigens and the myeloid differentiation antigens CD15 and CDw65 [1, 2]. The cell line RS4;11, which was the first t(4;11) cell line described, can be induced to differentiate into the myeloid cell lineage [8]. These data led to the hypothesis that a common B-lymphoid and myeloid progenitor cell undergoes malignant transformation in t(4;11) leukemias.

The genes involved in the t(4;11) translocation have been characterized recently. The gene MLL (HRX, Htrx, ALL-1) is located on chromosome 11q23 and forms a fusion transcript with the gene AF-4 on chromosome 4q21. Both genes most likely represent DNA binding and transactivating genes whose physiologic function in normal human embryogenesis and lymphohematopoiesis remains to elucidated. The MLL gene contains functional domains as AT hooks for minor groove DNA binding and zinc fingers in the amino-terminal part of the protein. MLL is highly conserved between *Drosophila*, mouse, and man. In *Drosophila* it is involved in thoracic segmentation; in the mouse MLL may have a function in osteogenesis. The function of MLL in human embryogenesis and hematopoiesis is unknown. AF4 is a serine-proline-rich potential DNA-binding protein of unknown function [9–12]. 11q23 translocations occur in at least 30 different fusion partterns, some of which have been characterized and sequenced, such as AF4 at 4q21, AF-6 at 6p27, ENL at 19p13.3, ELL at 19p13.1, AF-9 at 9p22, AF-17 at 17q25, and AF-X at Xq13 [13]. In addition to de novo acute leukemias, 11q23 translocations have been found in patients after topoisomerase II inhibitor therapy [14, 15] Interestingly, an intragenic duplication of MLL fusing exon 6 to a duplicated exon 2 to 6 cassette has been found in a significant number of AML cases [16]. The common feature of all fusion transcripts in disruption of 5′ protein domains out of the physiologic configuration, which may lend transforming potential to the MLL fusion gene product. MLL fusion genes are not restricted to specific hematopoietic cell lineages; for example, the t(4;11) has been observed both in AML and ALL. Furthermore, MLL fusion genes do not show restriction to specific stages of differentiation; for example, MLL-AF4 fusion genes have been described both in pre-pre-B-ALL and in rare cases if c-ALL and pre-B-ALL. This review covers some of the biologic and molecular aspects of t(4;11) leukemias reported in the literature and studied by our group (Table 1) with a focus on the various types of MLL-AF-4 fusion genes described so far.

Composite Immunophenotype of MLL-AF4 Positive ALL

T(4;11) leukemias almost invariably express the immunophenotype of pre-pre-B-ALL, i.e., coexpression of B-lymphoid differentiation antigens CD19, CD22, and lacking surface expression of CD10 [2]. Furthermore, coexpression of CD15 had been reported [1]. There is evidence that t(4;11) ALL frequently coexpresses the CDw65 differentiation antigen [2,17]. In the latter study 18 pre-pre-B-ALL carrying the MLL-AF4 fusion transcript and 26 pre-pre-B-ALL without the MLL-AF4 fusion transcript were stained with monoclonal antibodies detecting the CDw65, CD13, and CD33 antigens. Twelve of 18 MLL-AF4 positive pre-pre-B-ALL were CDw65 positive, while 24 of 26 MLL-AF4 negative pre-pre-B-ALL were negative for the CDw65 antigen. None of the 18MLL-AF4 positive pre-pre-B-ALL coexpressed the myeloid differentiation antigens CD13 and CD33, while 3 of 26 MLL-AF4 negative pre-pre-B-ALL expressed these antigens. These studies suggest a good predictive value of CDw65 expression in pre-pre-B-ALL for the presence of the t(4;11) (Table 2).

In our own series of pre-pre-B-ALL [18] (Table 1) 21 samples were stained with anti-CDw65; all 17 t(4;11) pre-pre-B-ALL were positive for CDw65, while none of the 4 MLL-AF4 negative pre-pre-B-ALL expressed the CDw65 differentiation antigen. Twenty-three pre-pre-B-

Table 1. Patient characteristics, including sample number (#), phenotype karyatype, and presence of *HRX-FEL* fusion gene transcript. All leukemic samples studied were β-actin positive

Pat, #	Phenotype	CD15+%	CD15+%	Karyotype	*HRX/FEL*
Adult pre-pre-B-ALL with cytogenetic detection of t(4:11)					
14	Pre-pre-B	10	49	46,XY[6]/46,XY,t(4;11)(q21;q23)[16]	Pos
20	Pre-pre-B	89	45	46,XX,t(4;11)(q21;q23)[2]	Pos
27	Pre-pre-B	10	45	46,XY[1]/46,XY,t(4;11)(q21;q23)[15]	Pos
32	Pre-pre-B	57	77	44,XY, – 12, – 16[1]/45,XY, – 16[1]/45,XY, – 12[1]/ 46,XY[9]/44XY, – 9, – 16,t(4;11)(q21;q23)[1]/ 45,XY, – 19,t(4;11)(q21;q23)[1]/ 46,XY,t(4;11)(q21;q23)[5]/ 47,XY,-A, +2mar, t(4;11)(q21;q23)[1]	Pos
33	Pre-pre-B	43	61	46,XY, t(4;11)(q21;q23)[13]	Pos
MV 4;11	Pre-pre-B	nd	ND	Chen et al. (1993)	Pos
RS 4;11	Pre-pre-B	nd	ND	Stong et al. (1985)	Pos
Infant pre-pre-B-ALL with cytogenetic detection of t(4;11)					
17	Pre-pre-B	31	50	46,XX, t(4;11)(q21;q23)[5]	Pos
29	Pre-pre-B	39	49	46,XX,t(4;11)(q21;q23)[3]	Pos
31	Pre-pre-B	19	75	46,XX,t(4;11)(q21;q23),1(7q10), del (11)(q23)[5]	Pos
1.1	Pre-pre-B	30	ND	46,XX,t(4;11)(q21;q23)	Pos
1.2	Pre-pre-B	33	ND	46,XX,t(4;11)(q21;q23)	Pos
1.3	Pre-pre-B	66	ND	46,XX,t(4;11)(q21;q23)	Pos
Adult pre-pre-B-ALL without cytogenetic detection of t(4;11)					
1	Pre-pre-B	59	30	46,XY[33]	Pos
7	Pre-pre-B	5	15	46,XX[6]	Pos
8	Pre-pre-B	90	83	46,XY[14]	Pos
10	Pre-pre-B	nd	55	46,XX[18]/47,XX+C[2]	Pos
12	Pre-pre-B	52	8	46,XY[13]/52–55,XY, +X,dup(1)(q32q21), +4 +6, +8, +10, – 13, +14, +15, +21,mar[30]	Neg
18	Pre-pre-B	84	89	46,XX[14]	Pos
22	Pre-pre-B	58	52	ND	Pos
24	Pre-pre-B	17	30	ND	Pos
28	Pre-pre-B	28	15	ND	Pos
Infant pre-pre-B-ALL without cytogenetic detection of t(4;11)					
1.4	Pre-pre-B	45	15	nd	Pos

Table 2. Association of myeloid antigens and of CDw65 and CD15 with MLL-AF4 Fusion transcripts (from [27])

	MLL-AF4$^+$	MLL-AF^4
Myeloid antigens		
CDw65$^+$	12/18	2/26
CD13$^+$	0/18	3/26
CD33$^+$	0/18	3/26
CDw65 and CD15		
CDw65$^+$	17/17	0/0
CDw65$^-$	0/0	4/4
CD15$^+$	16/20	4/20
CD15$^-$	3/3	0/0

[a]Selected for pre-pre-B-ALL.
[b]Selected for pre-pre-B-ALL coexpressing CD15 and CDw65.

ALL were stained with anti-CD15: of the 20 CD15$^+$pre-pre-B-ALL only 16 carried the t(4;11), while 4 of 20 CD15$^+$pre-pre-B-ALL were negative for the MLL-AF4 transcript. Furthermore, in three pre-pre-B-ALL negative for CD15 surface expression the MLL-AF4 transcript was detected (Table 2). In conclusion, our data suggest that CDw65 is a better discriminator for the presence of the t(4;11)/MLL-AF4 fusion transcript than CD15 expression. The different results may be due to the fact that three-color flow-cytometry allowed us to lower the threshold for detection of a positive leukemic population to 5%.

Detection of Fusion Genes in pre-pre-B-ALL Without Demonstration of t(4;11)

In our series of 13 pre-pre-B-ALL with cytogenetic demonstration of t(4;11) (group A) we detected a fusion transcript in all cases using an MLL exon 5 primer and an AF-4 exon c primer. Thus this primer combination may be able to detect all MLL-AF-4 fusion transcripts with high sensitivity (see Table 1)

Group B consisted of nine adult and one infant pre-pre-B-ALL selected upon pre-pre-B-ALL phenotype and coexpression of CD15 and/or CDw65 in whom either karyotype analysis was not carried out, no metaphases were obtained, or cytogenetics did not pick up the t(4;11) translocation. In nine of ten leukemias reverse-transcriptase polymerase chain reaction analysis demonstrated the transcription of a MLL-AF-4 fusion gene. Molecular methods thus detect the presence of t(4;11) in a significant number of pre-pre-B-ALL which are not detected by cytogenetics in a multicenter setting. These results are in line with other large multicenter trials in which detection of a MLL rearrangement in cytogenetically normal ALL was found to be in the range of 30%–50% [4–6,19,20].

Types of Fusion Transcripts

The genomic breakpoints within the MLL gene are clustered in a small area of 8.3 kb between introns 5 and 9. Various genomic breakpoints and differential splicing leads to a number of various fusion transcripts that were observed both in our series (Tables 3, 4) and in those of others (Table 5). Of special interest is the fact that differential splicing of transcripts may occur in one individual leukemia, leading to more than one transcript. Differential splicing led to the detection of two MLL-AF4 transcripts in cases 1.4, 17, and RS4;11 and to that of three transcripts in case 1.2 (Table 4). The most frequently observed fusion sites were MLL exon 7 in 10, exon 6 in 7, and exon 8 in 2 MLL-AF4 transcripts. AF4 exon usage was not evenly distributed, as exon a was found to be involved in 16 MLL-AF4 fusion transcripts, while exon b was found only in 3 cases. Exon c usage seems to be rare; in our series no pre-pre-B-ALL was found to have this fusion.

Interestingly, MLL exon usage in fusion sites was not evenly distributed with respect to age. All infant ALL MLL-AF4 transcripts used either exon 7 or exon 8, while 7 of 13 adult ALL used exon 6 (Table 3). No obvious age-related bias was detected relative to AF4 exon usage (Table 3).

Table 3. Distribution of MLL and AF-4 Fusion sites

MLL	e6	e7	e8	Total
Infants	0	4	2	6
Adults	7	6	0	13
Total	7	10	2	19
AF4[a]	a	b	c	Total
Infants	6	0	0	6
Adults	10	3	0	13
Total	16	3	0	19

[a]AF4-exon assignment accouding to [18], [25], and this manuscript.

Table 4. Sequences of *HRX-FEL* genes

Pats, # 10, #24, #27, #32			
	Exon 6	Exon 7	
HRX germline	AAAACCAAAAGAAAAG	GAAAAACCACCT...	
Fusion Gene	AAAACCAAAAGAAAAG		CAGACCTACTCCAATGAAGTCC
FEL Germline			CAGACCTACTCCAATGAAGTCC
			FEL(exon a) nt: 1413
MV 4;11, pt#1, #20			
	Exon 6	Exon 7	
HRX germline	AAAACCAAAAGAAAAG	GAAAAAACCACCT...	
Fusion *GENE*	AAAACCAAAAGAAAAG		GAAATGACCCATTCATG
FEL germline			TCGAAGGAAATGACCCATTCATG
			FEL (exon b) nt: 1458
RS 4;11, pats. #8, #14, #22, #28, #33, #1.2*, #1.4*			
	Exon 7	Exon 8	
HRX-germline	ATCAGAGTGGACTTTAAG	GAGGATTGTGAA...	
Fusion GENE	ATCAGAGTGGACTTTAAG		ACCTACTCCAATGAAGTCC
FEL germline			CAGACCTACTCCAATGAAGTCC
			FEL (exon a) nt: 1416
RS 4;11, #17*, #1.2*, #1.3*, #1.4*			
	Exon 7	Exon 8	
HRX germline	ATCAGAGTGGACTTTAAG	GAGGATTGTGAA...	
Fusion GENE	ATCAGAGTGGACTTTAAG		CAGACCTACTCCAATGAAGTCC
FEL germline			CAGACCTACTCCAATGAAGTCC
			FEL (exon a) nt: 1413
Pt #17*, #1.2*			
	Exon 8	Exon 9	
HRX germline	AGTGGGCATGTAGAG	GTTTGTGTATTG...	
Fusion GENE	AGTGGGCATGTAGAG		CAGACCTACTCCAATGAAGTCC
FEL germline			CAGACCTACTCCAATGAAGTCC
			FEL (exon a) nt: 1413

Assignment of nucleotides to the *HRX* and *FEL* genes was based on the published intron/exon boundaries, *FEL* exons "a" and "b" according to Downing et al., Blood 1994. The numbering of nucleotides is according to [10], [11], and [25].

Table 5. Distribution of MLL and AF4 Fusion sites (from [11, 17-23])

MLL	Infants		Children		Adults		Total	
	n	%	*n*	%	*n*	%	*n*	%
e6	10	34	2	28.5	18	51	30	42
e7	5	17	3	43	16	46	24	34
e8	14	48	2	28.5	1	3	17	24
Total	29	41	7	10	35	49	71	100
AF4								
ea	20	69	6	86	29	83	55	77
eb	8	28	1	14	5	14	14	20
ec	1	3	0	0	1	3	2	3
Total	29	41	7	10	35	49	71	100

A review of the literature analyzing MLL usage in all sequenced MLL-AF4 fusion transcripts reveals a trend toward 3′ MLL exon usage in infant ALL, as 66% of all infant pre-pre-B-ALL cases use either exon 7 or exon 8, while 51% of all adult pre-pre-B-ALL show exon 6 fusion sites. The difference in the usage of exon 8 is striking, as 48% of all infant ALL display an exon 8 fusion while only 3% of adult ALL had an exon 8 fusion (Table 5) [11, 18-23]. Whether different exon usage reflects different genomic breakpoints cannot be answered at this time. However, the hypothesis that genomic breakpoints differ in infant and adult ALL is of interest in light of the significant differences in clinical outcome. Specifically, genomic breakpoints in infant pre-pre-B-ALL may be localized in the 3′ area of the breakpoint cluster region in the vicinty of topoisomerase II binding sites and therefore may be similar to breakpoints observed in topoismerase II inhibitor induced secondary leukemias (see Rowley, this volume)

Prognosis of Leukemias and Possible Relationship to Induction Mechanisms

The prognosis of infant pre-pre-B-ALL carrying a t(4;11) seems to be dismal with chemotherapy alone [4, 5]. Pre-pre-B-ALL represents a high risk factor in the German adult ALL study. Since 1993 adults diagnosed with pre-pre-B-ALL receive an intensive induction regimen with high-dose arabinose-C starting at week 5, and the prognosis of adult pre-pre-B-ALL carrying a t(4;11) has considerably improved [24]; see also Hoelzer, this volume). Whether different types of MLL-AF4 fusion transcript may be associated with different outcomes is presently unclear. Therefore we asked whether 3′ MLL exon usage ("infant type" fusion transcript) is associated with a poorer prognosis than 5′ MLL exon usage ("adult type" fusion transcript). While 3 of 5 infant pre-pre-B-ALL individuals with MLL exon 6 fusion transcripts were long-term survivors, 8 of 11 infant ALL with MLL exon 8 fusions died. Of 16 ALL adults carrying MLL exon 6 fusion transcripts to were treated after 1991 and received high-dose arabinose-C. Five of these 10 ALL adults were long-term survivors (Table 6). These very premilinary data warrant a thorough analysis of treatment outcome relative to the types of fusion transcripts in a homogeneously treated population.

Table 6. Survival of MLL-AF4^{+}, ALL and type of fusion transcript

	Infants	Children	Adults
e6	3/5	1/2	5/10 (5/16)
e7	0/1	1/2	4/13
e8	3/11	0/1	0/0

References

1. Borowitz MJ, Carroll AJ, Shuster JJ, Look AT, Behm FG, Pullen DJ, Land VJ, Steuber P, Crist WM (1993) Use of clinical and laboratory features of define prognostic subgroups in B-precursor acute lymphoblastic leukemia: experience of the Pediatric Oncology Group. In: Ludwig W-D, Theil E (eds) Recent results in cancer research. Recent advances in cell biology of acute leukemia Springer, Berlin Heidelberg New York, pp 257-267

2. Ludwig W-D, Harbott J, Bartram CR, Komischke B, Sperling C, Teichman JV, Seibt-Jung H, Notter M, Odenwald E, Nehmer A, Thiel E, Riehm H (1993) Incidence and prognistic significance of immunophenotypic subgroups in childhood acute lymphoblastic leukemia: experience of the BFM Study 86. In: Ludwig W-D, Thiel E (eds) Recent results in cancer research. Recent advances in cell biology of acute leukemia Springer, Berlin Heidelberg New York, pp 269–282
3. Arthur DC, Bloomfield CD, Lindquist LL, Nesbit ME Jr (1982) Translocation 4;11 in acute lymphoblastic leukemia: clinical characteristics and prognostic significance. Blood 59: 96–101
4. Rubnitz JE, Link MP, Shuster JJ, Carroll AJ, Hakami N, Frankel LS, Pullen DJ, Cleary ML (1994) Frequency and prognostic significance of HRX rearrangements in infant acute lymphoblastic leukemia: a Pediatric Oncology Group study. Blood 84: 570–573
5. Chen C-S, Sorensen PHB, Domer PH, Reaman GH, Korsmeyer SJ, Heerema NA, Hammond FD, Kersey JH (1993) Molecular rearrangements on chromosome 11q23 predominate in infant acute lymphoblastic leukemia and are associated with specific biologic variables and poor outcome. Blood 81: 2386–2393
6. Thiman MJ, Gill HJ, Burnett RC, Mbangkollo D, McCabe NR, Kobayashi H, Ziemen-car der Poel S, Kanek Y, Morgan R, Sandberg AA, Chaganti RSK, Larson RA, Le Beau MM, Diaz MO, Rowley JD (1993) Rearrangements of the MLL gene in acute lymphoblastic and acute myeloid leukemias with 11q23 chromosomal translocations New Engl J Med 329: 909–914
7. Ludwig W-D, Rieder H, Bartram CR, Griesinger F, Hossfeld DK, Heinze B, Gökbuget N, Herrmann F, Hiddemann W, Löffler H, Fonatsch C, Thiel E, Hoelzer D (1994) Immunophenotypic and genotypic heterogeneity of adult pre-pre-B acute lymphoblastic leukemia (ALL): experience of the German multicenter tirals (GMALL 3/87 and 04/89). Blood 84: 516a (abstract 2049)
8. Stong RC, Korsmeyer SJ, Parkin JL, Arthur DC, Kersey JH (1985). Human acute leukemia cell line with the t(4;11) chromosomal rearrangement exhibits B lineage and monocytic characteristics. Blood 65: 21–31
9. Gu Y, Nakamura T, Alder H, Prasad R, Canaani O, Cimino G, Croce CM, Canaani E (1992) The t(4;11) chromosome translocation of human acute leukemias fuses in ALL-1 gene. related Drosophila trithorax, to the AF-4 gene. Cell 71: 701–708
10. Tkachuk DC, Kohler S, Cleary ML, (1992) Involvement of a homolog of Drosophila trithorax by 11q23 chromosomal translocations in acute leukemias Cell 71: 691–700
11. Morrissey J, Tkachuk DC, Milatovich A, Francke U, Link M, Cleary ML (1993) A serine rich-proline protein is fused to HRX in t(4;11) acute leukemias. Blood 81: 1124–1131
12. Ma Q, Alder H, Nelson KK, Chatterjee D, Gu Y, Nakamura T, Canaani E, Croce CM, Siracusa LD, Buchberg AM (1993) Analysis of the murine ALL-1 gene reveals conserved domains with human ALL-1 and identifies a motif shared with DNA methytransferases Proc Natl Acad Sci USA 90: 6350–6354
13. Kobayashi H, Espinosa F, Thirman MJ, Gill HJ, Fernald AA, Diaz MO, Le Beau MM, Rowley JD (1993) Heterogeneity of breakpoints of 11q23 rearrangments in hematologic malignancies identified with fluorescence in situ hybridization. Blood 82: 547–551
14. Pui C-H, Ribeiro RC, Hancock ML, Rivera GK, Evans WE, Raimondi SC, Head DR, Behm FG, Mahmoud MH, Sandlund JT, Crist WM (1991) Acute myeloid leukimia in children treated with epipodophyllotoxins for acute lymphoblastic leukemia. N Eng J Med 325: 1682–1687
15. Bower M, Parry P, Gibbons B, Amess J, Lister TA, Young BD, Evans GA, (1994) Human trithorax gene rearrangements in therapy-related acute leukemia after episode treatment Leukemia 8: 226–229
16. Schichman SA, Caligiuri MA, Gu Y, Strout MP, Canaani E, Bloomfield CD, Croce CM (1994) ALL-1 partial duplication in acute leukemia Proc Natl Acad Sci USA 91: 6236–6239
17. Janssen JWG, Ludwig W-D, Borkhardt A, Spadinger U, Rieder H, Fonatsch C, Hossfeld DK, Harbott J, Schulz AS, Repp R, Sykora KW, Hoelzer D, Bartram CR (1994) Pre-pre-B-acute lymphoblastic leukemia: high frequency of alternatively spliced ALL-1-AF-4 transcripts and absence of minimal residual disease during complete remission. Blood 84: 3835–3842
18. Griesinger F, Elfers H, Ludwig W-D, Falk M, Rieder H, Harbott J, Lampert F, Heinze B, Hoelzer D, Thiel E, Riehm H, Wormann B, Fonatsch C, Hiddemann W (1994) Detection of HRX FEL fusion transcripts in pre-pre-B-ALL with and without cytogenetic demonstration of t(4;11) Leukemia 8: 542–548
19. Biondi A, Rambaldi A, Roßi V, Elia L, Caslini C, Baßo G, Battista R, Barbui T, Mandelli F, Masera G, Croce C, Canaani E, Cimino G (1993) Detection of ALL-1/AF4 fusion transcript by reverse transcription PCR for diagnosis and monitoring of acute leukemias with the t(4;11) translocation Blood 82: 2943
20. Borkhardt A, Repp R, Haupt E, Brettreich S, Buchen U, Lampert F (1994) Molecular analysis of MLL-1/AF4 recombination in infant acute lymphoblastic leukemia. Leukemia 8: 549–553
21. Corral J, Forster A, Thompson S, Lampert F, Kaneko Y, Slater R, Kroes WG, van der Schoot CE, Ludwig W-D, Karpas A, Pocock C, Cotter F, Rabbitts RH (1993) Acute leukemias of different lineages have similar MLL gene fusions encoding related chimeric proteins resulting from chromosomal translocations Proc Natl Acad Sci USA 90: 8538–8542
22. Hilden JM, Chen C-S, Moore R, Frestedt J, Kersey JH, (1993) Heterogeneity in MLL/AF-4 fusion messenger RNA detected by the polymerase chain reaction in t(4;11) acute leukemia. Cancer Res 53: 8538–8542

23. Yamamoto K, Seto M, Iida S, Komatsu H, Kamada N, Kojima S, Kodera Y, Nakazawa S, Takahashi T, Ueda R (1994) A reverse transcriptase-polymerase chain reaction detects heterogeneous chimeric mRNAs in leukemia with 11q23 abnormalities. Blood 83: 2912–2921
24. Hoelzer D, Arnold R, Büchner T, Freund M, GassmannW, Gökbuget N, Hiddemann W, Koch P, Löffler H, Ludwig W-D, Maschmeyer G, Thiel E, Völkers B, Messerer D, for the German Adult ALL Study Group (1995) Ann Hematol 70 [Suppl II] A104
25. Downing JR, Head DR, Raimondi SC, Carroll AJ, Curico-Brint AM, Motroni TA, Hulshof MG, Pullen DJ, Domer PH (1994) The der (11) encoded MLL/AF-4 fusion transcript is consistently detected in t(4;11)(q21;q23) containing acute lymphoblastic leukemia. Blood 83: 330–335

Acute Leukemias VI
Prognostic Factors
and Treatment Strategies
Büchner et al. (eds)

Homozygous Deletion of the p16 Gene in Childhood Acute Lymphoblastic Leukemia

T. Seriu[1], S. Takeuchi[2], C.W. Miller[2], A. Tobler[3], J.W.G. Janssen[1], A. Reiter[4], W.-D. Ludwig[5], M. Zimmermann[4], J. Schwaller[3], E. Lee[2], I. Miyoshi[6], H.P. Koeffler[2], and C. R. Bartram[1]

Abstract. p16/MTS1 (multiple tumor suppressor)/CDK4I (cyclin-dependent kinase 4 inhibitor) is a putative tumor suppressor gene involved in carcinogenesis in a wide variety of tissues. To study the involvement of the p16 gene in leukemogenesis, we performed Southern blot analyses in chilhood acute lymphoblastic leukemia (ALL) DNA sample from 110 children with primary ALL (22 T-ALL, 88 precursor-B ALL) revealed homozygous deletions in 29/110 cases (26%), and showed a significant association with the T-lineage [17/22 T-ALL (77%) versus 12/88 precursor-B ALL (14%); 0.001]. Additionally, hemizygous deletions were observed in 2 cases of T-ALL and 9 of precursor-B ALL. None of 19 cases with p16 deletions showed evidence of germline alterations. This study demonstrates that homozygous loss of the p16 gene represents the most frequent genetic alteration in childhood ALL, and suggests that inactivation of p16 is a critical event in leukemogenesis.

Introduction

Significant progress has been made in our knowledge of the regulatory system of the cell cycle. Cyclin-dependent kinases (CDKs) phosphorylate substrates that are critical for the transition between different cell cycle phases [1, 2]. Numerous stimulatory and inhibitory signals for cell division are coordinated by CDKs in co-operation with cyclins or CDK inhibitor proteins. One of the CDKs, CDK4, forms complexes with cyclin D1, and drives cells through G1 into S via phosphorylation of the Rb protein in late G1 phase [3]. A 16 kDa protein, p16, competes with cyclin D1, inactivates the kinase function of CDK4, and thus regulates the cell cycle negatively [4]. The p16 gene was mapped to chromosome 9p21, where cytogenetic aberrations frequently occur in ALL [5] as well as various solid tumors [6–8]. In fact, the p16 locus is homozygously deleted or mutated in the majority of tumor cell lines investigated thus far [9, 10]. This result suggests that the loss of p16 plays a pivotal role in carcinogenesis. Along the same line, homozygous deletions or mutations of the p16 gene were recently reported in several types of primary tumors [11–14].

We report on Southern blot and polymerase chain reaction – single strand conformational polymorphism (PCR-SSCP) analyses of the p16 gene in primary childhood ALL, and discuss the relation between the mutational p16 status and clinical characteristics.

[1] Section of Molecular Biology, Department of Pediatrics II, University of Ulm, Germany
[2] Division of Hematology/ Oncology, Cedars-Sinai Medical Center, UCLA School of Medicine, USA
[3] Central Hematology Laboratory, University of Bern, Switzerland
[4] Department of Pediatrics IV, Hanover Medical School, Germany
[5] Department of Medical Oncology and Applied Molecular Biology, Robert-Rössle-Klinik, Free University of Berlin, Germany
[6] Department of Internal Medicine, Kochi Medical School, Japan

Materials and Methods

Cells

Bone marrow (BM) and peripheral blood (PB) were obtained after informed consent from 110 children with ALL enrolled in the multicenter ALL trials ALL/NHL-BFM 86 and ALL-BFM 90 of the German Berlin-Frankfurt-Münster (BFM) study group. These patients were selected by the availability in the central laboratory of cryopreserved cell samples from initial diagnosis and partly complete remission for immunophenotyping in addition to the needs of routine programs. Cell-surface and cytoplasmic antigens were detected by a standard indirect or direct immunofluorescence assay, and the ALL samples were classified according to their immunophenotypes, as previously described [15, 16]. The definitions for the immunophenotyping and subclassification of the ALL samples in this study were as follows: 10 precursor-B ALL (TdT and CD19;+), 61 common ALL (TdT,CD19 and CD10;+, cy-IgM;−), 17 precursor-B ALL (TdT CD19 and cy-IgM; +,CD10; +/−, s-IgM;-), 7 early T-ALL(TdT,CD7 and cy-CD3;+,CD1 and s-CD3; -), 14 intermediate T-ALL (TdT,CD1 and CD7;+), 1 mature T-ALL (TdT;+/−, s-CD3 and CD7; +,CD1; −). Leukemia cell samples contained more than 90% of blasts.

Southern Blot Analysis

High-molecular-weight genomic DNA was prepared from BM or PB cells. Ten micrograms of each DNA were digested with EcoRI, separated on 0.6% agarose gel, and transferred onto nylon membranes (Nytran 13N; Schleicher & Schuell, Dassel, Germany). After hybridization the filters were washed and exposed on X-ray film using intensifying screens. A *Kpnl* fragment from the 3′ half of exon 2 was isolated from a full length p16 cDNA and used as a probe [4]. The blots were hybridized with a 1.9-kb *Eco*RI fragment of Tal-1 gene to ensure that equal amounts of DNA were applied on each lane [17]. Southern blot analysis was confirmed by quantification of au-toradiographic signals using a laser densitometer (Ultrascan XL; Pharmacia/LKB, Freiburg, Germany).

Polymerase Chain Reaction-Single Strand Conformational Polymorphism

Each PCR reaction contained 25 ng DNA, 0.7 pmol primers, 5 pmol dNTP, 0.5 U Taq DNA polymerase, 3 µCi (α-^{32}P)dCTP in 20 µl specified buffer with 1.5 m*M* $MgCl_2$. Samples were amplified by 35 cycles of denaturing for 40 s at 94°C, annealing for 30 s at 55°C, and extending for 2 min at 72°C in a programmable thermal controller. Primers for amplification of p16 were as follows: p16-X1S4 (GGAGAGGGGGAGAACAGACAACGG) and p16-X1MTSA1 (GCGCTACCTGATTCCAATTC) for exon p16X2S2 (ACCCT GGCTCTGACCATTCTGTTCT) and p16X2IA1 (CAGGCATCGCGCACGTCCAG) for the 5 half of exon 2 and p16X2IS1 (CTTCCTGGACACGCTGGTGGTGCTG) and p16X2A2 (GTACAAATTCAGATCATCAGTCC) for the 3 half of exon 2. One microliter of each reaction was added to 9 µl formamide, denatured at 95°C for 5 min, and subjected to electrophoresis through MDE gels (J.T. Baker Inc, Phillipsburg, NJ, USA). The gel was dried and exposed on X-ray film.

Statistical Analysis

Differences in the distribution of variables among patients who did and those who did not have homozygous deletions of the p16 were analyzed using Fisher's exact test for catergorical variables and the Wilcoxon rank sum test for continuous variables.

Results

Southern blot analysis showed that 17 of the 22 T-ALL patients (77%, i.e, 6/7 early T-ALL and 11/14 intermediate T-ALL) and 12 of the 88 precursor-B ALL patients (14%) had homozygous deletions of the p16 gene (Fig. 1, Table 1). Hemizygous deletions of the p16 gene were found in 2 T-ALL and 9 precursor-B ALL samples. The PCR-SSCP analysis of exon 1 and exon 2 revealed that none of 54 samples exhibited p16 point mutations. The matched normal DNAs obtained from these 54 ALL patients after suc-

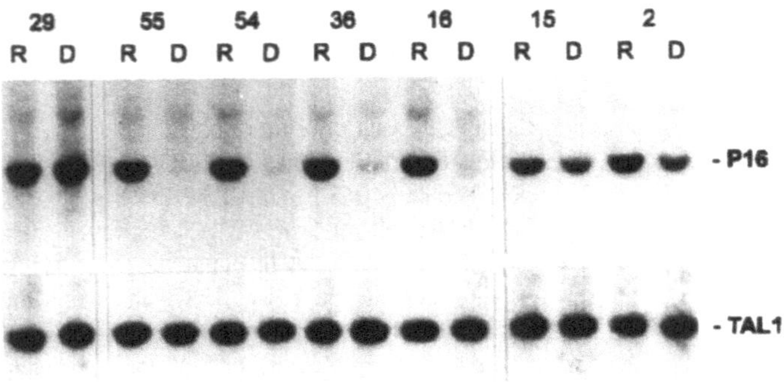

Fig. 1. Southern blot analysis of the p16 gene in depresentative samples from children with acute lymphoblastic leukemia. Filters were hybridized consecutively with p16 and TAL-1 probes. Homozygous deletions of the p16 gene are observed in samples nos. 16, 36, 55. Hemizygous deletions are seen in samples nos. 2 and 15. D, DNA obtained at initial diagnosis; *R*, DNA obtained in complete remission

Table 1. Southern blot analysis of p16 gene in samples from 110 children with primary acute lymphoblastic leukemia (ALL)

	No. with homozygous p16 deletion		No. with hemizygous p16 deletion		No. with p16 germline	Total
	n	%	*n*	%		
T-ALL	17	77	2	9	3	22
Precursor B-ALL	12	14	9	10	67	88
Total	29	26	11	10	70	110

cessful induction of remission showed a germline status of the p16 gene.

The clinical characteristics of the 97 patients from the multicenter ALL trials ALL/NHL 86 and ALL-BFM 90 were compared with the mutational status of the p16 gene (Table 2). Homozygous deletions of the p16 gene were significantly more frequent in T-ALL samples (16 of 20) than in precursor-B ALL samples (11 of 77; $p < 0.001$). Patients with homozygous deletions of the p16 gene were also older ($p = 0.03$), had increased white blood cell counts (WBC) at diagnosis ($p = 0.04$), and more frequently had a mediastinal mass at presentation ($p < 0.001$). However, logistic regression analysis revealed that only the T-cell phenotype was independently associated with homozygous p16 deletions. No statistically significant associations were found between homozygous deletions of the p16 gene and either gender or clinical course. Concerning the treatment outcome of these 97 patients, 17 did not respond to therapy (relapse or failure remission): 5 of 27 patients with homozygous deletions, 2 of 8 patients with hemizygous deletions, and 10 of 62 without deletions of p16 gene.

Discussion

A much lower frequency of p16 mutations was initially reported in primary tumors than in tumor cell lines, leading to speculation that p16 mutations represent secondary events in tumor cell lines [18, 19]. Recent studies, however, have demonstrated that the p16 gene was also deleted or mutated in several types of primary tumors [11-14]. Here we show that homozygous deletions of the p16 gene are found in 29 (26%) of 110 primary ALL samples. A remarkably high incidence (77%) is observed in T-ALL patients. None of 19 cases with p16 deletions showed evidence of germline alterations of the p16 gene. The frequency of homozygous p16 deletions is much higher than that of the interferon-α, -β1 genes which are also located in 9p21[20, 21].

Table 2. Clinical characteristics of 97 patients with ALL and their mutational status of their p16 gene

	No. with Homozygous p16 deletion	No. with hemizygous p16 deletion	No. with p16 germline	p value (homozyg. deletion vs germline)
Total	27	8	62	
Sex				
Male	14	3	27	N.S.
Female	13	5	35	
Age (median, years)	6.3	4.6	4.3	0.03
WBC median, $\times 10^9$/l	32.4	32.0	15.8	0.04
T-ALL	16	1	3	< 0.001
Precursor-B ALL	11	7	59	
Mediastinal mass present	13	0	1	< 0.001
Response ($\geqslant 1000/\mu l$ blasts on day 8)	3	1	3	n.s.
Nonresponse or relapse	5	2	10	n.s.

Mutations of known tumor suppressors such as the p53 gene and Rb gene occur infrequently in ALL [22, 23]. Cytogenetically, chromosomal deletions have been observed in ALL at 6q, 9p, 12p, and 19p with frequencies of 8%–17%, 7%–16%, 10%, and 9%, respectively [24]. Taken together, our data show that deletions of the p16 gene are the most frequent genetic alteration in primary ALL cells, particularly in T-ALL, reported to date, and suggest that inactivation of p16 represents an important step in leukemogenesis.

Eleven of 110 ALL samples had hemizygous p16 deletions. However, we found no point mutations at the second p16 allele in these cases. This suggests that the p16 might not be the sole target gene for the deletion event of chromosome 9p, and an unknown tumor suppressor gene may lie near the p16 locus on 9p.

The association of p16 deletions with various clinical and laboratory features was analyzed in 97 patients. However, only the correlation between T-ALL and a homozygous deletion of the p16 gene was statistically significant; the association of a deletion of p16 with increased age and an increased WBC at diagnosis might be due to the correlation of T-ALL with increased age and WBC at diagnosis.

After completion of our investigation, homozygous deletions of the p16 gene were reported in four of 14 ALL samples by Ogawa et al. [25]. In the study of Hebert et al. [26], the p16 gene was homozygously deleted in 20 of 24 T-ALL and 2 of 31 B-lineage ALL samples. Taken together, these data suggest that homozygous loss of the p16 gene plays a crucial role in childhood ALL.

Acknowledgments. We are grateful to Dr.D. Beach for providing the p16^{ink4} cDNA clone. We also thank the participants of the BFM study for their cooperation, Dr.T. E. Hansen-Hagge for valuable discussions, and D.Erz for expert technical assistance. This work was supported in part by grants from the Deutsche Forschungsgemeinschaft and Deutsche Krebshifle.

References

1. Hunter T, Pines J. Cyclins and cancer II: cyclin D and CDK inhibitors come of age. Cell 1994; 79: 573–582.
2. Sherr CJ.G1 phase progression: cycling on cue. Cell 1994; 79: 551–555.
3. Kato J, Matsushime, Hiebert SW, Ewen ME, Sherr CJ. Direct binding of cyclin D to the retinoblastoma gene product (pRb) and, pRb phosphorylation by the cyclin D-dependent kinase CDK4. Genes Dev.1993; 7: 331–342.
4. Serrano M, Hannon GJ, Beach D.A new regulatory motif in cell-cycle control causing specific inhibition of cyclin D/CDK4. Nature 1993; 366: 704–707.
5. Raimondi SC. Current status of cytogenetic research in childhood acute lymphoblastic leukemia. Blood 1993; 81: 2237–2251.
6. Fountain JW, Karayiorgou M, Ernstoff MS, Kirkwood JM, Vlock DR, Titus-Ernstoff L, Bouchard B, Vijayasaradhi S, Houghton AN, Lahti J, Kidd VJ, Housman DE, Dracopoli N. Homozygous deletions of human chromosome 9p21 in melanoma. Proc Natl Acad Sci USA 1992; 89: 10557–10561.
7. Ichimura K, Schmidt EE, Yamaguchi N, Jammes CJ,Collins VP. A common region of homozygous deletion in malignant human gliomas lies between the IFN α/ω gene cluster and the D9S171 locus. Cancer Res 1994; 54: 3127–3130.

8. Merlo A, Gabrielson E, Askin F, Sidranski D. Frequent loss of chromosome 9 in human primary non-small cell lung cancer. Cancer Res 1994; 54: 640–642.
9. Kamb A, Gruis NA, Weaver-Feldhaus J, Liu Q, Harshman K, Tavtigian SV, Stockert E, Day RSI, Johnson BE, Skolnick MH. A cell cycle regulator potentially involved in genesis of many tumor types. Science 1994; 264: 436–440.
10. Nobori T, Miura K, W DJ, Lois A, Takabayahsi K, Carson AD. Deletions of the cyclindependent kinase-4 inhibitor gene in multiple human cancers. Nature 1994; 368: 753–756.
11. Hussussian CJ, Struewing JP, Goldstein AM, Higgin PAT, Ally DS, Sheahan D, Clark WHJ, Tucker MA, Dracopoli NC. Germline p16 mutations in familial melanoma. Nature Genet 1994; 8: 15–21.
12. Mori T, Miura K, Aoki T, Nishihira T, Mori S; Nakanura Y.Frequent somatic mutation of the MTS1/CDK41 (multiple tumor suppressor/cyclin-dependent kinase 4 inhibitor) gene in esophageal squamous cell carcinoma. Cancer Res 1994; 54: 3396–3397.
13. Hayashi N, Sugimot Y, Tsuchiya E, Ogawa M, Nakamura Y. Somatic mutations of the MTS (multiple tumor suppressor) 1/CDK41 (cyclin-dependent kinase-4 inhibitor) gene in human primary non-small cell lung carcinomas. Biochem Biophys Res Commun 1994; 202; 1426–1430.
14. Caldas C, Hahn SA, da Costa LT, Redston MS, Schutte M, Seymour AB, Weinstein CL, Hruban RH, Yeo CJ, Kern SE. Frequent somatic mutations and homozygous deletions of the p16 (MTS1) gene in pancreatic adenocarcinoma. Nature Genet 1994; 8: 27–32.
15. Ludwig W-D, Bartram CR, Ritter J, Raghavachar A, Hiddeman W, Heil G, Harbott J, Seibt-Jung H, Teichmann JV, Riehm H. Ambiguous phenotypes and genotypes in 16 children with acute leukemia as characterized by multiparameter analysis. Blood 1988; 71: 1518–1528.
16. Van der Does-van den Berg A, Bartram CR, Basso G, Benoit YCM, Biondi A, Debatin KM, Haas OA, Harbott J, Kamps WA, Köller U, Lampert F, Ludwig W-D, Niemeyer CM, van Wering ER. Minimal requirements for the diagnosis, classification, and evaluation of the treatment of chilhood acute lymphoblastic leukemia (ALL) in the "BFM family" cooperative group. Med Pediatr Oncol 1992; 20: 497–505.
17. Bernard O, Lecointe N, Jonveaux P, Souyri M, Mauchauffe M, Berger R, Larsen CJ, Mathieu-Mahul D. Two site-specific deletion and t(1; 14) translocation restricted to human T-cell actue leukemia disrupt the 5′ part of the tal-1 gene. Oncogene 1991; 6: 1477–1488.
18. Cairns P, Mao L, Merlo A, Lee DJ, Schwab D, Eby Y, Tokino K, van der Riet P, Blaugrund JE, Sidranski D.Rates of p16 (MTS1) mutations in primary tumors with 9p loss. Science 1994; 265:415–416.
19. Spruck III CH, Gonzalez-Zulueta M, Shibata A, Simoneau AR. Lin M-F, Gonzales F, Tsai YC, Joans PA. P16 gene in uncultured tumors. Nature 1994; 370: 183–184.
20. Diaz MO, Ziemin S, Le Beau MM, Pitha P, Smith SD, Chilcote RR, Rowely JD. Homozygous deletion of α- and β1-interferon genes in human leukemia and derived cell lines. Proc Natl Acad Sci USA 1988; 85: 5259–5263.
21. Diaz MO, Rubin CM, Harden A, Ziemin S, Larson RA, Le Beau MM, Rowley JD. Deletion of interferon genes in acute lymphoblastic leukemia. N Engl J Med 1990; 322: 77–82.
22. Wada M, Bartram CR, Nakamura H, Hachiya M, Chen D-L, Borenstein J, Miller CW, Ludwig L, Hansen-Hagge TE, Ludwig W-D, Reiter A, Mizoguchi H, Koeffler HP. Analysis of p53 mutations in a large series of lymphoid hematologic malignancies of childhood. Blood 1993; 82: 3163–3169.
23. Chen Y-C, Chen P-J, Yeh S-H, Tien H-F, Wang C-H, Tang J-L, Hong R-L. Deletion of human retinoblastoma gene in primary leukemia. Blood 1990; 76: 2060–2064.
24. Johansson B, Mertens F, Mitelman F. Cytogenetic deletion maps of hematologic neoplasm: circumstantial evidence for tumor suppressor loci. Genes Chrom and Cancer 1993; 8: 205–218.
25. Ogawa S, Hirano N, Sato N, Takahashi T, Hangaishi A, Tanaka K, Kurokawa M, Tanaka T, Mitani K, Yazaki Y, Hirai H. Homozygous loss of the cyclin-dependent kinase 4-inhibitor (p16) gene in human leukemias. Blood 1994; 84: 2431–2435.
26. Hebert J, Cayuela M, Berkeley J, Sigaux F. Candidate tumor-suppressor genes MTS1 ($p16^{INK4A}$) and MTS2($p15^{INK4B}$) display frequent homozygous deletions in primary cells from T-but not from B-cell lineage acute lymphoblastic leukemias. Blood 1994; 84: 4038–4044.

Acute Leukemias VI
Prognostic Factors
and Treatment Strategies
Büchner et al. (eds)

CDKN2 Deletions in Leukemia-Derived Cell Lines: Detection by Fluorescence In Situ Hybridization with Interphase Cells

M.H. Dreyling, O.I. Olopade, and S.K. Bohlander

Abstract. Hemizygous and homozygous deletions of chromosomal band 9p21 have been detected in various tumor types as well as in more than 20% of acute lymphoblastic leukemia. Recently, the *CDKN2* gene (p16^{INK4A}, MTS I, *CDK4I*) has been proposed as a candidate tumor suppressor gene because it is frequently deleted in cell lines derived from multiple tumor types. We examined 18 leukemia-derived cell lines (13 T-ALL, 3 B-cell-precursor ALL,1 AML,1 CML-blast crisis) by polymerase chain reaction and Southern blot analysis to further define the frequency and size of 9p deletions in hematological malignancies. Homozygous *CDKN2* deletions were detected in 16 cell lines (89%). Interphase fluorescence in situ hybridization (FISH) is a powerful method to detect chromosomal rearrangements, including submicroscopic deletions. Using a cosmid contig of the *CDKN2* region, we performed interphase FISH in nine cell lines to study the accuracy of this method in detecting 9p deletions. Interphase FISH determined accurately all deletions of the tumor suppressor region previously detected by Southern blot or PCR. In six cell lines the cosmid contig was completely deleted. In one cell line, the intensity of the hybridization signals was significantly reduced, indicating a partial deletion of the hybridization region. One cell line had a hemizygous deletion which is difficult to detect by molecular techniques. Genomic deletions seem to be the predominant mechanism of *CDKN2* inactivation in acute leukemias. Interphase FISH will play an important role in defining the frequency of *CDKN2* deletions in primary tumors, because it is able reliably to analyze clinical samples that are contaminated by normal cells.

Introduction

Cytogenetic deletions of chromosomal band 9p21 have been observed frequently in lymphoid malignancies and in various solid tumors [1–3]. Our group as well as others have observed homozygous deletions of the interferon typeI (*IFN*) gene cluster, which maps to 9p21–22, in different tumor types [4–8]. Recently, the *CDKN2* gene (*p16*^{INK4A}, *MTS I, CDK4I*) has been proposed as a candidate tumor suppressor gene because it is deleted in cell lines derived from multiple tumor types [3, 9, 10]. The reported incidence of *CDKN2* deletions in leukemic cell lines ranges between 25% and 64% [1, 10]. p15(*MTS2, CDKN2B*), a TGF-β regulated member of the p16 family which maps 20 kb centromeric to *CDKN2*, is often deleted as well [3, 11]. We analyzed 18 leukemia-derived cell lines to further define the frequency and size of 9p deletions. In nine of these cell lines, we performed fluorescence in situ hybridization (FISH) Fish with interphase cells to determine the accuracy of this method in detecting 9p deletions. Interphase FISH is a well-established method for identifying genetic alterations at single cell level. It reliably detects hemizygous deletions as well as deletions in subpopulations of cells. Thus, this method is especially suited to analyze clinical samples which have admixtures of normal cells.

Department of Medicine, Section of Hematology/Oncology, The University of Chicago, 5841 S. Maryland, Box 2115, Chicago, IL 60637, USA

Materials and Methods

Cell Lines

Eighteen cell lines were studied: 13 T-ALL, 3 B-cell precursor ALL, 1 AML, and 1 cell line derived from a CML-blast crisis. The cell lines were obtained from the investigator who had established them or from the American Type Culture Collection (Rockville, MD).

Southern Blot Analysis

High-moleculer-weight DNA was isolated as previously described [12]. The purified DNA was treated with restriction enzyme(*Hind*III), electrophoresed on a 1% agarose gel, and transferred to a nylon membrane (Gene Screen plus, NEN, Boston). The filters were hybridized with ^{32}P-labeled probes from 9p21 and exposed to X-ray film [13]. The chromosomal localization of the 9p probes REY24,M1.4 (the 3′ untranslated region of methylthioadenosinephosphorylase), *CDKN2*(cDNA), p15(exon 1), D9S966, and D9S963 is shown in Fig. 1 [1, 14, 15]. Equal DNA loading was verified by visual inspection of ethidium-bromide-stained gels and by control hybridizations to a transferrin receptor probe located on chromosome 3 [16].

Polymerase Chain Reaction

The *IFN* gene cluster, 1063.7, *CDKN2* exon 1–3, and the sequence-tagged sites D9S96 and D9S963 were amplified by polymerase chain reaction(PCR) as previously described [3, 10, 14, 17]. p15 exon 1 was amplified with 10% DMSO using the previously published primers (94°C–30 s; 52°C–45 s, 72°C–45 s) [3]. The position of the molecular markers is shown in Fig. 1.

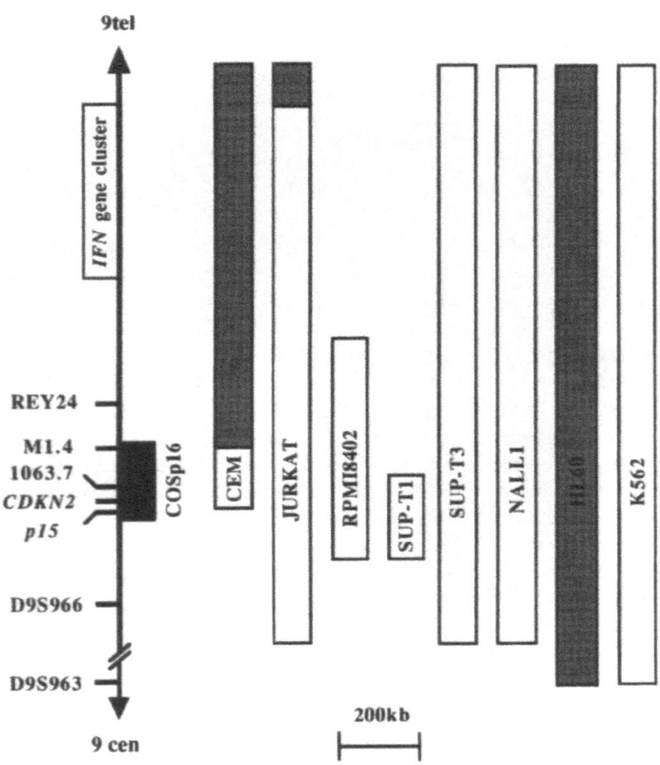

Fig. 1. Deletions of 9p in leukemia cell lines. Homozygous deletions are shown as *white bars*, hemizygous deletions as *gray bars*

Fluorescence In Situ Hybridization

Nine cell lines and normal peripheral blood cells were grown in short-term culture and harvested using standard cell culture techniques [18]. A contig of six cosmids (COSp16) encompassing a 200-kb region around *CDKN2* and *p15* was assembled by screening a flow-sorted human chromosome 9 library (Lawrence Livermore Laboratories) with probes from a YAC contig of the region [15, 19]. YAC 284D6(320 kb), later referred to as YAC 10/2, from chromosomal band 8q22 was used as a control probe [20]. pHuR98, a variant satellite 3 sequence, was used to determine the copy number of chromosome 9 [21]. FISH probes were prepared using sequence-independent amplification (SIA) as described previously [22]. The copy number of chromosome 8 was determined by a centromeric FISH probe CEP 8 Spectrum Orange (Imagenetics, Framingham, Mass). Two-color FISH with a YAC or cosmid probe and a centromeric probe was performed as previously described [23]. Briefly, the hybridization solution contained approx. 0.1 μg of each probe, 1 μg human Cot1-DNA (BRL), 0.6 μg human placental DNA, and 3 μg salmon sperm DNA/slide in a 10 μl volume. The biotinylated probes were detected with fluorescein-isothiocyanate(FITC)-conjugated avidin. The slides were counterstained with 4′,6′-diamidino-2-phenylindole dihydrochloride(DAPI), and were analyzed using epifluorescence and a single pass filter (Chroma Technology) to avoid superimposition of the centromeric and the cosmid signals.

For each cell line, 250 single, intact cells were analyzed. For Fig. 2, separate gray scale images of DAPI-stained cells and fluorescence signals were captured using a cooled charge-coupled device camera (Photometrics, Tucson, Ariz) and were merged using the NIH Image or Abode Photoshop software.

Results

Homozygous 9p deletions were detected in 16 cell lines (89%, Table 1). In 8 cell lines (44%), the proximal *IFN* gene cluster, which is approximately 500 kb telomeric to the *CDKN2* gene, was deleted (Fig. 1). Eleven deletions (61%) included

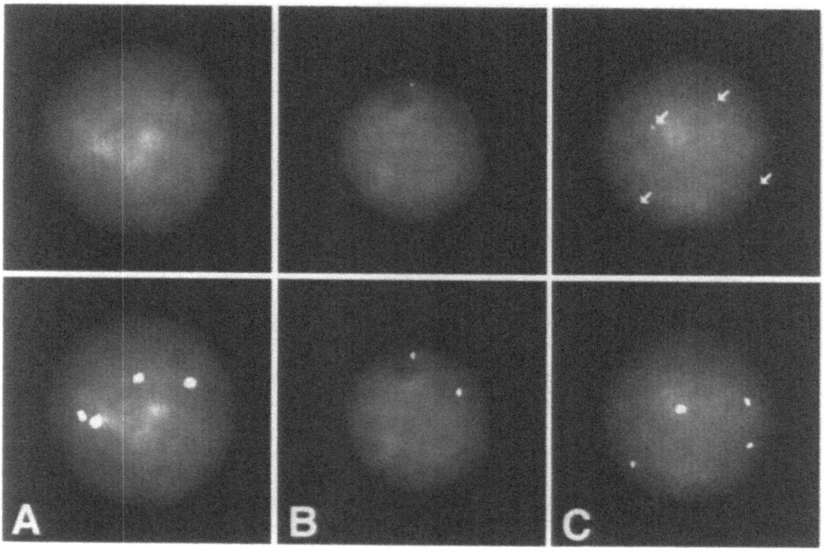

Fig. 2A–C. Interphase FISH with COSp16 and pHuR98. **A** CEM, a tetraploid cell line with homozygous 9p deletion. An interphase cell with four centromere 9 signals (*lower panel*) and no COSp16 signal (*upper panel*) is shown. **B** HL60, a near-diploid cell line with hemizygous 9p deletion. One COSp16 signal (*upper panel*) and two centromere 9 signals (*lower panel*) are detectable. **C** SUP-T1, a tetraploid cell line with a small homozygous 9p deletion. An interphase cell with four centromeric (*lower panel*) and four faint COSp16 signals (*arrows, upper panel*) is shown

Table 1. Homozygous 9p deletions in 18 leukemia cell lines (%)

IFN A[a,b,c]	REY 24[b]	M1.4[b]	1063.7[c]	*CDKN2*[b,2]	*p15*[c] exon 2	p15[b] exon 1	D9S966[b,c]	D9S963[b,c]
44	50	61	89	89	78	67	44	22

[a]Published by Diaz et al. [4].
[b]southern blot.
[c]Polymerase chain reaction.

MTAP1.4, and 14 deletions (78%) involved *p*15. These two molecular markers flanked the smallest region of deletion, which included *CDKN2* as well as 1067.9, which is 30 kb further telomeric.

As most of the 9p deletions extended over 200 kb and more, we tested the accuracy of interphase FISH to detect 9p deletions using a cosmid contig of the *CDKN2* region (COSp16, Fig. 1). In at least five test hybridizations of peripheral blood cells from normal individuals, both cosmid contig and YAC control probes showed an almost identical distribution of signals per cell, comparable to previously published results for centromeric probes. In 500 nuclei scored, two signals were detected in 92%–97% of the cells.

In nine cell lines selected on the basis of the availability of cell material, FISH with interphase cells was able to diagnose accurately all deletions of the tumor suppressor region detected by molecular techniques. In six cell lines the cosmid contig was completely deleted. In $99.7 \pm 0.4\%$ of the cells there was no COSp16 signal, while only $0.16 \pm 0.40\%$ of the cells showed no signal of the control YAC (Fig. 3). In one cell line, the intensity of the hybridization signals was significantly reduced, indicating a partial deletion of the cosmid contig (Sup-T1, Fig. 2). This result was later confirmed by the Southern blot analysis of this cell line (Table 1). In another cell line (HL60) interphase FISH identified a hemizygous deletion which was not detectable by PCR (Fig. 3). However, in the Southern blot analysis the intensity of the bands of the 9p probes was significantly reduced in comparison to the control probe.

Discussion

Our results underline the importance of *CDKN2* deletions in leukemia-derived cell lines. In 89% of the studied cell lines, we detected a homozygous deletion of the *CDKN2* region. The initial studies reported a significantly lower frequency of 9p deletions (25–64%) [3, 10, 24]. However, these studies included only a small number of leukemic cell lines. The high frequency of 9p deletions in our study may also reflect the fact

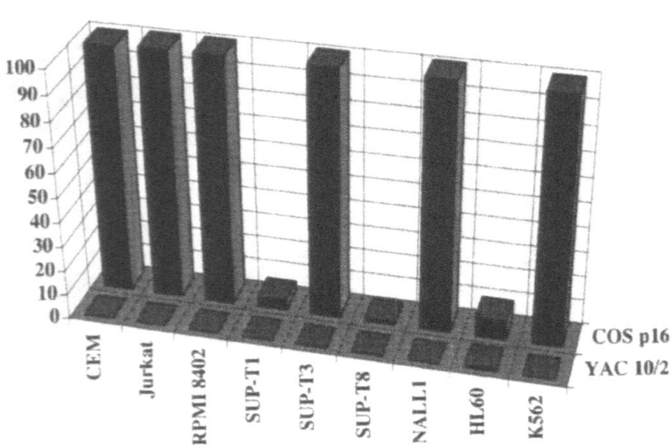

Fig. 3. Cells without hybridization signal (%)

that the majority of cell lines were derived from ALL, especially T-ALL. Recently, other groups have shown that 9p deletions are rather rare in myeloid leukemias, whereas most T-ALL cell lines have *CDKN2* deletions [24, 25].

The deletion analysis confirms that *CDKN2* is included in the minimal deletion region on 9p which is flanked by the molecular markers M1.4 and *p*15. Both exons of *p*15 were retained in two cell lines with 9p deletions. However, as 1063.7 is included in all deletions, our deletion mapping does not exclude the possibility that genes telomeric to *CDKN2* may contribute to the malignant phenotype.

If *CDKN2* is the target of 9p deletions in leukemia-derived cell lines, the remaining allele in HL60, a cell line with hemizygous 9p deletions, should be inactivated as well. In fact, our group as well others detected a point mutation in exon 2 of *CDKN2* (M.H.Dreyling et al., unpublished material) [26]. Therefore, our data strongly suggest that the inactivation of *CDKN2* is a critical event in leukemia-derived cell lines.

In contrast, point mutation of *CDKN2* rarely occurs in various primary solid tumors [27–30]. Recently, Quesnel et al. [31] detected only one *CDKN2* point mutation in 88 cases of ALL. These data indicate that homozygous genomic deletions are the predominant mechanism of inactivation of *CDKN2* in primary tumors. It may well be that the deletion of either *p*15 or other genes in the region may contribute to the malignant phenotype as well. Large homozygous genomic deletions would inactivate both genes in one step.

So far, it has been difficult to evaluate the importance of *CDKN2* deletions in clinical samples, because conventional molecular techniques like PCR and Southern blot analysis are not able to identify deletions in subpopulations of cells. Interphase FISH is a well-established technique for identifying genetic alterations at a single-cell level. It is especially suited to detecting losses of one allele or to analyze clinical tumor samples which have admixtures of normal cells. Stilgenbauer et al. [32] were able reliably to detect *RB* deletions in CLL using a phage contig of the *RB* region. In our study, we used a cosmid contig probe of the *CDKN2* region which was generated by sequence-independent amplification [22,23]. In contrast to FISH probes generated by Alu-PCR, this technique does not rely on the presence of any particular sequence in the template DNA and therefore generates probes which represent the template evenly [34,35]. Thus, in one cell line (Sup-T1) we were able to detect a partial deletion of the cosmid contig which was later confirmed by Southern blot analysis.

Interphase FISH analysis is able reliably to detect hemizygous 9p deletions. Using a similar cosmid contig of the *CDKN2* region we were able to detect hemizygous deletions in six cases of primary ALL (M.H.Dreyling et al., unpublished material). Southern blot analysis failed to detect these deletions because only subpopulations of cells (43%–86%) were involved. Further analysis of point mutations in these cases may help to illuminate the role of *CDKN2* in hematological malignancies.

In conclusion, our study shows that interphase FISH using a cosmid contig is a reliable method to detect 9p deletions. It will play an important role in defining the frequency of 9p deletions in primary malignancies because the method is especially well suited to the analysis of clinical samples.

Acknowledgments. We thank Janet D. Rowley for her generous support of this project, Lise Sveen, Fitsum Hagos and Donna Fackenthal for technical assistance, and David Beach for providing the *CDKN2* and *p*15 cDNAs. The work was supported in part by the J.S. McDonnell Foundation grant no.92-51 (O.I.O.), DOE grant DE-FE02-86ER60408 (Janet D. Rowley), and a training grant from the Deutsche Forschurgsgemeinschaft (M.H.D.).

References

1. Chilcote, R.R., Brown, E., and Rowley, J.D. Lymphoblastic leukemia with lymphomatous features associated with abnormalities of the short arm of chromosome 9.N Engl J Med, 313: 286–291, 1985.
2. Murphy, S.B., Raimondi, S.C., Rivera, G.K., Crone, M., Dodge, R.K., Behm. F.G., Pui, C.H., and Williams, D.L. Nonrandom abnormalities of chromosome 9p in childhood acute lymphoblastic leukemia. Blood, 74: 409–415, 1989.
3. Kamb, A., Gruis, N.A., Weaver, F.J., Liu, Q., Harshman, K., Tavtigian, S.V., Strockert, E., Day III, R., Johnson, B.E., and Skolnick, M.H. A cell cycle regulator potentially involved in genesis of many tumor types. Science, 264: 436–40, 1994.
4. Diaz, M.O., Ziemin, S., Le Beau, M.M., Pitha, P., Smith, S.D., Chilcote, .R.R., and Rowley, J.D. Homozygous deletion of the α- and β-interferon genes in human leukemia and derived cell lines. Proc Natl Acad Sci USA, 85: 5259–5263, 1988.

5. Diaz, M.O., Rubin, C.M., Harden, A., Ziemin, S., Larson, R.A., LeBeau, M.M., and Rowley, J.D. Deletions of interferon genes in acute lymphoblastic leukemia. N Engl J Med, 322: 77–82, 1990.
6. James, C.D., J., C., Caarlbom, E., Nordenskjold, M., Cavenee, W.K., and Collins, V.P. Chromosome 9 deletion mapping reveals interferon A and interferon B gene deletions in human glial tumors. Cancer Res, 51: 1684–1688, 1991.
7. Olopade, O.I., Jenkins, R.B., Ransom, D.T., Malik, K., Pomykala, H., Nobori, T., Cowan, J.M., Rowley, J.D., and Diaz, M.O. Molecular analysis of deletions of the short arm of chromosome 9 in human gliomas. Cancer Res, 52: 2523–2529, 1992.
8. Olopade, O.I., Buchhagen, D.L., Malik, K., Sherman, J., Nobori, T., Bader, S., Nau, M.M., Gazdar, A.F., Minna, J.D., and Diaz, M.O., Homozygous loss of the interferon genes defines the critical region on 9p that is deleted in lung cancers. Cancer Res, 53: 2410–2415, 1993.
9. Serrano, M., Hannon, G.J., and Beach, D. A new regulatory motif in cell-cycle control causing specific inhibition of cyclin D/CDK4. Nature, 366: 704–707, 1993.
10. Nobori, T., Miura, K., Wu, D.J., Lois, A., Takabayashi, K., and Carson, D.A. Deletions of the cyclin-dependent kinase-4 inhibitor gene in multiple human cancers. Nature, 368: 753–756, 1994.
11. Hannon, G.J. and Beach, D.p15^{INK4B} is a potential effector of TGF-β-induced cell cycle arrest. Nature, 371: 257–261, 1994.
12. James, C.D., Carlboom, E., Dumanski, J.D., Hansen, M., Nordenskjold, M., Collins, V.P., and Cavenee, W.K. Clonal genomic alterations in glioma malignancy stages. Cancer Res, 48: 5546–5551, 1988.
13. Feinberg, A.P., and Vogelstein, B. A technique for radiolabeling DNA restriction endonuclease fragments to high specific activity. Anal Biochem, 132: 6–13, 1983.
14. Bohlander, S.K., Dreyling, M.H., Hagos, F., Sveen, L., Olopade, O.I., and Diaz, M.O. Mapping of a putative tumor suppressor gene on chromosome 9 band p21–22 with microdissection probes. Genomics, 24: 211–217, 1994.
15. Olopade, O.I., Pomykala, H.M., Hagos, F., Sveen, L.W., Espinosa III, R., Dreyling, M.H., Gursky, S., Stadler, W.M., Le Beau, M.M., and Bohlander, S.K. Construction of a 2.8 megabase YAC contig and cloning of the methyladenosine phosphorylase (MTAP) gene from the tumor suppressor region on 9p2. Proc Natl Acad Sci USA, in press.
16. Schneider, C., Owen, M.J., Banville, D., and Williams, J.G. Primary structure of the human transferrin receptor deduced from the mRNA sequence. Nature, 311: 675–678, 1984.
17. Henco, K., Brosius, J., Fujisawa, J.I., Haynes, J.R., Hochstadt, J., Kovacic, T., Pasek, M., Schambock, A., Schmid, S., Todokoro, K., Wälchli, M., Nagata, S., and Weissmann, C. Structural relationship of human interferon alpha genes and pseudogenes. J Med Biol, 185: 227–260, 1988.
18. Le Beau, M.M. Cytogenetic analysis of hematological malignant diseases. In: M.J.Barch, The ACT cytogenetics laboratory manual, pp.395–445. New York: Raven Press, 1994.
19. Dreyling, M., Olopade, O.I., and Bohlander, S.K. A method for screening arrayed cosmid libraries with mega insert yeast artificial chromosomes. Nucl Acids Res, in press.
20. Erickson, P., Gao, J., Chang, K.S., Look, T., Whisenant, E., Raimondi, S., Lasher, R., Trujillo, J., Rowley, J.D., and Drabkin, H. Identification of breakpoints in t(8;21) acute myelogenous leukemia and isolation of a fusion transcript AML1/ETO, with similarity to drosophila segmentation gene, runt. Blood, 80: 1825–831, 1992.
21. Moyzis, R.K., Albright, K.L., Bartholdi, M.F., Cram, L.S., Deaven, L.L., Hildebrand, C.E., Joste, N.E., Longmire, J.L., Meyne, J., and Schwarzacher-Robinson, T. Human chromosome-specific repetitive DNA sequences: Novel marker for genetic analysis Chromosoma, 95: 375–386, 1987.
22. Bohlander, S.K., Espinosa III, R., Fernald, A.A., Rowley, J.D., Le Beau, M.M., and Diaz, M.O. Sequence-independent amplification and labeling of yeast artificial chromosomes for fluorescence in situ hybridization. Cytogenet Cell Genet, 65: 108–110, 1994.
23. Rowley, J.D., Diaz, M.O., Espinosa III, R., Patel, Y.D., van Melle, E., Ziemin, S., Taillon-Miller, P., Lichter, P., Evans, G.A., Kersey, J.H., Ward, D.C. Domer, P.H., and Le Beau, M.M. Mapping chromosome band 11q23 im human acute leukemia with biotinylated probes: Identification of 11q23 translocation breakpoints with a yeast artificial chromosome. Proc Natl Acad Sci USA 87: 9358–9362, 1990.
24. Ogawa, S., Hirano, N., Sato, N., Takahashi, T., Hangaishi, A., Tanaka, K., Kurokawa, M., Tanaka, T., Mitani, K., Yazaki, Y., and Hirai, H. Homozygous loss of the cyclin-dependent kinase 4-inhibitor (p16) gene in human leukemias. Blood, 84: 2431–2435, 1994.
25. Nakamaki, T., Tobler, A., Schwaller, J., Tsuruoka, N., Miller, C.W., and Koeffler, H.P. p16-alterations in myeloid leukemias. Blood, 84(Suppl 1): 48a, 1994(abstract).
26. Gombart, A.F., Shintaku, I.P., Said, J.W., Miller, C.W., and Koeffler, H.P. Alterations of the CDK4/MTS1 (cyclin-dependent kinase 4 inhibitor/multiple tumor suppressor 1) gene in uncultured B-cell lymphoma. Blood, 84 (Suppl 1): 445a, 1994(abstract).
27. Cairns, P., Mao, L., Merlo, A., Lee, D.J., Schwab, D., Ebry, Y., Tokino, K., van der Riet, P., Blaugrund, J.E., and Sidransky, D. Rates of p16 (MTS1) mutations in primary tumors with 9p loss. Science, 265: 415–416, 11994(letter).
28. Giani, C. and Finocchiaro, G. Mutation rate of the *CDKN2* gene in malignant gliomas. Cancer Res, 54: 6338–6339, 1994.
29. Jen, J., Harper, J.W., Bigner, S.H., Bigner, D.D., Papadopoulos, N., Markowitz, S., Willson, J.K.V., Kinzler, K.W., and Vogelstein, B. Deletion of p16

and p15 genes in brain tumors. Cancer Res, 54: 6353–6358, 1994.
30. Okamoto, A., Demetrick, D.J., Spillare, E.A., Hagiwara, K., Hussain, S.P., Bennett, W.P., Forrester, K., Gerwin, B., Serrano, M., Beach, D.H., and Harris, C.C. Mutations and altered expression of $p16^{INK4}$ in human cancer. Proc Natl Acad Sci USA, 91: 11045–11049, 1994.
31. Quesnel, B., Preudhomme, C., Philippe, N., Vanrumbeke, M., Dervite, I., Lai, J.L., Bauters, F., Wattel, E., and Fenaux, P. p16 gene homozygous deletions in acute lymphoblastic leukemia. Blood, 85: 657–663, 1995.
32. Stilgenbauer, S., Döhner, H., Bulgay-Mörschel, M., Weitz, S., Bentz, M., and Lichter, P. High frequency of monoallelic retinoblastoma gene deletion in B-cell chronic lymphoid leukemia shown by interphase cytogenetics. Blood, 81: 2118–2124, 1993.
33. Bohlander, S.K., Espinosa III, R., Le Beau, M.M., Rowley, J.D., and Diaz, M.O. A method for the rapid sequence-independent amplification of microdissected chromosomal material. Genomics, 13: 1322–1324, 1992.
34. Nelson, D.L., Ledbetter, S.A., Corbo, L., Victoria, M.F., Ramirez-Solis, R., Webster, T.D., Ledbetter, D.H., and Caskey, C.T. Alu polymerase chain reaction: A method for rapid isolation of human-specific sequences from complex DNA sources. Proc Natl Acad Sci USA, 86: 6686–6690, 1989.
35. Tocharentanaphol, C., Cremer, M., Schröck, E., Blonden, L., Kilian, K., Cremer, T., and Ried, T. Multicolor fluorescence in situ hybridization on metaphase chromosomes and interphase Halo-preparations using cosmid and YAC clones for the simultaneous high resolution mapping of deletions in the dystrophin gene. Hum Genet, 93: 229–235, 1994.

Acute Leukemias VI
Prognostic Factors
and Treatment Strategies
Büchner et al. (eds)

Diversity of the TcR-d Gene Rearrangements Indicates Subclone Formation in Acute B Cell Precursor Leukemias

E.R. Panzer-Grümayer[1], D. Ghali[1], S. Panzer[2], S. Fischer[1], A. Argyriou-Tirita[1], O.A. Haas[1], H. Kovar[1], and H. Gadner[1]

Abstract. Acute B cell precursor leukemias (B-ALLs) have been demonstrated by Southern blot hybridization to be oligoclonal at the IgH gene level in up to 40% of cases. In contrast, oligoclonality as deduced from diversity of the TcR-d gene rearrangements of the immature types has not been reported so far. In 4 of 20 cases of childhood BCP-ALL we detected oligoclonality characterized by the coexistence of different junctional regions varying in size by 3–25 nucleotides of identical Vd2-Dd3 rearrangements. No variation was found in the IgH and TcR-g gene status. Two cases displayed the variants in an unequal proportion, while in the last two, in which similar quantities of the coexisting rearrangements were detected, single-cell nuclei (PCR) revealed two separate leukemic populations. The variants arose independently of each other as deduced from their individual sequences. We postulate that in these leukemic cell populations TcR-d gene diversity arose after rearrangements of the IgH genes, resulting in apparent clonality at the IgH gene level. However, cells are oligoclonal if the TcR-d gene rearrangements are taken into account.

Introduction

Precursor B-ALLs are thought to represent the clonal expansion of a precursor cell arrested at an early stage of differentiation [1]. TcR-d genes have one or two alleles rearranged in about 50% of precursor B-ALLs [2, 3]. By Southern blot studies, the number of rearranged bands of the TcR-d genes have therefore been used in addition to IgH gene rearrangement to study clonality in these leukemias, and discrete faint TcR-d rearrangements in addition to more prominent bands have been described on Southern blots, suggesting oligoclonality [3, 4]. Preferential usage of the Vd2-Dd3 rearrangement in 72%, and of the most "immature" Dd2-Dd3 re-arrangement in 10% of all rearrangements in precursor B-ALLs has been reported [3, 5]. This limited recombinatorial repertoire is compensated by an extensive diversity of the junctional region [6, 7]. Oligoclonality resulting from identical rearranging of TcR-d regions has not been reported so far.

Materials and Methods

Samples from 20 children consecutively diagnosed as having precursor B-ALLs were analyzed in this study. Bone marrow samples at diagnosis contined >95% leukemic blasts. All children were treated according to the BFM-90 protocal.

Chromosome preparations were performed according to standard routine cytogenetic techniques. Slides were R- and C- banded with chromomycin A3 and distamycin A/DAPI.

High-molecular-weight DNA was extracted from MNC. Southern blotting and hybridization of high-molecular-weight DNA digested to completion with the restriction enzymes *Eco*RI,

[1]Children's Cancer Research Institute, St. Anna Kinderspital, Vienna, Austria
[2]Department of Blood Group Serology, University of Vienna, Vienna, Austria

*Hind*III, *Bam*HI, *Bgl*II, or a combination of *Bam*HI/*Hind*III (Boehringer Mannheim, Mannheim, Germany) were performed according to standard methods. TcR-d chain gene configuration was investigated with the TCRDJ1 probe (provided by Dr. J.J.M. van Dongen, Rotterdam, Netherlands). The status of the TcR-b genes was analyzed with a cDNA C region probe (provided by Dr. T.W. Mak, Toronto, Canada) and of the TcR-g genes with a Jg1.3 probe (provided by Dr. J.G. Seidman, Boston, Mass). Rearrangements of IgH genes were detected with a IgHJ6 probe (Dr. J.J.M. van Dongen, Rotterdam, Netherlands).

Polymerase chain reaction (PCR) was essentially performed as described by Saiki et al.[8]. Primers are listed in Table 1 (1 and 2 for the first round, nested primers 3 and 4 for the second round). PCR products were electrophoresed on a 15% nondenaturing polyacrylamide gel and stained with ethidiumbromide. Isolation of relevant DNA fragments from polyacrylamide gel was performed in an elution buffer. DNA was precipitated in ethanol and redissolved in Tris, 10 m*M*, pH7.4, 0.1m*M* EDTA, pH8.0, H_2O.

Direct dideoxynucleotide sequencing of double-stranded PCR products was performed using the fmolTM DNA sequencing system (Promega Corporation, Woods Hollow Road, Mass) with internal sequencing primers (primers 5 and 6).

Microdissection was performed as described by Meltzer et al. [10].

Results

Configuration of TcR-d Genes in 20 Precursor B-ALL samples

At diagnosis, 15 of 20 precursor B-ALLs showed a TcR-d chain gene rearrangement as evaluated by Southern blot hybridization. Fourteen of the 15 leukemias with a rearrangement showed only one rearranged band: a Vd2-Dd3 rearrangement in 12 cases and a Dd2-Dd3 in two. In one leukemia, two rearranged bands were visible, representing a Vd2-Dd3 and a Dd2-Dd3 rearrangement. Seven leukemias presented with a germline band in addition to a Vd2-Dd3 rearrangement. One of these germline bands was very weak, reflecting about 5% of normal cells.

Table 1. Sequence of oligomers used for PCR analysis

1.[a] 5′	ACC CAA GGA AGA ACA GCA GTG AG	3′
2.[a] 5′	ACC TGG TAC AGG AAG ACC CAA GG	3′
3.[a] 5′	TCA GCA GCT GTG GTC ATC TCC CT	3′
4.[a] 5′	GGA CAT CTA TGG CCC TGG TTT CA	3′
5. 5′	GCA CTT TTG CCC CTG CAG TTT TTG	3′
6. 5′	TGA TAT TGC AAA GAA CCT GGC TGT ACT	3′

[a] As published previously [9].

Sequence Analysis of Rearranged TcR-d Chain Genes

The Vd2-Dd3 and Dd2-Dd3 rearrangements in all 15 leukemias were amplified by PCR and the amplification products were used for direct sequence analysis. The sequence of the junctional region was sufficiently readable for 11 leukemias confirming their homogeneity in the TcR-d gene. In the remaining 4 leukemias with a Vd2-Dd3 rearrangement, however, the sequence of the junctional region could not be analyzed. Consequently, amplified DNA was electrophoresed through a 15% high-resolution polyacrylamide gel. All four leukemias now showed two (leukemia #1, #2, #4) or three (leukemia #3) bands of different size varying from approximately 30 to 40 bp (Fig. 1). The densities of bands obtained from each of the two PCR products were similar for leukemias #1 and #2, whereas those of the three bands of leukemia #3 and the two bands of leukemias #4 were different. The separated PCR products were isolated for sequencing and the results are shown in Table 2.

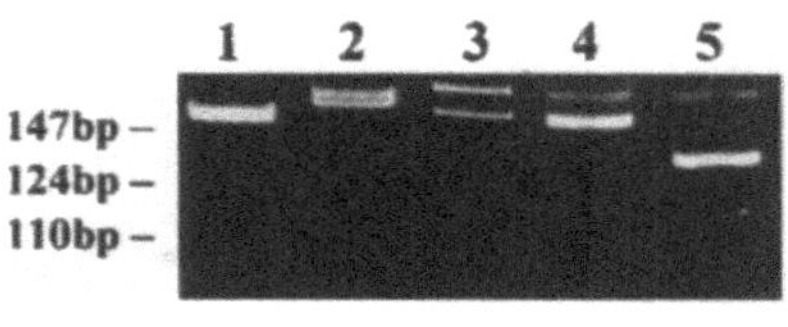

Fig. 1. Polyacrylamide gel electrophoresis (PAGE) analysis of PCR-amplified Vd2-Dd3 rearrangements from the four leukemias at diagnosis. *Lane 1,* Single PCR product of a monoclonal leukemia; *lanes 2–5,* PCR products of leukemias #1 to #4

Bioligoclonal Vd2-Dd3 Rearrangements Result from Subclone Formation

The different PCR products from Vd2-Dd3 rearrangements in precursor B-ALLs may have resulted from (i) bioligoclonal leukemias as defined by IgH gene rearrangements, (ii) two or

Table 2. Sequence of junctional region of Vd2-Dd3 rearrangements in four precursor B-ALLs

		Vd2	N	Dd3	Heptamer Spacer
Germline		GGTCTTACTACTGTGCCTGTGACACC		ACTGGGGGATACG	cacagtgctacaaaaccta
Leukemia #1	PCR-P. 1	GGTCTTACTACTGTGCCTGTGAC	CTCCTTT	ACTGGGGGATACG	cacagtgctacaaaaccta
	PCR-P. 2	GGTCTTACTACTGTGCCTGTG	TCTCCTC	CTGGGGGATACG	cacagtgctacaaaaccta
Leukemia #2	PCR-P. 1	GGTCTTACTACTGTGCCTGTGAC	TCCCCCTGGGGGATGG	GGGGGATACG	cacagtgctacaaaaccta
	PCR-P. 2	GGTCTTACTACTGTGCCTGTGA	TACGGGG	TGGGGGATACG	cacagtgctacaaaaccta
Leukemia #3	PCR-P. 1	GGTCTTACTACTGTGCCTGTGACACC	GGAAAAAGTAACGAG	CG	cacagtgctacaaaaccta
	PCR-P. 2	GGTCTTACTACTGTGCCTGTGACA	GG	GGGGGATACG	cacagtgctacaaaaccta
	PCR-P. 3	GGTCTT		GGATACG	cacagtgctacaaaaccta
Leukemia #4	PCR-P. 1	GGTCTTACTACTGTGCCTGTGACA	GGGGG	GGGGGATACG	cacagtgctacaaaaccta
	PCR-P. 2	GGTCTTACTACTGTGCC	CGGTAGG		*caaaac*cta

N, Nongermline nucleotides, PCR-P., PCR product.
Germline sequences of Vd2 (3′ end) and Dd3 gene segments are in capital letters; heptamer motif of the recombination signal at the 3′ end of Dd3 and 5′ end of the 23-bp spacer in lower-case characters; D-derived nucleotides in the N-region in italics; sequences of subclone-specific probes underlined.

more Vd2-Dd3 rearrangements in a clonal population including hyperdiploid leukemias, or (iii) formation of subclones. These possibilities were differentiated by evaluation of TcR-b, TcR-g and IgH gene configuration by Southern blotting (Table 3), by cytogenetic analysis and measurement of DNA content (Table 4). All leukemias were clonal by the above methods. By Southern blot analysis we found three rearranged IgH bands of similar density in leukemia #2, compatible with the presence of three chromosomes 14 in cytogenetic analysis. A weak band corresponding to the germline configuration of the IgH genes resulted presumably from normal hematopoietic cells (Table 3). Single-cell PCR was performed in leukemias #1 and #2 to differentiate whether the presence of two different Vd2-Dd3 PCR products resulted from biallelic rearrangements or separate subclones. The results indicate the presence of two different cell populations (Fig. 2).

Discussion

We demonstrated subclone formation leading to bioligoclonality in precursor B-ALLs at the TcR-d gene level. This bioligoclonality resulted from identical Vd2-Dd3 rearrangements but diverse junctional regions. Therefore, it was only detectable after PCR amplification of the rearranged TcR-d gene segments and separation of the PCR products by poly acrylamide gel electrophoresis.

Previously, Southern blot analysis of Ig and TcR gene rearrangements has been used to define clonality. It has been assumed that both rearrangements of alleles and bioligoclonal rearrangements can be differentiated by the number and the density of the rearranged bands [11]. Therefore, bioligoclonal populations in leukemias are associated with three or more bands, which cannot be explained by chromosomal translocations or extra copies of chromosomes, whereas biallelic rearrangements are thought to be represented by two bands of similar densities in the absence of a germline band [11]. According to this interpretation, our four leukemias were clonal at the IgH gene level.

In precursor B-ALLs about 50% of all recombinatorial events are Vd2-Dd3 rearrangements. Therefore, bioligoclonal rearrangements are likely to be composed of the same rearranging segments and will therefore be missed by

Table 3. IgH and TcR gene patterns in four precursor B-ALLs

Leukemia no.	Southern blot analysis				No. of Vd2-Dd3 PCR products
	IgH	TcR-b	TcR-g	TcR-d	
1	G^a/R	G	G/R	G^a/R	2^b
2	G^a/R/R/R	G	G	G^a/R	2^b
3	R/R	G	G	R	3^c
4	R/R	G	G/R	R	2^c

G, Germline; R, rearrangement.
[a] Weak germline bands resulting from normal hematopoietic cells.
[b] PCR products of similar densities.
[c] PCR products of different densities.

Table 4. Clinical, immunophenotypic, and cytogenetic data, and DNA content of four patients with oligoclonal precursor B-ALL

Leukemia no.	Age (years)	Sex	WBC ($\times 10^9$/l)	Immuno-phenotype	Cytogenetic analysis	DNA content[a]	Clinical outcome
1	2.4	F	24.3	Pre B-ALL	46,XX, [4]	1.00	CCR 32 months
2	3.9	F	18.2	CALLA$^+$	56,XX,+X,del(1) (p34),+4,+6,+7,+8, +14,+15,+18,+21,+22,[6]	$1.00^b + 1.23$	CCR 20 months
3	1.8	M	1.3	CALLA$^+$	n.d.	1.00	CCR 33 months
4	2.4	M	15.8	CALLA$^+$	46,XY,[8]	1.00	CCR 25 months

CCR, Complete continuous remission; n.d., not done.
[a]Ratio of diploid cells (1.00) to cell populations with aneuploid DNA content.
[b]Diploid population of about 8% resulting from normal hematopoietic cells.

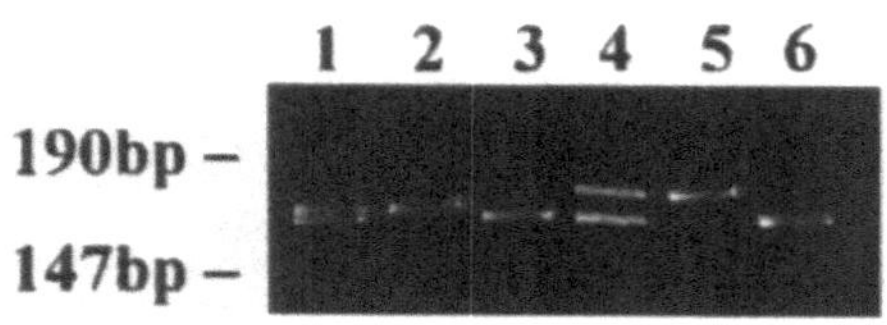

Fig. 2. PAGE analysis of PCR-amplified Vd2-Dd3 rearrangements of single cell nuclei from leukemias #1 and #2 at diagnosis. *Lanes 1-3*: leukemia #1; *lanes 4-6*; leukemia #2; *lanes 1,4*: PCR products from unselected cells; *lanes 2,3,5,6*: PCR products of single cell nuclei. The two single bands resulting from single cell nuclei PCR can be assigned to the two bands seen in the whole leukemic population

Southern blot analysis. These rearrangements could be detected after PCR amplification, however, provided the junctional regions vary in size. In the presence of multiple rearrangements the PCR becomes competitive [12], with a sensitivity for detection of about 5%, comparable to that of Southern blot analysis.

We have performed titration experiments to define the detection limits for subclones. Biclonality of the Vd2-Dd3 rearrangement after two rounds of PCR amplification was discernible with a sensitivity comparable to that of Southern blot analysis (5%–20%). By this approach, we were able to assign subclone formation to leukemias #3 and #4. In the remaining two leukemias, #1 and #2, the densities of bands were similar, compatible with either a biallelic rearrangement, as no germline band was visible by Southern blot analysis, or with subclone formation. In particular, in leukemia #2 we expected that the two Vd2-Dd3 rearrangements would represent a biallelic rearrangement in a leukemic cell population, which is characterized by a trisomy 14 and three rearranged IgH genes. By PCR from single cell nuclei, we were able to demonstrate that these rearrangements occured in individual cells. Two alleles of the TcR-d genes were deleted in each cell. These results confirm the presence of different clones. Subclone formation was also demonstrated by single cell-nuclei PCR in leukemia #1, where one allele of the TcR-d gene was deleted in each cell. In leukemia #3 we found three bands, two with similar density and one of higher density. These bands could have been derived from either three subclones, each with an individual Vd2-Dd3 rearrangement, or from two subclones with a biallelic rearrangement in the smaller clone.

There are conflicting data about the influence of oligoclonal leukemias on the prognosis in these children [13–15]. Whether the differences in oligoclonality/subclone formation between the IgH and the TcR-d gene level occur in leukemias with different immunophenotypes needs to be investigated in larger series of leukemias. All four patients were regarded as being at higher than standard risk for relapse and responded well to chemotherapy.

References

1. Arnold A, Cossman J, Bakhshi A, Jaffe ES, Waldmann TA, Korsmeyer SJ: Immunoglobulin gene rearrangements as unique clonal markers in human lymphoid neoplasms. N Engl J Med 309: 1593, 1983
2. Yokota S, Hansen-Hagge TE, Bartram CR: T-cell receptor d gene recombination in common acute lymphoblastic leukemia: Preferential usage of Vd2 and frequent involvement of the Ja cluster. Blood 77: 141, 1991
3. Breit TM, Wolvers-Tettero ILM, Beishuizen A, Verhoeven MAJ, Van Wering ER, Van Dongen JJM: Southern blot patterns, frequencies, and junctional diversity of T-cell receptor-d gene rearrangements in acute lymphoblastic leukemia. Blood 82: 3063, 1993
4. Felix CA, Poplack DG, Reaman GH, Steinberg SM, Cole DE, Taylor BJ, Begley CG, Kirsch IR: Characterization of immunoglobulin and T-cell receptor gene patterns in B-cell precursor acute lymphoblastic leukemia of childhood. J Clin Oncol 8: 431, 1990
5. Biondi A, Di Celle PF, Rossi V, Casorati G, Matullo G, Giudici G, Foa R, Migone N: High prevalence of T-cell receptor Vd2-(D)-Dd3 or Dd1/2-Dd3 rearrangements in B-precursor acute lymphoblastic leukemias. Blood 75: 1834, 1990
6. Lafaille JJ, De Cloux A, Bonneville M, Takagaki Y, Tonegawa S: Junctional sequences of Tcell receptor g/d genes: Implications for g/d T cell lineages and for a novel intermediate of V-(D)-J joining. Cell 59: 859, 1989
7. Loh EY, Cwirla S, Serafini AT, Phillips JH, Lanier LL: Human T-Cell-receptor d chain: Genomic organization, diversity, and expression in population of cells. Proc Natl Acad Sci USA 85: 9714, 1988
8. Saiki RK, Gelfand DH, Stoffel S, Scharf SJ, Higuchi R, Horn GT, Mullis KB, Erlich HA: Primer-directed enzymatic amplification of DNA with a thermostable DNA polymerase; Science 239: 487, 1988.
9. Griesinger F, Grümayer ER, Van Ness B, Kersey JH: Rearrangement and diversification of T-cell receptor delta genes in acute lymphoblastic leukemia. Leukemia 6: 1054, 1992
10. Meltzer PS, Guan XY, Burgess A, Trent JM: Rapid generation of region specfic probes by chromosome microdissection and their application. Nature Genet 1: 24, 1992
11. Van Dongen JJM, Wolvers-Tettero ILM: Analysis of imunoglobulin and T cell receptor genes. Clin Chim Acta 198: 1, 1991
12. Gilliland G, Perrin S, Blanchard K, Bunn HF: Analysis of cytokine mRNA and DNA: Detection and quantitation by competitive polymerase chain reaction. Proc Natl Acad Sci USA 87: 2725, 1990
13. Kitchingman GR, Mirro J, Stass S, Rovigatti U, Melvin SL, Williams DL, Raimondi SC, Murphy SB: Biologic and prognostic significance of the presence of more than two µ heavychain genes in childhood acute lymphoblastic leukemia of B precursor cell origin. Blood 67: 698, 1986
14. Katz F, Ball L, Gibbons B, Chessells J: The use of DNA probes to monitor minimal residual disease in childhood acute lymphoblastic leukaemia. Br J Haematol 73: 173, 1989
15. Beishuizen A, Hählen K, Hagemeijer A, Verhoeven MAJ, Hooijkaas H, Adriaansen HJ, Wolvers-Tettero ILM, Van Wering ER, Van Dongen JJM: Multiple rearranged immunoglobulin genes in childhood acute lymphoblastic leukemia of precursor B-cell origin. Leukemia 5: 657, 1991

Acute Leukemias VI
Prognostic Factors
and Treatment Strategies
Büchner et al. (eds)

Molecular Genetic Detection of Chromosomal Abnormalities at 11q23 in Patients with De Novo and Secondary Acute Leukemia

A. Borkhardt, R. Repp, S. Schlieben, J. Harbott, J. Kreuder, S. Brettreich, M. Mitteis, and F. Lampert

Abstract. The MLL gene on chromosome 11q23 undergoes chromosomal translocations in a substantial proportion of patients with acute lymphoblastic leukemia (ALL), acute myelogeneous leukemia (AML), as well as in cases of biphenotypic and secondary acute leukemias. Abnormalities at 11q23 have generally been considered to carry a poor prognosis in both AML and ALL. By the RT-PCR technique we investigated 89 patients with ALL, AML, and secondary leukemia for the presence of a chimeric mRNA known to be the equivalent of the various chromosomal translocations involving 11q23. We found eight different MLL fusion mRNAs, corresponding to the chromosomal translocations t(1;11), t(4;11), t(6;11), t(9;11), t(10;11), t(11;17), t(11;19) and t(X;11). This indicates that the RT-PCR technique is suitable to identify such gene rearrangements and can prospectively be used in order to define patients with acute leukemia belonging to a higher risk group.

Introduction

Cytogenetic studies have previously identified abnormalities of chromosome band 11q23 in a substantial part of de novo and secondary acute leukemias. Most of these abnormalities are reciprocal translocations between chromosome 11 and a variety of partner chromosomes (for review see [1]). These chromosomal translocations involving 11q23 are mostly associated with a poor clinical prognosis despite the improvements in present-day chemotherapy protocols. Many chromosomal breakpoints at 11q23 affect a *Drosophilatrithorax* gene homologue called MLL, or HRX, or ALL-1 [2]. The translocations result in a formation of a chimeric gene which is part MLL and part a gene on the reciprocating chromosome. The resulting fusion mRNA enables the molecular genetic detection of these aberrations by RT-PCR. In the view of their biological, clinical, and prognostic relevance, the detection of MLL gene fusions is of paramount importance in the clinical setting. In the present study, we used the RT-PCR approach in order to detect the molecular equivalents of various translocations involving 11q23, i.e., t(1;11)(p32;q23), t(4;11)(q21;q23), t(6;11)(q27;q23), t(9;11), (p22, q23) t(10;11)(p12;q23), t(11;17) (q23;q21), t(11;19)(q23;p13) and t(X;11) (q13;q23).

Material and Methods

Bone marrow or peripheral blood samples were most frequently sent by mail to the Central Cytogenetic Laboratory of the BFM and CoALL study group, i.e., our laboratory in Giessen, Germany. All patients' samples were fractionated on a Ficoll gradient and cryopreserved before use. The permanent leukemic cell lines were used directly. The selection of these leukemic cell lines was based on publications by Drexler et al. [3,4].Total RNA was prepared by the guanidium thiocyanate method as described previously [5]. In a total volume of 20 µl, 10 µg of RNA

Department of Pediatrics, University Hospital, Feulgenstr. 12, 35385 Giessen, Germany was reverse transcribed to cDNA with random hexamer primers (Boehringer, Mannheim, Germany) by a standard protocol [6]. For PCR amplification 2 μl of the cDNA conversion mixture was used. PCR primers were synthesized on a Applied Biosystems oligonucleotide synthesizer (Applied Biosystems, Weiterstadt, Germany) and purified by high-performance liquid chromatography. To achieve maximal sensitivity and specificity, a nested PCR protocol was used. The PCR primers were selected as described previously and in accordance with the published cDNA sequence data [7–15]. PCR amplification was generally performed with the "hot-start" technique. After an initial melting step (5 min at 94°C) the taq polymerase (Perkin Elmer, Langen, Germany) was added and 35 amplification cycles of 60 s at 94°C, 120 s at 60°C, and 120 s at 74°C were carried out in 50 μl final volume containing 4 pmol of each primer during the first round of the nested PCR. One microliter of the first round product was subjected to the second round of PCR. This differed from the first round in the number of cycles, which was reduced to 25, and the amount of primer (20 pmol each). Cycling was performed in a Bio-Med Thermocycler (Bio-Med, Theres, Germany) using a GeneAmp kit (Perkin Elmer). PCR products were analyzed on a 2% agarose gel and visualized by ethidium bromide staining. As a positive control template for the various MLL rearrangements we used in vitro synthesized chimeric RNA generated for each specific MLL rearrangement by a method published recently [16].

Results

To estimate the frequency of the various MLL rearrangements we retrospectively analyzed 89 patients with de novo and secondary acute leukemia as well as a panel of permanent leukemic cell lines (Fig. 1). The cell lines which were identified as having a MLL rearrangement are MV4;11, RS4;11, (both MLL/AF4 rearrangement), ML-2 (MLL/AF6 rearrangement), THP-1, Mono-Mac6 (both MLL/AF9 rearrangement), and Karpas 45 (MLL/AFX rearrangement). We did not find a permanent cell line expressing a MLL/AF1p, MLL/AF10, MLL/AF17, MLL/ENL, or MLL/ELL fusion transcript. The results of the screening procedure performed on the patient samples are summarized in Table 1.

After identification of the cell lines with the different MLL gene rearrangements we evaluated the sensitivity of our nested PCR protocol by dilution series of the corresponding cells mixed with an increasing amount of HL60 cells. Our PCR assay was shown to be able to detect at least one MLL rearranged cell in 10 000 unrearranged HL60 cells. In the case of the MLL/AF4 and MLL/AF9 rearrangement, moreover, even one rearranged cell per 100 000 unrearranged cells was detectable (data not shown).

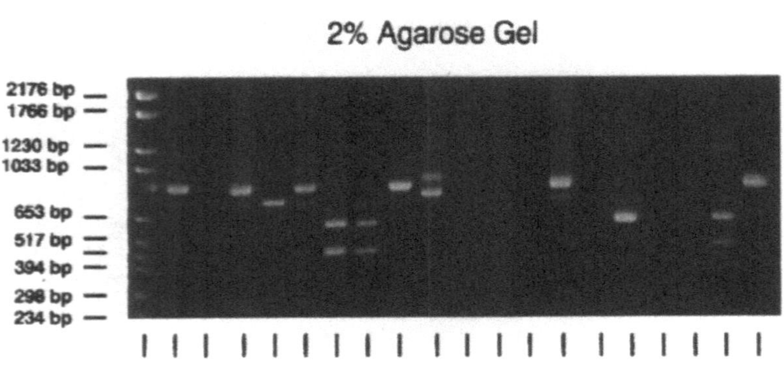

Fig. 1. PCR products of different MLL gene rearrangements separated over an 2.0% agarose gel. *Lane 1* molecular weight marker VI (Boehringer, Mannheim, Germany). *Lanes 2, 4, 6,* and *9* show a MLL/AF4 rearrangement. *Lanes 5 and 19* MLL/ENL rearrangement. *Lanes 7* and *8, 9* MLL/AF9 rearrangement. Note the identical splicing sites in these lanes. *Lane 10* MLL/AF1p rearrangement. *Lane 14* MLL/AF6 rearrangement, *Lane 20* MLL/AF10 rearrangement. Lane 16MLL/AFX rearrangement as amplified from cDNA of the Karpas 45 cell line

Table 1. Numbers of the different MLL fusion transcripts found in our patients

Disease	MLL/ AFIp	MLL/ AF4	MLL/ AF6	MLL/ AF9	MLL/ AF10	MLL/ AF17	MLL/ ENL	MLL/ ELL	MLL/ AFX
ALL($n=34$)	0	2	0	0	0	0	1	0	0
Infant ALL ($n=18$)	0	6	0	0	0	0	4	0	0
AML ($n=24$)	1	0	1	2	1	1	0	0	1
Secondary leukemia ($n=13$)	1	2	0	3	0	0	1	0	0

ALL, Acute Lymphoblastic leukemia; AML, acute myeloblastic leukemia.

Discussion

Different groups have cloned and sequenced the MLL gene at 11q23 as well as the various partner gene on chromosomes 1, 4, 6, 9, 10, 17, 19, and X. In this report, we have shown that the RT-PCR technique is suitable for diagnosis of these rearrangements as a fusion mRNA, transcribed from MLL and the corresponding partner gene, is expressed in the leukemic cells. This enables a rapid and sensitive diagnosis of these particular rearrangements. In our series we found 27 patients with different MLL rearrangements, with a remarkably high incidence in infant and secondary leukemias. In the light of the high frequency and the prognostic significance of MLL rearrangements we recommend prospective screening for MLL/AF4 and MLL/ENL rearrangements in infants with ALL at diagnosis. The MLL rearrangement can also be identified by Southern blotting [11], but the partner gene remains unknown with this technique. Heerema et al. recently reported that the specific translocation t(4;11) and not an 11q23 per se may be associated with a poor prognosis in infants with ALL [17]. This finding further emphasizes the need for an identification of the translocation partner of 11q23.

It should be kept in mind that two different chromosomal regions at chromosome 19p have been described cytogenetically. The breakpoint at 19p13.3 was found in patients suffering from ALL, biphenotypic leukemia, and infants or very young children with AML. The other breakpoint, at 19p13.1, was found in older children or adults having AML of the myelomonocytic or monoblastic subtype.

The gene that fuses to MLL in patients with t(11;19)(q23;p13.1) was named ELL [13]. The corresponding MLL/ENL mRNA has not been detected in any of our patients so far.

In secondary leukemias it has previously been shown that especially patients previously treated by topoisomerase II-reactive drugs, i.e., teniposide or etoposide, have an increased risk of seondary acute leukemia with aberrations at 11q23 [18]. Our data indicate that the MLL rearrangements in these patients were identical to those commonly found in de novo ALL or AML cases, at least on the cDNA level. Whether the exact breakpoints of MLL on the genomic DNA level differ significantly between de novo and secondary leukemia however, remains unknown to date.

In summary, we have shown that RT-PCR is a rapid and sensitive tool to detect the molecular equivalents of chromosomal translocations involving the breakpoint 11q23. The high sensitivity of RT-PCR enables the monitoring of minimal residual disease by amplification of the MLL fusion transcripts.

Acknowledgments. These studies were supported by Forschungshilfe Station Peiper. We thank Claudia Keller and Ursula Buchen for excellent technical assistance.

References

1. Rowley, J.D. 1993. Rearrangements involving chromosome band 11q23 in acute leukemia. *Seminars in Cancer Biology* 4: 377–385.
2. Ziemin-van der Poel, S., N.R. McCabe, H.J. Gill, R. Espinosa, III, Y. Patel, A. Harden, P. Rubinelli, S.D. Smith, M.M. LeBeau, J.D. Rowley, and M.O. Diaz. 1991. Identification of a gene, MLL, that spans the breakpoint in 11q23 translocations associated with human leukemias. *Proc. Natl. Acad. Sci. USA* 88: 10735–10739.

3. Drexler, H.G., R.A.F. MacLeod, A. Borkhardt, and J.W.G. Janssen. 1995. Recurrent translocations and fusion genes in leukemia-lymphoma cell lines. *Leukemia* 9: 480–500.
4. Drexler, H.G., R.A.F. MacLeod, H. Quentmeier, and H.Steube. 1994. DSM Catalogue of Human and Animal Cell Lines. Braunschweig.
5. Chomczynski, P. and N.Sacchi. 1987. Single-step method of RNA isolation by guanidium thiocyanate-phenol-chloroform extraction. *Anal. Biochem.* 162: 156–159.
6. Sambrock, J., E.F. Fritsch, and T. Maniatis. 1989. Molecular cloning: A laboratory manual. Cold Spring Harbor University Press, Cold Spring Harbor.
7. Bernard, O.A., M.Mauchauffe, C. Mecucci, H. Van den Berghe, and R. Berger, 1994. A novel gene, AF-1p, fused to HRX in t(1;11)(p32;q23), is not related to AF-4, AF-9 nor ENL. *Oncogene* 9: 1039–1045.
8. Gu, Y., T. Nakamura, H. Alder, R. Prasad, O. Canaani, G. Cimino, C.M. Croce, and E. Canaani. 1992. The t(4;11) chromosome translocation of human acute leukemias fuses the ALL-1 gene, related to *Drosophila trithorax,* to the AF4 gene. Cell7 1: 701–708.
9. Prasad, R., Y. Gu, H. Alder, T. Nakamura, O. Canaani, H. Saito, K. Huebner, R.P. Gale, P.C. Nowell, K. Kuriyama, Y. Miyazaki, C.M. Croce, and E. Canaani. 1993. Cloning of the ALL-1 fusion partner, the AF-6 gene, involved in acute myeloid leukemias with t(6;11) chromosome translocation. *Cancer Res.* 53: 5624–5628.
10. Nakamura, T., H. Alder, Y. Gu, R. Prasad, O. Canaani, N. Kamada, R.P Gale, B. Lange, W.M. Crist, P.C. Nowell, C.M. Croce, and E. Canaani. 1993. Genes on chromosomes 4,9 and 19 involved in 11q23 abnormalities in acute leukemia share sequence homology and/or common motifs. *Proc. Natl. Acad. Sci. USA* 90: 4631–4635.
11. Chaplin, T., P. Ayton, O.A. Bernard, V. Saha, V. Della Valle, J. Hillion, A. Gregorini, D. Lillington, R. Berger, and B.D. Young. 1995. A novel class of zinc finger/leucine zipper genes identified from molecular cloning of the t(10;11) translocation in acute leukemia. *Blood* 85: 1435–1441.
12. Prasad, R., D. Leshkowitz, Y. Gu, H. Alder, T. Nakamura, H. Saito, K. Huebner, R. Berger, C.M. Croce, and E. Canaani. 1994. Leucine-zipper dimerization motif encoded by the AF17 gene fused to ALL-1 (MLL) in acute leukemia. *Proc. Natl. Acad. Sci. USA* 91: 8107–8111.
13. Thirman, M.J., D.A. Levitan, H. Kobayashi, M.C. Simon, and J.D. Rowley. 1994. Cloning of ELL, a gene that fuses to MLL in a t(11;19)(q23;p13.1) in acute myeloid leukemia. *Proc. Natl. Acad. Sci.* USA 91:12110–12114.
14. Corral, J., A. Forster, S. Thompson, F. Lampert, Y. Kaneko, R. Slater, C.E. van der Schoot, W.D. Ludwig, C. Pocock, F. Cotter, and T.H. Rabbitts. 1993. Acute leukaemias of different lineages have similar MLL gene fusions encoding related chimeric proteins resulting from chromosomal translocation. *Proc. Natl. Acad. Sci. USA* 90: 8538–8542.
15. Repp, R., A. Borkhardt, E. Haupt, J.Kreuder, S. Brettreich, J. Hammermann, K. Nishida, J. Harbott, and F. Lampert. 1995. Detection of four different 11q23 chromosomal abnormalities by multiplex PCR and fluorescence-based automatic DNA fragment analysis. *Leukemia* 9: 210–215.
16. Borkhardt, A., M. Mitteis, S. Brettreich, S. Schlieben, J. Hammermann, R. Repp, J. Kreuder, U. Buchen, and F. Lampert. 1995. Rapid synthesis of hybrid RNA molecules associated with leukemia-specific chromosomal translocations. *Leukemia* 9: 719–722.
17. Heerema, N.A., D.C. Arthur, H. Sather, V. Albo, J. Feusner, B.J. Lange, P.G. Steinherz, P. Zeltzer, D. Hammond, and G.H. Reaman. 1994. Cytogenetic features of infants less than 12 months of age at diagnosis of acute lymphoblastic leukemia: impact of the 11q23 breakpoint on outcome: a report of the childrens cancer group. *Blood* 83: 2274–2284.
18. Pedersen-Bjergaard, J. and P. Philip. 1991. Balanced translocations involving chromosome bands 11q23 and 21q22 are highly characteristic of myelodysplasia and leukemia following therapy with cytostatic agents targeting at DNA-topoisomerase II. *Blood* 78: 1147–1148.

Acute Leukemias VI
Prognostic Factors
and Treatment Strategies
Büchner et al. (eds)

Sequence Analysis of the GAP-Related Domain of the NFI-Gene and All Three RAS Protooncogenes in Patients with Secondary Acute Leukemia

S. Brettreich, A. Borkhardt, J. Hammermann, A.K. Borkhardt, J. Kreuder, R. Repp, and F. Lampert

Abstract. We analyzed the N-RAS, K-RAS, H-RAS and FLR exon of the neurofibromatosis 1 (NF1) gene in 11 patients at the time of diagnosis of a secondary acute leukemia. Eight of these patients suffered from secondary acute myelogeneous leukemia (AML) and three patients had a secondary acute lymphoblastic leukemia (ALL). After isolation of genomic DNA we selectively amplified codons 12,13 or 60,61 of the RAS genes and the FLR exon of NF1 by polymerase chain reaction (PCR). Afterwards, all PCR products were directly sequenced by the chain termination method. We found only one point mutation in codon 13 of the K-RAS gene (GGC to GAC) leading to an amino acid exchange from glycine to aspartic acid. All other RAS genes as well as the FLR exon of NF1 were found to be of wild-type DNA sequence. We conclude that the RAS protooncogenes and the NF1 gene do not play a major role in the development of secondary leukemias.

Introduction

Although the RAS protooncogenes are frequently described as having mutated in a wide range of human malignancies, the frequency with which mutations are found varies enormously. A central role of RAS genes in the malignant transformation process was described in about 30% of primary AML and in about 5%–10% of ALL[1]. Point mutation within the hotspots of the RAS genes prevents hydrolysis of the active guanosine triphosphate-bound state of RAS (RAS-GTP) to the inactive guanosine diphosphate-bound state (GDP-RAS), leading to permanent activation of the pathway. Another oncogenic mechanism interacting with the RAS-mediated signaling pathway was recently demonstrated [2–4]. The neurofibromatosis 1 gene (NF1) encodes for neurofibromin, a GTPase-activating protein that is capable of down-regulating RAS by stimulating its intrinsic GTPase activity. Loss of function of the NF1 gene may result, therefore, in the same effect as point mutation of the RAS genes. While both RAS genes and the GTPase activating domain of NF1 (GAP) have already been analyzed in primary myeloid leukemias, no analysis of the involvement of these genes in secondary leukemias after radio and/or chemotherapy has been reported. In 11 children with secondary acute leukemia here we investigated all three RAS genes (K-RAS, H-RAS, and N-RAS) as well as the so-called FLR exon of NF1, in which mutations have previously been described in 1 out of 28 patients with a myelodysplastic syndrome [5].

Materials and Methods

Patients

Eleven children who fulfilled the criteria for diagnosis of secondary acute leukemia were enrolled in the present study. All bone marrow samples were taken at diagnosis of secondary leukemia and the amount of blast cells was generally higher than 70%. The clinical data of the patients are summarized in Table 1.

Department of Pediatrics, University Hospital, Feulgenstr. 12, 35385 Giessen, Germany

Table 1. Clinical characteristics and DNA sequence data of patients with secondary acute leukemia

Patient No.	Primary malignancy	Latency period (years, months)	Age[a] (years)	Sex	Secondary leukemia type	Out-come	N-RAS	K-RAS	H-RAS of NF1	FLR exon
1	ALL	4,6	7	m	AML	Died	wt	wt	wt	wt
2	Hepatoblastoma	2,3	4	m	AML	Died	wt	wt	wt	wt
3	ALL	4,10	19	m	AML	Died	wt	wt	wt	wt
4	B-NHL	1,9	11	m	AML	Died	wt	wt	wt	wt
5	Ewing Sarcoma	1,5	14	f	AML	Died	wt	codon 13 GGC to GAC	wt	wt
6	T-NHL	8,8	22	m	AML	Died	wt	wt	wt	wt
7	Astro-cytoma	17,0	23	m	ALL	Died	wt	wt	wt	wt
8	Neuro-blastoma	21,6	22	f	ALL	Died	wt	wt	wt	wt
9	Wilms tumor	9,7	13	m	AML	Died	wt	wt	wt	wt
10	Rhabdomyo-sarcoma	2,3	10	m	ALL	Died	wt	wt	wt	wt
11	ALL	1,3	5	f	AML	Died	wt	wt	wt	wt

[a]At diagnosis of secondary leukemia.
wt, Wild-type DNA sequence.

DNA Extraction and PCR Amplification

DNA was extracted from the bone marrow of the 11 children with secondary leukemia with the help of a Quiagen 20 column (Diagen, Düsseldorf, Germany) according to the manufacturer's protocol. In order to improve sensitivity and specificity, we followed a nested PCR protocol for amplification of the RAS genes. Primer sequences for selective amplification of gene fragments spanning codon 12, 13 or 60, 61 of H-RAS, K-RAS, and N-RAS have been described previously [6].

For amplification of the NF1-FLR exon we used primers described by Li et al. [5] and performed only a single PCR run. PCR was carried out in a Biomed 60 thermocycler (Biomed, Theres, Germany) and was essentially performed as described by Saiki et al. [7]. In order to enable the purification of PCR products by magnetic bead technology (Dynal, Oslo, Norway), we labeled the downstream PCR primers within biotin.

Direct DNA Sequencing

Direct sequencing of all PCR products was performed by solid-phase sequencing [8]. Briefly, double-stranded PCR products amplified by biotin-labeled primers were captured using streptavidin-coated magnetic beads and a neodymium-iron-boron permanent magnet, MPC 96 (Dynal, Oslo, Norway). After immobilization, the DNA was converted to single strands by 0.2*M* NaOH. The supernatant with the nonbiotinylated DNA strand was precipitated and both DNA strands were subjected to the chain termination reaction [9]. The sequencing procedure was carried out with the help of a Sequenase PRISM kit and the automatic sequencing system 373A from AB1 (Applied Biosystems, Weiterstadt, Germany). By dilution experiments we proved that we were able to detect 10% of mutated cells in 90% of wild-type sequences.

Results

Only one of our 11 patients (9%) with secondary leukemia revealed a heterozygous point mutation in codon 13 of the K-RAS protooncogene (GGC-GAC). The mutation leads to an amino-acid exchange from neutral glycine to aspartic acid in the corresponding RAS protein. This patient suffered from secondary AML occuring 17 months after diagnosis of a Ewing sarcoma. All other patients revealed wild-type sequenes of N-RAS, K-RAS, or H-RAS, as well as in the GAP-related domain of the neurofibromatosis 1 gene (Table 1).

Discussion

The comparatively low frequency of RAS gene mutations and the absence of mutations of the FLR exon of NF1 led to the conclusion that these genes do not play a major role in the development of secondary leukemia.

Secondary malignant tumors occurring after treatment of a primary malignant disease are one of the most important side effects of chemo- and/or radiotherapy. Among secondary leukemias, more than 90% have been reported to be myelogeneous, whereas only a small subset of secondary leukemias belong to the lymphoid lineage [10–12]. In our series, in which the selection of cases was based only on the availability of cryopreserved bone marrow samples, we also found predominantly secondary AML cases (8 out of 11).

In de novo AML cases, RAS protooncogenes mutations are one of the most commonly observed molecular alterations, with the reported incidence ranging from 20% to 30% in AML [1, 13]. Studies in de novo AML, furthermore, suggest that a mutational status of RAS may be a predictor for improved survival, correlating with a better cytogenetic category and a lower leukemic cell burden [14]. The rare occurrence as well as the extraordinarily poor prognosis of patients with secondary AML, however, makes it difficult to study the biologic influence of RAS gene mutations in these patients.

It has also been suggested that RAS gene mutations found in hematologically normal patients after chemotheraphy for childhood ALL may be predictive of early secondary leukemia [15]. Our data show that RAS gene mutations are a rare event in secondary leukemias and therefore do not support this hypothesis.

Acknowledgment. These studies were supported by Forschungshilfe Station Peiper. S. B. was supported by a Graduiertenstipendium, Justus-Liebig University, Giessen.

We thank Mrs. Claudia Keller and Mrs. Ursula Buchen for excellent technical assistance.

References

1. Bos, J.L. 1989. ras oncogenes in human cancer: A review. *Cancer Res.* 49: 4682–4689.
2. DeClue, J.E., A.G. Papageorge, J.A. Fletcher, S.R. Diehl, N. Ratner, W.C. Vass, and D.R. Lowy. 1992. Abnormal regulation of mammalian p21ras contributes to malignant tumor growth in von Recklinghausen (type 1) neurofibromatosis. *Cell* 69: 265–273.
3. Shannon, K.M., P. O'Connell, G.A. Martin, D. Paderanga, K. Olson, P. Dinndorf, and F. McCormick. 1994. Loss of the normal NF1 allele from the bone marrow of children with type 1 neurofibromatosis and malignant myeloid disorders. *N. Engl. J. Med.* 330: 597–601.
4. Martin, G.A., D. Viskochil, G. Bollag, P.C. McCabe, W.J. Crosier, H. Haubruck, L. Conroy, R. Clark, P. O'Connell, R.M. Cawthon, M.A. Innis, and F. McCormick. 1990. The GAP-related domain of the neurofibromatosis type 1 gene product interacts with ras p21. *Cell* 63: 843–849.
5. Li, Y., G. Bollag, R. Clark, J. Stevens, L. Conroy, D. Fults, K. Ward, E. Friedman, W. Samowitz, M. Robertson, P. Bradley, F. McCormick, R. White, and R. Cawthon. 1992. Somatic mutations in the neurofibromatosis 1 gene in human tumors. *Cell* 69: 275–281.
6. Bohle, R.M., S. Brettreich, R. Repp, A. Borkhardt, W. Kosmehl, F. Lampert, and H.M. Altmannsberger. 1995. Unique somatic point mutation of ras genes in malignant fibrous histiocytomas. *Am. J. Pathol.* in press.
7. Saiki, R.K., D.H. Gelfand, S. Stoffel, S.J. Scharf, R. Higuchi, G.T. Horn, K.B. Mullis, and H.A. Erlich. 1988. Primer-directed enzymatic amplification of DNA with a thermostable DNA polymerase. *Science* 239: 487–491.
8. Kaneoka, H., D.R. Lee, K.C. Hsu, G.C. Sharp, and R.W. Hoffmann. 1991. Solid-phase direct DNA sequencing of allele-specific polymerase chain reaction-amplified HLA-DR genes. *Bio Techniques* 10: 30–34.
9. Sanger, F., S. Nicklen, and A.R. Coulson. 1977. DNA sequencing with chain terminating inhibitors. *Proc. Natl. Acad. Sci.* USA 74: 5463–5467.
10. Hunger, S.P., J. Sklar, and M.P. Link. 1992. Acute lymphoblastic leukemia occurring as a second malignant neoplasm in childhood: report of three cases and review of the literature. *J. Clin. Oncol.* 10: 156.
11. Lennard, A., G.H. Jackson, P.J. Carey, N. Bown, P. Middleton, and S.J. Proctor. 1991. Secondary acute lymphoblastic leukaemia with 4: 11 translocation following treatment for Hodgkin's disease: Case report and review of the literature. *Leukemia* 5: 624–627.
12. Zaccaria, A., G. Alimena, M. Baccarani, R. Billström, F. Carbonell, G.L. Castoldi, K. Fuscaldo, F. Hecht, D.K. Hossfeld, F. Mitelman, G. Rosti, A.A. Sandberg, A. Tassinari, N. Testoni, and S. Tura. 1987. Cytogenetic analyses in 89 patients with secondary hematologic disorders-Results of a cooperative study. *Cancer Genet. Cytogenet.* 26: 65–74.
13. Radich, R.P., K.J. Kopecky, C.L. Willman, J. Weick, D. Head, F. Appelbaum, and S.J. Collins. 1990. N-ras mutations in adult de novo acute myelogeneous leukemia: Prevalence and clinical significance. *Blood* 76: 801–804.
14. Neubauer, A., R.K. Dodge, S.L. George, F.R. Davey, R.T. Silver, C.A. Schiffer, R.J. Mayer, E.D. Ball, D. Wurster-Hill, C.D. Bloomfield, and E.T. Liu. 1994. Prognostic importance of mutations in the ras protoncogenes in de novo acute myeloid leukemia. *Blood* 83: 1603–1611.
15. Taylor, C., H. McGlynn, G. Carter, A.H. Baker, N. Warren, S.A. Ridge, G. Owen, E. Thompson, P.W. Thompson, A. Jacobs, and R.A. Padua. 1995. RAS and FMS mutations following cytotoxic therapy for childhood acute lymphoblastic leukaemia. *Leukemia* 9: 466–470.

Acute Leukemias VI
Prognostic Factors
and Treatment Strategies
Büchner et al. (eds)

Molecular Genetic Screening of Children with Acute Leukemia by RT-PCR

S. Schlieben, I. Reinisch, A. Borkhardt, F. Lampert, and J. Harbott

Introduction

A variety of oncogenes are activated by specific chromosomal translocations, which are associated with distinct subtypes of leukemia. The identification of these rearrangements provides critical diagnostic and prognostic information which may contribute to the selection of specific antileukemia therapy. Of clinical importance are t(9;22) (2–5% of c- and pre-B-ALL) [1], t(4;11) (60% of infant and pre-pre-B-ALL) [2], t(11;19) (1% of biphenotypic leukemia) [3], and t(9;11) (20–30% of ANLL-M5) [4], which are characterized by a poor prognosis, whereas t(8;21) (40% of ANLL-M2) and inv(16) (8% of ANLL-M4eo) [6] seem to be more favorable [5, 6].

Molecular analysis of these chromosomal translocations occurring in human leukemias shows the interruption of two different genes and their fusion, forming a new chimeric gene. Genes fused in these rearrangements are *BCR* with *ABL* (t(9;22)), *MLL* with *AF*4 (t(4;11)), *MLL* with *LTG*19 (t(11;19)) or with *LTG*9 (t(9;11)), *AMLI* with ETO (t(8;21)), and finally *CBFß* with *MYH*11 (inv(16)).

We used RT-PCR to detect these six rearrangements. The application of this sensitive strategy has introduced a new standard for the diagnosis and monitoring of leukemia patients. The enormous sensitivity makes it necessary to establish precautions to minimize the danger of false positive results caused by contamination or false negative results caused by RNA degradation, focal disease, or limited sensitivity.

Patients

Heparinized bone marrow and/or blood samples of 942 children participating in one of the German multicenter therapy trials were sent in before treatment by more than 70 pediatric oncologic centers in Germany.

Molecular Detection of the Fusion Transcripts

Mononuclear cells were obtained by Ficoll centrifugation and stored at −70°C prior to use. Cell lines K 562, SUP B15, MV 4;11, MM6 Kasum (−1, and ME 1 were used as positive controls.

Total RNA was extracted from nucleated cells using the method of Chomczynski and Sacchi [8]. In vitro reverse trasnscription was performed with random hexamer priming using standard techniques.

Amplifications were performed using a Perkin Elmer thermocycler (9600) with primers synthesized from Roth, Karlsruhe, Germany. The sequences of the oligomers are summarized in Table 1.

Two amplifications were performed on each cDNA sample:

1. Control amplification of the ABL gene
2. Diagnostic amplification (nested or seminested) of fusion products.

The first round of nested PCR contained 1 µl cDNA, 1 × reaction buffer, 0.2 m*M* dNTP (Boehringer, Mannheim, Germany), 0.08 µ*M* of each external primer, 0.5 U *Taq* polymerase

Oncogenetic Laboratory, Department of Pediatrics, University Hospital, Feulgenstr. 12, 35392 Giessen, Germany

Table 1. Sequences of the primers used for the detection of rearrangements

Number	Position	Sequence 5′→3	
1	5′external-ABL	ccagtagcatctgactttgagcct	
2	3′external-ABL	ccagactgttgactggcgtgatt	
3	5′internal-ABL	tgagtgaagccgctcgttggaact	
4	3′internal-ABL	ttccacccattccccattgtgatt	
6	5′internal-m-BCR	atgacgagggcgccttccatggag	
7	5′external-M-BCR	cctctgactatgagcgtgcagatg	
8	5′internal-M-BCR	agaagtgtttcagaagcttctccct	
9	5′external-MLL	ctgaatccaaacaggccaccactc	[9]
10	3′external-AF4	gtcactgagctgaaggtcgtct	[9]
11	5′internal-MLL	ggtctcccagccagcactggtc	[9]
12	3′internal-AF4	agcatggatgacgttccttgctga	[9]
13	3′ext-int-LTG19	gacgaagagtcgtcctcgtcggact	[10]
14	3′ext-int-LTG19	accatccagtcgtgagtgaacccct	[10]
15	3′ext-int-LTG9	tcgtgatgtaggggtgaagaagcag	[4]
16	5′external-AML1	agcttcactctgaccatcac	[11]
17	5′internal-AML1	ttcacaaacccaccgcaagt	[11]
18	3′ext-int-ETO	tgaactggttcttggagctcc	[11]
19	5′ext-int-CBFβ	caggcaaggtatatttga	[12]
20	3′internal-MYH11	ctcctcttctcctcattctgctc	[12]
5	5′external-m-BCR	caacagtccttcgacagcagcagt	

(Gibco BRL, Eggenstein, Germany) and sterile double-distilled water to 20 µl. First amplification was obtained with 35 cycles at 94°C for 15 s, 65°C for 45 s and 72°C for 45 s. Nested PCR was carried out under the same conditions but with 30 cycles in the presence of 0.4 µ*M* internal primers using 1 µl amplification product of the first round. The samples were analyzed by gel electrophoresis (1% agarose) and visualized by ethidium bromide staining.

For cytogenetic investigations the samples of bone marrow or peripheral blood were prepared and GTG-banded using standard techniques [7]. Karyotyping followed the criteria of the ISCN [13]. Immunophenotyping was performed in two central laboratories (Berlin and Hamburg)

Results

Bone marrow and blood samples of 942 children treated by the protocol of one of the German multicenter therapy trials were analyzed in a prospective PCR study for chimeric transcripts (Fig. 1). The results are shown in Table 2. In 774 patients ALL de novo was diagnosed, 168 ALL patients were investigated at relapse, and a further 105 cases, first diagnosed as ALL, later

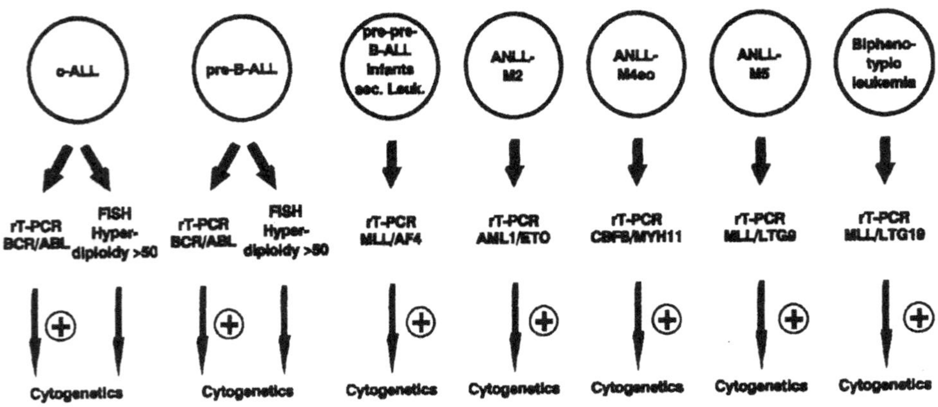

Fig. 1. Techniques in oncogenetic diagnosis

Table 2. Incidence of the investigated rearrangements in children with ALL and ANLL

Diagnosis	No. of Patients	BCR/ABL	MLL/AF4	MLL/LTG19	AML1/ETO	MLL/LTG9	CBFβ/MYH1
Pre-pre-B-ALL	42	–	1	1	–	–	–
c-ALL	529	18	–	1	–	–	–
Pre-B-ALL	112	2	–	–	–	–	–
B-ALL	1	–	–	–	–	–	–
T-ALL	69	1	–	–	–	–	–
AHL	12	2	–	–	–	–	–
Unclear	20	–	–	–	–	–	–
ALL(infants)	21	–	8	–	–	–	–
ANLL-M1/M2	32	–	–	–	6	–	–
ANLL-M4e0	3	–	–	–	–	–	1
ANLL-M5	6	–	–	–	–	2	–

changed to another type of malignant disease. Forty-one patients with ANLL-M1,-M2, -M4eo, and -M5 were also screened as well for the appropriate rearrangement. Figure 2 demonstrates a screening gel for all fusion transcripts. Altogether 96% of the samples were analyzed successfully. Of these successfully analyzed patients 3.3% with ALL de novo transcribed the

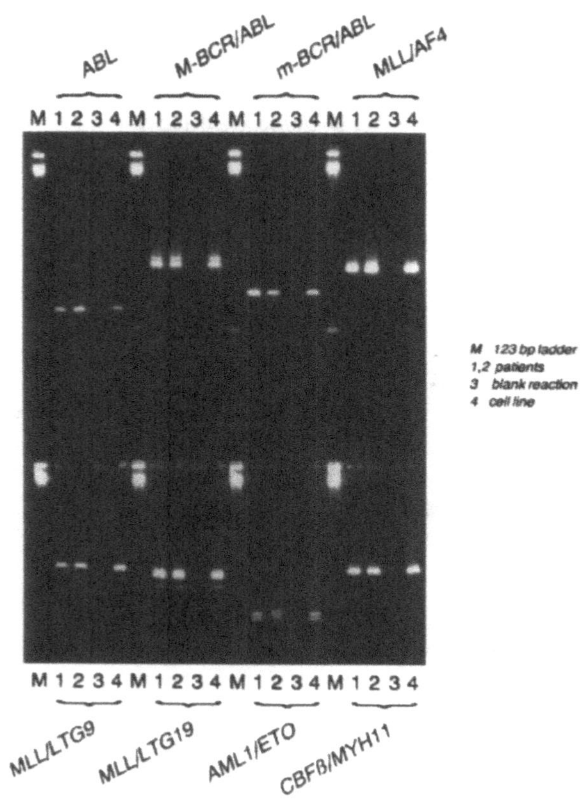

Fig. 2. Gel electrophoresis of the analyzed gene rearrangements

chimeric BCR/ABL gene, whereas 10.9% at relapse and 2 patients with AHL showed the fusion transcript.

In 8 of 21 infants (age <1 year) with ALL and in one of 21 older children with pre-pre-B-ALL the *MLL/A*F4 transcript was detected. Further screening for other aberrations in 11q23 as *MLL/LTG*19 was positive in 2 patients one with common ALL and one with pre-pre-B-ALL, and the *MLL/LTG*9 chimeric gene could be shown in 2 of 6 patients with *ANLL-M*5. The screening of 25 children with *ANLL-M*1/*M*2 for the *AML*1/*ETO* rearrangement detected 5 patients with the fusion transcript, whereas in 1 of 3 analyzed patients with ANLL-M4eo the *CBF*β/*MYH*11 transcript was demonstrated. Chimeric gene products detected by RT-PCR were confirmed by cytogenetics and/or a PCR analysis in an external laboratory (Fig. 3).

Discussion

The present study is a prospective analysis of the incidence of special rearrangements in children. We found an overall prevalence of the BCR/ABL fusion gene transcript detected by PCR of 3.3%; this is within the published range of 2%–5% [1, 14], whereas at the time of relapse the incidence increased up to 10.9%. BCR/ABL-positive patients present a homogeneous immunophenotype. The majority were found to have c- or pre-B-ALL, whereas the transcript was not detected in pre-pre-, B-, T-ALL, and myeloid cases. The predominance of the ela2 (m-BCR/ABL) transcript in children with ALL has previously been noted [16], but seems not to be associated with special clinical features [15].

Studying other rearrangements such as MLL/AF4, this has an occurrence of 39% in infants and is less frequent in older children. Another chimeric transcript with prognostic relevance [5], AML1/ETO, was detected in 20% of patients with AML-M1/M2. Screening for further rearrangements as MLL/LTG19, MLL/LTG9, and CBFβ/MYH11 did not result in statistically evaluable data because of the short time of screening.

Further prospective studies are therefore necessary, to determine the incidence and clinical outcome of the different rearrangements in children with ALL or AML.

Acknowledgments. We are indebted to Andrea Richter for excellent technical assistance. The study was supported by the Deutsche Krebshilfe–Mildred-Scheel Stifung, Parents' Initiative Giessen, and the Forschungshilfe Station Peiper.

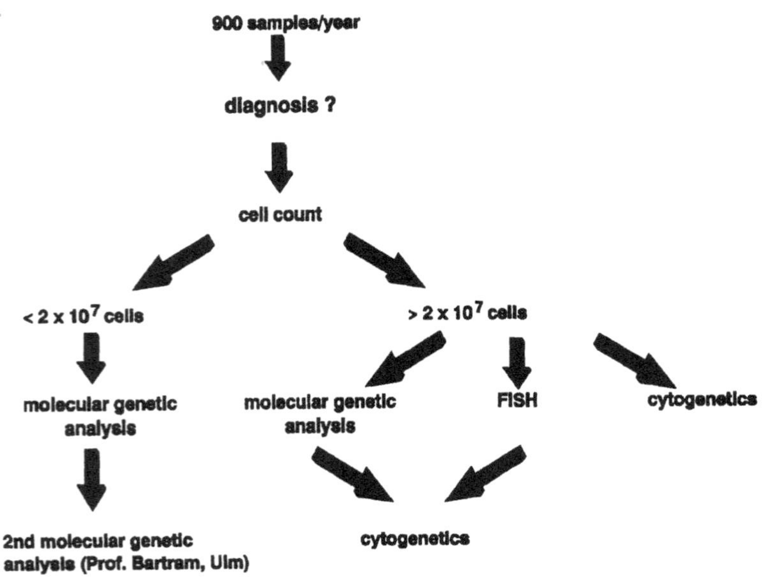

Fig. 3. Techniques applied in dependence on the diagnosis and cell count

References

1. Crist W, Caroll J, Shuster J (1990) Philadelphia chromosome positive childhood acute lymphoblastic leukemia: clinical and cytogenetic characteristics and treatment outcome. A Pediatric Oncology Group study. Blood 3: 489–494
2. Chen CS, Sorenson PHB, Domer PH, Reaman GH, Korsmeyer SJ, Heerema NA, Hammond GD, Kersey JH (1993) Molecular rearrangements on chromosome 11q23 predominate in infant acute lymphoblastic leukemia and are associated with t(11;19) specific biologic variables and poor outcome. Blood 81: 2386–2393
3. Iida S, Seto M, Yamamoto K, Komatsu H, Akao Y, Nakazawa S, Ariyoshi Y, Takahashi T, Ueda R (1993) Molecular cloning of 19p13 breakpoint region in infantile leukemia with t(11;19) (q123;p13) translocation. Jpn J Cancer Res 84, 532–537
4. Iida S, Seto M, Yamamoto K, Komatsu H, Tojo A, Asano S, Kamada N, Ariyoshi Y, Takahashi T, Ueda R (1993) MLL T3 gene on 9p22 involved in t(9;11) leukemia encodes a serine/proline rich protein homologous to MLL T1 on 19p13. Oncogene 8, 3085–3092
5. Nucifora G, Birn DJ, Erickson P, Gao J, Lebeau MM, Drabkin HA, Rowley JD (1993) Detection of DNA rearrangements in the AML1 and ETO loci and of an AML1/ETO fusion mRNA in patients with t(8;21) acute myeloid leukemia. Blood 81, 883–888
6. Liu P, Tarlé A, Hajra A, Claxton DF, Mariton P, Freedman M, Siciliano MJ, Collins FS (1993) Fusion between transcription factor CBFβ/PEBP2β and a myosin heavy chain in acute myeloid leukemia. Science 261, 1041–1044
7. Seabright M (1971) A rapid banding technique for human chromosomes. Lancet II, 971
8. Chomczynski P, Sacchi N (1987) Single-step method of RNA isolation by acid guanidinium thiocyanate-phenol-chloroform extraction. Anal Biochem 162, 156–159
9. Janssen JWG, Ludwig W-D, Borkhardt A, Spadinger U, Rieder H, Fonatsch C, Hossfeld DK, Harbott J, Schilz AS, Repp R, Sykora K-W, Hoelzer D, Bartram CR (1994) Pre-pre-B acute leukemia: High frequency of alternatively spliced ALL1-AF4 transcripts and absence of minimal residual disease during complete remission. Blood 84: 3835–3842
10. Yamamoto K, Seto M, Komatsu H, Iida S, Akao Y, Kojima S, Kodera Y, Nakazawa S, Ariyoshi Y, Takahashi T, Ueda R (1993) Two distinct portions of LTG19/ENL at 19p13 are involved in t(11;19) leukemia. Oncogene 8: 2617–2625
11. Maruyama F, Yang P, Stass SA, Cork A, Freireich EJ, Lee M-S, Chang K-S (1993) Detection of the AML1/ETO fusion transcript in the t(8;21) masked translocation in acute myelogenous leukemia. Cancer Res. 53, 4449–4451
12. Claxton DF, Liu P, Hsu HB, Marlton P, Hester J, Collins F, Deisseroth AB, Rowley JD, Siciliano MJ (1994) Detection of fusion transcripts generated by the inversion 16 chromosome in acute myelogenous leukemia. Blood 83, 1750–1756
13. ISCN (1991) Guideline for cancer cytogenetics, supplement to an International System for Human Cytogenetic Nomenclature. F. Mitelman (ed.); S. Karger, Basel
14. Ribeiro RC et Pui CH (1993) Prognostic factors in childhood acute lymphoblastic leukemia. Hematologic Pathology 7, 121–142
15. Radich JP, Kopecky KJ, Boldt DH, Head D, Slovak ML, Babu R, Kirk J, Lee A, Kessler P, Appelbaum F, Gehly G (1994) Detection of BCR-ABL fusion genes in adult acute lymphoblastic leukemia by the polymerase chain reaction. Leukemia 8, 1688–1695
16. Kantarjian HM, Talpaz M, Dhingra K, Estey E, Keating MJ, Ku S, Trujillo J, Huh Y, Stass S, Kurzrock R (1991) Significance of the p219 versus p195 molecular abnormalities in adults with Philadelphia chromosome-positive acute leukemia. Blood 78, 2411–2418

Acute Leukemias VI
Prognostic Factors
and Treatment Strategies
Büchner et al. (eds)

Detection of the Wilms Tumor Gene (wt-1) mRNA in Complete Remission of AML Frequently Precedes Relapse

J. Brieger, E. Weidmann, U. Maurer, P.S. Mitrou, D. Hoelzer, and L. Bergmann

Abstract. Leukemic blast cells taken from 83 patients with AML at time of diagnosis and 20 patients during follow-up in complete remission were examined for the expression of wt-1 mRNA. For this purpose blast cells were isolated from bone marrow or peripheral blood and total RNA was extracted. The wt-1 transcription was subsequently studied via RT-PCR. Mononuclear cells and bone marrow from healthy persons were used as controls. Wilms' tumor mRNA was detectable in 67 out of 83 cases of AML (81%). None of the 13 healthy controls expressed wt-1. After achieving cytological Complete Remission (CR) 14/20 patients studied lost wt-1 expression. In 7/8 patients in CR persistence or reappearance of wt-1 expression preceded relapse of the disease. Response to therapy and survival did not correlate with wt-1 mRNA expression in newly diagnosed AML before therapy. Our data show that expression of wt-1 mRNA is widely spread in AML and may be a useful marker for detection of minimal residual disease (MRD) in acute leukemia. The follow-up data strongly suggest that analysis of wt-1 gene expression via PCR in CR may be a sensitive technique for the early detection of relapse. Analysis of wt-1 expression accompanying routine bone marrow aspiration may be useful to define the quality of remission and early prediction of relapse of the disease. Its relevance to outcome, follow-up, and detection of MRD, however, as well as its potential role in the pathogenesis of acute leukemia, remain to be confirmed by ongoing studies.

Introduction

Early detection of relapse during complete remission (CR) from leukemia may be important for the initiation of appropriate therapy. Various translocations have been considered as genetic markers for different types of acute myelocytic leukemia (AML), but all have the disadvantage of only accompanying restricted groups of AML subtypes. Moreover, the sensitivity of the usual detection systems is not always satisfying [1, 2]. Therefore, we recently investigated the Wilms' tumor gene (wt-1) a proposed tumor suppressor gene [3, 4], as a molecular marker detectable with the sensitive PCR technique [5, 6]. The Wilm' tumor gene (wt-1) is generally expressed in the fetal kidneys, gonads, spleen, and in Wilms' tumor, a tumor of the kidneys. The gene encodes a zinc finger DNA binding protein that functions as a transcriptional suppressor of different growth and differentiation-related genes, such as insulin-like growth factor-2 (IGF-2) [7], platelet-derived growth factor α-chain (PGF)[8], and transforming growth factor β1[9]. Moreover, wt-1 is homologous to the early growth response genes 1 and 2 (EGRI,-2) [10–12] two other growth-related genes. Additionally, PGF gene expression can be upregulated by the wt-1 gene product [13]. Therefore, it seems likely that the mutated wt-1 gene product is involved in carcinogenesis [14, 15]. Recently the expression of wt-1 predominantly in blasts with immature phenotypes of the myeloid lineage has been demonstrated [16, 17].

Department of Internal Medicine, Division of Hematology and Oncology, Johann Wolfgang Goethe University, Frankfurt am Main, Germany

We initiated this study to evaluate the prognostic value of detecting the reappearance of wt-1 mRNA in CR from AML. For this purpose we analyzed wt-1 gene expression in untreated AML, in complete remission (CR), and in healthy persons. Patients with untreated AML expressed high levels of wt-1 mRNA, whereas wt-1 expression was undetectable or reduced in bone marrow cells of AML patients achieving CR. In several cases, relapse was preceded by reappearing and further increasing mRNA levels.

Materials and Methods

Samples

Blast cells from 83 patients with newly diagnosed AML, 20 AML patients in CR, and 13 healthy persons were analyzed for wt-1 mRNA expression. For this purpose bone marrow or peripheral blood mononuclear cells containing 35%–95% blast cells were recovered from heparinized bone marrow aspirated at time of diagnosis or heparinized peripheral blood. After density gradient sedimentation using Ficoll-Hypaque, the cells were washed twice with phosphate-buffered saline (PBS) and used for RNA extraction (Table 1).

Leukemias were classified using the morphological and cytochemical criteria of the French American-British (FAB) study group classification [18].

Table 1. Proportions of patients expressing wt-1 mRNA

	wt-1-positive patients	
	No.	%
AML de novo	57/70	81
AML secondary (MDS)	8/11	73
AML first relapse	2/2	100
FAB subtype		
M0	1/1	100
M1	5/5	100
M2	20/27	74
M3	5/5	100
M4	22/26	85
M5	5/9	56
M6	2/2	100
Age >60 years[a]	43/52	81
Age <60 years[a]	24/30	80

[a]Patients' median age: 51 years (range 21–75 years).

PCR and Southern Blot

Aliquots of 5 μg total RNA were reverse transcribed and used for amplification with wt-1 specific oligonucleotides, according to published sequences [19]. Amplification was performed as follows: 35 cycles starting with 5 min at 94°C before adding the enzyme. The cycles were initiated by denaturing the DNA at 94°C for 30 s, followed by an annealing reaction for 30 s at 64°C and extending at 72°C for 45 s. After the last cycle, we applied a final extension reaction at 72°C for 7 min. The amplification products (857 bp) were separated by electrophoresis and classified as not amplified (−) or weakly (+), moderately (++), or strongly amplified (+++), as described earlier [5, 6].

The specifity of amplification of representative samples was verified by chemoluminescent detection of the blotted and hybridized product according to the manufacturer's instructions (Tropix, Bedford, MA).

Results

Total mRNA from 83 patients with AML were analyzed by PCR for wt-1-specific transcripts. Mononuclear cells separated from healthy persons' bone marrow and peripheral blood were used as controls. None of the 13 healthy volunteers expressed detectable levels of wt-1 transcripts, whereas 67/83 (81%) of the studied AML samples expressed wt-1 (Table 1). No difference between de novo AML and AML after myelodysplastic syndrome could be determined (Table 1).

We correlated wt-1 expression at time of diagnosis and response to therapy. The achievement of CR was not related to the detection of wt-1 gene transcripts prior to treatment (Table 2).

Next, we studied the wt-1 expression during CR of patients who had been wt-1-positive before treatment. In 14 out of 20 cases evaluated, wt-1 mRNA was undetectable by ethidium bromide staining of the amplificates after achievement of CR. In three cases wt-1 expression was reduced and in two patients wt-1 disappeared after 3 months in CR. Only one patient had unaltered wt-1 m-RNA levels despite morphological and clinical CR. All patients in stable CR had very low or undetectable wt-1 mRNA levels, whereas seven of eight patients expressed wt-1 mRNA prior to morphologically detectable relapse or in partial remission. One of these

Table 2. Expression levels[a] of wt-1 mRNA in patients' blast cells in relation to FAB subtype and achievement of complete remission

	0	+	++	+++
CR, all	13/19 (68%)	9/19 (47%)	10/19 (53%)	16/22 (73%)
CR, de novo	12/18 (67%)	9/17 (53%)	8/15 (53%)	16/21 (76%)
Age (years)	52 (32–75)	45 (24–75)	52 (19–73)	49 (17–72)
FAB subtype				
M0		1		
M1	1	2	1	5
M2	7	6	4	6
M3		2	2	1
M4	6	5	5	4
M5	3	1	1	2
M6			1	
Undefined	1			3
MDS	1	1	5	
First relapse		1		1

[a]0 No expression, + weak, ++ moderate, and +++ strong expression MDS myelodysplastic syndrome

patients remained wt-1-positive in CR, but relapsed early. One other was wt-1-negative despite subsequent recurrence of disease (Table 3).

Discussion

In AML some chromosomal aberrations have been described as being related to prognosis. The most common abnormalities are a gain of chromosome 8 and a loss of chromosome 7, accounting for approximately 20% found in AML; other aberrations are rare, and most patients have a normal karyotype [20]. An important problem for the success of chemotherapy and autologous stem cell transplantation is the detection of minimal residual disease (MRD). The various chromosomal aberrations

Table 3. Course of wt-1 expression in CR

Patient	At diagnosis	After Chemotherapy	3 months	6 months	9 months	12 months	15 months	18 months	Present status
S.C.	+	0		0		0	0	0	CR
H.A.	+++	+	0	0	0	0	0	0	CR
E.R.	+	0		0	+	0	0	0	CR
B.G.	+	0	+	0		0			CR
T.J.	+++	+	0	0	0				CR
B.T.	++	0		0					CR
E.K.	+	+	0	0					CR
J.A.	++	0	0						CR
C.S.	++		0						CR
D.E.	+++	0							CR
G.E.	++	0							CR
M.F.	++	0							CR
V.H.	++	0	+++	+++					PR
H.A.	+++	0	0	0				+++	R
B.P.	+++	0	0	++	0	+++			R
M.P.	++	+	0		++	o			R
O.D.	+	+	++	+++					R
P.F.	+++	0	+	+					R
R.T.	+++	0	+++						R
J.G.	+++	0	+						R

PR, Partial remission; R, relapse.

may be used for detection of MRD on an individual basis, but they cannot generally be used as a common marker for AMLs as these various genetic markers occur only in a small proportion of AMLs.

As the Wilms' tumor gene (wt-1) is expressed in about 80% of AMLs, the present study was initiated to evaluate whether the detection of wt-1 mRNA may be helpful for the early detection of relapse in AML patients clinically in CR [5, 15, 16]. For this purpose we used a wt-1 RT-PCR assay earlier established and determined the incidence and strength of wt-1 expression in untreated AMLs and after achievement of CR [5, 6].

We found the expression of high levels of wt-1 mRNA to be associated with a higher CR rate of 76%, compared to 53% in patients with weak or moderate expression and 67% in those without detectable mRNA by PCR. However, the differences are not yet statistically significant (Table 2). Patient outcome was not related to the pretreatment wt-1 gene expression level, and so far there has been no difference in the probability of overall survival and disease-free survival in correlation to the mRNA levels in our series [6]. This is not surprising, because wt-1 seems to be a marker for malignant activity of the tumor, and in CR few leukemic blasts are present and active. Thus, the pretreatment activity—indicated by wt-1—is not necessarily related to the posttreatment expression of wt-1. However, it should be pointed out that the quantitation of PCR products is only semiquantitative and, therefore, has to be interpreted cautiously.

For the follow-up, wt-1 expression may be useful for early prediction of relapse. In 14/20 patients evaluable so far, the wt-1 signal disappeared immediately after achieving CR. The significance of persistance or intermittent reappearance of low levels wt-1 in CR for long-term remission is not yet defined. Here, prospective controlled trials are required to define the clinical relevance of these observations, especially, whether minimal residual blasts may be eliminated by autologous antileukemic activities [21, 22]. The reoccurrence of wt-1 expression, however, is highly associated with a following relapse. In our study. Meanwhile, seven out of eight patients in CR relapsed morphologically 3-6 months after reappearence of wt-1 transcripts.

In conclusion, the reported data strongly suggest wt-1 to be a useful marker for detection of MRD in acute leukemias. Analysis of wt-1 expression accompanying routine bone marrow aspiration may be useful to define the quality of remission and for early prediction of relapse of the disease. Its relevance to outcome, follow-up, and detection of MRD in autologous stem cell transplantation has still to be evaluated by ongoing studies, as does its potential role in the pathogenesis of acute leukemias.

Acknowledgments. Supported in part by the Deutsche Krebshilfe, grant w22/92.Be-1 and by the Adolf Messer Stiftung.

References

1. Maseki N, Miyoshi H, Shimizu K, Homma C, Ohki M, Sakurai M, Kaneko Y. The 8;21 chromosome translocation in acute myeloid leukemia is always detectable by molecular analysis using AML1. Blood 1993; 81: 1573-1579.
2. van Dongen JJM, Breit TM, Adriaansen HJ, Beishuizen A, Hooijkaas H. Detection of minimal residual disease in acute leukemia by immunological marker analysis and polymerase chain reaction. Leukemia 1992; Suppl 1: 47-59.
3. Call KM, Glaser T, Ito CY, Buckler AJ, Pelletier J, Haber DA, Rose EA, Kral A, Yeger H, Lewis WH, Jones C, Housman DE. Isolation and characterization of a zinc finger polypeptide gene at the human chromosome 11 Wilms' tumor locus. Cell 1990; 60: 509-520.
4. Gessler M, Poustka A, Cavenee W, Neve RL, Orkin SH, Bruns GAP. Homozygous deletion in Wilms' tumor of a zinc-finger gene identified by chromosome jumping. Nature 1990; 343: 774-778.
5. Brieger J., Weidmann E., Fenchel K., Mitrou P.S., Hoelzer D., Bergmann L: The expression of the Wilms' tumor gene in acute myelocytic leukemias as a possible marker for leukemic blast cells. Leukemia 1994; 8: 2138-2143.
6. Brieger J., Bergmann L., Weidmann E., Maurer U., Hoelzer D., Mitrou P.S.: The Wilms' tumor gene (WT-1) is frequently expressed in acute leukemias and may provide sensitive detection of residual blast cells by PCR. Ann. Oncol. (1995), in press
7. Drummond IA, Madden SL, Rohwer-Nutter P, Bell GI, Sukhatme VP, Rauscher FJ 3d. Repression of the insulin-like growth factor II gene by the Wilms' tumor suppressor wt-1. Science 1992; 257: 674-678.
8. Gashler AL, Bonthron DT, Madden SL, Rauscher FJ 3d, Collins T, Sukhatme VP. Human platelet-derived growth factor A chain is transcriptionally repressed by the Wilms tumor suppressor WT1. PNAS 1992; 89: 10984-10988.
9. Dey BR, Sukhatme VP, Roberts AB, Sporn MB, Rauscher FJ, KIM SJ: Repression of the transforming growth factor-beta 1 gene by the Wilms' tumor

suppressor WT1 gene product. Mol Endocrinol 1994; 8: 595–602.
10. Sukhatme VP, Cao X, Chang LC, Tasi-Moris C-H, Stamenkovich D, Ferreira PCP, Cohen DR, Edwards SA, Shows TB, Curran T, Le Beau MM, Adamson ED. A zinc finger-encoding gene coregulated with c-fos during growth and differentiation, and after cellular depolarization. Cell 1988; 53: 37–43.
11. Joseph LJ, Le Beau MM, Jamieson GA, Acharys S, Shows TB, Rowley JD, Sukhatme VP. Molecular cloning, sequencing, and mapping of EGR2, a human early growth response gene encoding a protein with 'zinc-binding finger' structure. PNAS 1988; 85: 7164–7168.
12. Madden SL, Cook DM, Morris JF, Gashler A, Sukhatme VP, Rauscher FJ III. Transcriptional repression mediated by the WT-1 Wilms' tumor gene product. Science 1991; 253: 1550–1553.
13. Wang ZY, Qiu QQ, Deuel TF. The Wilms' tumor gene product wt-1 activates or suppresses transcription through separate functional domains. J Biol Chem 1993; 268(13): 9172–9175.
14. Haber DA, Buckler AJ, Glaser T, Call KM, Pelletier J, Sohn RL, Douglass EC, Housman DE. An internal deletion within an 11p13 zinc finger gene contributes to the development of Wilms' tumor. Cell 1990; 61: 1257–1269.
15. Coppes MJ, Liefers GJ, Paul P, Yeger H, Williams BR. Homozygous somatic wt-1 point mutations in sporadic unilateral Wilms tumor. PNAS 1993; 90: 1416–1419.
16. Miwa H, Beran M, Saunders GF. Expression of the Wilms' tumor gene (wt-1) in human leukemias. Leukemia 1992; 6: 405-409.
17. Tatsushi M, Ahuja H, Kubota T, Kubonishi I, Koeffler HP, Miyoshi I. Expression of the Wilms' tumor gene, wt-1, in human leukemia cells. Leukemia 1993; 7: 970–977.
18. Bennet JM, Catovsky D, Daniel MT, Flandrin G, Galton DAG, Gralnick HR, Sultan C. Proposed revised criteria for the classification of acute myeloid leukemia. A report of the French-American-British Cooperative Group. Br J Haematol 1976; 33: 451–458.
19. Brenner B, Wildhardt G, Schneider S, Royer-Pokora B. RNA polymerase chain reaction detects different levels of four alternatively spliced wt-1 transcripts in Wilms' tumors. Oncogene 1992; 7: 1431–1433.
20. Lukens JN. Classification and differentiation of the acute leukemias. In Clinical Hematology (Lee GR, Bithell TC, Foerster J, Athens JW, Lukens JN; eds) Lea & F ebiger, Philadelphia, 1993, pp 1873–1919.
21. Bergmann L., Heil G., Kolbe K., Lengfelder E., Puzicha E., Martin H., Lohmeyer J., Mitrou P.S., Hoelzer D.: Interleukin-2 bolus infusion as late consolidation therapy in 2nd remission of acute myelocytic leukemia. Leuk. Lymphoma 1995, 16: 271–279.
22. Jahn B., Bergmann L., Weidmann E., Brieger J., Fenchel K., Schwulera U., Hoelzer D., Mitrou P.S.. Bone marrow derived T cell clones of previously untreated acute myelocytic leukemia exhibit blast directed autologous cytotoxicity. Leuk Res 1995, 19: 73–82.

Acute Leukemias VI
Prognostic Factors
and Treatment Strategies
Büchner et al. (eds)

CBFβ/MYH11 Rearrangement in M4Eo with Inversion 16: A Novel Marker for Diagnosis of Minimal Residual Disease by RT-PCR

E. Koller[1], M. Pfeilstöcker[1], B. Pavlova[1], H. Mühlberger[1], H. Nowotny[1], H. Kasparu[2], R. Heinz[1], E. Pittermann[1], and H. Karlic[1]

Abstract. The inversion of chromosome 16(p13-q22) is a characteristic cytogenetic marker for acute myelogenous leukemia subtype M4Eo. Recently the fusion gene product of this pericentric translocation was characterized. The CBFβ gene is translocated from 16q in the region of MYH11, a smooth muscle gene on the short arm of chromosome 16. This may result in altered regulation of transcription and subsequent leukemic transformation. We wanted to evaluate the potential of this rearrangement as a new target for minimal residual disease (MRD) diagnosis, which is routinely carried out by RT-PCR. BM and PB samples from six patients with M4Eo were analyzed at diagnosis, in clinical remission, and during relapse. The detection of inv(16) always correlated with a CBFβ/MYH11 rearrangement. Five patients showed a type A transcript and one patient a type B fusion. PCR negativity in remission was observed in one patient who has been relapse-free for more than 20 months. Samples from three other patients investigated in clinical and cytogenetic remision remained PCR-positive; two of them have relapsed so far. We conclude that the CBFβ/MYH11 rearrangement is highly sensitive, and residual leukemia can be detected during remission. The value of for MRD evaluation needs confirmation in a larger study of prospectively analyzed patients.

Introduction

The inversion of chromosome 16(p13q22) is the characteristic marker for acute myelogenous leukemia subtype M4Eo. Recently the fusion gene product of this translocation was characterized on the molecular level [1]. It has been shown that CBFβ/PEBP2β, a gene encoded at 16q22, is translocated to the region of MYH11, a smooth muscle gene, encoded at 16p13. The joining of a transcription factor with a housekeeping gene may result in altered regulation and subsequent leukemic transformation in these patients. We present data from RT-PCR analyses of chimeric transcripts consisting of upstream CBFβ fused to downstream MYH11 which present a novel diagnostic target for refined definition and minimal residual disease (MRD) evaluation of M4Eo [2].

Material and Methods

Cytogenetic analyses using the tristaining technique for simultaneous detection of R- and C- bands [3] and preparation of mRNA and cDNA using a commercially available system (Pharmacia) were performed during routine investigations according to institutional guidelines. PCR protocols were carried out as previously described using reagents from Boehringer Mannheim and a Techne PHC3 PCR processor

[1]Ludwig Boltzmann Institute for Leukemia Research and Hematology, Hanusch Hospital, Pav.4/4, Heinrich Collinstrasse 30, A-1140 Vienna, Austria
[2]Krankenhans Elisabethinen, Linz, Austria

Table 1. Patient data

Patient	Age/Sex	Karyotype	Status	Material	Date	PCR	Transcript type
F.J.	19/M	46,XY, inv(16)	Diagnosis	BM	14 Apr 93	+	A
			CR	PB+BM	4 Mar 93-		
B.J.	39/M	46,XY, inv(16)	Diagnosis	BM	3 Jan 92	+	B
			First CR	BM buffy	9 Sep 92	+/−	
			Second CR	PB	4 Mar 94	+	
R.A.	25/M	46,XY, inv(16)	Diagnosis	BM	18 Aug 89	+	A
			First CR	PSC	18 Nov 89	+	
			Second CR	BM buffy	23 Apr 90	+	
S.F.	46/M	46,XY, inv(16),+8	Relapse	PB	22 Feb 94	+	A
R.T.	66/F	46,XX, t(4; 17), inv(16), del(20q)	Diagnosis	BM	10 June 94	+	A
			PR	BM	26 July 94	+	
S.M.	44/F	46,XX, inv(16)	Relapse	BM	3 May 94	+	A
			Second CR	PB	14 June 94	+	

CR, Complete remission; PR, partial remission; BM, bone marrow; PB, peripheral blood.

[2, 4]. Aliquots of PCR products were sequenced on an Applied Biosciences Inc. automated sequencer.

Results and Discussion

At the time of diagnosis or relapse, detection of inv(16) correlated with a rearrangement of CBFβ/MYH11 in all six cases (see Table 1). Seven cases had a type A transcript, which has been shown to occur in the majority of patients reported so far [2]. One patient had a type B fusion. Five of our patients could be monitored during clinical and cytogenetic remission. In two cases enriched stem cells from BM or PB could be evaluated in addition. To date one patient with a negative RT-PCR result after chemotherapy has been in continuous complete remission for more than 20 months. Samples of three other patients investigated in remission remained PCR-positive at the MRD level (1 leukemic cell in 10^5 cells); two of them have relapsed so far. Our data confirm current observations by showing that RT-PCR is highly sensitive for the detection of leukemic cells during morphological and cytogenetic remission in M4Eo [2]. The CBFβ/MYH11 rearrangement may widen the panel of MRD markers in acute leukemia, but prospective studies in a larger number of patients are needed for confirmation.

References

1. Liu P, Tarl, SA, Hajra A, Claxton DF, Marlton P, Freedman M, Siciliano MJ, Collins FS. Fusion between transcription factor CBFβ/PEBP2β and a myosin heavy chain in acute myeloid leukemia. Science 1993; 261: 1041–1044.
2. Claxton DF, Liu P, Hsu HB, Marlton P, Hester J, Collins F, Deisseroth AB, Rowley JD, Siciliano MJ. Detection of fusion transcripts generated by the inversion 16 chromosome in acute myelogenous leukemia. Blood 1994; 83: 1750–1756.
3. Schweizer D. Counterstain enhanced chromosome banding. Hum Genet 1981; 57: 307–324.
4. Karlic H, Pavlova B, Koller E. Detection of CBFβ/MYH11 mRNA in bone marrow smears. Leukemia 1995 in press.

Acute Leukemias VI
Prognostic Factors
and Treatment Strategies
Büchner et al. (eds)

Detection of Minimal Residual Disease on Bone Marrow Smears by Reverse Transcriptase Polymerase Chain Reaction

R. Schoch[1], P. Schafhausen[1], S. Jenisch[2], T. Haferlach[1], W. Müller-Ruchholtz[2], W. Gassmann[1], and H. Löffler[1]

Abstract. The polymerase chain reaction (PCR) is now often used for the identification of the three most common chromosomal aberrations, t(8; 21), t(15; 17) and inv(16), in adult AML, which account for 30%–40% of chromosomal aberrations in de novo AML. In addition, the high sensitivity of this technique has provided a way to detect residual leukaemia at previously unobtainable levels. For primary diagnosis one bone marrow aspirate smear is sufficient for the reverse transcriptase (RT) PCR assay. This source has the advantage that no special handling and transport of the specimen is necessary. The aim of the present study was to detect minimal residual disease on bone marrow smears and to compare the results with the detection of the fusion transcript in bone marrow aspirates. In 21 patients with AML or ALL in complete clinical and haematological remission (7 Patients with t(15; 17), 4 Patients with t(8; 21), 7 Patients with inv(16) and 3 Patients with t(9; 22)) bone marrow smears as well as 3 ml bone marrow aspirate were investigated. The normal gene could be detected from the glass slide smear and the bone marrow aspirate in every case. The specific translocation as a marker for minimal residual disease was observed in 10 of the 21 cases from the bone marrow smear. In the control with the bone marrow aspirate the specific translocation was detectable in only 7 of these 10 cases. These results demonstrate that bone marrow smears are a suitable source for RT-PCR-based detection of minimal residual disease. Further studies should evaluate this possibility.

Introduction

Molecular analysis of chromosomal aberrations has become widespread in the diagnosis of haematopoietic malignancies. RT-PCR assays have been developed for the three most common chromosomal abnormalities in AML, translocations (8; 21) [1–8] and (15; 17) [9, 10] and inversion (16) [11, 12], defining subgroups with a good response to chemotherapy and a good prognosis. In ALL the PCR-based identification of the Philadelphia chromosome [t(9; 22)] is well established [13–15]. For the detection of these chromosomal aberrations, one bone marrow glass slide smear is a sufficient source [16–19].

In this study we compare bone marrow slide smears as a source for the detection of minimal residual disease with the standard procedures. We used a method for dissolving RNA directly on the glass slide and adapted the procedure to safely avoid cross contaminations between the samples [18].

Material And Methods

Patients and Samples

Bone marrow aspirates and bone marrow smears were obtained from 21 patients with

[1]Department of Internal Medicine II, Christian Albrecht University of Kiel, Kiel, Germany
[2]Department of Immunology, Christian Albrecht University of Kiel, Kiel, Germany

AML or ALL in complete clinical and haematological remission. At primary diagnosis seven patients were classified according to the FAB classification as FAB M_3 with t(15; 17), four as FAB M_2 with t(8; 21), seven as FAB M_{4eo} with inversion (16) and three had Philadelphia-chromosome-positive ALL. In every case 3 ml bone marrow aspirate and one unstained bone marrow smear were investigated.

RNA Preparation

The bone marrow aspirate was isolated on Ficoll-Hypaque. The RNA was extracted from the mononuclear cell fraction with a buffer containing guanidinium thiocyanate and phenol (RNAzol), followed by chloroform purification [20]. From the bone marrow smear RNA was dissolved directly on the glass slides with the described RNAzol buffer [18]. For both sources the RNA pellet was precipitated once in isopropanolol and a second time in ethanol and afterwards dissolved in 15 µl DEPC-treated water. The first-strand cDNA synthesis was carried out with 7 µl of the RNA solution with AMV-reverse transcriptase (cDNA-Kit Serva) using random primers in a total reaction volume of 15 µl. The reaction was performed for 45 min at 42°C.

PCR Amplification

PCR was performed with 1 µl of the cDNA product. In every case a single-step PCR of the ß-Actin gene was performed as a control for satisfactory sample cDNA. For t(15; 17) an amplification of the RARα gene was used additionally. The RARα gene and the PML-RARα fusion gene were amplified with primers as published [9]. For t(8; 21) the AML gene as a control and the AML-ETO fusion gene were used [1,21]. The CBFß-MYH11 fusion transcript, the counterpart of the inv(16), was detected with the primers published in [11]. For t(9; 22) the c-ABL gene and the BCR-ABL fusion gene were amplified as described [13]. PCR was performed with *Taq*-polymerase (Boehringer, Mannheim) in a total reaction volume of 20 µl at standard conditions with an annealing temperature between 50°C and 60°C, depending on the primers used. The PCR product was diluted 1: 100 in water and 1 µl of this solution was used for a second step of amplification with a second set of primers. The PCR products of the first and second steps were run on a 1.5% agarose gel, stained with ethidium bromide and visualised under UV light. Numerous precautions were taken to avoid contaminations [22].

Table 1. Detection of minimal residual leukaemia by RT-PCR in 21 patients with AML or ALL in complete clinical and haematological remission

Patient	Age (years)	FAB subtype	Bone marrow aspirate	Bone marrow smear
T. A.	61	AML M3	+	+
J. T.	25	AML M3	o	o
R. H.	34	AML M3	o	o
A. M.	33	AML M3	o	o
K. E.	38	AML M3	o	o
A. U.	66	AML M3	o	+
A. M.	47	AMLM3	o	o
P. L.	18	AML M2	o	o
L. M.	29	AML M2	o	o
H. B.	66	AML M2	+	+
B. R.	29	AML M2	o	o
M. H.	60	AML M_{4eo}	+	+
S. G.	22	AML M_{4eo}	+	+
		After BMT	o	o
S. A.	28	AML M_{4eo}	o	o
T. S.	5o	AML M_{4eo}	o	+
H. U.	45	AML M_{4eo}	o	o
S. A.	41	AML M_{4eo}	o	+
H. A	31	AML M_{4eo}	o	o

+, Correct amplification, o, no amplification product.

Results

In every case the β-Actin gene was detected as a control of intact RNA from the bone marrow aspirate and the bone marrow smear (Table 1). In the first group, consisting of seven patients with t(15; 17) at primary diagnosis, the RARα gene was detected in every sample. In one case the PML/RARα fusion transcript was amplified in the bone marrow aspirate and the bone marrow smear. Interestingly, the second case showed the fusion gene in the material obtained from the bone marrow smear only; the bone marrow aspirate was PCR-negative in this case. In all other patients, there was no PML-RARα fusion transcript amplification in the bone marrow aspirates or in the bone marrow smears.

In the second group, consisting of four patients t(8; 21), the aspirate and smear results were completely concordant: the AML/ETO fusion gene was found in while, in one case, both sources the three remaining cases showed no AML-ETO fusion gene.

In four patients with inv(16) minimal residual leukaemia was detected. In each case the CBFβ/MYH11 fusion transcript was amplified from the bone marrow smear. In only two of these cases was the fusion gene detectable from the bone marrow aspirate. One patient was PCR-negative in both sources after allogeneic bone marrow transplantation.

In all three cases of ALL the BCR-ABL fusion gene was detected concordantly from both sources. In one case no BCR/ABL fusion transcript was visible after allogeneic bone marrow transplantation.

Discussion

RT-PCR-based assays for a translocation-specific fusion message can be used as a disease-specific marker in patients with cytogenetic aberrations. In AML t(15; 17)(q22; q11-22) [9,23], t(8; 21)(q22;q22) [1,3-6,8], t(9,11) (p21-22; q23) [24], t(6; 9)(p23; q34) [25] and inv(16)(p13; q22) [11,12] can be detected by PCR-based analysis. These techniques allow detection of minimal residual disease at previously unobtained levels. Protocols for collection and processing of the samples for this approach have not yet been standardised [10, 26]. Usually 3-5 ml bone marrow aspirate are used. For primary diagnosis sufficient material can be obtained from one smear of a bone marrow aspirate or of peripheral blood [17-19]. In this study we investigated the possibility of detecting minimal residual disease using material obtained from unstained glass slide smears of bone marrow aspirates. Two sources for the detection of minimal residual disease were therefore compared: one unstained bone marrow smear and, according to the usual protocols, 3 ml bone marrow aspirate. In the method, developed the dried bone marrow aspirate was directly dissolved on the glass slide. The advantage of this procedure, compared to other protocols in which the material is scraped from the glass slide, is that it safely avoids cross-contaminations between the samples and minimises the loss of material [16-18].

In this small study we were able to demonstrate that material obtained from bone marrow smears gives comparable or even better results than bone marrow aspirates in the detection of residual leukaemia. Because of the small number of patients investigated, it is not yet possible to say if glass slide smears are a suitable source in every case. Smears could be an interesting alternative as a sample and would have several advantages over bone marrow aspirates: For one thing, the collecting and processing of the samples is much easier. It is not yet clear why glass slide smears are such an extraordinarily good source for PCR-based investigations. One explanation may be that the rapid inhibition of enzymes due to air drying on the glass slide prevents the RNA from degradation.

References

1. Nucifora G, Birn DJ, Erickson P, Gao J, LeBeau MM, Drabkin HA, Rowley JD (1993) Detection of DNA rearrangements in the AML1 and ETO loci and of an AML1/ETO fusion mRNA in patients with t(8; 21) acute myeloid leukemia. Blood 81: 883-888
2. Nisson PE, Watkins PC, Sacchi N (1992) Transcriptionally active chimeric gene derived from the fusion of the AML1 gene and a novel gene on chromosome 8 in t(8; 21) leukemic cells. Cancer Genet Cytogenet 63: 81-88
3. Nucifora G, Larson RA, Rowley JD (1993) Persistence of the 8; 21 translocation in patients with acute myeloid leukemia type M2 in long-term remission, Blood 82: 712-715
4. Downing JR, Head DR, Curcio-Brint AM, Hulshof MG, Motroni TA, Raimondi SC, Caroll AJ, Drabkin

HA, Willman C, Theli KS, Civin CI, Erickson P (1993) An AML1/ETO fusion transcript is consistently detected by RNA-based polymerase chain reaction in acute myelogenous leukemia containing the t(8; 21)(q22; q22) translocation. Blood 81: 2860–2865
5. Nucifora G, Dickstein JI, Torbenson V, Roulston D, Rowley JD (1994) Correlation between cell morphology and expression of the AML1/ETO chimeric transcript in patients with acute myeloid leukemia without the t(8;21). Leukemia 8: 1533–1538
6. Kwong YL, Chan V, Wong KF, Chan TK (1995) Use of the polymerase chain reaction in the detection of AML1/ETO fusion transcript in t(8; 21). Cancer 75: 821–825
7. Chang KS, Fan YH, Stass SA, Estey EH, Wang G, Trujillo JM, Erickson P, Drabkin HA (1993) Expression of AML-ETO fusion transcripts and detection of minimal residual disease in t(8; 21)-positive acute myeloid leukemia. Oncogene 8: 983–988
8. Kusec R, Laczika K, Knöbl P, Friedl J, Greinix H, Kahls P, Linkesch W, Schwarzinger I, Mitterbauer G, Purtscher B, Haas OA, Lechner K, Jaeger U (1994) AML1/ETO fusion mRNA can be detected in remission blood samples of all patients with t(8; 21) acute myeloid leukemia after chemotherapy or autologous bone marrow transplantation. Leukemia 8: 735–739
9. Biondi A, Rambaldi A, Pandolfi PP, Rossi V, Giudici G, Alcalay M,Lo Coco F,Diverio D, Pogliani EM, Lanzi EM, Mandelli F, Masera G, Barbui T, Pelicci PG (1992) Molecular monitoring of the myl/retinoic acid receptor-a fusion gene in acute promyelocytic by polymerase chain reaction. Blood 80: 492–497
10. Campana D, Pui CH (1995) Detection of minimal residual disease in acute leukemia: Methodologic advances and clinical significance. Blood 85: 1416–1434
11. Claxton DF, Liu P, Hsu HB, Marlton P, Hester J, Collins F, Deisseroth AB, Rowley JD, Siciliano MJ (1994) Detection of fusion transcripts generated by the inversion 16 chromosome in acute myelogenous leukemia. Blood 83: 1750–1756
12. Poirel H, Radford-Weiss I, Rack K, Troussard X, Veil A, Valensi F, Picard F, Guesnu M, Leboeuf D, Melle J, Dreyfus F, Flandrin G, Macintyre E (1995) Detection of the chromosome 16 CBFb-MYHll fusion transcript in myelomonocytic leukemias. Blood 85: 1313–1322
13. Maurer J, Janssen JWG, Thiel E, Van Denderen J, Ludwig WD, Aydemir Ü, Heinze B, Fonatsch C, Harbott J, Reiter A, Riehm H, Hoelzer D, Bartram CR (1991) Detection of BCR/ABL genes in acute lymphoblastic leukemia by polymerase chain reaction. Lancer 337: 1055–1058
14. Kawasaki ES, Clark SS, Coyne MY, Smith SD, Champlin R, Witte ON, McCormick FP (1988) Diagnosis of chronic myeloid and acute lymphatic leukemias by detection of leukemias specific mRNA sequences amplified in vitro. Proc Natl Acad Sci USA 58: 5698
15. Radich JP, Kopecky KJ, Boldt DH, Head D, Slovak ML, Babu R, Kirk J, Lee A, Kessler P, Appelbaum F (1994) Detection of BCR/ABL fusion genes in adult acute lymphoblastic leukemia by the polymerase chain reaction. Leukemia 8: 1688–1195
16. de Melo MB, Sales TSI, Lorand-Metze I, Costa FF (1992) Rapid method for isolation of DNA from glass slide smears for PCR. Acta Haematol 87: 214–215
17. Hanson CA, Holbrook EA, Sheldon S, Schnitzer B, Roth MS (1990) Detection of Philadelphia chromosome-positive cells from glass slide smears using the polymerase chain reaction. Am J Pathol 137: 1–6
18. Schoch R, Jenisch S, Haferlach T, et al: (1994) Detection of Philadelphia chromosome on stained smears of peripheral blood by reverse transcripptase polymerase chain reaction (RT-PCR). Onkologie 17 (Suppl 2): 133 (Abstract)
19. Yamashita S, Umemura T, Sadamura S, Yufu Y, Nishimura J, Natawa H (1994) Detection of bcr/abl in mRNA in in stained bone marrow smears. Leukemia 8: 1409–1410
20. Chomczynski P, Sacchi N (1987) Single step method of RNA isolation by acid guanidinium thiocyanate-phenol-chloroform extraction. Anal Biochem 162: 156–159
21. Kozu T, Miyoshi H, Shimizu K, Maseki N, Kanekok Y, Asou H, Kanada N, Ohki M (1993) Junctions of the AMLI/MTG8(ETO) fusion are constant in t(8; 21) acute myeloid leukemia detected by reverse transcriptase polymerase chain reaction. Blood 82: 1270–1276
22. Kwok S, Higuchi R (1989) Avoiding false positives with PCR. Nature 339: 2377–238
23. Miller WH, Jr, Levine K, DeBlasio A, Frankel SR, Dmitrovsky E, Warrell RP, Jr (1993) Detection of minimal residual disease in acute promyelocytic leukemia by a reverse transcriptase chain reaction assay for the PML/RAR-a fusion mRNA. Blood 82: 1689–1694
24. Yamamoto K, Seto M, lida D, Komatsu H, Kojima S, Kodera Y, Nakazawa S, Sito H, Takahashi T, Ueda R (1994) A reverse transcriptase polymerase chain reaction detects heterogenous chimeric mRNA in leukemias with 11q23 abnormalities. Blood 83: 2912
25. Soekarman D, von Lindern M, Daenen S, de Jong B, Fpnatsch C, Heinze B, Bartram C, Hagemeijer A, Grosveld G (1992) The translocation (6;9) (p23; q34) shows consistent rearrangements of two genes and defines a myeloproliferative disorder with specific clinical features. Blood 79: 2990–2997
26. Lin F, Goldman JM, Cross NCP (1994) A comparison of the sensitivity of blood and bone marrow for the detection of minimal residual disease in chronic myeloid leukemia. Br J Haematol 86: 683–68

Acute Leukemias VI
Prognostic Factors
and Treatment Strategies
Büchner et al. (eds)

Evaluation of Chimerism After Allogeneic Bone Marrow Transplantation Using Amplification of Hypervariable Regions of Human Genome by Polymerase Chain Reaction

I.A. Demidova, V.L. Surin, V.G. Savchenko, O.V. Smirnova, L.S. Lubimova, and L.P. Mendeleeva

Abstract. We used the polymerase chain reaction (PCR) as a novel and sensitive technique to evaluate posttransplant chimerism. Tandemly repetitive core sequences of regions with a variable number of tandem repeats (VNTR) served as genetic markers. Polymorphism of such loci results from allelic differences in the number of repeats. Primers flanking the repeat region of each of the corresponding VNTRs were used for amplification. Recipient and donor pretransplant DNA were amplified. The resultant fragments were analyzed after gel electrophoresis. Evaluation of four available cases indicated complete chimerism in three cases and mixed chimerism in one. The sensitivity of the method was determined by mixing various proportions of recipient and donor DNA; the limit of detection of the minor component in a mixture was 1%. PCR amplification of VNTR has advantages over other methods such as red blood cell phenotyping: high sensitivity, use of small amounts of blood or bone marrow, and the ability for early detection of posttransplant engraftment.

Introduction

Hypervariable regions (HVR) of human genome or regions with a variable number of tandem repeats (VNTR) can be used as highly polymorphic markers in human genome investigations. VNTRs can be characterized as highly polymorphic regions of human DNA consisting of tandemly repeated core sequences. The number of copies is variable and results from allelic differences in the number of repeats. These markers are inherited in a mendelian fashion and can be very informative when a locus has multiple alleles. These multiallele polymorphisms can be successfully used for the identification of DNA of different persons.

The recent development of DNA amplification based on polymerase chain reaction (PCR) has provided a powerful tool for analysis of human polymorphisms in many settings including the monitoring of engraftment in patients after allogeneic bone marrow transplanation (BMT) [1, 2]. This method is ideal for evaluating hematopoietic chimerism after allogeneic BMT between sibling pairs because several polymorphic loci can be analyzed, giving a high probability of having at least one informative locus.

Another advantage of the PCR method is its high sensitivity. It permits evaluation of a minor cell populations of DNA of donor or recipient origin, such as 1%.

The main goal of our study was to determine the genetic marker to distinguish donor and recipient cell populations and to provide longtime follow-up of engraftment dynamics after BMT.

Materials and Methods

Patients

Eight patients who underwent BMT for acute leukemia from histocompatible siblings at the

National Research Centre for Hematology, Moscow, Russia

National Research Centre for Hematology, Moscow, were investigated. Only these who survived for more than 90 days after BMT were included in the study. The conditioning regimens consisted of cyclophosphamide 120 mg/kg and total body irradiation 12 Gy in six fractions or cyclophosphamide and busulfan 16 mg/kg. Posttransplant bone marrow or peripheral blood were obtained on days +30, +60, +90 and every 3rd month after BMT during the 1st year. The longest period of observation was 3 years after BMT.

Isolation of Genomic DNA and PCR Amplification of VNTRs

High-molecular-weight DNA was extracted from blood or bone marrow as previously described [3]. In one case DNA was extracted from the patient, granulocytes isolated by Ficoll density centrifugation (this patient was treated by donor lymphocyte transfusions for posttransplant relapse). For our study we selected the following three VNTR regions: apolipoprotein B 3'hypervariable region (Apo B), DXS52 locus of X chromosome (DXS52), and VNTR in intron 40 of von Willebrand factor gene (vWF). The primers were synthesized and all reactions were performed according to methods previously described [3,7]. After amplification PCR products were separated by electrophoresis in 6%–12% polyacrylamide gel and tested under UV light after ethidium bromide staining.

Results

We tested donor/recipient eight pairs in order to evaluate marrow engraftment after BMT. Informative differences were found for four donor/recipient pairs. The others were non-informative. The results observed are usual for BMT when the donors and recipients are siblings and the number of the markers tested are less than 5.

The observed heterozygosity of the selected loci is shown in (Figs. 1, 2.)

The sensitivity of the method was determined using previous experiments by mixing of different proportions of recipient and donor DNA. The limit of detection of the minor component in a mixture was 1% (without using radiolabeling). The results are shown in (Fig. 3.)

Evaluating the results we used the following terms:

1) Complete chimera: only donor-type genetic markers detected in post-BMT samples
2) Mixed chimera: genetic markers of both donor and recipient detected

Evaluation of four available cases indicated three cases of complete chimerism. Two cases were detected using the ApoB genetic marker, one case using DXS52 (Figs. 4, 5). In all these cases the patients were in complete remission according to clinical and routine laboratory data.

In the case of mixed chimerism (Fig. 6) we detected both donor and recipient DNA from day +28 after BMT. On day +90 this patient

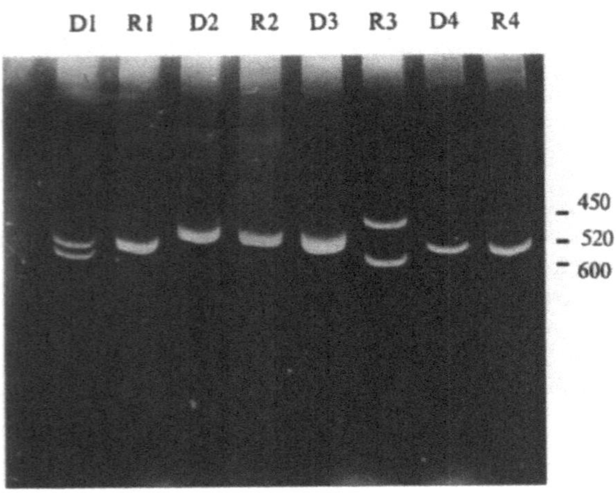

Fig. 1. Pre-BMT screening of four donor/recipient pairs by the PCR-VNTR method. Each lane contains the amplified DNA products using primers for ApoB Paris 1 and 3 are informative

Fig. 2. Analysis of amplified DNA products for four donor/recipient pairs using primers for the vWF locus

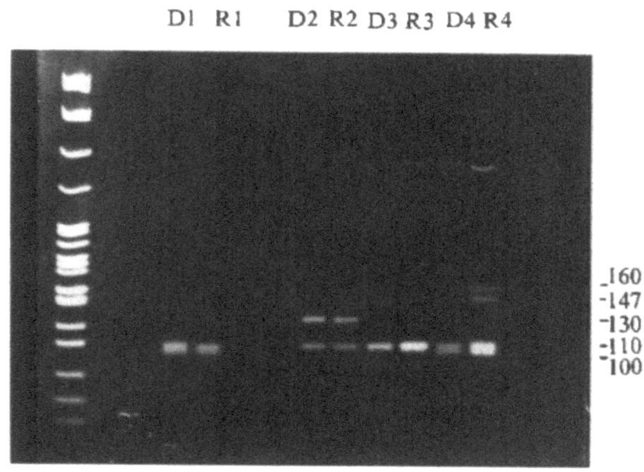

Fig. 3. Sensitivity of the PCR approach. The respective proportions of donor and recipient DNA are 20: 1, 50: 1, 100: 1 and 200: 1

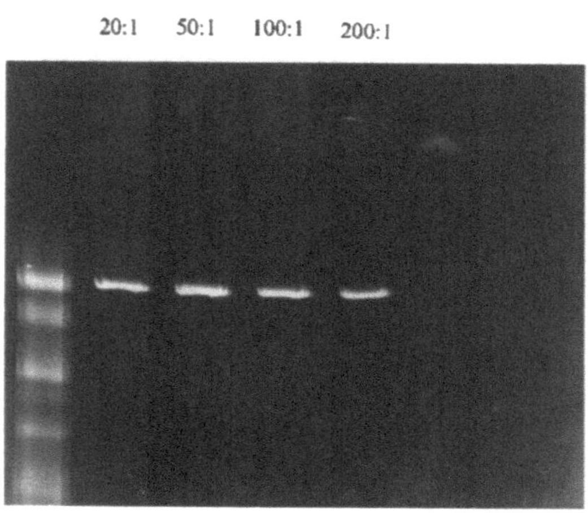

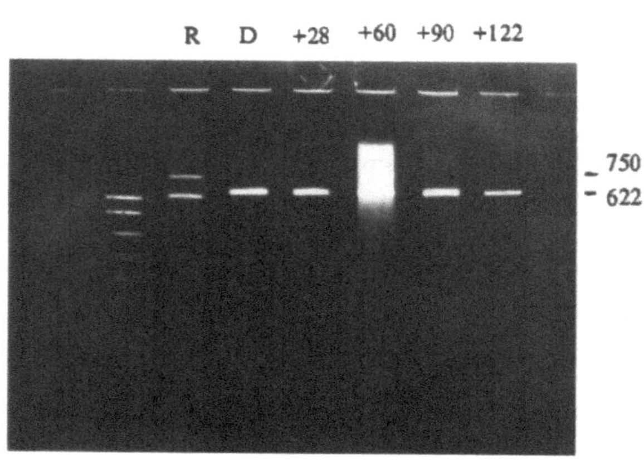

Fig. 4. A case of complete chimerism. DNA from recipient, donor and posttransplant DNA was amplified using ApoB primers. From day +28 after transplantation, only donor-specific fragment can be identified

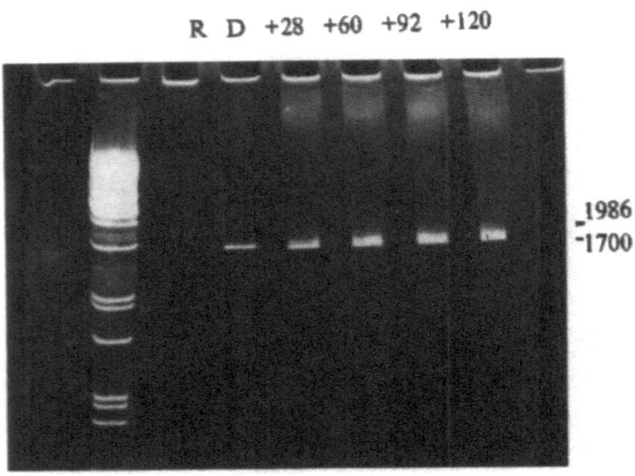

Fig. 5. The case of complete chimerism detected using DXS52 primers. Only donor-specific DNA is present after day +28

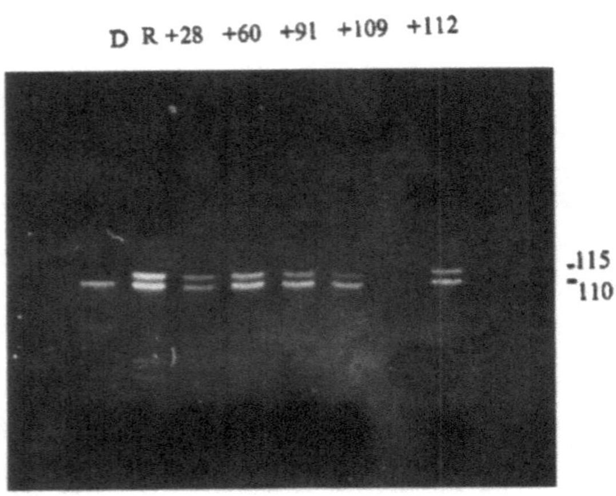

Fig. 6. The case of mixed chimerism. From day +28 both recipient and donor fragments are detectable. On days +91 and +109 the investigation was performed after transfusions of donor lymphocytes

relapsed and was treated by donor lymphocyte transfusions as immunotherapy. In this case the recipient DNA was isolated from the granulocytes of the patient after Ficoll density centrifugation. Mixed chimerism was observed during the whole course of treatment. This patient died of relapse on day +121 after BMT.

Discussion

Assessment of engraftment and chimerism after BMT requires the identification of both host and donor cells. This can be done by analysis of a number of different markers, including red cell antigen typing, karyotyping, and so on [8–10]. However, these methods have disadvantages during the early posttransplant period. In the very early stages of engraftment the peripheral blood and bone marrow are very hypocellular and it may be difficult to recover enough cells to perform karyotyping or any other method of chimerism detection. The polymerase chain reaction, which allows the amplification of specific DNA sequences, offers a way to overcome these problems, but it requires suitable polymorphic regions for amplification. We used the VNTR regions as highly polymorphic genetic markers, as described previously [4, 11].

Our results indicate that the PCR-VNTR technique can be used successfully for high sensitivity of the method reduces the number of cells required for analysis and allows detection of host cell repopulation in the early post-BMT period. In some cases it can predict relapse of the disease, as was demonstrated in our study. Surely, unlike the use of clonal markers such as bcr-abl [12] and T-cell receptor γ genes [13], this method detects the presence of any recipient DNA, regardless of the lineage of the cell containing this DNA. That is why it is so difficult to analyze the cases of mixed chimerism and to connect its occurrence with the probability of relapse [14].

An additional advantage of the PCR is the rapidity of the technique compared with the cytogenetic analysis, with results obtained within 24 h. In addition, compared with red blood cell phenotyping, the PCR-VNTR technique demonstrates the possibility of early detection of marrow engraftment, and is independent of erythrocyte transfusions.

We conclude that the PCR has already proved its value for monitoring the hemopoietic status of patients after BMT, and has important implications for studying engraftment kinetics.

References

1. Ugozzoli L, Yam P, Petz L.D. et al. Amplification by the polymerase chain reaction of hypervariable regions of human genome for evaluation of chimerism after bone marrow transplantation. Blood 1991, 77: 1607–1615.
2. van Leeuwen J.E.M, van Tol M.J.D, Bodzinga B.G, et al. Detection of mixed chimaerism in flow-sorted cell subpopulations by PCR-amplified VNTR markers after allogeneic bone marrow transplantation. Br J Haematol 1991, 79: 218–225.
3. A.V.Misyurin, V.L. Surin, G.Ya. Solov'ev, Determination of the frequency of allelic variants of the gene for von Willebrand factor on the basis of polymorphism of a number of tandem repeats in intron 40. Russian 1994, 30: 633–636.
4. Boerwinkle E, Xiang W, Fourest E, Chan L. Rapid typing of tandemly repeated hypervariable loci by the PCR. Application to the apolipoprotein B'3 HVR region. Pro Natl Acad Sci USA 1989, 86: 212–216.
5. A.I. Kaidalova, O.V. Smirnova, V.L. Surin, G. Ya. Solov'ev. Evaluation of frequencies of the polymorphic alleles of locus DX S52 of he human X-chromosome in the Moscow population. Russian Genet 1994, 30: 844–846.
6. Richards B, Heilig R, Oberle I, et al. Rapid PCR analysis of the ST 14 (DXS52) VNTR. Nucleic Acids Res 1991. 19: 1944.
7. Peake I, Bowen D, Bingnell P, et al. Family studies and prenatal diagnosis in severe von Willebrand disease by polymerase chain reaction amplification of a variable number tandem repeat region of the von Willebrand factor gene. Blood 1990, 76: 555–561.
8. van Dijk BA, Drenth-Schonk AM, Bloo A et al. Erythrocyte repopulation after allogeneic bone marrow transplantation. Transplantation 1987, 44: 650–654.
9. Bar Bmam, Schattenberg A, van Dijk BA et al. Host and donor erythrocyte repopulation patterns after allogeneic bone marrow transplantation analyzed with antibody coated fluorescent microspheres. Br J Haematol 1989, 72: 239–245.
10. Lawler SD, Harris H, Millar J et al. Cytogenetic follow-up studies of recipients of T-cell depleted allogeneic bone marrow. Br J Haematol 1987, 65: 143–150.
11. Nakamura Y, Leppert M, O'Connell P et al. Variable number of tandem repeat (VNTR) markers for human gene mapping. Science 1987, 235: 1616–1620.
12. Roth MS, Antin JH, Bingham EL, Ginsburg D. Detection of Philadelphia chromosome-positive cells by the polymerase chain reaction following bone marrow transplant for chronic myelogenous leukemia. Blood 1989: 74: 882–887.
13. Hansen-Hagge TE, Yokota S, Bartram CR. Detection of minimal residual disease in acute lymphoblastic leukemia by in vitro amplification of rearranged T-cell receptor delta chain sequeneces. Blood 1989, 74: 1762–1768.
14. Roy DC, Tantravahi R, Murray C, et al. Natural history of mixed chimerism after bone marrow transplantation with CD-6 depleted allogeneic marrow: A stable equilibrium. Blood 1990, 75: 296–304.

Leukemia Cell Biology: Cytokines

Acute Leukemias VI
Prognostic Factors
and Treatment Strategies
Büchner et al. (eds)

Truncated Granulocyte – Colony Stimulating Factor Receptors in Severe Congenital Neutropenia Terminating in Acute Myeloid Leukemia

F. Dong and I.P. Touw

Abstract. Severe congenital neutropenia (SCN) is a heterogeneous disease condition with a variable family history and a propensity to progress towards acute myeloblastic leukemia (AML). In collaboration with the SCN International Disease Registry, a study has been initiated aimed at the identification of abnormalities of G-CSF-R function in SCN. Among a series of 20 cases analyzed thus far, 5 patients have been found with point mutations in the G-CSF-R gene. These mutations were confined to cells of the myeloid lineage. They were all nonsense mutations, resulting in the truncation of the C-terminal cytoplasmic region, a subdomain that is crucial for G-CSF-mediated maturation signaling. In all cases, both the mutated and the normal allele were expressed. Three patients acquired cytogenetic abnormalities and developed AML. Of the two other patients, who are still neutropenic, one acquired a cytogenetic abnormality (monosomy 7). None of the 15 patients without G-CSF-R mutations (including 5 Swedish patients wlth a family history of neutropenia, the syndrome originally described by Kostmann) showed cytogenetic or clinical signs of progression to AML. Coexpression of mutant and wild-type G-CSF-R in murine maturation-competent myeloid cell systems indicated that the truncated G-CSF-R proteins interfered with G-CSF-induced maturation in a dominant negative fashion. We conclude that SCN patients with mutations in the G-CSF-R gene, resulting in the truncation of the C-terminal maturation domain, are predisposed to develop AML.

Severe Congenital Neutropenia

Severe congenital neutropenia (SCN) is a hematopoietic disorder characterized by profound absolute neutropenia and a maturation arrest of myeloid progenitor cells at the promyelocyte-myelocyte stage. As a result, patients suffer from life-threatening opportunistic infections and frequently die at under 10 years of age. The diagnosis of SCN is made in early infancy. SCN was originally described in 1956 by Kostmann [1] as an autosomal recessive disorder in several Swedish families. Subsequently, a number of other reports appeared in which a family history of SCN was not apparent [2]. Marrow cells from SCN patients often display a reduced responsiveness to granulocyte colony stimulating factor (G-CSF) in vitro, although neutrophilic colony formation can usually be induced with elevated G-CSF concentrations. Elevated levels of biologically active G-CSF (150–910 pg/ml) are frequently found in the serum of SCN patients. The administration of G-CSF in most cases improves granulopoiesis in vivo and is of therapeutic benefit [3, 4]. In agreement with in vitro observations, a considerable elevation of G-CSF levels is required to overcome the neutropenia in G-CSF-responsive SCN patients [3]. SCN patients have an increased probability of developing myelodysplastic syndrome or AML [3–7].

Department of Hematology, Daniel den Hoed Cancer Center and Erasmus University, Rotterdam, The Netherlands

G-CSF Receptor

G-CSF induces both proliferation and differentiation of myeloid precursor cells via activation of a single receptor (R) that belongs to the superfamily of hematopoietin receptors [8]. Activation of these receptors by their respective ligands is mediated through the formation of dimeric or oligomeric complexes of receptor structures. Some hematopoietin receptors form heteromeric receptor complexes, e.g., IL-2R, IL-3R, IL-5R, GM-CSF-R [9]. In contrast, G-CSF-R forms homodimeric complexes [10]. The extracellular region of the G-CSF-R is composed of an immunoglobulin (Ig)-like domain, the cytokine receptor homology (CRH) domain, and three fibronectin type III (FNIII) domains [11, 12]. The intracellular part of human G-CSF-R comprises 183 amino acids [12, 13]. Like other cytokine/hematopoietin receptors, the cytoplasmic domain of G-CSF-R lacks a kinase domain. Several stretches of amino acids in the G-CSF-R cytoplasmic domain show limited sequence homology to other members of the hematopoietin receptor superfamily. Two of these stretches, referred to as "box l" and "box 2", are positioned in the membrane-proximal region of G-CSF-R. Box 1 and box 2 are also present in several other hematopoietin receptors [10, 14]. The membrane-distal cytoplasmic region of the G-CSF-R contains a third segment, called "box 3", which is shared only with the IL-6 signal transducer gp130 [10].

The membrane-proximal cytoplasmic region is primarily involved in proliferative signaling [10]. The C-terminal (membrane-distal) region, on the other hand, is essential for transduction of maturation signals [15, 16]. Deletion of the C-terminus of G-CSF-R not only destroys the maturation signaling capacity but also removes a negative regulatory element inhibiting proliferative signaling [15]. Experiments by Fukunaga et al. [16] with a panel of G-CSF-R deletion mutants and chimeras of growth hormone receptor and G-CSF-R indicated that mutations in the membrane-proximal cytoplasmic region could also result in the abrogation of maturation induction by G-CSF. These data demonstrate that maturation signaling, although primarily controlled by the C-terminal region of G-CSF-R, is not independent of the function of the membrane-proximal region.

Defective Cytokine Receptors and Hematopoietic Disorders

Structure abnormalities of cytokine/hematopoietin receptors have been shown to contribute to different human diseases. A mutation in the receptor for erythropoietin (EPO-R), causing a truncation of a C-terminal negative-regulatory region, has been genetically linked to familial erythrocytosis [17]. Truncation of the common γ chain of the receptors for IL-2, IL-4, IL-7, and IL-15 is associated with X-linked severe combined immunodeficiency [18]. Finally, mutations in the receptor for growth hormone, also a member of the cytokine receptor superfamily, have been described in patients with Laron dwarfism [19–22]. Evidence for a possible role of abnormal cytokine receptors in leukemogenesis has been obtained in mice. A mutation in the extracellular domain of the murine EPO-R, causing constitutive homodimerization and activation of the EPO-R mutant protein, could be directly associated with the development of erythroleukemia [23]. Souyri et al. [24] found that myeloproliferative leukemia virus (MPLV) encodes a fusion product of virus envelope protein and the C-terminal part of the hematopoietin receptor structure MPL, recently identified as the receptor for thrombopoietin [25–27]. More recently, it was shown that a mutant form of the common-β chain (β_c) of the human IL-3/GM-CSF/IL-5 receptors, containing a duplication of 37 amino acids in the extracellular domain, confers growth factor independence on murine IL-3-dependent FDC-Pl cells [28]. The FDC-Pl transfectants expressing the mutant β_c protein gave rise to leukemic outgrowth upon injection into syngeneic mice, whereas FDC-Pl transfectants expressing the wild-type β_c protein, which remained factor-dependent, were nontumorigenic.

G-CSF-R Defects in SCN

Based upon the observation that G-CSF responses are frequently disturbed in SCN, it had been anticipated for some time that G-CSF-R dysfunction might be involved in the pathogenesis of the disease. This idea gained significant support when a somatic mutation in the G-CSF-R gene was found in a case of SCN [29]. This nonsense mutation resulted in the deletion of the C-terminal domain of G-CSF-R that been functionally linked to maturation signaling [15]. Indeed, upon its ectopic expression in murine myeloid cell lines, the mutant receptor protein was unable to transduce maturation signals. Because the normal allele was also expressed in the granulocytic cells of the patient, it appeared likely that the truncated receptor protein functioned in a dominant negative manner over the wild-type protein (Fig. 1). This notion was confirmed in cotransfection experiments in which truncated and wild-type G-CSF-R proteins were expressed at equal levels. These findings provided the first in vivo evidence that signals transduced by the G-CSF-R C-terminus are indispensable for the normal development of myeloid progenitor cells. Significantly, the mutation was found in the granulocytes of the patient (who received G-CSF treatment), but not in monocytes, erythroid colony cells, T and B lymphocytes, or skin fibroblasts. Apparently, progenitor cells committed to the granulocyte lineage had been the target population for the somatic mutation. Because committed progenitor cells are normally incapable of sustained self-renewal, the question arose how the affected progenitor cell population could persist in the patient. Given the fact that the truncated G-CSF-R protein, apart from lacking maturation signaling abilities, also lacks the C-terminal element that negatively regulates proliferation, it was suggested that expression of this mutant receptor contributed to immortalization/enhanced self-renewal capacity of the myeloid progenitor cells. On this basis, the neutropenia in this case was believed to reflect a preleukemic condition. In support of this notion, it was shown that the leukemic cells from two AML patients with a

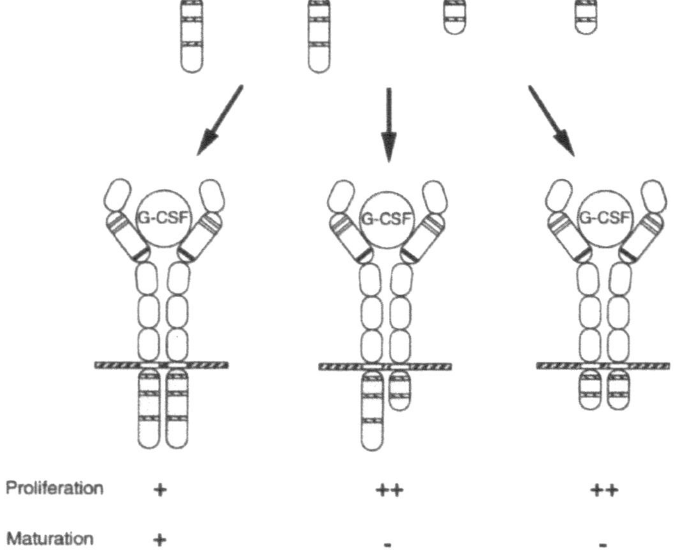

Fig. 1. Dominant negative action of truncated G-CSF-R on the maturation function of full-length (wild-type) G-CSF-R delection mutant interferes with maturation signaling by forming heteromers with wild-type G-CSF-R. Ig-like: Immunoglobulin-like domain; CRH: cytokine receptor homology domain; FNIII: Fibronectin-III domain. The *hatched* regions in the cytoplasmic domain mark boxes 1 (membrane-proximal) to 3 (membrane-distal)

history of SCN also had mutations in G-CSF-R, again truncating the C-terminal maturation-inducing region [30, 31]. In one of these patients, it could be demonstrated that the mutation was already present in the neutropenic phase of the disease. In collaboration with the SCN International Disease Registry, 20 patients with SCN have so far been studied for the presence of mutations in the G-CSF-R gene, including 5 cases with a family history of neutropenia (Fan Dong et al., in preparation). Mutations in the G-CSF-R, all resulting in the truncation of the C-terminal maturation domain, were found in 5 patients. Three of these had developed AML, whereas one had acquired a monosomy 7, a cytogenetic abnormality associated with myelodysplastic syndrome. These findings suggest that defects in the G-CSF-R are associated with disease progression from SCN towards myelodysplastic syndrome and AML.

G-CSF-R Abnormalities in De Novo AML

IN 25 cases of de novo AML that have been studied thus far, nonsense mutations in the G-CSF-R similar to those detected in SCN, and AML preceded by SCN, were not observed. In contrast, a different type of G-CSF-R mutation was found in the leukemic blasts of one de novo AML patient [32]. This mutation was discovered after performing reverse transcriptase-polymerase chain reaction (RT-PCR) analysis on the blast cells of 40 nonselected patients. The AML blasts of this patient showed high expression of a new mRNA splice variant, in which the C-terminus was altered due to a change in the reading frame. Analysis of cDNA and corresponding genomic sequences revealed a G-to-A transition next to a (cryptic) splice donor site involved in the alternative RNA splicing. The splice variant appeared unable to transduce proliferation and maturation signals upon transfer to murine cell systems [32]. In agreement with this, the primary AML blast cells of the patient failed to respond to G-CSF in proliferation assays, whereas the responsiveness to IL-3 or GM-CSF was maintained. This observation, although as yet anecdotal, further highlights G-CSF-R dysfunction, either caused by structural defects in the G-CSF-R itself, or by abnormalities in the maturation signaling function, as an important potential mechanism of neoplastic transformation in human AML.

Acknowledgments. This work was supported by The Dutch Cancer Society. The authors are grateful to Prof. B. Löwenberg for his continuous support and active contributions to this study.

References

1. Kostmann R., 1956. Infantile genetic agranulocytosis, Acta Paediatr. Scand., 45 (suppl.105), 1–78.
2. Dale D.C., Davis M., and Vincent M.E., 1994. Use of filgrastin (r-metHuG-CSF) in severe chronic neutropenia. In: Filgrastin in clinical practice. Morstyn G and Dexter TM (editors), pp 83-101, Marcel Dekker Inc., New York.
3. Gillio A.P., and Gabrilove J.L., 1993. Cytokine treatment of inherited bone marrow failure syndromes, Blood 81: 1669–1674.
4. Bonilla M.A, Dale D., Zeidler C., Last L., Reiter A., Ruggeiro M., Davis M., Koci B., Hammond W., Gillio A., and Welte K., 1994. Long-term safety of treatment with recombinant human granulocyte colony-stimulating factor (r-metHuG-CSF) in patients with severe congenital neutropenias. Br. J. Haematol. 88: 723–730.
5. Gilman P.A., Jackson D.P., Guild H.G., 1970. Congenital agranulocytosis: Prolonged survival and terminal acute leukemia, Blood 36: 576–585.
6. Rosen R.B., Kang S.J., 1979. Congenital agranulocytosis terminating in acute myelomonocytic leukemia, J. Pediatr. 94: 406–407.
7. Wong W.-Y., Williams D., Slovak M.L., Charak B., Mazumder A., Snyder D., Powars D.R., and Brynes R.K., 1993. Terminal acute myelogenous leukemia in a patient with congenital agranulocytosis, Amer. J. Hematol. 43: 133–138.
8. Bazan J.F., 1990. Structural design and molecular evolution of a cytokine receptor superfamily, Proc. Natl. Acad. Sci. USA 87: 6934–6938.
9. Miyajima A., Mui A.L.F., Ogorochi T., and Sakamaki K., 1993. Receptors for granulocyte-macrophage colony-stimulating factor, interleukin-3, and interleukin-5, Blood 82: 1960–1974.
10. Fukunaga R., Ishizaka-Ikeda E., Pan C.-X., Seto Y., and Nagata S., 1991. Functional domains of the granulocyte colony-stimulating factor receptor, EMBO J. 10: 2855–2865.
11. Fukunaga R., Ishizaka-Ikeda E., Seto Y., and Nagata S., 1990a. Expression cloning of a receptor for murine granulocyte colony-stimulating factor, Cell 61: 341–350.
12. Larsen A., Davis T., Curtis, B.M., Gimpel S., Sims J.E., Cosman D., Park L., Sorensen E., March C.J., and Smith C.A., 1990, Expression cloning of a human granulocyte colony stimulating factor receptor: a structural mosaic of hematopoietin receptor, immunoglobulin, and fibronectin domains, J. Exp. Med. 172: 1559–1570
13. Fukunaga R., Seto Y., Mizushima S., and Nagata S., 1990b, Three different mRNAs encoding human granulocyte colony-stimulating factor receptor, Proc. Natl. Acad, Sci. USA 87: 8702–8706

14. Murakami M., Narazaki M., Hibi M., Yawata H., Yasukawa K., Hamaguchi M., Taga T., and Kishimito T., Critical cytoplasmic region of the interleukin 6 signal transducer gp130 is conserved in the cytokine receptor family, 1991, Proc. Natl. Acad. Sci. USA. 88: 11349–11353
15. Dong F., Van Buitenen C., Pouwels K., Hoefsloot L.H., Löwenberg, and Touw I.P., 1993, Distinct cytoplasmic regions of the granulocyte colony-stimulating factor receptor involved in induction of proliferation and maturation, Mol. Cell. Biol. 13: 7774–7781
16. Fukunaga R., Ishizaka-Ikeda E., and Nagata S., 1993, Growth and differentiation signals mediated by different regions in the cytoplasmic domain of granulocyte colony stimulating factor receptor, Cell 74: 1079–1087
17. De la Chapelle A., Träskelin A.L., and Juvonen E., 1993, Truncated erythropoietin receptor causes dominantly inherited benign human erythrocytosis, Proc. Natl. Acad. Sci. USA. 90: 4495–4499.
18. Noguchi M., Yi H., Rosenblatt H.M., Filipovich A.H., Adelstein S., Modi W.S., McBride O.W., and Leonard W.J., 1993. Interleukin-2 receptor τ chain mutation results in X-linked severe combined immunodeficiency in humans, Cell 73: 147–157.
19. Amselem S., Duquesnoy P., Attree O., Novelli G., Bousnina S., Postel-Vinay M.C., and Goossens M., 1989. Laron dwarfism and mutations of the growth hormone receptor gene, N. Engl. J. Med. 321: 989–995.
20. Amselem S., Sobrier M.L., Duquesnoy P., Rappaport R., and Postel-Vinay M.C., 1991. Recurrent nonsense mutations in the growth hormone receptor from patients with Laron dwarfism J. Clin. Invest. 87: 1098–1102.
21. Duquesnoy P., Sobrier M.L., Amselem S., and Goossens M., 1991. Defective membrane expression of human growth hormone (GH) receptor causes Laron-type GH insensitivity syndrome, Proc. Natl. Acad. Sci. USA. 88: 10272–10276.
22. Berg M.A., Guevara-Aguirre J., Rosenbloom A.L., Rosenfeld R.G., and Francke U., 1992. Mutation creating a new splice site in the growth hormone receptor genes of 37 Ecuadorean patients with Laron syndrome, Hum. Mutat. 1: 24–
23. Longmore G.D., and Lodish H.F., 1991. An activating mutation in the murine erythropoietin receptor induces erythroleukemia in mice: A cytokine receptor superfamily oncogene, Cell 67: 1089–1102.
24. Sourzyi M., Vigon I., Penciolelli J.-F., Heard J.-M., Tambourin P., and Wendling F., 1990. A putative truncated cytokine receptor gene transduced by the myeloproliferative leukemia virus immortalizes hematopoietic progenitors, Cell 63: 1137–1147.
25. Lok S., Kaushansky K., Holly R.D., Kuijper J.L., Lofton Day C.E., Oort P.J., Grant F.J., Heipel M.D., Burkhead S.K., Kramer J.M., Bell L.A., Sprecher C.A., Blumberg H., Johnson R., Prunkard D., Ching A.F.T., Mathewes S.L., Bailey M.C., Forstrom J.W., Buddle M.M., Osborn S.G., Evans S.J., Sheppard P.O., Presnell S.R., O'Hara, P.J., Hagen, F.S., Roth, G.J. and Foster, D.C., 1994. Cloning and expression of murine thrombopoietin cDNA and stimulation of platelet production in vivo, Nature 369: 565–568.
26. Kaushansky K., Lok S., Holly R.D., Broudy V.C., Lin N., Baily M.C., Forstrom J.W., Buddle M.M. Oort P.J., Hagen F.S., Roth G.J., Papayannopoulou T., and Foster D.C., 1994. Promotion of megakaryocyte progenitor expansion and differentiation by the c-Mpl ligand thrombopoietin, Nature 369: 568–571.
27. Bartley T.D., Bogenberger J., Hunt P., Li Y.S., Lu H.S., Martin F., Chang M.S., Samal B., Nichol J.L., Swift S., Johnson M.J., Hsu R.Y., Parker V.P., Suggs S., Skrine J.D., Merewether L.A., Clogston C., Hsu E., Hokom M.M., Hornkohi A., Choi E., Pangelinan M., Sun Y., Mar V., McNinch J., Simonet L., Jacobsen F., Xie C., Shutter J., Chute H., Basu R., Selander L., Trollinger D., Sieu L., Padilla D., Trail G., Elliott, G., Izumi R., Covey T., Crouse J., Garcia A., Xu W., Castillo J.D., Biron J., Cole S., Hu M.C.T., Pacifici R., Ponting I., Saris C., Wen D., Yung Y.P., Lin H., and Bosselman R.A., 1994. Identification and cloning of a megakaryocyte growth and development factor that is a ligand for the cytokine receptor Mpl. Cell 77: 1117–1124.
28. D'Andrea R., Rayner J., Moretti P., Lopez A., Goodall G.J., Gonda T.J., and Vadas M., 1994. A mutation of the common receptor subunit for interleukin-3 (IL-3), granulocyte macrophage colony-stimulating factor, and IL-5 that leads to ligand independence and tumorigenicity, Blood 83: 2802–2808.
29. Dong F., Hoefsloot L.H., Schelen A.M., Broeders L.C.A.M., Meijer Y., Veerman A.J.P., Touw I.P., and Löwenberg B. 1994a. Identification of a nonsense mutation in the granulocyte-colony-stimulating factor receptor in severe congenital neutropenia, Proc. Natl. Acad. Sci. USA 91: 4480–4484.
30. Dong F., Brynes, R.K., Tidow, N., Welte K., Löwenberg, B., and Touw I.P., 1995. Mutations truncating the C-terminal maturation region of the G-CSF receptor in acute myeloid leukemia preceded by severe congenital neutropenia N. Engl. J. Med., in press (August 24 issue).
31. Touw I.P., Schelen, A., Brynes, R.K., Tidow, N., Welte K., Löwenberg, B., and Dong, F., 1994. Point mutations in the G-CSF-R gene in severe congenital neutropenia terminating in acute myeloid leukemia, Blood, 84 Suppl. 1, 375a (abstract).
32. Dong F., Van Paassen, M., Van Buitenen, C., Hoefsloot, L.H., Löwenberg, B., and Touw I.P., 1994. A point mutation in the granulocyte colony-stimulating factor receptor (G-CSF-R) gene in a case of acute myeloid leukemia results in the overexpression of a novel G-CSF-R isoform, Blood 85: 902–911.

Acute Leukemias VI
Prognostic Factors
and Treatment Strategies
Büchner et al. (eds)

BCR/ABL and Signal Transduction Pathways

R. Salgia, K. Okuda, N. Carlesso, and J.D. Griffin

Abstract. BCR/ABL transforms hematopoietic cells in vitro and in vivo and exerts a wide variety of biological effects, including induction of factor independence, reduction of apoptosis, and altering adhesion of CML cells to marrow stroma. However, at a biochemical level, the mechanisms by which BCR/ABL transforms myeloid cells are poorly understood. p210BCR/ABL has elevated ABL tyrosine kinase activity, relocates to the cytoskeleton, and phosphorylates several cellular proteins, including c-BCR, p120rasGAP, c-CBL, p52SHC, p93FES, p95VAV, p125FAK, p68paxillin, and p72SH PTP2. In addition, BCR/ABL has been shown to bind directly to GRB2 at Y177 of BCR, therefore potentially activating p21ras. However, it has been difficult to determine the significance of any of these potential BCR/ABL substrates, in part due to the complexity of studying a large protein with many potential signaling motifs, and in part due to the fact that there are so many BCR/ABL substrates in these cell lines. One approach to simplifying BCR/ABL biology has been to examine primary human CML cells, rather than cell lines made to overexpress BCR/ABL. Interestingly, in primary leukemic cells, there are only a few proteins which either intereact with BCR/ABL or are phosphorylated by BCR/ABL. This suggests that studies in primary CML cells, rather than tissue culture cell lines, may be more reliable in terms of identifying important signaling pathways. One of the major tyrosine phosphoproteins complexed with BCR/ABL in CML neutrophils has recently been identified as CRKL, an SH2/SH3 "adapter" protein. CRKL binds to BCR/ABL at least partly through its SH3 domain, and in cell lines may link BCR/ABL to some cytoskeletal proteins. The hypothesis hypothesis is set forth that BCR/ABL functions in part to disrupt signals going to, or coming from integrins in hematopoietic cells, and that this event is important in the pathogenesis of stable phase CML.

Chronic Myeloid Leukemia

CML was the first neoplasm associated with a specific chromosomal translocation, the Philadelphia chromosome, t(9;22)(q34;q11)[1]. The molecular basis for CML has been worked out in elegant detail by a number of laboratories (for reviews see [2, 3]), and it is now clear that virtually all cases are the result of fusion of the c-ABL tyrosine kinase with BCR, a ubiquitously expressed gene probably normally involved in regulating p21rac activity. Two major translocations exist, producing two related fusion proteins,a shorter form associated with Ph(+) ALL, $p190^{BCR/ABL}$, and the more common $p210^{BCR/ABL}$ associated with CML. The difference between the two forms is in the amount of BCR fused with ABL. The $p190^{BCR/ABL}$ form has several-fold higher tyrosine kinase activity than $p210^{BCR/ABL}$, and both forms have higher tyrosine kinase activity than c-ABL[4].

CML is characterized by massive expansion of myeloid cells in the marrow and blood, splenomegaly, extramedullary hematopoiesis, basophilia, hypermetabolism, and a high propensity to convert to acute leukemia. In many respects, the "stable" phase of CML is a preleukemic disorder, but it appears that virtually all patients

Division of Hematologic Malignancies, Dana-Farber Cancer Institute, 44 Binney St., Boston, MA 02115, USA

with CML will progress to acute leukemia if they do not succumb to an intervening illness. "Transformation" to acute phase is an event of dire significance as CML "blast crisis" is an aggressive acute leukemia with uniformly short survival. The blast crisis phase is characterized by the emergence of poorly differentiated primitive subclones, which typically have acquired new genetic mutations in addition to the Ph chromosome.

The BCR/ABL Oncogene

BCR/ABL is unique to CML and Ph(+) ALL, and does not transform most nonhematopoietic cells effectively, even in tissue culture [5]. The activation of the tyrosine kinase of ABL is critical for transformation [6], but the actual mechanism of transformation is largely unknown. c-ABL is ubiquitously expressed, both as a nuclear and a cytoplasmic protein [7, 8]. Recent studies suggest that nuclear c-ABL is likely to function as a negative regulator of growth, possibly through binding to known growth regulatory proteins in the nucleus such as Rb[9], although the significance of these observations is unknown. In contrast, $p210^{BCR/ABL}$ is exclusively cytoplasmic, with about 70% of the protein associated with the cytoskeleton [10]. Two groups have shown that $p210^{BCR/ABL}$ has a specific actin-binding domain [11–13], and studies from our laboratry show that $p210^{BCR/ABL}$ colocalizes with vinculin and paxillin in focal adhesion plaque-like stuctures in myeloid cells (R. Salgia and J. Griffin, unpublished, 1995).

Many domains in $p210^{BCR/ABL}$ have been shown to play a functional role in transformation, dependent on the type of assay used to measure function. BCR has been shown to be important for cytoplasmic localization, multimer formation [14], activation of the ABL kinase [15], and has also been shown to have some unique activities, including a serine/threonine kinase activity [16], and a domain which binds to the ABL SH2 domain in a phosphotyrosine-independent manner [17]. The racGAP domain of BCR is not part of the BCR/ABL fusion protein. In ABL, the tyrosine kinase domain is required for transformation, but not for actin binding [11]. The SH3 domain of ABL is inhibitory to kinase activity, and deletion of the SH3 domain makes c-ABL transform, suggesting that an unknown cellular protein or proteins bind to the SH3 domain and downregulate c-ABL. One potential ABL-SH3 binding protein has been identified [18]. The SH3 domain is deleted in v-ABL. The C-terminus of c-ABL is not strictly required for transformation, but is required for actin binding [11,13]. Deletion of sequences distal to ABL aa 585 does not prevent transformation by an SH3-deleted c-ABL. The ABL SH2 domain binds to cellular phosphoproteins in ABL-transformed cells [19], and may be important for transformation in some assays [12, 13, 20]. A point mutation in the conserved FLVRES motif in the SH2 domain inhibits transformation of Rat-1 cells and autokinase activity [21]. BCR/ABL and v-ABL are heavily tyrosine phosphorylated, but only some of the sites are known. For example, BCR/ABL has over 40 tyrosines and systematic mutagenesis of the tyrosines has not been undertaken. Tyr 177 has been shown to be part of a binding site for the SH2 domain of GRB2, and this site has been shown to be important for transformation in some assays [22, 23]. The major phosphorylation site within the kinase domain of p190 is important for transformation [6, 21]. There is a penta-lysine nuclear localization sequence C-terminal to the SH1 domain which is likely to be important in c-ABL function in the nucleus [8, 9, 24], but activated ABL oncogenes are universally in the cytoplasm, membrane, or cytoskeleton.

There are many fundamental biological questions about BCR/ABL that have not yet been answered. These include: (1) How does BCR increase the kinase activity of ABL? (2) Is autophosphorylation of BCR/ABL important and at which sites? (3) Which of the signaling proteins bound to BCR/ABL, if any, are important? (4) Which substrates of the BCR\ABL kinase (other than itself) are important for leukemia? (5) Which signaling pathways are important for stable phase? For blast phase? (6) What actually causes stable phase CML? A mitogenic signal? Decreased adhesion and early release from the marrow? Reduced apoptosis and prolonged life span? (7) What are the differences between p190 and p210BCR/ABL? Why is p190 primarily associated with acute lymphid leukemias and p210 rarely or never associated with acute lymphoid leukemias (until evolution to blast crisis)? As noted above, progress in understanding stable phase disease has been hampered by the fact that existing animal models are not ideal and transformation of cell lines generally produces a phenotype more similar to acute leukemia. No cell lines exist which have the phenotype of stable phase CML cells. In part, this is due to the fact that activated ABL oncogenes are associated with a high rate of mutations in cell lines [25]. For example, new chromosomal abnormalities occur extremely rapidly following the introduction of BCR/ABL [25].

Biological Effects of BCR/ABL

It has been remarkably difficult to determine exactly what the biological effects of BCR/ABL are. The stable (early) phase of CML differs from virtually all other human leukemias in that there is no apparent block in cell differentiation. In this phase, CML might more accurately be called a clonal myeloproliferative disorder. There is a striking tendency of CML to evolve, however, and acute leukemias will eventually supervene in most patients. The actual causes of the massive accumulation of myeloid cells characteristic of CML remains unclear. CML progenitor cells are actively cycling, probably more so than normal progenitor cells, but are entirely factor-dependent for proliferation in vitro [26, 27]. There are some reports of decreased sensitivity to inhibitory cytokines, such as MIP1α, but the significance of these observations remains unclear. In tissue culture, introduction of BCR/ABL into factor-dependent cell lines or murine marrow cells typically generates cell lines which evolve from hypersensitivity to growth factors to full factor independence, but again, the significance of this prominent tissue culture effect for the pathogenesis of CML is unclear [28]. Even modest hypersensitivity to growth factors is not a common feature of CML progenitor cells, except in more advances stages of the disease (J.D. Griffin, unpublished).

Several other biological effects have been reported and may be important. First, BCR/ABL may affect the sensitivity of CML cells to apoptosis [29, 32]. Normal hematopoietic cells are in a delicate balance of life and death. Most of the known hematopoietic growth factors induce cells to proliferate, differentiate, and/or activate but almost all factors also support viability. In the absence of growth factors, hematopoietic cells die at a very rapid rate, up to 1%–2% per hour. Most factor-dependent cell lines, such as 32Dcl3 or FDCP1 cells, also die rapidly, starting at about 18 h after removal of growth factors such as IL-3 or GM-CSF. BCR/ABL has a strong antiapoptotic activity in myeloid and lymphoid cells, and recent studies from several groups, including our own, suggest that this a primary and potentially important activity of this oncogene [29–33]. In an effort to generate cell lines which were biochemically more similar to primary CML cells, we made mutants of BCR/ABL which were temperature-sensitive for ABL kinase activity [33]. The best mutant, p210BCR/ABLts-1, has two point mutations (aa 457 R-H and aa 469 Y-H) and has low kinase activity at the non-permissive temperature (39°C) and high kinase activity at the permissive temperature (33°C). At the nonpermissive temperature, the cells are wild-type (IL-3-dependent for growth and viability/while at the permissive temperature the cells require IL-3 for proliferation, but no longer need IL-3 for viability. Thus, BCR/ABL dramatically reduces cell death in the absence of growth factors, at least in cell lines. Similar results were obtained by several groups with its mutants of v-ABL[30] and with primary CML neutrophils and progenitor cells [29].

Recent studies have also shown that CML cells have altered adhesion to marrow stromal cells and some extracellular matrix proteins, notably reduced adhesion of fibronectin [34]. The potential significance of this is substantial, as CML cells leave the marrow when immature, circulate in the blood in high numbers, and proliferate actively in tissues such as the spleen and liver which are not normally hematopoietic in adult humans. This phenomenon is likely to be explained in part by changes in adhesion molecule expression or function in CML progenitor cells, and there is growing evidence that CML cells have altered integrin expression and function.

It has recently been proposed that IFN-α may overcome the defective adhesion of CML progenitors to stromal cells by altering the neuraminic acid composition of stromal layer [35], and an in vitro culture system has been established to study this phenomenon [36], or by increasing the expression of the adhesion molocule LFA-3, which is decreased in CML cells [37]. Verfaillie et al. have shown decreased adhesion to stroma and fibronectin but increased adhesion to the basement membrane components laminin and collagen type IV of malignant progenitors in CML [34]. Defects in β1 integrins have been described and also shown to be corrected by IFN-α [38]. CML progenitors express α2 and α6 integrin chains, receptors for laminin and collagen, respectively, whereas these receptors are absent from normal progenitors. These observations suggest that the premature release of malignant CML progenitors may be caused by loss of adhesive interactions with stroma and/or fibronectin and acquisition of adhesive interactions with basement membrane components.

Integrins and Adhesion of Myeloid Cells

Integrins are expressed on almost every cell type and are important in linking the extracellular matrix to the cytoskeleton [39]. Each integrin consists of noncovalently linked, heterodimeric α β chains. Integrins are typicallu grouped according to the subunits. The β2 leukocyte integrins (CD18 β chain) have been demonstrated to be important in neutrophil functioning [40]. There are three α subunits which are associated with CD18: CD11a (LFA-1), CD11b (Mac-1, Mo-1), and CD11c (p150,95). The significance of the β2 leukocyte integrins has been characterized in leukocyte adhesion deficiency (LAD) type I syndrome, in which there is a partial or total absence of expression of the β2 chain (CD18) in leukocytes [41]. There are several ligands for β2 integrin family members, including ICAM-1 (intercellular adhesion molecule 1), fibrinogen, coagulation factor X, and iC3b. CD11b/CD18 is upregulated by tumor necrosis factor, C5a, platelet activating factor, fMLP, and phorbol esters.

There is a rapidly growing body of evidence showing that integrins send signals back to the cell when they in are contact with an appropriate ligand [39, 42–44]. For example, cross-linking of CD11b/CD18 in normal neutrophils leads to rapid tyrosine phosphorylation of several new cytoplasmic proteins. Recent studies have suggested that one biological effect mediated by integrin-initiated signaling may be inhibition of apoptosis for some cell types, and augmentation of apoptosis for others. Integrin signaling and control of integrin expression and function are poorly understood events. It is clear that in adherent cells, integrins and probably other adhesion proteins are not dispersed equally over the cell surface, but congregate in "patches" or groups at sites of attachment to the extracellular matrix [45]. On the inside of the cell membrane, specialized structures termed "focal adhesion plaques" (FAP) contain a unique set of proteins which are believed to be involved in linking the cytoskeleton to integrins and in sending and receiving messages from integrins [45].

Focal Adhesions, FAP Components, and Integrin Function

Focal adhesions are the site at which actin fibers are linked to integrins, and are essential for cell adherence to extracellular matrix components [46, 47]. Actin filaments form the cortical actin network, actin stress fibers, and membrane ruffles. New stress fibers and membrane ruffles are known to be stimulated by various growth factors in fibroblasts, such as platelet-derived growth factor and epidermal growth factor. Focal adhesions or focal contacts were first identified when electron micrographs revealed electron-dense areas of plasma membrane where tissue culture cells contacted the surface. In vivo, many types of cells are believed to form specialized regions that are structurally and functionally similar to focal contacts. A growing number of focal adhesion components have been identified [42, 46, 47]. These components are either extracellular (such as the extracellular matrix (ECM) proteins fibronectin and vitronectin), transmembrane (integrins), or cytoplasmic (such as actin, vinculin, tensin, paxillin, and other molecules). Focal adhesions function as anchors for actin fibers, and play a role in regulating actin assembly. It is still not clear which proteins bind directly to integrins, although p125FAK, tensin, vinculin, and paxillin are strong candidates. Recent studies have shown that cross-linking of integrins, sends signals into the cell through FAP components [42, 44, 45, 48, 49]. For example, after ECM molecules bind to integrins, there are several proteins which have been shown to be phosphorylated, including tensin, talin, and p125FAK. p125FAK is a tyrosine kinase which is unique to the FAP, and may be responsible for phosphorylating some of the other FAP proteins after activation. It is likely that these phosphorylations are associated with transient alterations in FAP structure and function. Activation of FAK has been shown to induce binding of the GRB2 adapter protein, thus linking integrin activation to the p21ras pathway [50]. It is also evident that the FAP can receive signals from other receptors in the cell. For example, phosphorylation of FAP components is also observed after activation of many different growth factor receptors or oncogenes

[44, 51], and it is possible that such signals cause or are associated with changes in integrin affinity for ligand or level of expression.

Another FAP protein which appears to be involved in signaling is paxillin. Paxillin is a 68 kDa focal contact protein which is tyrosine phosphorylated in response to many different stimuli, including intergrin cross-linking, growth factor signaling, and several oncogenes [52]. Paxillin was initially identified by Glenny during experiments in which antibodies were made blindly to phosphotyrosine-containing proteins in RSV-transformed chick embryo fibroblasts [53]. Up to 20%–30% of paxillin is phosphorylated on tyrosine in RSV-transformed cells and in embryonal tissues [43,54]. The significance of tyrosine phosphorylation is unknown, although the phosphorylation of this protein appears to be a consequence of signal transduction from membrane receptors in normal fibroblasts. Importantly, paxillin has recently been recognized to interact with FAK, vinculin, and $pp60^{v\text{-}Src}$ [52, 55] and recent data suggests that it may interact with the ß chains of some integrins. Paxillin, therefore, is potentially involved in mediating interaction of FAP components with integrins in a regulated manner.

In summary, FAP structures appear to be important in structural support of the cell and transmitting signals from cell receptors and various oncogenes to the cell membrane (Fig. 1).

Oncogenes and the FAP

The focal adhesion and focal adhesion proteins are also known to be strikingly modified by several oncogenes [44]. V-Src and V-Crk proteins are concentrated in focal adhesions. Also, several tyrosine kinase oncogenes (such as $p60^{v\text{-}Src}$, $p160^{v\text{-}ABL}$, $p60^{v\text{-}YES}$, and $p210^{BCR/ABL}$ induce phosphorylation of one or more proteins such as vinculin, talin, and tensin [56,57]. The interaction of oncogenes with FAP proteins has been implicated in transformation and particularly in changing adhesion to ECM proteins, decreased contact inhibition, and ability to metastasize [47, 51]. The effects of v-Src on the cytoskeleton are illustrative. After Rous sarcoma virus (RSV) infection (with most, but not all strains of virus), the v-Src protein localizes to FAP. The earliest manifestation is membrane ruffling, observed within minutes of induction of Src in a temperature-sensitive mutant [58]. In contrast to normal fibroblasts, RSV-infected cells round up, become refractile, and fail to undergo contact inhibition. There is a pronounced disorganization of the actin microfilaments associated with dramatic increases in the phosphotyrosine content of FAP proteins.

BCR/ABL, v-Src, and v-Crk Induce Tyrosine Phosphorylation of an Overlapping Set of Cellular Proteins

v-Src and v-Crk are known to induce tyrosine phosphorylation of some of the same cellular proteins [55, 56, 59–64]. Two of these, paxillin and p130CAS, are also prominent substrates of BCR/ABL [65]. Paxillin is one of the major tyrosine phosphoproteins in cells transformed by v-Src or v-Crk [55, 59]. Paxillin interacts directly with both v-Src and v-Crk proteins, through the

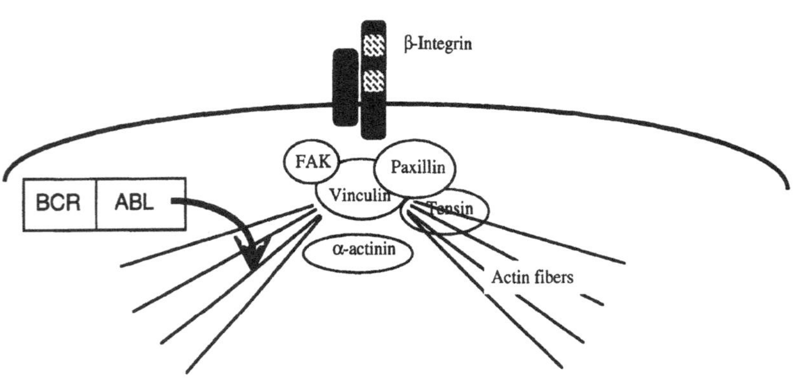

Fig. 1. A model of the interaction of BCR/ABL with the cytoskeleton

SH2 and SH3 domains of Src, and the SH2 domain of Crk, on the basis of in vitro binding studies. Binding of v-Src and v-Crk to paxillin may be important in concentrating both of these oncogenes in focal adhesions, and therefore could be important in the altered cytoskeletal structure and adhesive properties that accompany transformation by both viral oncogenes. However, there are no direct data to prove that binding to paxillin is important. Deletions in the SH2 domain, but not the SH3 domain, of v-Src eliminate binding to the cytoskeleton [57]. v-Crk is an adapter protein and does not have intrinsic tyrosine kinase activity. Recent studies form Hanafusa's laboratory have linked transformation by v-Crk to activation of the c-ABL tyrosine kinase [66]. This unanticipated finding may be relevant to understanding some of the interactions between BCR/ABL and proteins of the cytoskeleton described below.

CRK and CRKL

In primary neutrophils from CML patients in stable phase, there is only a single prominently phosphorylated cellular protein, p39, and there is no detectable activation of p21ras, c-myc, or other pathways. We and others have identified the p39 tyrosine phosphorylated protein in BCR/ABL-containing cells as CRKL (CRK-like) [64, 67, 68]. The CRKL gene has an overall homology of 60% to CRK, the human homologue of the v-Crk oncogene [69]. v-Crk is the oncogene in the avian retrovirus CT10, and has a deletion of the C-terminal SH3 domain (Fig. 2). v-Crk, CRK and CRKL each have one SH2 domain, an SH2′ domain, and two SH3 domains, without other known functional domains [69,70]. A summary of the structure of CRK and related proteins in shown in Fig. 2

Since several proteins in v-Crk transformed cells are heavily phosphorylated on tyrosyl residues, it has been suggested that v-Crk and c-CRK may serve as regulatory subunits of a tyrosine kinase [56, 71]. Recently, c-ABL has been identified as a possible CRK-associated tyrosine kinase [66]. c-ABL binds in vitro to the first CRK SH3 domain and phosphorylates CRK on tyrosine 221 (Y221). The phosphorylation on CRK (Y221) creates a binding site for the CRK SH2 domain, possibly inhibiting its binding to other proteins. Activation of CRK signal transduction is possibly linked to dephosphorylation of CRK Y221 by a cellular phosphatase, although there is no direct proof of this hypothesies [66]. It is not known if ABL and CRK interact in vivo. Activation of c-Src has also been observed in some cells by v-Crk[72]. Like GRB2, CRK and CRKL are likely to function as "adapter proteins," linking different proteins in a regulated manner. As described above, two other CRK-binding proteins are known, paxillin and p130 CAS [59, 62, 73]. Paxillin is prominently tyrosine-phosphorylated during transformation by v-Crk and has been shown to have a binding site for the SH2 domain of CRK in vitro [59]. Paxillin has recently been cloned by two groups including our own and shown to contain multiple protein-protein interaction domains [65, 74]. P130 CAS (for CRK-associated substrate) has recently been identified as a common cellular target of tyrosine phosphorylation via v-Crk and v-Src oncogenes [62]. p130CAS has recently been cloned and shown to contain an SH3 domain and multiple potential SH2 binding sites [62], including nine potential CRK SH2 binding motifs, YDXP.

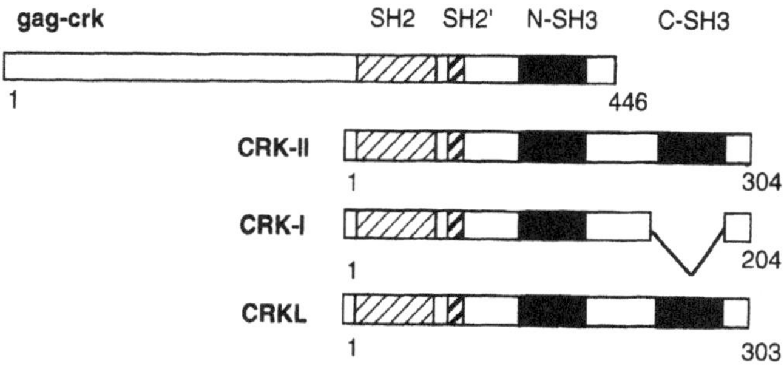

Fig. 2. CRK Proteins. (Adapted from [69, 70])

A Model Linking BCR/ABL to Signal Transduction Pathways in the Cytoskeleton

In stable phase CML neutrophils, we have identified a prominent $p210^{BCR/ABL}$ binding protein to be CRKL, an adapter protein, which may bind to BCR/ABL primarily via its SH3 domain. We hypothesize that this interaction would have several effects.

First, it would disrupt the normal function of CRKL in the cell. Second, it would potentially allow the SH2 domain of CRKL to bind to other cellular proteins, bringing them into close proximity with BCR/ABL. This could activate signaling pathways that are normally quiescent in resting myeloid cells. Based on studies with v-Src, v-Crk, and c-CRK, it would be reasonable to predict that the SH2 domain of CRKL could bind to either paxillin, p130CAS, or both, and this hypothesis is currently being tested. Paxillin would be of potential interest because it is linked to signaling to (and from) integrins.

One hypothesis that emerges from these observations is that BCR/ABL is likely to interfere with signaling in FAP-like structures in myeloid cells. The consequences of this inteference could be significant. For example, it is known that both the level of expression and the affinity of some integrins for their ligands is regulated by signals from other receptors in the cell. BCR/ABL may block the signals that regulate either expression or affinity, thus altering the ability of the cell to change its adhesive profile. This could easily change the ability of the cell to bind to critical ECM components.

Another intriguing possibility is that BCR/ABL inteferes with signals that are initiated by integrins when they are either bound to their ligand or aggregated. Such signals are known to involve rapid activation of the focal adhesion kinase FAK, and tyrosine phosphorylation of FAP proteins such as paxillin. The role of integrin signalling into the cell is not clear, but several themes are emerging. First, in addition to simply providing adhesion to the proper substratum, some cells are likely to need to know that they are in the right microenvironment. One way in which this could occur is to have integrins (and/or other adhesion molecules and cell surface receptors) send signals into the cell when they are appropriately activated by ligand. In this way, cells would sense when they are in the right microenvironment for proliferation of different functions. Such a sensing mechanism may be particularly important for highly migratory hematopoietic cells. Although immature hematopoietic stem cells are found in the blood and circulate through all organs, proliferation of these cells is observed almost exclusively (in humans) in the bone marrow. In conditions of extreme hematopoietic stress, proliferation can be seen in a few other organs, such as the spleen or liver. This could be due primarily to a lack of growth factors in nonmarrow tissues. Indeed, chronic administration of G-CSF has been shown to induce mild splenomegaly due to myelopoiesis, but this is not generally observed in other tissues. It is possible that multiple signals through cell surface receptors would be integrins. If so, BCR/ABL could confuse the cell dramatically. The data cited above, in fact, would suggest that BCR/ABL would initiate signals that could indicate that integrins are "activated", even when they are not. Thus, activation of FAK, paxillin, CRKL and other proteins in the cytoskeleton would potentially send signals to the cell that the cell may be attached even when it is not. One theoretical outcome would be the ability of CML cells to proliferate in locations (such as blood and other tissues) where normal hematolpoietic progenitor cells cannot – a prominent feature of stable phase CML cells. There is no compelling reason why this must involve cytoskeletal proteins, and weak mitogenic signals from BCR/ABL may also be sufficient to allow this phenotype to be observed in vivo. Clearly, however, some new avenues of research are opening on BCR/ABL biology that will be worth pursuit.

References

1. Nowell, P.C. and Hungerford, D.A. A minute chromosome in human chronic granulocytic leukemia, J Natl Cancer Inst. 25: 85–109, 1960.
2. Kurzrock, R., Gutterman, J.U., and Talpaz, M. The molecular genetics of Philadelphia chromosome-positive leukemias, N Engl J Med. 319: 990–998, 1988.
3. Witte, O.N. Role of the BCR-ABL oncogene in human leukemia: fifteenth Richard and Hinda Rosenthal Foundation Award Lecture. [Review], Cancer Res. 53: 485–9, 1993.
4. Lugo, T.G., Pendergast, A.M., Muller, A.J., and Witte, O.N. Tyrosine kinase activity and transformation potency of bcr-abl oncogene products, Science. 247: 1079–82, 1990.

5. Daley, G.Q., McLaughlin, J., Witte, O.N., and Baltimore, D. The CML-specific p210bcr/abl protein, unlike v-abl, does not transform NIH/3T3 fibrobalsts, Science. 237: 532–538, 1987.
6. Pendergast, A.M., Gishizky, M.L., Havlik, M.H., and Witte, O.N. SH1 domain autophosphorylation of P210 BCR/ABL is required for transformation but not growth factor independence, Mol Cell Biol. 13: 1728–36, 1993.
7. Kipreos, E.T. and Wang, J.Y. Differential phosphorylation of c-Abl in cell cycle determined by cdc2 kinase and phosphatase activity, Science. 248: 217–20, 1990.
8. Kipreos, E.T. and Wang, J.Y. Cell cycle-regulated binding of c-Abl tyrosine kinase to DNA, Science. 256: 382–5, 1992.
9. Welch, P.J. and Wang, J.Y. A C-terminal protein-binding domain in the retinoblastoma protein regulates nuclear c-Abl tyrosine kinase in the cell cycle, Cell. 75: 779–90, 1993.
10. Wetzler, M., Talpaz, M., Van Etten, R.A., Hirsh-Ginsberg, C., Beran, M., and Kurzrock, R. Subcellular localization of Bcr, Abl, and Bcr-Abl proteins in normal and leukemic cells and correlation of expression with myeloid differentiation, J Clin Invest. 92: 1925–39, 1993.
11. Van Etten, R.A., Jackson, P.K., Baltimore, D., Sanders, M.C., Matsudaira, P.T., and Janmey, P.A. The COOH terminus of the c-Abl tyrosine kinase contains distinct F- and G-actin binding domains with bunding activity [published erratum appears in J Cell Biol 1994 Mar;124(5):865], J Cell Biol. 124: 325–40, 1994.
12. MacKenzie, E., Stewart, E., and Birnie, G.D. ABL-BCR mRNAs transcribed from chromosome 9q+ in Philadelphia-chromosome-positive chronic myeloid leukaemia, Leukemia. 7: 702–6, 1993.
13. McWhirter, J.R. and Wang, J.Y. An actin-binding function contributes to transformation by the Bcr-Abl oncoprotein of Philadelphia chromosome-positive human leukemias, EMBO J. 12: 1533–46, 1993.
14. McWhirter, J.R., Galasso, D.L., and Wang, J.Y. A coiled-coil oligomerization domain of Bcr is essential for the transforming function of Bcr-Abl oncoproteins, Mol Cell Biol. 13: 7587–95, 1993.
15. Muller, A.J., Young, J.C., Pendergast, A.M., Pondel, M., Landau, N.R., Littman, D.R., and Witte, O.N. BCR first exon sequences specifically activate the BCR/ABL tyrosine kinase oncogene of Philadelphia chromosome-positive human leukemias, Mol Cell Biol. 11: 1785–92, 1991.
16. Maru, Y. and Witte, O.N. The BCR gene encodes a novel serine/theonine kinase activity within a single exon, Cell. 67: 459–68, 1991.
17. Pendergast, A.M., Muller, A.J., Havlik, M.H., Maru, Y., and Witte, O.N. BCR sequences essential for transformation by the BCR-ABL oncogene bind to the ABL SH2 regulatory domain in a non-phosphotyrosine-dependent manner, Cell. 66: 161–71, 1991.
18. Cicchetti, P., Mayer, B.J., Thiel, G., and Baltimore, D. Identification of a protein that binds to the SH3 region of Abl and is similar to Bcr and GAP-rho, Science. 257: 803–6, 1992.
19. Mayer, B.J., Jackson, P.K., and Baltimore, D. The noncatalytic src homology region 2 segment of abl tyrosine kinase binds to tyrosine-phosphorylated cellular proteins with high affinity, Proc Natl Acad Sci USA. 88: 627–31, 1991.
20. Mayer, B.J., Jackson, P.K., Van Etten, R.A., and Baltimore, D. Point mutations in the abl SH2 domain coordinately impair phosphotyrosine binding in vitro and transforming activity in vivo, Mol Cell Biol. 12: 609–18, 1992.
21. Afar, D.E.A., Goga, A., McLaughlin, J., Witte, O.N., and Sawyers, C. Differential complementation of Bcr-Abl point mutants with c-Myc, Science. 264: 424–426, 1994.
22. Pendergast, A.M., Quilliam, L.A., Cripe, L.D., Bassing, C.H., Dai, Z., Li, N., Batzer, A., Rabun, K.M., Der, C.J., Schlessinger, J., and et al. BCR-ABL-induced oncogenesis is mediated by direct interaction with the SH2 domain of the GRB-2 adaptor protein, Cell. 75: 175–85, 1993.
23. Puil, L., Liu, J., Gish, G., Mbamalu, G., Bowtell, D., Pelicci, T.G., Arlinghaus, R., and Pawson, T. Bcr-Abl oncoproteins bind directly to activators of the ras signalling pathway, EMBO J. 13: 764–773, 1994.
24. Wang, J.Y. Abl tyrosine kinase in signal transduction and cell-cycle regulation. [Review], Curr Opin Gene Dev. 3: 35–43, 1993.
25. Laneuville, P., Sun, G., Timm, M., and Vekemans, M. Clonal evolution in a myeloid cell line transformed to interleukin-3 independent growth by retroviral transduction and expression of p210bcr/abl, Blood. 80: 1788–97, 1992.
26. Metcalf, D., Moore, M.A., Sheridan, J.W., and Spitzer, G. Responsiveness of human granulocytic leukemic cells to colony-stimulating factor, Blood. 43: 847-59, 1974.
27. Metcalf, D. and Moore, M.A. Growth and responsiveness of human granulocytic leukemic cells in vitro, Bibl Haemato. 40: 235-41, 1975.
28. Daley, G. and Baltimore, D. Transformation of an interleukin-3-dependent hematopoietic cell line by the chronic myelogenous leukemia-specific p210 BCR/ABL protein, Proc Natl Acad Sci USA. 85: 9312, 1988.
29. Bedi, A., Zehnbauer, B.A., Barber, J.P., Sharkis, S.J., and Jones, R.J. Inhibition of apoptosis by BCR-ABL in chronic myeloid leukemia, Blood. 83: 2038–44, 1994.
30. Evans, C.A., Owen-Lynch, P.J., Whetton, A.D., and Dive, C. Activation of the Abelson tyrosine kinase activity is associated with suppression of apoptosis in hemopoietic cells, Cancer Res. 53: 1735–8, 1993.
31. Laneuville, P., Timm, M., and Hudson, A.T. bcr/abl expression in 32D cl3(G) cells inhibits apoptosis induced by protein tyrosine kinase inhibitors, Cancer Res. 54: 1360–6, 1994.
32. Smetsers, T.F., Skorski, T., van de Locht, L.T., Wessels, H.M., Pennings, A.H., de Witte, T., Calabretta, B., and Mensink, E.J. Antisense BCR-ABL oligonucleotides induce apoptosis in the

Philadelphia chromosome-positive cell line BV173, Leukemia. 8: 129-40, 1994.
33. Carlesso, N., Griffin, J.D., and Druker, B.J. Use of a temperature sensitive mutant to define the biological effects of the p210bcr/abl tyrosine kinase on proliferation of a factor-dependent murine myeloid cell line, Oncogene. 9: 149-56, 1994.
34. Verfaillie, C.M., McCarthy, J.B., and McGlave, P.B. Mechanisms underlying abnormal trafficking of malignant progenitors in chronic myelogenous leukemia, J Clin Invest. 90: 1232-1241, 1992.
35. Dowding, C., Guo, A.P., Osterholz, J., Siczkowski, M., Goldman, J., and Gordon, M. Interferon-alpha overrides the deficient adhesion of chronic myeloid leukemia primitive progenitor cells to bone marrow stromal cells, Blood. 78: 499-505, 1991.
36. Osterholz, J., Dowding, C., Guo, A.P., Siczkowski, M., and Goldman, J.M. Interferon-alpha alters the distribution of CFU-GM between the adherent and nonadherent compartments in long-term cultures of chronic myeloid leukemia marrow, Exp Hematol. 19: 326-31, 1991.
37. Guba, S.C. and Emerson, S.G. Hematopoietic regulation of stem cell cynamics in chronic myelogenous leukemia, p. 337-347. New York: Marcel Dekker, 1991.
38. Bhatia, R., Wayner, E.A., McGlave, P.B., and Verfaillie, C.M. Interferon-alpha restores normal adhesion of chronic myelogenous leukemia hematopoietic progenitors to bone marrow stroma by correcting impaired beta 1 integrin receptor function [see comments], J Clin Invest. 94: 384-91, 1994.
39. Hynes, R.O. Integrin: versatility, modulation, and signaling in cell adhesion, Cell. 69: 11-25, 1992.
40. Larson, R. and Springer, T. Structure and function of leukocyte integrins, Immunol. Rev. 114: 181-217, 1990.
41. Kishimoto, T.K., Hollander, N., Roberts, T.M., Anderson, D.C., and Springer, T.A. Heterogeneous mutations in the beta subunit common to the LFA-1, Mac-1, and gp150,95 glycoproteins cause leukocyte adhesion deficiency, Cell. 50: 193-202, 1987.
42. Romer, L., Burridge, K., and Turner, C. Signalling between the extracellular matrix and the cytoskeleton: tyrosine phosphorylation and focal adhesion assembly, Cold Spring Harbor Symp Quant Biol. 62: 193-201, 1993.
43. Burridge, K., Turner, C.E., and Romer, L.H. Tyrosine phosphorylation of paxillin and pp125FAK accompanies cell adhesion to extracellular matrix: a role in cytoskeletal assembly, J Cell Biol. 119: 893-903, 1992.
44. Guan, J.-L. and Shaloway, D. Regulation of focal adhesion-associated protein tyrosine kinase by both cellular adhesion and oncogenic transformation, Nature. 358: 690-692, 1992.
45. Kornberg, L., Earp, H., Parsons, J., Schaller, M., and Juliano, R. Cell adhesion or integrin clustering increases phosphorylation of a focal adhesion-associated tyrosine kinase, J biol Chem. 267: 23439-23442, 1992.
46. Burridge, K., Fath, K., Kelly, T., Nuckolls, G., and Turner, C. Focal adhesions: Transmembrane junctions between the extracellular matrix and the cytoskeleton, Ann Rev Cell Biol. 4: 487-525, 1988.
47. Lo, S. and Chen, L. Focal adhesion as a signal tranduction organelle, Cancer Metastasis Rev. 13: 9-24, 1994.
48. Schaller, M., Borgman, C., Cobb, B., Vines, R., Reynolds, A., and Parsons, J. pp125^{FAK}, a structurally distinctive protein-tyrosine kinase associated with focal adhesions, Proc. Natl. Acad. Sci. USA. 89: 5192-5196, 1992.
49. Hanks, S., Calalb, M., Harper, M., and Patel, S. Focal adhesion-protein kinase phosphorylated in response to cell attachment to fibronectin, Proc Natl Acad Sci USA. 89: 8487-8491, 1992.
50. Schlaepfer, D.D., Hanks, S.K., Hunter, T., and van der Geer, P. Integrin-mediated signal transduction linked to ras pathway by GRB2 binding to focal adhesion kinase, Nature. 372: 786-791, 1994.
51. Zachary, I. and Rozengurt, E. Focal adhesion kinase (p125^{FAK}): a point of convergence in the action of neuropeptides, integrins, and oncogenes, Cell. 71: 891-894, 1992.
52. Turner, C.E. Paxillin: a cytoskeletal target for tyrosine kinases. [Review], Bioessays. 16: 47-52, 1994.
53. Glenney, J. and Zokas, L. Novel tyrosine kinase substrates from Rous sarcoma virus-transformed cells are present in the membrane skeleton, J Cell Biol. 108: 2401-2408, 1989.
54. Turner, C. Paxillin is a major phosphotyrosine-containing protein during embryonic development, J Cell Biol. 115: 201-207, 1991.
55. Weng, Z., Taylor, J., Turner, C., Brugge, J., and Seidel-Dugan, C. Detection of src-SH3 binding proteins, including paxillin, in normal and v-src-transformed BALB/c3T3 cells, J Biol Chem. 268: 14956-14963, 1993.
56. Mayer, B.J. and Hanafusa, H. Association of the v-crk oncogene product with phosphotyrosine-containing proteins and protein kinase activity, Proc Natl Acad Sci USA. 87: 2638-42, 1990.
57. Fukai, Y., O'Brien, M.C., and Hanafusa, H. Deletions in the SH2 domain of p60v-src prevent association with the detergent-insoluble cellular matrix, Mol Cell Biol. 11: 1207-1213, 1991.
58. Wang, E. and Goldberg, A.R. Changes in microfilament organization and surface topography upon transformation of chick embryo fibroblasts with Rous sarcoma virus, Proc Natl Acad Sci. USA. 73: 4065-69, 1976.
59. Birge, R.B., Fajardo, J.E., Reichman, C., Shoelson, S.E., Songyang, Z., Cantley, L.C., and Hanafusa, H. Identification and characterization of a high-affinity interaction between v-Crk and tyrosine-phosphorylated paxillin in CT10-transformed fibroblasts, Mol Cell Biol. 13: 4648-56, 1993.
60. Koch, C.A., Moran, M.F., Anderson, D., Liu, X.Q., Mbamalu, G., and Pawson, T. Multiple SH2-mediated interactions in v-src-transformed cells, Mol Cell Biol. 12: 1366-74, 1992.
61. Matsuda, M., Mayer, B.J., Fukui, Y., and Hanafusa, H. Binding of transforming protein, P47gag-crk, to

a broad range of phosphotyrosine-containing proteins, Science. 248: 1537-9, 1990.

62. Sakai, R., Iwamatsu, A., Hirano, N., Ogawa, S., Tanaka, T., Mano, H., Yazaki, Y., and Hirai, H. A novel signaling molecule, p130, forms stable complexes in vivo with v-Crk and v-Src in a tyrosine phosphorylation-dependent manner, EMBO J. 13: 3748-56, 1994.
63. Hamguchi, M., Matsuda, M., and Hanafusa, H. A glycoprotein in the plasma membrane matrix as a major potential substrate of p60v-src, Mol Cell Biol. 10: 830-836, 1990.
64. ten Hoeve, J., Kaartinen, V., Fioretos, T., Haataja, L., Voncken, J.W., Heisterkamp, N., and Groffen, J. Cellular interactions of CRKL, and SH2-SH3 adaptor protein, Cancer Res. 54: 2563-7, 1994.
65. Salgia, R., Li, J.-L., Lo, S.H., Brunkhorst, B., Kansas, G.S., Sobhany, E.S., Sun, Y., Pisick, E., Hallek, M., Ernst, T., Tantravahi, R., Chen, L.B., and Griffin, J.D. Molecular cloning of human paxillin, a focal adhesion protein phosphorylated by p210bcr/abl., J Biol Chem. 270: 5039-47, 1995.
66. Feller, S.M., Knudsen, B., and Hanafusa, H. c-Abl kinase regulates the protein binding activity of c-Crk, EMBO J. 13: 2341-51, 1994.
67. ten Hoeve, J., Arlinghaus, R.B., Guo, J.Q., Heisterkamp, N., and Groffen, J. Tyrosine phosphorylation of CRKL in Philadelphia+ leukemia, Blood. 84: 1731-6, 1994.
68. Oda, T., Heaney, C., Hagopian, J.R., Okuda, K., Griffin, J.D., and Druker, B.J. Crkl is the major tyrosine-phosphorylated protein in neutrophils from patients with chronic myelogenous leukemia, J Biol Chem. 269: 22925-8, 1994.
69. ten Hoeve, J., Morris, C., Heisterkamp, N., and Groffen, J. Isolation and chromosomal localization of CRKL, a human crk-like gene, Oncogene. 8: 2469-74, 1993.
70. Matsuda, M., Mayer, B.J., and Hanafusa, H. Identification of domains of the v-crk oncogene product sufficient for association with phosphotyrosine-containing proteins, Mol Cell Biol. 11: 1607-13, 1991.
71. Mayer, B.J. and Hanafusa, H. Mutagenic analysis of the v-crk oncogene: requirement for SH2 and SH3 domains and correlation between increased cellular phosphotyrosine and transformation, J Virol. 64: 3581-9, 1990.
72. Sabe, H., Okada, M., Nakagawa, H., and Hanafusa, H. Activation of c-Src in cells bearing v-Crk and its suppression by Csk, Mol Cell Biol. 12: 4706-13, 1992.
73. Ogawa, S., Toyoshima, H., Kozutsumi, H., Hagiwara, K., Sakai, R., Tanaka, T., Hirano, N., Mano, H., Yazaki, Y., and Hirai, H. The C-terminal SH3 domain of the mouse c-Crk protein negatively regulates tyrosine-phosphorylation of Crk associated p130 in rat 3Y1 cells, Oncogene. 9: 1669-78, 1994.
74. Turner, C.E. and Miller, J.T. Primary sequence of paxillin contains putative SH2 and SH3 domain binding motifs and multiple LIM domains: identification of a vinculin and $pp125^{Fak}$ binding region, J Cell Sci. 107: 1583-1591, 1994.

Acute Leukemias VI
Prognostic Factors
and Treatment Strategies
Büchner et al. (eds)

Interleukins (IL-1, IL-2, IL-4, IL6) and TNF Production in Children with Acute Lymphoblastic Leukemia

A. Chybicka[1], J. Salwa[2], W. Jaworski[3], Cz. Radzikowski[2], and J. Boguslawska-Jaworska[1]

Abstract. This study was undertaken to establish the role of cytokines (IL-1, IL-2, IL-4, IL-6, and TNF) in the pathogenesis and the clinical course of childhood ALL. A total of 150 children with ALL (88 boys and 62 girls, aged from 0.5 to 15 years) were included in the study. TNF production was studied in supernatants deriving from 24-h PBSC mononuclear culture using the method based on growth inhibition of mice fibroblasts sensitive to TNF α 929, IL-1 production using a method based on inhibition of autologous rosette formation by CBA mouse thymocytes, and IL-2, IL-4, and IL-6 production using a conventional ELISA Genzyme test. Thirty-nine healthy children served as the control group. TNF and IL-1 production decreased after starting chemotherapy for ALL, while a relative increase of IL-6 was observed. It was found that, in children with ALL, IL-1 production, was significantly lower during the whole of therapy than that observed in the control group of healthy children ($p = 0.005$). No IL-2 and IL-4 production was observed in children with ALL during the 2.5-year period of observation. After cessation of therapy IL-1 and TNF production rose, while IL-6 production remained on the same level. During the 10-year period after the end of therapy IL-1 median values did not reach the values of the control group. EFS at 73 months in ALL children with IL-1 production < 10 units before therapy was better than that observed in children with production >10 units (90.48% v 76.19%; $p = 0.005$). EFS at 65 months in ALL children with no detectable TNF production before therapy was better than that observed in children with detectable TNF production (92.31% v 72.73%; n.s.). EFS at 55 months in ALL children with IL-4 production >400 pg/ml before therapy was better than that observed in children with production < 400 pg/ml (80% v 64.26%; n.s.). IL-1, IL-4, and TNF production could be useful prognostic factors.

Introduction

Acute lymphoblastic leukemia (ALL) is a malignant process characterized by unrestricted growth and maturation arrest of hematopoietic precursor cells, possibly due to abnormal cytokine production or abnormal cytokine receptor expression [1–5]. Despite the recent progress in our understanding of the role of cytokines in the origin of cancer cells, their biological significance for malignant cell proliferation is far from clear. The network of cytokines (e.g., G-CSF, TGFβ, MIPα) can stimulate as well as inhibit the proliferation of hematopoietic stem cells and leukemic cells together with the bone marrow stromal complex, including the cellular and extracellular components of the hematopoietic micorenvironment, which support direct hematopoiesis and leukemic proliferation [6–9]. TNF, IL-1, IL-2, IL-4, and IL-6 cooperation in the neoplastics process has not yet been finally elucidated [10–14]. Inadequate

[1]Department of Pediatric Hematology and Oncology, Wroclaw University of Medicine, Wroclaw, Poland
[2]Department of Tumor Immunology, Institute of Immunology and Experimental Therapy Polish Academy of Science, Wroclaw, Poland
[3]Department of Pediatric Surgery, Wroclaw University of Medicine, Wroclaw, Poland

cooperation between cytokines in the cytokine network also plays an important role in the clinical course of the disease [15–17]. We have previously reported the disturbances in IL-1, IL-6, and TNF production, in lymphocyte subset numbers, and in the cytotoxic activity of natural killer cells during the course of cytostatic therapy in children with ALL [18,19]. Therefore, we were interested to find out whether production of cytokines IL-2 and IL-4 is impaired. The aim of this study was to establish the role of IL-1, IL-2, IL-4, IL-6, and TNF in the pathogenesis and clinical course of childhood ALL.

Patients

Between 1988 and 1995, 150 children (88 boys and 62 girls) ranging in age from 0.5 to 15 years (median 9 years) were treated according to the German BFM protocol, which consisted of aggressive chemotherapy combined with radiotherapy. All children were treated in the Department of Pediatric Hematology and Oncology, Faculty of Medicine, in Wroclaw. Thirty-nine healthy children of the same age served as controls for IL-1 level examinations, 20 for TNF production, and 22 for IL-1, IL-2, IL-4, and IL-6 activity. The initial characteristics of the children with ALL are presented in Table 1.

Table 1. Clinical characteristics of children with ALL

	n	%
Sex		
Boys	88	58.67
Girls	62	41.33
Age		
< 2years	8	5.33
2–10 years	130	86.67
> 10 years	12	8.00
Clinical classification		
LRG	45	30.00
MRG	92	61.33
HRG	13	8.67
FAB classification		
L1	123	82.00
L2	25	16.67
L3	2	1.33
Immunological classification		
Pre-B	45/62	72.58
B	2/62	3.23
T	5/62	8.06
Non-T, non-B	10/62	16.13

Methods

Heparinized venous blood samples were drawn from the children at the time of diagnosis, during intensive therapy (induction, consolidation), during maintenance therapy, and after completion of the treatment. Serum IL-4 was examined. Other cytokines in supernatants from 24-h cell culture were studied. Mononuclear cells were isolated on a Lymphoprep (Nesco) gradient.

Isolation of Mononuclear Cells

Mononuclears were counted, resuspended in Eagle's medium containing 10% FCS and placed in an incubator (37°C, 5% CO_2) at a concentration 2×10^6 cells/ml for 24 hours. After 24 hours of incubation the supernatants were removed and used as a source of TNF and IL-1 IL-2 IL-6.

IL-1 Determination

The method used to determine of IL-1 activity was that described by Zimecki and Wieczorek [32], based on inhibition of the number of thymocytes forming autologous rosettes. The thymocytes in 10^7 cells/1.8 ml RPMI, supplemented with 10% FCS and antibotics, were incubated with 0.2 ml of supernatant at various dilutions for 24 h in a CO_2 incubator. For the rosette assay, the cells were resuspended in Eagle's medium at a concentration of 3×10^6 cells/ml, supplemented with 10% mouse serum (preabsorbed with syngenic erythrocytes). To 0.1 ml cell suspension, 0.1 ml 12% syngenic erythrocytes was added, mixed, and centrifuged for 5 min 200 g at 4°C. After 24 h incubation at 4°C, 0.5 ml Hank's medium and 0.1 ml of 0.1% acridine orange solution was added, and the cells were gently resuspended and kept in an ice bath. The percentage of autologous rosettes formed by thymocytes from 2-month-old CBA mice were counted and varied from 28% to 33%. Control samples consisted of referential r-IL-1 dilution. All the results were expressed in units of IL-1. One unit of IL-1 inhibited 50% of rosette formation.

TNF Assay [17]

5×10^4 mice fibroblasts/200 ml per well were incubated for 4 h at 37°C. After washing with 100 RPMI, 640+2% FCS+actinomycin D 1mg/ml and different dilutions of supernatants

(20%, 10%, 5%, 1.0%, and 0.5%) were added. Control samples consisted of referential r-TNF dilution. After a further 18 h incubation (37°C, 5% CO_2), nonadherent cells were removed by washing in PBS, then crystal violet was used to color the cells. After that, violet was extracted and absorbency values of the cell suspension were read at 570 nm. Accurate sample concentrations of TNF were determined by comparing their respective absorbencies with those obtained for the standards plotted on a standard curve.

IL-2, IL-4 and IL-6 Assay [22]

For IL-2, IL-4, and IL-6 specific measurement commercially available antibody "sandwich" ELISA assay was used (TM Interleukin-2, 4, 6 Genzyme Elisa kit). First samples, standards, and control were incubated with a solid phase monoclonal antibody supplied precoated on microtiter wells and used to capture the IL-2, 4, 6 present. The solid phase bound IL-2, 4, 6 was then incubated with a second antibody, biotinylated mouse antihuman IL-2, 4, 6 polyclonal. The resulting immune complexes were then incubated with avidin peroxidase conjugate. The substrate (peroxide) and the chromogen (tetramethylbenzidine) were added. Resulting color developments were directly proportional to the amount of IL-2, IL-4, IL-6. Absorbance values were read at 450 nm for IL-2 and IL-6 and 490 nm for IL-4, using ELISA readers. Accurate sample concentrations of IL-2, 4, 6 were determined by comparing their respective absorbancies with those obtained for the standards plotted on a standard curve.

Results

The results of our studies on IL-1, IL-2, IL-4, and IL-6 and TNF production in various phases of therapy are shown in Table 2. At the time of diagnosis, before any treatment was started, we found a decrease of median values of IL-6, parallel with deficient IL-1 production, compared with the values in the control group of healthy children. Median TNF and IL-4 production was higher than in children from the control group (0.188U v 0U; 330 pg/ml v 122 pg/ml). No IL-2 presence in 24-h supernatants was observed during the whole period of therapy.

Event-free survival (EFS) at 73 months in ALL children with IL-1 production <10 units before therapy was better than that observed in children with production >10 units (90.48% v 76.19%; $p=0.005$; Fig. 1).

EFS at 65 months in ALL Children with no detectable TNF production before therapy was better than that observed in children with detectable TNF production (92.31% v 72.73%; n.s; Fig. 1).

EFS at 55 months in ALL children with IL-4 production >400 pg/ml before therapy was better than that observed in children with production <400 pg/ml (80% v 64.26; n.s.; Fig. 1).

There was no difference between EFS at 56 months in ALL children with IL-6 production <450 pg/ml before therapy and those with production >450 pg/ml (87.5% v 83.33%; Fig. 1).

TNF, IL-1, and IL-4 production decreased after starting chemotherapy and remained low during the whole period of treatment (Fig. 2), while a relative increase of IL-6 was observed.

After the end of therapy an increase in TNF and IL-1 production was noticed, and a decrease in IL-4 production, while IL-6 values remained at the same level. For 5 years after the end of therapy IL-1 median values did not reach the values of the control group of healthy children, while IL-6 and TNF production were within normal limits or even above.

Discussion

The reduction in production of IL-1 in patients with cancer was previously found by ourselves and Herman et al. [24]. As an extension of that observation [18, 19], we hypothesize that impaired IL-1, TNF, and IL-6 production observed in children with ALL may be connected with the impaired production of IL-2 and IL-4. In the present study we investigated IL-1, IL-2, IL-4, IL-6, and TNF in children with ALL before, during and after chemotherapy. The results obtained before therapy suggest that IL-1, IL-4, and TNF production could be used as additional prognostic factors, while IL-6 cannot (Fig. 1).

Our findings suggest that TNF, IL-1, and IL-6 may be released by cancer cells in some patients. It seems to be proven that IL-1, IL-6, and TNF play the important role in myeloma and plasmocytoma cells proliferation [20–22]. Malignant cell growth influenced by IL-6 and its production is stimulated by IL-1 [17].

Table 2. IL-1, IL-4, IL-6 and TNF production in children with ALL during various phases of treatment

	Before therapy			During cytostatic therapy			After cytostatic therapy			Control group		
	Median	Mean	Range	Median	Mean	Range	Median	Mean	Range	Median	Mean	Range
IL-I (units)	14.60	23.27	0–64	4	10.57	0–64	10	19.10	0–72	15	26.21	2–64
IL-4 (pg/ml)	330	408.38	100–840	20	66	0–590	0	125.8	0–600	122.5	137.5	0–470
IL-6 (pg/ml)	405	402	0–954	1800	1218	0–1800	1800	1800	0–1800	1320	1230	0–1800
TNF (units)	0.188	0.798	0–5.3	0	0.43	0–6.2	0.178	0.8	0–3.2	0	0.344	0–1.23

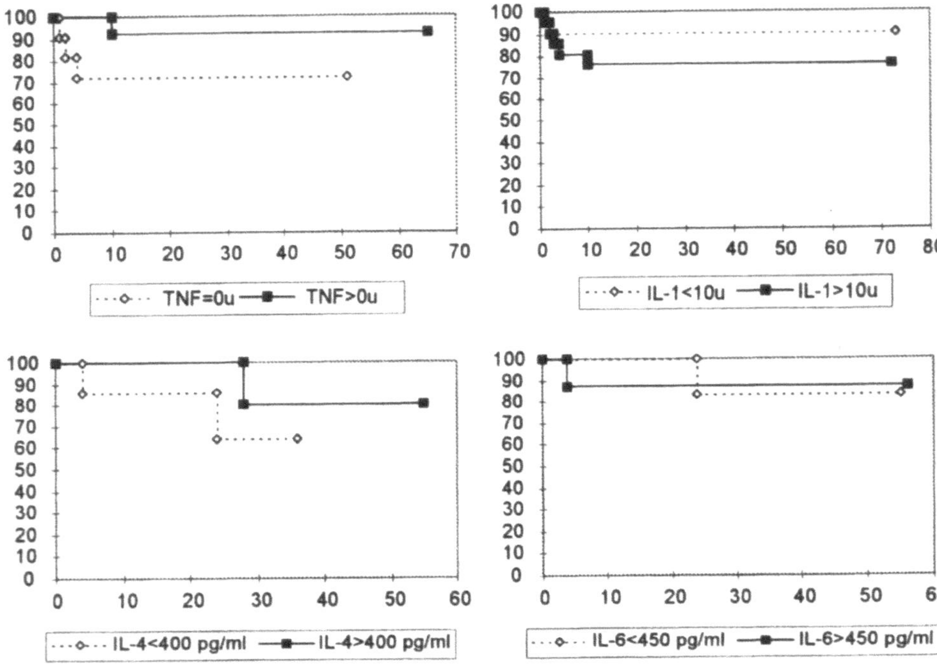

Fig. 1. Event-free survival in children with (ALL) in relation to IL-1, IL-4, IL-6, and TNF production before therapy was started.

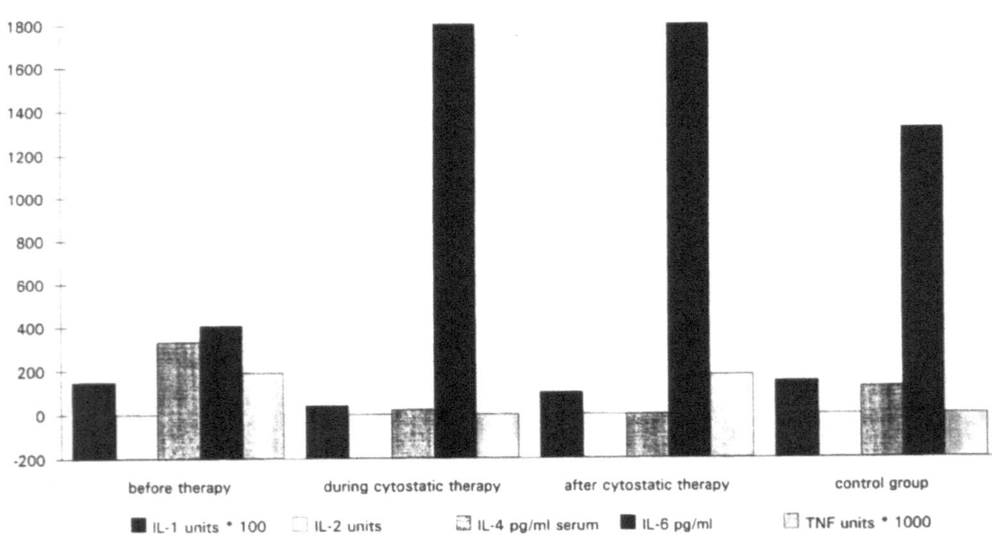

Fig. 2. IL-1, IL-2, IL-4, IL-6, and TNF production in children with ALL during various phases of treatment (median values)

Another point for discussion is the influence of chemotherapy administered to children with ALL on TNF, IL-1, IL-4, and IL-6 production. Chemotherapy may damage the mechanisms which lead to defective production of cytokines TNF, IL-1, and IL-4. This deficit may contribute to the increased risk of life-threatening infection in these patients [23]. Balkwill et al. have reported similar results in patients with difference types of cancer during chemotherapy [13].

Our studies revealed that IL-6 production during the whole period of therapy was higher than in normal healthy controls, which does not correlate with the impaired IL-1, IL-4 activity, and TNF production (n.s.). This observation can be explained by data of Schindler et al., who found that IL-6 suppresses both TNF and IL-1 production [28].

It is to be noted after the end of chemotherapy IL-1 and IL-4 production remain decreased. The reason for this decrease is not clear. The possible role of specific IL-1 inhibitors needs experimental confirmation [21, 23, 27]. After the end of chemotherapy IL-6 and TNF production were found to be highly elevated. It seems that high IL-6 and TNF activity could be explained by concomitant infection with hepatitis B and C viruses, recorded in some of the children [25, 26, 29–31]. However, the reason for the increased IL-6 and TNF activity after successful chemotherapy requires further studies and observation.

Acknowledgments. This work was supported by grant no.4S405 079 07.

References

1. Minamishima I., Ohga S., Ishii E., Matsuzaki A., Kai T., Akazawa K., Ueda K. (1993) Serum interleukin-6 and fever at diagnosis in children with acute leukemia. Am J Pediatr Hematol Oncol, Vol.15, No. 2,1993
2. Ouazz F., Menz F., Mossalayi M.D., Schmitt C., Michel A., Debre P., Guillosson J-J, Merle-Beral H., Arock M. (1994) Interleukin 4 inhibits the proliferation and promotes the maturation of human leukemic early B cells. Eur J Haematol: 51: 276–281.
3. Ferrajoli A., Zipf T.F., Talpaz M., Felix E.A., Estrov Z. (1993) Growth factors controlling interleukin-4 action on hematopoietic progenitors. Ann Hematol 67: 277–284
4. Jewell A.P., Yong K.L., Worman C.P., Giles F.J., Goldstone A.H., Lydyard P.M. (1992) Cytokine induction of leucocyte adhesion molecule-1 (LAM-1) expression on chronic lymphocytic leuukaemia cells. Leukemia, 6,5:400–404
5. Janssen R.A., Mulder N.H., Hauw The T., de Leij L. (1994) The immunobiological effects of interleukin-2 in vivo. Cancer Immunol Immunother 39: 207–216
6. Griffiths S.D., Cawley J.C. (1990) The effect of cytokines, including IL-1, IL-4, and IL-6, in hairy cell proliferation/differentation. Leukemia, 4, 5: 337-340
7. Namunaitis J. (1994) Growth factors of the future. Leuke Lymphoma, 9: 329–336
8. Carter A., Haddad N., Draxler I., Tatarsky I. (1994) Effects of soluble interleukin-1 receptor and tumor-necrosis factor receptor, respectively, on the IL-1 and TNF-α-induced DNA synthesis of acute myeloblastic leukemia blasts in vitro. Eur J Haematol: 53: 38-45.
9. Börset M., Waage A., Brekke O.L., Helseth E. (1994) TNF and IL-6 are potent growth factors for OH-2, a novel human myeloma cell line. Eur J Haematol; 53: 31–37.
10. Aguilar-Santelises M., Magnusson R., Svenson, S.B., Loftennuis A., Anderson B., Mellstedt H., Jondal M., (1991) Expression of interleukin 1 alfa, interleukin 1 beta and interleukin -6 in chronic B lymphocytic leukaemia -B-CLL) cells from patients at different stages of disease progression. Clin. Exp. Immunol, 84, 422–428
11. Akira S., Kishmoto T., (1992) IL-6 and TNF IL-6 in acute phase response and viral infection. Immunol. Rev. 127, 25–50.
12. Baigrie R.J, lamont P.M, Dallman M., Morris P.J, (1991) The release of interleukin-1 beta (IL-1) precedes that of interleukin-6 (IL-6) in patients undergoing major surgery. Lymphokine Cytokine Res, 10, 4 253–256
13. Balkwill F., Burke F., Talbot D., Tavernier J., Osborne R., Naylor S., Durbin H., Fiers W. (1987): Evidence for tumor necrosis factor/cachectin production in cancer. Lancet 28: 1229–1232.
14. Bauer J., Herrman F. (1991) Interleukin-6 in clinical medicine. Ann Hematol 62, 203–210
15. Bocci V., (1991) Interleukins. Clinical pharmacokinetics and practical implications. Clin. Pharmacokinet. 21, 274–284
16. Boer E.C., Jong H.W, Steerengberg P.A., Aarden L.A., Tetteroo E., Groot E.R., Van der Mejden A.P.M., Vegt P.D, J, Degruyne F.M, Ruitenberg E.J., (1992) Induction of urinary interleukin -1(IL-1), IL-2, IL-6 and tumor necrosis factor during intravesical immunotherapy with bacillus Calmette-Guerin in superficial bladder cancer. Cancer Immunol. Immunother. 34, 306–312
17. Carter A., Merchav S., Silvian-Draxler I., Tatarsky I. (1990): The role of interleukin-1 and tumor necrosis factor-a in human multiple myeloma. Br.J. Haematol. 74: 424–431.
18. Chybicka A., Boguslawska-Jaworska J. (1990): Interleukin-1 Production in Childhood Acute Lymphoblastic Leukemia During Chemo- and Radiotherapy According to BFM protocols. In: Acute Leukemia II. Ed: Büchner T., Schellong G.,

Hiddemann W., Ritter J. Hematology and Blood Transf. Springer-Verlag 133: 72–75.
19. Chybicka A, Boguslawska-Jaworska J., Budzynski W., Radzikowski Cz., Jaworski W. (1992), IL-1 production by mononuclear cell and NK cell activity in children with ALL Hematol. and Blood Transf.- Acute Leukemias ed Kusche/Hiddemann Springer-Verlag
20. Danis V.A., Franic G,M, Rathjen D.A., Brooks P.M. (1991) Effects of granulocyte macrophage colony stimulating factor (GM-CSF), IL-2, interferon gamma (IFNgamma), tumor necrososis factor alfa (TNF alfa) and IL-6 on the production of immunoreactive IL-1 and TNF alfa by human monocytes. Clin. Exp. Immunol. 85, 143–150
21. Fibbe E., Schaafsma M.R., Falkenburg F.J., Willemze R. (1989) The biological activities of interleukin 1. Blut, 59: 147.
22. Grau G.E. (1990): Implications of cytokines in immunopathology experimental and clinical data. Eur. Cytokine Net., 1, 203–210
23. Hamilton J,A. (1993) Colony stimulating factors, cytokines and monocyte-macrophages-some contronversies. Immunol. Today 14,1,18–23
24. Herman J.A., Kew M.C., Rabson A.R. (1984). Defective interleukin-1 production by monocytes from patients with malignant diseases: interferon increases IL-1 production. Cancer Immunol. Immunotherap 16: 182–5.
25. Hirano T., Akira S., Taga T. Hishimoto T. (1990) Biological and clinical aspects of interleukin 6. Immunology Today 11, (12) 443–449
26. Kastan J.B., Strauss L.C., Civin C.I. (1989) The role of hematopoietic growth factors and oncogenes in leukemogenesis. Am. J. Ped. Hem/Oncol. 11, 249–267.
27. Rosenstreich D., Haimovitz A., Brown K., Liao Z. (1987) Human interleukin 1 inhibitors. Lymphokines, ed. Edger Pick Academic Press inc 14,64
28. Schindler R., Mancilla J., Endres S., Ghorbani R., Clark S.C., Dinarello C.A. (1990) Correlations and interactions in the production of interleukin-6 (IL-6), IL-1 and tumor necrosis factor (TNF) in human blood mononuclear cells: IL-6 suppresses IL-1 and TNF. Blood 75, 40–47
29. Tosato G., Jones K.D. (1990) Interleukin 1 induces interleukin-6 production in peripheral blood monocytes. Blood 75,(6), 1305–1310
30. Wardrop C.C.J., Holland B. (1992) Hematopoietic growth factors. Curr Opin Pediatr 4,84-91
31. Wong G.C., Clark S.C., (1988) Multiple actions of interleukin 6 within a cytokine network. Immunology Today 9,(5)
32. Zimecki M., Wieczorek Z. (1987) IL-1 decreases the level of thymocytes forming rosettes with autologous erythrocytes, a new method of determination of IL-1 activity. Arch Immunol Ther Exp (Warsz) 355: 371.

Acute Leukemias VI
Prognostic Factors
and Treatment Strategies
Büchner et al. (eds)

Insulin-Like Growth Factors and Their Specific Binding Proteins in Leukemia (ALL) and Non-Hodgkin Lymphoma

P. Vorwerk[1], K. Mohnike[1], W.F. Blum[2], U. Kluba[1], V. Aumann[1], and U. Mittler[1]

Abstract. Insulin-like growth factors (IGF) are potent mitogens both in normal growth and in tumor proliferation. The bioavailability of both IGF-I and IGF-II is regulated by at least six specific IGF-binding proteins (IGFBP). IGFBP-3 is growth hormone dependent and part of the predominant circulating IGF carrier in serum. During fetal life IGFBP-2 is found ubiquitously. In addition it is expressed in a range of tumor cell lines and lymphoblasts. We studied serum levels of IGF-I, IGF-II, IGFBP-2, and IGFBP-3 in 25 children with acute lymphoblastic leukemia or non-Hodgkin lymphoma. Serum levels of IGF-I (mean/range: −2.3/−0.7 to −9.9 standard deviation score, SDS), IGF-II (−2.6 / 0.3 to −5.6 SDS) and IGFBP-3 (−1.6/0.7 to −6.8 SDS) were significantly decreased, comparable to levels in growth hormone deficiency or during starvation. On the other hand, IGFBP-2 levels (+3.5/−2.7 to +8.3 SDS) were found to be markedly elevated. After hematological remission upon chemotherapy, IGF-I, IGF-II, and both IGFBP-2 and IGFBP-3 had normalized. We conclude that (1) malignant lymphoblasts proliferate despite decreased serum levels of IGF-I, IGF-II, and IGFBP-3; (2) changes in IGFBP-2 far exceeded those that would be expected in patients with growth hormone deficiency; and (3) chemotherapy led to normalization of serum IGF-I, IGF-II, and IGFBP-3.

Introduction

Insulin-like growth factors (IGF)-I and IGF-II are thought to be significant mitogenic factors [1]. IGF-II has been described as a fetal growth factor [2, 3], and high level expression is also found in Wilms' tumor [4,5], sarcomas, and a variety of other tumors [6]. IGFs share a significant structural homology with insulin. In contrast to insulin, IGF-I and IGF-II are bound to specific IGF-binding proteins (IGFBPs), which regulate their bioavailability [7–9]. Six different peptides have been classified as IGFBP-1 to −6 according to an international nomenclature [10, 11]. Postnatally a ternary complex consisting of IGFBP-3, IGF-I or IGF-II, and a third protein, "ALS" (acid-labile subunit), is the predominant circulating carrier. During fetal life the most abundant binding protein is IGFBP-2 [2, 12]. Elevated serum levels of IGFBP-2 have been found in patients with prostate cancer [13], Wilms' tumor [14], and other tumors [9]. However, only limited information is currently available on the IGF regulatory system in leukemia. Therefore, the principal objective of this study was to characterize serum levels of IGF-I, IGF-II, IGFBP-2, and IGFBP-3 at diagnosis and during therapy.

Patients and Methods

All blood samples were obtained from patients with acute lymphoblastic leukemia (ALL) or non-Hodgkin lymphoma (NHL) who were referred to our oncological unit (Table 1). Diagnoses were based on the definition of the BFM cooperative study group [15]. Twenty-five children were followed during chemotherapy

[1]Otto-van-Guericke-Universität Magdeburg, Zentrum für Kinderheilkunde, Halberstadter Str. 13, 39120 Magdeburg, Germany
[2]Endokrinlogisches Forschungslabor der Universitätsklinik, Feulgenstr. 12, 35385 Giessen, Germany

Table 1. Disease classification of patients enrolled in the study

Immunophenotype	Number of patients	age range (years)
Pre-B-ALL	5	0.9–8.3
B-ALL/B-NHL	3/3	5.5–9.2
C-ALL	5	1.5–8.4
T-NHL	4	3.4–15.9
T-ALL	4	6.3–12.3

ALL, Acute lymphoblastic leukemia; NHL, non-Hodgkin lymphoma.

using protocol BFM 90 [16]. Serum was stored at −20°C until analysis. IGF-I, IGF-II, IGFBP-2, and IGFBP-3 were determined by radioimmunoassay as described previously [17,18], except that recombinant hIGFBP-2 (the kind gift of Sandoz, Basel, Switzerland) was used for tracer and standard preparation [19]. IGF-I and IGF-II were measured after acid ethanol extraction. Because of the age dependence of the normal ranges during childhood, the values of IGF-I, IGF-II, IGFBP-2, and IGFBP-3 were age-adjusted [20] by calculating the standard deviation score (SDS).

Statistical evaluation was done with the statistical package SPSS for Windows, using the Wilcoxon test and correlation analysis. p values below 0.05 were considered as significant.

Results

Initial Data at Diagnosis

Serum levels of IGF-I, IGF-II, IGFBP-3, and IGFBP-2 at diagnosis of ALL or NHL were compared with the age-dependent normal range (Fig. 1). Levels of IGF-I (13 patients out of 25), IGF-II (14/22), and IGFBP-3 (9/25) were found to be below the 5th percentile of the controls [20]. Serum concentrations of IGFBP-2 were on average above the 95th percentile (19/23). IGFBP-3 showed a positive correlation with IGF-I ($r=0.50$, $p=0.012$) and IGF-II ($r=0.78$, ($p<0.0001$), and a negative correlation with IGF-I IGFBP-2 ($r=-0.46$, $p=0.027$). No differences were found with respect to mean IGF-I, IGF-II, IGFBP-2, and IGFBP-3 levels in patients with NHL or ALL, different immunophenotypes, age groups, or ALL risk factor.

Influence of Treatment

Figure 2 shows individual serum SDS values of IGF-I, IGF-II, IGFBP-2, and IGFBP-3 during chemotherapy. A significant increase in the low values of IGF-I ($z=-4.01$, $p=0.0001$), IGF-II ($z=-2.35$, $p=0.019$), and IGFBP-3 ($z=-3.12$, $p=0.0018$) occurred with the hematological remission. Correspondingly, the elevated IGFBP

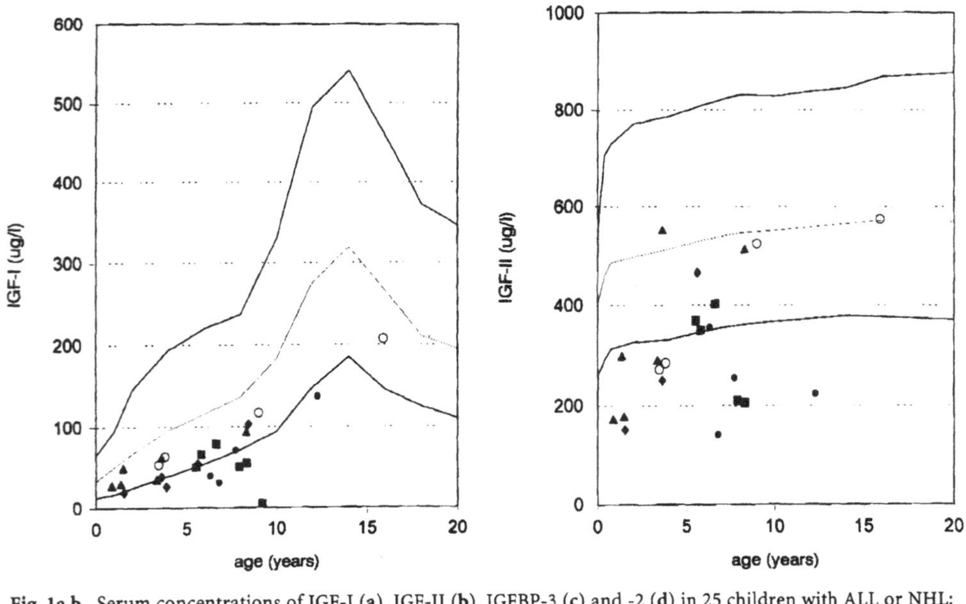

Fig. 1a,b. Serum concentrations of IGF-I (**a**), IGF-II (**b**), IGFBP-3 (**c**) and -2 (**d**) in 25 children with ALL or NHL: B-cell-precursor ALL (▲), C-ALL (◆), B-ALL/B-NHL (■), T-NHL, (○), and T-ALL (●). The age-dependent normal range is given for the 5th, 50th, and 95th percentiles

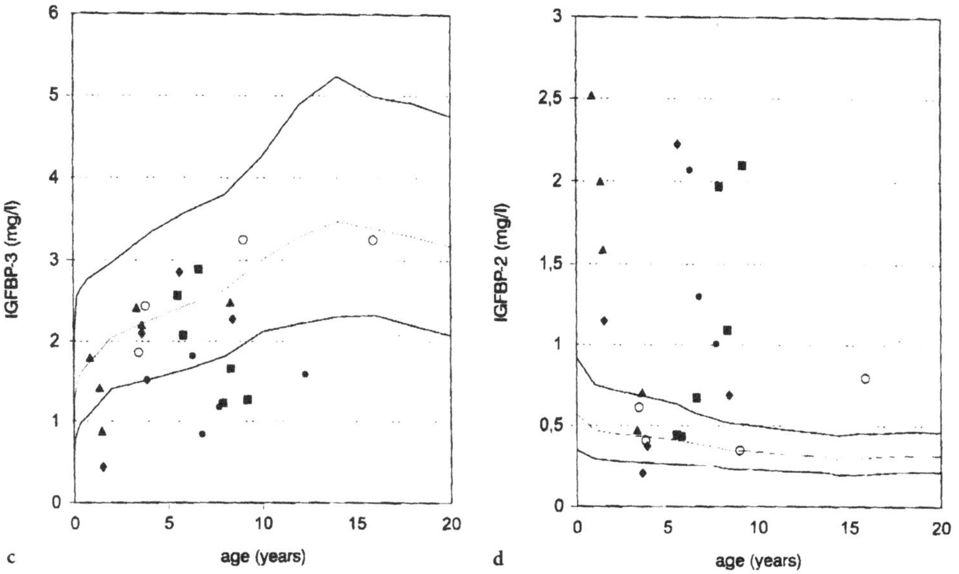

Fig. 1c,d

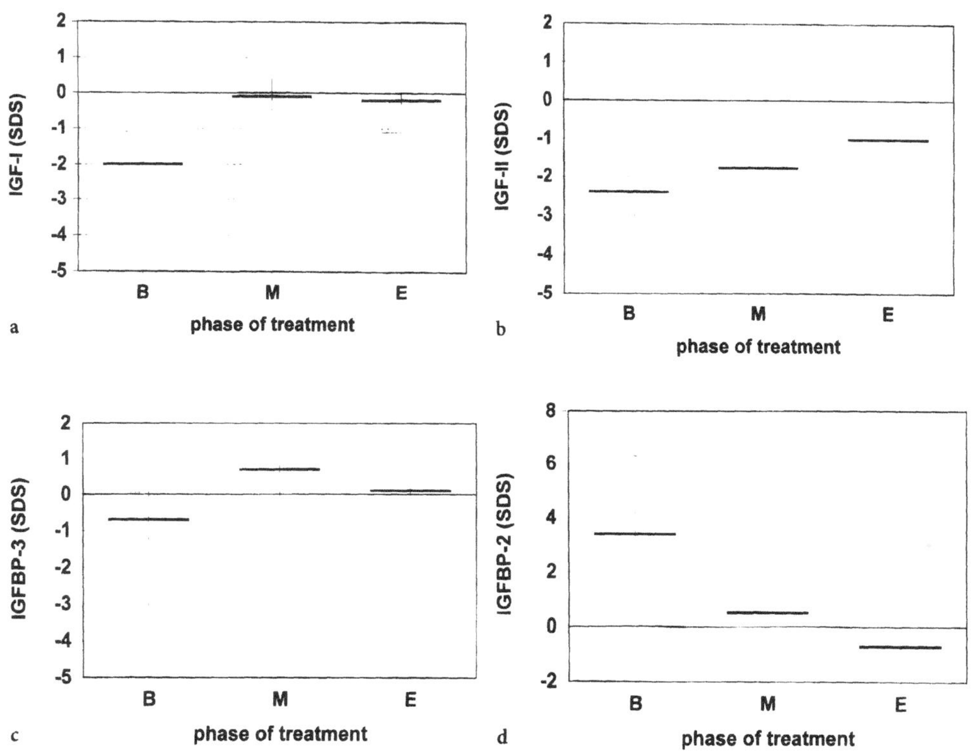

Fig. 2a–d. Serum levels (SDS) of IGF-1 (**a**), IGF-II (**b**), IGFBP-3 (**c**), and -2 (**d**) during treatment according to BFM 90 (B: before therapy, M: protocol M, E: after treatment). The 25th, 50th, and 75th percentiles are shown

−2 levels declined into the normal range ($z = -2.53, p = 0.011$).

A relapse was diagnosed in four additional patients. At the time of relapse all four parameters were within normal limits in three of four children. However, in one boy with leukemic meningiosis the serum levels were altered, showing a similar pattern as in patients at diagnosis (IGF-I: −5.3 SDS; IGF-II: −2.6 SDS; IGFBP-3: 1.1 SDS; IGFBP-2: +5.4 SDS).

Discussion

It has recently become clear that the IGF regulatory pathway is of major impact in solid tumors. In patients with prostate cancer Kanety et al. [13] have by Western ligand blotting found elevated serum levels of IGFBP-2 and decreased levels of IGFBP-3, whereas IGF-I and IGF-II values were within the normal range. Elevated serum levels of IGFBP-2 were described in Wilms' tumor [14], and in addition, in endometrial cancer, significantly lower values of IGF-I, IGF-II, and IGFBP-3 [21]. Moreover, the present study shows that in ALL the IGF regulatory pathway is altered in a similar way, as reflected by serum levels of IGFs and IGFBPs. Thus, taken together these data allow several conclusions to be drawn. First, proliferation of malignant lymphoblasts occurs despite decreased serum levels of the mitogenic peptides IGF-I and IGF-II. Second, two major serum IGFBPs are regulated in opposite directions [9, 22]. Third, these data indicate that serum levels of IGFBP-2 may be directly related to the proliferation of lymphoblasts. Although IGFBPs are known to regulate the bioavailability of IGF-I and/or IGF-II [1, 9] their precise overall function is not yet known. From the data of the present study it might be speculated that IGFBP-2 may be involved in the proliferation of leukemic cell clones. Two possible explanations might explain the observed changes in serum levels of IGFBP-2: production by the malignant lymphoblast clones or upregulation of common synthetic pathways in response to the disease. In favor of the first hypothesis is the finding that normal lymphoblasts respond to the mitogen PHA with an extensive increase in the IGFBP-2 gene expression [23]. Also, malignant lymphoblasts express and release IGFBP-2 [24]. However, the second hypothesis cannot be excluded in view of the existence of a variety of pathological conditions where IGF-I is low and free IGF-II is expected to be high and elevated IGFBP-2 levels have been found [25]. Basal levels of IGF-I and IGF-II were low and are comparable to those in patients with growth hormone (GH) deficiency or starvation. So far, little information is available on GH secretion in these patients, and in this study GH secretion was not evaluated. Serum levels of IGFBP-3 in GH deficiency are below the 5th percentile [17], whereas in our patients only a small group was below this limit. However, it remains an open question whether or not low GH secretion accounts for low IGF-I, IGF-II, and IGFBP-3 levels. Starvation does not seem to play a role in these patients at diagnosis. Surprisingly, during treatment all measured IGF parameters normalized, despite the fact that in a number of patients severe nutritional problems occurred due to chemotherapy and cytotoxicity. Therefore, nutrition does not appear to be a major regulator in such situations.

On the other hand, it cannot be ruled out that the influence of cytokines, i.e., IL-1, IL-6, or TNFα may be responsible for downregulation of these parameters [26]. In septicemia there is a massive resistance to GH action with respect to IGF-I production [27], and IL-1 has been shown to suppress IGF-1 production. The course of IGF-I, IGF-II, and IGFBP-3, which are thought to be important for growth, parallel the changes in growth velocity as observed by us in a corresponding group of patients [28]. Therefore it appears that these parameters are major determinants of growth in leukemic patients. In addition, IGFBP-2 may be useful for monitoring therapy; it remains an objective for future research to determine whether or not it is a useful parameter for early detection of a relapse of leukemia.

References

1. Cohick WS, Clemmons DR: The insulin-like growth factors. Annu Rev Physiol 1993;55: 131–153.
2. Orlowski CC, Brown AL, Ooi GT, et al.: Tissue, developmental, and metabolic regulation of messenger ribonucleic acid encoding a rat insulin-like growth factor-binding protein. Endocrinology 1990; 126: 644–652.
3. Han VK, D'Ercole AJ, Lund PK; Cellular localization of somatomedin (insulin-like growth factor) messenger RNA in the human fetus. Science 1987; 236: 193–197.

4. Ren-Qiu Q, Ruelicke T, Hassam S, et al.: Systemic effects of insulin-like growth factor-II produced and released from Wilms tumour tissue. Eur J Pediatr 1993; 152: 102–106.
5. Ogawa O, Eccles MR, Szeto J, et al.: Relaxation of insulin-like growth factor II gene imprinting implicated in Wilms' tumor. Nature 1993; 362: 749–751.
6. Daughaday WH, Deuel TF: Tumor secretion of growth factors. Endocrinol Metab Clin North Am 1991; 20: 539–563.
7. Binoux M, Roghani M, Hossenlopp P, et al.: Molecular forms of human IGF binding proteins: physiological implications. Acta Endocrinol (Copenh) 1991; 124 Suppl 2: 41–47.
8. Clemmons DR: Insulinlike growth factor binding proteins; in LeRoith D (ed): Insulin-like growth factors: molecular and cellular aspects. Boca Raton, CRC Press, 1991, pp 151–180.
9. Rechler MM: Insulin-like growth factor binding proteins. Vitam Horm 1993; 47: 1–114.
10. Ballard J, Baxter R, Binoux M, et al.: On the nomenclature of the IGF binding proteins [letter]. Acta Endocrinol (Copenh) 1989; 121: 751–752.
11. Drop SL: Report on the nomenclature of the IGF binding proteins. Acta Endocrinol (Copenh) 1991; 125: 707–708.
12. Wood TL, Streck RD, Pintar JE: Expression of the IGFBP-2 gene in post-implantation rat embryos. Development 1992; 114: 59-66.
13. Kanety H, Madjar Y, Dagan Y, et al.: Serum insulin-like growth factor-binding protein-2 (IGFBP-2) is increased and IGFBP-3 is decreased in patients with prostate cancer: correlation with serum prostate-specific antigen. J Clin Endocrinol Metab 1993; 77: 229–233.
14. Zumkeller W, Schwander J, Mitchell CD, et al.: Insulin-like growth factor (IGF)-I, -II, and IGF binding protein-2 (IGFBP-2) in the plasma of children with Wilms' tumour. Eur J Cancer 1993; 29A: 73–77.
15. van der Does-van den Berg A, Bartram CR, Basso G, et al: Minimal requirements for the diagnosis, classification, and evaluation of the treatment of childhood acute lymphoblastic leukemia (ALL) in the "BFM Family" Cooperative Group. Med Pediatr Oncol 1992; 20: 497–505.
16. Sauerbrey A, Zintl F, Malke H, et al.: [Results and experiences with a modified BFM protocol for treatment of recurrences in children with acute lymphoblastic leukemia in East German areas]. Klin Padiatr 1993; 205: 281–287.
17. Blum WF, Ranke MB, Kietzmann K, et al.: A specific radioimmunoassay for the growth hormone (GH)-dependent somatomedin-binding protein: its use for diagnosis of GH deficiency. J Clin Endocrinol Metab 1990; 70: 1992–1298.
18. Blum WF, Ranke MB, Bierich JR: A specific radioimmunoassay for insulin-like growth factor II: the interference of IGF binding proteins can be blocked by excess IGF-I. Acta Endocrinol (Copenh) 1988; 118: 374–380.
19. Chard T, Blum WF, Brunjes J, et al.: Levels of insulin-like growth factor-binding protein-2 and insulin-like growth factor-II in maternal serum, amniotic fluid and extraembryonic coelomic fluid at 9-20 weeks to pregnancy. J Endocrinol 1994; 142: 379–383.
20. Blum WF: Insulin-like growth factors and their binding proteins; in Ranke MB (ed): Functional endocrinologic diagnostics in children and adolescents. Mannheim, J & J Verlag, 1992, pp 102–118.
21. Rutanen EM, Stenman S, Blum WF, et al.: Relationship between carbohydrate metabolism and serum insulin-like growth factor system in postmenopausal women: comparison of endometrial cancer patients with healthy controls. J Clin Endocrinol Metab 1993; 77: 199–204.
22. Clemmons DR, Jones JI, Busby WH, et al.: Role of insulin-like growth factor binding proteins in modifying IGF actions. Ann N Y Acad Sci 1993; 692: 10–21.
23. Nyman T, Pekonen F: The expression of insulin-like growth factors and their binding proteins in normal human lymphocytes. Acta Endocrinol (Copenh) 1993; 128: 168–172.
24. Lee PD, Rosenfeld RG, Hintz RL, et al.: Characterization of insulin, insulin-like growth factors I and II, and growth hormone receptors on human leukemic lymphoblasts. J Clin Endocrinol Metab 1986; 62: 28–35.
25. Blum WF, Horn N, Kratzsch J, et al.: Clinical studies of IGFBP-2 by radioimmunoassay. Growth Regul 1993; 3: 100–104.
26. Yateman ME, Claffey DC, Cwyfan Hughes SC, et al.: Cytokines modulate the sensitivity of human fibroblasts to stimulation with insulin-like growth factor-I (IGF-I) by altering endogenous IGF-binding protein production. J Endocrinol 1993; 137: 151–159.
27. Dahn MS, Lange MP, Jacobs LA: Insulinlike growth factor 1 production is inhibited in human sepsis. Arch Surg 1988; 123: 1409–1414.
28. Timme J, Mittler U, Mohnike K: Einfluss verschiedener Therapieprotokolle auf das Wachstum und die Endgrösse von Kindern mit akuter lymphoblastischer Leukamie oder Non-Hodgkin-Lymphom. Klin Pädiatr 1994; (in press)

Acute Leukemias VI
Prognostic Factors
and Treatment Strategies
Büchner et al. (eds)

IFN-α Is an Inhibitory Cytokine of Leukemic B-Cell Precursors

C. Buske, H. Schotte , M. Feuring-Buske, S. Könemann, W. Hiddemann, and B. Wörmann

Abstract. For the development of new therapeutic strategies in B-cell precursor acute lymphoblastic leukemia (BCP-ALL), the identification of negative growth regulators of leukemic BCP is of great importance. Recently, the establishment of stromal-cell-dependent coculture systems allowed the in vitro culture of normal and leukemic BCP. We used a cross-species feeder-cell-dependent coculture system for the identification of inhibitory cytokines of leukemic BCP. The leukemic pre-B cell line BLIN-1 was selected for establishment and standardization of experimental conditions. Apoptosis of BLIN-1 was reduced from 22% to 3.6% by the murine fibroblast subclone C58 in the coculture system. Leukemic BCP were tested in nine patients. The murine feeder cells efficiently reduced apoptosis in six samples with a mean reduction of 57%. Thus murine fibroblasts can substitute for human bone marrow stromal cells and block the rapid spontaneous cell death of leukemic blasts in vitro. Next we investigated the influence of IFN-α on cell viability and apoptosis of leukemic blasts from patients with the diagnosis BCP-ALL and of the cell line BLIN-1 in the feeder-cell-dependent coculture system. Cell viability of 5/5 samples tested was reduced by IFN-α Loss of cell viability was 35% (range 51–23.5). IFN-α enhanced apoptosis in 3/5 samples with a 34% increase (range 5.6–85.6) in the responder compared to the control. There was great interindividual heterogeneity in IFN-α response. In 2/3 samples tested IL-7 blocked IFN-α induced apoptosis. BLIN-1 showed an increase of the apoptotic cell fraction from 11% in the control to 25% with IFN-α. The results characterize IFN-α as an inhibitory cytokine of leukemic BCP. The use of murine feeder-cell-dependent coculture systems may help analysis of the growth regulation of leukemic BCP in vitro.

Introduction

One potential option for novel therapeutic approaches in B-cell precursor Acute Lymphoblastic Leukemia (BCP-ALL) is the identification of negative growth signals for the leukemic blasts. Studies on the regulation of proliferation and growth inhibition in normal and leukemic human pre-B cells have long been hampered by the rapid death of the cell population ex vivo and the lack of a reproducible in vitro assay [1]. Murine long-term culture systems were not easily transferable to the human system [2, 3]. Recently, several groups have suceeded in maintaining in vitro viability and inducing some proliferation of fetal pre-B cells [4, 5] as well as leukemic blasts from patients with B-lineage ALL [6]. These assays are stromal-cell-based and open the way for in-depth analysis of pre-B cell regulation. The effect of bone marrow stromal cells can partially be substituted by murine fibroblasts [7]. One of the major candidates for negative regulation are the interferons [8, 9]. In the murine system IFN-γ blocks IL-7-induced proliferation of normal pre-B cells [8]. IFN-α reduced cell viability of Ph+-ALL cell lines at high concentrations [10].

Department of Internal Medicine, Division of Hematology Oncology, University Hospital, Robert-Koch-Str. 40, 37075 Göttingen, Germany

In vivo IFN-α was investigated as maintenance therapy in Ph+-ALL [11] and has already been introduced in clinical medicine for treatment of low-grade non Hodgkin's lymphoma, hairy cell leukemia, multiple myeloma, and chronic myelogenous leukemia.

We have used a recently developed murine feeder-cell-dependent coculture system which prevents the rapid death of leukemic BCP in vitro [7] to address the question whether IFN-α is a relevant negative growth regulator in BCP-ALL. We used the cytokine-sensitive leukemic pre-B cell line BLIN-1 as a model for establishment and standardization of experimental conditions[12] and analyzed five leukemic samples of patients with the diagnosis BCP-ALL.

Material and Methods

Human Leukemic BCP

Mononuclear bone marrow cells of seven children with C-ALL and of two children with pre-pre-B cell ALL were isolated by Ficoll density gradient and stained with CD10-FITC and CD19 -PE. Quantification of leukemic blasts was performed by FACS analysis, defining cells with the typical lymphoid scatter profile and positivity for CD10/CD19 as leukemic(BCP). Between 70% and 90% of mononuclear cells belonged to the leukemic cell population.

Cell Lines

BLIN-1 is a human leukemic cytokine-sensitive pre-B cell line, established from a patient with ALL [12]. BLIN-1 grows spontaneously only at a high cell concentration. C58 is a subclone of the murine fibroblast cell line L929 [7]. Cells were cultured in RPMI 1640 (Gibco, Germany) supplemented with 5% or 10% FCS (HyClone, USA), 100 U penicillin/ml, and 100 µg streptomycin/ml (Sigma, Germany) in humidified air with 5% CO_2 at 37°C. Confluent C58 layers were passaged by treatment with 0.1% trypsin-EDTA. HL-60 cells incubated with 100 µmol Ara-C (Pfizer, Germany) for 24 h served as positive control for apoptosis.

Coculture Systems

BLIN-1 cells (1×10^4 cells/ml) were seeded on subconfluent human bone marrow stromal cells or irradiated (40 Gy) confluent C58 layers. For analysis of cell morplhology, 1×10^4 cells were sppun onto glass slides using a cytospin (Cytospin 2, Shandon, UK) and stained with May-Grunwald/Giemsa. 1×10^6 mononuclear cells/ml bone marrow aspirate of patients with the diagnosis BCP-ALL were seeded on irradiated confluent C58 feeder layers and cocultured at 37°C and 5% CO_2. Viability was assessed by trypan blue assay. Specificity was partly confirmed by staining with CD10 and CD19 on day 6. In all samples tested surviving cells were CD10/CD19-positive.

Cytokines

The following cytokines were used: IL-7 (10 ng/ml); (Genzyme, Germany), IFN-α (100–1000 U/ml); (Hoffmann LaRoche, Germany).

Propidium Iodide Staining

Propidium Iodide staining was performed as previously described [13]. Briefly, 1×10^5 – 5×10^5 BLIN-1 cells or 1×10^4 human pre-B cells were washed in PBS once and gently mixed with 1.5 ml hypotonic fluorochrome solution consisting of 50 µg PI/ml (Sigma, Germany) in 0.1% Triton-X (Sigma, Germany) and 0.1% sodium citrate. Cells were incubated overnight in the dark at 4°C and analyzed on a FACScan (Becton Dickinson, USA) equipped with a 488 nm argon laser. Acquisition was performed at a flow rate lower than 200 nuclei. Five thousand nuclei were measured per sample. Analysis was performed using FACS research software. Apoptosis was quantified by measuring signals in the hypodiploid region, excluding cell debris of low red fluorescence. Histogrames were smoothed five times for presentation in the figures.

DNA Gel Electrophoresis

Gel electrophoresis for analysis of DNA fragmentation was performed as previously described. Briefly, 5×10^6 BLIN-1 cells were washed once in PBS. The cell pellet was gently mixed in 2 ml TNE buffer and lysed by adding 200 µl 10% SDS and 1 mg Proteinase K (Boehringer Mannheim, Germany) at 55°C for 12 h. The lysate was heated at 85°C for 15 min, DNA was extraced twice using phenol/chloroform-isomylethanol and precipated in ice-cold ethanol. DNA was dried overhight at 55°C and dissolved in TE buffer at

37°C overnight. Then 5–15 μg DNA per sample was separated by electrophoresis for 3 h at 60 V using a 1% agarose gel stained with 5 μl ethidium bromide (10 g/ml). Results were documented by polaroid photograph.

Results

Leukemic BCP Die by Apoptosis In Vitro

The leukemic pre-B cell line BLIN-1 was cultured at low cell concentration (1×10^5/ml). The cells failed to proliferate under these growth conditions. Light microscopic evaluation showed the characteristic features of apoptosis (data not shown). This was confirmed by using DNA gel electrophoresis, showing the typical "ladder pattern" caused by DNA fragmentation (Fig. 1) Quantification was performed using PI staining. The apoptotic cell fraction after 48 h represented 22 ± 4% of all stained a rapid apopototic cell death ex vivo. In nine samples tested the apoptotic cell fraction was 61% (range 35%–87%) after 4 days.

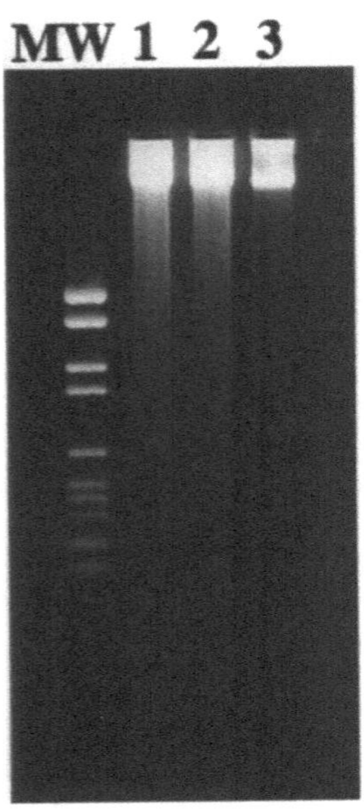

Fig. 1. BLIN-1 cells were cultured with medium alone (lane 1) with IL-7 (lane 2), or with subconfluent human bone marrow stromal cells (lane 3) for 48 h. Apoptosis was tested by DNA gel electrophoresis. MW Molecular weight marker from 2176 bp to 154 bp

Human Bone Marrow Stromal Cells and Murine Fibroblasts Reduce Apoptosis

BLIN-1 cells were cultured with human bone marrow stromal cells for 48 h or 144 h. S-phase and apoptosis were assessed by PI staining. The percentage of cells in the hypodiploid region was reduced from 22% to 5% after 48 h. Figure 2 shows the reduction of apoptosis by stromal cells on day 6 in the histogram analysis. DNA gel electrophoresis confirmed the significant and almost complete reduction of DNA fragmentation. IL-7 only moderately reduced apoptosis compared to bone marrow stromal cells (Fig. 1). The percentage of cells in S-phase was not significantly different. Conculturing with murine fibroblasts reduced the percentage of apoptotic cells to 3.6±1.5%. When leukemic BCP were cocultured on murine C58 fibroblasts six nine samples analyzed showed a significant reduction of apoptosis, with a median of 56.5% (range 91.9%–20.8%) compared to the control.

IFN-α Reduces Cell Viability

Leukemic BCP of five patients with BCP-ALL were cocultured on C58 fibroblasts in medium alone (control) or with IFN-α (1000 U/ml). IFN-α reduced cell viability in five of five samples tested. Loss of cell viability was 35±11% of the control (range 51%–23.5%) (Fig. 3).

IFN-α Enhances Apoptosis

BLIN-1 cells were incubated for 48 h with 100 or 1000 U/ml IFN-α IFN-α reduced the percentage in S-phase from 36% to 26% or 20% at concentrations of 100 U/ml or 1000 U/ml, respectively. In addition, IFN-α triggered apoptosis, with an increase from 11% control to 25% (1000 U/ml). To analyze the influence of IFN-α on apoptosis of leukemic BCP, five samples from patients with BCP-ALL were cocultured on C58 fibroblasts in medium alone (control) or with 1000 U/ml IFN-α. In three samples IFN-α enhanced the apoptotic cell fraction with a 34% increase (range 5.6%–85.6%) compared to the control. There was great interindividual heterogeneity in the IFN-α response. In two samples 5 and 11 IL-7 blocked IFN-α induced apoptosis, whereas in sample 4 IL-7 has no effect (Fig. 5).

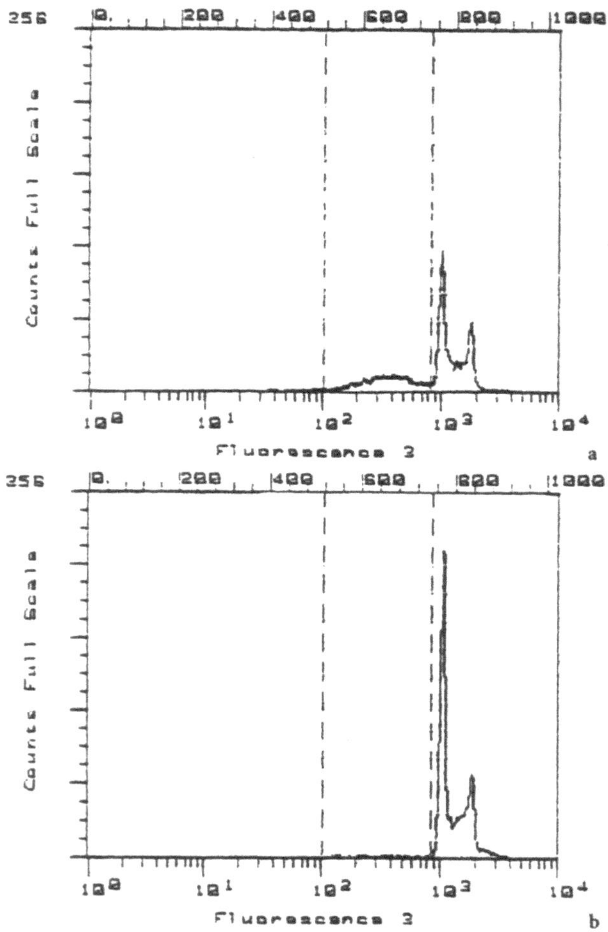

Fig. 2a,b. BLIN-1 was cultured in RPMI 1640 with 5% FCS at a cell concentration of 1×10^5 for 6 days alone or with human bone marrow stromal cells. The percentage of apoptotic cells was measured by Propodium Iodide staining. This figure represents one of the three independent measurements

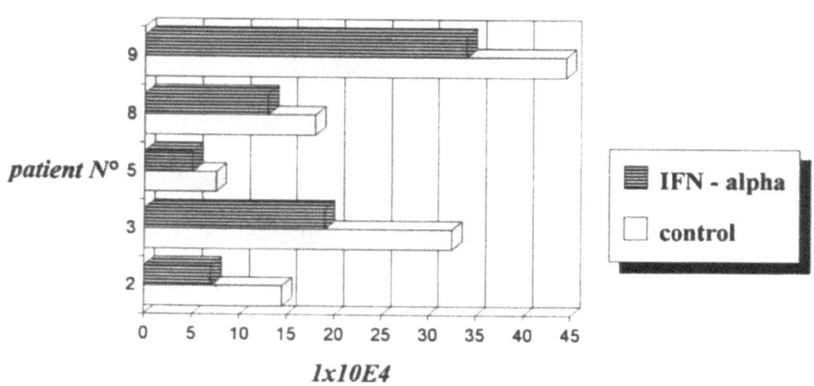

Fig. 3. Leukemic B-cell precursors 1×10^6/ml were cultured on irradiated C58 fibroblasts in RPMI 1640 with 10% FCS alone or with 1000 U/ml IFN-α Cell viability was tested by trypan blue exclusion on day 4. Results represent the mean of two independent measurements. The horizontal scale is viability of cells excluding trypan blue

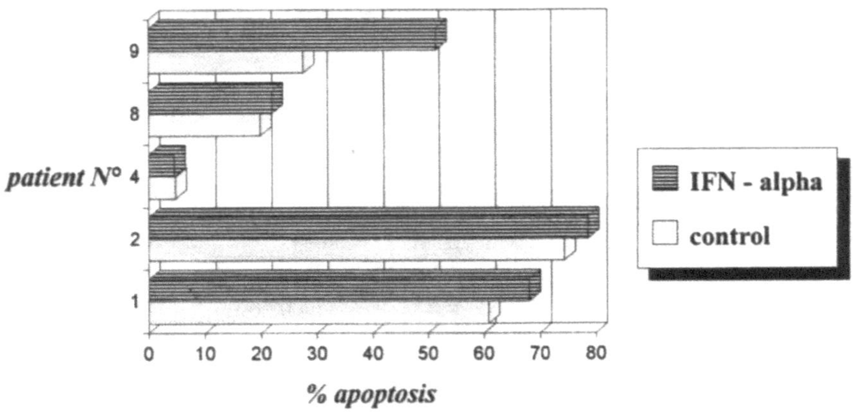

Fig. 4. Leukemic B-cell precursors 1×10^6/ml were cultured on irradiated C58 fibroblasts in RPMI 1640 with 10% FCS alone or with 1000 U/ml IFN-α apoptosis was quantified by PI staining on day 4. Results represent the mean of two independent measurements

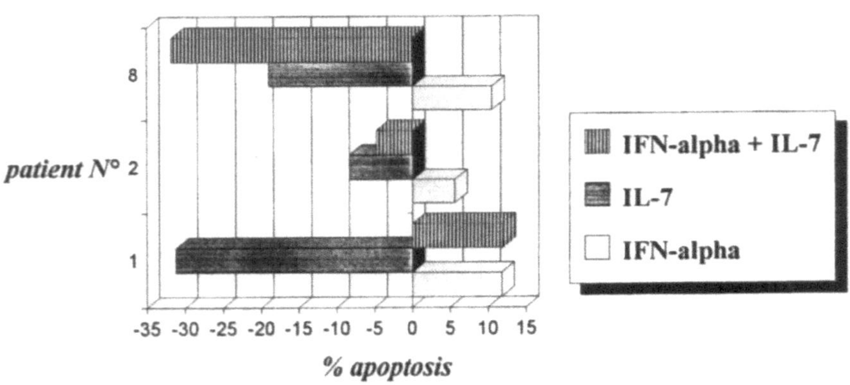

Fig. 5. Leukemic B-cell precursors 1×10^6/ml were cultures on irradiated C58 fibroblasts in RPMI 1640 with 10% FCS alone (control), with 1000 U/ml IFN-a with 10 ng/ml IL-7, or with IFN-α and IL-7. Apoptosis was quantified by PI staining on day 4. The relative increase/reduction of apoptosis compared to the control is shown. Results represent the mean of two independent measurements

Discussion

The identification of negative growth regulators of leukemic BCP has been a frustrating experience in the past because of the rapid spontaneous death of the leukemic blasts ex vivo. The methodological basis for investigations into the growth regulation at the BCP stage was the establishment of a reproducible in vitro culture system. Recently, successful culturing of normal and leukemic pre-B cells in stromal cell assays has ended the search of almost two decades for reproducible in vitro systems [4, 6]. One of the key elements in the murine assay for normal pre-B cells and the human assays for leukemic pre-B cells is prevention of apoptosis by the feeder cells [6]. We recently developed a cross-species coculture system, in which the murine fibroblast subclone C58 as a substitute for human bone marrow stromal cells induces proliferation of the human leukemic pre-B cell line BLIN-1 and enhances viability of leukemic BCP of patients with the diagnosis BCP-ALL [7]. Here we show that the murine fibroblasts are equipotent in blocking apoptosis of the pre-B cell line BLIN-1. In addition, the high spontaneous apoptotic death rate of leukemic BCP from patients with BCP-ALL was also efficiently reduced to C58 fibroblasts. Interestingly, samples of three patients were refractory to the stimulative effect of C58.

These data underline the possibility of replacing human bone marrow stromal cells by murine fibroblasts, which simplifies the methodological approach and facilities the standardization of the culture system. The exact mechanisms of prevention of apoptosis of leukemic BCP have not been elucidated so far. For normal pre-B cells adhesion via VLA-4 is an important element [14]. Decreased adhesion has been postulated as a mechanism of delayed regeneration of B-lymphocytopoiesis after bone marrow transplantation. Further mechanisms may be release of cytokines from stromal cells or from extracellular matrix. A prime candidate is IL-7. In our experiments, IL-77 has only a moderate effect in preventing of apoptosis of the leukemic pre-B cell line BLIN-1.

In the second set of experiments we used the cross-species coculture system for identification of negative regulators of leukemic BCP and focused of IFN-α. The dominant effect of IFN in this cell model seems to be induction of apoptosis. Our observations agree with previous data, which show a loss of cells in S-phase and induction of apoptosis in IL-7-stimulated pre-B cells in mice by IFN-α [15], as well as higher rates of apoptosis in human ALL blasts treated with IFN-α in vitro [16]. When leukemic blasts of patients with the diagnosis of BCP-ALL were incubated with IFN-α on C58 fibroblasts, cell viability was reduced in all samples. In three of five samples IFN-α induced apoptosis, with a 34% increase. Our data are consistent with the IFN-induced loss of cell viability of leukemic pre-B cells cultured on human bone marrow stromal cells [16]. The responsiveness to IFN does not seen to reflect an altered cytokine sensitivity of the leukemic clone since normal human pre-B cell lines are also inhibited by IFN [9]. There was a remarkable heterogenity of the sensitivity to IFN-α, which might reflect a different receptor profile of the different leukemic clones. Although there was no obvious correlation between IFN response and the relative number of non leukemic cells in the sample, the differences might be caused by indirect modification of the IFN effect by accessory cells. This may be addressed in future experiments, using highly purified leukemic cell populations. IL-7 blocked the IFN-induced apoptosis in two of three samples. These results with leukemic BCP have to be compared with normal lymphocytopoiesis. Our previous data on the similarity of normal and leukemic BCP in their responsiveness to cytokines suggest that IFN-α and IL-77 are physiological antagonists in the growth regulation of early BCP. In mice IL-7 does not reduce IFN-γ-induced apoptosis of normal pre-B cells [15]. The mechanism of IFN-α which is responsible for growth inhibition by shortening the half-life of mRNA transcripts of stimulating cytokines as it has been shown for TNF-α and IL-6 in B-CLL and hairy cell leukemia [17].

Our experiments characterize IFN-α as an inhibitory cytokine of leukemic B-cell precursors and indicate the relevance of feeder-cell-dependent coculture systems in the analysis of growth regulation in BCP-ALL.

Acknowledgment. This work was supported by the Deutsche Forschungsgemeinschaft wo35522.

References

1. LeBien TW (1986) Growing human B cell precursors in vitro: the continuing challenge. Immunol. Today 10: 296–298
2. Dexter M (1989) Regulation of hemopoietic cell growth and development Experimental and clinical studies. Leukemia 3: 469–474
4. Wolf ML, Buckley JA, Goldfarb A, Law CL, LeBien TW (1991) Development of a bone marrow culture for maintenance and growth of normal human B cell precursors. J. Immunol. 1477: 3324–3330
5. Moreau I, Duvert V, Banchereau J, Saeland S (1993) Culture of human fetal B cell precursors on bone marrow stroma maintains highly proliferative CD20 cells. Blood 81: 1170–1178
6. Manabe A, Coustan-Smith E, Behm FG, Raimondi SC, Campana D (1992) Bone marrow derived stromal cells prevent apoptotic cell death in B-lineage acute lymphoblastic leukemia. Blood 9: 2370–2377
7. Buske C, Hiddemann W, Wörmann B (1994) Proliferation of human leukemic pre-B cells induced by human bone marrow stromal cells and murine fibroblasts. Cell Biol Int. 18: 1049–1058
8. Grawunder U, Melchers F, Rolink A (1993) Interferon-γ arrests proliferation and causes apoptosis in stromal cell/interleukin-7-dependent normal murine pre-B cell lines and clones in vitro, but does not induce differentiation to surface immunoglobulin-positive B cells. Eur. J. Immunol. 23: 544–551
9. Blomhoff HK, Davies C, Ruud E, Funderud S, Global T (1985) Distinct effects of γ-interferon on

human precursor cell lines. Scan. J. Immunol 1985. 22: 611–6618
10. Okabe M, Kunieda Y, Sugiwura T, Tanaka M, Miyagishima T, Saiki I, Minagawa T, Kurosawa M, Itaya T, Miyazaki T (1991) Inhibitory effect of interleukin - 4 on the in vitro growth of Ph1-positive acute lymphoblastic leukemia cells. Blood 78: 1574–80
11. Ohyashiki K, Ohyashiki JH, Tauchi T, Fujieda H, Hojo H, Ohtaka M, Saito M, Nakazawa S, Toyama K (1991) Treatment of Philadelphia chromosome-positive acute lymphoblastic leukemia: a pilot study which raises important questions. Leukemia 5: 611–4
12. Wörmann B, Anderson JM, Liberty JA, Gajl-Peczalska K, Brunning RD, Silberman TL, Arthur DC, LeBien TW (1989) Establishment of a leukemic cell model for studying human pre-B to B cell differentiation. J. Immunol 142: 110–11735.
13. Nicoletti I, Migliorati G, Pafliacci MC, Grignani F, Riccardi C (1991) A rapid and simple method for measuring thymocyte apoptosis by propiduium iodide staining and flow cutometry. J. Immunol. Methods 139: 271–279
14. Dittel BN, McCarthy JB, Wayner EA, LeBien TW (1993) Regulation of human B-Cell precursor adhesion to bone marrow stromal cells by cytokines that exert opposing effects on the expression of vascular cell adhesion molecule-1 (VCAM-1). Blood 81: 2272–2282
15. Garvy BA, Riley RL(1994) IFN-γ abrogates IL-7 dependent proliferation in pre-B cells, coinciding with oneset of apoptosis. Immunology 81: 381–388
16. Manabe A., Yi T., Kumagai M., Campana D. 1993. Use of stroma-supported cultures of leukemic cells to assess antileukemic drugs. I. Cytoxicity of interferon alpha in acute lymphoblastic leukemia. Leukemia 7: 1990–1995
17. Heslop HE, Bianchi ACM, Cordingley FT, Turner M, De Mel WCP, Hoffbrand AV, Brenner MK (1990) Effects of interferon α on autocrine growth factor loops in B lymphoproliferative disorders. J. Exp. Med. 172: 1729–1734)

Acute Leukemias VI
Prognostic Factors
and Treatment Strategies
Büchner et al. (eds)

Cytokine Serum Levels During the Course of Acute Myeloid Leukemia

M. Stauch, D. Fritsche, and K. Höffken

Abstract. Cytokines are a group of hormone-like regulatory polypeptides. Several investigators have shown that cytokines, while essential for in vitro proliferation and differentiation of normal hematopoietic cells, may also be involved in the process of malignant transformation of hematopoietic cells. The role of the in vivo production of cytokines in the transformational process of acute myeloid leukemia (AML) remains uncertain. We studied the serum levels of interleukin-1 (IL-1), IL-1β IL-2, soluble IL-2 receptor (IL-2R), IL-6, tumor necrosis factor-α (TNFα), granulocyte-macrophage colony-stimulating factor (GM-CSF), granulocyte colony-stimulating factor (G-CSF), and erythropoietin (EPO), using enzyme-linked immunosorbent assays, in 45 patients with de novo AML (AML/BT), during hematological reconstitution following induction chemotherapy (AML/I) and 12 weeks after treatment (AML/AT), and in 40 healthy volunteers (NP). We found a significant increase in the serum levels of the cytokines studied in patients with de novo AML compared with the control group. In patients with AML, a positive linear correlation was found between the elevated serum concentrations of IL-6 and G-CSF and the C-reactive protein (CRP). The elevated serum level of EPO did not correlate with the decreased hemoglobin and hematocrit. The increased serum concentration of soluble IL-2R correlated in an indirect linear fashion with the absolute number of AML blast cells as well as a direct linear fashion with the number of PMN in peripheral blood. After induction chemotherapy the serum levels of IL-2, IL-2R, IL-6, G-CSF, GM-CSF, EPO and CRP remained increased. IL-6 and G-CSF correlated with the serum CRP, too. In addition, IL-6 showed a direct correlation to the WBC and PMN count of the blood. Normal cytokine serum levels were observed 12 weeks after treatment. The data presented here show that the increase in the endogenous cytokines studied in patients with de novo AML was not only due to the underlying disease: The cytokines studied seem to be involved in the hematological reconstitution after chemotherapy.

Introduction

Cytokines are a group of hormone-like regulatory polypeptides that are defined by their ability to support the clonogenic growth of hematopoietic progenitor cells in vitro. They are known to be involved in the complex physiological regulation of normal hematopoiesis and the immune system.

Besides their physiological roles, cytokines may also be involved in the process of the malignant transformation of hematopoietic cells. Several investigators have shown that cytokines, such as stem cell factor (SCF) [56], granulocyte-macrophage colony-stimulating factor (GM-CSF) [3, 10, 32, 78, 48, 82, 89], interleukin-3 (IL-3) [10, 74, 82, 97], granulocyte colony-stimulating factor (G-CSF) [74, 89, 90, 97, 113] and erythropieten (EPO) [72] stimulate the proliferation and/or differentiation of human acute myeloid leukemia (AML) cells in vitro. In con-

Department of Internal Medicine II, Division of Oncology Hematology, Friedrich Schiller University of Jena, 07740 Jena, Germany

trast, monocyte colony-stimulating factor (M-CSF) [90] was shown to inhibit the self-renewal of leukemic blast cell cultures. Tumor necrosis factor-α (TNFα) [24, 31, 69], interleukin-1 (IL-1) [7, 20, 25] and IL-6 [61, 99] act synergistically with the stimulative effects of GM-CSF and IL-3 on the proliferation of the malignant clone from AML patients in vitro. This multifactorial effect is not limited to AML blasts; it is also documented for the growth of hematopoietic progenitor cells in vitro. In constrast to normal hematopoietic stem cells, blast cells from some patients with AML have been shown to grow autonomously in vitro, independently of exogenous growth factor stimulation. These AML blast cells produce multiple cytokines in culture, such as GM-CSF, G-CSF, M-CSF, IL-6, IL-1, and TNF [8, 9, 40, 54, 57, 88]. The in vivo role of cytokines in the physiological regulation of hematopoiesis and the immune system as well as in the process of the malignant transformation of hematopoietic cells remains unknown.

We studied the serum levels of IL-1, IL-1β, IL-2, soluble IL-2 receptor (IL-2R), IL-6, TNF-α, GM-CSF, G-CSF, and EPO, in 45 patients with de novo AML, during hematological reconstitution following induction chemotherapy and 12 weeks after treatment, and in 40 normal individuals, using an enzyme-linked immunosorbent assay. The results were correlated with the level of C-reactive protein (CRP) in the serum, a measure of acute inflammatory processes and the measured blood parameters.

Material and Methods

Forty five patients with newly diagnosed AML were studied. Their clinical characteristics are shown in Table 1.

Table 1. Clinical characteristics of 45 patients with AML

	No. of Patients
Males	27
Females	18
Median age (years)	49.9
Age range (years)	22–68
FAB classification	
M0	1
M1	10
M2	13
M3	2
M4	8
M5a	2
M5b	4
M6	2
M7	1

At the time of diagnosis of patients, during hematological reconstitution following induction chemotherapy, 12 weeks after treatment and in 40 healthy individuals, blood was obtained, centrifuged, and the serum frozen at −20°C until cytokine analysis was performed. Simultaneously, blood was collected for determination of WBC count, differential count, hemoglobin, hematocrit, reticulocytes, platelets, and CRP concentration.

Serum Cytokine Assay

We used a sandwich enzyme immunoassay technique to determine IL-1, IL-1b, IL-2, IL-6, G-CSF, TNF-α (Quantikine kits, R&D System), soluble IL-2R (T-cell Diagnostics), GM-CSF (Medgenix Diagnostics), and EPO (Medac-Diagnostika) serum levels.

CRP levels were determined with a nephelometric method.

Statistical Evaluation

Statistical comparsions were done using the nonparametric Mann-Whitney test (U-test). The data are shown as mean ± SE. Linear regression analysis was employed to analyze the relationship between cytokine levels and CRP in the serum and between cytokine levels and blood parameters.

A p level of < 0.05 was accepted as statistically significant.

Results

The serum levels of IL-1, IL-1β, IL-2, IL-2R, IL-6, G-CSF, GM-CSF, TNF-α and EPO were determined in 45 patients at diagnosis of de novo AML, in 42 patients following induction treatment in 22 patients 12 weeks after treatment, and in 40 healthy controls. The results are shown in Fig. 1 and 2 and in Tables 2–5.

In patients newly diagnosed with AML a significant increase in serum levels of IL-1 (p=0.048), IL-1β (p=0.004), IL-2 (p=0.007), IL-2R ($p < 0.0001$), IL-6 ($p < 0.0001$), G-CSF ($p < 0.0001$), GM-CSF(p=0.011), TNF-α ($p < 0.0001$), EPO ($p < 0.000$) and CRP ($p < 0.000$) was found compared to healthy controls (Fig. 1, Table 3). In

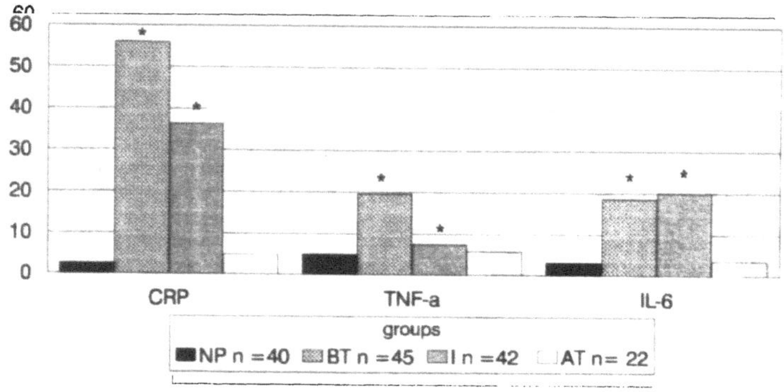

Fig. 1. CRP(mg/ml), TNF-α(pg/ml), and IL-6 (pg-ml) concentrations in AML before treatment (BT), following induction therapy (I), after treatment (AT), and in healthy controls (NP), $*p < 0.05$ versus control

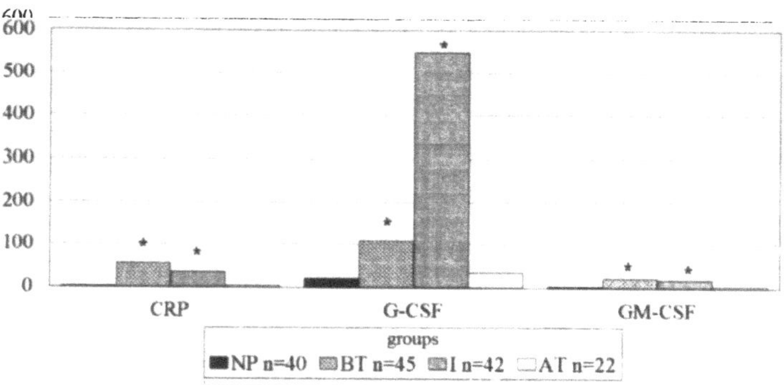

Fig. 2. CRP(mg/ml), G-CSF (pg/ml) and GM-CSF (pg/ml) concentration in AML before treatment (BT), following induction therapy (I), after treatment (AT) and in healthy controls (NP), $*p < 0.05$ versus control

Table 2. Blood parameters in healthy control and patients with AML (mean ± SE)

	Controls	Patients		
	($n = 40$)	($n = 45$)	($n = 42$)	($n = 22$)
Hemoglobin (Gpt/l)	8.5 ± 0.4	5.4 ± 0.2	6.2 ± 1.3	8.0 ± 0.4
Hematocrit %	48.2 ± 6.6	27.8 ± 0.9	31.5 ± 2.9	38.1 ± 1.6
WBC (Gpt/l)	6.2 ± 0.3	26.5 ± 5.2	7.7 ± 1.8	4.7 ± 0.6
PMN (Gpt/l)	3.5 ± 0.2	3.6 ± 1.0	2.8 ± 0.7	2.7 ± 0.5
Lymphocytes (Gpt/l)	1.8 ± 0.1	4.0 ± 0.8	1.8 ± 0.3	1.4 ± 0.2
Monocytes (Gpt/l)	0.4 ± 0.04	3.7 ± 1.6	0.7 ± 0.4	0.4 ± 0.1
Platelets (Gpt/l)	233.5 ± 12.0	62.6 ± 12.5	128.6 ± 19.4	135.2 ± 15.9

BT, Before treatment; I, following induction therapy; AT, after treatment.

these patients significant correlations existed between the elevated serum concentrations of several cytokines, shown in Table 4. The increased values of IL-6 and G-CSF correlated with the increased level of C-reactive protein (Table 4). In patients with newly diagnosed AML no statistically significant correlation was found between the elevated serum concentration of EPO and the diminished hemoglobin and hematocrit (Tables 2, 5). In these patients with AML no significant correlation was found between the WBC count of the peripheral blood and any of

Table 3. Cytokine serum levels of healthy controls and patients with AML (means+SE)

	Controls	Patients		
	($n=40$)	($n=45$)	($n=42$)	($n=22$)
IL-1 (pg/ml)	1.01±0.01	1.5±0.4	1.0±0.2	1.01±0.01
IL-Iß (pg/ml)	1.6±0.4	4.1±0.6	0.9±0.3	0.1±0.04
IL-2 (pg/ml)	3.0±0.01	3.1±0.1	3.5±0.4	3.0±0.01
IL-2R (U/ml)	507.6±30.0	1678.0±346.8	1739.2±247.8	443.9±54.4
IL-6 (pg/ml)	3.1±0.1	18.7±3.9	20.1±5.7	3.6±0.4
G-GSF (pg.ml)	3.0±2.3	107.0±32.6	566.2±173.5	34.6±8.8
GM-CSF (pg/ml)	3.6±0.2	22.6±12.6	19.5±11.9	24.6±6.6
TNF-α (pg/ml)	5.0±0.03	19.6±5.2	7.4±1.5	5.8±0.8
EPO (mU/ml)	8.4±1.6	56.3±8.8	41.3±10.7	24.5±9.1
CRP (mg/ml)	2.5±0.3	56.2±12.0	36.2±10.3	4.8±1.7

EPO, Eythropoietin; CRP, C-reactive protein.

Table 4. Correlations between serum levels of cytokine patients with AML

	BT ($n=45$)		I ($n=42$)		AT ($n=22$)	
IL-1	IL-6	$r=0.522$ $p=0.002$	IL-1β	$r=0.6273$ $p=0.048$	None	
IL-1β	None		IL-1	$r=0.6273$ $p=0.048$	None	
			IL-2	$r=0.5742$ $p=0.032$		
IL-2	None		IL-1β	$r=0.5742$ $p=0.032$	None	
IL-2R	TNF-α	$r=0.4370$ $p=0.024$	GM-CSF	$r=0.6423$ $p<0.000$	G-CSF	$r=0.6556$ $p=0.14$
			EPO	$r=0.5703$ $p=0.0006$		
IL-6	G-CSF	$r=0.4622$ $p=0.005$	G-CSF	$r=0.4592$ $p=0.002$	GM-CSF	$r=0.5105$ $p=0.037$
G-CSF	IL-6	$r=0.4622$ $p=0.005$	IL-6	$r=0.4592$ $p=0.006$	IL-2R	$r=0.6556$ $p=0.0014$
			TNF-α	$r=0.3906$ $p=0.006$	TNF-α	$r=0.7116$ $p=0.007$
GM-CSF	EPO	$r=0.3522$ $p=0.039$	IL-2R	$r=0.6423$ $p<0.000$	IL-6	$r=0.5105$ $p=0.037$
					EPO	$r=0.5573$ $p=0.037$
TNF-α	IL-2R	$r=0.4370$ $p=0.024$	G-CSF	$r=0.3906$ $p=0.02$	G-CSF	$r=0.7116$ $p=0.007$
	EPO	$r=0.4386$ $p=0.016$				
EPO	GM-CSF	$r=0.3522$ $p=0.039$	IL-2R	$r=0.5703$ $p=0.002$	GM-CSF	$r=0.5573$ $p=0.037$
	TNF-α	$r=0.4386$ $p=0.016$				
CRP	IL-6	$r=0.5222$ $p=0.0010$	IL-6	$r=0.9309$ $p<0.000$	None	
	G-CSF	$r=0.5977$ $p<0.000$	G-CSF	$r=0.4703$ $p=0.016$		

Table 5. Correlations between blood parameters and serum levels of cytokines in patients with AML

	BT ($n=45$)		I ($n=42$)		AT ($n=22$)	
Hemoglobin	None		IL-1	$-r=0.3440$ $p=0.037$	IL-1β	$-r=0.6766$ $p=0.033$
			IL-6	$-r=0.4475$ $p=-0.006$		
Hematoait	TNF-α	$r=0.3331$ $p=0.042$	IL-6	$-r=0.4006$ $p=0.013$	IL-1β	$-r=0.6425$ $p=0.033$
					G-CSF	$-r=0.5917$ $p=0.028$
WBC	None		IL-6 $p=0.032$	$-r=0.3025$	G-CSF	$r=0.5370$ $p=0.044$
					TNF-α $p=0.03$	$-r=0.5344$
					IL-6 $p=0.017$	$r=0.5877$
PMN	IL-2R	$r=0.4370$ $p=0.024$	IL-6 $p=0.003$	$r=0.4812$	None	
	IL-6	$r=0.4339$ $p=0.007$				
Blast cells	IL-2R	$-r=0.3834$ $p=0.029$	IL-6	$r=0.3848$ $p=0.016$	IL-1	$r=0.7649$ $p=0.014$
	IL-6	$-r=0.3706$ $p=0.018$				
Platelets	IL-1b	$-r=0.8290$ $p=0.041$	IL-2R	$-r=0.3715$ $p=0.022$	None	
			IL-6	$-r=0.3025$ $p=0.049$		
			G-CSF	$-r=0.3474$ $p=0.032$		

the cytokines studied. The absolute number of PMN showed a direct linear correlation with the serum levels of IL-6 and IL2R (Table 5). In addition, an indirect linear correlation was found between the number of AML blast cells and the IL-6 serum level and a direct linear correlation with the serum IL-2R (Table 5).

After induction chemotherapy, the serum levels of IL-2 ($p=0.04$), IL-2R ($p<0.0001$), G-CSF ($p<0.001$) , GM-CSF ($p=0.001$), IL-6 ($p<0.0001$), TNF-α ($p<0.0001$), EPO ($p<0.0001$) and CRP ($p<$ 0.0001) remained increased compared to controls (Fig. 1,2, Table 3). IL-6 and G-CSF correlated also in this phase of the disease with serum CRP (Table 5). Furthermore, there were statistically significant correlations between the decreased number of PMN and an elevated endogenous IL-6 (Tables 2, 3, 5). The absolute number of AML blast cells showed in this phase of the disease a direct linear correlation with the IL-6 serum level. There were also statistically significant correlations between the serum value of IL-6 and WBC and PMN of the peripheral blood. The decreased number of platelets correlated with the elevated serum levels of IL-2R, IL-6, and G-CSF (Tables 2, 5).

There were normal serum levels of IL-2, IL-2, IL-2R, IL-6, G-CSF, GM-CSF TNF-α EPO, and CRP 12 weeks after treatment (Fig. 1, Tab. 3). The serum level of IL-1β was statistically significantly decreased compared to healthy controls. The decreased IL-1β correlated indirectly linearly with the Hb and Hct but not with the WBC and PMN of the peripheral blood. In these patients with AML we did detect any statistically significant correlations between the PMN and the cytokines measured (Table 5). In addition, the WBC count showed an indirect linear correlation with G-CSF and TNF-α and a direct correlation with IL-6 (Table 5).

As to remission rates, only the GM-CSF serum level at the time of diagnosis was statistically significantly higher in patients who achieved partial remission (67.56 +49.47 pg/ml, $p=0.003$) than in patients who achieved complete remission (3.74 +0.54 pg/ml).

Discussion

We studied the serum levels of various cytokines in different states during AML and compared the results with those of healthy controls.

We demonstrated that patients with de novo AML have significantly elevated serum levels of IL-1, IL-1β, IL-2, IL-2R, IL-6, G-CSF, GM-CSF TNF-α EPO, and CRP compared to the control group. These results confirm the data observed in various in vitro systems suggesting the involvement of these cytokines, which are essential for in vitro proliferation of normal hematopoietic cells [2, 14, 27, 35–38, 41, 43–45, 46, 66, 77, 80, 81, 86, 100, 105] and also in the clonogenic growth of leukemic blast cells [39,40]. In these studies it has been demonstrated that most of AML progenitor cells require exogenous cytokines for survival and proliferation [31, 32, 39, 42, 62, 107, 108]. Several investigators have shown that in the majority of cases exogenous IL-3, GM-CSF, and G-CSF stimulated the proliferation and differentiation of clonogenic leukemic cells or activated DNA synthesis [20, 32, 51, 74, 108]. Miauchy et al. [69, 70] have demonstrated that the responsiveness to one of these cytokines as well as their activities varies among individual cases. The involvement of IL-6 and TNF-α in the clonogenic growth or differentiation of leukemic blast cells in vitro was also recognized [5, 6, 24, 26, 29, 31, 33, 55, 59, 69, 70, 93]. In addition, Motoji et al. [72] have described the influence of EPO in leukemic blast cell proliferation in cell culture. It was shown that the proliferative response to EPO when used together with PHA-LCM is not restricted to erythroid lineage only, but also to other clonogenic myeloid cells. The role of IL-1 as an exogenous stimulator of leukemic blast cell growth in culture has also been described [16, 44, 73, 106]. In addition to these observations, IL-2 has been shown to be an inducer of blast cell proliferation in vitro. Carron and Carley [12] demonstrated that the proliferative activity of IL-2 is restricted only to clonogenic cells with monocytic differentiation. Cimino et al. [13] found elevated serum concentrations of IL-2 only with respect to the M4-M5 group. In contrast to these findings we demonstrated elevated serum levels of IL-2 in other cases of de novo AML also. This is consistent with our own results of a significant increase of serum levels of the soluble IL-2R recently described in patients with newly diagnosed AML. [13] Furthermore, a few leukemic blast cells proliferate independently of exogenous cytokines in culture. In several studies it has been shown that these blast cells may produce endogenous cytokines, including IL-1, IL-6, G-CSF, GM-CSF and TNF-α in an autocrine or paracrine manner [8–10, 39, 40, 54, 78, 106]. In addition, several recent reports have described different cytokines acting synergistically or additively to induce blast colony formation in vitro [51, 90, 107]. Confirming these results in vitro, we demonstrated that in patients with de novo AML direct linear correlations exist in vivo between IL-1 and IL-6; and IL-6 and G-CSF; GM-CSF and EPO; TNF-α IL-2R, and EPO; and EPO, GM-CSF, and TNF-α. Furthermore, our data suggest the involvement of these cytokines in the multifactoral process of leukemic blast cell proliferation in vivo.

Studies in vivo and in vitro have shown that TNF-α [1, 21, 22, 28, 53, 60, 64, 65, 67, 68, 84, 103, 104, 109–112], IL-1 [85, 87, 94, 96, 115], IL-6 [11, 23, 30, 63, 79, 101, 102], G-CSF [50, 63], GM-CSF [78,95], and IL-2R [49] are capable of acting as inflammatory cytokines, too. In our study, we found a clear correlation between the elevated serum levels of G-CSF and IL-6 and the C-reacative protein as a mediator of the acute inflammatory response. In addition, our findings of a direct linear correlation between IL-6 and the absolute number of PNM and as a negative correlation between IL-6 and absolute blast cell count, in patients with de novo AML suggest the involvement of this cytokine not only in the growth of the malignant leukemic cell clone, but also in the regulation of the host defense.

Furthermore, studies previously conducted in vitro have shown that various cytokines including IL-1, IL-3, IL-6, G-CSF, and GM-CSF may also be included during hematological recovery following intensive chemotherapy [71]. In vivo administration of these cytokines accelerates myeloregeneration following cytoreductive treatment [75, 83]. In autologous bone marrow transplantation and peripheral blood stem cell transplantation (PBSCT), treatment with recombinant G-CSF or GM-CSF results in faster engraftment of transplanted autologous stem cells and reduction of the duration and severity of neutropenia [4]. However, little is known about the production of endogenous cytokines in vivo during the process of hematological recovery after intensive cytoreductive chemotherapy. The present study demonstrates significantly elevated serum levels of IL-2, IL-2R,

G-CSF, GM-CSF, TNF-α and EPO in patients with AML following induction chemotherapy compared to healthy controls. This provides evidence for the involvement of these cytokines in the in vivo regulation of the hematological reconstitution after administration of cytotoxic drugs as well. These results are consistent with those of Takamatsu et al. [98] who also found elevated serum levels of IL-6 and G-CSF in the recovery phase following intensive chemotherapy. In contrast to them, we were unable to detect any increase in endogenous IL-1 in this phase of the disease. Baiocchi et al. [4] evaluated the kinetics of the release of endogenous cytokines in patients with advanced ovarian cancer following high-dose chemotherapy and PBSCT. They demonstrated sequential coordinated release of GM-CSF, IL-1α, G-CSF, and IL-8 after myeloablative chemotherapy and PBSCT. We found direct linear correlations between IL-1β and IL-2, IL-6 and G-CSF, TNF-α and G-CSF, GM-CSF and IL-2R, and EPO and IL-2R, which indicates a combination interaction of different cytokines in the process of myeloregeneration. Our findings of indirect linear correlations between PMN and IL-6 support the hypothesis that the production of endogenous cytokines will be supported by cells other than PMN. We and others [47, 76] did not find any correlations between the elevated serum levels of EPO and the hemoglobin and hematocrit of the peripheral blood. Schapira et al. [91] demonstrated elevated serum levels of EPO in 31 patients undergoing bone marrow transplantation following intensive chemotherapy. Our results suggest that the EPO increase in the recovery phase after intensive chemotherapy was caused by a mechanism other than increasing anemia and oxygen triggering in the kidney. This process may be indirectly supported by IL-6 and IL-1, which were shown to be negatively linearly correlated with the diminished hemoglobin in this phase of the disease.

Normal cytokine serum levels were found 12 weeks after treatment. Only the endogenous level of IL-1β was statistically significantly decreased compared to healthy volunteers. Further studies are necessary to prove the role of this parameter for prognosis and survival of patients with AML.

In conclusion, our results indicate that the increase of endogenous cytokines demonstrated in patients with AML was not only due to the underlying disease. In addition, the endogenous cytokines studied in patients with AML seem to be involved in the hematological reconstitution following chemotherapy as well as in the host defense. The use of cytokines as stimulators of the hematological recovery in the treatment of AML leukemias should be considered with greater caution, since their involvement in leukemogenesis remains obscure. Further studies are required in order to select the most appropriate treatment strategies for the administration of cytokines in AML patients.

References

1. Abrahamsson, J., Carlsson, B., Mellander, L.: Tumor necrosis factor-alpha in malignant disease. Am. J. Pediatr. Hematol. Oncol. 15: 364–369, 1993.
2. Aggarwal, B., Pocsik, E.: Cytokines: from clone to clinic: Arch. Biochem. Biophys. 292: 335–359, 1992.
3. Andreeff, M., Welte, K.: Hematopoietic colony-stimulating factors. Sem. Oncol. 16: 211–229, 1989.
4. Baiocchi, G., Scambia, G, Benedetti, P., Menichella, G., Testa, U., Pierelli, L., Martucci, R., Foddai, M. L., Bizzi, B., Mancuso, S., Peschle, C.: Autologous stem cell transplantation: sequential production of hematopoietic cytokines underlying granulocyte recovery. Cancer Res. 53: 1297–1303, 1993.
5. Bergamaschi, G., Carlo-Stella, C., Cazzola, M., De Fazio, P., Pedrazzoli, P., Peverali, F. A., Valle, G. D.: Tumor necrosis factor alpha down-regulates c-myc mRNA expression and induces in vitro monocytic differentiation in fresh blast cells from patients with acute myeloblastic leukemia. Leukemia 4: 426–430, 1990.
6. Bloch, A.: Dynamics of interaction between DNA-specific antitumor agents and serum-contained cytokines in the initiation of ML-1 human myeloblastic leukemia cell differentiation. Leukemia 7: 1219–1224, 1993.
7. Bot, F. J., Schipper, P., Broeders, L., Delewel, R., Kaushansky, K., Löwenberg, B.: Interleukin-1 alpha also induces granulocyte-macrophage colony-stimulating factor in immature normal bone marrow cells. Blood 76: 307–311, 1990.
8. Bradbury, D., Bowen, G., Kozlowski, R., Reilly, I., Russel, N. H.: Endogenous interleukin-1 can regulate the autonomous growth of blast cells of acute myeloblastic leukemia by induction of autocrine secretion of GM-CSF. Leukemia 4: 44–47, 1990.
9. Bradbury, D., Rogers, S., Kozlowski, R., Bowen, G., Reilly, I. A., Russell, N. H.: Interleukin-1 is one factor which regulates autocrine production of GM-CSF by the blast cells of acute myeloblastic leukaemia. Br. J. Haematol. 78: 488–493, 1990.

10. Budel, L. M., Touw, I. P., Delwel, R., Clark, S. C., Löwenberg, B.: Interleukin-3 and granulocyte-monocyte colony-stimulating factor receptors on human acute myelocytic leukemia cells and relationship to the proliferative response. Blood 74: 565–571, 1989.
11. Calandra, T., Gerain, J., Heumann, D., Baumgartner, J. D., Glauser, M. P.: High circulating levels of interleukin-6 in patients with septic shock: evolution during sepsis, prognostic value and interplay with other cytokines. Am. J. Med. 91: 23–29, 1991.
12. Carron, J. A., Cawley, J. C.: IL-2 and myelopoiesis: IL-2 induced blast cell proliferation in some cases of acute myeloid leukemia. Br. J. Haematol. 73: 168–172, 1989.
13. Cimino, G., Amadori, S., Cava, M. C., De Sanctis, V., Petti, M. C., Di-Gregorio, A. O., Sgadari, C., Vegna, L., Cimino, G., Mandelli, F.: Serum interleukin-2 (IL-2), soluble IL-2 receptors and tumor necrosis factor-alfa levels are significantly increased in acute myeloid leukemia patients. Leukemia 5: 32–35, 1991.
14. Clark, S.C., Kamen, R.: The human hematopoietic colony-stimulating factors. Science 236: 1229–1237, 1987.
15. Coutinho, L. H., Will, A., Radford, J., Schiro, R., Testa, N. G., Dexter, T. M.: Effects of recombinant human granulocyte colony-stimulating factor (CSF), human granulocyte-macrophage-CSF and gibbon interleukin-3 on hematopoiesis in human long-term bone marrow culture. Blood 75: 2118–2129, 1990.
16. Cozzolino, F., Rubartelli, A., Aldinucci, D., Sitia, R., Torcia, M., Shaw, A., Di Gugliemo, R.: Interleukin-1 as an autocrine growth factor for acute myeloid leukemia cells. Proc. Nat. Acad. Sci. USA 86: 2369–2373, 1989.
17. Danis, V. A., Kulesz, A. J., Nelson, D. S., Brooks, P. M. Cytokine regulation of human monocyte interleukin-1 (IL-1) production in vitro. Enhancement of IL-1 production by interferon (IFN) gamma, tumor necrosis factor-alpha, IL-2 and IL-1, and inhibition by IFN-alpha. Clin. Exp. Immunol. 80: 435–443, 1990.
18. Debili, N., Massé J.-M., Katz, A., Guichard, J., Breton-Gorius, J., Vainchenker, W.: Effects of the recombinant hematopoietic growth factors interleukin-3, interleukin-6, stem cell factor, and leukemia inhibitory factor on megakaryocytic differentiation of CD34+cells. Blood 82: 84–95, 1993.
19. Delwel, R., Dorssers, L., Touw, I., Wagemakjer, G., Löwenberg, B.: Human recombinant multilineage colony stimulating factor (interleukin-3): stimulator of acute myelocytic leukemia progenitor cells in vitro. Blood 70: 333–336, 1987.
20. Delwel, R., Van Buitenem, C., Salem, M., Bot, F., Gillis, S., Kaushansky, A., Altrock, B., Löwenberg, B.: Interleukin-1 stimulates proliferation of acute myeloblastic leukemia cells by induction of endogenous granulocyte-macrophage colony-stimulating factor (GM-CSF) release. Blood 74 586–593, 1989.
21. Djeu, J. Y., Blanchard, D. K., Richards, A. L., Friedman, H.: Tumor necrosis factor induction by Candida albicans from human natural killer-cells and monocytes. J. Immunol. 141: 4047–4052, 1988.
22. Djeu, J. Y., Serbousek, D., Blanchard, D. K.: Release of tumor necrosis factor by human polymorphonuclear leukocytes. Blood 76: 1405–1409, 1990.
23. Dofferhoff, A. S., Bom, V. J., de Vries-Hospers, H. G., van Ingen, J., v.d. Meer, J., Hazenberg, B. P., Mulder, P. O., Weits, J.: Patterns of cytokines, plasma endotoxin, plasminogen activator inhibitor, and acute-phase proteins during the treatment of severe sepsis in humans. Crit. Care Med. 20: 185–192, 1992.
24. Elbaz, O., Budel, L. M., Hoogerbrugge, H., Touw, I. P., Delwel, R., Mahmoud, L. A., Löwenberg, B.: Tumor necrosis factor regulates the expression of granulocyte-macrophage colony-stimulating factor and interleukin-3 receptors on human acute myeloid leukemia cells. Blood 77: 989–995, 1991.
25. Estrov, Z., Kurzrock, R., Estey, E., Wetzler, M., Ferrajoli, A., Harris, D., Blake, M., Guttermann, J. U., Talpaz, M.: Inhibition of acute myelogenous leukemia blast proliferation by interleukin-1 (IL-1) receptor antagonist and soluble IL-1 receptors. Blood, 79: 1938–1945, 1992.
26. Evans, R., Fong, M., Fuller, J., Kamdar, S., Myerhardt, J., Strasssmann, G.: Tumor cell IL-6 gene expression is regulated by IL-1 alpha/beta and TNF alpha: proposed feedback mechanisms induced by interaction of tumor cells and macrophages. J. Leukoc. Biol. 52: 463–468, 1992.
27. Fibbe, W. E., van Damme, J., Billiau, A., Goselnik, H. M., Voogt, P. J., van Eeden, G., Ralph, P., Altrock, B. W., Falkenburg, J. H. F.: Interleukin-1 induces human marrow stromal cells in long-term culture to produce granulocyte colony-stimulating factor and macrophage colony-stimulating factor. Blood 71: 430–436, 1988.
28. Foss, N. T., de-Oliveira, E. B., Silva, C.-L.: Correlation between TNF production, increase of plasma C-reactive protein level and suppression of T-lymphocyte response to concanavalin A during erythema nodosum leprosum. Int. J. Lepr. Other Mycobact. Dis. 61: 218–226, 1993.
29. Fujii, Y., Takuma, T., Bloch, A.: A regulatory role for tumor necrosis factor (TNF) in ML-1 human myeloblastic leukemia cell maturation. Leuk. Res. 14: 941–947, 1990.
30. Geisterfer, M., Richards, C., Baumann, M., Fey, G., Gywnne, D., Gauldie, J.: Regulation of IL-6 and the hepatic IL-6 receptor in acute inflammation in vivo. Cytokine 5: 1–7, 1993.
31. Griffin, J. D., Löwenberg, B.: Clonogenic cells in acute myeloblastic leukemia. Blood 68: 1185–1195, 1986.
32. Griffin, J. D., Young, D. C., Herrmann D., Wiper, K., Wagner, K., Sabbath, K.: Effects of recombinant human GM-CSF on proliferation of clonogenic cells in acute myeloblastic leukemia. Blood 76: 1448–1453, 1986.

33. Guan, X. P., Hromchak, R. A., Takuma, T., Denstman. S. C., Bloch, A.: Tumor necrosis factor-alpha, transforming growth factor-beta, and tetradecanoylphorbol acetate: competence factors for ML-1 human myeloblastic leukemia cell differentiation. Cancer Commun. 3: 11–14, 1991.
34. Hammerle, A. F., Poschl, G., Kirnbauer, R., Trautinger, F., Micksche, M., Mayrhofer, O.: Serum proteins and cytokines for prediction of sepsis? Prog. Clin. Biol. Res. 308: 715–718, 1989.
35. Herrmann, F., Mertelsmann, R.: Polypeptides controlling hematopoietic cell development and activation: I. In vitro results: Blut 58: 117–128, 1989.
36. Herrmann, F., Gebauer, G., Lindemann, A., Brach, M., Mertelsmann, R.: Interleukin-2 and interferon-gamma recruit different subsets of human peripheral blood monocytes to secrete interleukin-1 beta and tumor necrosis factor-alpha. Clin. Exp. Immunol. 77: 97–100, 1989.
37. Herrmann, F., Cannistra, A., Lindemann, A., Mertelsmann, R.: Griffin, J. D.: Functional consequences of monocytes interleukin-2 receptor expression: Induction of interleukin-1 secretion by gamma-Interferon and interleukin-2. J. Immunol. 1989.
38. Herrmann, F., W., Lindemann, A., Mertelsmann, R.: Polypeptides controlling hematopoietic blood cell development and activation: II. Clinical results. Blut 58: 173–179, 1989.
39. Herrmann, F., Oster, W., Lindemann, A., Ganser, A., Dölken, B., Knapp, W., Griffin, J. D., Mertelsmann, R.: Leukemic colony forming cells in acute myeloblastic leukemia: Maturation hierarchy and growth conditions. Hematol. Blood Transf. 31: 185–190, 1987.
40. Herrmann, F., Oster, W., Mertelsmann, R.: Control of blast cell proliferation and differentiation in acute myelogenous leukemia by soluble polypeptide growth factors. Klin. Pädiatr. 202: 212–217, 1990.
41. Herrmann, F., Oster, W., Meurer, S. C., Lindemann, A., Mertelsmann, R.: Interleukin-1 stimulates T-lymphocytes to produce granulocyte-macrophage colony-stimulating factor. J. Clin. Invest. 81: 1415–1418, 1988.
42. Herrmann, F., Vellenga, E.: The role of colony-stimulating factors in acute leukemia. J. Cancer Res. Clin. Oncol. 16: 275–282, 1990.
43. Hestdal, K., Ruscetti, F. W., Chizzonite, R., Ortiz, M., Gooya, M. J., Longo, D. L., Keller, J. R.: Interleukin-1 (IL-1) directly and indirectly promotes hematopoietic cell growth through type I IL-1 receptor. Blood 84: 125–132, 1994.
44. Hoang, T., Haman, A., Goncalves, O., Letendre, F., Mathieu, M., Wong, G., Clark, S C.: Interleukin-1 enhances growth factor-dependent proliferation of the clonogenic cells in acute myeloblastic leukemia and of normal human primitive hemopoietic precursors. J. Exp. Med. 168: 463–474, 1988.
45. Jablonsons, D.M., Mulé, J.J., McIntosh, J.K., Sehgal, P.B., May, L.T., Huang, C.M., Rosenberg, S.A., Lotze, M.T.: IL-6/IFN-beta-2 as a circulating hormone: Induction by cytokine administration in humans. J. Immunol. 142: 1542–1547, 1989.
46. Jayaraman, S., Martin, C.A., Dorf, M.E.: Enhancement of in vivo cell mediated immune response by three distinct cytokines. J. Immunol. 144: 942–951, 1990.
47. Jelkmann, W., Johannsen, H., Wiedemann, G., Otte, W., Wagner, T.: Dependence of serum erythropoietin level on erythropoiesis in leukemia. Hämatol. Bluttransfus. 33: 83–86, 1990.
48. Kanakura, Y., Druker, B., Cannistra, S. A., Furukawa, Y., Torimoto, Y., Griffin, J.: Signal transduction of the human granulocytemacrophage colony-stimulating factor and interleukin-3 receptors involves tyrosine phosphorylation of a common set of cytoplasmatic proteins. Blood 76: 706–715, 1990.
49. Karrer, U., Aeschlimann, A., Fassbender, K., Vogt, P., Müller, W.: Interleukin-6 (IL-6), löslicher Interleukin-2-Rezeptor (sIL-2R) und Mikroheterogenität des alpha-1 sauren Glykoproteins (AGP): neue Marker der Akut-Phase-Reaktion? Schweiz Med. Wschenschr. 122: 233–236, 1992.
50. Kawakami, M., H. Tsutsumi, T. Kumakawa, H. Abe, M. Hirai, Sh. Kurosawa, M. Mori and M. Fukushima: Levels of serum granulocyte colony-stimulating factor in patients with infections. Blood 76: 1962–1964, 1990.
51. Kelleher, C., Miyauchi, J., Wong, G., Clark, S., Minden, M. D., McCulloch, E. A.: Synergism between recombinant growth factors, GM-CSF, and G-CSF, activity on the blast cells of acute myeloblastic leukemia. Blood 69: 1498–1503, 1987.
52. Kharazmi, A., Nielsen, H., Bendtzen, K.,: Modulation of human neutrophil and monocyte chemotaxis and superoxide response by recombinant TNF-alpha and GM-CSF. Immunobiology 177: 363–370, 1988.
53. Kiener, P. A., Marek, F., Rodgers, G., Lin, P.-F., Warr, G., Desiderio, J.: Induction of tumor necrosis factor, IFN-gamma and acute lethality in mice by toxic and non-toxic forms of lipid A. J. Immunol. 141: 870–874, 1988.
54. Kindler, V., Shields, J., Ayer, D., Mazzei, G. J.: Growth regulation of the AML-193 leukemic cell line: evidence for autocrine production of granulocyte-macrophage colony-stimulating factor (GM-CSF), and inhibition of GM-CSF-dependent cell proliferation by interleukin-1 (IL-1) and tumor necrosis factor. Int. J. Cancer 47: 450–454. 1991.
55. Kishimoto, T.: The biology of interleukin-6. Blood 74: 1–10, 1989.
56. Kiss, C., Cesano, A., Zsebo, K. M., Clark, S. C., Santoli, D.: Human stem cell factor (c-kit ligand) induces an autocrine loop of growth in a GM-CSF dependent megakaryocytic leukemia cell line. Leukemia 7: 235–240, 1993.
57. Kobara, L., Weil, D., Lemoine, F. M., Dubois, C., Thiam, D., Baillou, C., Guigon, M., Gorin, N. C., Najman, A.: Secretion of tumor necrosis factor-alpha by fresh human acute nonlymphoblastic leukemic cells: role in the disappearance of nor-

mal CFU-GM progenitors. Exp. Hematol. 18: 1187-1992, 1990.
58. Krantz, S. B.: Erythropoietin. Blood 77: 419-434, 1991.
59. Kubin, M., Chow, J. M., Trinchieri, G.: Differential regulation of interleukin-12 (IL-12), tumor necrosis factor alpha, and IL-1beta production in human myeloid leukemia cell lines and peripheral blood mononuclear cells. Blood 83: 1847-1855, 1994.
60. Kumaratilake, L. M., Ferrante, A., Jaeger, T., Rzepczyk, C. M.: Effects of cytokines, complement, and antibody on the neutrophil respiratory burst and phagocytic response to Plasmodium falciparum merozoites. Infect. Immun. 60: 3731-3738, 1992.
61. Lopez, M., Maroc, N., Kerangueven, F., Bardin, F., Courcoul, M., Lavezzi, C., Birg, F., Mannoni, P.: Coexpression of the genes for interleukin 6 and its receptor without apparent involvement in the proliferation of acute myeloid leukemia cells. Exp. Hematol. 19: 797-803, 1991.
62. Löwenberg, B., Touw, I. P.: Hematopoietic growth factors and their receptors in acute leukemia. Blood 81: 281-292, 1993.
63. Mackensen, A., Galanos, C., Engelhardt, R.,: Treatment of cancer patients with endotoxin induces release of endgenous cytokines. Pathobiology 59: 264-267, 1991.
64. Mänel, D. N., Northoff, H., Bauss, F., Falk, W.: Tumor necrosis factor: a cytokine involved in toxic effects of endotoxin. Rev. Infect. Dis. 9 Suppl. 5: 602-606, 1987.
65. Martich, G. D., Danner, R. L., Ceska, M., Suffredini, A. F.: Detection of IL-8 and TNF in normal humans after intravenous endotoxin. The effect of antiinflammatory agents. J. Exp. Med. 173: 1021-1024, 1991.
66. Metcalf, D.: The molecular biology and functions of the granulocyte-macrophage colony-stimulating factors. Blood 67: 257-268, 1986.
67. Michie, H. R., Manogue, K. R., Spriggs, D. R., Revhaug, A., O'Dwyer, S. T., Dinarello, C. A., Cerami, A., Wolff, S. M., Wilmore D. W.: Detection of circulating tumor necrosis factor after endotoxin administration. N Engl. J. Med. 318: 1481-1486: 1988.
68. Minamishima, I., Ohga, S., Ishii, E., Matsuzaki, A., Kai, T., Akazawa, K., Ueda, K.: Serum interleukin-6 and fever at diagnosis in children with acute leukemia. Am. J. Pediatr. Hematol. Oncol. 15: 239-244, 1993.
69. Miyauchi, J., Kelleher, C., A., Yang, Y.-C., Wong, G., Clark, S. C., Minden, M. D., Minkin, S., McCulloch, E. A.: The effects of three recombinant growth factors, IL-3, GM-CSF, and G-CSF, on the blast cells of acute myeloblastic leukemia maintained in short-term suspension culture. Blood 3: 657-663, 1987.
70. Miyauchi, J., Wang, C., Kelleher, C. A., Wong, G., Clark, S. C., Minden, M. D., Minkin, S., McCulloch, E. A.: The effects of recombinant CSF-1 on blast cells of acute myeloblastic leukemia in suspension culture. J. Cell. Physiol. 135: 55-62, 1988.
71. Moore, M. A. S.: Clinical implications of positive and negative hematopoietic stem cell regulators. Blood 78: 1-19, 1991.
72. Motoji, T., Hishino, S., Ueda, M., Takanashi, M., Masuda, M., Nakayama, K., Oshimi, K., Mizoguchi, H.: Enhanced growth of clonogenic cells from acute myeloblastic leukemia by erythropoietin. Br. J. Haematol. 75: 60-67, 1990.
73. Murohashi, I., Tohda, S., Suzuki, T., Nagata, K., Yamashita, Y., Nara, N.: Mechanism of action of interleukin 1 on the progenitors of blast cells in acute myeloblastic leukemia. Exp. Hematol. 18: 133-137, 1990.
74. Nomoto, N., Shibata, A.: Capability of various cytokines to induce quiescent myeloid leukemia cells to the proliferative stage. Leuk. Lymphoma 71: 143-150, 1992.
75. Ohno, R., Tomonaga, M., Kobayashi, T., Kanamaru, A., Shirakawa, S., Masaoka, T., Omine, M., Oh, H., Nomura, T., Sakai, Y., Hirano, M., Yokomaku, H., Nakayama, S., Yoshida, Y., Miura, A. B., Morishima, Y., Dohy, H., Niho, Y., Hamajima, N., Takaku, F.: Effect of granulocyte colony-stimulating factor after intensive induction therapy in relapsed or refractory acute leukemia. N Engl J Med 323: 871-877, 1990.
76. Ohno, R., Tomonaga, M., Kobayashi, T., Kanamaru, A., Shirakawa, S., Masaoka, T., Omine, M., Oh, H., Nomura, T., Sakai, Y., Hirano, M., Yokomaku, R., Nakayama, S., Yoshida, Y., Miura, A. B., Morishima, Y., Dohy, H., Niho, Y., Hamajima, N., Takaku, F.: Circulating erythropoietin levels after bone marrow transplantation: inappropriate response to anemia in allogenic transplants. Blood 77: 868-873, 1991.
77. Okabe, M., Asano, M., Kuga, T., Komatsu, Y., Yamasaki, M., Yokoo, Y., Itho, S., Morimoto, M., Oka, T.: In vitro and in vivo hematopoietic effect of mutant human granulocyte colony-stimulating factor. Blood 75: 1788-1793, 1990.
78. Okamura, S., Hayashi, S., Kawasaki, C., Kondo, S., Asano, Y., Omori, F., Otsuka, T., Shibuya, T., Harada, M., Niho, Y.: Expression of cytokine genes in hematological malignancies. Acta Haematol. 52: 1424-1432, 1989.
79. Oldenburg, H. S., Rogy, M. A., Lazarus, D. D., Van-Zee, K. J., Leeler, B. P., Chizzonite, R. A., Lowry, S. F., Moldawer, L. L.: Cachexia and acute-phase protein response in inflammation are regulated by interleukin-6. Eur. J. Immunol. 23: 1889-1894, 1993.
80. Oldham, R. K.: Biological response modifiers. J. Natl. Cancer Inst. 70: 789-796, 1983.
81. Ostensen, M., E., Thiele, D. L., Lipsky, P. E.: Tumor necrosis factor-alpha enhances cytolytic activity of human natural killer cells. J. Immunol. 138: 4185-4191, 1987.
82. Oval, J., Taetle, R.: Factor-dependent human leukemia cell lines: new models for regulation of acute non lymphocytic leukemia cell growth and differentiation. Blood Rev. 4: 270-279, 1990.

83. Patchen, M. L., MacVittie, T. J., Williams, J. L., Schwartz, G. N., Souza, L. M.: Administration of interleukin-6 stimulates multilineage hematopoiesis and accelerates recovery from radiation induced hematopoietic depression. Blood 77: 472-489, 1991.
84. Pinsky, M. R., Vincent, J. L., Deviere, J., Alegre, M., Kahn, R. J., Dupont, E.: Serum cytokine levels in human septic shock. Relation to multiple-system organ failure and mortality. Chest. 103: 565-575, 1993.
85. Ramadori, G., Van Damme, J., Rieder, H., Meyer zum Buschenfelde, K. H.: Interleukin 6, the third mediator of acute-phase reaction, modulates hepatic protein synthesis in human and mouse. Comparison with interleukin 1 beta and tumor necrosis factor-alpha. Eur. J. Immunol. 18: 1259-1264, 1988.
86. Rambaldi, A., Young, D. C., Griffin, J. D.: Expression of the M-CSF-gene by human monocytes. Blood 69: 1409-1413, 1987.
87. Riikonen, P., Saarinen, U. M., Teppo, A. M., Mets_rinne, K., Fyhrquist, F., Jalanko, H.: Cytokine and acute-phase reactant levels in serum of children with cancer admitted for fever and neutropenia. J. Infect. Dis. 166: 432-436, 1992.
88. Rodriguez-Cimadevilla, J. C., Beauchemin, V., Villeneuve, L., Letendre, F., Shaw, A., Hoang, T.: Coordinate secretion of interleukin-1 beta and granulocyte-macrophage colony-stimulating factor by the blast cells of acute myeloblastic leukemia: Role of interleukin-1 as an endogenous inducer. Blood 76: 1481-1489, 1990.
89. Sallerfors, B., Olofsson, T.: Granulocyte-macrophage colony-stimulating factor (GM-CSF) and granulocyte colony-stimulating factor (G-CSF) in serum during induction treatment of acute leukemia. Br. J. Haematol. 78: 342-351, 1991.
90. Santoli, D., Yang, Y. C., Clark, S. C., Kreider, B. L., Caracciolo, D., Rovera, G.: Synergistic and antagonistic effects of recombinant human interleukin (IL) 3, IL-1 alpha granulocyte and macrophage colony stimulating factors (G-CSF and M-CSF) on the growth of GM-CSF-dependent leukemic cell lines. J. Immunol. 139: 3348-3354, 1987.
91. Schapira, L., Antin, J. H., Ransil, B. J., Antman, K. H., Eder, J. P., McGarigle, C. J., Goldberg, M. A.: Serum erythropoietin levels in patients receiving intensive chemotherapy and radiotherapy. Blood 76: 2354-2359, 1990.
92. Schiller, J. H., Hank, J., Storer, B., Borchert, A. A., Moore, K. H., Albertini, M., Bechhofer, R., Wesley, O., Brown, R. R., Bastin, A. M., et al.: A direct comparison of immunological and clinical effects of interleukin 2 with and without interferon-alpha in humans. Cancer Res. 53: 1286-1292, 1993.
93. Sgadari, C., Vegna, L., Cimino, G., Mandelli, F.: Serum interleukin-2 (IL-2), soluble IL-2 receptors and tumor necrosis factor-alfa levels are significantly increased in acute leukemia patients. Leukemia 5: 32-35, 1991.
94. Shalaby, M. R., Waage, A., Aarden, L., Espevik, T.: Endotoxin, tumor necrosis factor-alpha and interleukin 1 induce interleukin 6 production in vivo. Clin. Immunol. Immunpathol. 53: 488-498, 1989.
95. Shimoda, K., S. Okamura, F. Omori, Y Mizuno, T. Hara, T. Aoki, H. Akeda, K. Ueda and Y. Niho: Detection of granulocyte-macrophage colony-stimulating factor in cerebrospinal fluid of patients with aseptic meningitis. Acta Haematol 86: 36-39, 1991.
96. Spinas, G. A., Bloesch, D., Kaufmann, M. T., Keller, U., Dayer, J. M.: Induction of plasma inhibitors of interleukin 1 and TMF-alpha activity by endotoxin administration to normal humans. Am. J. Physiol. 259: R 993-997, 1990.
97. Suzuki, T., Bessho, M., Hirashima, K., Tohda, S., Nagata, K., Imai, Y., Nara, N.: Interleukin-6 reduces the optimal growth in vitro of leukemic blast progenitors from acute myeloblastic leukemia patients. Acta Haematol. 87: 63-68, 1992.
98. Takamatsu, Y., Akashi, K., Harada, M., Teshima, T., Inaba, S., Shimoda, K., Eto, T., Shibuya, T., Okamura, S., Niho, Y.: Cytokine production by peripheral blood monocytes and T cells during haematopoietic recovery after intensive chemotherapy. Br. J. Haematol. 83: 21-27, 1993.
99. Takanashi, M., Motoji, T., Masuda, M., Oshimi, K., Mizoguchi, H.: The effects of leukemia inhibitory factor and interleukin 6 on the growth of acute myeloid leukemia cells. Leuk. Res. 17: 217-222, 1993.
100. Takaue, Y., Y. Kawano, Ch. L. Reading, T. Watanabe, T. Abe, T. Ninomiya, E. Shimizu, T. Ogura, Y. Kuroda, A. Yokobayashi, T. Nakahata, Sh. Asano and G. Ventura: Effects of recombinant human G-CSF, GM-CSF, IL-3 and IL-1 alpha on the growth of purified human peripheral blood progenitors. Blood 76: 330-335, 1990.
101. Tilg, H., Trehu, E., Atkins, M. B., Dinarello, C. A., Mier, J. W.: Interleukin-6 (IL-6) as an anti-inflammatory cytokine: Induction of circulating IL-1 receptor antagonist and soluble tumor necrosis factor receptor p55. Blood 83: 113-118, 1994.
102. Ulich, T. R., Guo, K. Z., Remick, D., del Castillo, J., Yin, S. M.: Endotoxin-induced cytokine gene expression in vivo. III. IL-6 mRNA and serum protein expression and the in vivo hematologic effects of IL-6. J. Immunol. 146: 2316-2323. 1991.
103. Ulich, T. R., Guo, K., delCastillo, J.: Endotoxin-induced cytokine gene expression in vivo. I. Expression of tumor necrosis factor mRNA in visceral organs under physiologic conditions and during endotoxemia. Am. J. Pathol. 134: 11-14, 1989.
104. Urbaschek, R, Urbaschek, B.: Tumor necrosis factor and interleukin 1 as mediators of endotoxin-induced beneficial effects. Rev. Infect. Dis. 9, Suppl. 5: 607-615, 1987.

105. Valtiere, M., Tweardy, D. J., Caracciolo, D., Johnson, K., Mavilio, F., Altmann, S., Santoli, D., Rovera, G.: Cytokine-dependent granulocytic differentiation. Regulation of proliferative and differentiative response in a murine progenitor cell line. J. Immunol. 138: 3829-2835, 1987.
106. Van der Schoot, C. E., Jansen, P., Poorter, M., Wester, M. R., von de Borne, A. E. G-K., Aarden, L. A., van Oers, R. H. J.: Interleukin-6 and interleukin-1 production in acute leukemia with monocytoid differentiation. Blood, 74: 2081-2087, 1989.
107. Vellenga, E., Ostaporicz, B., O'Rourke, J., Griffin, J. D.: Effects of recombinant IL-3, G-CSF, and G-CSF on proliferation of leukemic clonogenic cells in short-term and long-term cultures. Leukemia 1: 584-589, 1987.
108. Vellenga, E., Young, D. C., Wagner, K., Wiper, D., Ostraporicz, D., Griffin, J. D.: The effects of GM-CSF and G-CSF in promoting growth of clonogenic cells in acute myeloid leukemia. Blood 69: 1771-1776, 1987.
109. Waage, A., Aasen, A. O.: Different role of cytokine mediators in septic shock related to meningococcal disease and surgery/polytrauma. Immunol. Rev. 127: 221-230, 1992.
110. Waage, A., Brandtzaeg, P., Espevik, T., Halstensen, A.: Current understanding of the pathogenesis of gram-negative shock. Infect. Dis. North. Am. 5: 781-791, 1991.
111. Waage, A., Halstensen, A., Espevik, T.: Association between tumor necrosis factor in serum and fatal outcome in patients with meningococcal disease. Lancet 14: 355-357, 1987.
112. Waage, A., Steinmann, S.: Cytokine mediators of septic infections in the normal and granulocytopenic host.Eur. J. Haematol. 50: 243-249, 1993.
113. Watari, K., Asano, S., Shirafuji, N., Kódo, H., Ozawa, K., Takaku, F., Kamachi, S.: Serum granulocyte colony-stimulating factor levels in healthy volunteers and patients with various disorders as estimated by enzyme immonoassay. Blood 73: 117-122, 1989.
114. Weller, M., Stevens, A., Sommer, N., Melms, A., Dichgans, J., Wiethölter, H.: Comparative analysis of cytokine patterns in immunological, infectious, and oncological neurological disorders. J. Neurol. Sci. 104: 215-221, 1991.
115. Zuckerman, S. H., Evans, G. H.: Endotoxin tolerance: in vivo regulation of tumor necrosis factor and interleukin-1 synthesis is at the transcriptional level. Cell. Immunol. 140: 513-519, 1992.

Acute Leukemias VI
Prognostic Factors
and Treatment Strategies
Büchner et al. (eds)

Expression of FLT3 and FLT3 Ligand in Human Leukemia-Lymphoma Cell Lines

G. Meierhoff[1], U. Dehmel[1], H.J. Gruss[2], W. Dirks[1], and H.G. Drexler[1]

Abstract. The FLT3 gene encodes a receptor tyrosine kinase that is closely realted to two well-known receptors, KIT and FMS, which regulate with their respective ligands, stem cell factor (SCF) and macrophage colony-stimulating factor (M-CSF), proliferation and differentiation of hematopoietic cells. The ligand for FLT3, FL, is active in both soluble and membrane-bound forms. We examined expression of FL and FLT3 mRNA in a panel of some 110 continuous human leukemia-lymphoma cell lines from all major hematopoietic cell lineages by Northern blot analysis. FLT3 mRNA is expressed primarily in pre B-cell lines and myeloid and monocytic cell lines, whereas FL and mRNA was detected in most cell lines from all cell lineages. Forty of 110 cell lines displayed both receptor and ligand mRNA, suggesting a possible autocrine or intracrine stimulation. In normal hematopoietic cells expression of FLT3 was reported to be associated with positivity for CD34, a cell surface marker of immature and precursor cells. No correlation between FLT3 and CD34 expression was found in the cell lines analyzed. Gene transfection of an FL expression construct in BHK21 cells led to the production and secretion of a functional FL protein. Four out of 21 cell lines tested responded to incubation with this FL protein by enhanced proliferation (160%–500% of control cells grown without FL); all four cell lines were of myeloid origin. FL-induced proliferation was not enhanced by constimulation with interleukin-3 (IL-3), granulocyte-macrophage CSF (GM-CSF), or SCF. Transforming growth factor-β (TGF-β) inhibited FL-promoted proliferation in one cell line. These studies serve to further illustrate the importance of the FLT3-FL receptor-ligand system in the regulation of hematopoietic cells.

Introduction

Proliferation and differentiation of hematopoietic cells is controlled by a series of souble and membrane-bound regulators [1]. Besides the classical hematopoietic growth factors (or colony-stimulating factors, CSFs), a vast and ever increasing range of polypeptides has been discovered that together with the growth factors are now collectively termed cytokines. Cytokines participate not only in the stimulation of proliferation and differentiation of normal as well as malignant hematopoietic cells, but also in a variety of cellular responses, e.g., regulation of the immune system [2]. These hematopoietic regulators act through specific receptors [3]. Cytokine receptors belong to two different groups: those with intrinsic tyrosine kinase domains (termed receptor tyrosine kinase, RTK) and those lacking such sequences, e.g., interleukin-2 (IL-2), IL-3, IL-4, IL-5, IL-6, IL-7, granulocyte CSF (GM-CSF), and granulocyte-macrophage CSF (GM-CSF). These RTKs are divided into subclasses according to their amino acid sequences [4]. A role for RTKs in hematopoiesis, both at the level of the undifferentiated stem cell and in committed cell lineage precursors, has been clearly demonstrated by

[1]German Collection of Microorganisms and Cell Cultures, Braunschweig, Germay
[2]Immunex Research and Development Co., Seattle, Washington, USA

signalling through the KIT RTK and its cognate ligand, KIT-ligand or stem cell factor (SCF).

A search to detect further RTKs led to the discovery of a murine gene termed *fetal liver kinase 2* (flk2) [5]; the human gene was designated *FMS-like tyrosine kinase 3* (FLT3) [6–8]. Another acronym for FLT3/flk2 is STK-1 (for *stem cell tyrosine kinase 1*) [9]; but the gene is clearly different from the recently cloned gene STK (for *stem cell-derived tyrosine kinase*) [10]. The FLT3 RTK, located on chromosome 13q12, shares structural homology with the subclass III RTKs PDGF (platelet-derived growth factor receptor), KIT and FMS (or CSF1, receptor for the macrophage-CSF/M-CSF) [11]. Both the human and murine ligands for FLT3 (FL) were cloned and found to encode a type I transmembrane and a soluble protein [12–14]. FL protein stimulates proliferation of hematopoietic precursor cells, for instance CD34+ cells [12, 13]. These early studies on the physiological expression of FLT3 and on the type of normal cells that are responsive to FL suggest that FL and FLT3 may function as a growth factor receptor-ligand system on hematopoietic stem and/or progenitor cells.

Analysis of normal hematopoietic progenitors is hampered by their spurious occurrence in blood and bone marrow; homogenous populations of hematopoietic cells of any given lineage or stage of differentiation are not readily accessible. On the other hand, established leukemia-lymphoma cell lines represent clonal cell populations continuously available for experimental manipulations. Therefore, we analyzed expression of FLT3 and FL by cells from a large group of continuous leukemia-lymphoma cell lines. These cell lines constitute an extensive, well-characterized panel of different hematopoietic malignancies including specimens from the major cell lineages. The specific aims of the present analysis were: (1) to determine the incidence of FLT3 and FL expression in the various types of cell lines: (2) to examine the relationship of FLT3 expression to positivity for the stem cell surface marker CD34, as it has been suggested that FLT3/STK-1 is selectively expressed in CD34+ bone marrow cells [9]; and (3) to investigate the effects of FL protein on FLT3+ cell lines.

Materials and Methods

Cells

Cell line were grown and maintained by serial passages in appropriate media (Gibco BRL, Eggenstein, Germany) supplemented with 10%–20% (v/v) heat-inactivated fetal bovine serum (FBS;Sigma, Deisenhofen, Germany). Cells were cultured in tissue culture flasks or 24-well plates (Nunc, Wiesbaden, Germany) at 37°C in an atmosphere of 5% CO_2 in air. Some cell lines were taken from the DSM Cell Culture Bank [15], others were generously provided by the original investigators for research purpose only [16–19]. References and details for these cell lines will be provided upon request from the senior author. The growth factor-dependent cell lines F-36EGM, M-07e, OCI-AML-1, OCI-AML-5, TF-1, UCSD/AML-1, and UT-7 were cultured with supernatant from the bladder carcinoma cell lines 5637 producing GM-CSF, IL-3, and other cytokines; U-1996 needed IL-6 for continuous growth. All cultures were free of mycoplasma contamination. Cells were harvested in their logarithmic growth phase with viabilities of higher than 90% as examined by trypan blue exclusion. Normal mononuclear cells were purified from the peripheral blood of healthy volunteers by standard Ficoll-Hypaque density gradient centrifugation (Lymphoprep, Nycomed, Oslo, Norway); monocytes were obtained by adherence to plastic Petri dishes; tonsillar B-lymphocytes were separated from T-cells by sheep red blood cell rosetting.

RNA Preparation and Northern Blot Analysis

For Northern blot analysis, total RNA was prepared using the guanidinium isothiocyanate-CsCl method. Equal quantities of total RNA (10 µg) were separated on 1.0% formaldehyde agarose gels. The fractionated RNA was transferred to nylon filters (Gene Screen, DuPont, Bad Homburg, Germany) which were subsequently cross-linked with ultraviolet light. The gels were stained with ethidium bromide to ensure that equal amounts of RNA were analyzed and that no degradation had occurred. After prehybridization at 62°C overnight, the RNA was hybridized to random primed [α-^{32}P]dCTP (Amersham-Buchler, Braunschweig, Germany)-labeled cDNA probes at 62°C overnight. After stringent washing steps with 6X

SSC, 3X SSC, and 0.05X SSC, the blots were exposed to X-ray films with an intensifying screen at −80 °C. The same filters were subsequently rehybridized with a ß-actin probe. The following specific cDNA probes were used: for the human FLT3 gene (a 2.8 kb *PvuI/BamHI* cDNA cloned in λgt10, kindly provided by Dr. Daniel Birnbaum, Marseille, France) [7], for the human FL gene (a 0.9 kb *Eco*RI cDNA in Bluescript) [13], and for the actin control (a 1.4 kb *Pst*I fragment in pUC19).

Proliferation Assay

An FL expression vector was prepared using standard recombinant DNA methods. Briefly, a 983-bp FL cDNA excised from the plasmid Bluescript was added for cloning into the *Eco*RI site of the eukaryotic expression vector pSBC2 (20) and transformed into *E. coli* XL Blue (pSBC2-FL). pSV-2pac (for puromycin resistance) and pAG-60 (for gentamycin resistance) were employed as selection markers in BHK21 cells using a standard calcium chloride cotransfection protocol in order to obtain stable transfectants. After a 3-week incubation with puromycin and gentamycin, conditioned medium(CM) of a successfully transfected BHK21 clone (BHK21-FL) as shown by Northern blot analysis of BHK21-FL mRNA and hybridization with a specific probile was collected. The proliferative response of a panel of FLT3+ cell lines to BHK21-FL CM was seeded in duplicate at 0.5 × 10^6 cells/ml in 100 μl complete medium in 96-well plates and incubated for 40 and 64 h in the presence of 25% (v/v) BHK21-FL CM, 100 U/ml IL-3, 100 U/ml IL-7, 400 U/ml GM-CSF, 10 ng/ml SCF, or 10 ng/ml TGF-ß1 (Boehringer Mannheim, Germany); for the last 4 h of incubation 1 μCi methyl-[3H]thymidine (Amersham) was added to each well. Cell lines constitutively dependent on externally added growth factors were washed extensively prior to incubation with the specific cytokines and then cultured without these additives.

Results

Expression of FLT3 mRNA

FLT3 mRNA expression was examined by Northern blot analysis in 110 continuous human leukemia-lymphoma cell lines (Table 1): 10/11

Table 1. Expression of FLT3 and FL mRNA in leukemia-lymphoma cell lines

Cell line	Type/origin[a]	FLT3[b]	FL[b]
Pre B-cell lines:			
697	Pre B-ALL	+	(+)
ALL-1	Pre B-ALL	+++	(+)
BAY-91	ALL	+	(+)
EU-1	ALL	+	+
IARC-318	Pre B-ALL	++	+
LAZ-221	ALL	++	(+)
NALM-1	CML-lym BC	++	+
NALM-6	ALL	–	(+)
NALM-16	ALL	+++	+
PRE-ALP	Pre B-ALL	++	+
REH	ALL	++	+
B-cell lines:			
1E8	B-ALL	(+)	(+)
BALL-1	B-ALL	–	+
BALM-1	B-ALL	–	+
BJAB	Burkitt	–	+
BONNA-12	HCL	–	+
EB-1	Burkitt	(+)	+
EHEB	B-CLL	–	+
HAIR-M	HCL	–	+
KARPAS-231	B-ALL	–	+
KARPAS-353	B-ALL	–	+
WSU-NHL	B-NHL	++	–
Myeloma cell lines:			
EJM	Myeloma	–	+
KARPAS-707	Myeloma	–	+
L-363	PCL	–	+
LP-1	Myeloma	–	+
MM-1	Myeloma	–	+
MM-S1	Myeloma	–	(+)
NCI-H929	Myeloma	–	+
OPM-2	Myeloma	–	(+)
U-266	Myeloma	–	+
U-1996	Myeloma	–	(+)
T-cell lines:			
CTV-1	AML M5?	–	++
DU-528	T-ALL	–	++
HPB-ALL	T-ALL	–	+
JM	T-ALL	–	+
MDS	CML	–	+
MOLT-3	T-ALL	–	+
MOLT-16	T-ALL	–	+
MOLT-17	T-ALL	–	+
P12/ICHIK	ALL	–	+
PF-382	ALL	–	–
PFI-285	T-cell lymphoma	–	+
NK cell lines:			
NK-92	NHL with LGL	–	+++
YT	NHL	–	++
Myeloid cell lines:			
EM-2	CML-my BC	++	+
EM-3	CML-my BC	++	+
EOL-1	AML-eosino	+++	+
EOL-3	AML-eosino	+	+

Table 1. (*contd.*)

Cell line	Type/origin[a]	FLT3[b]	FL[b]
GDM-1	CML-my BC	–	+
HL-60	AML M2	+	+
KASUMI-1	AML M2	+	+
KBM-7	CML-my BC	–	+
KCL-22	CML-my BC	–	(+)
KG-1	AML	(+)	(+)
KG-1a	AML	–	+
MOLM-7	CML-my BC	++	+
MOLM-8	CML-my BC	+	(+)
MR-87	AML	(+)	(+)
NB-4	AML M3	+	+
OCI-AML-5	AML	(+)	+
PL-21	AML M3?	+	+
TI-1	AML M2	–	+
UCSD/AMLI	AML	–	+
YOS-M	CML-my BC	+	+
Monocytic cell lines:			
DD	Histocytic lymph.	–	(+)
JOSK-I	AML M4	(+)	+
JOSK-M	AML M4	–	(+)
KBM-3	AML M4	++	+
KBM-5	CML-mono BC	++	+
ML-2	AML M4	+	+
MOBS-1	AML M5	+	+
MV4-11	AML M5	+++	+
OCI-AML-1	AML M4	–	+
OCI-AML-3	AML M4	+	+
PLB-985	AML M4	+	+
SKM-1	AML M5	++	(+)
U-937	Histiocytic lymph.	–	(+)
X-376	AML	(+)	(+)
Megakaryocytic cell lines:			
CHRF288–11	AML M7	–	+
CMK	AML M7	–	++
DAMI	AML M7	–	+
LAMA-84	CML-BC	–	+
M-07e	AML M7	–	(+)
MEG-01	CML-BC	–	+
MEGAL	AML M7	+	+
MHH-225	AML M7	–	+
MKPL-1	AML M7	– –	
MOLM-1	CML-BC	++	+
T-33	CML-BC	–	+
TS9;22	CML-my BC	–	+
UT-7	AML M7	(+)	+
Erythroid cell lines:			
F-36EGM	AML MM	–	+
HEL	AML M6	–	+
JK-1	CML-BC	–	+
K-562	CML-BC	–	+
KH-88	CML-BC	–	+
KMOW-02	AML M6	–	+
OCI-M1	AML M6	–	+
OCI-M2	AML M6	–	+
TF-1	AML M6	–	+
Hodgkin/ALCL cell lines:			
CO (T-cell like)	Hodgkin	–	+
HDLM-1 (T)	Hodgkin	–	+
HDLM-2 (T)	Hodgkin	–	++
HD-MY-Z (Mono)	Hodgkin	–	(+)
JB-6	ALCL	–	++
KM-H2 (B)	Hodgkin	–	+
L-428 (B)	Hodgkin	–	+
L-540 (T)	Hodgkin	–	+
SUP-HDI (B)	Hodgkin	–	(+)
Normal cells:			
Monocytes (PB)		–	–
B-cells (tonsils)		+	–
Mononuclear cell fraction (PB)		+	+++

ALCL, anaplastic large cell lymphoma: ALL, acute lymphoblastics leukemia; AML, acute myeloid leukemia; B, B-cell; Burkitt, Burkitt's lymphoma; CLL, chronic lymphocytic leukemia; CML-BC, chronic myeloid leukemia in blast crisis; HCL, hairy cell leukemia; Hodgkin, Hodgkin's lymphoma; LGL, large granular lymphocyte leukemia; NHL, Non-Hodgkin's lymphoma; PB, peripheral blood; PCL, plasma cell leukemia; pre B, pre B-cell; T, T-cell.

[a]Cell lines were assigned to the respective categories based on their origin and their phenotypic and functional characteristics;
subtypes are given as indicated in the original publications (for review see [15–19]).

[b]Intensity of bands on Northern blots: –, negative; (+), weakly positive;+, ++, +++, various degrees of positivity. Equal loading of lanes and integrity of RNAs were verified by ethidium bromide staining of the gel and rehybridization with β-actin.

pre B-cell lines were positive; 3/11 B-cell lines; 0/10 myeloma cell lines; 0/11 T-cell lines; 0/2 NK cell lines; 14/20 myeloid cell lines; 10/14 monocytic cell lines; 3/13 megakaryocytic cell lines; 0/9 erythroid cell lines; and 0/9 Hodgkin or anaplastic large cell lymphoma-derived cell lines. Normal purified monocytes were negative; B-cells and the mononuclear cell fraction were positive. Thus, FLT3 mRNA is expressed primarily in pre B-cell lines, and myeloid and monocytic cell lines (Fig. 1).

Correlation of FLT3 Expression with CD34 Positivity

A previously suggested association of FLT3 expression with CD34 positivity [9] could not be confirmed in the panel of cell lines investigated here. The CD34– status was known for 64 cell lines. The correlation can be detailed as follows: 13 cell lines were FLT3+CD34+ (20%); 9 cell

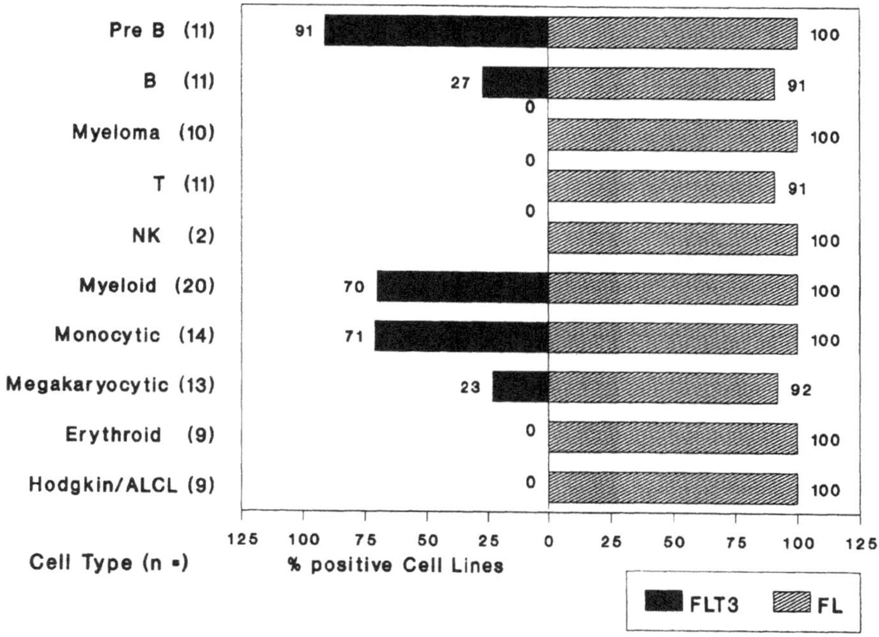

Fig. 1. Summary of expression of FLT3 and FL mRNA in the various subtypes of leukemia-lymphoma cell lines. The percentage of positive cell lines for each subtype are shown. For details see Table 1

lines were FLT3+ CD34− (14%); 19 cell lines were FLT3− CD34+ (30%); 23 cell lines were FLT3− CD34− (36%).

Expression of FLT3-Ligand mRNA

Northern blots showed widespread, but rather weak expression of the FL mRNA transcripts in most cell lines studied (Table 1): 10/10 pre B-cell lines were positive; 10/11 B-cell lines; 10/10 myeloma cell lines; 10/11 T-cell lines; 2/2 NK cell lines; 20/20 myeloid cell lines; 14/14 monocytic cell lines; 12/13 megakaryocytic cell lines; 9/9 erythroid cell lines; and 9/9 Hodgkin anaplastic large cell lymphoma cell lines. Normal monocytes and B-cell were negative; a positive signal was seen in the mononuclear cell fraction. Furthr, 40/110 cell lines expressed both receptor and ligand mRNA, suggesting a possible autocrine, intracrine, or paracrine stimulation. Taken together, FL mRNA is widely expressed in all cell lineages.

Proliferation Induced by FLT3 Ligand

Twenty-one cell lines were incubated with supernatant from BHK21 cells transfected with FL cDNA for 40 and 64 h. BHK21-FL CM enhanced proliferation in the four myeloid cell lines HL-60, EOL-1, OCI-AML-5, and MUTZ-2 by 160%–500% of control cultures (Fig. 2). ^{3}H-thymidine uptake of responsive cells was parallelled by increases in the actual number of cells as determined by cell counting in hematocytometer chambers and trypan blue dye staining. OCI-AML5 and MUTZ-2 are growth factor-dependent cell lines cultured routinely with 5637 CM. Coincubation with IL-3, IL-7, GM-CSF, or SCF singly or in combination did not have additive or synergistic effects on any of the cell lines studied. TGF-ß abrogated the proliferative stimulus of BHK21-FL CM on MUTZ-2 cells (TGF-β1;96% of ^{3}H-thymidine uptake of control cells at 64 h; FL: 645%;TGF-β1+FL: 317%). TGF-β was cytotoxic on OCI-AML-5 cells both in the presence and absence of FL (TGF-β1: 38% of control cells; FL: 383%;TGF-β1+FL: 34%).

Discussion

FLT3 is a member of the type III RTK family which also includes KIT, FMS and PDGF [5, 6, 9, 21]. FLT3 was reported to be expressed mainly

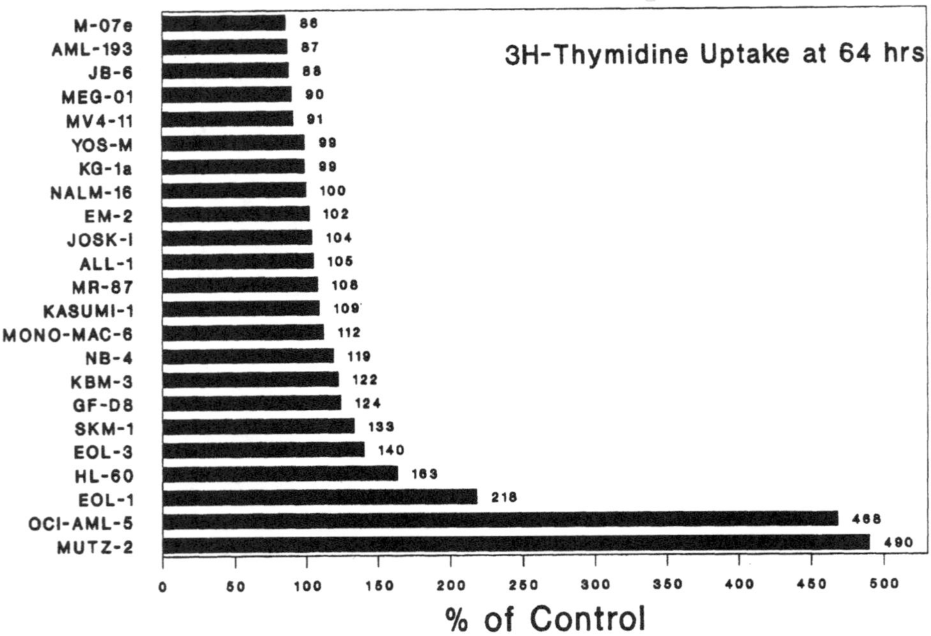

Fig. 2. Proliferative response of cell lines to BHK21-FL conditioned medium. Results of ^{3}H-thymidine uptake are shown as a percentage of control cells incubated with medium only. Cell lines were incubated with 25% (v/v) BHK21-FL CM for 64 h; the data obtained at 40 h showed similar values

in immature, both normal and malignant hematopoietic cells, including murine and human stem and progenitor cells [5–9]. These receptors have been documented to play important roles in the growth and/or differentiation of a variety of cells in which they are expressed [11]. Similar to the ligands for the KIT and FMS receptors, SCF and M-SCF, respectively, the FLT3 receptor is activated by a cognate molecule, termed FLT3 ligand [FL] [12–14]. Here, analysis of the mRNA expression of the FLT3 and FL genes in a large panel of well-characterized continuous human leukemia-lymphoma cell lines from all major cell lineages showed opposite expression patterns: widespread expression of the ligand FL in nearly all cell lines and cell lineages contrasts with an expression profile of the receptor FLT3 that is basically limited to immature B-cell lines and myelomonocytic cell lines. These findings suggest that selective expression of the receptor may be the restrictive factor in the regulation of the ligand-receptor interaction. As anti-FLT3 monoclonal antibodies were not available to us, transcript levels and surface expression of the FLT3 molecule could not be correlated. The assumption that physiological FLT3 expression is limited to the CD34+cell fraction of normal human bone marrow was not corroborated by the present results as there were no clear-cut differences between CD34+ and CD34− cell lines with regard to FLT3 mRNA expression.

Previous results showed that the ligand is capable of functioning as a proliferation factor on primitive hematopoietic cells [12–14, 22]. Furthermore, FL enhanced the response of stem and progenitor cells to other growth factors, as illustrated by the synergistic effects of combinations with IL-3, GM-CSF, PIXY-321 (the GM-CSF/IL-3 fusion protein), and to a limited extent also with SCF or IL-7, depending on the type of cells tested; no synergy was observed with erythropoietin [12–14]. Both native and recombinant FL induced tyrosine autophosphorylation of the FLT3 receptor [12, 14]. Here, stable transfection of the human FL gene into BHK21 cells led to the production of soluble activities that induced significant proliferation in four myeloid leukemia cell lines. The stimulatory effect of this crude native ligand could not be augmented additively or synergistically by IL-3, IL-7, GM-CSF, or SCF. In the absence of cytotoxic effects

TGF-β1 inhibited the proliferative activity of FL in one cell line, which while this factor caused extensive cell death in a second FL-responsive cell line.

We have identified the expression patterns of the FLT3 receptor gene and of its cognate ligand FL and have shown that some myeloid leukemia cells are biologically responsive to the ligand. Clearly, important biological processes such as proliferation and possibly other cellular events such as differentiation are controlled by this receptor-ligand pair. Our results indicate that the ligand may not only control specifically the growth response of hematopoietic progenitor and stem cell populations, but the unique FL-FLT3 ligand-receptor interaction may also be involved in the pathobiology of certain leukemia cells. Availability of the cloned genes, of native and recombinant ligand, of antibodies against the ligand and the receptor molecules, and of cell lines as readily available model systems will facilitate studies on the physiological and pathological rolls of this new cytokine-receptor system.

References

1. Metcalf D: Hematopoietic regulators: Redundancy or subtlety? Blood 82: 3515-3523, 1993
2. Löwenberg B, Touw I: Hematopoietic growth factors and their receptors in acute leukemia. Blood 81: 281-292, 1993
3. Metcalf D: The molecular control of cell division, differentiation commitment and maturation in haemppoietic cells. Nature 339: 27-30, 1989
4. Ullrich A, Schlessinger J: Signal transduction by receptors with tyrosine kinase activity. Cell 61: 203-212, 1990
5. Matthew W, Jordan CT, Wiegand GW, Pardoll D, Lemischka IR: A receptor tyrosine kinase specific to hematopoietic stem and progenitor cell-enriched populations. Cell 65: 1143-1152
6. Rosnet O, Marchetto S, DeLapeyriere O, Birnbaum D: Murine Flt3, a gene encoding a novel tyrosine kinase receptor of the *PDGFR/CSFRI* family. Oncogene 6: 1641-1650, 1991
7. Rosnet O, Schiff C, Pebusque MJ, Marchetto S, Tonnelle C, Toiron Y, Birg F, Birnbaum D: Human *FLT3/FLK2* gene: cDNA cloning and expression in hematopoietic cells. Blood 82: 1110-1119, 1993
8. Birg F, Courcoul M, Rosnet O, Bardin F, Pebusque MJ, Marchetto S, Tabilio A, Mannoni P, Birnbaum D: Expression of the *FMS/KIT* -like gene *FLT3* in human acute leukemias of the myeloid and lymphoid lineages. Blood 80: 2584-2593, 1992
9. Small D, Levenstein M, Kim E, Carow C, Amin S, Rockwell P, Witte L, Burrow C, Ratajczak MZ, Gewirtz AM, Civin CI: STK-1, the human homolog of Flk-2/Flt-3, is selectively expressed in CD34+ human bone marrow cells and is involved in the proliferation of early progenitor stem cells. Proc Natl Acad Sci USA 91: 459-463, 1993
10. Iwama A, Okano K, Sudo T, Matsuda Y, Suda T: Molecular cloning of a novel receptor tyrosine kinase gene, STK, derived from enriched hematopoietic stem cells. Blood 83: 3160-3169, 1994
11. Birg F, Rosnet O, Carbuccia N, Birnbaum D: The expression of *FMS, KIT* and *FLT3* in hematopoietic malignancies. Leukemia Lymphoma 13: 223-227, 1994
12. Lyman SD, James L, Vanden Bos T, De Vries P, Brasel K, Gliniak B, Hollingsworth LT, Picha KS, McKenna HJ, Splett RR, Fletcher FA, Maraskovsky E, Farrah T, Foxworthe D, Williams DE, Beckmann MP: Molecular cloning of a ligand for the flt3/flk-2 tyrosine kinase receptor: A proliferative factor for primitive hematopoietic cells. Cell 75: 1157-1167, 1993
13. Lyman SD, James L, Johnson L, Brasel K, de Vries P, Escobar SS, Downey H, Splett RR, Beckmann MP, McKenna HJ: Cloining of the human homologue of the murine flt3 ligand: A growth factor for early hematopoietic progenitor cells. Blood 83: 2795-2801, 1994
14. Hannum C, Culpepper J, Campbell D, McClanahan T, Zurawski S, Bazan JF, Kastelein R, Hudak S, Wagner J, Mattson J, Luh J, Duda G, Martina N, Peterson D, Menson S, Shanafelt A, Muench M, Keiner G, Namikawa R, Rennick D, Roncarolo MG, Zlotnik A, Rosnet O, Dubreuil P, Birnhaum D, Lee F: Ligand for FLT3/FLK2 receptor tyrosine kinase regulates growth of haematopoietic stem cells and is encoded by variant RNAs. Nature 368: 643-648, 1994
15. Drexler HG, MacLeod RAF, Quentmeier H, Steube K (eds): DSM Catalogue of Human and Animal Cell Lines, 4th Edition, Braunschweig, Germany, 1994
16. Drexler HG: Leukemia cell lines: In vitro models for the study of chronic myelodi leukemia. Leukemia Res 18: 919-927, 1994
17. Drexler HG, Gignac SM, Minowada J: Hematopoietic cell lines. In: Atlas of Human Tumor Cell Lines, Hay RJ, Park JG, Gazdar A (eds), pp. 213-250, 1994. Orlando: Academic Press
18. Drexler HG, Quentmeier H, MacLeod RAF, Uphoff CC, Hu ZB: Leukemia cell lines: In vitro models for the study of acute promyelocytic leukemia. Leukemia Res (in press)
19. Hassan HT, Drexler HG: Interleukins in human myeloid leukemia cell lines. Leukemia Lymphoma 20:1-15, 1995
20. Dirks W, Wirth M, Hauser H: Bicistronic transcription units for gene expression in mammalian cells. Gene 128: 247-249, 1993
21. Agnes F, Shamoon B, Dina C, Rosnet O, Birnbaum D, Galibert F: Genomic structure of the downstream part of the human *FLT3* gene: Exon/intron structure conservation among genes encoding

receptor tyrosine kinases (RTK) of subclass III. Gene 145:283–288, 1994
22. Zeigler FC, Bennett BD, Jordan CT, Spencer SD, Baumhueter S, Carroll KJ, Hooley J, Bauer K, Matthews W: Cellular and molecular characterization of the role of the FLK-2/FLT-3 receptor tyrosine kinase in hematopoietic stem cells. Blood 84: 2422–2430, 1994

Acute Leukemias VI
Prognostic Factors
and Treatment Strategies
Büchner et al. (eds)

GM-CSF Dose Response Curves in Priming of AML Progenitors for Ara-C

M. Zühlsdorf, V. Skobin, and T. Büchner

Abstract. Myeloid leukemic progenitors can be primed for ara-C cytotoxicity by hemopoietic growth factors such as GM-CSF. This effect is highly variable for different AML samples. Previous studies have used saturating concentrations of GM-CSF for priming. In this study, we sought to establish dose response curves for GM-CSF for samples. Seven samples were evaluated. AML blasts were isolated by Ficoll-Hypaque gradients and adherence depletion. Pretreatment with 0, 1, 10 and 100 U/ml GM/CSF was done for 48 h in IMDM, 10% FBS. Ara-C was added at 0–100 μM for 12 h. Cells were washed three times and seeded into a serum-free colony assay based on methylcellulose. Leukemic colonies were scored on day 14. For each GM-CSF dose, a D_{50} for ara-C was calculated using the median effect principle. A dose-response relation was found for each sample. However, the extent of priming was highly variable for different samples. A half maximal effect was reached at between 1 and 10 U/ml GM-CSF.

Introduction

The concept of priming leukemic blasts from AML patients with recombinant growth factors has been investigated in vitro and in vivo [1–9]. Most studies have used saturating doses of growth factors and short-term-exposures to ara-C, with the exception of one [9]. Apart from the choice of the particular growth factor, the dosage should be investigated in preclinical studies. The objective of this study was to establish does-response curves for rhGM-CSF priming prior to ara-C exposure.

Materials and Methods

Bone marrow aspirates were obtained with informed consent from patients with newly diagnosed AML. Mononuclear cells were isolated on Ficoll-Hypaque gradients, washed with IMDM, 2% BSA and adherence-depleted overnight in IMDM, 10% FBS (Boehringer). Cells were washed, adjusted to 0.5×10^6/ml, and pretreated with GM-CSF (0–100 U/ml), as indicated, in IMDM, 10% FBS for 48 h at 370°C, 5% CO_2 in a fully humidified atmosphere. Cells were then washed three times, counted, and seeded at 50,000/ml in a serum-free CFU-L assay based on methylcellulose with 20 mg/ml BSA (Sigma), 15 μM water-soluble cholesterol (Sigma), 500 μM water-soluble linoleic acid (Sigma), 2 μg/ml insulin, 50 nM transferrin, Fesaturated, 100 ng/ml SCF (Amgen), 2 ng/ml G-CSF (Amgen), GM-CSF (Behring), IL-1 (Boehringer), IL-3 (Behring), IL-6 (Genzyme), 2 U/ml EPO (Cilag), and 50 μM β-mercaptoethanlo (Biorad). On day 14, colonies were scored under an inverted microscope. Does-responses yielded D_{50} values for ara-C using the median effect priniciple [10, 11]. The fraction unaffected by ara-C (surviving colonies) is c/c_0. the formula used for linear

$$\log\left(\frac{c_0}{c} - 1\right) = m \log D - m \log D_{50}$$

$$y = a\,x + b$$

Division of Hematology and Oncology, Department of Internal Medicine Albert, University of Münster, Schweitzer.-Str. 33, 48129 Münster, Germany

where m is a scaling factor and D is the actual dose of ara-C for each data point. The second row indicates the interpretation of the formula for regression analysis. D_{50} values of ara-C were evaluated as a function of the GM-CSF concentration used for priming.

Result

The D_{50} values are summarized for the seven samples in Table 1. GM-CSF exerts a priming effect in a dose-dependent fashion. Individual samples vary in their susceptbility. The results for individual samples varied greatly.

Figure 1 depicts the individual D_{50} values observed in the dose-response curves. Figure 2 shows the cumulative frequency distribution of D_{50} values and their shift with various doses of GM-CSF. A clear dose-effect relationship can be found, which is statistically significant with $p<0.05$. A t-test may be used for this purpose, since the points are on straight lines in a normit-plot. A non parametric test confirms these data. All dose levels differ statistically from each other.

Table 1. Summary of D_{50} values in the seven AML samples

GM-CSF dose	Sample						
	1	2	3	4	5	6	7
0	0.825	0.7341	3.969	1.134	0.2611	0.1482	0.0676
1 U/ml	0.483	0.2944	0.7324	0.895	0.1974	0.1258	0.0651
10 U/ml	0.4185		0.1673	0.6352	0.0772	0.0971	0.0554
100 U/ml	0.1052	0.3362	0.014	0.3844	0.0707	0.0635	0.0266

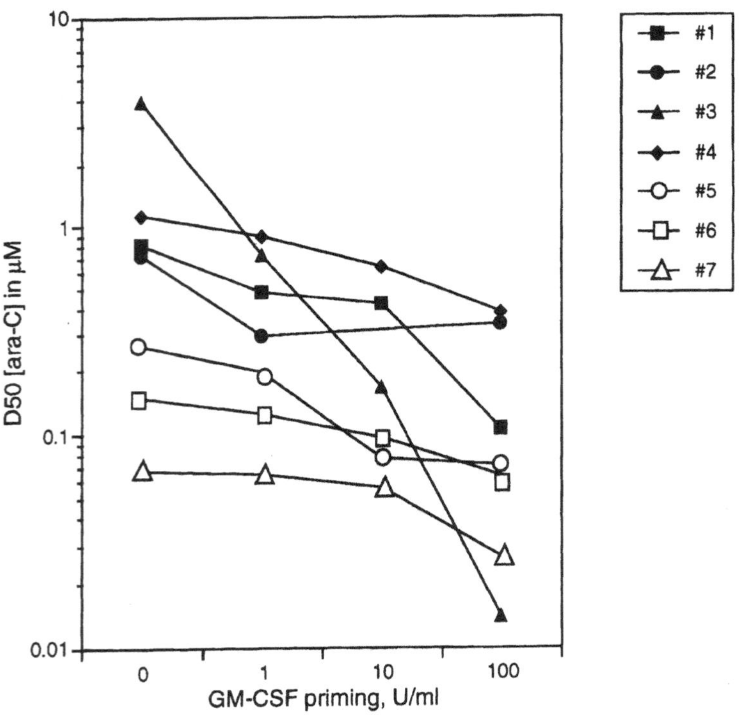

Fig. 1. Individual dose-response curves after Priming AML progenitors with GM-CSF for ara-C. Bone marrow mononuclear cells were isolated from patients with de novo AML, pretreated with GM-CSF for 48 h in the doses given by the x-axis and assayed for ara-C sensitivity. The median effective does, D50, is plotted on the y-axis

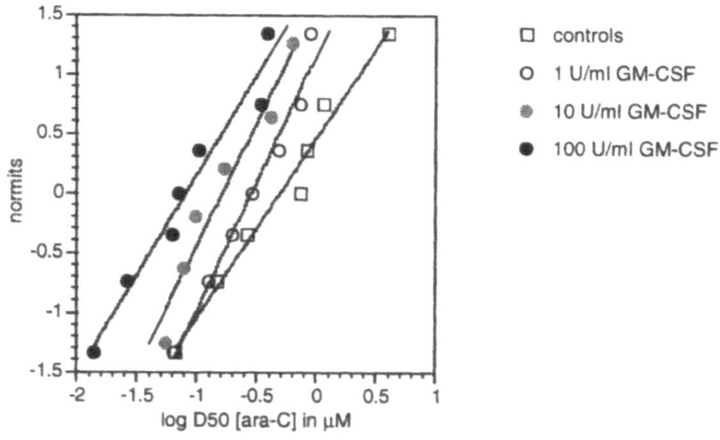

Fig. 2. Cumulative frequency distributions of ara-C sensitivity after priming with different GM-CSF concentrations. Seven samples from bone marrow mononuclear cells of patients with de novo AML were assayed for their ara-C sensitivity following GM-CSF priming at the concentrations given. The cumulative frequencies are plotted on a normit scale (y-axis). The log-normal distribution ($r^2 > 0.95$) of ara-C sensitivities (given as median effective dose, D50) is shifed left by priming with GM-CSF in a dose-dependent fashion. The distributions differ from each other with $p = 0.05$

Discussion

The dose dependency of GM-CSF priming resembles the dose range for induction of cell proliferation, with a saturation between 10 and 100 U/ml GM-CSF. Qualitatively, the induction of proliferation seems to be one possible mechanism of priming [12]. However, the degree of proliferation inducible by growth factors has not always been found to correlate with the degree of priming, but rather with metabolic changes within the leukemic population [7]. In our own series of 18 patients, proliferation and priming showed a significant, yet moderate correlation, explaining about 50% of the variation observed [13].

References

1. W. Hiddemann, E. Schleyer, M. Unterhalt, M. Zühlsdorf, C. Rolf, C. Reuter, U. Kewer, C. Uhrmeister, B. Wörmann and T. Büchner (1992) Differences in the Intracellular Pharmacokinetics of Cytosine Arabinoside (Ara-C) between Circulating Leukemic Blasts and Normal Mononuclear Blood Cells. Leukemia, 6: 1273–1280.
2. W. Hiddemann M. Zühlsodorf, B. Wörmann, M. Koenigsmann and T. Büchner (1990) Changing Response of Clonogenic Myeloid Leukemia Blasts to Granulocyte-Macrophage Colony-Stimulating Factor (GM-CSF) During Antileukemic Therapy—A Case Report on the Basis of a Clinical Phase II Trial. Leukemia Research, 14: 347–352
3. T. de Witte, P. Muus, C. Haanen, N. Van der Lely, E. Koekman, A. van der Locht, G. Blankenborg and J. Wessels (1988) GM-CSF Enhances Sensitivity of Leukemic Clonogenic Cells to Long-Term Low Dose Cytosine Arabinoside with Sparing of the Normal Clonogenic Cells. Behring Institute Mitteilungen, 83: 301–0307
4. T. Büchner, W. Hiddemann, B. Wörmann, R. Rottmann, M. Zühlsdorf, M. Koenigsmann, K. Buntkirchen, A. Sander, J. Frisch and G. Schulz (1991) Recombinant Human GM-CSF Priming And Long-Term Administration Together With Multiple Course Chemotherapy (CT) vs. CT Alone in Newly Diagnosed Acute Myeloid Leukemia. Blood, 78: abstr. 641
5. M.. Andreeff, A. Tafuri and S. Hegewisch-Becker (1989) Colony Stimulating Factors (rhG-CSF, rhGM-CSF, rhIL-3, and BCGF) Recruit Myeloblastic and Lymphoblastic Leukemic Cells and Enhance the Cytotoxice Effects of Cytosine Arabinoside. In: Acute Leukemias II-Prognostic Factors and Treatment Strategies. T. Büchner et al., ed. Springer, Berlin
6. J.M. Nørgaard, S.T. Langkjer, J. Ellegaard, T. Palshof, N. Clausen and P. Hokland (1993) Synergistic And Antagonistic Effects of Myeloid Growth Factors on In Vitro Cellular Killing by Cytotoxic Drugs. Leukemia Research, 17: 689–694
7. C. Reuter, U. Auf der Landwehr, E. Schleyer, M. Zühlsdorf, C. Ameling, C. Rolf, B. Wörmann, T. Büchner and W. Hiddemann (1994) Modulation of

Intracellualr Metabolism of Cytosine Arabinoside in Acute Myeloid Leukemia by Granulocyte-Macrophage Colony-Stimulating Factor. Leukemia, 8: 217–225
8. P.A. te Boekhorst, B. Löwenberg, M. Vlastuin and P. Sonneveld (1993) Enhanced Chemosensitivity of Clonogenic Blasts From Patients With Acute Myeloid Leukemia by G-CSF, IL-3 or GM-CSF Stimulation. Leukemia, 7: 1191–1198
9. N. van der Lely, T. de Witte, P. Muus, R. Raymakers, F. Preijers and C. Haanen (1991) Prolonged Exposure to Cytosine Arabinoside in the Presence of Hematopoietic Growth Factors Preferentially Kills Leukemic versus Normal Clonogenic Cells. Experimental Hematology, 19: 267–272
10. T.C. Chou and P. Talalay (1977) A Simple Generalized Equation for the Analysis of Multiple Inhibitions of Michaelis-Menten Kinetic Systems. Journal of Biological Chemistry, 252: 6438–6442
11. T.C. Chou, and P. Talalay (1984) Quantitative Analysis of Dose-Effect Relationships: The Combined Effects of Multiple Drugs or Enzyme Inhibitors. Advances in Enzyme Regulation, 22: 27–55
12. N. Van der Lely, T. De-Witte, J. Wessels, R. Raymakers, P. Muus and F. Preijers (1994) In vitro Response of Blasts to IL-3, GM-CSF, and G-CSF is Different for Individual AML Patients: Factors That Stimulate Leukemic Clonogenic Cells also Enhance Ara-C Cytotoxicity. Annals of Hematology, 68: 225–32
13. M. Zühlsdorf C. Ameling, S. Weißfennig, C. Busemann, W. Hiddemann and T. Büchner (1993) Correlation of Growth-Stimulation by rhGM-CSF for AML Progenitors and Priming Effects on Ara-C-Toxicity. Annals of Hematology, 67: A 142

Acute Leukemias VI
Prognostic Factors
and Treatment Strategies
Büchner et al. (eds)

Different Potential of G-CSF, GM-CSF, and pIXY in Priming of Myeloid Leukemic Progenitors for Ara-C

M. Zühlsdorf, M. Brandt, V. Skobin, and T. Büchner

Abstract. Cell kinect or metabolic resistance of myeloid leukemic cells to cycle-specific cytostatics, such as cytosine arabinoside (ara-C), may be overcome by priming with growth factors. The extent of priming with GM-CSF and IL-3 has been highly variable for meyloid leukemic progenitors in previous studies. We tested nine different AML samples for their ara-C sensitivity and the priming effects of G-CSF, GM-CSF, GM-CSF plus IL-3 and pIXY321. Bone marrow mononuclear cells were isolated from patients with newly diagnosed AML. All factors were used at 100 U/ml for 48 h, controls were incubated in medium only (IMDM, 10% FBS). Ara-C was added for 12 h at concentrations from 0 to 100 μ*M*. Cells were washed and seeded into a colony assay based on methylcellulose with serum-free conditions using a mixture of hemopoietic growth factors. After 14 days colonies were scored. From the dose-response curves for ara-C, D_{50} values were calculated with confidence limits and compared for different pretreatments, showing shifts in ara-C sensitivity due to priming. D_{50} values for ara-C covered a range of 1 log, in previous studies over 2 logs with a larger sample size. Priming with various factors decreased the D_{50} values for the majority of samples, The largest shifts were obtained with pIXY321 or the equimolar mixture of GM-CSF and IL-3 at a factor of 1:1500. Samples unresponsive to priming with one growht factor responded to another factor. Therefore, priming with a combination of factors, triggering different signal transduction pathways, might be more promising.

Introduction

The concept of priming leukemic cells for cytostatic therapy was introduced on the basis of cell kinectic considerations [1]. There is now evidence for a whole spectrum of mechanisms responsible for priming. The metabolism of ara-C within leukemic blasts is changed by G-CSF, GM-CSF, and Il-3 [2-5]. While a number of steps in ara-C uptake and activation as well as inactivation may be affected, this does not translate into a higher suceptability to ara-C toxicity in all samples. Ara-CMP incorporation into DNA may also be enhanced [6] increased the rate of apoptosis inducible by high-dose ara-C [7]. Cell kinetic parameters were shifted significantly in a smaller fraction of samples compared with metabolic changes [5]. Yet priming with a given factor or combination of factors does correlate moderately with the ability of this pretreatment to induce proliferation [8]. At present priming may be thought of as an activation of leukemic cells via signal transduction, which may include only minor changes in gene activation or may extend far enough to allow a higher rate of proliferation and measurable cell kinetic changes. The response to growth fractors shows great interindividual variation.

Clinical trials on priming in AML have yielded conflicting results [9-16]. At best, a trend towards longer remission was observed [17].

The objective of this study was to compare different factors available for clinical trials with respect to their priming potential. One study comparing G-CSF and GM-CSF did not include

Division of Hematology and Oncology, Department of Internal Medicine, University of Münster, Albert-Schweitzer.-Str. 33, 48129 Münster, Germany

controls without pretreatment [18]. In this series, samples were analyzed in a uniform assay allowing for untreated controls. The colony assay was adjusted to serum-free conditions, giving an improved growth of leukemic colonies versus macrophage colonies. Bone marrow samples were only used when their blast content exceeded 80%, to further reduce the possibility of normal CFU-GM formation.

Materials and Methods

Bone marrow aspirates were obtained with informed consent from adult patients with newly diagnosed AML. Mononuclear cells were isolated from the interface of Ficoll-Hypaque gradients, washed with IMDM, 2% BSA and adherence-depleted overnight in IMDM, 10% FBS (Boehringer). Cells were washed, adjusted to 0.5×10^6/ml, and pretreated with 100 U/ml of either factor in IMDM, 10% FBS for 48 h at 37°C, at 5% CO_2 in a fully humidified atmosphere. Factors were r-metHuG-CSF (Amgen), or rhGM-CSF (Behring, *E. coli* product), GM-CSF plus rhIL-3 (Behring), and pIXY321 (Immunex). Cells were then washed three times, countered, and seeded at 50 000/ml in a serum-free CFU-L assay based on methylcellulose with 20 mg/ml BSA (Sigma), 15 μ*M* "water-solubale cholesterol" (Sigma), 50 μ*M* "water-soluble linoleic acid" (Sigma), 2 μg/ml insulin, 50 n*M* ransferrin, Fe-saturated, 100 ng/ml SCF (Amgen), 2 ng/ml each of G-CSF, GM-CSF, rhIL-1β (Boehringer), IL-3, IL-6 (Genzyme, CHO-product), 2 U/ml Epo (Cilag), and 50 μ*M* 1β-mercaptoethanol (Biorad). After 14 days, colonies were scored on an inverted microscope.

Dose-responses yielded D50 values for ara-C using the median effect-principle [19,20]. The colony number obtained without ara-C is c_0, the number at the given ara-C concentration is c. The formula used to regression analysis is

$$\log\left(\frac{c_0}{c} - 1\right) = m \log \mathrm{D} - m \log \mathrm{D}_{50}$$

$$y = a\,x + b$$

where m is a scaling factor and D is the actual dose of ara-C for each data point. The second line shows the interpretation of this formula for a linear regression analysis. With respect to the colony numbers c this is a logistic regression. Confidence limits for the D_{50} values were obtained from the regression analysis [21].

Results

Table 1 shows the results with different pretreatments on the median D_{50} (ara-C).

Figure 1 depicts the individual D_{50} values observed by their cumulative frequencies. Figure 2 shows the same data in box plots, calculated on a log scale for D_{50} values. The number of responsive samples is evaluated comparing the confidence limits of D_{50} values after pretreatment with the values for unprimed controls in a t-test for samples with different standard deviations.

The results for individual samples varied greatly. The ara-C sensitivity of controls covered a range of approximately 1 log. Few samples showed an increase in ara-C sensitivity exceeding 1 log, yet these samples contributed to the value of the median D_{50}. The box plot shows a more moderate shift in the mean D_{50} values. pIXY321 and an eqimolar mixture of GM-CSF and Il-3 showed similar effects with the exception of two samples. Samples with a marked proliferative response to a particular factor or combination tended to show a significant priming effect with this pretreatment. This could not be shown in a statistically meaningful way with this small number of samples.

Table 1. Effects of different pretreatments on median D50 (ara-c)

Pretreatment	control	G-CSF	GM-CSF	GM+IL-3	pIXY321
No. of Samples	9	9	8	7	7
Median D50(μM)	0.287	0.086*	0.199	0.078	0.027*
x-fold change	–	3.32	1.44	3.66	10.4
No of responsive samples	–	7 of 9	3 of 8	3 of 7	5 of 7

*$p < 0.05$

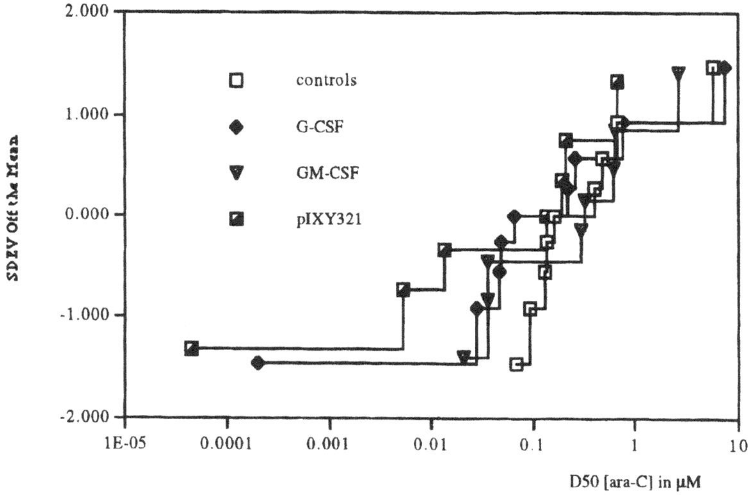

Fig. 1. Cumulative frequency distribution of D50 (ara-C) after different pretreatments. The sensitivity of AML progenitor cells was measured in a colony assay after different types of pretreatment for 48 h with the growth factors as given. The D_{50} for ara-C is the median effective dose. D_{50} values are shifted by most priming methods. Significant shifts are seen for r-metHu G-CSF and for pIXY321

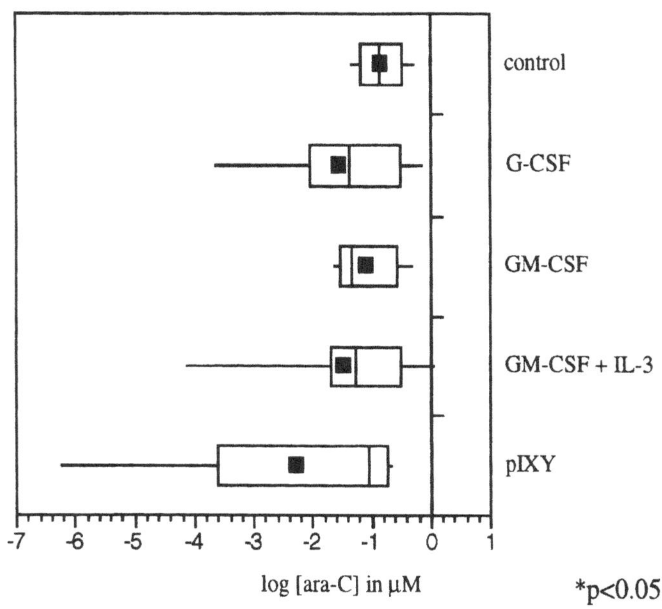

Fig. 2. Distribution of D_{50} (ara-C) for AML progenitor cells after different pretreatments. The sensitivity of AML progenitors to ara-C is depicted here by the median effective dose (D_{50}) after priming with various growth factors. The box plots show the mean, median, and standard deviation for each pretreatment. Shifts are significant for r-metHu G-CSF and PIXY321

Discussion

G-CSF and pIXY321 gave a higher priming effect in this study than GM-CSF. A similar result was found by other investigators comparing G-CSF with GM-CSF in another assay system which did not allow for unprimed conrols [18]. A negative effect of GM-CSF, as postulated as a common phenomenon by others [18, 22], could not be demonstrated. However, there is high interindividual variability within the ara-C sensitivity as well as the shifts obtained with particular factors. This also includes the possibility of shifs towards lower ara-C sensitivity in individual samples.

We conclude from the present data that G-CSF or pIXY321 may be better candidates for priming in clinical trials than GM-CSF.

References

1. S.A. Cannistra, P. Groshek and J. D. Griffin (1989) Granulocyte-Macrophage Colony-Stimulating Factor Enhances the Cytotoxic Effects of Cytosine-Arabinoside in Acute Myeloblastic Leukemia and in the Myeloid Blast Crisis Phase of Chronic Myeloid Leukemia. Leukemia, 3: 328–334
2. J.M. Norgaard, S.T. Langkjer, J. Ellegaard, T. Palshof, N. Clausen and P. Hokland (1993) Synergistic And Antagonistic Effects of Myeloid Growth Factors on In Vitro Cellular Killing by Cytotoxic Drugs. Leukemia Research, 17: 689–694
3. P. Lista, P.Porcu, G.C. Avanci and L. Pegoraro (1988) Interluekin 3 Enhances the Cytotoxic Activity of 1-ß-d-arabinofuranosylcytosine (ara-C) on Acute Myeloblastic Leukeamia (AML) cells. British Journal of Haematology, 69: 121–123
4. M. Brach, H. Klein, E. Platzer, R. Mertelsmann and F. Hermann (1990) Effect of Interleukin 3 on Cytosine Arabinoside-Mediated Cytotoxicity of Leukemic Myeloblats. Experimental Hematology, 18: 748–753
5. C. Reuter, U. Auf der Landwehr, E. Schleyer, M. Zühlsdorf, C. Ameling, C. Rolf, B. Wörmann, T. Büchner and W. Hiddemann (1994) Modulation of Intracellular Metabolism of Cytosine Arabinoside in Acute Myeloid Leukemia by Granulocyte-Macrophage Colony-Stimulating Factor. Leukemia, 8: 217–225
6. M. Tanaka (1993) Recombinant GM-CSF Modulates The Metabolism of Cytosine Arabinoside In Leukemic Cells In Bone Marrow. Leukemia Research, 17: 585–592
7. K. Bhalla, C. Tang, A.M. Ibrado, S. Grant, E. Tourkina, C. Holladay, M. Hughes, M.E. Mahoney and Y. Haung (1992) Granulocyte-Macrophage Colony-Stimulating Factor/Interleukin-3 Fusion Protein (pIXY321) Enhances High-Dose Ara-C-Induced Programmed Cell Death or Apoptosis in Human Myeloid Leukemia Cells. Blood, 80: 2883–2890
8. N. van der Lely, T. De-Witte, J. Wessels, R. Raymakers, P. Muus and F. Preijers (1994) In vitro Response of Blasts to IL-3, GM-CSF, and G-CSF is Different for Individual Aml Patients: Factors That Stimulate Leukemic Clonogenic Cells also Enhance Ara-C Cytotoxicity. Annals of Hematology, 68: 225–32
9. E. Estey, D. Dixon, H.M. Kantarjian, M.J. Keating, K. McCredie, G.P. Bodey, R. Kurzrock, M. Talpaz, E.J. Freireich, A.B. Deisseroth and J.U. Gutterman (1990) Treatment of Poor-Prognosis, Newly Diagnosed Acute Myeloid Leukemia With Ara-C and Recombinant Human Granulocyte-Macrophage Colony-Stimulating Factor. Blood, 75: 1766–1769
10. E. Estey, P.F. Thall, H.M. Kantarjian S, O'Brien, C.A. Koller, M. Beran J. Gutterman, A. Deisseroth and M. Keating (1992) Treatment of Newly Diagnosed Acute Myelogenous Leukemia With Granuloyte-Macrophage Colony-Stimulating Factor (GM-CSF) Before and During Continuous-Infusion High-Dose ara-C + Daunorubicin: Comparison to Patients Treated Without GM-CSF. Blood, 79: 2246–2255
11. G. Heil, L. Chadid, G. Seipelt, P. Mitrou, D, Hoelzer, K. Kolbe, C. Huber, A. Lindemann, R. Mertelsmann, J. Frisch, N.W. Gaus and H. Heimpel (1993) GM-CSF in a Double-Blind Randomized Placebo-Controlled Trial in Therapy of Adult Patients with De Novo Acute Myeloid Leukemia. In: Acute Leukemias IV - Prognostic Factors. T. Büchner et al., ed. Springer, Berlin
12. T. Büchner (1994) Hematopoietic Growth Factors in Cancer Treatment. Stem Cells, 12: 241–252
13. R. Ohno, T. Naoe, A. Kanamura, M. Yoshida, A. Hiraoka, T. Kobayashi, T. Ueda, S. Minami, Y. Morishima, Y. Saito, S. Furusawa, K. Imai, Y. Takemoto, Y. Miura, H. Teshima, N. Hamajima and K.L.S. Group (1994) A Double-Blind Controlled Study of Granulocyte Colony-Stimulating Factor Started Two Days Before Induction Chemotherapy in Refractory Acute Myeloid Leukemia. Blood, 83: 2086–2092
14. E. Archimbaud, P. Fenaux, J. Reiffers, C. Cordonnier, V. Leblond, P. Travade, X. Troussard, H. Tilly, G. Auzanneau, J.P. Marie, M. Ffrench and E. Berger (1993) Granuloyte-Macrophage Colony-Stimulating Factor in Association to Timed-Sequential Chemotherapy with Mitoxanthrone, Etoposide, and Cytarabine for Refractory Acute Myelogenous Leukemia. Leukemia, 7: 372–377
15. P. Bettelheim, P. Valent, M. Andreeff, a. Tafuri, J. Haimi, C. Gorischek, M. Muhum, C. Sillaber, O. Haas, L. Vieder, D. Maurer, G. Schulz, W. Speiser, K. Geissler, P. Kier, W. Hinterberger and K. Lechner (1991) Recombinant Human Granulocyte Macrophage Colony-Stimulating Factor in Combination with Standard Induction Chemotherapy in De Novo Acute Myeloid Leukemia. Blood, 77: 700–711
16. M. Andreeff, J. Drach, S. Zhao, U. Consoli, S. Escudier, G. Sanchez-Williams, Y. Liu, A. Goodacre, D. Drach, C. Dunne, A. Tafuri, E. Estey and A. Deisseroth (1994) Cell Kinetic, Molecular and Clinical Analysis of Growht Factor Sensitization of Myeloid Leukemia. In Hemopoietic Growth Factors, Oncogenes and Cytokines in Clinical Hematology. E. Cacciola, C.E. Deisseroth and R. Guistolisi, eds. Karger, Basel. pp 112–136
17. T. Büchner, W. Hiddemann, B. Wörmann, R. Rottmann, G. Maschmeyer, W.-D. Ludwig, M.Zühlsdorf, K. Buntkirchen, A, Sander, J, Aswald,

I. Binder, S. Prisett and M.-C. Sauerland (1993) The Role of GM-CSF in the Treatment of Acute Myeloid Leukemia. Leukemia and Lymphoma, 11: 21–24
18. P. Koistinen, C. Wang, J.E. Curtis and E.A. McCulloch (1991) Granulocyte-Macrophage Colony-Stimulating Factor and Interleukin-3 Protect Leukemic Blast Cells from Ara-C Toxicity. Leukemia, 5: 789–795
19. T.C. Chou and P. Talalay (1977) A Simple Generalized Equation for the Analysis of Multiple Inhibitions of Michaelis-Menten Kinetic Systems. Journal of Biological Chemistry, 252: 6438–6442
20. T.C. Chou and P. Talalay (1984) Quantitative Analysis of Dose-Effect Relationships: The Combined Effects of Multiple Drugs or Enzyme Inhibitors. Advances in Enzyme Regulation, 22: 27–55
21. G.W. Snedecor and W.G. Cochran (1980) Statistical Methods. 7th ed. Iowa State University Press, Ames, Iowa
22. J. Miyauchi, C.A. Kelleher, C. Wang, S. Minkin and E.A. McCulloch (1989) Growth Factors Influence the Sensitivity of Leukemic Stem Cells to Cytosine Arabinoside in Culture. Blood, 73: 1272–1278

Leukemia Cell Biology

Acute Leukemias VI
Prognostic Factors
and Treatment Strategies
Büchner et al. (eds)

An Alternative Transcript of the Human GM-CSF Receptor Alpha Chain Lacking the Signal Sequence Is Found in AML Blasts and Normal Controls

H.M. Wagner[1], R.E. Gale[2], D.C. Linch[2], and R. Andreesen[1]

Abstract. Blast cells from 70% of patients with acute myeloid leukaemia (AML) show autonomous growth characteristics. One of the autocrine growth factors involved is granulocyte-macrophage colony-stimulating factor (GM-CSF). The receptor for GM-CSF (GM-CSFR) is composed of at least 2 chains. The alpha chain binds GM-CSF specifically but with low affinity. The beta chain confers high affinity binding when associated with the alpha chain. So far at least 6 alternative transcripts of the alpha chain have been described which differ from each other in the 3' end of the coding sequence. Using RT-PCR of RNA from normal bone marrow mononuclear cells and blast cells from patients with AML we have found an mRNA transcript with a deletion of 102 nucleotides (nt) between nt 123 and 226 of the published sequence. This deletion removes the original initiation codon and the signal peptide sequence. Translation would still be possible starting from ATG (nt 282–284), creating an alpha chain lacking the signal peptide and the first 22 amino acids of the extracellular protein sequence. In RNAse protection assays transcripts carrying the 102 nt deletion were expressed at levels of about 20% of the total alpha chain message in normal bone marrow cells. In blasts from AML patients expression varied between 5 and 60%. Full length GM-CSFR alpha RT-PCR products from a patient with AML showed that transcripts carrying the 102 nt deletion also lack the sequence coding for the transmembrane domain. Translation of this mRNA transcript would therefore produce a signal peptide deficient, soluble GM-CSFR alpha isoform that might be confined to the cytosol. It is possible that such a cytosolic receptor chain could be involved in intracellular autocrine loops.

Introduction

Acute myeloid leukaemia (AML) is characterized by the excessive proliferation of maligant blast cells. AML blasts proliferate in response to haematopoietic growth factors which may be provided by the blast cells themselves in an autocrine fashion [1, 2]. Granulocyte-macrophage colony-stimulating factor (GM-CSF) appears to be involved in autocrine growth cycles [3]. The receptor for GM-CSF consists of 2 chains, an alpha and a beta chain. The alpha chain binds GM-CSF specifically but with low affinity. Association of the beta chain confers high affinity binding [4, 5, 6]. The GM-CSFR alpha chain as described by Gearing [4] is composed of a signal peptide of 22 amino acids (aa), an extracellular domain of 297 aa, a transmembrane anchor of 27 aa and an intracytoplasmic tail of 54 aa. To date, at least 6 different isoforms of the alpha chain have been found. All are generated by alternative splicing at the 3' end of the cDNA. They include the originally isolated low affinity receptor [4], a serine-rich insertion of 10 aa at the cytoplasmic end of the receptor [7], two soluble isoforms [8, 9, 10], an isoform with a novel 62 a carboxy-terminus with an alternative membrane anchor

[1]Abt. Hämatologie/Onkologie, Klinik und Poliklinik für Innere Medizin I, Universität Regensburg, 93042 Regensburg, Germany
[2]Dept. of Haematology, University College London Medical School, London, UK

[10] and finally an isoform that contains an insertion of 34 aa in the membrane-proximal area of the extracellular domain [11]. The biological function of these various isoforms has yet to be elucidated. We focussed our attention on the 5' end of the cDNA, where alternative splicing might be involved in translational control of receptor expression. In this report we describe a novel RNA transcript encoding a signal peptide deficient GM-CSFR alpha isoform. It is found in normal primary cells and with increased relative expression in AML blast cells.

Material and Methods

Bone marrow samples were obtained from adult patients with AML ($n = 10$). They were classified according to the FAB criteria: M12 patients (pts), M22 pts, M42 pts, M53 pts, M61 pt. Non-AML control marrows were obtained from 3 normal donors, 2 patients with Non-Hodgkin's lymphoma in complete remission and 1 patient with multiple myeloma with less than 5% plasma cells in the bone marrow aspirate.

The mononuclear cells, including leukaemic blast cells, were seperated by standard density gradient centrifugation. Total cellular RNA was prepared by lysis in guanidine thiocyanate and ultracentrifugation in caesium chloride.

RT-PCR and sequencing were performed as described in detail elsewhere [12]. In brief, 1 μg total cellular RNA was reverse transcribed using oligo dT as primer in a total volume of 20 μl. Reactions were incubated at 42°C for 1 h and at 99°C for 5 min. Then 4 μl of reverse transcription reaction was used for PCR in a total volume of 20 μl containing 0.5 U Taq polymerase. Thirty-five cycles of 95°C for 30 s, 62°C for 30 s, and 72°C for 1 min were performed. 5'primer A:GTAGAACCCTGTACGTGCTT and 3' primer B: GCACGAACATTCGTTGTTAC for fragment 1 (nucleotide 90–392) and 3' primer C:AGAAAACAGTTCCCCCGTGT for the entire GM-CSFR alpha cDNA (nucleotide 90–1416). PCR products were purified by electrophoresis through low melting point agarose and then sequenced using the chain termination method with modified T7 DNA polymerase.

The RNAse protection protocol has been described previously [13]. PCR product fragment 1 was subcloned into a pGem vector (Promega, USA) and digested with Rsa 1 to produce a 379 bp fragment containing the T7 polymerase promoter and nucleotides 102–392 of the alpha chain cDNA. A radioactive anti-sense probe was then transcribed off the T7 primer. Next, 5–20 μg of total RNA and 1 μl radioactive probe were added to a total of 25 μl hybridisation buffer. The hybridisation reaction was denatured at 90°C for 10 min. and then transferred to 50°C overnight to allow annealing between probe and relevant sequence. After hybridisation the reaction was treated with RNAse A and RNAse T1 at 30°C for 1 h and then with proteinase K at 37°C for 30 min. After phenol/chloroform/ehanol precipitation the samples were electrophoresed in denaturing 6% polyacrylamide gels. The dried gels were exposed to X-AR film or phosphorimager plates and evaluated on a Fujimax bas 1000 phosphorimager (Fuji, Japan). The signals were quantified using Millipore Whole Band Analyzer software (Millipore, UK) run on a Sun Sparc workstation. The signals were corrected for GTP content to obtain relative percentages of the different isoforms.

Results

In order to examine the 5' end of the GM-CSFR alpha cDNA for alternative splicing we used RT-PCR with a pair of primers (A+B) that cover the 5' end of the untranslated sequence, the signal peptide sequence and the amino-terminus of the mature receptor (Fig. 1). According to the Gearing sequence [4] a PCR product of 303 bp was expected. In addition, however a smaller band of 201 bp was found in TF-1 cells, in normal bone marrow mononuclear cells and in leukaemic blast cells (data not shown).

Direct sequencing of the 201 bp PCR product revealed that the 201 bp band is caused by a deletion of 102 nucleotides between nt 123 and 226 representing exon 3 [14]. This deletion removes the original initiation codon and the signal peptide sequence. Further downstream after the deletion there is another potential start codon at methionine 45 (Fig. 2). If this initiation codon were used a GM-CSFR alpha chain would be created that lacks the signal peptide and the first 22 amino-terminal amino acids of the mature alpha chain. In the following the signal peptide deficient isoform will be referred to as SPD.

To study the whole SPD-mRNA total RNA was subjected to RT-PCR using primers (A+C)

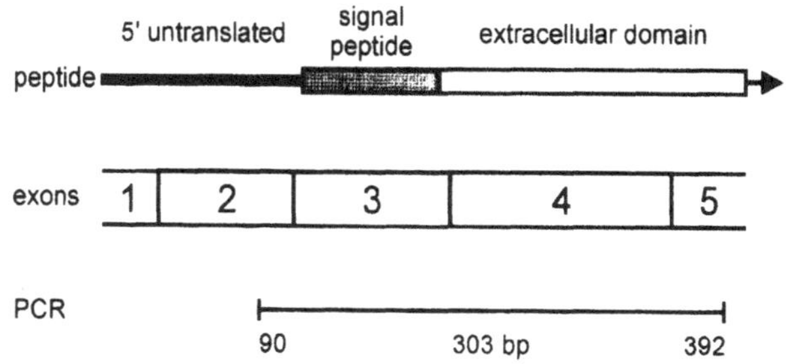

Fig. 1. Exon and peptide structure of the 5' end of GM-CSFR alpha. PCR fragment 1 is indicated

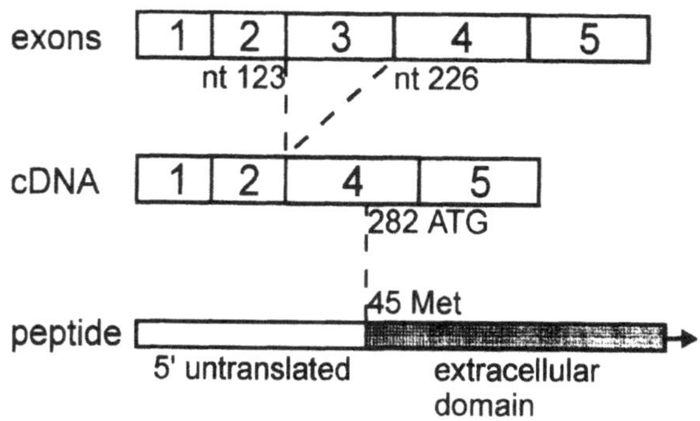

Fig. 2. Deletion of exon 3. Exon, cDNA and peptide structure of the transcript with deletion of 102 nt. New potential start codon at Met 45 creating a signal peptide deficient isoform

in the untranslated regions on either side of the coding sequence. The full length products of approximately 1.3 kb length were sub-cloned into a plasmid vector. Individual clones were examined by PCR for signal peptide depletion and alterations around the transmembrane region. Twelve clones derived from 1 AML patient were screened. Three clones were signal peptide deficient; 1 of the 3 contained the transmembrane region as in the Gearing sequence [4], 2 lacked the transmembrane region as in the Ashworth/Raines sequence [8, 9].

RNAse protection assays were performed to assess the relative expression of the SPD isoform and to exclude the possibility that the deletion is an RT-PCR artefact due to secondary RNA structure (Fig. 3). The probe protects a 291 bp fragment (nt 102–392) of the Gearing sequence. The SPD isoform yields a fragment of 167 bp (nt 226–392). The deletion of exon 2 causes the 269 bp band [15]. On the RNAse protection autorads a phosphorimager was used to quantify the relative expression of the SPD isoform. In neutrophils and normal bone marrow cells the SPD isoform accounted for about 20% of the total alpha message. In 10 AML samples the relative expression varied between 5 and 65% (Fig. 4).

Discussion

GM-CSF is an important growth factor for AML blast cells. For the alpha chain of its receptor (GM-CSFR alpha) multiple isoforms have been described [4, 7–11]. They are all created by alternative splicing at the 3' end of the alpha chain cDNA and result in alterations around the transmembrane anchor or in the cytoplasmic domain of the receptor molecule. Here, we demonstrate a new receptor isoform that codes for an SPD, soluble GM-CSFR alpha chain. The SPD transcript is generated by splicing out exon 3 at the 5' end of the gene. The deletion of exon 3 removes the original initiation site. Further downstream codon $A_{282}TG$ represents a potential start codon. It lies within a suboptimal initiation context, but translation appears still possible [16]. $A_{282}TG$ codes for Met_{45} of the mature receptor alpha chain. If $A_{282}TG$ were used as an initiation codon, a receptor would be generated that starts at Met_{45} of the alpha chain in frame with the Gearing sequence. This alpha chain would lack the signal peptide and the 22 amino-terminal aminoacids of the mature receptor. We found two SPD transcripts; one represents the Gearing sequence except for deletion of exon 3, the other lacks the transmembrane anchor in addition to exon 3

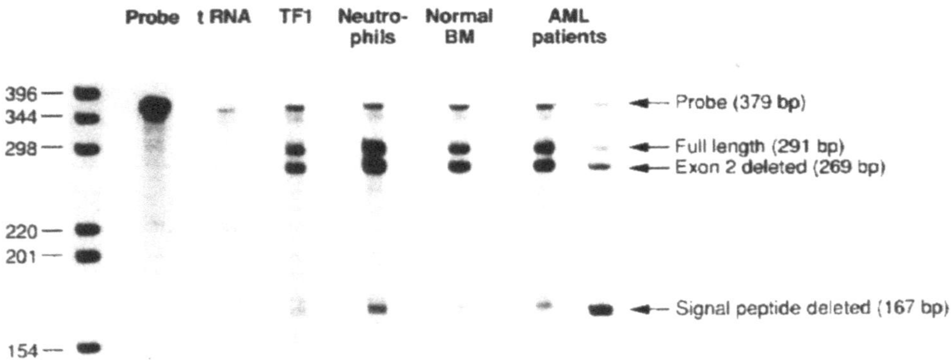

Fig. 3. RNAse protection analysis of the GM-CSFR alpha using total RNA from TF1 cells, normal neutrophils, normal bone marrow cells and AML blast. The full length probe (379 bp) protects a fragment of 291 bp of the Gearing sequence and a fragment of 167 bp of the SPD isoform. Deletion of exon 2 yields a fragment of 269 bp

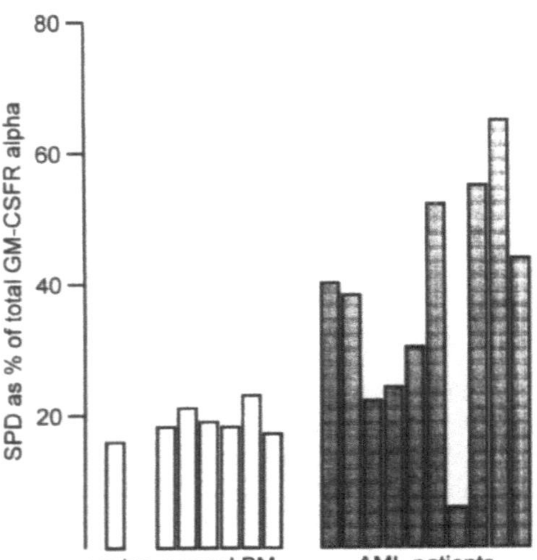

Fig. 4. Relative expression of SPD mRNA in normal bone marrow cells and AML blats. RNAse protection assays were performed on total RNA from neutrophils, normal bone marrow cells (*open bars*) and AML blast cells (*Shaded bars*). Autorads were scanned by a phosphorimager. For each sample the intensity of the band representing the SPD transcript was expressed as percentage of the total GM-CSFR alpha message

equivalent to the soluble receptor as described by Ashworth and Raines [8, 9]. Thus the latter transcript encodes a polypeptide deficient of signal peptide and transmembrane anchor. Since it is the function of the signal peptide to guide a newly synthesized polypeptide chain out of the cytosol through the membrane via the ER lumen to the cell surface, a receptor lacking the signal peptide and the transmembrane anchor is therefore expected to remain in the cytosol as an unglycosylated polypeptide [17].

SPD mRNA is expressed in normal neutrophils and bone marrow cells at a level of approximately 20% of the total alpha chain message. In blast cells from some AML patients the levels of SPD mRNA expression are increased to up to 65% of the total message.

Blast cells from a proportion of AML patients show an autocrine growth pattern and proliferate in culture without addition of exogenous growth factors [1, 18]. The autocrine growth can be inhibited by addition of antibodies against growth factors. This suggests a model where the blast cells secrete the growth factor into the extracellular space. The growth factor then binds to the specific receptor expressed on the cell surface (Fig. 5a). In some cases the autocrine growth cycle cannot be interrupted by antibodies. However, proliferation can be suppressed by inhibiting the synthesis of growth factor with antisense DNA against growth factor message [3]. This could be explained by a model where the growth factor remains within the cell and binds to an intracellular receptor (Fig. 5b). A signal peptide deficient, cytosolic GM-CSFR alpha chain might be involved in such an intracellular autocrine growth cycle. Up to now SPD GM-CSFR alpha has only been shown as an mRNA transcript. Studies on the expression of this isoform as a protein are in progress.

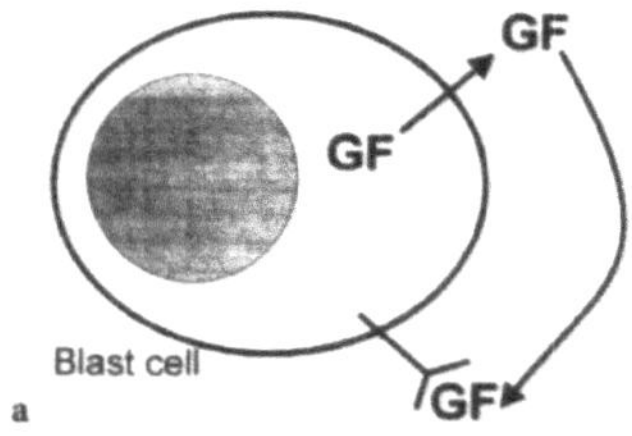

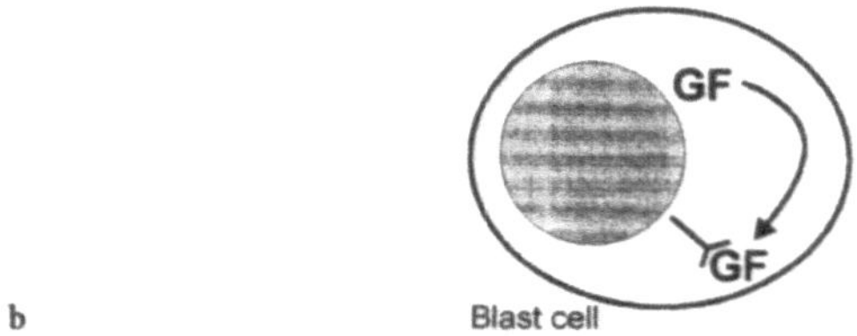

Fig. 5. Model of extracellular (**a**) and intracellular (**b**) autocine growth loops. *GF*; growth factor

References

1. Russell NH. 1992. Autocrine growth factors and leukaemic haemopoiesis. Blood Rev. 6: 149–156.
2. Löwenberg B, Touw IP. 1993. Hematopoietic growth factors and their receptors in acute leukemia. Blood 81: 281–292.
3. Rogers SY, Bradbury D, Kozlowski R, Russell NH. 1994. Evidence for internal autocrine regulation of growth in acute myeloblastic leukemia cells. Exp. Hematol. 22: 593–598.
4. Gearing DP, King JA, Gough NM, Nicola NA. 1989. Expression cloning of a receptor for human granulocyte-macrophage colony-stimulating factor. EMBO J. 8: 3667–3676.
5. Hayashida K, Kitamura T, Gorman DM, Arai KI, Yokota T, Miyajima A. 1990. Molecular cloning of a second subunit of the receptor for human granulocyte-macrophage colony-stimulating factor (GM-CSF): Reconstitution of a high-affinity GM-CSF receptor. Proc. Natl. Acad. Sci. USA. 87: 9655–9659.
6. Kitamura T, Sato N, Arai KI, Miyajima A. 1991. Expression cloning of the human IL-3 receptor cDNA reveals a shared beta subunit for the human IL-3 and GM-CSF receptors. Cell 66: 1165–1174.
7. Crosier KE, Wong GG, Mathey-Prevot B, Nathan DG, Sieff CA. 1991. A functional isoform of the human granulocyte-macrophage colony-stimulating factor receptor has an unusual cytoplasmic domain. Proc. Natl. Acad. Sci. USA. 88: 7744–7748.
8. Ashworth A, Kraft A. 1990. Cloning of a potentially soluble receptor for human GM-CSF. Nucl. Acid. Res. 18: 7178.
9. Raines MA, Liu L, Quan SG, Joe V, DiPersio JF, Golde DW. 1991. Identification and molecular cloning of a soluble human granulocyte-macrophage colony-stimulating factor receptor. Proc. Natl. Acad. Sci. USA. 88: 8203–8207.
10. Hu X, Emanuel PD, Zuckerman KS. 1994. Cloning and sequencing of the cDNAs encoding two alternative splicing derived variants of the alpha subunit of the granulocyte-macrophage colony-stimulating factor receptor. Biochim. Biophys. Acta. 1223: 306.
11. Devereux S, Wagner HM, Khwaja A, McMillan AK, Linch DC. 1993. A novel isoform of the low affinity granulocyte-macrophage colony-stimulating factor receptor. Brit. J. Haematol. 84, Suppl, 1: 21.
12 Wagner HM, Gale RE, Freeburn RW, Devereux S, Linch DC. 1994. Analysis of mutations in the GM-CSF receptor alpha coding sequence in patients with acute myeloid leukaemia and haematologically normal individuals by RT-PCR-SSCP. Leukemia 8: 1527–1532.
13. Devalia V, Thomas NS, Roberts PJ, Jones HM, Linch DC. 1992. Down-regulation of human protein kinase C alpha is associated with terminal neutrophil differentiation. Blood 80: 68–76.
14. Nakagawa Y, Kosugi H, Miyajima A, Arai KI, Yokota T. 1994. Structure of the gene encoding the alpha subunit of the human granulocyte-macrophage colony-stimulating factor receptor. J. Biol. Chem. 269: 10905–10912.
15. Chopra R, Kendall G, Gale RE, Thomas NSB, Linch DC. 1995. Expression of two alternatively spliced forms of the 5' untranslated region of the granulocyte-macrophage colony-stimulating factor receptor alpha chain mRNA. Submitted for publication.
16 Kozak M. 1984. Selection of initiation sites by eukaryotic ribosomes: Effect of inserting AUG triplets upstream from the coding sequence for preproinsulin. Nucl. Acid. Res. 12: 3873.
17. Rapoport TA. 1990. Protein transport across the ER membrane. TIBS 15: 355–358.
18. Löwenberg B, van Putten WLJ, Touw IP, Delwel R, Santini V. 1993. Autonomous proliferation of leukemic cells in vitro as a determinant of prognosis in adult acute myeloid leukemia. New Engl. J. Med. 328: 614–619.

Acute Leukemias VI
Prognostic Factors
and Treatment Strategies
Büchner et al. (eds)

Marked Effect of the Combination of a Novel Vitamin D_3 Analog, KH 1060, and 9-cis-RA on Inhibition of Clonal Growth, Decreases of bcl-2 Level and Induction of Apoptosis in HL-60 Cells

E. Elstner[1], T. Umiel[1], J. Said[2], J. Lee[1], L. Binderup[3], and H.P. Koeffler[1]

Abstract. All-trans retinoic acid (RA) is the first highly effective differentiation-inducing agent for remission induction in patients with APL, but remissions are short-lived because the treatment fails to eliminate the malignant clone and clinical resistance develops rapidly. Another retinoic acid compound, 9-cis-RA, unlike all-trans-RA—which binds only retinoic acid receptors (RARs)—is a high affinity ligand for both RARs and RXRs. To prevent or overcome resistance and to eliminate the malignant clone, in analogy with chemotherapy, combinations of new potent differentiation-inducing drugs working through different receptors and signal pathways may be useful. The active form of vitamin D_3 [1,25 dihydroxyvitamin D_3 (1, 25D)] is an inhibitor of proliferation and effector of differentiation of myeloid leukemic cells to monocytes. The 20-epi-22oxa-24a, 26a, 27a-tri-homo-1α,25(OH)$_2$D$_3$ (KH 1060) belongs to the family of 20-epi-vitamin D_3 analogs and is considerably more potent in vitro than 1,25D as a regulator of growth of the HL-60 cell line. The aim of this study was to evaluate the affect of the combination of KH 1060 with 9-cis-RA on proliferation of the human promyelocytic leukemia cell line HL-60. The 9-cis-RA (10^{-8}M) produced a 30% inhibition of clonal proliferation of HL-60, and KH 1060 at 10^{-9} M resulted in 50% inhibition of clonal proliferation of the leukemic cells. No colonies were detectable after incubation with 10^{-7} MKH 1060. The combination of 9-cis-RA (10^{-8}M) with KH 1060 (10^{-9}M) produced a 95% inhibition of clonal growth. When the HL-60 clonogenic cells were cultured in liquid medium with either 10^{-7} M of KH 1060 or 9-cis-RA for 3 days, washed and plated in soft agar, KH 1060 and 9-cis-RA inhibited 54% and 30% of the HL-60 cells, respectively. In constrast, when the cells were cultured in liquid culture with 10^{-7} M KH 1060 and 9-cis-RA together for 3 days, washed and plated in soft agar, no colonies were detectable. In order to gain insight into the remarkable antileukemic effect of the combination of these analogs, apoptosis and expression of bcl-2 were examined. After 3 days of culture of HL-60 cells with the combination of KH 1060 (10^{-7} M) and 9-cis-RA (10^{-7} M), apoptosis was induced in 62% of cells, as detected by measurement of morphological changes. Also after 3 days, bcl-2 protein, as analyzed by immuno-histochemistry, became nearly undetectable when cells were cultured with both KH 1060 and 9-cis-RA (10^{-7} M). When cultured over the same period with either KH 1060 or 9-cis-RA (10^{-7} M), 26% and 36% of cells expressed bcl-2, respectively, and 100% of wild-type HL-60 expressed bcl-2. In summary, our data demonstrate that the combination of KH 1060 and 9-cis-RA ireversibly and synergistically inhibited clonal growth and induced apoptosis of HL-60 cells concomitantly with a very marked decrease expression of bcl-2.

Introduction

All-trans retinoic acid (RA) is the first highly effective differentiation-inducing agent for

[1]Division of Hematology-Oncology, Depts. of Medicine, Pathology
[2]UCLA School of Medicine, Cedars-Sinai Medical Center, Los Angeles, California, USA
[3]Dept. of Biology, Leo Pharmaceutical Products, Ballerup, Denmark

remission induction in patients with APL, but remissions are short-lived because the treatment fails to eliminate the malignant clone and clinical resistance develops rapidly [1]. Another retinoic acid compound, 9-cis-RA—unlike all-trans-RA, which binds only retinoic acid receptors (RARs)—is a high affinity ligand for both RARs and retinoid "X" receptors (RXRs). In the presence of 9-cis-RA, RXRs from RAR/RXR heterodimers and/or RXR/RXR homodimers [2, 3]. 9-cis-RA was slightly more potent than all-trans-RA in inducing myeloid differentiation in HL-60 cells in vitro [4, 5] but does not reverse clinically acquired retinoid resistance [6].

The active vitamin D_3 metabolite, $1,25(OH)_2$ vitamin D_3 (1,25D), is another differentiation-inducing agent and an important modulator of cellular proliferation in a number of malignant cell types. This biological response is mediated by binding to nuclear receptors for 1,25D [vitamin D3 receptor (VDR)] which belong to the same steroid receptor superfamily as RARs and RXRs [7]. This ligand-inducible transcription factor mediates the 1,25D signaling pathway by binding to specific response elements in the prometer region of 1,25D regulated genes. The VDR can function as a homodimer VDR-VDR), but also heterodimerizes with RXR [8, 9, 10, 11]. The ligand concentration is an additional regulatory guide to help discriminate between signaling pathways involving homo-and heterodimeric hormone receptors [12]. The clinical use of 1,25D for leukemia is, however, limited, not only because of its calcemic side effects, but because 1,25D fails alone to eliminate the malignant clone and its induction of differentiation is a reversible process [13, 14, 15].

The KH 1060 [20-epi-22oxa-24a,26a,27a-trihomo-$1,25(OH)_2D_3$] belongs to the family of 20-epi-vitamin D_3 analogs, which are considerably more potent than 1,25D as an inhibitor of clonal growth of leukemic cell lines [16,17], breast cancer cell lines [18] and prostate cancer cell lines in vitro, with low potential for inducing hypercalcemia in vivo [19].

Recently, evidence has accumulated that ligands that bind to RARs are sufficient to inhibit proliferation and to induce myelocytic differentiation of HL-60 cells, but can not cause apoptosis. Data have suggested that the induction of apoptosis requires ligand activation of RXRs [20, 21], and the commitment to apoptosis requires an initial progression to differentiation. The possibility of inducing programmed cell death of promyelocytic cells during the early stages of induced granulocytic differentiation should therefore be explored.

The aim of this study was to evaluate the effects of the combination of two potent secosteroids which achieve their affects by two independent but interrelated pathways. We examined the antileukemic action of 9-cis-RA and KH 1060 on the promyelocytic cell line HL60 in vitro. Cell cycle analysis, apoptosis and expression of bcl-2 were also examined.

Material and Methods

Cell Lines

HL-60 cells are promyelocytes established from a patient with acute myeloid leukemia [22]. The cells were cultured according to ATCC recommendations in culture flasks with vented filter caps (Costar, Cambridge, Mass).

Vitamin Analogs

KH 1060 (synthesized in the Department of Chemical Research, Leo Pharmaceutical Products, Denmark) was dissolved in is propanol at 4×10^{-3} *M* as a stock solution, which was stored at $-20°C$ and protected from light. 9-cis-RA (a generous gift of Dr. H. Klaus, Hoffmann-LA Roche, Basel, Switzerland) was dissolved in DMSO to 10^{-2} *M* stored at $-80°C$ and protected from light.

Studies of Induction of Differentiation

Differentiation of HL-60 was assessed by ability of the cells to produce superoxide as measured by reduction of nitroblue tetrazolium (NBT) [23], to stain with α-naphthyl acetate esterase (NSE) (Sigma, St. Louis, Mo.) and by morphology, detected on cytospin preparations stained with Diff-Quick Stain Set (Baxter Healthcare Corporation, Miami, Fla.) after 3 days, cultivation of HL-60 cells in suspension with and without analogs.

Cell Cycle Analysis by Flow Cytometry

The cell cycle was analyzed after 3 days of incubation of HL-60 cells cultured with and without analogs (10^{-7} *M*). The cells were fixed in methanol and incubated for 30 min at 4°C in the dark with a solution of 5 μg/ml propidium iodide, 1 mg/ml RNase (Sigma), and 0.1% Nonidet P-40 (Sigma). Analysis was performed immediately after staining using the CELLFit program (Becton Dickinson), whereby the S-Phase was calculated with an RFit model.

Clonogenic Assay in Soft Agar

HL-60 cells were cultured in a two-layer soft agar system for 10 days without adding any growth factors, as previously described [24]. The analogs were added on day 0 in the agar. For the reversibility of clonogenic assay the cells were cultured in suspension with analogs. After 3 days the culture flasks were gently shaken to loose adherent cells; the cells were washed two times in medium with 10% serum to remove the test drugs, and the clonogenic assay was performed.

Apoptosis

Apoptosis was assessed by changes in cell morphology and by analysis of DNA fragmentation after 3 days of incubation of HL-60 cell lines without and with compounds (10^{-7} *M*). Morphologically, cells undergoing apoptosis possess many prominent features such as intense, staining, highly condensed chromatin, fragmented nuclear chromatin, a general decrease in overall cell size, and cellular fragmentation into apoptotic bodies [25]. These features make apoptotic cells relatively easy to distinguish from necrotic cells. These changes are conveniently detected on cytospin preparations stained with Diff-Quick Stain Set. Enumeration of apoptotic cells was performed by evaluation of about 300 cells by light microscopy.

The extent of DNA fragmentation was determined by a modification of the method of Sellins and Cohen which relies on labeling of DNA strand breaks [26]. As a positive control for DNA fragmentation, a human T-cell leukemia cell line (CEM) was treated for 8 h with anti-CD3 mAb (OK T3) (Ortho Biotech, Raritan, NJ) (Umiel et al., submitted).

Immunostaining for bcl-2

Immunostaining of HL-60 cells for bcl-2 was performed on HL-60 cells which had been grown in suspension culture with and without analogs (10^{-7} *M*) for 3 days. Intracellular bcl-2 protein was detected with a mouse monoclonal antibcl-2 antibody (DAKO, Carpinteria, Calif). Antibody localization for bcl-2 was performed with 3,3'-diaminobenzidene hydrochloride (Sigma, St. Louis) 5 mg/10ml to which 0.03% hydrogen peroxide was added just before use. Slides were counterstained with methyl green and mounted with Permount.

Results

Effect of Analogs on Clonal Proliferation of HL-60 Cells

HL-60 cells were cloned in soft agar in the presence of KH 1060 or 9-cis-RA at 10^{-12} to 10^{-6} M and in the combination of 10^{-8} M 9-cis-RA with KH 1060 (10^{-12}–10^{-6} *M*) (Fig.1). The 9-cis-RA (10^{-8} *M*) alone produced a 30% inhibition of clonal proliferation of HL-60, and KH 1060 (10^{-9} *M*) alone inhibited about 50% of the clonal proliferation of HL-60 cells. No colonies were detectable after incubation with 10^{-7} *M* KH 1060. The combination of 9-cis-RA (10^{-8} *M*) with KH 1060 (10^{-9} *M*) produced a 95% inhibition of clonal growth (Fig. 1). When the HL-60 cells were cultured in liquid medium for 3 days with either 10^{-7} *M* of KH 1060 or 9-cis-RA, washed and plated in soft agar, inhibition of clonal proliferaton of the HL-60 cells was 54% and 30%, respectively. In contrast, when the cells were cultured in liquid culture for 3 days with either 10^{-7} *M* of KH 1060 or 9-cis-RA, washed and plated in soft agar, inhibition of clonal proliferation of the HL-60 cells was 54% and 30%, respectively. In constrast, when the cells were cultured in liquid culture for 3 days with 10^{-7} *M* KH 1060 and 10^{-7} *M* 9-cis-RA together, washed and plated in soft agar, no colonies were detectable (Table 1). These latter results suggest that exposure to both analogs, but not to either alone, resulted in an irreversible inhibition of clonogenic growth after removal of these drugs.

Induction of Differentiation of HL-60 Cells

The functional capacity of HL-60 cells to differentiate was tested via the NBT reduction test, NSE and morphology. The NBT test is rather nonspecific, since cells undergoing either monocytic or granulocytic differentiation will stain positively. NSE is a monocytic specific test. Our data for NBT and NSE staining after 3 days of suspension culture of HL-60 cell are shown in Table 1. Differentiation of HL-60 cells was additively enhanced by the combination of KH 1060

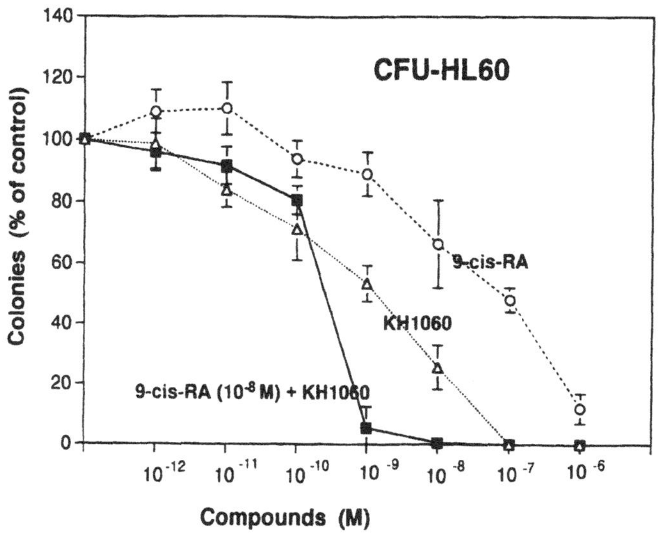

Fig. 1. Dose-response effects of KH 1060, 9-cis-RA and the combination of both on clonal proliferation of HL-60 cells in soft agar culture. The compounds were added to the cells on day 0

Table 1. Effects of KH 1060 and 9-cis-RA after 3 days cultivation in suspension culture on HL-60 cells

Analogs	Inhibition of clonal proliferation (%)	NSE (%)	NBT (%)	Cell cycle analysis (%)		Expression of bcl-2	Apoptosis (%)
				G0/G1	S		
(-)	0	3±2	1±0.5	58±1	34±5	100	5±2
KH 1060	54±10	22±9	20±10	70±10	24±10	32±5	3±1
9-cis-RA	30±9	4±3	12±4	72±11	24±10	27±5	20±6
KH 1060+ 9-cis-RA	>95	8±3	70±4	80*±6	20*±8	0	62±8

Results represent the mean ± SD of 3 independent experiments.
*$p < 0.05$ as determined by Students-test.

and 9-cis-RA (70% NBT positive cells; KH 1060 alone 20% NBT positive cells; 9-cis-RA alone 10% NBT positive cells). The KH 1060 alone differentiates the HL-60 cells down the monycytic pathway (22% NSE positive cells). The combination of both analogs induced the differentiation of the cell population towards granulocytes (NSE 8%, NBT 70%). Neither macrophage-like cells or granulocytes were observed morphologically after 3 days of culture of HL-60 with either KH 1060 or 9-cis-RA alone or in combination.

Cell Cycle Analysis

HL-60 had a increase in the number of cells in G0/G1 phase of the cycle after exposure to KH 1060, 9-cis-RA or the combination of both compared to control unexposed HL-60 cells (Table 1). The combination of both analogs showed an additive increase in arrest in G0/G1.

Decreased Level of bcl-2 Induced by Exposure of HL-60 to Analogs

Expression of bcl-2 protein, as analyzed by immuno-histochemistry, became nearly undetectable when cells were cultured with both KH 1060 and 9-cis-RA (10^{-7} *M*) for 3 days. When cultured over the same period with either KH 1060 or 9-cis-RA (10^{-7} *M*), 27% and 32% of cells expressed bcl-2, respectively; 100% of wild-type HL-60 expressed bcl-2 (Table 1).

Induction of Apoptosis

The strong antiproliferative effects of the combination of KH 1060 and 9-cis-RA on HL-60 cells in Vitro may be caused by induction apoptosis. To test this hypothesis, we examined cellular morphology (Table 1) and DNA fragmentation (Fig. 2) as markers for apoptosis. Apoptosis was induced in 20% and < 1% of HL-60 cells after 3 days of culture with 9-cis-RA or KH 1060, respectively. Apoptosis synergistically increased to greater than 60% when the cells were cultured in the combination of both KH 1060 and 9-cis-RA. Apoptosis was confirmed by DNA ladder formation (Fig. 2), and these changes were observed before terminally differentiated cells were detected.

Discussion

All-trans-RA is the first differentiation agent which is able to induce complete remission in patients with acute promyelocytic leukemia (APL). APL is characterized by reciprocal translocations of chromosomes 15 and 17 that fuse a portion of a gene encoding a protein associated with the nuclear matrix known as PML with a gene coding the nuclear receptor for retinoic acid (RAR-α). Administration of this agent can not, however, cure APL because most patients become resistant after several months. This limitation has prompted as search for additional APL-differentiation-inducing agents having different pharmacological and biological properties. 9-cis-RA could prove slightly more useful than all-trans-RA at initial diagnosis, but it can not overcome clinically acquired resistance to all-trans-RA in patients with APl [6].

To eliminate the malignant clone quickly and completely before the resistance can develop, in analogy with chemotherapy, the combination of new, potent differentiation and/or apoptosis-inducing drugs working through different receptors and signal pathways may be useful.

We tested both KH 1060 and 9-cis-RA individually and in combination to inhibit clonal proliferation and induce cellular differentiation of HL-60 cells. Our previous data suggested that the HL-60 cell line is a good model for APL even though HL-60 does not express PML/RARα [27]. In this study we have shown that the combination of KH 1060 and 9-cis-RA results in a more than additive inhibition of clonal growth (Fig. 1). For example, 9-cis-RA ($10^{-9}M$) caused inhibition, KH 1060 (10^{-9}) produced about 40% inhibition, and both together (10^{-9} M) caused nearly 95% clonal inhibition. Importantly clonogenic growth arrest of each compound alone was in part reversible, while the combination of the compounds resulted in irreversible clonal arrest of proliferation (Fig. 1, Table 1).

In order to evaluate the effect of KH 1060 and 9-cis-RA on differentiation, we measured induction of superoxide production in individual cells as measured histochemically by NBT reduction. An additional marker of differentiation that was measured was the acquisition of NSE, an enzyme detected in cells undergoing monocyte-macrophage differentiation: it is absent in cells undergoing granulocytic differentiation. The treatment of HL-60 cells with KH 1060 (10^{-7} M) for 3 days increased monocytic differentiation (20% NBT and 22% NSE positive), while exposure to 9-cis-RA led to slight granulocytic differentiation (12% NBT and 4% NSE positive) under the same conditions (Table 1). The combination of both analogs produced a synergistic

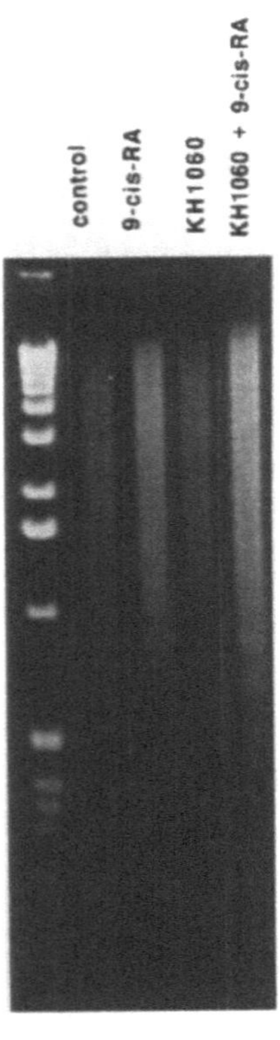

Fig. 2. DNA fragmentationof HL-60 cells. DNA fragmentation of low molecular weight DNA from HL-60 cells treated with KH 1060 (10^{-7}M). 9-cis-RA (10^{-7}M) or the combinationof both (10^{-7}M) was examined after 50 h of culture. Fragmented DNA, the hallmark of apoptosis, is shown in a ladder pattern in multiples of 180 base pairs

increase of differentiation, which indirectly was shown to be granulocytic because 70% of the cells were NBT positive cells but less than 8% of the cells were NSE positive (Table 1). Our data regarding the direction of differentiation differ from that of another group [28], who demonstrated that the combination of 1,25D with either 9-cis-RA or all trans-RA induced monocytic differentiation in 100% of HL-60 cells. KH 1060 belongs to the 20-epi family of vitamin D_3 analogs, which differ markedly from 1,25D in their conformational distribution [29]. The side-chain of the 20-epi-vitamin D_3 analogs is directed to the left, while it is directed to the right in the "normal" isomers. This can induce significant changes in the conformation of the receptor upon ligand-binding and thereby produce differences in the biological selectivity of various compounds. The 20-epi analogs can efficiently enhance homo- and heterodimerization of VDR with VDR and RXR compared to 1,25 D_3 [8, 12, 30]. The competition between the RAR and VDR for association with RXR may provide an additional important control step for the effects of these ligands [9].

In order to gain insight into the remarkable antileukemic effect of the combination of the two analogs, apoptosis and expression of bcl-2 were examined. The bcl-2 protein became nearly undectable when cells were cultured with the combination of KH 1060 and 9-cis-RA (10^{-7} *M*) (Table 1). When cultured over the same period with either KH 1060 or 9-cis-RA (10^{-7}*M*), 27% and 32% of cells, respectively, expressed bcl-2; 100% of wild-type HL-60 cells expressed bcl-2; (Table 1). A positive correlation existed between inhibition of clonal growth and decreased levels of bcl-2 in HL-60 cells cultured with KH 1060 combined with 9-cis-RA.

Therapeutic agents can induce regression of leukemic cells through inhibition of clonal proliferation, activation of programmed cell death (apoptosis), or both. Apoptosis is an active process which contributes to the shaping of organs during embryogenesis; to the maintenance, growth or involution of tissues; to the elimination of damaged cells; and to carcinogenesis. Chromatin condensation, DNA fragmentation, cell volume reduction, and cytoplasmic budding are the main characteristics of the early stages of the process. Apoptosis seems to play a critical role in white blood cell count regulation [31, 32]. Apoptosis depends on expression or lack of expression of a specific set of genes, including bcl-2. Brief exposure of HL-60 to 1,25D has been shown to protect cells from undergoing an apoptotic death. The protective effect of 1,25 D treatment was apparent before phenotypic evidence of differentiation [33]. The rapidity of the protective effect of 1,25D is consistent with the hypothesis that the activation of the monocytic differentiation program is sufficient to interfere with programs that lead to cell death by apoptosis [33, 34, 35]. Data with antisense inhibition of VDR suggested that in the monocytic lineage, VDR expression after 1,25D treatment may act as a protective mechanism against apoptosis. Parodoxically, the expression of the bcl-2 proto-oncogene is rapidly reduced by 1,25D, which excludes the involvement of this gene in the protective effect [33]. In contrast, all-trans-RA can induce apoptosis and this event may be secondary to the induction of terminal granulocytic differentiation [36], although maturation is not completely and is partially defective [37]. Although granulocytic differentiation and apoptosis occur concomitantly, they appear to be regulated independently in myeloid cells [38]. Our data demonstrated that apoptosis was induced in 20% and less than 5% of HL-60 cells after 3 days of culture with either 9-cis-RA or KH 1060, respectively. In contrast, 62% of HL-60 cells underwent apoptosis when treated for 3 days with the combination of KH 1060 and 9-cis-RA. These effects were observed during the early stages of induction of granulocytic differentiation before terminally differentiated cells were morphologically detected. The mechanism of strong apoptosis after treatment of HL-60 cells with the combination of KH1060 and 9-cis-RA is unclear. The combination of 9-cis-RA and KH 1060 can cause the activation of RAR/RAR, RXR/RXR and VDR/VDR homodimers and VDR/RXR, VDR/RAR and RAR/RXR heterodimers [10,11]. Moreover, the concentration of ligands is an additional regulatory level in the discrimination between signaling pathways involving homo-and heterodimeric hormone receptors in the presence of these ligands [12].

Recently, evidence has accumulated that ligand bound RARs are sufficient to inhibit the proliferation and induce myelocytic differentiation of HL-60 cells, but can not cause apoptosis. Data have suggested that the induction of apoptosis requires ligand activation of RXRs [20, 21] and the commitment to apoptosis requires an initial progression to granulocytic differentiation. Further studies are required to establish how 9-cis-RA and KH 1060 inhibit leukemic cell growth.

In conclusion, our data demonstrate that the combination of KH1060 and 9-cis-RA irreversibly and synergistically inhibits clonal growth and induces apoptosis of HL-60 cells concomitantly with a very marked decreased expression of bcl-2. These effects were observed during the early stages of granulocytic differentiation, before terminally differentiated granulocytes were morphlogically detectable. This combination may be useful in the treatment of APL.

References

1. Warrell, R.P Jr.: Retinoid resistance in acute promyelocytic leukemia: new mechanisms, strategies, and implications. Blood [editorial] 82: 1949–1953, 1993.
2. Heyman, R, Mangelsdorf D, Dyck J, Stein R.B, Eichele G, Evans R.M: 9-cis retinoic acid is a high affinity ligand for the retinoid X receptor. Cell 68: 397–406, 1992.
3. Levin A, Strzenbecker L, Kazmer S, Bosakowski T, Huselton C, Allenby G, Speck J, Kratzeisen C, Rosenberger M, Lovery A, Grippo J.F: 9-cis retinoic acid sterioisomer binds and activates the nuclear receptor RXR-α. Nature 335: 359–361, 1992.
4. Kizaki M, Ikeda Y, Tanosaki R, Nikajama H, Morikawa M, Sakashita A, Koeffler H.P: Effects of novel retinoic acid compound, 9-cis-retinoic acid, on proliferation, differentiation and expression of retinoic acid receptor RNA by HL-60 cells. Blood 83: 3592–3599, 1993.
5. Sakashita A, Kizaki M, Pakkala S, Schiller G, Tsuroka N, Tomosaki R, Cameron, Dawson MI, Koeffler H.P: 9-cis-retinoic acid: effects on normal and leukemic hematopoiesis in vitro. Blood 81: 1009–1016, 1993.
6. Warrell RP Jr., Miller WH Jr., Tong WP, Jakubowski A, Miller V, Rigas JR, Benedetti F,. Gill G, Truglia J. 9-cis retinoic (LG 1057) yields sustained plasma drug concentration but does not reverse clinically acquired retinoid resistance in acute promyelocytic leukemia. Blood 84(Suppl 1): 379a, 1994.
7. Baker AR, McDonnell D.P, Hughes M, Crisp T.M, Mangelsdorf DJ, Haussler MR, Pike JW, Shine J, O'Malley BW: Cloning and expression of full-length cDNA encoding human vitamin D receptor. Proc Natl Acad Sci USA 85: 3294, 1988.
8. Imai Y, Pike JW, Koeffler HP: Potent vitamin D3 analogs their abilities to enhance transactivation and to bind the vitamin D3 response element. Leukemia Res 19: 147–158, 1995.
9. Carlberg C, Bendik I, Wyss A, Meier E, Sturzenbecker LJ, Grippo JF, Hunziter W. Two nuclear signalling pathways for vitamin D. Nature 361: 657–660, 1993.
10. Schräder M, Benedik I, Becker-André M, Carlberg C. Interaction between retinoic acid and vitamin D signalling pathways J Biol Chem 268: 17830–17836, 1993.
11. Schräder M, Müller KM, Carlberg C. Specificity and flexibility of vitamin D signaling. J Biol Chem 269: 5501–5505, 1994.
12. Carlberg C, Mathiasen YS, Saurat Y-H, Binderup L. The 1,25- dyhydroxyvitamin D3 (VD) analog MC903, EB1089 and KH1060 activate the VD receptor: homodimers show higher ligand sensitivity than heterodimers with retinoid X receptors. J Steroid Biochem Molec Biol: 51: 137–142, 1994.
13. Koeffler, HP, Hirji K, Itri L. Southern California Leukemic Group: 1,25-dhydroxyvitamin D3: In vivo and in vitro effects on human preleukemic and leukemic cells. Cancer Treat Rep 69: 1399, 1985.
14. Bar-Shavit Z, Kahn AJ, Stone KR, Trial J, Hilliard T, Reitsma P, Teitebaum SL. Reversibility of vitamin D-induced human leukemia cell maturation. Endocrinology: 118: 679–686, 1986.
15. Studzinski GP, Brelvi ZS: Changes in proto-oncogene expression associated with reversal of macrophage-like differentiation of HL-60 cells. J. Natl Cancer Inst.: 79: 67–76, 1987.
16. Binderup L, Latini S, Binderup E, Bretting C, Calverley M, Hansen K. 20-epi-vitamin D3 analogues: a novel class of potent regulators of cell growth and immune responses. Biochem. Pharmac 42: 1569–1575, 1991.
17. Elstner E, Lee YY, Hashiya M, Pakkala S, Binderup L, Norman AW, Okamura WH, Koeffler HP. 1α 25-dihydroxy-20-epi-vitamin D3: an extraordinarily potent inhibitor of leukemic cell growth in vitro. Blood: 84: 1960–1968, 1994.
18. Elstner E, Linker-Israeli M, Said J, Umiel T, de Vos S, Shintaku IP, Heber D, Binderup K, Uskokovic M, Koeffler PH: 20-epi-vitamin D3 analogs: a novel class of potent inhibitors of proliferation and inducers of differentiation of human breast cancer cells lines. Cancer Res, in press 1995.
19. de Vos S, Holden S, Heber D, Elstner E, Binderup L, Uskokovich M, Rude B, Chen DL, Cho SK, Koeffler HP: In vitro effects of potent vitamin D3 analogs on clonal proliferation of human prostate cancer cell lines (submitted, 1995).
20. Davis PJA: Retinoid-regulated gene expression during myeloid cell apoptosis (Abstract) Mechanism of action of retinoids, vitamin D, and steroid hormones. AACR special conference, Whistler, Canada, January 14–19, 1995.
21. Nagy L, Thomzy V, Syka P, Heyman R, Chandraratna R, Davies P: Activation of Retinoid-X-Receptors induces apoptosis in myeloblastic leukemia cells. (Abstract) Mechanism of action of retinoids, vitamin D, and steroid hormones. AACR special conference, Whistler, Canada, January 14–19, 1995.

22. Collins SJ, Gallo RC, Gallagher RE: Continuous growth of human myeloid leukemic cells in suspension culture Nature 270: 347, 1977.
23. Collins SJ, Ruscetti FW, Gallagher RE, Gallo RC: Normal functional characteristics of cultured human promyelocytic leukemia cells (HL-60) after induction of differentiation by dimethylsulfoxide. J Exp Med 149: 969, 1979.
24. Munker R, Norman AW, Koeffler HP: D. Vitamin compounds: Effects on clonal proliferation and differentiation of human myeloid cells. J. Clin Invest 87: 424–430, 1986.
25. Martin SJ, Cotter TG: Apoptosis of human leukemia induction, morphology, and molecular mechanisms. In: Apoptosis II: Molecular basis of apoptosis in disease. Cold Spring Harbor Laboratory Press, p.1, 1994.
26. Sellins KS, Cohen JJ: Gene induction by Gamma-irradiation leads to DNA fragmentation in lymphocytes. J. Immunology 139: 3199–3206, 1987.
27. Kizaki M, Dawson MI, Heyman R, Elster E, Marosetti R, Pakkala S, Chen D-L, Ueno H, Morikawaq M, Ikeda Y, Pfahl M, Koeffler HP. Effects of novel retinoic X receptor (RXR) specific ligands on myeloid leukemic differentiation and proliferation in vitro (submitted, 1995).
28. Verstuyf A, Mathieu C, Bouillon R: Terminal differentiation of human leukemia cells (HL60) by a combination of 1,25-dihydroxyvitamin D3 and retinoic acid (all trans or 9-cis) (abstract). Ninth Workshop on Vitamin D, May 28-June 2, Orlando, p. 138, 1994.
29. Midland MM, Plumet Y, Okamura WH: Effect of C20 sterochemistry on the conformational profile of the side chains of vitamin D analogs. Bioorganic and Medicinal Chemistry Letters: 3: 1799–1804, 1993.
30. Peleg S, Sastry M, Collinst E, Bishop YE, Norman AW. Distinct conformational changes induced by 20-epi analogs of 1, 25- dyhydroxyvitamin D3 are associated with enhanced activation of the vitamin D receptor. J Biol Chem: 270: 3–8, 1995.
31. Savil JS, Wylie AH, Henson JE, Walport MJ,Henson PM, Haslett C. Macrophage phageocytosis of neutrophils in inflammation. J Clin Invest: 83: 865–75, 1989.
32. Whyte MK, Meager LC, MacDemot, J, Haslett C. Impairment of function in agian neutrophils is associated with apoptosis. J Immunol: 150: 5124–34, 1993.
33. Xu H.M, Tepper CG, Jones JB, Fernandez CE,Studzinski GP: 1,25-Dihydroxyvitamin D3 protects HL-60 cells against apoptosis but down-regulates the expression of the bcl-2 gene. Exp Cell Res 209: 367–374, 1993.
34. Solary E, Bertrand R, Pommier Y. Differential induction of apoptosis in undifferentiated and differentiated HL-60 cells by DNA topoisomerase I and II inhibitors. Blood: 81: 1359–68, 1993.
35. Slary E, Bertrand R, Pommier Y: Apoptosis of human leukemic HL-60 cells induced to differentiate by phorbol ester treatment. Leukemia 8: 792–97, 1994.
36. Martin SJ, Bradley JG, Cotter TG: HL-60 cells induced to differentiated towards neutrophils subsequently die via apoptosis. Clin. Exp. Immunol.: 79: 448–453, 1990.
37. Brackman D, Lund-Johansen F, and Aarskog D: Expression of cell surface antigens during differentiation of HL-60 cellsinduced by 1,m25-dihydroxyvitamin D3, retinoic acid and DMSO. Leukemia Research: 19: 57–64, 1995.
38. Naumovski L, and Cleary ML: Bcl-2 inhibits apoptosis associated with terminal differentiation of HL-60 myeloid leukemia cell. Blood: 83: 2261–2267, 1994.

Acute Leukemias VI
Prognostic Factors
and Treatment Strategies
Büchner et al. (eds)

Adoptive Transfer of NK Cells Can Eradicate Residual Leukemia After BMT

M. Zeis[1,3], L. Uharek[1], B. Glass[1], J. Steinmann[2], H. Löffler[1], and W. Gassmann[1]

Abstract. The transfer of allogeneic lymphocytes given after allogeneic bone marrow transplantation (BMT) provides a beneficial antileukemic effect, the so-called graft-versus-leukemia (GVL) effect. However, T cell mediated severe graft-vs-host-disease (GVHD) remains a major problem. The aim of the present study was to determine the antileukemic potential of IL-2 activated NK cells given shortly after BMT. BALBC/mice were given a lethal dose of A20 (H-2^d, B cell leukemia) cells 2 days prior to lethal total body irradiation (TBI) and transplantation of either syngeneic or allogeneic bone marrow cells. After depletion of Thy-1.2-positive T cells, either syngeneic or allogeneic IL-2 activated spleen cells were given 24 h after BMT. Injection of A20 leukemia led to death after a median of 30 days. A lethal dose of TBI followed by either syngeneic or allogeneic Thy 1.2 depleted BMT resulted in a slight antileukemic effect. The adoptive transfer of syngeneic enriched and IL-2 preincubated NK cells at the time of BMT exerted a significant GVL effect. Although the animals demonstrated no signs of GvHD, the strongest GVL effect was observed after infusion of allogeneic MHC-mismatched NK cells. The results clearly demonstrate that allogeneic NK cells offer superior antileukemic activity without mediating GVHD.

Introduction

Allogeneic bone marrow transplantation (BMT) is an effective treatment for a large number of patients suffering from several malignant hematologic disorders. Treated patients benefit from the combined advantages derived from high dose chemoradiotherapy and an additional immune-mediated graft-versus-leukemia (GVL) effect. However, the cellular and humoral immune mechanisms underlying this GVL phenomenon are not yet precisely characterized.

Despite improvements, graft-vs-host disease (GVHD) and leukemia relapse remain major problems in allogeneic BMT. In patients undergoing autologous or T cell depleted allogeneic transplantation, the primary cause of failure is relapse of the underlying malignancy. Recently, it has been demonstrated that the administration of donor leukocyte infusions at the time of leukemia relapse after allogeneic BMT can produce hematologic and cytogenetic remissions [1–3]. The high incidence of severe GVHD and marrow aplasia, however, represents an obstacle to this type of therapy [4]. Unfortunately, the infusion of immunocompetent donor T lymphocytes is responsible for the antileukemic effect as well as for GVHD-related morbidity and mortality.

However, T cells are not the only antileukemic effect cells. GVL effects are also mediated by MHC nonrestricted natural killer (NK) cells and lymphokine activated killer cells [5–8]. Activated Nk cells are capable of lysing fresh leukemia blasts in vitro [8] as well as inhibiting the growth of myeloid leukemia cells [9]. Furthermore, NK cells have been shown to engraft quickly after BMT and can represent the majority of PBL during the first few weeks posttransplant.

[1]Department of Internal Medicine II and [2]Institute of Immunology, University of Kiel, Germany
[3]Present address: II. Medizinische Klinik der Christian-Albrechts-Universität zu Kiel, Chemnitzstr. 33, 24116 Kiel, Germany

Using a murine model, we have previously described GVL effects independent from GVHD and correlated with the donor's NK activity [7]. In this study we show that both allogeneic MHC mismatched and syngeneic enriched NK cells given after BMT can induce substantial GVL activity independent form GVHD.

Materials and Methods

Animals

BALB/c (H-2^d), and C57B6 (H-2^b) mice were bred and kept at the animal facitilities of our institute. All animals were housed in conventional cages, 7 to 10 animals to a cage, and were given non-sterilized food and water ad libitum. Cotrimoxazole was given for 40 days after bone marrow transplantation.

Tumor Cells

A20 is a nonimmunogeneic B cell leukemia/lymphoma of Balb/c origin that occurred spontaneously in a 15 month old mouse [5]. The cells were continuosly maintained in culture in RPMI 1640 + 5% FCS at 37°C and 5% CO_2. These cells were injected i.v. into Balb/c animals. After developing hepato-splenomegaly the mice were killed in the terminal stage of their disease and their spleens were removed. Spleen cell suspensions containing nearly 100% of leukemia/lymphoma cells were stored in liquid nitrogen and used for further experiments.

Tumor Diagnosis

The animals were examined daily and necropsied after death. Death due to leukemic relapse was defined as death with macroscopic evidence of tumor and liver weight > 1.5 g and spleen weight > 0.15 g. For some animals in each group histologic examination of liver and spleen was performed. Animals with hepato-splenomegaly were found to have infiltrations in any case. Healthy mice of the same age were found to have a liver weight of 1.3 g ± 0.2 g and a spleen weight of 0.1 g ± 0.02 g.

Bone Marrow Transplantation

A Cs^{137} source was used for total body irradiation (TBI). 7.5 Gy TBI was chosen as the dose for allogeneic BMT. Bone marrow was collected by flushing the femurs and tibias with RPMI, and a single cell suspension was prepared by passing the BM through a nylon mesh. Experiments with graded numbers of allogeneic BM cells revealed that 2×10^7 cells were sufficient to ensure engraftment [5].

Spleen Cell Preparation and T Cell Depletion

To obtain syngeneic (Balb/c H-2^d) and allogeneic (C57B6, H-2^b) donor lymphocytes mice were killed under ether anesthesia. The spleens were removed and pressed through wire mesh screens to obtain single cell suspensions. The mononucleated cells were isolated by Ficoll-Hypaque gradient centrifugation. T cells were removed by immunomagnetic separation technique.

IL-2 Treatment

Donor strain marrow or spleen cells (5×10^6/ml) were incubated with 200 U/ml IL-2 (Genzyme, Munich, Germany) in RPMI 1640 +5% FCS for 24 h at 37°C with 5% CO_2. Effector cells were harvested, washed two times with RPMI, and resuspended appropriately in RPMI.

Blood Cell Counts

Blood was drawn from the lateral tail vein of the mice and collected in a leukocyte pipette. The total white cell count was obtained by counting the cells in a Thoma Chamber. The percentage of lymphocytes and granulocytes was determined on Pappenheim stained blood smears.

NK Cell Assay

Effector cells were prepared by density gradient centrifugation of spleen cell suspensions of syngeneic Balb/c and allogeneic GVH-nonreactive (C57 × Balb/c) F1 mice. Target cells were obtained from cell culture and were labeled with 200 μCi of $NaCrO_4$ (Amersham-Buchler, Braunschweig, Germany) in 0.5 ml complete medium of 1 h. They were washed 3 times with complete medium and added at a concentration of 1×10^4 cells/well in round bottomed microtiter plates (Nunc, Denmark). Effector cells were added at various effector: target ratios in a final volume of 200 μl/well. The plates were incubated for 4 h at 37°C in a humid atmosphere with 5% CO_2. Maximum chromium release was ensured by addition of 10% Triton-X, and spontaneous release was allowed by addition of CM to the target cells. The culture supernatant was harvested with a Scatron Titertek System (Scatron, Suffolk, UK) and counted in a gamma counter (Beckmann, Heidelberg, Germany) The percetage of specific lysis was calculated as

$$\frac{\text{Experimental cpm} - \text{spontaneous cpm}}{\text{Maximum cpm} - \text{spontaneous cpm}} \times 100$$

All determinations were made in hexaplicate and data were calculated as mean ±SE. Each experiment was done seven times.

Immunophenotyping

For marker analysis, spleen cells were incubated with the appropriate primary and secondary antibodies, as previously described [7]. The primary antibodies used were: 2C11 (anti-CD3), anti-Lyt-2 (anti-CD8), anti-L3T4 (anti-CD4), 30-H12 (anti-Thy1.2), PK136 (anti-NK1.1), 5E6 (NK), anti-asialo-GM-1.

Experimental Design

100–200 day old female Balb/c mice were injected i.v. with 1×10^5 A20 cells 2 days prior to BMT. After conditioning with 7.5 Gy TBI, 2×10^7 bone marrow cells of Balb/c or T-cell-depleted C57B6 origin were transplanted i.v. Some experimental groups were additionally treated with donor-derived 1×10^7 CD-3 depleted and Il-2 stimulated spleen cells given 24 h post BMT.

Results

Phenotypical Characteristics of Transferred Effector Cells

CD3-positive T cells were removed from splenocytes of Balb/c and C57B6 mice by immunomagnetic separation. As shown in Fig. 1 the resulting cell population consisted of up to 50% NK cells and showed less than 2% T cells. The short term incubation of effector cells with IL-2 did not significantly alter this pattern (data not shown).

Significant Cytotoxicity of Allogenic and Syngeneic NK-Enriched Cell Population In Vitro

Enriched NK cells used for cellular immunotherapy were tested for in vitro cytotoxicity against A20

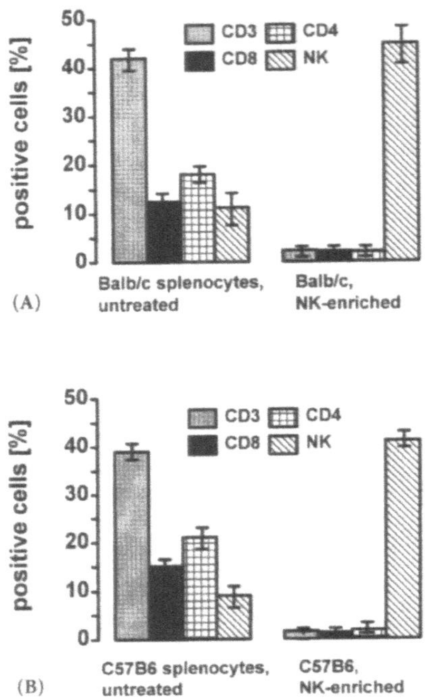

Fig. 1. Immunophenotypic analysis of syngeneic Balb/c (A) and C57B6(B) splenocytes used for cellular immunotherapy. Data from at least 6 different experiments were pooled

leukemia (H-2^d) targets in a 4-h 51Cr release assay. As shown in Fig. 2, syngeneic (Balb/c, H-2^d) and allogeneic (C57B6, H-2^b) NK cells demonstrate significantly higher lytic activity than untreated splenocytes. This effect could be markedly enhanced by pretreatment with IL-2. Interestingly, allogeneic IL-2 activated NK cells generated higher cytolytic activity than activated syngeneic effector cells.

GVL Effects of Syngeneic NK-Enriched Splenocytes In Vivo

As shown in Fig. 3, Balb/c recipients inoculated with 1×10^5 A20 leukemia cells died with a median survival time of 30 days. After TBI followed by syngeneic BMT only 10% survived for more than 120 days and were apparently cured from disease. Treatment with 1×10^7 syngeneic IL-2 activated NK-enriched effector cells at the time of BMT resulted in significantly lower relapse rates than with syngeneic BMT alone (50% vs. 90%).

Fig. 2. Cytotoxic activity of IL-2 pretreated enriched NK cells derived Balb/c and C57BL/6 mice used for cellular immunotherapy. A20 leukemia was used as a target in a 4 h ^{51}Cr release assay

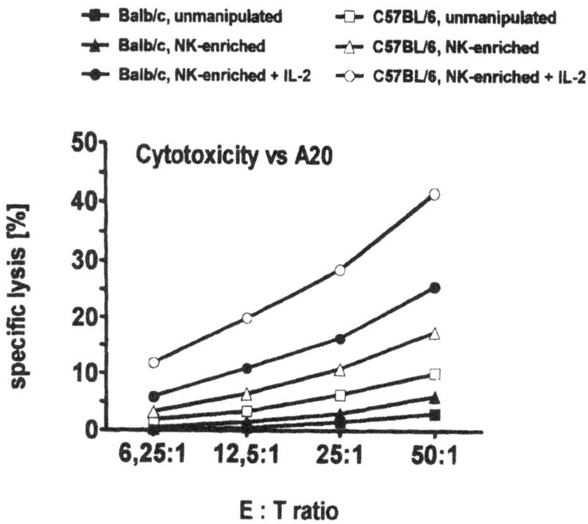

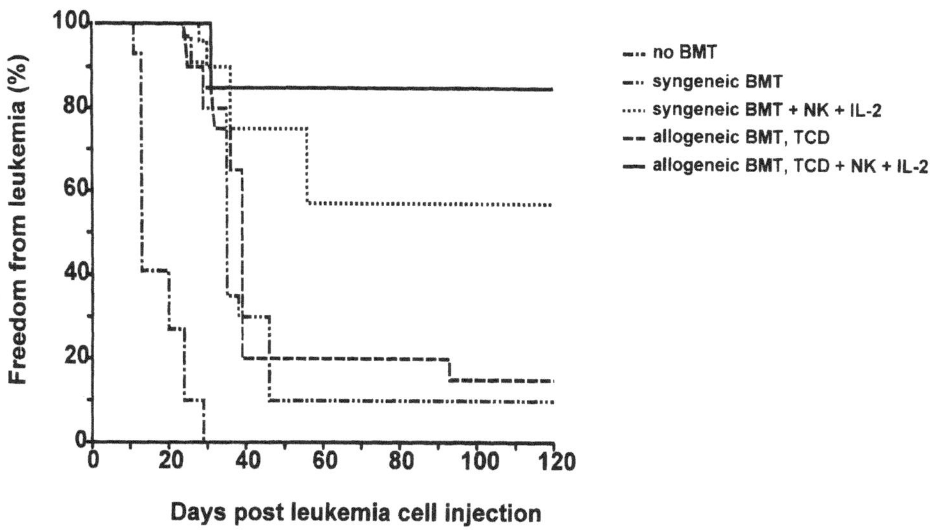

Fig. 3. Freedom from leukemia after lethal irradiation with 7.5 Gy of TBI and treatment with either syngeneic or allogeneic MHC mismatched C57B6 BM prior pretreated with anti-Thy 1.2 + complement. Some experimental groups were additionally treated with donor-derived 1×10^7 IL-2 stimulated CD3 depleted splenocytes from either syngeneic or allogeneic origin. The differences between animals receiving syngeneic BMT only and additional treatment with activated enriched NK cells and between animals receiving allogeneic Thy 1.2-pretreated C57B6 only and adoptive therapy with activated allogeneic NK cells are statistically significant ($p < 0.05$). The difference between adoptive transfer of activated allogeneic enriched NK cells and syngeneic enriched NK cells is also statistically significant ($p < 0.05$)

GVL Effects Induced by Allogeneic Enriched NK Cells

After injection A20 leukemia cells, the pretreatment of allogeneic MHC-mismatched BM cells with anti Thyl.2 resulted only in a slight antileukemic effect. As shown in Fig. 3, only 20% of the animals were cured and median survival time was only slightly prolonged compared to untreated animals (14 days vs. 38 days, $p < 0.05$). Transplantation of allogeneic C57B6 marrow graft led to severe graft-vs-host disease with high mortality (data not shown).

Administration of 1×10^7 donor-type allogeneic enriched NK cells given shortly after BMT resulted in a significant augmentation of GVL activity: the incidence of leukemia relapse decreased from 80% to 15% ($p < 0.05$). Thus, GVL activity of allogeneic NK cells is significantly ($p < 0.05$) greater than that of syngeneic NK-cells (Fig. 3).

Transfer of Enriched NK Cells Did Not Influence Engraftment

To asceretain the influence of aktivated NK cells on hematopoietic recovery, differential blood cell counts were determined after infusion of syngeneic or allogeneic cells post BMT. There was no obvious difference in the absolute number of white blood cells between the experimental groups (Table 1).

Discussion

We have previously shown that NK cells can play an important role in mediating GVL activity [5, 7]. Strong antileukemic activity was induced by NK cells of semiallogeneic donor strains, although the cells were unable to induce GVHD because of immunogenetic reasons. The experiments reported here were undertaken to determine the capacity of allogeneic MHC-mismatched NK cells to induce GVHD-independent GVL activity.

To investigate the antileukemic potential of syngeneic and allogeneic NK cells in a phase of minimal residual disease, we administered IL-2 stimulated NK-enriched cell fractions shortly post BMT. Our data show significant GVL activity of both syngeneic and allogeneic NK cells. However, allogeneic NK cells are superior to syngeneic NK cells in the effectiveness of their eradication of residual leukemia cells after BMT.

A number of experimental and clinical studies have demonstrated that infusions of donor peripheral mononuclear cells (PBMC) can result in complete hematological and cytogenetic remissions in patients with relapsed leukemia [1–3]. However, this type of cellular immunotherapy was associated with severe GVHD and myelosuppression. Our experimental data demonstrate that treatment with activated NK cells exerts GVL activity without mediating GVHD. First clinical reports also show evidence for NK cells involved in GVL phenomena [10].

Furthermore, our data reveal that the administration of allogeneic NK cells can provide a stronger antileukemic effect than that of sy geneic NK cells. This in vivo observation correlates with donor NK activity determined in vitro. However, the cellular mechanisms involved in this phenomenon are not yet clear.

Adoptive immunotherapy with IL-2 activated NK cells given post BMT is capable of restoring GVL activity after T cell depleted BMT. Although low numbers of IL-2 pretreated allogeneic T cells (2%) were injected, no GVHD resulted in these recipients, suggesting that donor NK cell may suppress GVHD. Several mechanisms, possibly working in concert, may be responsible. Murphy et al. [11] demonstrated that activated NK cells can produce TGF-β, and this may also be a mechanism for suppressing the alloreactive T cells responsible for mediating GVHD. However,

Table 1. Reconstitution of white blood cells following syngeneic and allogeneic BMT and additional transfer of NK cells

	Days post transplant							
	7	10	13	16	19	22	25	50
WBC count ($\times 10^9$/l)[a]								
Balb/c	0.3 ± 0.3	1.6 ± 0.2	3.0 ± 0.1	4.5 ± 0.1	3.5 ± 0.3	4.6 ± 0.3	4.7 ± 0.2	3.5 ± 0.1
Balb/c + NK+IL-2	0.4 ± 0.1	1.5 ± 0.3	2.9 ± 0.1	4.3 ± 0.2	4.2 ± 0.1	4.2 ± 0.2	4.2 ± 0.1	4.2 ± 0.1
C57,TCD	0.2 ± 0.5	1.9 ± 0.1	3.3 ± 0.2	4.1 ± 0.4	3.1 ± 0.4	5.3 ± 0.1	4.6 ± 0.1	4.7 ± 0.2
C57, TCD + NK+IL-2	0.5 ± 0.2	1.8 ± 0.3	2.8 ± 0.3	4.1 ± 0.2	3.8 ± 0.2	4.9 ± 0.2	5.4 ± 0.2	4,4 ± 0,1

TCD, T cell depletion.
After conditioning with TBI (7.5 Gy), Balb/c mice received 2×10^7 bone marrow cells of Balb/c or C57. Some experimental groups received 1×10^7 enriched IL-2 stimulated NK cells post BMT. [a]There is no difference between experimental groups receiving BMT only and groups additionally treated with IL-2 activated NK-cells at any data point.

evidence exists that NK cells may be a potential effector cell type capable of inducing GVHD. While donor T cells are clearly involved as the primary cause of GVHD in allogeneic transplantation, it may be that they can recruit donor NK cells which participate in tissue damage.

There are contradictory data with regard to the role of NK cells in BM engraftment [11-13]. While some data suggest that NK cells inhibited hematopoiesis [12], Murphy [13] reported that the addition of NK cells promoted hematopoietic growth. However, our data indicate that the transfer of IL-2 stimulated NK cells does not influence hematopoietic recovery in vivo.

This report shows that adoptive immunotherapy with IL-2 activated enriched NK cells can restore or even enhance GVL effects after transplantation of autologous or allogeneic T cell depleted marrow grafts without mediating GVHD or any other side effects.

References

1. Kolb H.J., Mittermuller J., Clemm C. Donor leucocyte transfusion for treatment of recurrent chronic myelogenous leukemia in marrow transplant patients. Blood 1990; 76: 2462.
2. Porter D.L., Mark S.R., McGarigle C., Ferrara J.L.M., Antin J.H. Induction of graft-versus-host disease as immunotherapy for relapsed chronic myeloid leukemia. N Engl J Med 1994330: 100.
3. Drobyski W.R., Keever C.A., Roth M.S., Koethe S., Hanson G., McFadden P., Gottschall J.L., Ash R.C., van Tuinen P., Horowitz M.M., Flomenberg N. Salvage immunotherapy using donor leucocyte infusions as treatment for relapsed chronic myelogenous leukemia after allogeneic bone marrow transplantation: efficacy and toxicity of a defined T-cell dose. Blood 1993; 82 : 23100
4. Antin J.H. Graft-versus-leukemia: no longer an epiphenomenon. Blood 1993; 82: 2273.
5. Uharek L., Glass B., Gaska T., Zeis M., Gassmann W., Loeffler H., et al. Natural killer cells as effector cells of graft-versus-leukemia activity in a murine transplantation model. Bone Marrow Transplant 1993; 12: 57.
6. Glass B., Uharek L., Gassmann W., Focks B., Bolouri H., Loefflertt., Mueller-Ruchholtz W. Graft-versus-leukemia activity after bone marrow transplantation does not require graft-versus-host disease. Ann Hematol 1992; 64: 255.
7. Zeis M., Uharek L., Glass B., Gaska T., Gassmann W., Loeffler H., et al. Allogeneic NK-cells as potent antileukemic effector cells after allogeneic bone marrow transplantation in mice. Transplantation in press.
8. Hauch M., Gazzola M.V., Small T., Bordignon C., Barnett L., Cunningham I., Castro Malaspinia H., O'Reilly R.J., Keever C.A. Anti-leukemia potential of interleukin-2 activated natural killer cells after bone marrow transplantation for chronic myelogenous leukemia. Blood 1990; 75: 2250.
9. Lotzová E., Savary C.A., Herberman R.B. (1987). Inhibition of clonogeneic growth of fresh leukemia cells by unstimulated and IL-2 stimulated NK cells of normal donors. Leukemia Res. 11, 1059.
10. Jiang YZ, Cullis JO, Kanfer EJ, Goldman JM, Barrett AJ. T cell and NK cell mediated graft-versus-leukemia reactivity following donor buffy coat transfusion to treat relapse after marrow transplantation for chronic myeloid leukemia. Bone Marrow Transplant. 1993; 11: 133.
11. Murphy J.M., Bennett M., Kumar V., Longo D.L. Donor-type activated natural killer cells promote marrow engraftment and B cell development during allogeneic bone marrow transplantation. J. Immunol. 1992; 148: 2953.
12. Fujimori Y., Hara H., Nagai K. Effect of lymphokine-activated killer cell fraction on the development of human hematopoietic progenitor cells. Cancer Res. 1987; 48: 534.
13. Murphy JM, Reynolds C.W., Tiberghien P., Longo DL. Natural killer cells and bone marrow transplantation. J. Natl Cancer Inst 1993; 85, 1475.

Acute Leukemias VI
Prognostic Factors
and Treatment Strategies
Büchner et al. (eds)

Characterization of Normal and Leukemic Lymphohematopoietic Precursor Cells by Three-Color Flow Cytometry and Detection of Clone-Specific Leukemia-Associated T-Cell Receptor δ Rearrangements

F. Griesinger, N. Kaib, S. Könemann, B. Maecker, M. Piró-Noack, M. Falk, J. Ritter, T. Büchner, W. Hiddemann, L.W.M.M. Terstappen, and B. Wörmann

Abstract. Acute lymphoblastic leukemias (ALL) represent the clonal expansion of malignant, transformed lymphohematopoietic progenitors (LPH). The molecular genetic basis of ALL is unfolding and progress has been made in deducing distinct stages of differentiation of leukemic cells based on expression patterns of differentiation antigens. However, although normal LHP compartments have been defined functionally and immunologically, very few direct data exist on the leukemogenic "stem" cell in ALL. Its identification would lay the basis for targeted gene therapy as well as for exclusion strategies in autologous stem cell retransfusion. We have previously demonstrated an incidence of 92% of leukemia-associated phenotypes (LAP), i.e., asynchronous and/or aberrant expression patterns of differentiation antigens (DAg) in 220 consecutive ALLs. The detection of LAP+cells in remission bone marrow is potentially useful for the prediction of relapse in 4/4 relapsing ALL patients, >0.1% of cells carrying the LAP were detected in remission bone marrow at more than one time point. In an analysis of 32 c-ALL and 6 pre-pre-B-ALL, the median percentages of the most immature (CD34++ CD38-DR-) "stem cells" were 0.02% and 0.01%, respectively. CD34+CD38+DR+ or CD34-CD38+DR+ populations represented the predominant leukemic populations. Two c-ALL carried a clone-specific, leukemia-associated genetic marker, i.e., a TCR delta rearrangement. Highly purified CD34++CD38- and CD34+ CD38++ lymphohematopoietic progenitors were isolated by sorting with a FACStar Vantage and Vδ2-Dδ3 rearrangements were amplified by polymerase chain reaction from a minimum of 200 cells. The clone-specific genetic marker was present in the CD34+CD38++ compartment in two successfully sorted c-ALL. In 1/2 c-ALL, it was absent in the CD34++CD38- progenitors, while it was present in the other c-ALL. These data suggest that at least in some c-ALL, malignant transformation may occur at later stage of differentiation than the most immature identifiable hematopoietic progenitors. Thus, it may be possible to exclude leukemic cells from stem cells harvested for autotransplant based on CD34 and CD38 expression. However, in some c-ALL, it may be necessary to further dissect the "stem" cell compartments in order to be able to distinguish between normal and leukemic progenitor cells. With respect to the detection of minimal residual disease, it may not be sufficient to monitor cells with the leukemia-associated phenotype derived from the leukemic bulk population at diagnosis. Instead, it may be necessary, to expand monitoring for MRD to the stem cell compartment to show, that CD34+ CD38− cells are not involved in the leukemic clone by molecular genetic methods.

Introduction

Acute lymphoblastic leukemias (ALL) are clonal expansions of malignant transformed lymphohematopoietic progenitor cells. The detection of differentiation antigens by monoclonal antibod-

Departments of Internal Medicine, University of Göttingen and Münster, Department of Pediatrics, University of Münster, 37075 Göttingen, Germany.

ies has led to the characterization of various stages of differentiation in ALL [1, 2]. These studies have been based principally on the orderly acquistion of differentiation antigens in normal hematopoietic precursor cells. Although the acquisition of lineage-unrestricted and lineage-restricted differentiation antigens has been found to be recapitulated to a certain extent in ALL [3–10], it has also been recognized that ALL may coexpress differentiation antigens normally observed in different lineage (aberrant leukemia-associated phenotype, (LAP) [11–15]. Alternatively, differentiation antigens restricted to distinct stages of differentiation may be coexpressed in the leukemic population (asynchronous LAP) [8–10]. Therefore the incidence of LAP was studied in a large number of 220 consecutive ALL cases. LAP was established in 92% of ALL. To study the prognostic value of detecting LAP1cells in remission marrow for the prediction of relapse, four relapsing ALL patients were studied in whom at least three follow-up marrows were obtained.

Although it may be possible to predict clinical relapse by the detection of LAP^+ cells in remission marrow, it is still unclear from which leukemic subset relapses originate. This is due in part to the fact that leukemic stem cells in ALL are poorly defined. The definition of leukemic stem cells in ALL is of great interest, regarding which leukemic subset should be monitored for the detection of residual leukemic disease. Furthermore, the definition of leukemic stem cells and the discrimination of leukemic versus normal progenitor cells are prerequisites for innovative therapeutic approaches in relapsing ALL such as autologous stem cell retransfusion and genemodifying strategies.

The earliest currently identifiable normal progenitor cells are characterized by the expression of CD34, the lack of expression of lineage-unrestricted differentiation antigens CD38 and HLA-DR [12, 16, 17], and the lack of lineage-restricted differentiation antigens, i.e., CD7, CD19 and CD33. While some data exist concerning "stem cell" involvement of the most immature progenitor compartment ($CD34^+$ $CD38^-$) in acute (AML) and chronic myeloid (CML) [7,8–23], this question is still unresolved in ALL. Therefore, the second aim of our study was defined—the incidence of the most immature progenitor cells in diagnostic bone marrow of common-type acute lymphatic leukemia (c-ALL) and pre-pre-B-ALL and to study the clonal relationship of $CD34^+$ $CD38^-$ and $CD34^+$ $CD38^+$ progenitor cell compartment to the malignant clone using junctional region probes of leukemic clone specific Vδ2-Dδ3 rearrangements.

Material and Methods

Three-Color Flow Cytometry

Mononuclear cells (Ficoll gradient) were incubated for 20 min at 4°C with antibodies conjugated directly with Fluorescein isothiocyanate (FITC), PE (phycoerythrin), or peridin chlorophyll (Per CP; Cy 5; Becton and Dickinson, CA). After three washes the cells were analyzed with a FACSScan, data were analyzed using Paint-a-Gate software. Results are shown as two-dimensional contour plots with a lymphocyte/-blast gate [19,20,24]. The expression of differentiation antigens was defined as "asynchronous" if differentiation antigens restricted to different stages of differentiation were coexpressed on the leukemic cell population, as "aberrant" if differentiation antigens restricted to distinct cell lineages (i.e., B-lymphoid and myeloid) were coexpressed, and as "aberrant + asynchronous" if both of the above were the case. Time points for the detection of cells expressing the leukemia-associated phenotype were before induction therapy, during consolidation therapy, at reinduction, during consolidation, during maintenance therapy, before relapse therapy, and during relapse therapy.

Analysis of Progenitor Populations in ALL

Seventeen consecutive c-ALL cases were selected for cell sorting based on the presence of an amplifiable Vδ2-Dδ3 rearrangements. Polymerase chain reaction analysis was performed under stringent conditions using published Vδ2 framework and a 3' of Dδ3-intronic primers. Between one and ten cells were incubated with 40 ml monoclonal antibodies CD34-FITC, CD38-PE, and CD3-PerCP and sorted with a FACSStar Vantage (Becton Dickinson). Reanalysis of cells confirmed a sorting purity greater than 99% [19, 20]. DNA was extracted by a modified (volumes scaled down) method using polymerase chain reaction buffer, proteinase K, and triton X, as described [25, 26].

Vδ2-Dδ3 rearrangements were amplified from the subpopulations using the same primers as above, blotted on nylon membranes.

Amplification products were subjected to hybridization with clone-specific digoxigenin-labeled oligonucleotides complementary to the junctional region of Vδ2-Dδ3 rearrangements, as shown. Nucleotide sequence were obtained from directly sequenced amplification products of the diagnostic bone marrow by cycle sequencing on an automated sequencer (ABI) [26].

Results and Discussion

Detection of LAP⁺ Cells in Remission Bone Marrow of ALL Patients

A previous study of 220 consecutive ALL established LAP in 92% of ALL cases studied. LAP was defined either by asynchronous expression of differentiation antigens, i.e., the coexpression of antigens physiologically restricted to distinct stages of differentiation, or aberrant expression of differentiation antigens, i.e., the coexpression of antigens physiologically restricted to distinct cell lineages. To determine how reliable the expression of specific LAP is, the first aim of the study was to investigate the significance of detecting LAP^+ cells in remission marrows for the prediction of relapse. For this, bone marrow samples obtained in morphologic complete remission in four patients who subsequently relapsed were studied by three-color flow cytometry detecting cells coexpressing the LAP (Figs. 1–4). LAP^+ cells were observed with a frequency higher than 0.1% at more than one time point in all four relapsing patients. LAP^+ cells were detected 12, 7, 6 and 2 months before overt morphologic relapse in patients 1, 3, 2, and 4 respectively. Significantly, $CD34^+$ $CD22^+$ $CD20^-$ cells were observed at a frequency greater than 0.1% in two relapsing c-ALL patients with this LAP (patients 1 and 4), while the incidence of this population was less than 0.1% in two patients in continuous complete remission with a $CD34^+$ $CD22^+$ $CD20^-$ LAP (data not shown). These findings are important in light of the fact that cells with the identical immunophenotype have been described in regenerating bone marrow [8–10]. At least with the chemotherapy given in the German childhood and adult chemotherapy protocols the most frequently observed asynchronous LAP $CD34^+$ $CD22^+$ $CD20^-$ seems to be useful for monitoring minimal residual leukemic disease in c-ALL. However, confirmation in a larger number of ALL patients expressing this specific LAP is required. Furthermore, the incidence of $CD34^+$ $CD22^+$ $CD20^-$ cells in regenerating bone marrow after the identical chemotherapy for ALL not expressing this LAP needs to be analyzed systematically. These data indicate that detection of LAP varieties may be of clinical relevance for predicting relapse in ALL.

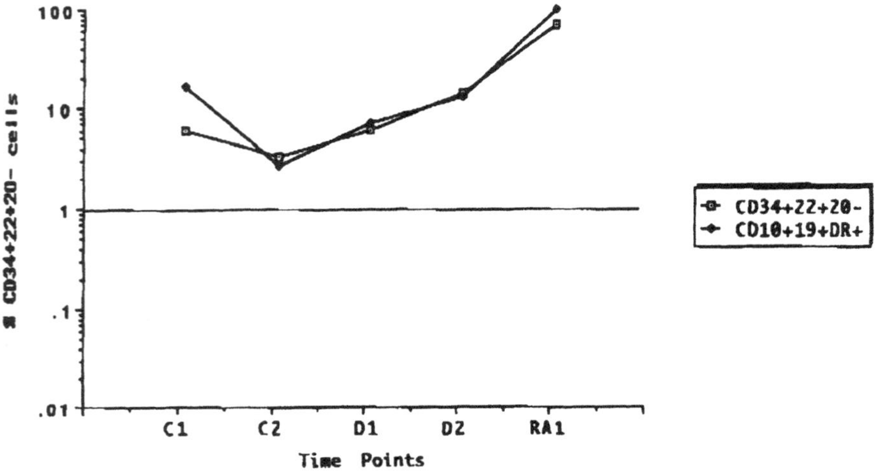

Fig. 1. Relapsing $CD34^+$ $CD22^+$ CD^- C-ALL (Pat. 1)

Frequency of Progenitor Cell Subsets in Diagnostic Bone Marrow of ALL and Their Clonal Relationship to the Leukemic Clone

We next analyzed the frequency of CD34$^+$ CD38$^-$ DR$^-$, CD34$^+$ CD38$^-$ DR$^+$ and CD34$^+$ CD38$^+$ DR$^+$ progenitor subsets in 31 B-lineage ALL (6 pre-pre-B-ALL, 25 c-ALL). The median frequencies of the most immature definable compartment were 0.03% and 0.01% in c-ALL and pre-pre-B-ALL, respectively (Table 1). In 7/25 c-ALL and 3/6 pre-pre-B-ALL the predominant leukemic population were triple-positive cells, while in 18/25 c-ALL and 3/6 pre-pre-B-ALL, the predominant leukemic population expressed CD38 and HLA-DR but no CD34. In 10/25 c-ALL and 2/3 pre-pre-B-ALL the frequency of CD34$^+$ CD38$^-$ DR-cells was below 10^{-5}. The incidence of the most immature progenitor cells seems to be lower in ALL than in AML [19, 20]; however, CD34$^+$ CD38$^-$ HLADR–cells were detected in diagnostic bone marrows in each case analyzed. Whether these immature subpopulations are clonally related to the malignant leukemic clone is currently unknown. Our group and others have shown the presence of

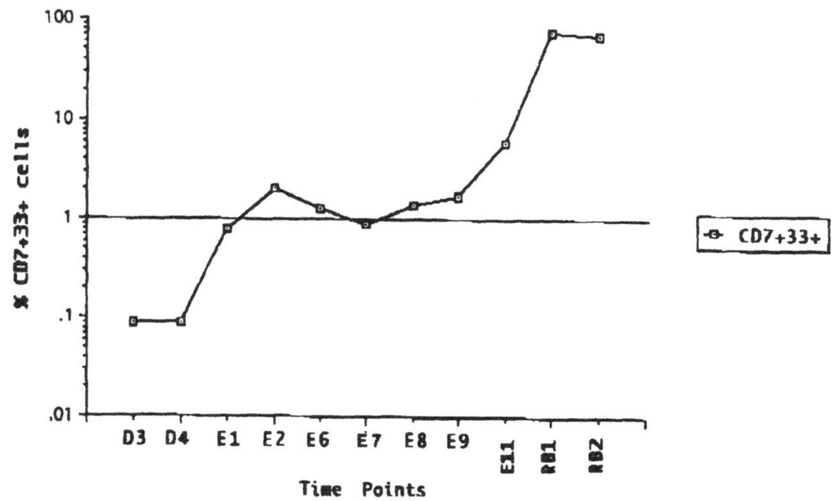

Fig. 2. Relapsing CD7$^+$ CD33$^+$ T-ALL (Pat. 2)

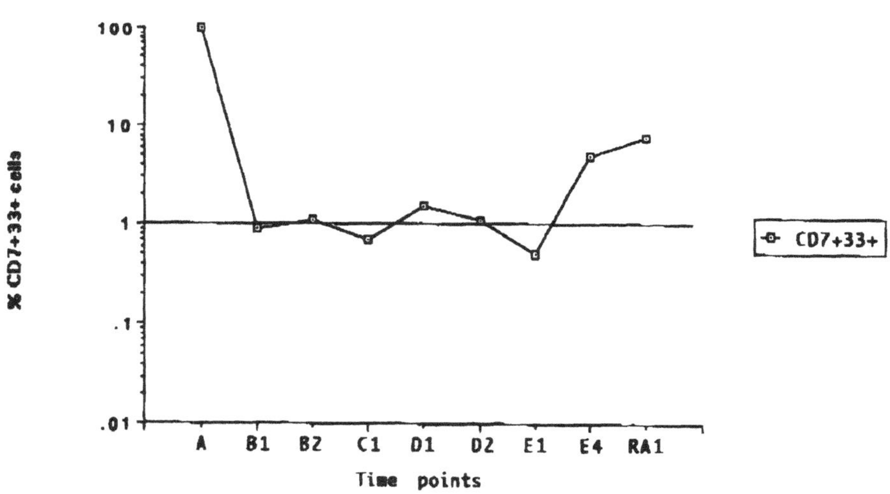

Fig. 3. Relapsing CD7$^+$ CD33$^+$ T-ALL (Pat. 3)

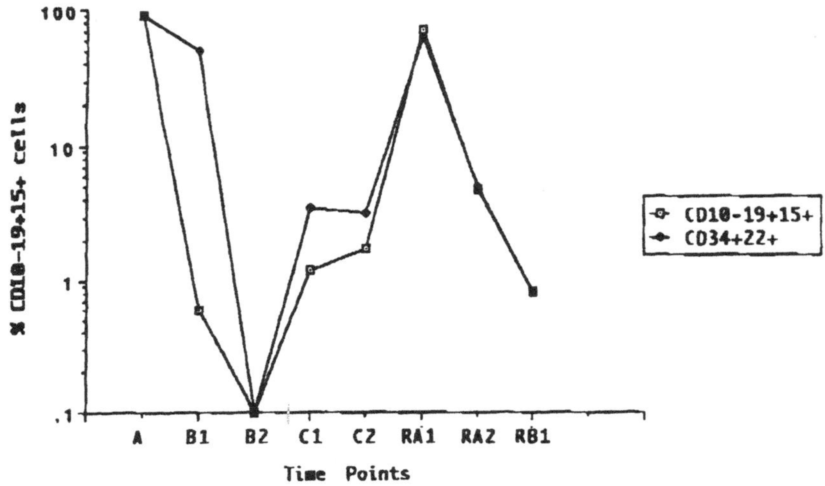

Fig. 4. Relapsing pre-pre-B-ALL (Pat. 4)

Table 1. Frequency of hematopoietic stem cell marker expression in B-lineage-ALL

c-All	$CD34^+$	$CD38^-$	DR^-
1	0.1	0.2	20
2	< 0.01	0.2	65
3	0.01	0.1	0.1
4	0.1	0.3	32
5	< 0.01	0.6	21
6	< 0.01	< 0.01	11
7	0.1	0.3	40
8	0.03	0.1	7
9	< 0.01	0.2	58
10	0.1	3	42
11	0.2	46	23
12	0.03	0.2	9
13	< 0.01	0.1	20
14	< 0.01	< 0.01	14
15	0.1	0.4	75
16	0.2	0.2	2
17	0.02	0.2	56
18	< 0.01	< 0.01	47
19	< 0.01	< 0.01	81
20	< 0.01	0.1	10
21	0.03	0.3	28
22	< 0.01	0.01	39
23	0.1	0.9	90
24	0.1	0.4	75
25	0.02	0.04	30
Median	0.02	0.2	30
pre-pre-B-ALL			
1	< 0.01	0.2	2
2	0.01	0.04	1
3	0.02	2	79
4	1	2	81
5	< 0.01	0.1	1
6	0.03		66
median	0.01	0.2	2

known cytogenetic abnormalities in the CD34$^+$ CD38$^-$ stem cell compartment in subsets of AML which were highly purified by cell sorting [19-23]. Therefore our initial approach was a combined cytogenetic and molecular genetic analysis of sorted progenitor subpopulations in c-ALL. However, sufficient metaphases were not readily obtained in sorted ALL. This may be explained by the rapid induction of apoptosis ex vivo, which has long hampered successful in vitro culture of ALL cells. They may be overcome using stromal cell based culture systems. Because of these limitations polymerase chain reaction analysis of Vδ2-(D)-Dδ3 rearrangements, which is a frequent and stable marker in B-lineage ALL, was selected for this study. Other groups [26–29] and our own [25,30] have found 65%-90% cross-lineage TCR rearrangements. The genomic repertoire of the TCR gene is limited, and the TCR gene arrangement most frequently found in c-ALL is an incomplete Vδ-(D)-δ3 join occuring in 40%–50% of c-ALL. As junctional regions are highly diversified, Vδ2-(D)-Dδ3 rearrangements have been widely used as leukemic clone-specific genetic markers for diagnosis and detection of minimal residualleukemic disease.

In two c-ALL cases CD34$^+$ CD38$^-$ and CD34$^+$ CD38$^+$ progenitor cells were sorted and their clonal relationship with the malignant leukemic clone was analyzed. Both c-ALL cases had a Vδ2–Dδ3 rearrangement, and sequence information allowed the establishment of a leukemic clone-specific oligonucleotide probe. Hybridization of the CD34$^+$ CD38$^+$ cell with the clone-specific probe gave a positive signal in both c-ALL; the negative control population (CD3$^+$ mature lymphocytes) were negative. In one c-ALL the most immature compartment yielded a positive signal, while in the other case the CD34$^+$ CD38$^-$ population did not hybridize to the junctional region probe.

If these data hold true in a large number of patients, they will have a significant impact on our understanding of the biology and mechanisms of maligant transformation of ALL as well as in the area of novel treatment approaches in ALL. As new therapeutic approaches are being tested for the treatment of resistant disease, such as autologous stem cell transplantation, the discrimination of normal and leukemic progenitor cells is paramount. While progenitor cell compartments in AML and CML have been found to be clonally related to the malignant clone, no such data exist in ALL. Our data indicated that at least in some ALL cases the most immature "stem" cell compartment is clonally related to the malignant clone. Thus, new strategies to further dissect the stem cell compartment in order to discriminate normal and leukemic progenitor cells are needed. Furthermore, it may not suffice to monitor cells with a LAP derived from the bulk population at diagnosis, as is currently being done for the prediction of relapse [15]. Instead it may be necessary to study immature progenitor cells in remission marrows for the presence of cells carrying the leukemic clone-specific genetic marker.

The results in the second c-ALL, in which no hybridization signal was obtained in the most immature stem cell compartment, suggest that no leukemic cells were present within the CD34$^+$ CD38$^-$ stem cell subset above the detection level of the polymerase chain reaction.Thus it may be possible to discriminate normal from leukemic progenitor cells based on the expression of CD34 and CD38 differentiation antigens. This conclusion is correct only if malignant transformation occurs in a progenitor cell which has already rearranged its TCR δ locus. However, some data relative to clonal evolution indicate that TCR δ rearrangements may also occur as a posttransformational event [31–37]. If this is the case, a lymphohematopoietic progenitor may already have undergone malignant transformation but may have not yet rearranged its TCR δ gene. Alternatively, the bulk leukemic population, from which the TCR δ junctional region is derived, may carry a different TCR δ rearrangements than the leukemic stem cell. Therefore our studies need to be expanded to the analysis of progenitor subsets using genetic markers which are directly involved in a optimally single-step malignant transformation such as MLL-AF4 fusion genes in pre-pre-B-ALL or B-cell receptor ABL in c-ALL.

References

1. Borowitz MJ, Carroll AJ, Shuster JJ, Look AT, Behm FG, Pullen DJ, Land VJ, Steuber P, Crist WM (1993) Use of clinical and laboratory features to define prognostic subgroups in B-precursor acute lymphoblastic leukemia: experience of the Pediatric Oncology Group. In: Ludwig W-D, Theil E (eds) Recent results in cancer research.

Recent advances in cell biology of acute leukemia. Springer, Berlin Heidelberg New York, pp 257–267
2. Ludwig W-D, Harbott J, Bartram CR, Komischke B, Sperling C, Teichmann JV, Seibt-Jung H, Notter M, Odenwald E, Nehmer A, Thiel E, Riehm H (1993) Incidence and prognistic significance of immunophenotypic subgroups in chilodhood acute lymphoblastic leukemia: experience of the BFM Study 86. In: Ludwig W-D, Thiel E (eds) Recent results in cancer research. Recent advances in cell biology of acute leukemia. Springer, Berlin Heidelberg New York, pp 269–282
3. Civin I, Trischmann TM, Fackler MJ, Bernstein ID, Bühring H, Campos L, Greves MF, Kamoun M, Katz DR, Lansdorp PM, Look AT, Seed B, Sutherland DR, Tindle RW, Uchanska-Ziegler B (1990) Report on CD34 cluster workshop. In: Knapp W, Dörken B, Gilks WR, Rieber EP, Schmidt RE, Stein H, von dem Borne AEGK (eds) Leukocyte typing IV: white cell differentiation Antigens. Oxford University Press, Oxford, p 818
4. Terstappen LWMM, Loken MR (1990) Myeloid cell differentiation in normal bone marrow and acute myeloid leukemia assessed by multi-dimensional flow cytometry. Anal Cell Pathol 2: 229–240
5. Verfaillie CM, Miller JS (1994) $CD34^+$ $CD33^-$ cells reselected from macrophage inflammatory protein 1alpha+interleukin-3-supplemented "stroma non-contact" cultures are highly enriched for long-term bone marrow culture initiating cells. Blood 84: 1442–1449
6. Verfaillie CM, Catanzarro PM, Li WN (1994) Macrophage inflammatory protein 1 alpha, interleukin 3 and diffusible marrow stromal factors maintain human hematopoietic stem cells for at least eight weeks in vitro. J Exp Med 179: 643-649
7. Verfaillie CM, Miller WJ, Boylan K, McGlave PB (1992) Selection of benign primitive hematopoietic progenitors in chronic myelogenous leukemia on the basis of HLA-DR antigen expression. Blood 79: 1003–1010
8. Hurwitz CA, Loken MR, Graham ML, Karp JE, Borowitz MJ, Pullen DJ, Civin CI (1989) Aynchronous antigen expression in B lineage acute lymphoblastic leukemia. Blood 72: 299-307
9. Re GG, Estrov Z, Antoun GR, Felix EA, Pinkel DP Zipf TF (1991) Differentiation in B-precursor acute lymphoblastic leukemia cell populations with CD34 positive subpopulations. Blood 78: 575–580
10. Hurwitz CA, Gore SD, Stone KD, Civin CI (1992) Flow cytometric detection of rare normal human marrow cells with immunophenotypes characteritic of acute lymphoblastic leukemia cells. Leukemia 6: 233–239
11. Drexler HG, Thiel E, Ludwig W-D (1991) Review of the incidence and clinical relevance of myeloid antigen-positive acute lymphoblastic leukemia. Leukemia 5: 637–645
12. Pui CH, Behm FG, Crist WM (1993) Clinical and biologic relevance of immunologic marker studies in childhood acute lymphoblastic leukemia. Blood 82: 343–362
13. Janssen JWG, Ludwig W-D, Borkhardt A, Spadinger U, Rieder H, Fonatsch C, Hossfeld DK, Harbott J, Schulz AS, Repp R, Sykora KW, Hoelzer D, Bartram CR (1994) Pre-pre-B-acute lymphoblastic leukemia: high frequency of alternatively spliced ALL-1-AF-4 transcripts and absence of minimal residual disease during complete remission. Blood 84: 3835–3842
14. Griesinger F, Elfers H, Ludwig W-D, Falk M, Rieder H, Harbott J, Lampert F, Heinze B, Hoelzer D, Thiel E, Riehm H, Wörmann B, Fonatsch C, Hiddemann W (1994) Detection of HRX-FEL fusion transcripts in pre-pre-B-ALL with and without cytogenetic demonstration of t(4;11). Leukemia 8: 542–548
15. Orfao A, Ciudad J, Lopez-Berges MC, Lopez A, Vidriales B, Caballero MD, Valverde B, Gonzalez M, San Miguel JF (1994) Acute lymphoblastic leukemia (ALL) detection of minimal residual disease (MRD) at flow cytometry. Leuk Lymphoma 13: 87–90.
16. Greaves MF (1986) Differentiation-linked leukemogenesis in lymphoctes. Science, 234: 697–704.
17. Loken MR, Shah VO, Dattilio KL, Civin CI (1987). Flow cytometric analysis of human bone marrow II. Normal B lymphocyte development. Blood 70: 1316–1324.
18. Verfaillie CM, Miller W, Miller JS, Bhatia R, McGlave PB (1994) Benign primitive progenitors can be selected on the basis of the $CD34^+$ HLA^- DR^- phenotype in early chronic phase (ECP) but not advanced phase (AP) CML. Blood 84: 382a (abstract 1515)
19. Haase D, Feuring-Buske M, Könemann S, Troff C, Verbeek W, Hiddemann W, Wörmann B (1995) Evidence for malignant transformation in acute myeloid leukemia at the level of early hematopoietic stem cells by cytogenetic analysis of $CD34^+$ subpopulations. Blood 86; 2906–2912.
20. Feuring-Buske M, Haase D, Könemann S, Troff C, Grove D, Hiddemann W, Wörmann B (1995) Trisomy 4 in "stem cell like" leukemic cells of a patient with AML. Leukemia 9: 1918–1920.
21. Engel H, Drach J, Keyhani A, Jiang S, Sanchez-Williams G, Andreeff M (1994) Detection of high proliferative minimal residual disease in all patients with AML and MDS in complete remission with monosomy 7 by FACS/FISH. Blood 84: 300a (abstract 1185)
22. Lapidot T, Sirad C, Vormoor J, Murdoch B, Hoang T, Caceres-Cortes J, Minden M, Paterson B, Caligiuri MA, Dick JE (1994) A cell initiating human acute myeloid leukaemia after transplantation into SCID mouse. Nature 367: 645–648.
23. Turhan AG, Lemoine FM, Debert C, Bonnet ML, Baillou C, Picard F, Macintyre EA, Varet B (1995) Highly purified primitive hematopoietic stem cells are PML-RARA negative and generate nonclonal progenitors in acute promyelocytic leukemia. Blood 85: 2154–2161.
24. Wörmann B, Grove D, Terstappen LWMM (1994) Mlutiparametrische Charaktersierung von Leukämie-und Lymphomzellen. In: Schmitz G, Rothe

G, Durchflußzytometrie in der klinischen Zelldiagnostik. Schattauer, Stuttgart, pp. 105–115.
25. Griesinger F, Grümayer ER, Van Ness B, Kersey JH (1992) Rearrangement and diversification of T-cell receptor delta genes in acute lymphoblastic leukemia. Leukemia 6: 1054–1062.
26. Griesinger F, Elfers H, Ludwig W-D, Flak M, Rieder H, Harbott J, Lampert F, Heinze B, Hoelzer D, Thiel E, Riehm H, Wörmann B, Fonatsch C, Hiddemann W (1994) Detection of HRX-FEL fusion transcripts in pre-pre-B-ALL with and without cytogenetic demonstration of t(4; 11). Leukemia 8: 542–548.
27. Biondi A, Yokota S, Hansen Hagge TE, Rossi V, Fiudici G, Maglia O, Basso G, Tell C, Masera G, Bartram CR (1992) Minimal residual disease in childhood acute lymphoblastic leukemia: analysis of patients in continuous completeremission or with consecutive relapse. Leukemia 6: 282–288
28. van Dongen JJM, Breit TM, Adriaansen, HJ, Beishuiyen A, Hooijkaas H (1992) Detection of minimal residual disease in acute leukemia by immunological marker analysis and polymerase chain reaction. Leukemia 6: 47–59
29. Yokota S, Hansen-Hagge RE, Ludwig W-D. Reiter A, Raghavachar A, Kleihauer E, Bartram CR. (1991) Use of polymerase chain reactions to monitor minimal residual disease in acute lymphoblastic leukemia patients. Blood 77: 331–339
30. Griesinger F, Greenberg JM, Kersey JH (1989) T-cell receptor gamma and delta rearrangements in hematological malignancies: relationship to lymphoid differentiation. J. Clin. Invest. 84: 506–516
31. Beishuizen A, Hahlen K, Hagemeijer A, Verhoeven MA, Hooijkaas H, Adriaansen HJ, Wovers-Tettero IL, van Wering ER, van Dongen JJM (1991) Multiple rearranged immunoglobulin genes in childhood acute lymphobastic leukemia of precursor B-cell origin. Leukemia 5: 657–667
32. Tycko B, Ritz J, Sallan S, Sklar J (1992) Changing antigen receptor gene rearrangements in a case of early pre-B cell implications for monitoring residual disease. Blood 79: 418–488
33. Beishuizen A, Verhoeven M-AJ, van Wering ER, Hählen K, Hooijkaas H, van Dongen JJM (1994) Analysis of immunoglobulin and T-cell receptor genes in 40 childhood acute lymphoblastic leukemias at diagnosis and subsequent relapse: implications for the detection of minimal residual disease by polymerase chain reaction analysis. Blood 83: 2238–2247
34. Wörmann B, Anderson JM, Liberty JA, Gajl-Peczalzka K, Brunning RD, Silberman TL, Arthur DC, LeBien TW (1989) Establishment of a leukemic cell model for studying human pre-B to B cell differentiation, J. Immunol 142: 110–117
35. Hansen-Hagge TE, Yokota S, Teuter HJ, Schwarz K, Bartram CR (1992) Human common acute lymphoblastic leukemia-derived cell lines are competent to recombine their T-cell receptor delta/alpha regions along a hierarchically ordered pathway. Blood 80: 2353–2362
36. Gill-Super HJ, Rothberg PG, Kobayashi H, Freeman AI, Diaz MO, Rowley JD (1994) Clonal, nonconstitutional rearrangements of the MLL gene in infant twins with acute lymphoblastic leukemia: in utero chromosome rearrangement of 11q23. Blood 83: 641–644
37. Griesinger F, Janeszek H, Breukelmann D, Englert M, Humpe A, Büchner T, Hiddemann W, Wörmann B (1993) High incidence of RAG-1 and RAG-2 transcripts in ALL and ANLL. Correlation to cross-lineage TCR and IgH rearrangements. Blood 82: 525a, (abstract 2084)

Acute Leukemias VI
Prognostic Factors
and Treatment Strategies
Büchner et al. (eds)

Monitoring Leukemic Cells During the Course of Acute Leukemia by Immunophenotyping and Genotyping

K. Pachmann[1], U. Goehly[1], J.U. Walther[2], and B. Emmerich[1]

Abstract. Leukemic blasts and cells carrying the bcr/abl translocation were monitored in the bone marrow of a patient with acute leukemia during the course of disease by immunophenotyping, Southern blot analysis and in situ amplification of the bcr/abl translocation. The blasts initially had a cALLa positive, CD19 positive phenotype and the Philadelphia chromosome was detected at diagnosis. From the initial bone marrow aspirate there was not sufficient material for Southern blot analysis, but the bcr/abl translocation could be verified by the polymerase chain reaction. In situ amplification of the bcr/abl mRNA showed that not all cells identified as blasts were positive, but, in contrast, some cells with lymphoid morphology were labeled. After phase I of the induction therapy no translocation was seen in Southern blot analysis, complete remission was diagnosed morphologically, but cALLA positive cells were still detectable and an increased fraction of cells expressed HLA-DR and CD19. After the beginning of the consolidation therapy Southern blot analysis showed a rearranged band and labeled cells were frequent on in situ amplification. Morphologically blasts were detected and expressed cALL antigen but Southern blot analysis of this and the subsequent aspirations was consistenly negative even with increasing numbers of blasts. In accordance with the negative results of the Southern blot analysis the cells with amplifiable bcr/abl mRNA remained rare Moreover, the blasts growing aggressively after therapeutic intervention were obviously those negative for the translocation, as Southern blot analysis and in situ amplification suggest. Thus in this leukemia, although it was positive for the bcr/abl translocation, already the bcr/abl was either not expressed in all leukemic blasts or was not present in all cells of the malignant clone as shown by in situ amplification, although expressing the cALL antigen.

Therefore, even if the polymerase chain reaction for a genetic marker such as the bcr/abl translocation remains positive during the course of disease, it is not necessarily a consistent feature of all tumor cells and, above all, may not be selected against by therapy.

Introduction

Immunophenotyping is a valuable tool complementary to morphology and cytochemistry for unequivocal classification of most acute leukemias [1] based on the surface antigen pattern of the leukemic cells [2] However,until now no antigen or antigen combinations unique for leukemic cells have been observed. All of the antigens used for classification of leukemias appear during normal maturation, too [3, 4]. Therefore it is difficult to distinguish leukemic blasts from regenerating hematopoesis during remission or early during relapse.

Genetic aberrations, in contrast, are rarely found in normal cells [5], but are frequently detected in leukemias and are assumed to contribute the initial step in leukemogenesis [6, 7]. During clonal growth such genetic aberrations are transferred from the transformed cell to the

[1]Medizinishe Klinik and [2]Kinderpoliklinik, Klinikum Innenstadt der Ludwig Maximilians-Universität München, Munich, Germany

daughter cells and can serve as markers for cells belonging to the malignant clone. There exist different methods to detect clonal aberrations, such as cytogenetics [8] or restriction fragment length analysis using Southern blotting, which requires prior isolation of the DNA in sufficient amounts from the cells [9]. If the respective adjacent gene sequences are known, polymerase chain amplification can be used to detect aberrant genes even if they are present only in minute amounts [10]. All of these methods supply only equivocal information about the number of cells belonging to the clone, despite some attempts to develop semiquantitative PCR [11], and yield no information at all about the morphology of the cells. Amplification of gene sequences directly in individual cells [12] and subsequent relocalization allows one to determine the nature of the cells concerned and might help to estimate the amount of remnant clonal cells after therapy. In the present report, the immunophenotype of the lymphoid cells from the bone marrow was monitored during the course of disease of an acute lymphoblastic Philadelphia chromosome positive leukemia, and bone marrow smears prepared at different times during therapy [13] were analyzed for blasts and cells expressing the hybrid bcr/abl mRNA by morphological analysis as well as by immunophenotyping and in situ amplification in order to identify and estimate the amount of clonal cells. Comparison of the results obtained shows the advantages but also the limitations of these methods.

Patient and Methods

The patient was a 52 year old woman who presented in May 1992 with peripheral leukopenia. The bone marrow aspirate showed an infiltration with immature blasts which amounted to 50% of the nucleated cells. The blasts were negative for the peroxidase and the esterase reaction, and only very few blasts showed fine granular staining for PAS. Cytogenetic analysis showed a Philadelphia chromosome. The patient was treated according to the BMFT protocol for adults [13].

Cells from bone marrow aspirates obtained at the indicated times during therapy were analyzed for their surface antigen pattern of the antigens CD7, CD3, CD10 (cALLA), CD19, CD20 and HLA-DR, CD13, CD33, CD34 (all antibodies from Immunotech, Dianova, Hamburg). For this purpose 100 µl of heparinized whole blood or bone marrow aspirate was mixed with 10 ml of directly fluorochrome-labeled antiserum and incubated for a least 10 min. Subsequently the cells were treated according to the Coulter Q-prep method (Coulter, Dreieich), which includes addition of a lysis buffer, a stabilizer and a fixing agent. As a control the cells were incubated with a control serum of the same isotype. The cells were then analyzed by means of flow cytometry 2–24 h later in an Epics Profile (Coulter). Whole blood analysis allowed estimation of the proportion of all cell types present by their forward and side scatter properties, but only the cells of the lymphoid population were analyzed for surface antigen pattern. Positivity was defined as fluorescence intensity exceeding the 99% threshold of the population stained with the control serum.

In situ amplification was performed as described earlier [12]. In short, small pieces were cut from slides carrying the smears in question to fit into conventional PCR vials. Reverse transcription was performed as described in the CML Primer Set (Oncogene Science, Dianova, Hamburg) [14], in a fourfold volume using cell bound RNA as template with no additional RNA added. The pieces of slides were then removed from the first reaction mixture, washed once with 1 × SSC and subsequently added to a fourfold volume of the first amplification reaction. Then the cell bound cDNA was used as a template and one nucleotide was added as ^{3}H dNTP (Amersham). After amplification the pieces of slides were removed, washed in 0.1 × SSC, reattached to their original position on the slide, covered with nuclear track emulsion (NTB), exposed for 24–72 h in the dark and developed. The second amplification was performed from 4 µl of the supernatant from the first amplification and the amplification product examined on an ethidium bromide stained gel. Relocalization was performed as described [15]. For Southern blot analysis DNA was extracted from 2 ml of bone marrow aspirate according to standard methods and digested with the following enzymes: *Bam*HI, *Bgl*II and *Hind*III. DNA was electrophoresed, transferred to a blotting membrane and hybridized with a probe complementary to the abl gene (Oncogene Science, Dianova, Hamburg).

Results

Analysis of the cells from the bone marrow aspiration drawn for initial diagnosis showed an increased proportion of cells of blastoid appearance. Some 50% of the cells in the lymphoid gate showed reactivity with monoclonal antibodies against CD10, CD19 and HLA DR, whereas only 30% were reactive with anti-CD7 and anti-CD3, indicating that the normal lymphocytes had to a significant extent been replaced by cALLA positive blasts (Fig. 1). Cytogenetic analysis revealed a Philadelphia chromosome. The 9; 22 translocation in fact affected the abl gene as verified by Southern blot analysis where a rearranged band was detected and by the polymerase chain reaction (Fig.2–4).

In situ amplification of the bcr/abl RNA directly on the diagnostic bone marrow smear showed labeled cells mingled with unlabeled cells (Fig. 4a, b). When morphologically defined cells (Fig. 4a) were relocalized after the amplification step it could be demonstrated, that not all cells, morphologically appearing as blasts, were labeled (see arrows in Fig. 4), and cells considered as normal lymphocytes were labeled too.

Cells from bone marow aspirations obtained at the indicated times during therapy were analyzed for their immunophenotype (Fig. 1). After the onset of the induction therapy, a rapid decrease of cALLA positive cells and a more delayed decrease in HLA DR and CD19 positive cells was observed, accompanied by an increase in CD7 and CD3 positive cells. There was a transitory slight increase in cALLA positive cells, with simultaneously some blasts appearing in bone marow following the consolidation therapy. CD3 positive cells, however, continued to fall below the normal range. Before reinduction the cALLA positive cells reappeared, accompanied by an even more pronounced increase in HLA DR and CD19 positive cells. Reinduction therapy again reduced the cALLA positive as well as the blast cells but was not capable of completely eliminating them. T-cells once again recovered.

Subsequently, however, a sharp rise in cells carying the tumor associated antigens was observed, accompanied by an increase in bone marrow blasts and a disappearance of mature T-cells. Now also blast cells were observed in the periphery, leading rapidly to leukocytosis. The ALL recurrence protocol once again reduced the blast population, but again remnant blasts were detected on morphological analysis as well as by immunophenotyping. The AML recurrence protocol again was able to reduce the peripheral blasts, but bone marrow status was no longer monitored and the patient died on day 403 after diagnosis.

In situ amplification of the bcr/abl translocation in cells from smears of bone marrow with cytologically diagnosed complete remission (day 46 and day 203) still detected unequivocally labeled cells. On day 46 such cells were preferentially detected captured in the filamentous material (Fig. 5a, b). At relapse (day 245), although only 20% of the cells were identified as blasts, labeled cells densely infiltrated the bone marrow smears (Fig. 5c). However, on day 340, when most of the bone marrow cells were blasts, bcr/abl mRNA could be demonstrated only in a very restricted population of cells (Fig. 5d). Southern blot analysis was positive only at one instance and remained negative later during relapse, even with increasing numbers of blasts, indicating that these cells were negative for the rearrangement, whereas the polymerase chain reaction remained positive at all instances.

Discussion

Although immunophenotyping has now a firm place in the initial diagnosis of leukemia [16] it is difficult to discriminate regenerating hematopoesis from reappearing blasts by this method [17] since classification of the leukemic cells is performed according to antigenic markers also normally occurring on immature cells. Moreover, the sensitivity of the method is not much above the sensitivity of conventional bone marrow cytology.

Longitudinal immunologic observation of the subpopulations may contribute additional information. In the present case we have monitored an acute lymphatic leukemia, which at diagnosis presented with only 50% blasts in the bone marrow and peripheral leukopenia during the course of disease by immunophenotyping bone marrow cells at every occasion of bone marrow aspiration. The percentage of cALLA positive cells correlated well with the percentage of blasts detected morphologically. The concomitant decrease in cALLA positive, CD19 positive and HLADR positive cells in response to therapy indicated that all three markers were expressed on the malignant clone. Obviously normal T-

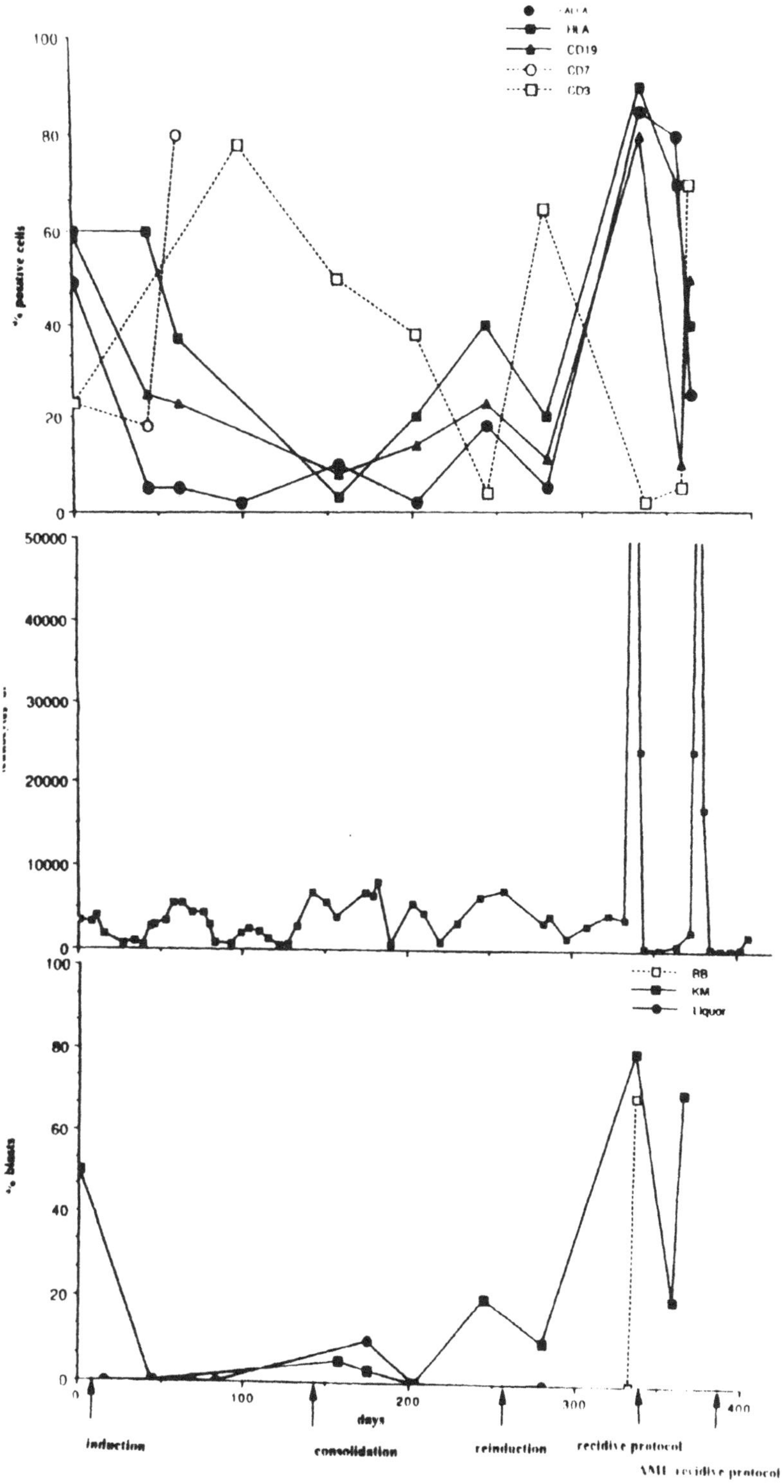

Fig. 1. Immunphenotype, peripheral leukocyte count and percentage of blasts in bone marrow during the course of disease

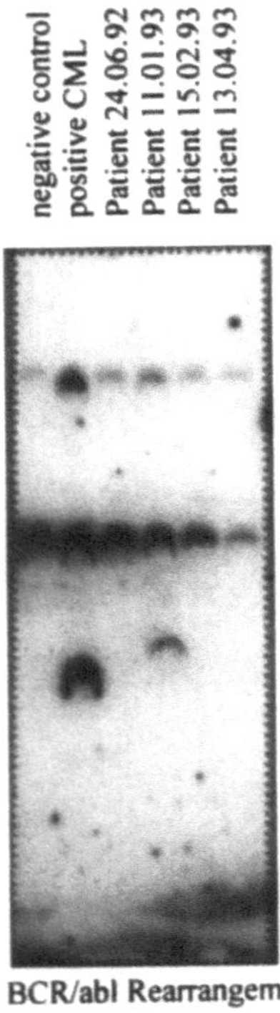

Fig. 2. Southern blot analysis of the bcr/all translocation of the bone marrow cells at diagnosis. Lane 1 negative control; lane 2, CML; lanes 3–6, patient's cells from the indicated times

Fig. 3. Amplification of the bcr/abl RNA from cells of a bone marrow smear at the time of diagnosis and at different times during the course of disease

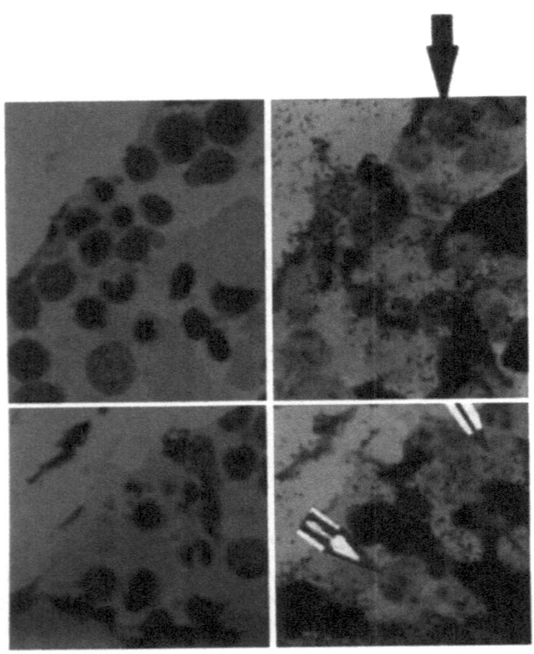

a b

Fig. 4. a Panoptically stained area and **b** relocalization of the same area after in situ amplification of the bcr/abl RNA in the cells, filled arrows, labeled blasts; empty arrow, unlabeled blasts; thin arrows, labeled lymphocytes

cells increased in response to therapy. Subsequently the proportion of T-cells in the lymphoid population in the bone marrow dropped again below normal values, accompanied by the reappearance of a small percentage of blasts and of cALLA positive cells. This transient appearance of cALLA positive cells by itself would not have been proof of relapse of the ALL by itself, since such phenomena have been observed during chemotherapy of other diseases too. Retrospectively, however, the combined immunophenotype may be interpreted as indicative of disease relapse even if the marker pattern was equivocal at that time.

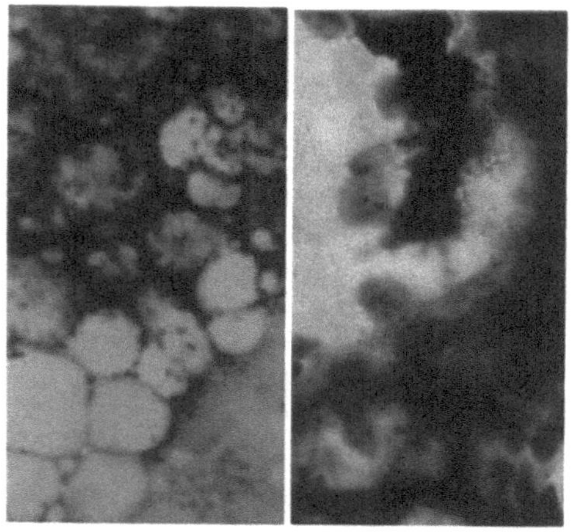

a

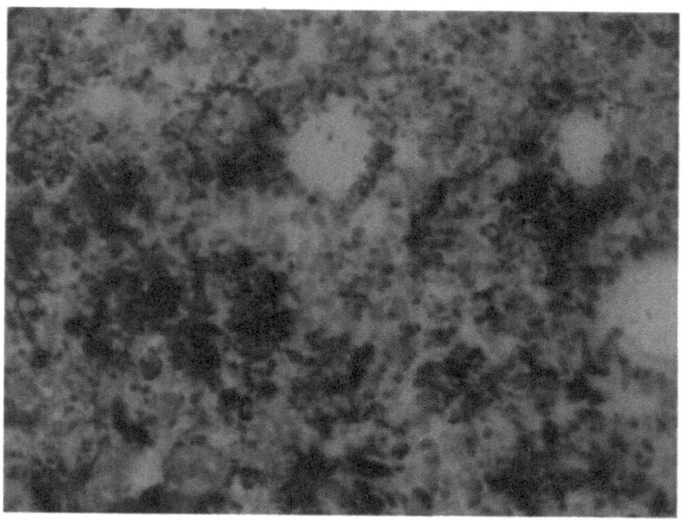

b

Fig. 5. Labeled cells after in situ amplification in bone marrow smears in remission (**a**) and on day 46, (**b**) day 203 (**c**) day 245

In contrast to immunological markers, genetic aberrations may be regarded as clonal markers, allowing one to distinguish the clonally expanded cells from all other "germline" cells. Thus the bcr/abl translocation, observed in about 60% of cALLA positive lymphatic leukemias of adults [18–19], was used in the present case as a marker of clonal cells in such a leukemia. We could show by Southern blot analysis that the abl gene was rearranged. The hybrid RNA as a result of the translocation could be detected in individual cells of the leukemia directly on the slides using reverse transcription and subsequent incorporation of radioactive nucleotides during amplification. Relocalization of the labeled cells and comparison with morphology, however, revealed that not all, and not only, cells diagnosed as blasts were labeled. Since in the present case the hybrid RNA is traced, the negativity of some blasts may be due to the fact that these cells do not transcribe the RNA although they do carry the translocation. On the other hand, cells with lymphoid appearance were labeled, too. This may indicate that cells of the leukemic clone still have limited maturational capacity.

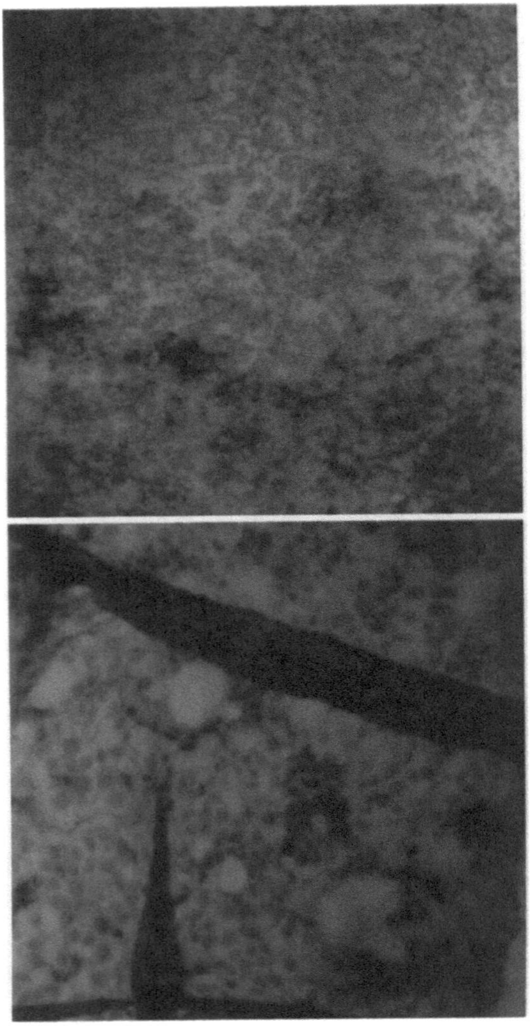

Fig. 5c

Monitoring of the proportion of cells carrying the translocation at different times revealed labeled cells even at points, when no leukemic cells were detectable either morphologically or by immunophenotyping. Thus this method can help to detect minimal amounts of leukemic cells. Cells which are labeled can be unequivocally assigned to the leukemic clone, even if they are morphologically in different stages of maturation. However, if the cells are not labeled, this does not preclude them from belonging to the clone, since with the bcr/abl translocation the detection is dependent on the transcriptional activity of the cells. During the final acceleration of the disease the reduced detection of labeled cells may on one hand have been due to a reduced transcriptional activity, or else, as Southern blot analysis suggests, a clone may have evolved lacking the translocation but with a very high proliferative activity. Thus we have shown that in situ amplification allows detection of cells with defined gene aberrations directly in bone marrow smears and to enumerate them. This method, in addition, is able to identify remnant cells, belonging to the malignant clone, even if they are no longer detectable by other methods. Conventional PCR is prone to false positive results due to contamination with external DNA, but this can be excluded in situ amplification because only cell related labeling is considered.

The significance of such minimal tumor load with respect to outcome has to be determined. This may depend not only on the amount of cells left after therapy but also on the proliferative capacity of remnant tumor cells. Thus, more immature cells may be more likely to regrow and produce a relapse. Further analysis of the proliferative potential of such remnant cells will be required.

Acknowledgment. This work was supported by Deutsche Forschungsgemeinschaft grant Pa 205/3-6.

References

1. Campana D, Coustain-Smith E, Janossy G. Immunphenotyping in hematological diagnosis. In: Cavill (ed) Advancing hematological techniques. Bailliere's clinical haematology (1990) Vol 3 number 4 Bailiere Tindall, London Philadelphia Sydney p889
2. Greaves MF. Differentiation linked leukemogenesis in lymphocytes. Science 1986; 234: 697
3. Self SE, Morgan S, Grush O. Significance of common acute lymphoblastic leukemia antigen (cALLA) positive cells in bone marrow of children off therapy in complete remission. Hematol Oncol 1990; 8: 91
4. Terstappen LWMM, Safford M, Könemann, S, Loken MR, Zurlutter K, Büchner T, Hiddemann W, Wörmann B Flow cytometric characterization of acute myeloid leukemia. PartII. Phenotypic heterogeneity at diagnosis. Leukemia 1991; 5: 757
5. Limpens J, de Jong D, van Krieken JHJM, Price CGA, Young BD, van Ommen G-JB, Kluin PM. Bcl2/JH rearrangements in benign lymphoid tissues with follicular hyperplasia. Oncogene 1991; 6: 2271
6. Fish P, Boehm T, Lavenir I, Larson T, Arno J, Foster A, Rabbitts TH. T-cell acute lymphoblastic lymphoma induced in trasngenic mice by the RTBNI and the RTBN2 LIM domain genes. Oncogene 1992; 7: 2389
7. Lewin B. Oncogene conversion by regulatory changes in transcription factors. Cell 1991; 64: 303
8. Arthur CK, Apperly JF, Guo AP, Rasool F, Gao LM, Goldman JH. Blood 1988; 71: 1179
9. Yunis JJ, Mayer MG, Arnesen MA, Aepply DP, Oken MM, Frizzera G. bcl-2 and other genomic alterationc in the prognosis of large cell lymphoma. N Engl J Med 1989; 320: 1047
10. Lee M, Chang K, Freireich EJ. Detection of minimal residual bcr/abl transcripts by a modified polymerase cchain reaction Blood 1988; 71: 893
11. Henn T, Gaiger A, Lion T. Frühzeitige Rezidiverkennung bei Patienten mit CML nach Knochenmarkstransplantation mittels quantitativer Polymerase Ketternreaktion. 5. Tumozytogenetische Arbeitstagung Wien 1992
12. Spann W, Pachmann K, Zabnienska H, Pielmeier A, Emmerich B. In situ amplification of single copy gene segments in individual cells by the polymerase chain reaction. Infection 1991; 19: 242
13. Hoelzer D, Gale RP. Acute lymphoblastic leukemia in adults: recent progress, further directions. Semin Hematol 1987;24:27
14. Blennerhasset GT, Furth ME, Anderson A, Burns JP, Changati RSK, Blick M, Talpaz M, Dev VG, Chan LC, Wiedemann LM, Greaves MF, Hagemeijer A, van der Plas D, Skuse G, Wang N, Stam K. Clinical evaluation of a DNA probe assay for the Philadelphia (Phl) translocation in chronic myelogenous leukemia. Leukemia 1988;2: 648
15. Pachmann K, Span W, Zabnienska H, Knizia M, Emmerich B. In situ Amplification of rearranged Gene sequences in individual cells for tracing clonal cells in smears from blood and bone marrow, In:Büchner et al (eds) Acute Leukemias IV Prognostic Factors Springer Verlag Berlin Heidelberg 1993; 501
16. Ludwig WD, Tiel E. Diagnostik der akuten Leukämien mit morphologischen, immunologischen und zytogenetischen Verfahren. Internist 1993; 34: 498
17. van Dongen JJM, Breit TM, Adriaansen HJ, Beihuisen A, Hooijkaas H. Detection of minimal residual disease in acute leukemia by immunological markers and polymerase chain reaction. Leukemia 1993; 6 (Suppl 1): 47
18. Maurer J, Janssen JWG, Thiel E, van Denderen J, Ludwig WD, Aydemir Ü, Heinze B, Fonatsch C, Harbott J, Reiter A, Riehm H, Hoelzer D, Bartram CR. Lancet 1991; 337: 1055
19. Götz G, Weh HJ, Walter TA, Kruse R, Kolbe K, Dölken G, Hellriegel KP, Hoelzer D, Hellriegel DK. Clinical and prognostic significance of the Philadelphia chromosome in adults with acute lymphoblastic leukemia. Ann Hematol 1992; 64: 67

Acute Leukemias VI
Prognostic Factors
and Treatment Strategies
Büchner et al. (eds)

Flowcytometric Detection of Aneuploidies in Acute Lymphoblastic Leukemia (ALL) Before and After Chemotherapy

U. Oelschlägel[1], R. Nowak[1], R. Hofmann[1], H. Zengler[1], R. Siegert[2], and G. Ehninger[1]

Abstract. We performed flowcytometric determination of DNA content in immunophenotyped ALL cells. With this method one can increase the certainty of detecting aneuploidies compared with the commonly used one-parameter DNA analysis. We had found aneuploidies in 37% (9 of 24) of ALL patients. The proposed method can be used for detecting residual aneuploid leukemia cells after chemotherapy. Therefore we carried out experiments in which we mixed diploid bone marrow cells with the leukemic aneuploid cells for evaluating the sensitivity of our method. The results show that the sensitivity of the described flowcytometric method is much higher than those of the microscopical evaluation to look for residual leukemic cells. Important factors which influence the aneuploidy detection are the DNA index of the aneuploid population and the coefficient of variation of the G0/G1 peak of the cells. It should be further investigated whether this method can be used in monitoring patients with aneuploid leukemia cells.

Introduction

There are several methods of detecting minimal residual disease, for example flowcytometric detection of aberrant antigen expression, PCR, T-cell receptor rearrangement, and in situ hybridization [1].

We take advantage of another characteristic of malignant disorders. A high percentage (ca. 30–40%) of acute lymphoblastic leukemia (ALL) patients show deviations from normal DNA content, so called aneuploidies. Especially in childhood, B-progenitor ALL patients with a DNA index greater than 1.16 have an excellent treatment outcome [2].

We performed flowcytometric determination of DNA content in immunophenotyped ALL cells with one-laser flowcytometer. With this two-parameter analysis it is possible to increase the certainty of aneuploidy detection because of differentiation between the DNA content of malignant cells and residual normal hematopoiesis.

The proposed method can be used for detecting residual aneuploid leukemia cells after chemotherapy [3]. We had found aneuploidies in 37% (9/24) of ALL patients at diagnosis and made follow-up investigations of seven patients.

Therefore we carried out experiments in which we mixed diploid bone marrow cells with leukemic aneuploid cells for evaluation of the sensitivity of our method. We obtained the diploid cells from leukemia patients in remission to simulate conditions in remission, i.e. regenerating bone marrow with the presence of a high proportion of cells in DNA synthesizing phase.

Material and Methods

Cell Separation Procedures

Bone marrow or peripheral blood cells were obtained at diagnosis or for evaluation of remis-

[1]Medical Clinic of Technical University Dresden, Dept. of Hematology, Dresden, Germany.
[2]Clinic of Pediatrics, Fetscherstr. 74, 01307 Dresden, Germany

sion after chemotherapy. Bone marrow cells were aspirated in a syringe with 1/ml PBS (Seromed) and 100 U/ml heparin (Seromed).

Cell suspensions were overlaid on a density gradient (1.077 g/ml: Nycomed) and centrifugated at 300 g; 30 min at 20°C. Thereafter mononuclear cells (MNC) were washed twice with PBS, resuspended and counted. For dilution assays MNC were stored in portions (1×10^7 cells) at −80°C.

Immunophenotyping

We performed an indirect immunofluorescence method. Cells were incubated with saturating concentrations of unconjugated monoclonal antibodies for 30 min at 4°C (for example anti CD3; anti CD19; anti CD10-DAKO; anti CD34-Becton Dickinson). Thereafter the cells were washed in PBS, incubated with goat-anti-mouse IgG F(ab)2 fragment (GAM-FITC; Coulter) for 10 min and washed twice in PBS. As a nonspecific fluorescence control, cells were incubated with an isotope specific monoclonal antibody and afterwards with GAM-FITC, as previously described.

Preparation of Cells for Cell Cycle Analysis

Cells were prepared as described by Nowak and Hietschald [4]. Briefly, after immunophenotyping cells were thoroughly resuspended and cold ethanol (−20°C) was added. The specimens were stored overnight at 4°C. After washing and resuspension in PBS the cells were incubated with RNAse (1.25 mg/ml; Sigma) at room temperature and after that in propidium iodide (50 µg/ml; Sigma).

Flowcytometric Two-Parameter Analysis

Cell samples were measured on a FACS can flow cytometer with serial filter configuration. Electronic compensation was used between the FITC and propidium iodide fluorescence channels to correct spectral overlay. Doublet discrimination mode was available to exclude cell doublets.

Dilution Assays for Testing the Sensitivity of Two-Parameter Analysis

Mononuclear cells from patients with an initial detected aneuploidy were mixed diploid cells of patients in complete remission after chemotherapy for determining the sensitivity of our DNA-quantification method. We dilute the original aneuploid cells so as to obtain the following concentrations: ca. 1%; 0.5%; 0.1%; 0.05% aneuploid cells. As many cells as possible were analyzed on the flow cytometer (max. 50 000 MNC).

Results

With the method of flowcytometric DNA analysis in immunophenotyped cells we detected aneuploidies in 9 of 24 ALL patients initially. In 7 of these patients we made one or more follow-up investigations, five of them reached a morphological complete remission, but we could detect aneuploid cells in the range between 0.01% and 1.08%. Data of a patient with pre-B-Cell ALL are shown in Fig. 1. One can see that the 0.59% aneuploid cells after chemotherapy were only detectable after additional immunophenotyping, just as in the other investigations after chemotherapy.

Moreover, we carried out dilution assays to investigate the sensitivity of the two-parameter DNA analysis. The aneuploid cells were mixed with diploid cells from leukemia patients in remission. In Table 1 is shown that we could determine amounts of less than 0.1% of aneuploid cells within the diploid MNC. One example of such an dilution experiment with aneuploid cells of a patient with common ALL is displayed in Fig. 2. The added bone marrow cells belonged to a patient with AML-M2 in complete remission who had no aneuploid cells. The minimal detected amount of aneuploid cells was in this case 0.06% of all MNC.

Discussion

We propose detection of DNA content in immunophenotyped cells for investigation of malignant lymphatic disorders.

There are some advantages in registration of aneuploidies compared with one-paramter analysis. At diagnosis of ALL we are able to look for residual normal cells to ascertain the G0/G1-peak of the diploid populaiton. In B-cell malignancies, the T-cells represent this internal standard [5], and vice versa.

Also, the detection of residual aneuploid cells after chemotherapy is only possible with addi-

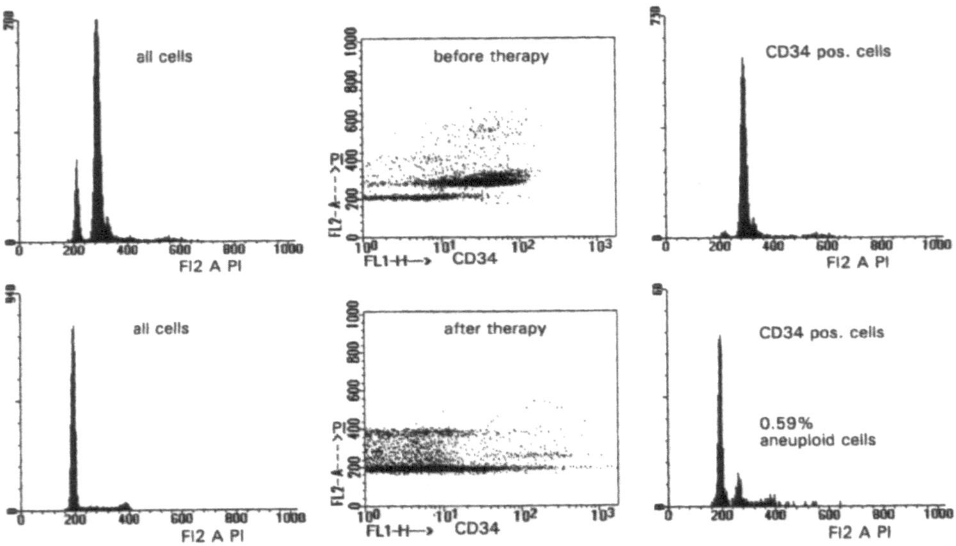

Fig. 1. Immunophenotyping and DNA content of an pre-B-cell ALL before therapy (top) and after therapy (bottom). Left histograms show, DNA content of all cells, right histograms of immunophenotyped cells. The dot plots in the middle demonstrate immunophenotyping on the *x*-axis and DNA content on the *y*-axis

Table 1. Dilution assays: percentage of aneuploid cells in original bone marow and minimal detected aneuploid cells after dilution with remission bone marrow, and DNA index

Test no.	Percentage of aneuploid cells Original bone marrow	Mixed bone marrow (minimal detected cells)	DNA index
1	5.03	0.06	1.50
2	73.80	0.19	1.36
3	96.10	0.06	1.18
4	95.80	0.03	1.18
5	96.30	0.06	1.18
6	82.60	0.10	1.37
7	95.60	0.10	1.18
8	82.60	0.03	1.37
9	85.05	0.07	1.18
10	85.05	0.04	1.18

tional immunophenotyping. If there only one-parameter analysis would not were carried out it is possible that the G0/G1 peak of a small aneuploid population be recognizable in the high S-phase of regenerating bone marrow. In our experiments the proportion of normal cells in S-phase was 3.9%–14.8%. Moreover, the DNA index plays an important role. If the deviation from normal DNA content refers only to one chromosome, the G0/G1 peak of these aneuploid cells could escape detection in view of the G0/G1 peak of the diploid cells. With additional immunophenotyping we could mostly differentiate between diploid and aneuploid populations. An important point for good measurement quality is the setting of optimal compensation between the two overlappping fluorescences to reach small coefficients of variation in G0/G1 peak.

In future, we have to investigate what role the 50–100 times higher sensitivity of detection of residual leukemic cells plays in remission as-

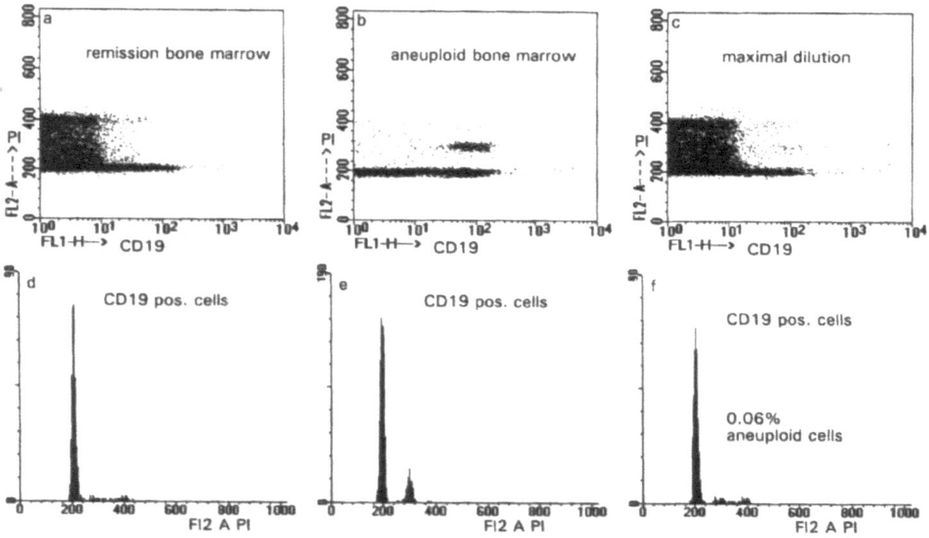

Fig. 2. Dilution experiment: aneuploid cALL bone marrow (**b, e**); diploid AML bone marrow in remission (**a, d**); results of maximal dilution (**c, f**). Top line, dot plots with immunophenotyping on *x*-axis and DNA-content on *y*-axis, bottom line, DNA histograms belonging to the dot plots

sessment, compared with the morpholoical 5% blasts limit for complete remission. Moreover, the determination of residual aneuploid cells after chemotherapy could possibly clarify whether the morphological registered blasts are leukemic or normal blasts which occur in regenerating phase after chemotherapy with other methods like PCR, in situ hybridization and T-cell receptor rearrangement, the described method could contribute, in particular, to the monitoring of aneuploid ALL concerning minimal residual disease.

References

1. Wörmann B. (1993) Implications of detection of minimal residual disease; Current opinion in oncology 5, 3–12
2. Truthworthy R., Shuster J., Look T., Crist W., Borowitz M., Caroll A., Frankel L., Harris M., Wagner H., Haggard M., Mosijczuk A., Pullen J., Steube P. and Land V. (1993) Ploidy of lymphoblasts is the strongest predictor of treatment outcome in B-progenitor cell acute lymphoblastic leukemia of childhood: a pediatric oncology group study; J. clin. Oncology 10, 606
3. Nowak R., Oelschlägel U., Hofmann R., Zengler H. and Huhn R. (1994) Detection of aneuploid cells in acute lymphoblastic leukemia with flow cytometry before and after chemotherapy (Concise report) Leuk. res. 18, 897
4. Nowak R., Hietschold V., (1991) Simultaneous analysis of cell membrane antigens and DNA-content in bone marrow cells-potential meaning for hematology Z. klin. Med. 46, 435
5. Jensen, I. M., Ellegaard, J. et al (1993) Differences in relative DNA-content between human peripheral blood and bone marrow subpopulations-consequences for DNA index calculations Cytometry 14, 936

Acute Leukemias VI
Prognostic Factors
and Treatment Strategies
Büchner et al. (eds)

Comparison of Growth Patterns of Acute Myeloid Leukemia Cells In Vitro and In Vivo by Flow Cytometry

R. Nowak, U. Oelschägel, R. Hofmann, M. Palitzsch, H. Zengler, and G. Ehninger

Abstract. Cells from patients with acute myeloid leukemia were analyzed by flow cytometric detection of PI staining for evaluation of proliferative activity. The distribution in cell cycle was measured immediately after bone marrow aspiration (as in vivo S-phase) and after 72 h cultivation without and with interleukin 3 (IL 3). As expected, in most cases (20/38) proliferation of blasts was stimulated with IL 3. But in four leukemias an increase was observed in control culture compared with in vivo S-phase. Interestingly, most cases of FAB M4 and M5 (9/13) were not sensitive to IL 3, but inversely most cases of FAB M1 and M2 showed a proliferation induction with IL 3 (13/18).

Introduction

Since the first cloning of complementary DNA for cytokines, these mediators have been subjects of clinical investigation. One approach is the acceleration of hematological reconstitution after chemotherapy in malignant disorders [1]. Another intention is to find out the influence of cytokines on chemotherapy results [2]. The proliferative activity of myeloid leukemia cells has been primed with G-CSF or IL 3, accompanied by increase of chemotherapy sensitivity. Recently there have been indications of cytokine influence in proneness of leukemia cells to apoptosis.

The acute myeloid leukemias are heterogeneous in cytomorphological and cytochemical characteristics. Whereas the immunologically defined subtypes of acute lymphatic leukemia have different therapeutic consequences, these cannot be derived from FAB classification or immunophenotyping in acute myeloid leukemia, apart from some entities, like promyelocytic leukemia.

In this contribution results from investigation of growth patterns of cells from acute myeloid leukemia with the nonexpensive flow cytometric DNA quantification are presented. The cell cycle phase analysis was done immediately after diagnostic bone marrow aspiration and in short term liquid culture for evaluation of interleukin 3 dependence of leukemia cells.

Material and Methods

Cell Separation Procedures

Patients with newly diagnosed acute myeloid leukemia were investigated. Bone marrow cells were obtained from the posterior iliacla crest. Mononuclear cells were yielded after density gradient separation (Ficoll gradient; 1.077 g/ml, Serva) and two washings steps in phosphate buffered solution (PBS, Seromed), resuspended in Iscoves modified Dulbeccos medium (ICN Biochemicals) and counted. At the latest 2 h after diagnostic intervention, cell separation was done.

Suspension Cultures

The mononuclear cells were deposited in 50 ml culture flasks (Falcon) in Iscoves' modified Dulbecco's medium supplemented with 10%

Dept. of Hematology, Medical Clinic of Technical University Dresden, Dresden, Germany

autologous plasma. The influence of IL 3 on proliferative activity was investigated in one culture with additional 500 U/ml IL 3. Cells were incubated for 72 h in a humified 5% CO_2 atmosphere at 37°C. Then the cells were counted and the viability was measured with acridine orange.

Preparation of the Cells for Cell Cycle Phase Analysis

The preparation of cells was as described [3]. After density gradient separation cold ethanol (−20°C, final concentration 33%) was added for overnight incubation of cells at 4°C. After washings in PBS the cells were thoroughly resuspended in PBS and incubated for 15 min in RNAse (1 mg/ml; Sigma) at room temperature and after that with propidium iodide (Becton Dickinson; final concentration 50 mg/ml).

Because of the more accurate assessment of leukemia cell population in the case of lower than 60% blasts as result of cytological examination, cells were indirectly immunophenotyped with saturating concentration of monoclonal antibodies for 30 min at 4°C (anti CD 34 or CD 13; Becton Dickinson). After washing in PBS and following incubation with goat antimouse IgG $F(ab)_2$ fragment (GAM fluorescein isothiocynate, FITC, Coulter Hialeah) for 10 min at room temperature, cells were prepared for cell cycle phase analysis.

Flow Cytometric Analysis

Cell samples were measured on a FACScan flow cytometer with serial filter configuration. In the case of simultaneous measurement of immunophenotype and propidium iodide, fluorescence electronic compensation was used between the green and red fluorescence channels to correct spectral overlay of signals. Cell cycle phase analysis was done in R-fit mode. At least 15 000 cells were evaluated. This was considered as neccessary for statistical analysis, especially in the cases of low S-phases.

Change of proliferative activity was arbitrarily defined as more than 50% increase or decrease of S-phase.

Results

In this study cells of 38 newly diagnosed AML patients were investigated. The distribution of FAB subtypes is shown in Table 1. The classification in growth patterns results from alterations in S-phases of more than 50%. In this way from 9 theoretically possible growth patterns only 6 were detected (Table 1). In most cases (20/30) blasts were stimulated with Il 3 as expected. From these cases 7 are clearly dependent on Il 3, because the S-phase decreased in control culture in comparison to "in vivo S-phase" and increased in culture with Il 3, drawing a comparison to the control culture. Most cases of FAB M4 or M5 (9/13) were not sensitive to IL 3 when evaluated with this method. In the group of FAB M1/2 leukemias, 13/18 cases show increase of S-phase in response to IL 3. Promyelocytic leukemia cells were investigated in 2 cases. In this group leukemic populations were also stimulated with interleukin 3. But in 4/38 leukemias an increase was observed in control group without additional acceleration of growth with IL 3.

Table 1. Distribution of FAB subtypes of acute myeloid leukemias in growth patterns. The first sign represents the comparison results between the control culture and S-phase in vivo, the second sign the comparison between the control culture and culture with IL 3: ⇓ = decrease of S-phase; ⇑ = increase of S-phase; ⇔ = no change in S-phase exceeding 50%

Growth pattern	FAB classification					
	M 0	M 1	M 2	M 3	M 4	M 5
⇔/⇔	4/5		3/13		2/6	3/7
⇑/⇔			1/13		1/6	2/7
⇓/⇔		1/5			1/6	
⇑/⇑			3/13		1/6	1/7
⇔/⇑		3/5	4/13	1/2		
⇓/⇑	1/5	1/5	2/13	1/2	1/6	1/7

Discussion

The described method for determination of cytokine sensitivity was kept as simple as possible. Another aim was the adjustment of culture conditions to in vivo circumstances. Therefore fetal calf serum was replaced with autologous serum. The viability of cells after short term culture, tested with acridine orange, was in average 83% and 85% in control culture and culture with IL 3 respectively.

The data show proliferation inducing activity of IL 3 in 20 of 38 investigated cases. These data are comparable with other assays for this interleukin 3 effects [4]. These sensitive cases are heterogeneously distributed among the FAB subgroups. In AML M1/M2, 72% of cases were shown as IL 3 sensitive. In contrast, only 31% (4 of 13) myelomonocytic leukemias M4 and monoblastic M5 responded with proliferation. This difference may be interesting for use of cytokines for increasing of cytostatic effects. There are some reports for cytokine induced increase of cytosine-arabinoside antileukemic effect [5, 6, 7]. This higher cytosine arabinoside cytotoxicity is connected with cytokine induced increase of proliferation.

The data of this paper show that a great part of acute myeloid leukemias has no proliferation inducing effect with the relative ubiquitous acting cytokine IL 3. These cases are mainly distributed in FAB M4 and 5 and also in FAB M0 (Table 1). One cause for this growth pattern may be the presence of intercellular autocrine loops, as described. Therefore patient specific investigation of cytokine effects is recommended in AML subgroups. The long term prognostic relevance of these data will be investigated.

References

1 Crawford, J., Ozer, H., Stoller, R., Johnson, D., Lyman, G., Tabara, I., Kris, M., Grous, J., Piozzi, J., Rausch, G., Smith, R., Gradishar, Yanhanda, A., Vincenth, M., Steward, M. and Glaspy, J.: Reduction by granulocyte colony stimulating factor of fever and neutropenia induced by chemotherapy in patients with small cell lung cancer N. England J. Med. 325 (1991) 167–174.

2 Bettelheim, P., Valent, P., Andreeff, M., Tafuri,A., Haimi, J., Gorischek, C., Muhm, M., Sillaber, C., Hass, O., Vieder, L., Maurer, D., Schulz, G., Speiser, K., Geissler, K., Kier, P., Hinterberger, W and K. Lesche.: Recombinant human granulocyte macrophage colony stimulating factor with standard induction chemotherapy in de novo acute myeloid leukemia Blood, (1991) 700–711.

3. Nowak, R., Hietschold, V., Koslowsky, R. and M. Plat: Simultaneous analysis of cell membrane antigens and DNA-content in bone marrow cells-potential importance for Hematology Z. Klin. Med. 46 (1991) 535–537.

4 Tafuri, A., Lemoli, R. M., Chen, R., Gulati, S. C., Clarkson, B. D. and M. Andreeff.: Combination of hemapoietic growth factors containing IL 3 induce acute myeloid leukemia cell sensitization to cycle specific and non cycle specific drugs Leukemia 8; (5) (1994), 749–757.

5 Van der Lely, N., De Witte, T., Wessels, J., Raymakers, R., Muus, P. and Preijers, F. In vitro response of blasts to IL-3, GM-CSF and G-CSF is different for individual AML patients: factors that stimulate leukemic clonogenic cells also enhance Ara C cytotoxicity: Ann. Hematol. 1994 68 (5) 225–232.

6. Reuter, C., Auf der Landwehr, U., Schleyer, E., Zuhlsdorf, M., Ameling, C., Rolf, C., Wormann, B., Buchner, T. and Hiddemann, W.: Modulation of intracellular metabolism of cytosine arabinoside in acute myeloid leukemia by granulocyte macrophage colony stimulating factor: Leukemia (1994) Feb 8 (2) 217–225.

7. Rogers, SY, Bradbury, D., Kozlowsky, P. and Russell Evidence for internal autocrine regulation of growth in acute myeloblastic cells: Exp. Hematol. 1994, 22; 593–608

Acute Leukemias VI
Prognostic Factors
and Treatment Strategies
Büchner et al. (eds)

The Influence of Short Term Liquid Culture of Leukemic Blasts on Their Phenotype

K. Kuliczokowski, S. Kotlarek-Haus, and K. Sedek

Abstract. The immunophenotyping of acute leukemia blasts is not always satisfactory regarding precise determination of the type of proliferating cells. An attempt was made to ascertain whether a short (3 days) culture of leukemic cells in RPMI 1640+10% FCS medium will disclose their additional featues. Blasts were classified according to FAB and phenotyped with the following monoclonal antibodies (DAKO): HLA-DR, CD10, TdT, CD3, CD19, CD33, CD13 and CD15 prior to and after the culture. Studies of 16 patients (13 with AML and 3 with ALL) showed an increase or, inversely, a decrease of percentage of the cell type which seemed to predominate before culture. In three cases cells were suspected to be bi-phenotypic on morphological and cytochemical grounds and this was confirmed after the culture (in two AML lymphoblasts appeared and in one ALL myeloblasts). Blasts of one case of AML Mo revealed lymphoblastic features after the culture, and in one case with bi-phenotypic cells (myeloblasts and lymphoblasts) only lymphoblasts proliferated. In conclusion it seems that 3-day culture of leukemic blasts may be helpful in diagnosing acute leukemias.

Introduction

The classification of a given case of acute leukemia (AL) is usually based on the morphological, cytochemical immunophenotypical features of the blasts. However, in a small subgroup of AL it is very difficult to establish the exact subgroup according to FAB or even to diagnose lymphoid or myeloid lineage. In AL there exists a maturation block, but it has been shown that some of the malignant cells in acute myeloid leukemia (AML) can differentiate but differentiation programs are expressed abnormally [1,2,3].

In the present study we tried to find whether there are any changes of leukemic blasts phenotype during 3 days' liquid culture in medium consisting of RPMI 1640 with 10% of FCS and whether some immunological features become more distinct, allowing more precise diagnosis of AL.

Material and Methods

Patients

A group of 16 leukemic patients (seven women and nine men) aged 17-71 years at the time of diagnosis, before therapy were examined. They were classified according to FAB criteria for acute leukemia: 3L2, 1Mo, 1M1, 3M2, 1M3, 6M4 and one with mixed lineage leukemia, myeloid and lymphoid type.

Methods

Bone marrow cells were recovered onto heparinized medium. The mononuclear cell fraction was separated by Ficoll density gradient, washed three times, and resuspended in phosphate-buffered saline. The leukemic cells were analyzed by indirect immunofluorescence under a fluorescent microcope (Jena-Lumar) using different sets of DAKO MoAbs (Table 1

Department of Hematology, Medical University of Wroclaw, Poland

Table 1. Hematological data of patients and cytochemical characteristics of blast cells

Patient no.	Type of AL	Age	Sex	WBC g/l	% of blasts Peripheral blood	Bone marrow	Cytochemistry: % of positive cells			
							PAS	Sudan B	NSE	ANAE
1	L2	29	M	306.0	89	91	0	10	0	59
2	L2	23	F	29.5	25	100	20	0	0	63
3	L	61	F	114.0	77	77	0	0	0	44[a]
4	M0	70	F	2.7	3	89	7	16	33	6
5	M1	20	F	2.6	38	54	0	66	86	76
6	M2	40	M	83.3	99	100	0	94	0	80
7	M2	18	M	10.3	13	42	39	71	0	74
8	M2	17	M	406.0	76	74	0	100	0	22
9	M3	56	M	29.2	82	92	0	55	0	37
10	M4	31	F	30.4	73	80.5	0	39	39	67
11	M4	60	M	46.4	70	80	0	10	0	100
12	M4	44	F	187.0	91	79	35	99	50	60
13	M4	30	M	14.6	55	48	52	58	70	70
14	M4	62	F	24.4	39	50.5	0	91	0	80
15	M4 E0	28	M	30.4	73	80.5	0	39	39	67
16	L/M	19	M	3.5	78	51 (26 Mbl, 25 Lbl)	0	0	4	39[a]

[a]Dot-like reaction characteristic of lymphoid cells.

and 2). Cells were considered positive when 10% blasts had positive markers according to proposals of the General Haematology Task Force BCSH 1994 [4].

Culture

The cells, 10^6 ml, were cultured for 3 days in RPMI 1640 supplemented with 10% heat inactivated FCS, 50 mg gentamicin in humidified 5% CO_2. After 3 days cells were counted, their viability examined by trypan blue dye exclusion and they were labelled with the same set of MoAbs.

Results

In two observed cases of ALL, cells expressed lymphoid marker CD3 only after 3 days' culture. In the third one both lymphoid (CD3, CD7, CD10, CD19) and myeloid markers (CD13, CD15, CD33) were present on cells before culture, but after culture the percentage of CD15 positive cells decreased.

In one case of Mo the cells after culture become TdT positive. In two out of three cases of M2 leukemia CD13 positive cells, appeared after culture while in one case the percentage of those cells decreased. In another case of M2 leukemia cells positive for CD14 disapeared.

Increase of percentage of positive CD13 and CD14 cells was observed in culture of M3 leukemia.

In all cases of M4 leukemia except one (no. 9), there was observed an increase of percentage of cells with myeloid markers: CD13 in 5/7 examined, CD14 in 2/2, CD15 in 3/7 and HLA-DR in 6/7. In two cases (nos. 12, 13) lymphoid markers CD7 and CD10 appeared after 3 days, accompanied by CD3. In one patient (no. 16) diagnosed already under light microscope as leukemia of two lineages, lymphoid and myeloid, the appropriate markers, CD13 and CD19, appeared on cells in culture after 3 days.

Discussion

Leukemia is characterized by the accumulation of blasts, which fail to differentiate and egress from the bone marrow. Differentiation of leukemic blasts into more mature forms has been demonstrated in liquid [2] and semiliquid [3] cultures. Other studies have shown absent or abnormal differentiation [1]. In vitro the maturation block of AML cells [5, 6, 7] as well as those of lymphoid leukemia [8, 9] can be overcome by a variety of chemical compounds including TPA. Also acute undifferentiated leukemia (AUL) may show differentiation on TPA treatment [7, 10, 11].

In the present study it was shown that changes of blast cell phenotype in myeloid as well as lymphoid leukemias can be observed. In most myeloid or myelo-monocytoid leukemia cases the number of cells with myeloid or monocytoid markers increased, but in some the cells previously showing these markers decreased or disappeared. Similar results were observed by van der Schoot et al. [7].

In one case of ALL, myeloid cells—CD13, CD15 and CD33 labelled cells—were found before culture, and after the culture the percentage of CD15 decreased. The presence of myeloid markers in lymphoid leukemia was also noted in adults by Sobol et al. [12] and van der School et al. [7] and in children by Hara et al. [13] and Tsuchiya et al. [14].

Lymphoid markers can appear also in myeloid leukemias. Mixed-lineage AML may carry a worse prognosis than routine AML with standard therapy, and may respond to ALL therapy if AML therapy fails [15]. In our material lymphoid markers appeared in two M4 cases in vitro after 3 days' culture.

Table 2. Different monoclonal antibodies used in phenotyping of the examined acute leukemias

Patient number	Type of leukemia	Monoclonal antibodies
1, 2	ALL	CD10, TdT, CD3, CD19
3	ALL	CD3, CD7, CD10, CD19, CD13, CD15, CD33
4–11,15	AML	CD13, CD14, CD15
12–14,16	AML	CD3, CD10, CD19, CD13 CD14, CD15, CD33

Table 3. Results of leukemic cell phenotyping before and after 3 days' culture (% of positive cells)

Patient no.	Type of AL	Monoclonal antibodies																			
		HLA-DR		TdT		CD3		CD7		CD10		CD13		CD14		CD15		CD19		CD33	
		1	2	1	2	1	2	1	2	1	2	1	2	1	2	1	2	1	2	1	2
1	L2	3	5	0	0	3	24	–	–	–	–	–	–	–	–	–	–	–	–	–	–
2	L2	0	0	0	0	2	25	–	–	–	–	–	–	–	–	–	–	–	–	–	–
3	L	65	70	–	–	57	47	27	35	65	40	21	17	–	–	–	–	–	–	–	–
4	M0	61	27	0	96	–	–	–	–	0	0	0	0	–	–	–	–	–	–	–	
5	M1	3	2	–	–	–	–	–	–	–	–	40	57	9	7	3	0	–	–	–	–
6	M2	1	14	–	–	–	–	–	–	–	–	0	35	0	0	0	0	–	–	–	–
7	M2	24	36	–	–	–	–	–	–	–	–	43	10	69	0	0	0	–	–	–	–
8	M2	13	4	–	–	–	–	–	–	–	–	0	70	50	87	0	0	–	–	–	–
9	M3	3	3	–	–	–	–	–	–	–	–	0	0	81	81	0	0	–	–	–	–
10	M4	12	11	–	–	–	–	–	–	–	–	30	78	0	33	35	0	–	–	–	–
11	M4	0	36	–	–	–	–	–	–	0	0	0	44	15	81	0	0	–	–	–	–
12	M4	43	80	–	–	2	13	0	14	5	5	8	14	–	–	0	2	2	7	–	–
13	M4	10	25	–	–	0	10	0	26	0	25	23	12	–	–	4	28	9	10	0	21
14	M4	11	45	–	–	0	22	0	14	0	22	3	26	–	–	2	15	1	30	0	17
15	M4 E0	29	66	–	–	–	–	–	–	–	–	2	48	11	13	0	0	–	–	–	–
16	L/M	35	90	–	–	0	5	0	7	1	7	0	10	0	7	15	7	8	20	0	9

Results obtained before culture; 2, results after 3 days' culture; –, not done.

In our only case of (AUL), negative for CD13, cells positive for TdT appeared after the culture. TdT positive cells may appear in myeloid leukemias as previously noted [16]. Van der Schoot et al. [7] observed in vitro after 3 days' blast culture of 8 cases of AUL appearance of cells with myeloid markers. These authors suggest that myeloid membrane phenotype after culture was not due to proliferation of normal bone marrow cells but to leukemic clone. The results of labelling of our single case of AUL would suggest a lymphoid origin of leukemia.

It seems that appearance of new markers on cells or increase of the percentage of cells with specific marker after 3 days' liquid culture may result from proliferation of blasts with specific marker; however, increased expression cannot be excluded. On the other hand, disappearance of some cell phenotypes could be explained by decrease of expression rather than their death.

Our preliminary results seem to justify the examination of leukemic cells' phenotype after 3 days' culture as a helpful tool in diagnosis of acute leukemias, but the method needs confirmation in larger groups of patients.

References

1. Touw I., Lowenberg, B.: Variable differentiation of human acute leukemia during colony formation in vitro: a membrane marker analysis with monoclonal antibodies. Brit. J. Haemotol. 59, 37-44, 1985-1983.
2. Hoelzer, D., Kurrle, E., Schmucker, H. Harris, E.B.: Evidence for differentiation of human leukemia blood cells in diffusion culture. Blood 49, 729-744, 1977.
3. Reid, M.M., Tantravaki, R., Grier, H.E., O'Toole, S., Miller, B.A., Lipton, J.M., Weinstein, M.J., and Nathan, D.G.: Detection of leukemic - related karyotypes in granulocyte\myelomonocytic leukemia. New Engl. J. Med. 308, 1324, 1983.
4. General Haematology Task Force of BCSH: Immunophenotyping in the diagnosis in the diagnosis of acute leukemias. J. Clin. Pathol. 47, 777-781, 1994.
5. Pegoraro, L., Abraham, J., Cooper, R.A., Levis, A., Lange, B., Meo, P. and Rovera, G.: Differentiation of human leukemias in response to 12-0-tetradecanoyl phorbol-13-acetate in vitro. Blood 55, 859-862, 1980.
6. Ohta, M., Saito, M., Suda, K., Sakamota, S., Kitagawa, S., Miura, Y. Takaku, F.: Differentiation of human leukemia cells and its usefulness for clinical diagnosis Leuk. Res. 7, 363-374, 1983.
7. Van der Schoot, C.E., Visser, F.J., Tetteroo, P.A.T. and von dem Borne, A.E.G.Kr.: In-vitro differentiation of cells of patients with acute undifferentiated leukemia. Brit. J. Haematol. 71, 351-355, 1989.
8. Flug, F., Dodson, L., Wolff, J., Guarini, L., Ransen, A., Wang, C.Y. and Knowles, D.M.: B-lymphocyte-associated differentiation antigen expression by "non-B, non-T" acute lymphoblastic leukemia. Leuk. Res. 9,1051-1058, 1985.
9. Efremedis, A.P., Haubenstock, H., Holland, J.F. Bekesi, J.G.,: TPA-induced maturation in secretory human B-leukemic cells in vitro: DNA synthesis, antigenic changes, and immunoglobulin secretion. Blood 66,953-960, 1985.
10. Gregg, S.L., Gaijl-Peczalska, K.J., LeBien, T.W., Bloomenfield, C.D., Brunning, R. and Sagawa,K.: Monoclonal antibody MCS-2 as the marker of phorbol diester-induced myeloid differentiation in acute undifferentiated leukemia. Cancer Res. 44, 2724-2730, 1984.
11. Skolnick, T., Schlossman, S.F., Griffin, J.D.: Acute undifferentiated leukemia: induction of partial differentiation by phorbol ester. Leuk. Res. 9, 11-17, 1985.
12. Sobol, R.E., Mick, R., Royston, I., Devey, F.R., Ellison, R.R., Newman, R., Cuttner, J., Griffin, J.D., Collins, H., Nelson, D.A. and Bloomenfield, C.D.: Clinical importance of myeloid antigen expression in adult acute lymphoblastic leukemia. New Engl. J. Med. 316, 1111-1117, 1987.
13. Hara, J., Kawa-Ha, K., Yumura-Yagi, K., Kurahashi, H., Taura, A., Ishihara, S., Inoue, M., Murayama, N., Okada, S.: In vivo and in vitro expression of myeloid antigens on B-lineage acute lymphoblastic leukemia cells. Leukemia 5, 19-23, 1991.
14. Tsuchiya, H., El-Sonbaty, S.S., Watanabe, M., Sozushima, H., Asou, N., Murakami, T., Takeda, T., Shimosaka, A., Takatsuki, K. and Matsuda, I.: Analysis of myeloid characteristics in acute lymphoblastic leukemia. Leuk. Res. 17, 809-813, 1993.
15. Pui, C.H., Raimondi, S.C., Head, D.R., Schell, M.J., Rivera, G.K., Mirro, J., Grist, W.M. Behm, F.G.: Characterization of childhood acute leukemia with mutiple myeloid and lymphoid markers at diagnosis and relapse. Blood 78, 1327-1337, 1991.
16. Graeves, M.F., Chana, L.C., Furley, A.J.W., Watt, S.M. and Molgaard, H.V.: Lineage promiscuity in hematopoietic differentiation and leukemia. Blood 67, 1-11, 1986.

Acute Leukemias VI
Prognostic Factors
and Treatment Strategies
Büchner et al. (eds)

Correlation of Deoxycytidine Deaminase, Thymidine Kinase and Polymerase Alpha Activity and Deoxycytidine Deaminase Gene Expression In Vivo with Clinical Response to TAD-9+GM-CSF Induction Therapy in Acute Myeloid Leukemia

G. Jahns-Streubel[1], M. Unterhalt[1], E. Schleyer[1], C. Reuter[2], B. Wörmann[1], T. Büchner[3], and W. Hiddemann[1]

Abstract. Although significant advances have been made in the treatment of acute myeloid leukemia with araC containing regimes, a considerable number of patients do not reach an adequate blast cell reduction after induction therapy. Therefore it is an important task to find sensitive and reliable prognostic parameters for clinical response in order to screen patients before the start of therapy and to optimize induction therapy.

Bone marrow cells from 32 patients with newly diagnosed AML were analyzed for the activities of the following enzymes relevant for the metabolism of araC: deoxycytidine kinase (DCK), thymidine kinase (TK), deoxycytidine deaminase (DCD), polymerase alpha (poly alpha) and overall polymerase. Median values and range were: for DCK 27.2 pmol/min/mg protein (3.8–196), for TK 3.1 pmol/min/mg protein (0.0–21.6), for DCD 1.64 nmol/min/mg protein (0.0–8.6), for overall polymerase 55.9 pmol/min/mg protein (17.3–131) and for poly alpha 1.22 pmol/min/mg protein (0.03–8.8).

The data of the enzyme activities were related to clinical response of TAD-9 +GM-CSF induction therapy in 29 patients, taking the blast cell reduction at day 10 or day 16 as a parameter of early response. A blast cell reduction to <5% blasts at this time point was considered as adequate response, while >5% blasts was classified as non-response. Neither DCK-nor overall polymerase activity was predictive for response. However, the (S-phase dependent) activities of TK and poly alpha were associated with an adequate blast cell reduction. Differences in TK and poly alpha activity between the responder group and the nonresponder group were statistically significant ($p = 0.0064$ for TK and $p = 0.0062$ for poly alpha). The DCD activity turned out to be the most sensitive parameter for clinical response to TAD-9 +GM-CSF induction therapy. The difference between the responder group (median) 0.333 nmol/min/mg protein, range 0.0–4.1) and the nonresponder group (median) 4.8 nmol/min/mg protein, range 0.11–8.45) was statisticallty significant ($p = 0.0012$). In order to gain an insight into the molecular mechanism underlying these varying enzyme activities, transcription of the DCD gene was investigated in leukemic blasts of 15 AML patients. Preparation of total RNA, cDNA synthesis by RT and PCR were done according to standard protocols. RT-PCR of ß-actin served as control for integrity of the RNA and as reference for quantification of DCD gene expression. Specificity was checked by direct DNA sequencing. It could be demonstrated that high DCD activity was associated with high transcription rate of the DCD gene and vice versa.

It can be concluded from this study that high activities of the S-phase-dependent enzymes TK and poly alpha and low activity of DCD are associated with good clinical outcome. The results demonstrate that these factors are valuable parameters for dividing patients into favorable and unfavourable prognosis groups for induction therapy, which is the basis for risk-adapted therapy protocols.

[1]Dept. of Hematology and Oncology, University of Göttingen, Germany
[2]Dept. of Microbiology and Cancer Center, University of Virginia, USA
[3]Dept. of Hematology and Oncology, University of Münster, Germany

Introduction

Although significant advances have been made in the treatment of acute myeloid leukemia with araC containing regimens, 20–40% of patients do not reach adequate blast cell reduction after induction therapy. This unresolved problem has stimulated many different studies trying to identify mechanisms that are responsible for sensitivity or resistance to araC based therapy and may determine final outcome. Extensive laboratory investigations focused on cell proliferative activity and determinants of araC metabolism as potential predictors of clinical response but no clear results emerged. The significance of proliferative patterns as an indicator of the efficacy of leukemic cell kill by araC has been debated for the past 20 years [1, 2, 3]. Studies on parameters of araC metabolism in human leukemic cells have led to different conclusions about the primary determinant of the therapeutic efficacy of araC. Some studies found a considerable overlap in araC metabolite formation among groups of araC sensitive and resistant patients [4], while other investigations revealed an association between remission duration and the intracellular retention of araCTP [5, 6]. Similarly, several studies revealed that the activity of DCK in leukemic bone marrow cells is predictive for therapeutic response [7, 8] while others suggested that some specific metabolic control, rather than the amount of the active enzyme, determines the maximum level of araC incorporation and cytotoxicity [9, 10]. Though higher DCD activities have been found in resistant patients by some authors [7, 11] this has not been confirmed by others [12, 13].

Few data are available about the regulation of the enzymes relevant for the metabolism of araC on the molecular level. A recent report [14] demonstrated that structural alterations in the coding region of the DCK gene occur at such a low frequency that this mechanism can scarcely account for cellular resistance to araC. Mutations in the sites within the genes coding for CTP synthetase do not appear to be a mechanism of resistance to araC, either [15]. A cDNA clone for human DCD has been identified [16] but no analyses of structural alterations or expression of the DCD gene have been performed in AML blasts. The current study was designed to measure both proliferative activity and parameters of araC metabolism in a representative group of patients with de novo AML and to evaluate their prognostic significance, taking the blast cell reduction after induction therapy as early indicator for adequate or inadequate response. In an approach to a better understanding of the regulation of DCD activity the mRNA levels in leukemic blasts were assessed by a semi-quantitative RT-PCR method.

Patients, Materials and Methods

AML Induction Therapy

Patients being included into the clinical evaluation of this study underwent the TAD-9 +GM-CSF regimen as first induction cycle. GM-CSF was given at a dose of 250 μg/m^2/day starting 24 h before and continuing during induction chemotherapy until recovery of blood counts. TAD-9 comprised 100 g/m^2/day araC given by continuous i.v. infusion on days 1 and 2 followed by short term infusions of araC 100 mg/m^2 every 12 h on days 3–8; 6-thioguanine 100 mg/m^2 every 12 h orally on days 3–9 and 60 min infusions of daunorubicin 60 mg/m^2 on days 3–5. Early response to therapy was assessed by a bone marrow examination on day 10 or 16 after the onset of therapy. A reduction of leukemic blasts below 5% at this time was considered as adequate blast cell reduction.

Cell and Cell Extract Preparation

Bone marrow aspirates were obtained from 32 patients with newly diagnosed AML. The diagnosis was based on FAB criteria and complementary cytochemical and immunological analyses. Leukemic cells comprised 90% of the total population at median with a range of 50–95%. 29 cases were evaluable for the assessment of clinical response.

Cells were subjected to Ficoll density gradient separation. Next 10^7 cells were resuspended in 100 μl 50 mM Tris-HCl, pH 7.4, and lysed by three freeze-thaw cycles, and cellular debris and unresolved proteins were pelleted by centrifugation at 12 000 *g* for 5 min at 4°C. The supernatant was assayed for enzyme activities and protein concentration.

Analysis of Cellular DNA Content

Cells were washed twice in 0.9% NaCl, drained through a nylon filter, fixed with ice-cold 96%

ethanol and centrifuged at 1000 g for 5 min. The pellet was resuspended in 1–2 ml of a 0.5% pepsin-HCl solution and stained with ethidium bromide and mithramycin. After 15–20 min of staining, DNA content was measured on a PAS II instrument (Partec, Münster, Germany).

Production and Purification of the Monoclonal Antibody (Mab) SJK 237-7 Against DNA Polymerase Alpha

The hybridoma cell line SJK 237–71 was obtained from the American Type Culture Collection, Rockville, Maryland, USA. Hybridoma cells were cultivated in minimal essential medium (MEM) supplemented with 10% heat inactivated fetal calf serum (FCS), glutamine (300 μg/ml) and antibiotics (penicillin 60 μg/ml; streptomycine 133 μg/ml) at 37° in a 5% CO_2 atmosphere. Monoclonal antibodies were isolated from the cell culture supernatants using the commerical Affi-Gel Protein A MAPS II (monoclonal antibody purification system) kit (Biorad, Munich, Germany) according to the manufacturer's instruction. The concentration of DNA polymerase alpha-Mab was assessed by ELISA, using as coating antibody 31500045 (Jackson Immuno Research, Baltimore, MD, USA) as detection antibody peroxidase conjugated 315035003 (Jackson), o-phenylendiamine dihydrochloride (OPD) (Jackson) as substrate and mouse IgG (Sigma) as internal standard.

DNA Polymerase Alpha Assay

DNase-activated calf thymus DNA, which served as a starter of the polymerase alpha assay was prepared as described by Aposhian and Kornberg [17]. The DNA polymerase alpha assay was performed according to Hammond et al. [18], with the following modifications: 20 μl cell extract was incubated with 4 mg protein A-Sepharose (Pharmacia, Freiburg, Germany), and 25 μl of purified MAB SJK 237–71 (0.1 mg/ml) in phosphate-buffered saline (PBS) for 2 h at 4°C. After washing of the immobilized immunocomplexes with 1 ml PBS and 1 ml reaction buffer [5 mM $MgCl_2$, 1 ml dithiothreitol (DTT) and 50 mM Tris-HCl pH 7.4], a final volume of 100 μl was added, containing 30 μg DNase-activated DNA, 10 μM dCTP, 10 μM dATP, 10 μM dGTP, 5mM $MgCl_2$, 1mM DTT, 50 mM Tris–HCl pH 7.4 and 1 μCi dCTP (26 Ci/mmol; Amersham Buchler). The reactions were incubated for 15 min at 37°C. Incorporation of ^{3}H-dCMP into DNA was determined by using DE81 filter paper (Whatman, UK) as previously described [19]. All experiments were performed in triplicate.

Overall Polymerase Assay

The DNA polymerase assay was performed according to Hammond et al. [18] with the following modifications: a final volume of 100 μl contained 30 μg DNase-activated DNA, 250 μM dGTP, 250 μM dCTP, 250 μM dATP, 5mM $MgCl_2$, 1 mM dithiothreitol (DTT), 50mM Tris-HCl pH 7.4 and 1 μCi ^{3}H-dCTP (26 Ci/mmol, Amersham Buchler). The reactions were incubated for 30 min at 37°C. Incorporation of ^{3}H-dCMP into DNA was determined by using DE 81 filter (Whatman, UK) as previously described [19]. All experiments were performed in triplicate.

Deoxycytidine Deaminase Assay

For DCD assay 90 μl of reaction buffer (final) concentrations: 1.9 mM Tris-HCl pH 8.0, 60 nM deoxycytidine) and deoxy (5-^{3}H) cytidine (0.006 μCi/ml, 22 Ci/mmol) were added to 10 μl cell extract and incubated at 37°C for 60 min. The reaction was terminated by addition of 50 μl 1.2 M trichloracetic acid, and the mixture was added to a 0.5 × 7 cm column of Dowex resin (AG 50W-XA), which was subsequently washed with distilled water (2 volumes). The product ^{3}H-deoxyuridine eluted with the void volume, and radioactivity was determined in a liquid scintillation counter.

Thymidine and Deoxycytidine Kinase Assays

For thymidine kinase (TK) and deoxycytidine kinase (DCK) assays [27], 100 μl reaction buffer (final concentrations: 100 mM Tris-HCl pH 8.0, 4.5 mM ATP, 5 mM Mg EDTA, 0.2 mM ^{3}H-TdR (5 Ci/mmol) or 0.1 mM ^{3}H-ara-C (35 Ci/mmol) was added to 100 μl cell extract and incubated at 37°C for 1 hour. The reaction was stopped by incubation of the samples at 100°C for 2 min. After precipitation of the proteins by centrifugation for 3 min at 2500 g and 4°C, 20 μl of the clarified reaction mixture was spotted on DE81 anion exchange filter discs (Whatman) and washed twice with 0.1 mM ammonium formiate (5 ml) and H_2O (5 ml) and once with 96% ethanol. Radioactivity of the phosphorylated mucleosides was counted in a LKB fluid scintillation counter. All experiments were performed in triplicate.

RNA Isolation and Reverse Transcription (RT)

For the preparation of cytoplasmic RNA a preparation method modified from Chomczynski [20] was adopted. In the reverse transcriptase step 1.5 µg of total RNA was employed in an incubation volume of 13 µl. C+DNA synthesis was performed using a commercially available kit (Superscript Preamplification System, Gibco). Final concentrations of buffer, deoxynucleotides, oligo-dT primer and reverse transcriptase were as recommended by the manufacturer. After an incubation time of 40 min at 42 °C, the reaction was stopped by heating to 95 °C for 5 min.

Polymerase Chain Reaction (PCR)

The subsequent PCR was performed on an automated thermocycler (Model 480, Perkin-Elmer Cetus, Emeryville, USA) with 2 µl of the reaction mixture from the RT step, 2.5 units of Taq polymerase (Gibco), 200 nmol of each specific primer, 10 nmol dNTP, 1.5 mM $MgCl_2$ and 10x buffer: 500 mM KCl, 100 mM Tris-HCl (pH 9.0), 1% Triton x-100, in a total volume of 50 µl. Standard cycle conditions were: 40 s at 95°C for denaturation of DNA, followed by an annealing reaction for 30 s at 60°C and extending at 72°C for 30 S. The last primer extension and the first denaturation step were extended to 5 min. Usually 25 cycles were sufficient to detect a signal in all cases of AML. Products were run on a 2% agarose gel (2% w/v Nusieve) and stained with ethidium bromide.

DNA Sequencing

Amplified DNA was purified using the Magic PCR Preps Purification System (Promega) according to the manufacturer's instructions. PCR products were directly sequenced by the Taq cycle sequencing method involving, in parallel, assay each of the specific primers and the Ready Reaction Dye Deoxy Terminator Cycle Sequencing kit (Applied Biosystems, Weiterstadt, Germany). Sequencing reaction products were analyzed on the automated DNA sequencer (Model 373A, Applied Biosystems) [21].

Statistical Methods

Comparisions between two groups of patients with adequate (<5% blasts) and inadequuate (>5% blasts) blast cell clearance after TAD-9 were made by the Wilcoxon test. The Fisher test was used to analyze contingency tables. For all tests, p values <0.05 were considered significant. Data were analyzed using the PC-Statistik programs (Lizenzagentur Lambda, Graz, Austria) and TopSoft (Version 2.05, 1990, Hanover, Germany).

Results

Response to TAD-9 + GM-CSF Induction Therapy

Bone marrow aspirates from 32 patients were analyzed; 29 patients were evaluable for response to TAD-9 + GM-CSF induction therapy. Patients characteristics are shown in Table 1. Adequate blast cell reduction to below 5% balsts at day 10 or 16 was achieved in 16 cases, while 13 patients had an inadequate early response. Blast cell reduction after the first induction course was not predictive for subsequent achievement of complete remission after the completion of double induction therapy (Table 2).

Proliferative Activity and Parameter of araC Metabolism In Vivo: Relation to Clinical Response

Results of pretreatment analyses of TK and % S phase as a reflection of proliferative activity and activities of DCD, DCK, Poly alpha and overall polymerase as determinants of araC metabolism are summarized in Table 3. The data reveal sub-

Table 1. Patient characteristics

Number of patients	32
Age (years)	range: 20–72 median: 50 age > 60: 8
Sex	male: 15 female: 17
FAB type	M0: 1 M1: 4 M2: 8 M3: 1 M4: 13 M5: 4 M6: 1 M7: 1

Table 2. Response to induction therapy

Blast cell clearance, day 10 or 16	$<5\%$:16 (55%)
	$>5\%$:13 (45%)
Complete remission	$<5\%$:14 (87.5%)
	$>5\%$:10 (77%)

Table 3. Proliferative activity and araC metabolism

Parameter	Median	Range
TK (pmol/min/mg protein)	3.1	0.0–21.6
%S phase	5.5	1.8–16.2
DCK (pmol/min/mg protein)	27.2	3.8–196.0
DCD (nmol/min/mg protein)	1.64	0.0–8.6
Overall polymerase (pmol/min/ mg protein)	55.9	17.3–131
Polymerase alpha (pmol/min/ mg protein)	1.22	0.03–8.81

stantial interpatient variablity. The respective parameters were related to early clinical response as determined by the reduction of blast cells at day 10 or 16. High TK activity but not % S phase was associated with adequate blast cell clearance. The median values of TK activity were 3.6 pmol/min/mg protein (range: 2.0–21.6) for patients responding to induction therapy as compared to 1.85 pmol/min/mg protein (0.0–7.2) for the nonresponders ($p = 0.0064$). In contrast to overall Polymerase activity, the poly alpha activity to leukemic blasts before the start of therapy was highly predictive for early response. Whereas median values and range were 2.17 pmol/min/mg protein (0.63–8.8) for the responders, the respective values for patients with inadequate blast cell reduction were 0.5 pmol/min/mg protein (0.03–6.7) ($p = 0.0062$). The activity of DCK before therapy was not related to clinical outcome after the first course of induction therapy. The DCD activity, however, was found to be the most sensitive parameter to predict an adequate blast cell clearance. Patients with DCD activity below the overall median of 1.64 nmol/min/mg protein achieved an adequate response in 10 of 12 cases (83%) whereas patients with higher than median values failed in 11 of 14 cases (79%) ($p = 0.002$). Median values and range for DCD activity were 0.33 nmol/min/mg protein (0.0–4.1) for patients with an adequate blast cell reduction, whereas the nonresponders revealed a median of 4.8 nmol/min/mg protein and a range of 0.11–9.45 ($p = 0.0012$) (Fig. 1).

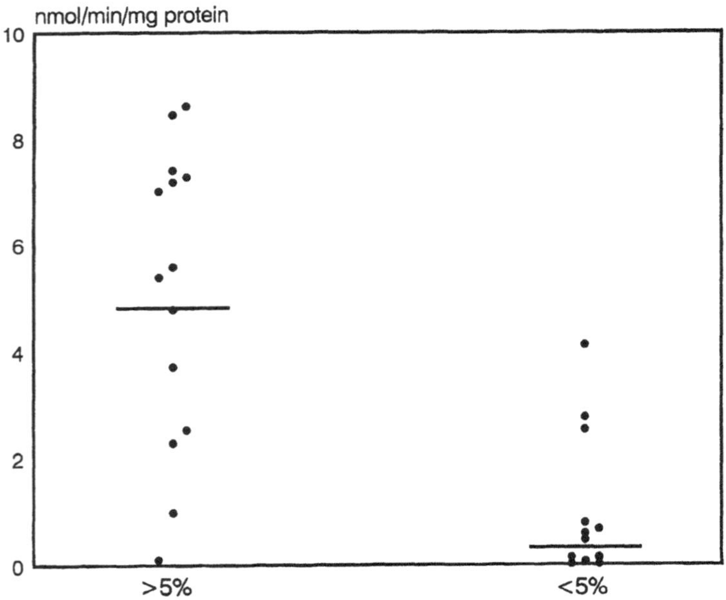

Fig. 1. Distibution of DCD activity for responders ($<5\%$) and non responders ($>5\%$) to induction therapy. Median values of the respective groups are indicated

Deoxycytidine Deaminase Expression in AML Blasts: Correlation with DCD Activity

Total RNA extracted from leukemic blasts from 15 patients with AML and from peripheral blood mononuclear cells (PBMNC) from healthy donors was tested for possible RNA degradation by amplification of a 484 base pair (bp) segment from ß-actin cDNA. Sterile water was used as negative, RNA from PBMNC as positive control. As shown in Fig. 2, a 546 b p PCR product was detected in all AML cases. Specificity of this amplification product for DCD gene expression was checked by direct DNA sequencing. In an approach to quantification of initial DCD mRNA amounts, the relative signal strength of the ethidium bromide stained bands was determined as compared to the signal intensity of the β-actin amplification product. Values for the relative optical densities (OD) provided the basis for dividing the amount of DCD gene expression into cases with high or low mRNA levels. Table 4 shows the respective enzyme activities for these subgroups of AML patients. Six of Seven patients with high transcription rate of DCD gene showed higher than median DCD enzyme activity, whereas in blast cells from all the seven patients with low DCD mRNA levels, low enzyme activity was detected. These data indicate that DCD activity is regulated by the transcription rate of the DCD gene and that a low transcription rate must be regulated at the gene level.

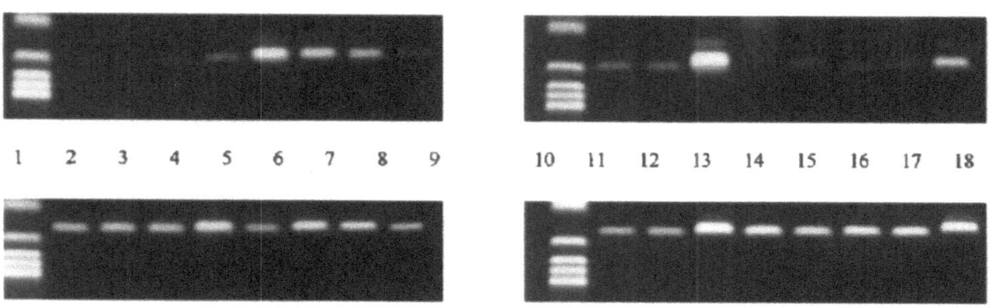

Fig. 2. RT-PCR products for DCD transcripts (*upper row*) and ß-actin transcripts (*lower row*) from leukemic blasts. PCR products were run in the following lanes: *2–9* and *11–17* AML patients (F.H.; E.S.; G.R.; I.W.; H.P.; H.H.; E.T.; H.V.; A.B.; S.S.; I.R.; B.K.; I.M.; H.F.; H.B.); 18 positive control; 1 and 10 molecular weight markers

Table 4. Correlation of DCD gene expression and DCD activity

Patient	DCD gene expression	DCD activity (nmol/min/mg protein)
E.S.	low	0.8
G.R.	low	0.02
I.W.	low	0.164
H.V.	low	0.8
H.B.	low	0.02
B.K.	low	0.13
H.F.	low	0.6
F.H.	median	1.0
H.P.	high	1.64
H.H.	high	2.7
T.E.	high	2.28
A.B.	high	0.215
S.S.	high	6.6
I.R.	high	2.4
I.M.	high	7.0

Discussion

In this study pretreatment analysis of TK activity as a reflection of proliferative activity and of poly alpha and DCD activities as determinants of araC metabolism provided important information about early response to induction therapy.

In cell culture and animal studies, the most prevalent mechanism of resistance to araC is the complete absence or a decrease of DCK activity [22, 23, 24]. However, there are only few clinical studies, some based on relatively small numbers of patients, that tackle the concept of DCK deficiency as a mechanism of resistance operative in leukemic blast cells [7, 8, 12, 13]. In the present study no relation between DCK activity and clinical outcome after induction therapy with standard doses of araC was observed.

The significance of high DCD activity for araC resistance has been suggested by several investigators. Stuart and Burke [11] found a high DCD activity in the leukemic cells of patients who did not respond to conventional dose araC therapy. Tattersall et al. [7] described high DCD activity in leukemic patients who did not respond to araC; however, a considerable overlap in enzyme activity with that of araC responsive patients was also observed.

Colley et al. [8] found in a group of 21 patients (11 patients with de novo AML) that therapy-resistant patients had either a very low DCK activity or an increased DCD activity. The distribution of ratios of araU/araC in plasma of patients with AML, ALL or CML was analyzed by Kreis et al. [25], who identified two groups of deaminators, but differences between both groups were not statistically significant. Nevertheless, the relevance of DCD as a determinant of araC resistance has been denied by other investigators [12, 13]. These discrepancies may reflect variability in study design, patient characteristics and laboratory techniques.

Our results clearly demonstrate that the level of DCD activity in leukemic blasts before therapy is a very sensitive parameter in predicting clinical response to standard induction therapy. These findings and their possible clinical implications are a challenge to investigate the regulation of DCD activity. We found that DCD activity correlated with the amount of mRNA in leukemic cells, in that for patients with low DCD gene expression in AML blasts low levels of enzyme activity were detected, and vice versa. Consequently DCD gene expression is thought to correlate with patient's response to induction therapy. Further studies with a larger group of patients and a more discriminative method for mRNA quantification are needed to substantiate these preliminary data. These studies are currently underway.

Acknowledgments. The authors express their thanks to PD Dr. M. Kneba, Dr. C. Pott and I. Bolz for various suggestions and help in DNA sequencing.

References

1. Hillen, H., Wessels, J., Haanen, C.: Bone-marrow-proliferation patterns in acute myeloblastic leukemia determined by pulse cytophotometry. Lancet, 15, 609–611, 1975
2. Kantarjian, H.M., Barlogie, B., Keating, M.J., Hall, R.R.: Pretreatment cytokinetics in acute myeloid leukemia. J. Clin Invest, 76, 319–324, 1985
3. Lacombe, F., Belloc, F., Dumain, P., Puntous, M., Makhoul, P.C., Saux, M.-C., Bernhard, P., Boisseau, M.R., Reiffers, J.: Detection of cytarabine resistance in patients with acute myelogenous leukemia using flow cytometry. Blood, 84, 716–723, 1994
4. Ross, D., Thompson, B.W., Joneckis, C.C., Akman, S.A., Schiffer, C.A., Metabolism, of araC by blast cells from patients with ANLL. Blood, 68, 76–82, 1986
5. Rustum, Y.M., Preisler, H.D.: Correlation between leukemic cell retention of 1-ß-D-arabinofuranosylcytosine 5'-triphosphate and response to therapy. Cancer Res 39, 42–49, 1979
6. Preisler, H.D., Rustum, Y., Priore, R.L.: Relationship between leukemic cell retention of cytosine arabinoside triphosphate and the duration of remission in patients with acute non-lymphocytic leukemia. Eur J Cancer Clin Oncol 21, 23–30, 1985.
7. Tattersall, M.H.N., Ganeshaguru, K., Hoffbrand, A.V.,: Mechanism of resistance of human acute leukemia cells to cytosine arabinoside. Br J Hematol 27, 390–046, 1974
8. Colly, L.P., Peters, W.G., Richel, D., Arentsen-Honder, M.W., Starrenburg, C.W., Willemze, R.: Deoxycytidine kinase and deoxycytidine deaminase values correspond closely to clinical response to cytosine arabinoside remission induction therapy in patients with acute myelogenous leukemia. Semin Oncol 14, 257–261, 1987
9. Lilienmark, J.O., Plunkett, W.: Regulation of 1-ß-D arabinofura-nosylcytosine 5'-triphosphate accumulation in human leukemic cells by deoxycytidine 5' triphosphate. Cancer Res 46, 1079–1083, 1986
10. Jamieson, G.P., Snook, M.B., Wiley, J.S.: Saturation of intracellular cytosine arabinoside triphosphate accumulation in human leukemic blast cells. Leukemia Res 14, 475–479, 1990
11. Stuart, D.C., Burke, P.J.: Cytidine deaminase and development of resistance to arabinosylcytosine. Nature New Biol 233, 109–110, 1971
12. Symth, J.F., Robins, A.B., Leese, C.L.: The metabolism of cytosine arabinoside as a predictive test for clinical response to the drug in acute myeloid leukemia. Eur J Cancer, 12, 567–573, 1976
13. Chiba, P., Tihan, T., Szekeres,T., Salamon,J., Kraupp,M., Eher,R., Köller,U., Knapp,W.: Concordant changes in pyrimidine metabolism in blasts of two cases of acute myeloid leukemia after repeated treatment with ara-C in vivo. Leukemia, 4, 761–765, 1990
14. Flasshove, M., Strumberg, D., Ayscue, L., Mitchell, B.S., Tirier, C., Heit, W., Seeber, S., Schütte, J.: Structural analysis of deoxycytidine kinase gene in patients with accute myeloid leukemia and resistance to cytosine arabinoside. Leukemia 8, 780–785.
15. Whelan, J., Smith, T., Phear, G., Rohatiner, A., Lister, A., Meuth, M.: Resistance to cytosine arabi-

noside in acute leukemia: the significance of mutations in CTP synthetase. Leukemia 1994. 8; 264-265
16. Kühn, K., Bertling, W.M., Emmrich, F.: Cloning of a functional cDNA for human cytidine deaminase (CDD) and its use as a marker of monocyte/ macrophage differentiation. Biochem Biophys Res Commun 1993, 190; 1-7
17. Aposhian, H.V., Kornberg, A.: Enzymatic synthesis of deoxyribonucleic acid J Biol Chem 237, 519-525, 1962
18. Hammond, R.A., Byrnes, J.J., Miller, M.R. : Identification of DNA polymerases in CV-1 cells: studies implicating both DNA polymerase alpha and DNA polymerase delta in DNA replication. Biochemistry 26, 6817-6824, 1987
19. Sambrook, J., Fritsch, E.F., Maniatis, T. In: Nolan, C., Ford, N., Ferguson, M (eds.). Molecular cloning. A laboratory manual. Cold Spring Harbor Laboratory Press 1989, E 19
20. Chomczynski, P., Cacchi, N. Single-step method for RNA isolation by acid guanidium thiocyanate-phenol-chloroform extraction. Anal Biochem 1987, 162; 156-159.
21. Linke, B., Bolz, I., Pott, C., Hiddemann, W., Kneba, M. A novel PCR based technique for identification of clonally rearranged immunoglobulin heavy chain genes. Onkologie 1994, 17 (suppl. 2); 91
22. Meyers, M.B., Kreis, W.: Structural comparison of deoxycytidine kinases purified from sensitive (P815) or resistant (P815/araC) to 1-ß-D-arabinofuranosylcytosine. Cancer Res 38, 1099-1104, 1978
23. Rogers, A.M., Hill, R., Lehman, A.R., Arlett, C.F., Burns, V.W.: The induction and characterisation of mouse lymphoma L 5178Y cell lines resistant to 1-ß-D arabinofuranosylcytosine. Mutat Res 69, 139-148, 1980
24. Bhalla, K., Nayak, R., Grant, S.: Isolation and characterization of a deoxycytidine kinase deficient human promyelocytic leukemic cell line highly resistant to 1-ß-D-arabinofuranosylcytosine. Cancer Res 44, 5029-5037, 1984
25. Kreis, W., Lesser, M., Budman, D.R., Arlin, Z., DeAngelis, L., Baskind, P., Feldman, E.J., Akerman, S.: Phenotypic analysis of 1-ß-D-arabinofuranosylcytosine deamination in patients treated with high doses and correlation with response. Cancer Chemother Pharmacol 30, 126-130, 1992

Acute Leukemias VI
Prognostic Factors
and Treatment Strategies
Büchner et al. (eds)

CD7+CD4-CD8-Blast Cells in Acute Leukemia

D.F. Gluzman, I.V. Abramenko, N.I. Belous, L.M. Sklyarenko, L.Y. Poludnenko, S.N. Gaidukova, V.D. Drozdova, S.B. Donskaya, and E.A. Lyvshits

Abstract. Immunocytochemical methods (PAP and APAAP) and monoclonal antibodies (MoAbs) were applied against leukocyte differentiation antigens. In 16 of 89 examined children and 112 adult patients with different forms of acute leukemias (AL), blasts with phenotype CD7+CD4−CD8− were revealed. Three cases were diagnosed as pre-T ALL 6 cases as AL of myeloid origin (AML M0, M1, M4 and M5a by FAB classification). In two biphenotypical AL, lymphoid (CD 10), myeloid (CD 33) and erythroid (glycophorin A) antigens or markers of lymphoid (CD10, CD37) and monocytes (CD14) were coexpressed on CD7+CD4−CD8− blast cells. CD7=CD4− CD8− blast cells of 5 patients had minimal cytochemical and immunological signs of differentiation.

Introduction

The study of morphological and cytochemical features of blast cells is the foundation of universally recognized FAB classification of acute leukemias. It is succesfully supplemented with immunophenotypical investigations using monoclonal antibodies (MoAbs) that allow distinction of different forms of acute lymphoblastic (ALL) and myeloblastic (AML) leukemias.

Owing to the immunophenotyping it was found that in some cases of leukemias certain lymphoid antigens were expressed on myeloid blast cells and vice versa [1,2]. It was supposed that these so-called biphenotypical leukemias arise from early hematological cell precursors [3]. Andrews et al. [4] identified, in human adult bone marrow, polypotential colony-forming cells expressing beside CD34 (antigen of stem cells), also CD7, the antigen of T-lymphocytes. Kurtzberg et al. [5] described the new form of acute leukemia with CD7+CD4−CD8− phenotype, arising from hematopoietic stem cells. Malignant transformed blast cells in this leukemia are capable of in vitro differentiation in myeloid and lymphoid directions. The aim of the present study is the characterization of immunophenotypical features of CD7+ CD4− CD8− acute leukemias (AL) and the detection of possible heterogeneity of this disease.

Materials and Methods

Sixteen of a total of 184 patients with AL for whom immunophenotypic analysis of blast cell antigens was carried out during 1991-1995 were included in the study. The diagnosis of AL was established on the basis of clinical and hematological data and morphological examination of bone marrow and peripheral blood smears. The recognition of AL forms was carried out according to FAB classification. Cytochemical reactions include the detection of activity of myeloperoxidase (MPO), nonspecific a-naphthyl acetate esterase (NE), acid phosphatase (AP), acid nonspecific esterase (ANAE) and PAS reaction [6] (Table 1). For detection of antigens on surface membrane of blast cells the immunocytochemical PAP and avidin-biotin-alkaline phosphatase methods were applied[7]. MoAbs used in the study are indicated in Table 2. In some cases the antigens CD38 [8], CD37 [9].

R.E. Kavetsky Institute of Experimental Pathology, Oncology and Radiobiology, Kiev, Ukraine

Table 1. Cytochemical sdigns of blast cells in CD7+ CD4− CD8− acute leukemias

Patient/FAB classification	Myelo-peroxidase	Acid phosphatase	Acid non-specific esterase	Non-Specific α-naphtyl acetate esterase	PAS reaction
1/M4	50%	diffuse	diffuse	strong, NaF-sensitive	diffuse
2/M4	35%	diffuse	diffuse	strong, NaF-sensitive	diffuse
3/M5	6%	diffuse	diffuse	strong, NaF-sensitive	diffuse
4/M5	1%	diffuse	diffuse	strong, NaF-sensitive	diffuse
5/M1	8%	negative	negative	weak, NaF-sensitive	granular 5%
6/M1	10%	negative	negative	weak, NaF-sensitive	negative
7/M0	0%	negative	negative	weak, NaF-sensitive	granular, 5%
8/ALL, pre-T	0%	local	negative	ND	negative
9/ALL, pre-T	0%	local	granular	weak	granular, 5%
10/ALL, pre-T	0%	local	granular	ND	granular, 10%
11/ALL, pre-T	0%	local	ND	ND	negative
12/AL	0%	diffuse, 50%	diffuse, 50%	ND	granular, 8%
13/AL	0%	granular, 50%	granular, 50%	ND	granular, 5%
14/AL	0%	granular, 50%	granular, 50%	weak	granular, 7%
15/AL	0%	granular, 50%	granular, 50%	weak	granular, 2%
16/AL	0%	granular, 30%	granular, 50%	weak	granular, 2%

ND, Activity of enzyme was not determined.

Table 2. Phenotypical signs of blast cells in CD7+ CD4− CD8− acute leukemias

Patients/FAB classification	ANTIGENS											
	CD7	HLA-DR	CD5	CD4	CD8	CD20	CD10	CD13	CD33	CD34	CD14	CD15
1/M4	+	−	−	−	−	−	±	ND	+	−	+	+
2/M4	+	+	−	−	−	−	−	±	+	−	+	+
3/M5	+	+	ND	−	−	−	−	ND	ND	ND	+	+
4/M5	+	±	−	−	−	−	−	±	±	−	+	+
5/M1	+	+	−	−	−	−	−	±	−	−		−
6/M1	+	−	−	−	−	−	−	−	−	−	−	−
7/M0	+	+	−	−	−	−	±	ND	+	+	±	−
8/Pre-T ALL	+	±	±	−	−	−	−	−	−	±	−	−
9/Pre-T ALL	+	−	±	−	−	−	−	−	−	−	−	−
10/Pre-T ALL	+	±	±	−	−	−	−	ND	ND	ND	−	−
11/PRE-T ALL	+	+	−	−	−	−	±	ND	±	ND	−	−
12/AL	+	+	ND	−	−	−	−	ND	−	−	−	+
13/AL	+	+	−	−	−	−	−	ND	ND	±	−	−
14/AL	+	−	−	−	−	−	−	−	−		−	−
15/AL	+		−	−	−	−	−	ND	ND	ND		−
16/AL	+	+	−	−	−	−	−	−	−	+	−	+

+, 80–100% of positive-reacting cells; ±, 40–50% of positive-reacting cells; − negative reaction with MoAbs; ND, antigen was not determined.

CD45RA [10], glycophorin A [11], receptors of CSF - GM and c-kit, proteins of myeloid cells p8 and p14 [12] were detected.

Results

Based on morphological and cytochemical features of blast cells, we distinguished the following variants of CD7+CD4−CD8− AL: acute monoblastic leukemia (AMonL M5), 2 patients; acute myelomonoblastic leukemia (AMMonL, M4), 2 patients, acute myeloblastic leukemia (AML; M0 and M1), 3 patients; acute lymphoblastic leukemia (ALL), 9 patients.

Blast cells from patients with AML M4 and AMonL M5 has the activity of AP, ANAE, NE and diffuse PAS reaction. The activity of NE was sensitive to NaF. Myeloid antigens CD33, CD14, and CD15 were expressed on surface membranes in addition to CD7 antigen.

Cases of CD7+ AML belonged to the less differentiated variants M1 and M0: most blast cells were peroxidase negative (>90%) and did not display AP and ANAE activity or PAS-positive substance; the activity of NE was detected as single fine granules. More differentiated myeloperoxidase positive blast cells of 14 patients of AML, M2 (used for comparison) were CD7−. On the surface membrane of CD7+ blast cells in AML, Ml, most of the studied linear-specific markers were not detected. The expression of CD13 antigen and receptors for CSF-GM and c-kit testified to the myeloid nature of blast cells from patient 5. Blast cells of patient 6 were still less differentiated: antigens CD13, CD33, CD34 receptors for CSF-GM and c-kit weren't expressed, but the highly specific markers of cells of myeloid origin, p8 and p14 [13] were detected in the cytoplasm of 15% of blast cells.

According to most phenotypical features, the blast cells of patient 7 corresponded to polypotential colony-forming unit cells (CFU-GEMM) [14]. The activity of enzymes was not detected; PAS reaction was negative; antigens CD34, CD33, HLA-DR and, CD45RA were expressed simultaneously. On this basis, supported by the myeloid orientation of blast cells, AML M0 was diagnosed.

The diagnosis of 4 patients (nos.8–11) on morphological and cytochemical features of blast cells (myeloperoxidase-negative, dot-line reaction on AP) was pre-T-ALL. Blast cells of patients 8 and 9 (2 and 10 years old) in this group had the most complete characterization. Using broad set of markers (including MoAbs to receptors to CSF-GM, c-kit, p8 and p14–all these reagents did not react with blast cells) we studied their phenotype (CD7+CD4−CD8−CD38+CD33−HLA−DR−CD45RA+CD45RO−) and thus detected one-way lymphoid direction of its differentiation. In contrast, the most malignant cells of patient 11 (45 years old) beside antigens CD7 and HLA-DR also expressed antigens CD10 and CD33 and small population of these blast cells reacted with MoAbs HAE3, directed to glycophorin A, i.e. coexpressed markers of different lines of hematopoiesis. In this connection the suggestion about the origin of adult ALL from cells that are common precursors of lympho- and myelopoiesis is worthy of note. At the same time, the target cells for leukemic transformation in pediatric (excluding infant leukemias) are considered to be the precursors of only lymphopoiesis [15].

In the separate group we picked out patients 12–16, whose blast cells had cytomorphological features of lymphoblasts, were myeloperoxidase - negative, and were AP and ANAE negative or the activities of AP and ANAE were detected in single blasts as fine granules or diffuse staining of cytoplasm. PAS reaction was observed in 2–8% of blast cells. Stable expression of CD7 on blast cells of these patients was combined with the absence of most studied antigens and, non-typical for ALL of T-cell origin,. activity of AP and ANAE. In cytoplasm of 11% of blast cells of patient 13, p8 was revealed, typical for cells of myeloid origin.

Discussion

The results of our study revealed that expression of CD7 antigen is detected on hematopoietic precursor cells of different lineages. Using a relatively wide set of MoAbs we picked out such variants of CD7+CD4−CD8−AL:

1. AL of myeloid origin - M1, M4 and M5 variants according to the FAB classification (patients 1–6). It should be taken into account that the expression of CD7 persisted on monoblasts of relatively late stage of differentiation (blast cells had strong activity of AC, ANAE, marked PAS positivity, expressed CD14 and CD15 antigens), whereas expression of CD7 on myeloblasts disappeared during its maturation (cases of CD7+ AML, M1 and CD7− AML, M2 correspondingly).

2. ALL of T-cell origin (patients 8–10).
3. biphenotypical AL - AL with blast cells coexpressing antigens of different linear specificity. In this group we included patients 7 and 11. In peripheral blood of the latter patient we revealed the presence of CD10, CD33 and glycophorin A positive blast cells. The phenotype of blast cells of the first patient corresponded in general to polypotential colony-forming units that served as a basis for diagnosis of AML, M0, but some lymphoid (CD10, CD37) and monocytic (CD14) antigens also were detected on 30-40% of blast cells.
4. AL with minimal cytochemical and immunological signs of differentiation of blast cells (patients 12–16).

Cases of AL classified as biphenotypic AL and AL with minimal signs of differentiation may possibly CD7+CD4−CD8− AL arising from hematopoietic stem cells, as described by Kurtzberg et al. [5]. In the first of the two cases blast cells has phenotypical indication of differentiation to different lines of hematopoiesis in vivo. In the second case we did not find any conclusive proof of the possible way of development of malignant transformed hematopoietic cells. Using the routine morphological and cytochemical criteria of the FAB classification, the primary diagnosis of these two patients was ALL. So we presume that the set of MoAbs for immunophenotyping of blast cells from myeloperoxidase negative AL, especially adult ALL, must include, without fail, MoAbs to myeloid, erythroid and megakaryocytic antigens.

The proposal of Kurtzberg et al. [5] to distinguish CD7+CD4−CD8− "stem cell" AL is apparently justified, but phenotypical features of blast cells of this form of AL are in need of more accurate definition.

References

1. Stass S A, Mirro J (1985) Lineage heterogeneity in acute leukemia: acute mixed lineage leukemia and lineage switch. Clin Hematol 15: 811–821.
2. Gale R P, Bassat I B (1987) Hybrid acute leukemia. Brit J Hematol 73: 261–264.
3. Zutter M M, Martin P J, Hanke D, Kidd P G (1990) CD7+acute non-lymphocytic leukemia: evidence for an early multipotential progenitor. Leukemia Res 14: 23–26.
4. Andrews R C, Singer J W, Bernstein I D (1986) Monoclonal antibody 12-8 recognizes a 115 kD molecule present on both unipotent and multipotent hematopoietic colony forming cells and other precursors. Blood 67: 342–344.
5. Kurtzberg J, Waldmann T A, Davey M P (1989) CD7+CD4−CD8− acute leukemia: a syndrome of malignant pluripotent lymphohematopoietic cells. Blood 73: 381–390.
6. Gluzman D F, Sidorenko S P, Nadgornaya V A (1982) Cytochemistry and immunocytology of malignant lymphoproliferative disorders. Kiev: Naukova dumka
7. Pinchouk V G, Gluzman D F, Nadgornaya V A (1990) Immunocytochemistry and monoclonal antibodies in oncohematology. Kiev: Naukova dumka.
8. Baryshnikov A Yu, Kadagidze Z G, Machnova L A, Tupytsin N N (1989) Immunological phenotype of leukemic cell. Moscow: Medizina.
9. Sidorenko S P, Vetrova E P, Yurchenko O V, Berdova A G, Gluzman D F (1992) Monoclonal antibodies of IPO series against B cell differentiation antigens in leukemia and lymphoma immunophenotyping. Neoplasma 39: 3–11.
10. Filatov A B, Bachurin P S, Alexeev L. (1988) Biotechnological methods in estimation of human immune status. J of D. I. Mendeleev all-Union Chemical society 23: 561–566.
11. Mechetner E B, Gluzman D F., Rosinova E N, Nadgornaya V A (1989) Immunoenzymatic cytochemical studies in oncohematology. Hematol Transfusiol 2: 57–60.
12. Leukocyte Typing V. Ed. Schlossman S., Boumsell L., Gilks W.R. - Oxford University Press, Oxford, 1994 -543p.
13. Imamichi T, Uchida I, Wahl S (1993) Expression and cloning of migration inhibitory factor - (MPR) related protein 8 and protein MRP 14 in arthritis-susceptible rats. Biochem Biophys Res Commun 194: 819–825.
14. Strobl H. Takimoto M, Majdic O (1993) Myeloperoxidase expression in CD34 normal human hematopoietic cells. Blood 82: 2069–2078.
15. Greaves M (1993) A natural history for pediatric acute leukemia. Blood 82: 1043–1050.

Acute Leukemias VI
Prognostic Factors
and Treatment Strategies
Büchner et al. (eds)

Lymphoid Antigen Expression in Acute Myeloid Leukemia

G. Specchia, G. Palumbo, A. Mestice, D. Mininni, M. Fiore, P. Carluccio, A. Quarta, G. Debellis, C. De Cillis, and V. Liso

Abstract. Leukemic blasts of some patients with AML display surface lymphoid-associated antigens (AML Ly+). The incidence of these lymphoid antigens in AML varies considerably among different studies (from 13% to 60%). Frequently, the presence of asynchronous and mixed-lineage antigen expression is associated with poor outcome in AL.

Immunophenotypes for 209 patients with AML were analyzed using a wide panel of monoclonal antibodies, and surface marker analysis was performed by immunofluorescence (APAAP). All cases expressed one or two myeloid-associated antigens (CD13, CD33, CD14, CD15). Of 209 cases, 91 (44%) expressed at least one lymphoid-associated antigen (CD7 21%, CD4 22%, CD2 12%, CD3 3%, CD19 5%, CD10 20%). The incidence of Ag Ly expression in FAB subgroups was 91% in M0 cases (10/11), 42% in M1 (6/13), 40% in M2 (32/81), 37% in M3 (11/30), 48% in M4 (16/33), 52% in M5 (14/27), 15% in M6 (2/13) and 0% in M7.

No significant differences were found between Ly+ and Ly- AML patients as regards presenting clinical features and complete remission rate. There was greater expression of CD7, CD4 and CD2 antigen in M0/M1, M4/M5 and M3 FAB types, respectively. We confirm the relevant frequency of lymphoid markers, particularly T (40%), less often B (4%), on the surface of AML blasts.

Introduction

The classification of AML has traditionally been based on a combination of morphological and cytochemical staining features [1, 2]. The use of a large panel of monoclonal antibodies (MoAb) for immunophenotyping AML has shown that antigens of different lineage (lymphoid antigens) are coexpressed by a significant percentage of leukemic blasts (Ly+ AML) [3–10]. The variable incidence of Ly+ AML (13%–60%) is probably related to different study populations (children vs adults), use of fresh or frozen samples, use of flow cytometry, immunofluorescence microscopy or immunoenzymatic staining, different cut-off levels of positivity, and different panels of MoAb [11]. In other reports, correlation with FAB morphology has been found for CD4 (with M4/M5) [12], CD7, (M0, M1, M2) [13–15], and CD2 (M3, M3v) [16]. Except for CD7+ AML, no consistent prognostic relevance of other LyAg has been shown [17–19], and no cytogenetic anomaly is specifically associated with these leukemias [18, 20].

The pathophysiological mechanism involved is controversial: some authors suppose that malignant transformation leads to aberrant gene expression ("lineage infidelity"); others that coexpression of lineage-specific antigens occurs normally in the differentiation of hematopoietic cells ("lineage promiscuity") [21].

In this study, we investigated the immunophenotype of 209 previously untreated patients with AML, in order to assess the incidence of lymphoid antigen expression, its correlation

Hematology Service, University of Bari, 70124 Bari, Italy

with the FAB classification and its possible clinical significance.

Materials and Methods

Patients

The study included 209 patients, all at onset of disease, with a median age of 60 years (range 15–87); their clinical and immunological features are shown in Table 1. The diagnosis of AML was on the basis of the morphologic and cytochemical criteria established by the FAB Cooperative Group [1].

Immunophenotype

Cell surface antigens were detected by standard direct or indirect immunofluorescence using the monoclonal antibodies to HLA-DR, CD11b, CD13, CD14, CD15, CD33, CD34, CD2, CD3, CD4, CD5, CD7, CD8, CD10, CD19. Staining of at least 20% of cells was considered positive for all antigens. Coexpression of lymphoid and myeloid antigens by single cells was confirmed by two-colour immunofluorescence and flow cytometric analysis, using phycoerythrin (PE)- and fluorescein isothiocyanate (FITC)-conjugated MoAb (FACScan, Becton Dickinson). The same MoAb were also evaluated by the immunocytochemical method (APAAP) on cytospins from freshly prepared mononuclear cells separated by Ficoll-Hypaque density centrifugation. Surface immunophenotyping was always performed on fresh samples.

Table 1. Clinical and immunological features of 209 AML cases

	Ly+	Ly-
No. of cases	91 (44%)	118 (56%)
Age	59 (15–82)	60 (15–87)
M/F	54/37	60/58
Hb (g/dl)	8.4 (4.05–15.3)	8.3 (4–14.7)
WBC ($\times 10^9$/l)	18.6 (0.7–241.7)	14 (0.3–222)
Plt ($\times 10^9$/l)	49 (7–574)	43 (3–296)
FAB		
M0	10 91%	1
M1	6 42%	7 58%
M2	32 40%	49 60%
M3	11 37%	19 63%
M4	16 48%	17 52%
M5	14 52%	13 48%
M6	2 15%	11 85%
M7	0	1

Statistical Analysis

A two-sample t-statistic was used to compare the means for clinical and immunophenotypic data of the two groups, LyAg+ and LyAg- AML. A probability value of < 0.05 was considered to be significant. Potential differences in lymphoid antigen expression in the FAB subgroups were evaluated using the chi squared test. We also used the chi squared test for evaluating differences in complete remission rate between Ly+ and Ly- AML cases.

Results

The laboratory features are shown in Table 1; the cases were classified as 11 M0, 13 M1, 81 M2, 30 M3, 33 M4, 27 M5, 13 M6 and 1 M7, according to the FAB criteria. No differences were observed between LyAg+ and LyAg- AML as regards age, hemoglobin content, WBC, and platelet count.

The incidence of antigen expression is reported in Table 2: the myeloid antigens CD13 and CD33 were expressed by 98% and 94% of

Table 2. Incidence of antigen expression

Antigen	No. of cases tested	Positive cases (%)
Myeloid-associated		
CD33	209	94
CD13	205	97
CD15	175	47
CD11b	159	47
CD14	204	22
Any myeloid	116	99
T-lymphoid-associated		
CD2	177	12
CD3	178	3
CD4	177	22
CD5	106	4
CD7	205	21
CD8	196	4
Any T	122	40
B-lymphoid-associated		
CD19	167	5
CD10	176	2
Any B	142	4
CD34	179	56
HLA-DR	184	80

patients, respectively, CD14 by 22% and the stem cell marker CD34 by 56%. The incidence of lymphoid antigen expression was 44% (91/209), subdivided into 40% (49/122) for T-and 4% (6/142) for B-lymphoid antigents.

The expression of lymphoid-associated markers in the morphologically defined subgroups was 91% in M0 cases (10/11), 42% in M1 (6/13), 40% in M2 (32/81), 37% in M3 (11/30), 48% in M4 (16/30), 52% in M5 (14/27), 15% in M6 (2/13), and 0% in M7 (Table 1). The most frequently expressed antigens, were CD4 (22%), CD7 (22%), and CD2 (12%). In particular, we found that CD4 was expressed in 39% (19/49) M4/M5 cases and 15% (19/128) of other types ($p<.005$); CD2 was expressed in 37% (10/27) M3 cases and in 7% (10/140) of other types; CD7 was expressed in 50% (12/24) M0/M1 cases and in 17% (30/181) of other FAB types (for these two antigens, x^2 could not be evaluated due to the small number of cases).

No significant differences were found between Ly+ and Ly- AML patients as regards presenting clinical features and complete remission rate.

Of the 209 patients included in this study, 108 were selected for age (<60 years) and homogeneous treatment schema, but 26 of these were excluded, having died of severe bone marrow hypoplasia during induction chemotherapy. Complete remission was achieved in 70% (57/82) of cases treated with GIMEMA protocols (AML 8A/B and AML 10) [22]: more precisely, the complete remission rate was 61% (23/38) in Ly+ and 77% (34/44) in Ly- AML patients (n.s) (Table 3).

Discussion

Although several studies have demonstrated that leukemic blasts simultaneously express markers of both the lymphoid and the myeloid lineage, the clinical and prognostic significance of mixed lineage expression remains uncertain. The incidence of "abnormal" antigen expression in AL is extremely variable, ranging from 13% to 60%; this large variability is related to different series (children or adults) and methods used (fresh or cryopreserved samples, MoAb, flow cytometry, immunofluorescence, immunocytochemistry) [11].

We reported the incidence and the clinical significance of myeloid antigens expression in acute lymphoblastic leukemia (ALL) in a previous study [23].

In the present study we have evaluated the expression of "lymphoid-associated" markers in AML, classified using FAB criteria. It is currently thought that some surface antigens (CD2, CD3, CD5, CD8, CD19, CD20, CD21, CD22) are displayed only by cells of the lymphoid lineage, while expression of other surface antigens, originally regarded as lymphoid-specific, has been clearly demonstrated on both lymphoid and myeloid cells: CD4, expressed by T cells and mobocytes [24], CD10, by preB cells and granulocytes [25], and CD7, by T cells and a subset of myeloid progenitors [26]. Thus it is necessary to evaluate the specificity of each marker before considering its significance.

In our study the incidence of lymphoid-associated antigens in AML was 44% (91/209), subdivided into 40% for T- and 4% for B-lymphoid antigens. The most frequently expressed were CD4 (22%), CD7 (21%), and CD2 (12%). As expected, CD4 positivity was found significantly more often in M4 and M5 cases (39% in M4/M5 cases vs 15% in other cytotypes). CD2 was expressed in 37% of M3 cases, all M3 variants, and in 7% of other types. Other authors have reported a high incidence of CD2 (adhesion molecule) in M3 variant promyelocytes, but the biological significance of this expression is unknown [16]. CD7 was most often detected in the less differentiated AML: in 50% of M0/M1 cases and in 17% of other FAB types. No significant differences were found between Ly+ and Ly- AML patients as regards expression of CD34 (progenitor cell antigen).

Although contradictory results are reported in the literature on the prognostic impact of expression of lymphoid-associated antigens in AML [17,18,27], CD7 seems to be associated with poor prognosis in AML [19]: CD7+ AML may represent a particular subset of immature

Table 3. Response to induction therapy in 108 Ly+ and Ly− patients

	Ly+	Ly−
No. of cases	48	60
CR	23 (61%)	34 (77%)
NR	15 (39%)	10 (23%)
Early death	10	16
Duration of CR (months)	9.5 (2–47)	8 (1–45)

AML (M0/M1) with a higher resistance to therapy than other differentiated subgroups of AML.

No significant differences were found between Ly+ and Ly- AML patients as regards presenting clinical features and complete remission rate (Table 3) (CR 61% in Ly+ and 77% in Ly-).

We consider that the presence of lymphoid-associated antigens in myeloid blasts does not confer "distinct clinical identity" but that further studies are needed to assess the biological significance of uncommon antigen expression in normal and leukemic myeloid cells.

References

1. Bennett JM, Catovsky D, Daniel MT, Flandrin G, Galtan DAG, Gralnik HR, Sultan G (1976) Proposal for the classification of the acute leukemias. Br J Haematol 33: 451-58.
2. Castoldi GL, Liso V, Fenu S, Vegna ML, Mandelli F (1993) Reproducibility of the morphological diagnostic criteria for acute myeloid leukemia: the GIMEMA group experience. Ann Hematol 66:171-74.
3. Greaves MF, Chan LC, Furley AJW, Watt SM, Molgaard HV (1986) Lineage promiscuity in hemopoietic differentiation and leukemia. Blood 67: 1-11.
4. Drexel HG (1987) Classification of acute myeloid leukemia-A comparison of FAB and immunophenotyping. Leukemia 1:697-705.
5. Mirro J Jr, Kitchingman GR (1989) The morphology, cytochemistry, molecular characteristics and clinical significance of acute mixed-lineage leukaemia. In Scott Cs, ed. Leukaemia cytochemistry. Chichester: Ellis Horwood, pp. 155-79.
6. Terstappen LWMM, Safford M, Konemann S, Loken MR, Zurlutter K, Buckner T, Hiddeman W, Wormann B (1991) Flow cytometric characterization of acute myeloid leukemia. Part II. Phenotypic heterogeneity at diagnosis. Leukemia 5: 757-67.
7. Griffin JD, Davis R, Nelson DA, Davey FR, Mayer RJ, Shiffer C, McIntyre OR, Bloomfield CD (1986) Use of surface marker analysis to predict outcome of adult acute myeloblastic leukemia. Blood 68: 1232-41.
8. Del Canizo C, San Miguel JF, Gonzales M, Anta JP, Orfao A, Lopez Borrasca A (1987) Discrepancies between morphologic, cytochemical and immunologic characteristics in acute myeloblastic leukemia. Am J Clinic Pathol 88: 38-42.
9. Neame PB, Soamboonsrup B, Browman GP, Meyer RM, Benger A, Wilson WEC, Walker IR, Saeed N, McBride JA (1986) Classifying acute leukemia by immuno-phenotyping: a combined FAB-immunologic classification of AML. Blood 68: 1355-62.
10. Oster W, Konig K, Ludwig WD, Ganser A, Lindemann A, Mertelsmann R, Herrmann F (1988) Incidence of lineage promiscuity in acute myeloblastic leukemia: diagnostic implication of immunoglobulin and T-cell receptor gene rearrangement analysis and immunological phenotyping. Leuk Res 12: 887-95.
11. Drexler HG, Thiel E, and Ludwig WD (1993) Acute myeloid leukemias expressing lymphoid-associated antigens: diagnostic incidence and prognostic significance. Leukemia 7 (4): 489-98.
12. Vidriales MB, Orfao A, Gonzales M, Hernandez JM, Lopez-Berges, Garcia MC, Caballero MD, Macedo A, Landolfi C, San Miguel (1993) Expression of NK and lymphoid associated antigens in blast cells of acute myeloblastic leukemia. Leukemia 7: 2026-29
13. Lo Coco F, De Rossi G, Pasqualetti D, Lopez M, Diverio D, Latagliata R, Fenu S, Mandelli F (1989) CD7 positive acute myeloid leukemia: a subtype associated with cell immaturity. B J Haematol 73: 480-85.
14. Auger MJ, Ross JA, Ross FM, Ford A, Rassel L, Graig JI, Mackie MJ (1992) CD7 positive acute myeloblastic leukaemia: an heterogenous leukaemic subtype. Leuk Lymphoma 6: 487-91.
15. Bassan R, Biondi A, Benvestito S, Tini ML, Abbate M, Viero P, Barbui T, Rambaldi A (1992) Acute undifferentiated leukemia with CD7+ and CD13+ immunophenotype. Cancer 69: 396-404.
16. Rovelli A, Biondi A, Cantù Rajnoldi, Conter V, Giudici G, Jankovic M, Locasciulli A, Rizzari C, Romitti L, Rossi MR, Schirò R, Tosi S, Uderzo C, Masera G (1992) Microgranular variant of acute promyelocytic leukemia in children. J Clin Oncol 10: 1413-18.
17. Smith FO, Lampkin B, Versteeg C, Flowers D, Dinndorf I, Buckley J, Woods W, Hammond D, Bernstein ID (1992) Expression of lymphoid-associated cell surface antigens by childhood acute myeloid leukemia cells lack prognostic significance. Blood 79: 2415-22.
18. Ball ED, Davis RB, Griffin JD, Mayer RJ, Davey FR, Arthur DC, Wurster-Hill D, Noll W, Elghetany MT, Allen SL, Rai K, Lee EJ, Schiffer CA, Bloomfield CD (1991) Prognostic value of lymphocytes surface markers in acute myeloid leukemia. Blood 77: 2242-50.
19. Kita K, Miwa H, Nakase K, Kawakami K, Kobayashi T, Shirakawa S, Tanaka I, Ohta C, Tsutani H, Oguma S, Kyo T, Dohy H, Kamada N, Nasu K, Uchino H (The Japan Cooperative Group of Leukemia/Lymphoma) (1993): Clinical importance of CD7 expression in acute myelocytic leukemia. Blood 81: 2399.
20. Cuneo A, Mecucci C, Kerim S, Vandenberghe E, Dal Cin P, Van Orshoven A, Rodhain J, Bosly A, Michaux JL, Martiat P, Boogaerts M, Carli MG, Castoldi G, Van den Berghe H (1989) Multipotent stem cell involvement in megakaryoblastic leukemia: cytologic and cytogenetic evidence in 15 patients. Blood 74: 1781-98.
21. Drexler HG, Thiel E, Ludwig WD (1991) Review of the incidence and clinical relevance of myeloid antigen-positive acute lymphoblastic leukemia. Leukemia 5: 637-45.

22. Zittoun R, Liso V, Mandelli F, Rotoli B, de Witte T et al. (1992) Intensive consolidation chemotherapy versus standard consolidation maintenance in acute myelogenous leukemia (AML) in first remission: an EORTC/GIMEMA phase III trial (AML 8B). Leukemia 6: Suppl 2: 120–3
23. Specchia G, Pansini N, Mininni D, Mestice A, Debellis G, Ditonno P, Cleopazzo E, Pastore D and Liso V (1994) Myeloid surface antigen expression in adult acute lymphoblastic leukemia. In Acute Leukemias IV Prognostic Factors Buchner et al. Eds: 442–46
24. Steward SJ, Fujimoto J, Levy RJ (1986) Human T-lymphocytes and monocytes bear the same Leu3 (T4) antigen. J Immunol 136: 3773–76.
25. Cossman J, Neckers LM, Leonard WJ, Greene WC (1983) Polymorphonuclear neutrophils express the common acute lymphoblastic leukemia antigen. J Exp Med 157: 1064–69.
26. Chabannon C, Wood P, Simmons PJ, Johnsons G, Torok-Storb B (1990) Normal expression of Cd7 is not restricted to lymphoid cells. Exp Hematol 18: 584.
27. Geller RB, Zahurak M, Hurwitz CA, Burke PJ, Karp JE, Piantadosi S, Civin CI (1990) Prognostic importance of immunophenotyping in adults with acute myelocytic leukaemia: The significance of the stem-cell glycoprotein CD34 (My10) Br J Haematol 76: 340–7.

Acute Leukemias VI
Prognostic Factors
and Treatment Strategies
Büchner et al. (eds)

CD54 Expression and Its Role in Homotypic Aggregation of the Blasts of Acute Myeloblastic (AML) and Acute Lymphoblastic Leukemia (ALL)

J. Krauter, K. Pompe, H. Heimpel, and G. Heil

Abstract. CD54 (ICAM-1) expression was studied on blasts of 13 cases of de novo AML and 10 cases of ALL prior to and after stimulation by interferon-gamma (IFN-γ). Furthermore, its functional activity was studied by analysis of the influence of CD54 on homologous interaction of the blasts. Prior to culture only a minority of the AML and ALL blasts displayed CD54 positivity. Timed incubation of the blasts in RPMI-1640/FCS or serum-free medium "spontaneously" increased the percentage of CD54 positive cells in 11/13 AML cases but only in 2/10 ALL cases. In AML, IFN-γ (500 IU/ml) further enhanced CD54 positivity in 6/11 cases. 2/13 cases showed no CD54 upregulation at all. In 6/10 ALL cases CD54 upregulation after IFN-γ stimulation was found. In AML ICAM-1 expression was paralleled by homologous aggregation of the blasts in that (1) in all but the two CD54 negative cases autologous cluster formation could be detected; (2) IFN-γ enhanced cluster formation in 5/6 cases in which it had enhanced CD54 upregulation; (3) incubation of the blasts in the presence of an anti-CD54 MoAb (clone 84H10) reduced the "spontaneous" and IFN-γ induced cluster formation in the majority of the cases. In ALL only 2/6 cases with CD54 upregulation showed homologous cell aggregation, which could be slightly enhanced by IFN-γ stimulation and inhibited by the anti-CD54 moAb. Taken together, CD54 expression on AML and ALL blasts is heterogeneous with respect to (1) its "constitutional" expression and (2) its "spontaneous" and IFN-γ induced upregulation. While on AML blasts CD54 seems to be funtionally active once expressed on the surface membrane, in at least some ALL cases its function seems to depend on additional activation.

Introduction

The glycoprotein ICAM-1 (intercellular adhesion molecule-1, CD54), is a member of the immunoglobulin superfamily, which is bound to the cell surface membrane with a tissue-specific glycosylation resulting in a molecular weight range of 70–120 kDa [1–3]. ICAM-1 is expressed on cells of both hematopoietic and non-hematopoietic origin, including lymphocytes, monocytes, fibroblasts, epithelial and endothelial cells. Its expression in vivo is low in normal but high in inflamed tissue [2, 3]. This low constitutional expression can be increased in vitro by stimulation with various cytokines, including interferon-gamma (IFN-γ), interleukin-1 (IL-1), tumor necrosis factor (TNF), by certain mitogens and by phorbol esters [3]. ICAM-1 is a ligand for the lymphocyte function associated antigen-1 (LFA-1, CD11a/CD18), a member of the integrin family [4], mediating LFA-1-dependent cell-cell adhesion interaction such as antigen independent conjugate formation, cell mediated cytotoxicity, antigen induced T-cell proliferation and cell-stromal interactions that regulate normal hematopoiesis [2,5–8].

CD54 has also been found on cells of various hemopoietic neoplasms, including acute myeloid leukemias (AML) and acute, lymphoblastic leukemias (ALL) [9, 10], while little is known

Department of Internal Medicine III, University of Ulm, 89081 Ulm, Germany about its regulation of and function in these cells. It was the aim of this study to investigate CD54 expression on AML and ALL blasts and its modulation by in vitro culturing, including stimulation with IFN-γ. Furthermore, its functional activity was studied by analysis of the influence of CD54 on homologous interaction of the blasts by a homotypic aggregation assay, in which homogeneous cell populations adhere to one another to form multicellular clusters [1, 3].

Material and Methods

Leukemic Blasts

Pretreatment leukemic blasts were isolated from peripheral blood or bone marrow of 13 patients with de novo AML and 10 patients with ALL by Ficoll-Isopaque gradient and stored in liquid nitrogen (−196°C) prior to the analysis. The AMLs were classified according to the FAB criteria, the ALL cases according to the immunophenotype (Table 1). After thawing the blasts were enriched by monocyte and T-cell depletion according to usual procedures, resulting in a percentage of blasts of more than 95% and a viability of more than 95% in all cases under study.

Suspension Cultures

The leukemic blasts were incubated in serum-free culture medium (SF medium [11] at a concentration of 1×10^6 cells/ml with or without IFN-γ, kindly provided by Ernst-Boehringer-Institut/Bender Vienna, Austria (final concentration 500 IU/ml), at 37°C, 5% CO_2 in a fully humidified atmosphere for various times. Thereafter the cells were washed three times in SF medium and analyzed by flow cytometry.

Cell Aggregation Assay

The monocyte and T-cell depleted blasts were washed twice with SF medium and resuspended to a concentration of 2×10^6 cells/ml. Aliquots of 100 μl of this cell suspension were added to each well to flat-bottomed, 96 well microtiter plates (Nunc, Wiesbaden, FRG) and incubated at 37°C for different time intervals (12–96 h).

In controls the SF medium was supplemented either with EDTA (final concentration 0.1%) or with the anti-ICAM-1 antibody (CD54, IgG1, Clone 84H10, Dianova, Hamburg, FRG) or with an isotype matched control antibody. The final concentration of the monoclonal antibodies used in this assay was 10% (v/v) or 20 μg protein/ml respectively. To analyze the influence of IFN-γ on homotypic aggregation it was added to the SF medium at a final concentration of 500 IU/ml. The cell aggregate formation was determined at different times by direct visualization of the plates with an inverted light microscope. For quantitative measurement of cell aggregation the number of free cells was counted. Within each well, at least three randomly chosen areas were counted. At least three different wells per analysis were studied. Percent aggregation was determined by the following equation: Percent aggregation = 100 times × (1 − [number of free cells]/[total number of cells]) [1]. The total number of cells was scored in wells where the aggregation had been inhibited by the addition of EDTA to the medium.

Immunophenotyping

Cells were stained with saturating concentrations of fluorescein isothiocyanate-or phycoerythrin-labelled monoclonal antibodies (MoAb) according to standard procedures, fixed in 0.5% paraformaldehyde and analyzed by flow cytometry with an EPICScan (Coulter Electronics, Krefeld, FRG), as described [12].

Results

CD54 Upregulation of the Leukemic Blasts in Suspension Culture

Prior to culture in AML and in ALL only a minority of the blasts displayed CD54 positivity (Table 1). In AML the incubation of the blasts in SF medium for 48 h led to a "spontaneous" upregulation of CD54 expression as detected by an at least twofold increase in the percentage of CD54 positive blasts in 11/13 cases (AML3-AML13). The addition of IFN-γ to the medium further increased CD54 positivity in 6/11 AMLs (AML6-AML11). In the remaining cases no effect of IFN-γ could be detected. 2/13 AMLs showed no CD54 upregulation at all.

In ALL "spontaneous" CD54 upregulation after incubation in SF medium was found only in 2/10 cases (ALL1 and ALL2), whereas in the other cases no CD54 upregulation could be detected even after a 96 h incubation period.

Table 1. Influence of in vitro stimulation on CD54 expression

Patient	Before culture	After 48 h suspension culture	
		Without IFN-γ	With IFN-γ
	% CD54 pos.	% CD54 pos.	% CD54 pos.
AML1 (FAB M2)	4	4	5
AML2 (FAB M3)	2	1	2
AML3 (FAB M5)	0	95	87
AML4 (FAB M5)	0	68	56
AML5 (FAB M4)	11	93	93
AML6 (FAB M1)	11	85	99
AML7 (FAB M4)	15	31	41
AML8 (FAB M4)	17	56	75
AML9 (FAB M4)	17	29	44
AML10 (FAB M2)	28	93	96
AML11 (FAB M4)	29	95	99
AML12 (FAB M5)	30	96	86
AML13 (FAB M1)	31	98	97
ALL1 (c-ALL)	3	75	81
ALL2 (c-ALL)	15	50	74
ALL3 (c-T-ALL)	11	7	14
ALL4 (pre-T-ALL)	65	68	78
ALL5 (c-ALL)	38	38	44
ALL6 (c-ALL)	23	18	35
ALL7 (c-ALL)	6	8	10
ALL8 (pre-pre-B-ALL)	1	8	10
ALL9 (pre-pre-B-ALL)	6	3	4
ALL10 (c-ALL)	2	1	2

Percentage of CD54-positive blasts in the 13 AML and 10 ALL cases directly after isolation and after 48 h incubation in SF medium +/− stimulation with 500 IU/ml IFN-γ. The FAB subtype of the AMLs and the immunophenotype of the ALLs are given in brackets FAB, French-American British classification of AML; c-ALL, $CD10^+$; c-T-ALL, $CD10^+$, $CD2^+$; pre-T-ALL, $CD10^-$, $CD2^-$, $CD5^+$, $CD7^+$; pre-pre-B-ALL, HLA-DR^+, $CD19^+$, $CD10^-$.

Stimulation with IFN-γ led to CD54 upregulation in 6/10 ALL cases (ALL1–ALL6). In 4/10 ALLs no CD54 upregulation was found (Table 1).

Homotypic Cell Aggregation

11/13 AMLs displayed "spontaneous" homotypic aggregation after 24- to 48-h incubation, while the size of the multicellular clusters showed considerable variation among the different leukemias (Table 2). The number and size of the multicellular clusters was markedly (≥10%) enhanced in 5/11 cases (AML7–AML11, Table 2) by the addition of IFN-γ to the medium. The anti-CD54 MoAb (Clone 84H10) substantially reduced both the "spontaneous" and the "IFN-γ induced" cluster formation in 8/11 cases, whereas in a further 3 cases (AML3, AML4, AML12) this MoAb had no detectable effect (Table 2).

In ALL, "spontaneous" cell aggregation was found in 3/10 (ALL2, ALL4, ALL9, Table 2) cases. Stimulation with IFN-γ enhanced cluster formation in 1/3 cases (ALL2) and additionally induced weak cell aggregation in ALL5 (Table 2). The anti CD54 moAb inhibited spontaneous and IFN-γ induced cluster formation in all but 1 case (ALL9). The addition of a control antibody to the medium had no effect on cluster formation of either AML or ALL blasts, whereas EDTA completely inhibited cluster formation in all cases under study.

Discussion

It was the aim of this study to analyze CD54 distribution on AML and ALL blasts prior to and after in vitro culture with or without IFN-γ. In a second set of experiments the influence of CD54

Table 2. Homotypic aggregation after 48 h incubation

Patient	Without IFN-γ			With IFN-γ (500 IU/ml)		
	Medium	Anti-CD54	Control	Medium	Anti-CD54	Control
AML1	8	3	5	8	7	7
AML2	12	13	11	14	12	12
AML3	58	58	46	62	68	60
AML4	63	56	60	68	74	70
AML5	66	20	64	72	25	72
AML6	64	12	61	72	20	79
AML7	56	6	50	72	14	75
AML8	44	17	45	76	15	75
AML9	63	6	60	75	8	80
AML10	55	24	55	75	25	76
AML11	65	14	70	75	17	70
AML12	86	75	80	87	85	83
AML13	70	25	76	70	25	73
ALL1	5	3	8	7	8	7
ALL2	27	7	30	44	6	42
ALL3	5	6	4	7	8	6
ALL4	23	3	25	30	5	32
ALL5	5	7	3	26	5	28
ALL6	5	4	6	5	5	7
ALL7	5	4	7	5	6	4
ALL8	4	6	7	5	5	6
ALL9	56	53	55	55	52	57
ALL10	5	6	4	7	5	8

Homotypic aggregation of the AML and ALL blasts after 48 h incubation in SF medium in the presence or absence of 500 IU/ml IFN-γ. The cells were incubated in SF medium alone (Medium), together with a monoclonal anti-CD54 antibody, clone 84H10 in a 1:10 (v/v) dilution (anti-CD54), or in the presence of a IgG control antibody in the same concentration (control). The aggregation score was calculated as described in Material and Methods.

on homotypic aggregation of the blasts was analyzed.

Prior to culture, AMLs and ALLs showed a low percentage of CD54 positive blasts, as observed by other investigators [9]. In agreement with previous reports [5, 13] and with our own experience with normal monocytes which served as a control [14] (data not shown), timed incubation of the AML blasts in SF medium led to a "spontaneous" upregulation of CD54 expression in 11/13 cases. IFN-g was chosen for stimulation of the leukemic cells because of its known stimulatory effect on CD54 expression in a wide variety of cells [2]. Compared to previous data obtained from normal monocytes [13, 14], IFN-γ exerted only a moderate effect on the AML blasts, in that CD54 upregulation was found only in those cases where also "spontaneous" CD54 upregulation had been observed. Furthermore, IFN-γ induced CD54 upregulation exceeded "spontaneous" CD54 upregulation only in a minority of the cases.

In contrast to AML, only 2/10 ALL cases showed "spontaneous" CD54 upregulation, in agreement with the fact that "spontaneous" CD54 upregulation does not occur in lymphocytes [13]. On the other hand, IFN-γ was more effective regarding CD54 upregulation in ALL than in AML, in that CD54 expression was also induced in cases without "spontaneous" CD54 upregulation. This might reflect different regulation mechanisms of CD54 expression in myeloblasts and lymphoblasts. In myeloblasts "spontaneous" CD54 upregulation may correspond to the maximal inducible CD54 expression, which cannot be exceeded by additional stimulation, e.g. by IFN-γ, whereas in lymphoblasts CD54 expression might be regulated at the mRNA level via cytokine stimulation [13].

In AML evidence for a major role of CD54 in homotypic cell aggregation was found, since (1) all leukemias which were or became CD54 positive displayed homotypic aggregation, whereas the two CD54 negative cases failed to do so; (2)

the homotypic aggregation was inhibited/ reduced by an anti-CD54 MoAb in 8/11 cases; (3) IFN-γ enhanced the homotypic aggregation in the majority of those cases in which an additional effect of IFN-γ on CD54 upregulation could be observed.

In ALL, however, correlation between CD54 expression and cell aggregation was less clear, since CD54 upregulation was not paralleled by cluster formation in 3/6 cases. Such discordance between CD54 surface expression and CD54 function has already been described for fibroblasts [15] and might indicate the need for additional activation of CD54 and/or its ligand(s) after surface expression of these molecules in order to facilitate cell-cell interaction.

In 3/11 AML and in 1/4 ALL cases, the homotypic aggregation remained unaffected by the anti-CD54 MoAb. This indicates that, as has been described, (an)other ligand(s) independent of the LFA-1/ICAM-1 system contribute(s) to the homotypic aggregation of the blasts [16].

Taken together, CD54 expression and its functional activity on AML and ALL blasts is heterogeneous with respect to (1) its "constitutional" expression, (2) its "spontaneous" and IFN-γ induced upregulation and (3) the ability of CD54 surface expression to induce cellular interaction. Since "spontaneous" CD54 upregulation has been described for monocytes but not for lymphocytes [13], the differences in CD54 expression in AML and ALL blasts may be at least in part explained by different regulation mechanisms for CD54 expression in their natural counterparts. The fact that in 2/13 AMLs and 4/10 ALLs no CD54 expression was found may lend support to the hypothesis that in some AML and ALL cases CD54 expression may be defective. Moreover, in AML but not in ALL, CD54 expression is closely correlated to homotypic cell aggregation. This indicates that while on AML blasts CD54 seems to be functionally active once expressed on the surface membrane, in at least some ALL cases its function seems to be dependent on additional activation.

Acknowledgments. The authors are indebted to Mrs. I. Eschmann, Mrs. C. Schöpflin and Mrs. H. Dieth for excellent technical assistance.

References

1. Rothlein R, M.L, Dustin, S.D. Marlin, T.A. Springer A human intercellular adhesion molecule (ICAM-1) distinct from LFA-1.J Immunol 1986; 137: 1270–1274.
2. Dustin ML, R. Rothlein, A.K. Bhan, C.A. Dinarello, T.A. Springer Induction by IL 1 and interferon-gamma: tissue distribution, biochemistry, and function of a natural adherence molecule (ICAM-1). J Immunol 1986; 137: 245–254.
3. Wawryk SO, J.R. Novotny, I.P. Wicks et al. The role of the LFA-1/ICAM-1 interaction in human leukocyte homing and adhesion. Immunol Rev 1989; 108: 135–161.
4. Marlin SD, T.A. Springer Purified intercellular adhesion molecule-1 (ICAM-1) is a ligand for lymphocyte function-associated antigen 1 (LFA-1). cell 1987; 51: 813–819.
5. Arkin S, B. Naprstek, L. Guarini, S. Ferrone, J.M. Lipton Expression of intercellular adhesion molecule-1 (CD54) on hematopoietic progenitors. Blood 1991; 77: 948–953.
6. Makgoba MW, M.E. Sanders, L. G.E. Ginther Luce, et al. ICAM-1 a ligand for LFA-1 dependent adhesion of B, T and myeloid cells. Nature 1988; 331: 86–88.
7. Dougherty GJ, S. Murdoch, N. Hogg The function of human intercellular adhesion molecule-1 (ICAM-1) in the generation of an immune response. Eur J Immunol 1988;18: 35–39.
8. Makgoba MW, M.E. Sanders, Ginther Luce GE, et al. Functional evidence that intercellular adhesion molecule-1 (ICAM-1) is a ligand for LFA-1-dependent adhesion in T cell-mediated cytotoxicity. Eur J Immunol 1988;18:637–640.
9. Maio M, A. Pinto, A. Carbone, et al. Differential expression of CD54/intercellular adhesion molecule-1 in myeloid leukemias and in lymphoproliferative disorders. Blood 1990; 76: 783–790.
10. Boyd AW, S.M. Dunn, J.V. Fecondo, et al. Regulation of expression of human intercellular adhesion molecule 1 (ICAM-1) during lymphohematopoietic differentiation. Blood 1989; 73: 1896–1903.
11. Migliaccio G, A.R. Migliaccio. Cloning of human erythroid progenitors (BFU-E) in the absence of fetal bovine serum. Br J Haematol 1987; 67: 129–133.
12. Heil G,E. Gunsilius, A. Raghavachar, et al. Ultrastructural demonstration of peroxidase expression in acute unclassified leukemias: Correlation to immunophenotype and treatment outcome. Blood 1991; 77: 1305–1312.
13. Möst J, W. Schwaeble, J. Drach, A. Sommerauer, M.P. Dierich. Regulation of the expression of ICAM-1 on human monocytes and mono-

cytic tumor cell lines. J. Immunol 1992; 148: 1635–1642.
14. Heil G, J. Krauter, E. Beyer-Johannböke, D. Bunjes, E. Kurrle, C. Westphal-Frösch, H. Heimpel. CD54 expression and its role in homotypic aggregation of the blasts of acute myeloblastic leukemia. Int J Hematol 1994; 60: 39–49.
15. Piela TH and J.H. Korn. ICAM-1-dependent fibroblast-lymphocyte adhesion: discordance between surface expression and function of ICAM-1. Cell Immunol 1990; 129; 125–137
16. Campanero MR, R. Pulido, M.A. Ursa, M. Rodriguez Moya, de M.O. Landazuri, F. Sanchez Madrid. An alternative leukocyte homotypic adhesion mechanism, LFA-1/ICAM-1-independent, triggered through the human VLA-4 integrin. J Cell Biol 1990; 110: 2157–21–65.

Acute Leukemias VI
Prognostic Factors
and Treatment Strategies
Büchner et al. (eds)

Adhesion Molecule Receptor Profile in Acute Leukemia

M. Reuss-Borst[1], G. Klein[2], H.D. Waller[1], and C.A. Müller[2]

Abstract. A large number of leukemic samples were investigated for the expression of β1-, β2-, β3-integrins, CD44 and 5 splice variants, the selectins and several molecules of the immunoglobulin superfamily in order to evaluate whether variant expression profiles of adhesion molecules are found on leukemic cells in comparison to normal CD34+ hematopoietic precursors. In summary, adhesion molecules such as CD44, LFA-3 (CD58), the β1-integrins VLA-4 and VLA-5 and the β2-integrin LFA-1 (CD11a/CD18) were found on >70% of blasts in most leukemias. Other adhesion molecules seemed to be restricted to specific differentiation stages and lineage. The β2-integrins Mac-1 (CD11b) and gp 150,95 (CD11c) were preferentially expressed on AMLs of the differentiated subtypes M4 and M5, and NCAM (CD56) was found only on a subset of acute myeloid leukemias. Unexpectedly, some adhesion molecules such as the β1-integrins VLA-1, VLA-2, VLA-3 and VLA-6 were expressed on >70% blasts on a subset of leukemias not characterized by a common phenotype. These molecules were not found on normal CD34+ hematopoietic precursors of the bone marrow. Simultaneously obtained blood and bone marrow samples generally revealed a higher percentage of positive blasts in the blood than in bone marrow, possibly due to the up-regulation of these antigens. The functional significance of antigen expression in these cases remains to be elucidated; however, our observations suggest that in leukemia these antigens are displayed in a non-adherent phenotype.

Introduction

Close interactions of hematopoietic cells with stromal cells and the extracellular matrix have been claimed to be of crucial importance for the specific homing of hematopoietic precursors to the bone marrow [1]. Such cell-cell and/ or cell-matrix interactions are mediated by membrane-bound adhesion molecules, which are subdivided into different families such as the integrin family, which comprises the β1- (very late activation-antigens, VLA), β2-(leukocyte integrins) and β3-(cytoadhesins) integrins defined by distinct β-chains [2]. The β2-integrins are exclusively expressed on leukocytes and are only involved in cell-cell interactions, while β1- and β3-integrins primarily mediate cell-matrix interactions [3, 4, 5]. The integrins consist of heterodimers of noncovalently linked alpha and beta chains, in contrast to the members of the immunoglobulin superfamily such as ICAM-1 (CD54), LFA-3 (CD58) and NCAM (CD56), which are characterized by the presence of at least one immunoglobulin-like domain found within two antiparallel β-strands [6]. The members of the selectin family, recently clustered as CD62L (L-Selectin), CD62P (P-selectin) and CD62E (E-selectin) comprise cell adhesion receptors that contain a single amino-terminal lectin-like domain [7].

Variant expression patterns of these adhesion molecules on hematopoietic cells were attributed to different maturational stages of normal hematopoietic precursors, suggesting differentiation dependent changes of adhesive properties

[1]Second Department of Internal Medicine
[2]Section of Transplantation Immunology and Immunohematology, Medical University Clinic, Tübingen, Germany

during normal hematopoiesis [8, 9, 10]. In leukemia, the egress of blasts into the peripheral blood might thus be facilitated by distinct alterations of the adhesive qualities of the leukemic cells and/or the stromal components. To evaluate this hypothesis, the expressions of various adhesion molecules of different families was investigated on a large number of leukemic samples and compared to their expression on CD34+ normal hematopoietic precursors.

Material and Methods

Clinical Samples

Blood and/or bone marrow samples were obtained from 42 patients with acute lymphoblastic leukemia (ALL) and 98 patients with acute myeloid leukemia (AML) as well as from 6 healthy adult bone marrow donors. The diagnosis of leukemia was based on routine morphological evaluation and cytochemical staining of smears using the French-American-British (FAB) classification as well as on routine immunophenotyping. Only samples with >70% blasts in the differential count were included.

Monoclonal Antibodies (Moabs)

Of the β1-integrins, the moab against VLA-1 (CD49a) was obtained from Biermann (Bad Nauheim, Germany). Moabs against the other β1-integrins VLA-2 (CD49b), VLA-3 (CD49c), VLA-4 (CD49d), VLA-5 (CD49e), VLA-6 (CD49e) and the common β1-chain (CD29), the β2-integrins LFA-1 (CD11a) and gp150/95 (CD11b), the β3-integrins VNR-alpha-chain (CD51) and GPIIIa-VNR-β-chain (CD61), the selection LECAM (CD62L), ELAM-1 (CD62E), GMP-140 (CD62P), the members of the immunoglobulin superfamily ICAM-1 (CD54), NCAM (CD56), LFA-3 (CD58 and HCAM (CD44) were all purchased from Immunotech (Marseille, France). Moabs against five CD44 splice variants (v5, v6, v7-v8, v10) were bought from Serva (Heidelberg, Germany). Antibodies against the β2-integrins CD11b (11C2E2) and CD18 (11H6) were derived from our laboratory.

FACS Analysis

Mononuclear cells were obtained by Ficoll-Hypaque density gradient centrifugation. Single staining was performed using the indirect immunofluorescence technique, with monoclonal antibodies as first antibody layer and $F(ab)_2$ fragments of fluorescein isothiocyanate (FITC)-conjugated goat-anti-mouse immunoglobulins (Dianova, Hamburg, Germany) as second antibody layer.

For double labeling experiments cells were first stained with the monoclonal antibody and developed with goat-anti-mouse FITC; subsequently, the cells were incubated with excess mouse IgG to block free binding sites of the FITC conjugate and labeled with the CD34-specific phycoerythrin (PE)-conjugated monoclonal antibody HPCA-2 (Becton Dickinson, San Joes, USA).

Fluorescence was evaluated on a FACS IV cell sorter (Becton Dickinson, San Jose, USA) as previously described [11]. Dual scatter gates (forward × 90° scatter) were set to electronically select the blast cell population, of which the fluorescence distribution was analyzed. Dual scatter gates were also set for gating of the progenitor cell population of the normal bone marrow specimens. The green fluorescence of the FITC-labeled cells was measured through a 530 nm band pass (bp) filter and the yellow fluorescence of PE-stained compounds through a 570 nm bp filter. After proper compensation with control beds the fluorescence intensities (log scale, 4 decades) and the scatter signals (linear scale) were analyzed by a data lister and evaluated on an IBM-AT computer using in-house programs.

Results

Adhesion Molecules on Normal CD34+ Bone Marrow Cells

The majority of CD34+ cells expressed CD49d (VLA-4) and the β1-subunit CD29. However, CD34+ cells did not carry CD49a (VLA-1), CD49b (VLA-2), CD49c (VLA-3) or CD49f (VLA-6). CD49e (VLA-5) was only weakly expressed on CD34+ cells. Of the β2-integrins, CD11a (LFA-1) and its β-chain CD18 were detected on >50–60% CD34+ cells in all investigated cases, while CD11b and CD11c were absent on normal CD34+ bone marrow cells. The β3-integrins CD51 and CD61 were not found on CD34+ cells.

The majority of CD34+ cells coexpressed CD54 (ICAM-1) and CD58 (LFA-3) while being negative for CD56 (NCAM) and CD106 (VCAM-1). All normal CD34+ bone marrow cells strongly stained with the antibody directed against CD44, but not with moabs against the five investigated CD44 splice variants. L-selectin was expressed on 50–60% CD34+ cells, while P- and E-selectin were absent from CD34+ cells (Figs. 1, 2).

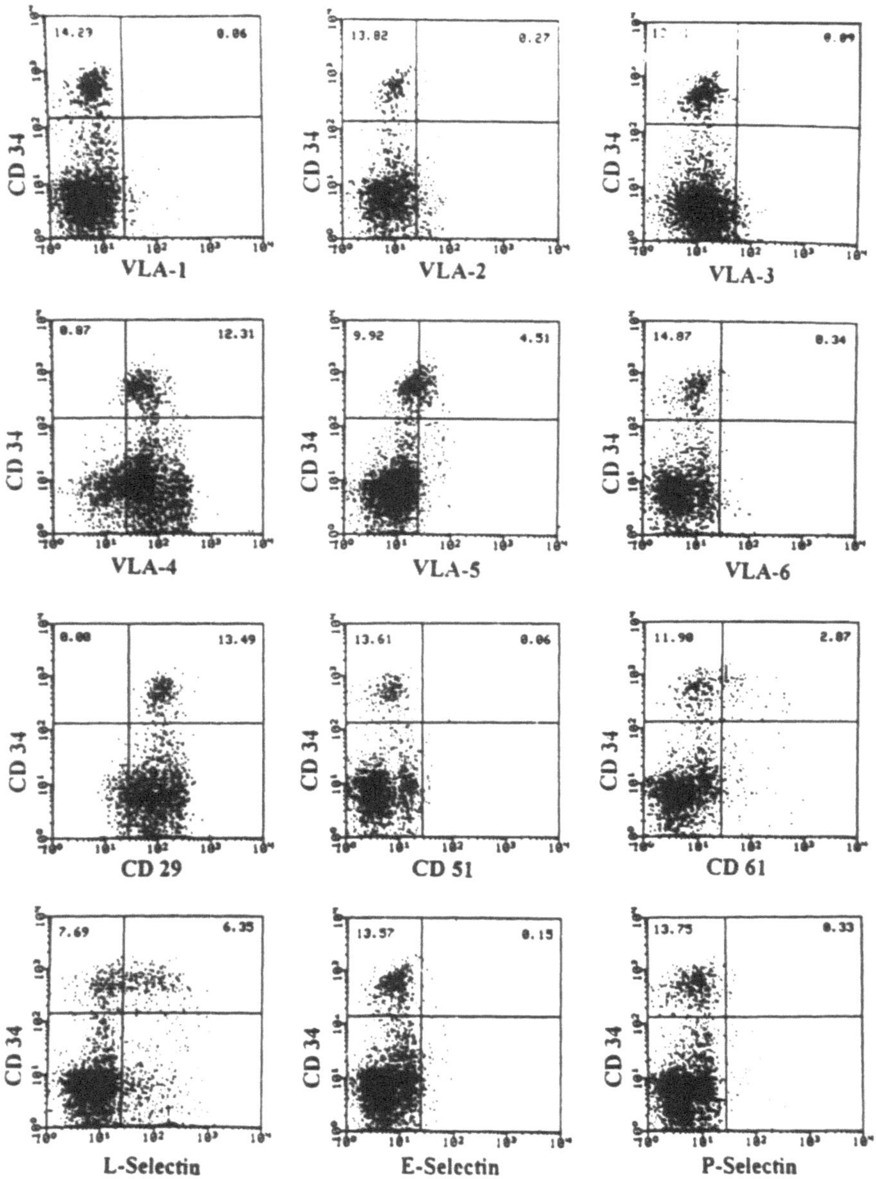

Fig. 1. Double fluorescence dot-plot display of CD341 normal bone marrow cells and the β1-integrins VLA-1, VLA-2, VLA-3, VLA-4, VLA-5, VLA-6, the β1-submit CD29, the β3-integrins CD51 and CD61 and the three selectins (in upper corners,% positive cells)

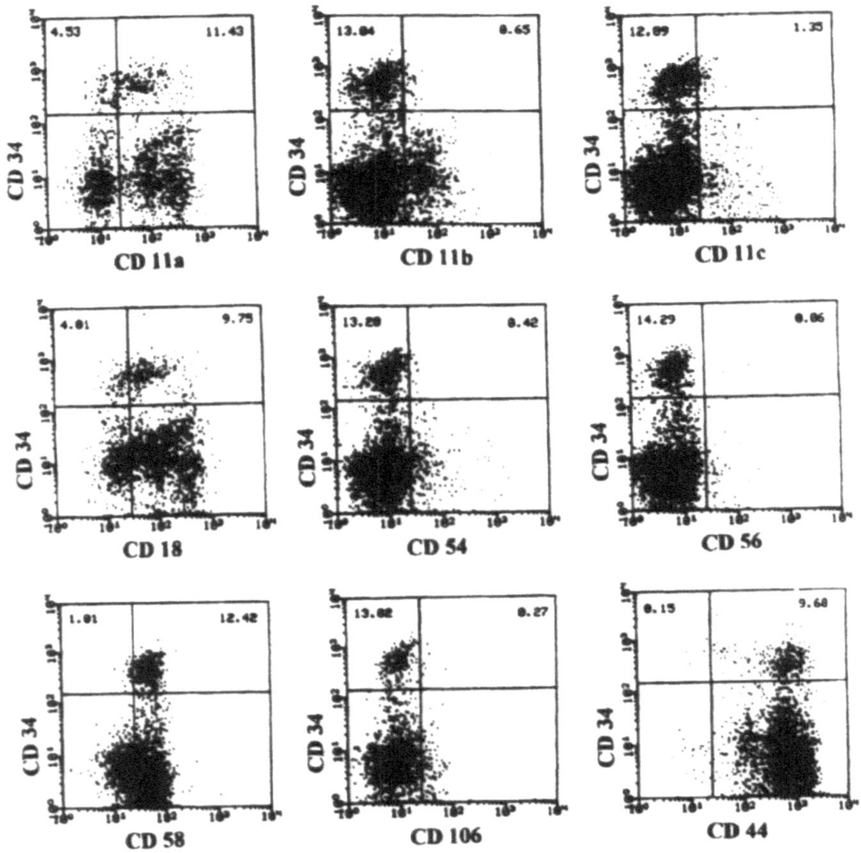

Fig. 2. Double fluorescence dot-plot display of CD341 normal bone marrow cells and the β2-integrins CD11a, CD11b, CD11c, CD18, the molecules of the immunoglobulin superfamily CD54 (ICAM-1), CD56 (NCAM), CD58 (LFA-3), CD106 (VCAM-1) and CD44 (in upper corners, % positive cells)

Adhesion Molecules in Acute Leukemia

Integrins (β1, β2, β3)

Cd49d (VLA-4) was positive on >70% of the blast cell population in 120/123 investigated samples. CD49e (VLA-5) and CD49f (VLA-6) were expressed on >70% of blasts in 45/51 and 15/29 samples. In only 5/43 samples >70% blasts carried VLA-3. VLA-1 was positive on >70% blasts in 1/51 and on 30–70% blasts in 3/51 leukemic samples classified as acute T-lymphoblastic leukemias. VLA-2 was observed on >70% blast cells in 18/123 investigated leukemic samples (Fig. 3). The VLA-2+, VLA-3+, VLA-5+ and VLA-6+ leukemias did not belong to a specific FAB subtype or to a particular immunophenotype. Intraindividual discordant expression between blood and bone marrow blasts was observed for VLA-2 in 11/33 cases with the specimens showing at least 15% more VLA-2+ blasts in the peripheral blood than in the bone marrow (Fig. 4). In addition, the four VLA-1+ samples were all blood derived; the simultaneously obtained bone marrow samples lacked VLA-1 expression.

CD11a and CD18 were expressed on the majority of cells from 149/157 leukemic samples irrespective of the subtype of leukemia. CD11b and CD11c were more heterogeneouly distributed, with a higher percentage of CD11b+ and CD11c+ cells in AML than in ALL. In addition, CD11b and CD11c were more frequently

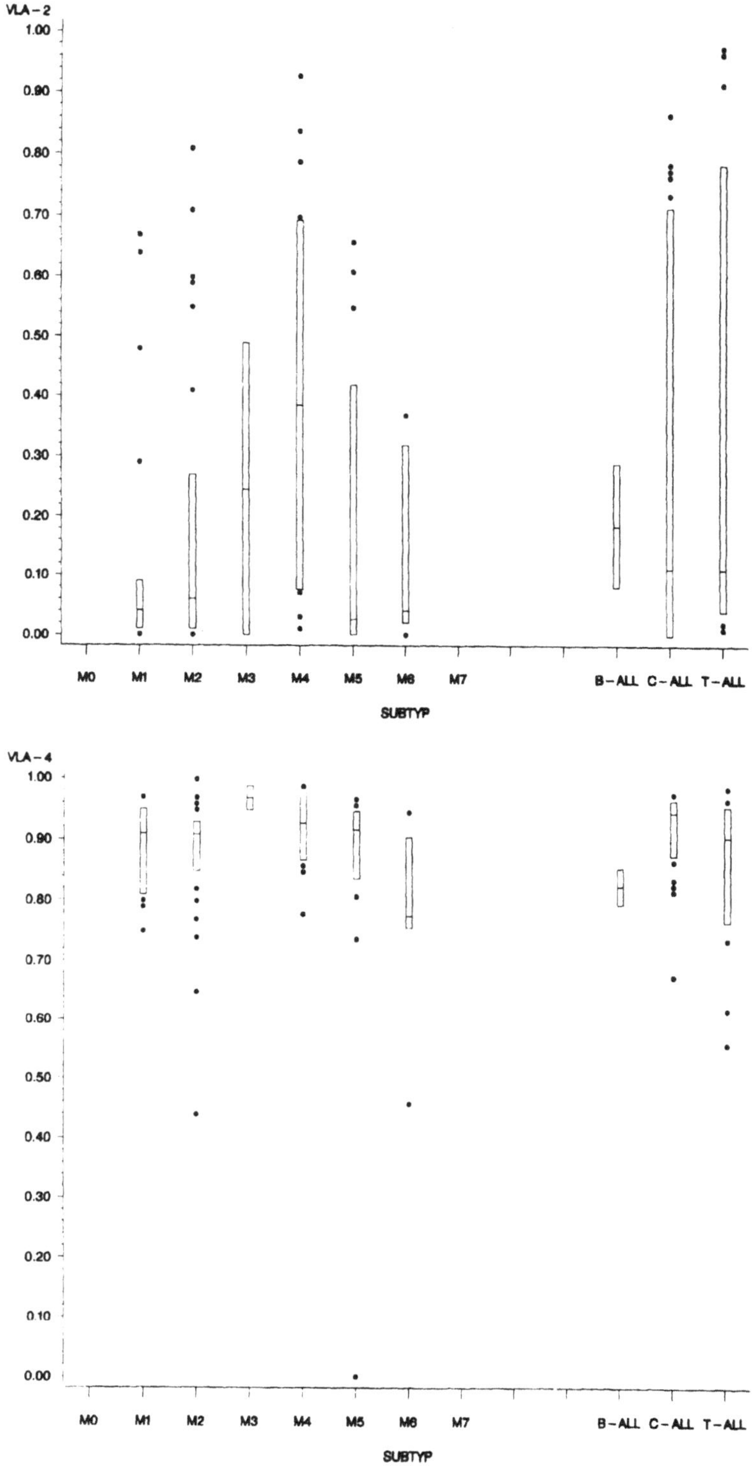

Fig. 3. Typical box-plot display of VLA-2 and VLA-4 expression on leukemic cells in acute leukemia according to different leukemic subtypes (median values and 25th and 75th percentiles are presented)

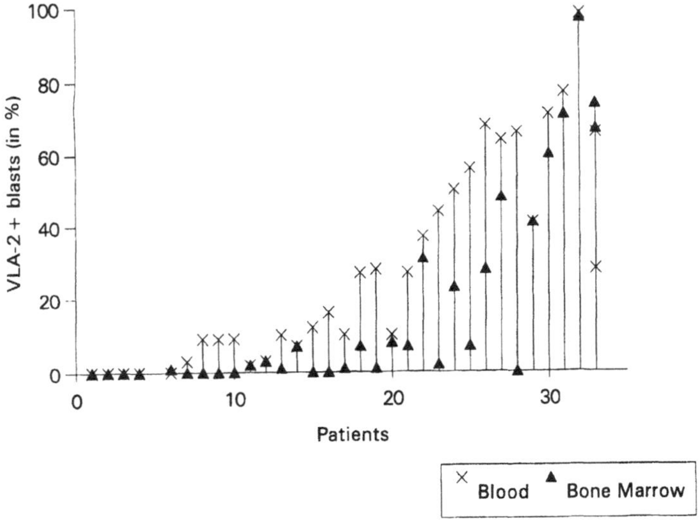

Fig. 4. Intraindividual differences in the expression of VLA-2 on bone-marrow and blood-derived blasts of 33 patients; for patient 33, values were obtained at first diagnosis and relapse

expressed on M4/M5 leukemias than on undifferentiated subtypes. The β3-integrins CD51 and CD61 were found only on a small proportion of cells in a few leukemias.

Adhesion Molecules of the Immunoglobulin Superfamily

CD58 was carried by >70% leukemic cells in 33/37 c-ALL and 13/17 T-ALL samples. The overwhelming majority of AML samples carried CD58 on >70% of the leukemic cells, with only 2/113 AML specimens being CD58 negative. CD54 (ICAM-1) was more heterogeneously expressed in leukemia with 13/56 ALL samples having >70% ICAM-1+ blasts. In AML, CD54 was expressed on >70% cells in 49/113 samples. The NK cell associated NCAM (CD56) was never observed on lymphoblastic cells, but 4/22 AML-M1, 7/30 AML-M2, 3/42 AML-M4 and 3/12 AML-M5 specimens carried CD56 on >70% of blasts.

CD44 and Splice Variants

HCAM (CD44) was expressed on >70% of leukemic cells in 167 investigated samples, being negative in only one AML-M5 and one c-ALL specimen. In contrast to normal CD34+ cells the CD44 variants were found in 3/9 AML specimens on a small percentage of leukemic cells.

Selectins

P-selectin was positive in 1 M7 leukemia out of 34 investigated AML specimens. E-selectin was observed on >70% of blasts in 2 leukemic samples of the AML-M5 subtype. In addition, E-selectin was carried by 10–50% of blasts in 7 AML specimens of the M1, M5 and M7 subtypes. The most widely distributed selectin, however, was L-selectin, which was detected on >70% blasts in 2/13 ALL and 9/34 AML samples.

Discussion

Some adhesion molecules were expressed on almost all investigated leukemic specimens, as well as on the majority of CD34+ normal bone marrow precursors. This applies for the lymphocyte-homing receptor HCAM (CD44), recently identified as a cell-surface receptor for hyaluronate and fibronectin, and the β1-integrins VLA-4 and VLA-5. In contrast to these ubiquitously expressed adhesion molecules, the β2-integrins CD11b and CD11c were restricted to the more differentiated M4 and M5 subtypes of myeloid leukemias, as previously suggested [12]. Remarkably, the NK cell associated antigen CD56, also known as neural-cell adhesion molecule (NCAM), was never observed on lymphoblastic leukemias, but it was expressed on a subset of myeloid leukemias not defined by a distinct clinical, phenotypic or FAB subtype [11]. The cytoadhesin CD51 and the common β3-chain (CD61) were only found on a limited percentage of blood-derived blasts in very few leukemias.

Interestingly, some β-integrins were variably expressed in leukemias but not on normal CD34+ hematopoietic precursors. These molecules were VLA-1 and VLA-2 with binding affinity to the extracellular matrix proteins laminin, collagen I and collagen IV, VLA-3 binding to collagen I, fibronectin and laminin and VLA-6, a receptor for laminin. Most of these variably expressed surface antigens are known to be regulated in their cellular and humoral environment by a wide range of cytokines which may be produced by the leukemic cells themselves [13]. Thus, the expression of VLA-1, VLA-2, VLA-3 and VLA-6 might be induced by local cytokine activity. Interestingly, analysis of simultaneously obtained blood and bone marrow samples from individual patients tended to reveal higher percentages of VLA-antigens on the blood-derived blasts, possibly due to the up-regulation of these antigens. Whether higher surface levels of these antigens in fact correspond to enhanced ligand binding remains to be elucidated. preliminary functional studies show that VLA antigen expression does not necessarily correlate with-binding affinity to the extracellular ligands. However, adhesiveness is a highly dynamic process, and cells that display adhesion molecules on their surface may rapidly convert from a non-adherent to an adherent phenotype by conformational changes without changes in the level of surface expression [14]. The observation that leukemic cells tend to express even more adhesion molecules than normal bond marrow precursors could therefore imply functional inactivity of these antigens.

References

1. Dorshkind K. (1990) Regulation of hemopoiesis by bone marrow stromal cells and their products. Annu. Rev. Immunol. 8, 111–137.
2. Long M.W. (1992) Blood cell cytoadhesion molecules. Exp. Hemat. 20, 288–301.
3. Larson R.S., T.A. Springer (1990) Structure and function of leukocyte integrins. Immunol. Rev. 114, 181–217.
4. Ruoslahti E. (1991) J. Integrins. Clin. Invest. 87, 1–5.
5. Hynes R.O. (1992) Integrins: versatility, modulation, and signaling in cell adhesion. Cell 69, 11–25.
6. Williams A.F., Barclay A.N. (1988) The immunoglobulin superfamily—domains for cell surface recognition. Annu. Rev. Immunol. 6, 381–405.
7. Vestweber D. (1992) Selectins: cell surface lectins which mediate the binding of leukocytes to endothelial cells. Semin. Cell. Biol. 3, 211–220
8. Miller L.J., R. Schwarting, T.A. Springer (1986) Regulated expression of the Mac-1, LFA-1, p150, 95 glycoprotein family during leukocyte differentiation. Immunology 137, 2891–2900
9. Campana D., B. Sheridan, N. Tidman, Hoffbrand A.V., Janossy G. (1986) Human leukocyte function-associated antigens on lymopho- hematopoietic precursor cells. Eur. J. Immunol. 16, 537–542
10. Kobayashi M., M. Imamura, T. Uede, K. Sakurada, S. Maeda, H. Iwasaki, Y. Tsuda, V. Musashi, T. Miyazaki (1994) Expression of adhesion molecules on human hematopoietic progenitor cells at different maturational stages. Stem Cells 12, 316–321
11. Reuss-Borst M.A., B. Steinke, H.D. Waller, H.J. Bühring, C.A. Müller (1992) Phenotypic and clinical heterogeneity of CD56- positive acute non-lymphoblastic leukemia. Ann. Hemat. 64, 78–82
12. Soligo D., R. Schiro, R. Luksch, G. Manara, N. Quirici, C. Parravicini, G.L. Deliliers(1990) Experssion of integrins in human bone marrow. Br.J. Haemat. 76, 323–332
13. Oster W., N.A. Cicco, H. Klein, T.Hirano, T. Kishimoto, A. Lindemann, R.H. Mertelsmann, F. Herrmann (1989) Participation of the cytokines interleukin-6, tumor necrosis factoralpha, and interleukin 1-beta secreted by acute myelogenous leukemia blasts in autocrine and paracrine leukemia growth control. J. Clin. Invest. 84, 451–457
14. Diamond M.S., T.A. Springer (1994) The dynamic regulation of integrin adhesiveness. Current Biology 4, 506–517

Acute Leukemias VI
Prognostic Factors
and Treatment Strategies
Büchner et al. (eds)

Expression of Adhesion Molecules on Blood Derived CD34 Positive Cells Immediately After Thawing and After Ex Vivo Incubation with Cytokines

Mi. Koenigsmann, Mo. Koenigsmann, M. Notter, C. Mücke, E. Thiel, and W.E. Berdel

Abstract. In order to understand the role of specific cell adhesion for stem cell engraftment after autologous transplantation we investigated the expression of adhesion molecules on blood derived CD34 positive cells from cancer patients immediately after thawing and after ex vivo incubation with or without cytokines. Peripheral blood progenitor cells were collected by leukapheresis after conventional chemotherapy and G-CSF given during the recovery phase. Aliquots were used for our study. The buffy coat cells were analyzed either fresh or after cryopreservation in liquid nitrogen. CD34 positive cells were enriched by immunomagnetic microbead seperation. CD34 and adhesion molecules were detected simultaneously by dual-color flow cytometry. Immediately after thawing we saw bright signal intensities for the integrin subunits CD29, CD18, CD49d, CD41, and for CD44. Dim intensity was found for CD49e, CD61 and for the selection CD62L. We did not detect CD49a, CD49b, CD49c, the beta 4 integrin subunit, CD51, CD62P, and the CD44 splice variants V6,V7,V7-8. On fresh cells, i.e. before cryopreservation, CD62L, CD49d, CD49e, CD29, and CD18 were brightly expressed on most CD34 positive cells. Some molecules were studied on thawed cells after 14 h of incubation in human AB serum. Without cytokine addition, an increase in signal intensity was seen for CD62L and CD29. The addition of a cytokine cocktail containing recombinant human G-CSF, SCF, IL-3, and IL-11, each at 100 ng/ml did not clearly change the signal intensities for these adhesion molecules. We conclude that: (1) immediately after thawing, the expression of some adhesion molecules like CD62L and CD49e on CD34 positive cells is decreased while it is maintained for others like CD18; (2) ex vivo incubation for 14 h leads to re-expression or increased expression of CD62L and CD29; (3) high concentrations of G-CSF, SCF, IL-3 and IL-11 do not clearly modulate rapid re-expression of these adhesion molecules.

Introduction

Specific cell adhesion is necessary for stem cell engraftment after transplantation. Similarly as for leukocyte emigration, a sequence of adhesion molecules might be involved from the moment of intravenous stem cell transfusion until the seeding of the cells within the bone marrow matrix [1]. Cytokines are known to regulate the expression of adhesion molecules [2] and at the same time to promote hematopoietic recovery in vivo[3]. In order to delineate the possible role of specific cell adhesion molecules for stem cell engraftment after autologous transplantation we investigated their expression on blood derived CD34 positive cells from cancer patients in four different situations: (1) immediately after thawing (the situation at transplantation); (2) before freezing (material freshly obtained from the patient); (3) after thawing and overnight incubation with AB serum; (4) after thawing and overnight incubation with a cytokine cocktail comprising G-CSF, IL-3, SCF and IL-11. The adhesion molecules investigated in this study are: the selection CD62L, the β1 through β4 inte-

Division of Hematology and Oncology, Benjamin Franklin Hospital of the Free University Berlin, Germany

grin subunits with respective α chains as well as CD44 and some of its splice variants.

Material and Methods

Peripheral blood progenitor cells from cancer patients were collected by leukapheresis (COBE Spectra) after conventional chemotherapy and 10 μg/kg/day s.c. G-CSF given during the recovery phase. Aliquots of fresh or frozen cells were used for our study with the patients, informed consent. CD34 positive cells were enriched to $74 \pm 14\%$ purity by immunomagnetic microbead separation (Miltenyi Biotech, Cologne, FRG) using the monoclonal antibody QBEND-10. The expression of CD34 (HPCA2) and adhesion molecules were detected simultaneously by dual color analysis using a FACScan flow cytometer with the Lysis II software (Becton & Dickinson). A 14-h incubation of enriched CD34 positive cells was done with 10% human AB serum alone or with addition of cytokines comprising recombinant human G-CSF (Rhone-Poulenc Rorer, Cologne, FRG), stem cell factor (Amgen GmbH, Munich, FRG), IL-3 (Behringwerke AG, Marburg, FRG), and IL-11 (R&D Systems, Abingdon, UK), each at concentration of 100 ng/ml.

The following adhesion molecules were assayed by FACS:

CD designation	Common name
CD62L	L-selectin
CD62P	P-selectin
CD29	β1 integrin subunit
CD49a–e	α1 through α5 integrin subunits
CD18	β2 integrin subunit
CD41	megakaryocyte glycoprotein IIb/IIIa
CD61	β3 integrin subunit gp IIIa
CD51	α_v integrin subunit (vitronectin receptor)
CD104	β4 integrin subunit
CD44	hyaluronic acid receptor

Results

Expression of Adhesion Molecules on CD34 Positive Cells Immediately After Thawing

Bright signal intensities were seen for the integrin subunits Cd29 (β1), CD18 (β2) , CD49d (α4) for CD41 (gpIIb/IIIa), and CD44. Dim intensity was found for the selectin CD62L and the integrin subunits CD49e (α5) and CD61 (β3 or gpIIIa). We did not detect expression of the integrin subunits CD49a (α1), Cd49b (α2), CD49c (α3), CD104(ß4), CD51 (αv), the selectin CD62P, and the CD44 splice variants V6, V7 and V7-8 (Fig. 1a,b).

Expression Before Freezing

On fresh leukapheresis samples a significantly higher expression was detected for CD62L (Fig. 2a) and CD49e when compared to cryopreserved samples. For CD49d and CD29 there was a small difference, however a similar trend was seen. (Fig. 2b).

Expression After Thawing and Overnight Incubation with AB Serum

Some molecules were studied after 14 h of incubation in human AB serum. Compared to time 0 immediately after thawing, a clear increase in signal intensity was seen for CD62L and CD29 (Fig. 3a and b).

Expression After Thawing and Overnight Incubation with a Cytokine Cocktail Comprising G-CSF, IL-3, SCF and IL-11

In comparison to AB serum alone the addition of the cytokine cocktail did not consistently further change the signal intensities for the adhesion molecules CD62L or CD29 (Fig. 3a, b).

Discussion

Immediately after thawing and enrichment of peripheral blood derived CD34 positive cells from cancer patients, several adhesion molecules like CD29, CD18, CD49d, CD41, and CD44 are brightly expressed. Dim intensity was found for the selectin CD62L, CD49e, and CD61. We did not detect CD49a, CD49b, CD49c, the beta 4 integrin subunit, CD51, CD62P, and CD44 splice variants V6, V7, V7-8.

Cryopreservation decreases the expression of some adhesion molecules like CD29, CD49e, and CD62L on CD34 positive cells, while expression-is maintained for others like CD18. Possible

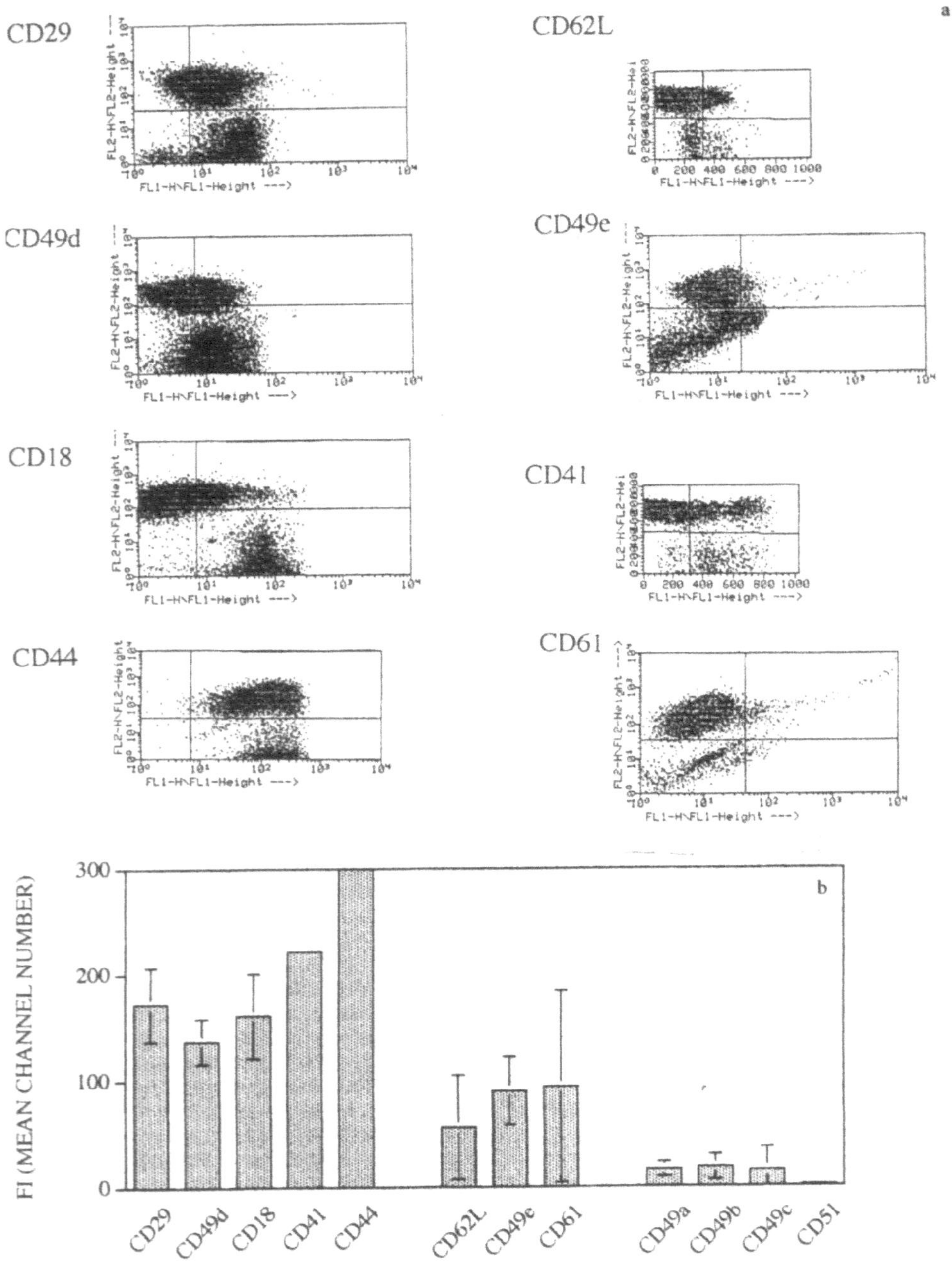

Fig. 1a,b. Expression of CD34 and adhesion molecules on mononuclear cells immediately after thawing and enrichment for CD34 positive cells. **a** Fluorescence intensity (*FI*) for CD34 on the *X*-axis (*FL*-1) versus the indicated adhesion molecules on the *Y*-axis (*FL*-2). **b** Cumulative data ± standard deviation from three or more repeat experiments

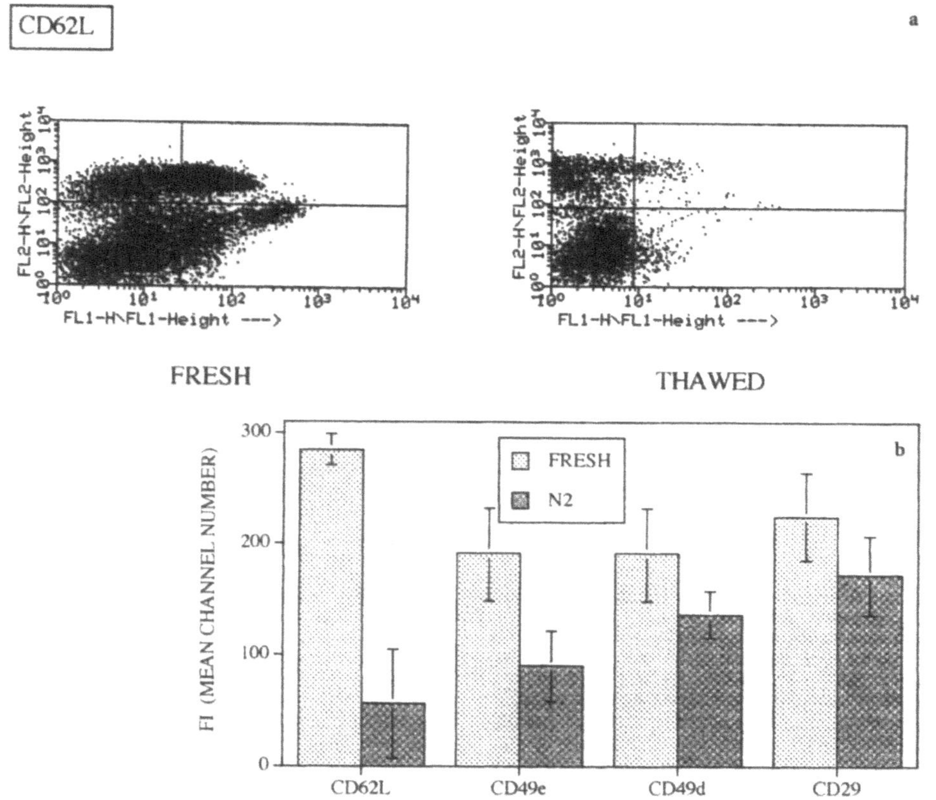

Fig. 2a,b. Effects of cryopreservation on adhesion molecule expression. **a** Freshly obtained vs thawed leukapheresis products from the same patient after enrichment for CD34 positive cells were analyzed for CD62L expression. Data are plotted as in Fig. 1a. The fraction as well as the mean channel number of CD62L positive cells was higher on fresh cells than on thawed CD34 positive cells. **b** Cumulative data from at least three experiments showing decreased expression for several adhesion molecules after cryopreservation

mechanisms leading to the decreased expression are physical destruction of the surface protein structure by cryopreservation, shedding of the protein from the surface, or internalization.

Ex vivo incubation in unsupplemented AB serum for 14 h leads to re-expression or increased expression of CD62L and CD29. These molecules are therefore candidates for playing a role during engraftment. However, the expression of adhesion molecules itself does not necessarily imply their activity. Additional stimuli might be required. For example, fibronectin binding of T cells by β1-integrin receptors can be increased by stimulating receptor avidity or by altering events after receptor occupancy [4]. Therefore, adhesion tests will show whether the expression of these receptors is associated with function.

Molecules like CD49a, CD49b, and CD49c might not contribute to the immediate phase of engraftment since they are not expressed either before cryopreservation or after 14 h of exvivo incubation. However, the possibility still exists that different cytokines or other factors might increase the expression of these molecules. Also, for times exceeding 14 h after transplantation these receptors could still play a role.

High concentrations of G-CSF, SCF, IL-3, and IL-11 do not consistently contribute to inducing rapid re-expression of these adhesion molecules. Therefore, ex vivo incubation of stem cells with these cytokines might not improve engraftment, at least not by the regulation of adhesion receptor expression. The potential effects of short-term ex vivo incubation of progenitor cells on

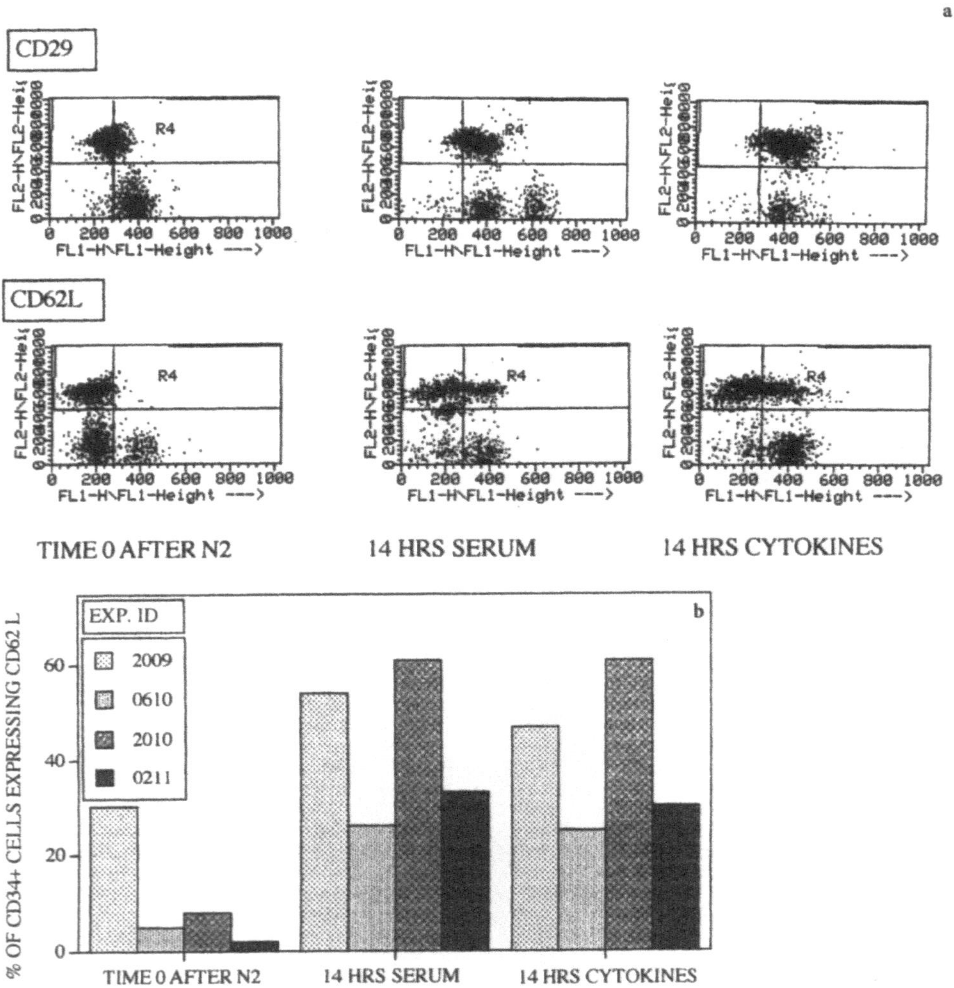

Fig. 3a,b. Re-expression of adhesion molecules on cryopreserved CD34 positive cells after ex vivo incubation with serum or cytokines. **a** Immediately after thawing *TIME* 0 the fraction of CD34 positive cells expressing CD29 and CD62L is relatively low. Re-expression is seen after 14 h ex vivo incubation with AB serum alone or with additional SCF, IL-3, IL-11, and G-CSF at 100 ng/ml each. **b** Increased expression of CD62L after serum incubation shown in four different experiments with cells from three different patients. No additional effect was seen after the addition of cytokines (SCF+IL-3+IL-11+G-CSF)

engraftment, however, have to be further explored by using different cytokines, by testing other adhesion molecules and by functional adhesion tests.

Acknowledgments. Supported by Dr. Mildred Scheel Foundation, grant No W27/92/Kol and by Rhone-Poulenc Rorer Inc, Paris, France.

References

1. Carlos TM, Harlan JM: Leukocyte-endothelial adhesion molecules. Blood 84: 2068, 1994
2. Griffin JD, Spertini O, Ernst TJ, Melvin MP Levine HB, Kanakura Y, Tedder TF: G-CSF and other cytokines regulate surface expression of the leukocyte adhesion molecule-1, on human neutrophils, monocytes, and their precursors. J Immunol 145: 576, 1990

3. Tavassoli M, Konno M, Shiota Y, Omoto E, Minguell JJ, Zanjani ED: Enhancement of the grafting efficiency of transplanted marrow cells by preincubation with interleukin -3 and granulocyte-macrophage colony-stimulating factor. Blood 77: 1599, 1991
4. Faull RJ, Kovach NL, Harlan JM, Ginsberg MH: Stimulation of integrin-mediated adhesion of T lymphocytes and monocytes: Two mechanisms with divergent biological consequences. J Exp Med 179: 1307, 1994

Acute Leukemias VI
Prognostic Factors
and Treatment Strategies
Büchner et al. (eds)

Cytomorphology and Clinical Outcome in 80 Patients with AML M4Eo and Inversion 16

T. Haferlach[1], H. Löffler[1], J.M. Bennett[2], J.W. Andersen[3], W. Gassmann[1], R. Schoch[1], E. Paietta[4], P.A. Cassileth[5], C. Fonatsch[6], C. Schoch[6], B. Schlegelberger[7], R. Becher[8], E. Thiel[9], W.-D. Ludwig[10], M.C. Sauerland[11], A. Heinecke[11], and T. Büchner[12] for the AML Cooperative Group and the ECOG

Abstract. We analyzed specific cytomorphological aspects and treatment results in 80 patients with AML M4Eo and inversion 16. All patients were treated according to protocols of the AMLCG ($n=60$) or the ECOG ($n=20$). Several morphological features, including myelodysplasia, did not influence the remission rate or prognosis in this cohort. The complete remission rate was 89%. Resistance to chemotherapy is therefore a rare event in AML M4Eo. For the AMLCG patients the relapse-free survival rate was 48.2% at 8 years. Thus, patients with AML M4Eo have a good prognosis in comparison to many other subtypes of AML. Allogeneic bone marrow transplantation should no longer be considered the treatment of choice in first complete remission in patients with AML M4Eo.

Introduction

Acute myelomonocytic leukemia with abnormal eosinophils (FAB AML M4Eo) is a distinct subtype of AML carrying specific clinical, morphological, cytogenetic, and prognostic features. It is characterized by a myeloblastic/monocytic infiltration of the bone marrow accompanied by a more or less prominent fraction of pathological eosinophils [1-3]. The abnormal eosinophils contain dysplastic immature granules, which are larger, more irregular, and more frequent than the basophilic granules of the normal eosinophilic precursors. These eosinophils usually make up 3-40% of the nucleated marrow cells and are positive for naphthol-AS-D-chloroacetate esterase staining, in contrast to normal eosinophils [4-6]. In 1983 cytogenetic analysis revealed a pericentric inversion of chromosome 16 in cases with the specific bone marrow morphology of M4Eo[7]. Thus, one can predict the cytogenetic result of inv(16) in almost any case of AML M4Eo and vice versa. Prognosis of AML M4Eo with inv(16) has been reported to be better than the prognosis of the other entities of AML combined AML M4Eo is considered to be one of the three subgroups of AML with the best prognosis, together with the FAB subtypes AML M3 with t(15;17) and AML M2(1) with t(8;21) [3, 8-11].

So far, in AML M4Eo most of the published data were collected from heterogenous patient

[1]University of Kiel, Second Medical Department, Kiel, Germany, (for the AML Cooperative Group)
[2]University of Rochester, Medical Oncology Unit, Cancer Center, Rochester NY, USA (for the ECOG)
[3]Division of Biostatistics, Dana Farber Cancer Institute, Boston, MA, USA
[4]Dpt. of Oncology, Montefiore Medical Center, Bronx, NY, USA
[5]University of Miami, Miami, FL, USA, (for the ECOG)
[6]University of Lübeck, Cooperative Group for Tumor Cytogenetics, Institute for Human Genetics, Lübeck, Germany
[7]University of Kiel, Institute for Human Genetics, Kiel, Germany
[8]University of Essen, Department of Internal Medicine, Essen, Germany
[9]University Steglitz, Department of Internal Medicine, Berlin, Germany
[10]Robert-Rössle-Hospital, Department for Medical Oncology and Molecular Biology, Berlin, Germany
[11]University of Münster, Institute for Medical Informatics and Biomathematics, Germany
[12]University of Münster, Department of Internal Medicine, Münster, Germany

populations treated with various chemotherapeutic regimens. We have analyzed treatment results for patients with AML M4Eo and detection of inv(16) in AMLCG and ECOG studies. Treatment schedules were comparable.

Material and Methods

We analyzed morphological features and treatment response of 80 patients with inversion 16 and the morphological appearance of AML M4Eo who underwent aggressive chemotherapy in two cooperative study groups (AMLCG: $n=60$; ECOG: $n=20$). All bone marrow smears were reviewed for this analysis by the authors (T.H. and H.L. for the AMLCG patients; T.H. and J.M.B. for the ECOG patients). Cytological examination included bone marrow smears and blood smears, if available, stained with the following cytochemical reactions according to standard procedures: Pappenheim (AMLCG) or Wright-Giemsa (ECOG), myeloperoxidase or sudan black B, non-specific esterase (NSE), and naphthol-AS-D-chloroacetate esterase[2]. FAB criteria were used for the definition of blasts type I, II, or III [12, 13] and for the definition of myelodysplasia [14]. Treatment schedules were comparable and included thioguanine, ARA-C, mitoxantrone, daunorubicin or idarubicin [15-18].

Median age was 44 years (range 19-73); 38 female and 42 male patients were studied. Remission data were available for all patients. Survival data were available only for patients treated bythe AMLCG. Relapse-free survival was calculated using the method of Kaplan and Meier [19]. The log-rank test was used for the comparison of survival curves [20].

Results

Cytomorphological Results

The percentage of blasts type I, II, and III combined, including monoblasts [12, 13] ranged between 45 and 90% (mean 66%); the percentage of monoblasts and monocytes ranged between 12 and 41% (mean 24%). Erythropoiesis was decreased to 3-25% (mean 8%). Auer rods were seen in Pappenheim (Wright-Giemsa) staining or with myeloperoxidase in 31% of the patients.

The number of abnormal eosinophils with basophilic granules in the bone marrow that led to the morphological diagnosis of AML M4Eo ranged between 1 and 31% (mean 10%). In contrast to normal eosinophils, some of these abnormal eosinophils were positive for chloroacetate esterase, as has been described as typical for AML MEo and inv(16). In 43 cases up to 10% of pathological eosinophils were observed in the bone marrow; in another 26 cases the percentage of eosinophils varied between 11 and 20%; in 11 cases more than 20% of abnormal eosinophils were detectable. Having in mind the diagnosis of AML M4Eo in the bone marrow, we were able to detect up to 10% of pathological eosinophils (mean 2%) in 29/59 available peripheral blood smears (49%). The NSE for monocytes and monoblasts was positive in 5-20% of the cells in 38% of the patients; in 29% it ranged between 21 and 30% and in one third it was positive for more than 30% of the bone marrow cells. Thus, the FAB criteria for AML M4—"more than 20% of the cells are of the monocytic lineage and positive for NSE" [1]—are not fulfilled in 38% of our cases with AML M4Eo. Therefore it is important that the result of the NSE staining should not lead to the diagnosis of AML "M2"Eo: one has to consider that NSE is sometimes very weak in cases with inv(16). With Pappenheim or Wright-Giemsa staining the calculated percentage of monoblasts and monocytes was higher (see above).

Dysplasia was analyzed according to standard criteria [14]. Dysgranulopoiesis (DysG) was observed in 14 patients (17%); two patients had DysG in combination with dysmegakaryopoiesis (DysM). 18 patients had only DysM. One patient had DysM combined with dyserythropoiesis. Only one patient had trilineage dysplasia. In the majority of all cases (43/80 patients, 54%) no dysplasia was detectable (Table 1).

Treatment Results

Response to chemotherapy was excellent in patients with AML M4Eo and inv(16): 71/80 patients (89%) achieved a complete remission, six patients experienced early death, and 3 patients no remission (Table 2).

Dysplastic features, the percentage of blasts, and the absence or presence of Auer rods did not influence the treatment results or survival data.

Table 1. Clinical and morphological data in 80 patients with AML M4Eo and inv(16)

	Number	Percentage of patients
Male	42	53
Female	38	47
Age (median 44 years)		
ECOG	20	25
AMLCG	60	75
AUER rods		
no	55	69
Yes	25	31
No dysplasia	43	54
Dysgranulopoiesis	14	17
Dyserythropoiesis	4	5
Dysmegakaryopoiesis	18	23
Trilineage dysplasia	1	1

Table 2. Treatment results in 80 patients with AML M4Eo and inv(16)

	Number	Percentage of patients
Complete remission	71	89
Early death	6	7.5
No remission	3	3.5

At the time of this analysis survival data were available only for patients treated in the AMLCG: The overall survival for the 60 patients in the AMLCG was 44.6% at 8 years, with no relapses observed in 13 patients after 3 years (Fig. 1). The corresponding relapse-free survival rate was 48.2% (Fig. 2). Four patients underwent allogeneic bone marrow transplantation. Survival data were censored at transplantation and did not influence the long-term results reported in this study.

In comparison to an AMLCG subgroup that excluded patients with AMLM4Eo, AML M3 and AML M1 or M2 with t(8;21) the survival was better for patients with AML M4Eo ($p = 0.0138$, Fig. 3).

Discussion

AML M4Eo with inversion 16 is a specific subtype of AML. Pathological eosinophils with distinct morphological and cytochemical characteristics are detectable in the bone marrow and allow one to predict that the inversion 16 should be present. These pathological eosinophils show positive reaction with naphthol-AS-D-chloroacetate-esterase staining in contrast to normal eosinophils. Several years ago this phenomenon led to the prediction that these

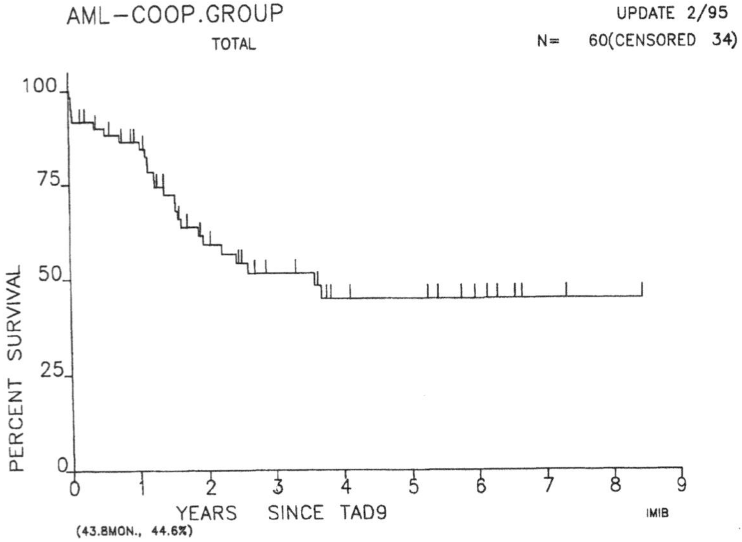

Fig. 1. Overall survival in 60 patients with AML M4Eo and inv(16) treated in the AMLCG. The remission rate was 90%

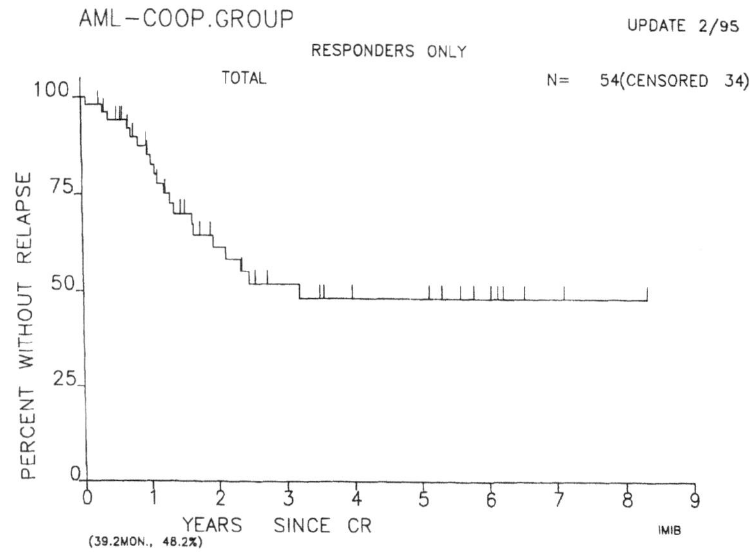

Fig. 2. Relapse-free survival in 54 patients with AML M4Eo and inv(16) treated in the AMLCG

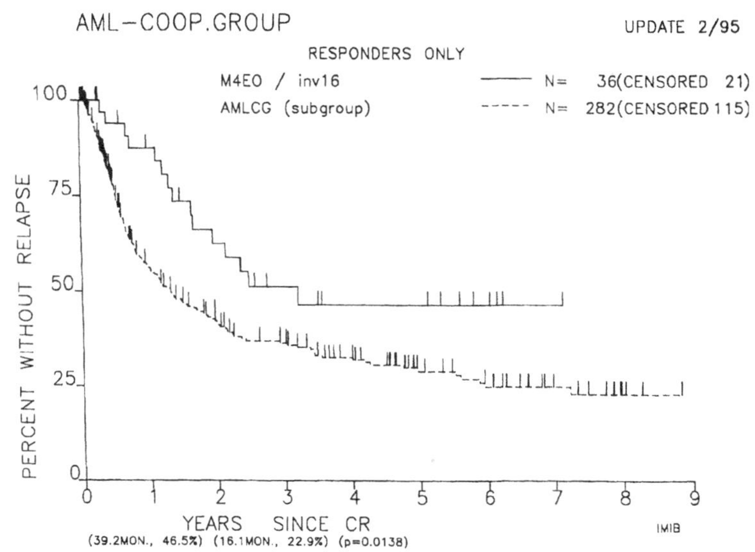

Fig. 3. Patients with AML M4Eo and inv(16) in comparison to an AMLCG subgroup that excluded patients with the following characteristics: AML M4Eo or AML M3 with t(15;17) and AML M2 or M1 with t(8;21) ($p = 0.0138$)

eosinophils define a specific subtype of acute leukemia [4]. In 1983 the detection of a specific chromosomal aberration—the inversion 16—was correlated with this specific morphology in cases of AML M4Eo [7].

In recent years several studies were able to demonstrate that patients with AML M4Eo and inv(16) had a better prognosis than patients with other subtypes of AML [8, 21–23]. Our analysis was performed to confirm treatment outcome in AML M4Eo in a group of patients with comparable treatment protocols.

The remission rate was 89% in 80 patients treated in the AMLCG and the ECOG. Primary resistance to chemotherapy was a rare event in AML M4Eo. Others also found the highest remission rate in AML in patients with AML M4Eo [7, 21, 24–26]. These corresponding results obviously demonstrate that patients with inv(16) normally achieved complete remission after the first course of chemotherapy or—in rare cases—experienced early death. Thus, very intensive supportive care may lead to even better results.

Although some patients relapsed, the 8 year relapse-free survival rate for 60 patients treated in the AMLCG was 48.2%. This is comparable to the survival rates of patients with AML and t(8;21) and with t(15;17) before ATRA and is much higher than in all other subtypes of AML combined [3, 10].

Specific bone marrow features such as dysplasia, percentage of blasts, presence of Auer rods, and percentage of pathological eosinophils did not influence the prognosis in our patients.

In conclusion, AML M4Eo with inv(16) is a subtype of AML with specific cytomorphological features and a corresponding cytogenetic aberration. The remission rate is very high, and the relapse-free survival is better than in many other subtypes of AML. Our results should lead to a modification of the treatment approach in AML M4Eo: if clinical, hematological, and cytogenetic analysis reveal a complete remission in patients with AML M4Eo, allogeneic bone marrow transplantation should no longer be considered the treatment of choice in first complete remission. Recently, monitoring for minimal residual disease in AML M4Eo has become possible using the polymerase chain reaction [27–31] or flourescence in situ hybridization [27, 28, 32, 33]. These techniques should be included in the diagnosis and for the detection of minimal residual disease and may help to modify treatment strategies for every patient in the future as well.

References

1. Bennett, J.M., Catovsky, D., Daniel, M.T., Flandrin, G., Galton, D.A.G., Gralnick, H.R., Sultan, C.: Proposed revised criteria for the classification of acute myeloid leukemia: A report of the French-American-British Cooperative Group. Ann Intern Med 103, 626–629 (1985)
2. Löffler, H.: Zytochemische Methoden. In: Huber, H., Löffler, H., Faber, V. (Hrsg.): Methoden der diagnostischern Hämatologie. Berlin u.a.O.: 125–136 (1991)
3. Haferlach, T., Gassmann, W., Löffler, H., Jürgensen, C., Noak, J., Ludwig, W.-D., Thiel, E., Haase, D., Fonatsch, C., Becher, R., Schlegelberger, B., Nowrousian, M.R., Lengfelder, E., Eimermacher, H., Weh, H.J., Braumann, D., Maschmeyer, G., Koch, P., Heinecke, A., Sauerland, M.C., Büchner, Th.: Clinical aspects of acute myeloid leukemias of the FAB types M3 and M4Eo. Ann Hematol 66, 165–170 (1993)
4. Löffler, H.: Zytochemische Klassifizierung der akuten Leukosen.In: Stacher, A. (Hrsg.): Chemo- und Immuntherapie der Leukosen und malignen Lymphome. Ludwig Boltzmann-Gesellschaft, Wien 1969, S. 120–127
5. Löffler, H.: Indications and limits of cytochemistry in acute leukemia. Rec Res Canc Res 43, 57–62 (1973)
6. Leder, L.D.: Akute myelo-monozytäre Leukämie mit atypischen Naphtol-AS-D-Chloroacetat-Esterase-positiven Eosinophilen. Acta Haematol 44, 52–62 (1970)
7. Le Beau, M.M., Larson, R.A., Bitter, M.A., Vardiman, J.W., Golomb, H.M., Rowley, J.D.: Association of an inversion of chromosome 16 with abnormal marrow eosinophils in acute myelomonocytic leukemia: A unique cytogenetic-clinicopathological association. N Engl J Med 309, 630–636 (1983)
8. Keating, M.J., Cork, A., Broch, Y., Smith, T., Waltes, R.S., McCredie, K.B., Trujillo, J., Freireich, E.J.: Toward a clinically relevant cytogenetic classification of acute myelogenous leukemia. Leukemia Res 11(2), 119–133 (1987)
9. Keating, M.J., Smith, T.L., Kantarjian, H.,Cork, A., Walters, R., Trujillo, J.M., McCredie, K.B., Gehan, E.A., Freireich, E.J.: Cytogenetic pattern in acute myelogenous leukemia: a major reproducible determinant of outcome. Leukemia 2, 403–412 (1988)
10. Haferlach, T., Bennett, J.M., Löffler, H., Gassmann, W., Andersen, J., Tuzuner, N., Cassileth, P.A., Fonatsch, C., Schlegelberger, B., Theil, E., Ludwig, W.-D., Sauerland, M.C., Heinecke, A., Büchner, T. for AML Cooperative Group and ECOG: Cytomorphology results and dysplastic features as prognostic factors in 41 cases with acute myeloid leukemia (AML) and translocation (8;21). Leuk Res 18 Suppl, 45 (1994)
11. Haferlach, T., Löffler, H., Gassmann, W., Bennett, J.M., Ludwig, W.-D., Maschmeyer, G.,. Thiel, E, Nowrousian, M.R., Lang, R., Kubica, U., Weiss, A., Lengfelder, E., Koch, P., Weh, H.J., Tirier, C., Sauerland, M.C., Heinecke, A., Büchner, T. for the German AML Cooperative Group: Cytomorphology features and prognostic factors in 33 patients with acute myeloid leukemia (AML) and translocation (8;21). Blood 84 Suppl 1, 308a (1994)
12. Cheson, B.D., Cassileth, P.A., Head, D.R., Schiffer, C.A., Bennett, J.M., Bloomfield, C.D., Brunning, R., Gale, R.P., Grever, M.R., Keating, M.J., Sawitsky, A., Stass, S., Weinstein, H., Woods, W.G.: Report of the National Cancer Institute-sponsered Workshop on the definitions of the diagnosis and

response in acute myeloid leukemia. J Clin Oncol 8, 813-819 (1990)
13. Goasguen, J.E., Bennett, J.M., Cox, C., Hambley, H., Mufti, G., Flandrin, G.: Prognostic implication and characterization of the blast cell population in the myelodysplastic syndrome. Leuk Res 15, 1159-1165 (1991)
14. Goasguen, J.E., Matsuo, T., Cox, C., Bennett, J.M.: Evaluation of the dysmyelopoiesis in 336 patients with de novo acute myeloid leukemia: Major importance of dysgranulopoiesis for remission and survival. Leukemia 6, 520-525 (1992)
15. Büchner, T., Urbanitz, D., Hiddemann, W., Rühl, H., Ludwig, W.-D., Fischer, J., AUI, H.C., Vaupel, H.A., Kuse, R., Zeile, G., Nowrousian, M.R., König, H.J., Walter, M., Wendt, F.C., Sodomann, H., Hossfeld, D.K., von Paleske, A., Löffler, H., Gassmann, W., Hellriegel, K.-P., Fülle, H.H., Lunscken, C.h., Emmerich, b., Pralle, H., Pees, H.W., Pfreundschuh, M., Bartels, H., Koeppen, K.-M., Schwerdtfeger, R., Donhuijsen-Ant, R., Mainzer, K., Bonfert, B., Köppler, H., Zurborn, K.-H., Ranft, K., Thiel, E., Heinecke, A.: Intensified induction and consolidation with or without maintenance chemotherapy for acute myeloid leukemia (AML): Two multicenter studies of the German AML Cooperative Group. J Clin Oncol 3, 1583-1588 (1985)
16. Büchner, T., Hiddemann, W.: Treatment strategies in acute myeloid leukemia (AML). Blut 60, 61-67 (1990)
17. Büchner, T., Hiddemann, W., Schaefer, U.W., Löffler, H., Maschmeyer, G., Ludwig, W.-D., Aul, C., Lathan, B., Heinecke, A.: Combined effect of early intensification and prolonged post-remission chemotherapy in patients with AML. Leukemia 6 Suppl. 4, 68-70 (1992)
18. Cassileth, P.A., Harrington, D.P., Hines, J.D., Oken, M.M., Mazza, J.J., McGlave, P., Bennett, J.M., O'Connell, M.J: Maintenance chemotherapy prolongs remission duration in adult nonlymphocytic leukemia. J Clin Oncol 6, 583-587 (1988)
19. Kaplan, E.L., Meier, P.: Nonparametric estimation from incomplete observations. Am Stat Assoc J 53, 457-481 (1958)
20. Peto, R., Pike, M.C., Armitage, P., Breslow, N.E., Cox, D.R., Howard, S., Mantel, N., McPherson, K., Peto, J., Smith, P.G.: Design and analysis of randomized clinical trials requiring prolonged observation of each patient. Br J Cancer 35, 1-39 (1977)
21. Holmes, R.I., Keating, M.J., Cork, A., Broach, Y., Trujillo, J., Dalton, W.T., McCredie, K.B., Freireich, E.J.: A unique pattern of central nervous system leukemia in acute myelomonocytic leukemia associated with inv(16) (p13q22). Blood 65, 1071-1078 (1985)
22. Fenaux, P., Preudhomme, C., Lay, J.L., Morel, P., Beuscart, R., Bauters, F.: Cytogenetics and their prognostic value in de novo acute myeloid leukaemia: A report on 283 cases. Br J Haematol 73, 61-67 (1989)
23. Plantier-Colcher, I., Lai, J.L., Wattel, E., Bauters, F., Fenaux, P.: inv(16) may be one of the only 'favorable' factors in acute myeloid leukemia: A report on 19 cases with prolonged follow-up. Leuk Res 18(12), 885-888 (1994)
24. Larson, R.A., Williams, S.F., Le Beau, M.M., Bitter, M.A., Vardiman, J.W., Rowley, J.D.: Acute myelomonocytic leukemia with abnormal eosinophils and inv(16) or t(16;16) has a favorable prognosis. Blood 68, 1242 (1986)
25. Schiffer, C.A., Lee, E.J., Tomiyasu, T., Wiernik, P.H., Testa, J.R.: Prognostic impact of cytogenetic abnormalities in patients with de novo acute nonlymphocytic leukemia. Blood 73, 263-270 (1989)
26. Kalwinsky D.K., Raimondi, S.C., Schell, M.J., Mirro J., Santana, V.M., Behm, F., Dahl, G.V., Williams, D.: Prognostic importance of cytogenetic subgroups in de novo pediatric acute nonlymphocytic leukemia. J Clin Oncol 8, 75-83 (1990)
27. Liu, P., Claxton, D.F., Marlton, P., Hajra, A., Siciliano, J., Freedman, M., Chandrasekharappa, S.C., Yanagisawa, K., Stallings, R.L., Collins, F.S., Siciliano, M.J.: Identification of yeast artificial chromosomes containing the inversion 16 p-arm breakpoint associated with acute myelomonocytic leukemia. Blood 82, 716-721 (1993)
28. Liu, P.P., Wijmenga, C., Collins, F.S.: Molecular pathogenesis of chromosome 16 inversion in the M4Eo subtype of acute myeloid leukemia. Blood 85, 2289-2302 (1995)
29. Claxton, D.F., Liu, P., Hsu, H.B., Marlton, P., Hester, J., Collins, F., Deisseroth, A.B., Rowley, J.D., Siciliano, M.J.: Detection of fusion transcripts generated by the inversion 16 chromosome in acute myelogenous leukemia. Blood 83, 1750-1756 (1994)
30. Hébert, J., Cayuela, J.M., Daniel, M.T., Berger, R., Sigaux, F.: Detection of minimal residual disease in acute myelomonocytic leukemia with abnormal marrow eosinophils by nested polymerase chain reaction with allele specific amplification. Blood 84, 2291-2296 (1994)
31. Poirel, H., Radford-Weiss, I., Rack, K., Troussard, X., Veil, A., Valensi, F., Picard, F., Guesnu, M., Leboeuf, D., Melle, J., Dreyfus, F., Flandrin, G., Macintyre, E.: Detection of the chromosome 16 CBFβ-MYH11 fusion transcript in myelomonocytic leukemias. Blood 85, 1313-1322 (1995)
32. Gad, S.G., Callen, D.F., Kuss, B., Downing, J.R., Behm, F., Head, D., Ribeiro, R.C., Raimondie, S.C.:Identification of an inversion 16 coexisting with an isochromosome 22q by *in situ* hybridization in a case of childhood AML M4e. Leukemia 7, 1658-1662 (1993)
33. Berger, R., Derré, J., le Conniat, M., Hébert, P., Romana, S., Jonveaux, P.: Inversion-associated translocations in acute myelomonocytic leukemia with eosinophilia. Genes, Chromosomes & Cancer 12, 58-62 (1995)

Acute Leukemias VI
Prognostic Factors
and Treatment Strategies
Büchner et al. (eds)

Prognostic Relevance of Proteolytically Inactivated Alpha$_1$-Antitrypsin Excreted in the Urine of Patients with Acute Myeloid Leukemia

R. Dengler[1], A. Plewan[2], C. Suss [1], R. Busch[2], G. Eger[3], and B. Emmerich[1]

Abstract. During remission induction chemotherapy, a fragment of α_1-antitrypsin (α_1-AT) can be observed in the urine of patients with acute myeloid leukemia (AML). By using immunoblotting, patients with various hemato-oncological diseases were screened for this inhibitor fragment. In 74% of AML patients, the protein was detected. Mean peak excretion was found to be 6.7 µg/mg creatinine (cr). The protein could also be detected in one out of 10 ALL and three out of 15 lymphoma pateints, but not in patients with solid tumors, infections, kidney diseases or healthy donors. Among the AML patients, those who responded completely to induction chemotherapy exhibited significantly higher concentrations of this protein than the non-responders (9.5 vs. 1.5 µg/mg cr). The probability of median time to reach remission was significantly shorter in patients excreting the inhibitor fragment than in the non-excreters (40 vs 100 days). In addition, Kaplan-Meier analysis revealed that overall survival differed significantly when using a best cut-off strategy, which showed that patients with >3 µg/mg cr had a median survival of 28 months compared with 10 months in the group with <3 µg/mg cr. The data presented here are the findings of a pilot study with a limited number of patients. Future studies with larger patient numbers are required to confirm whether or not the excretion of proteolyzed α_1-AT could be a marker for response and prognosis in AML patients.

Introduction

Although progress has been made in the treatment of acute myeloid leukemia (AML) during the past 20 years in that the percentage of patients entering remission has increased, more than 50% still relapse within the first 3 years after diagnosis, and most of these patients eventually succumb to their disease. Therefore, a stratification of subgroups by means of indicators for high or low risk would aid in the choice of the most appropriate treatment for an individual patient. Prognostic factors in AML are, however, limited, with age and FAB-subtype-associated cytogenetics being the only discriminators currently used in clinical practice [1, 2]. These parameters are, moreover, applicable to only a minority of patients. As stated in a recent article, "the use of prognostic factors in therapeutic decision making for patients with AML is still in its infancy" [3].

The response to induction chemotherapy, i.e. the extent of cytoreduction and the time to reach remission, seems to be one of the most powerful indicators for prognosis [4]. However, there are hardly any parameters predictive for achievement of remission [5].

[1]Medizinische Klinik, Klinikum Innenstadt der Universität München, Abteilung für Hämatologie und Onkologie, 80336 Munich, Germany
[2]Medizinische Klinik and Institut für Medizinische Statistik und Epidemiologie der Technischen Universität München, 81675 Munich, Germany
[3]Medizinische Klinik III der Universität Erlangen-Nürnberg, 91054 Erlangen, Germany

It was therefore our intention to develop a marker which could be detected easily, non-invasively and sequentially. We have thus screened the urine of AML patients for proteins and found that a 41-kDa glycoprotein appears during remission induction chemotherapy [6]. This molecule was purified to homogeneity and specific monoclonal antibodies raised against it which showed crossreactivity with α_1-antitrypsin (α_1-AT), also termed α_1-proteinase inhibitor [7]. Molecular characterization revealed that the inhibitor was proteolytically inactivated [8]. By using immunoblotting we have recently screened the urines of AML patients and found that the excretion of this protein (α_1-AT^{41}) correlates with therapy response [9]. In the study presented here we investigated whether the inhibitor fragment can be used as a prognostic marker.

Materials and Methods

Patients

Urine samples of 27 AML patients were investigated. In addition, 10 patients with ALL, 18 with non-Hodgkin's lymphomas, 2 with hodgkin's disease, 13 with solid tumors, including gonadal teratocarcinoma, synovial sarcoma, neuroblastoma, rhabdomyosarcoma, breast cancer, colorectal cancer, and non-small cell lung cancer, 7 with kidney diseases, including nephrotic syndrome, and 20 healthy subjects were screened for the α_1-AT fragment.

Treatment

Twenty four patients with AML received chemotherapy according to the German AML Cooperative group [10], by induction chemotherapy with TAD. Patients under the age of 60 years were treated with early intensification with HAM, and all patients received a second course of TAD. Three patients received the DAV regimen [11]. ALL patients were treated within the German ALL Multicenter study [12]. High-grade lymphoma patients received COPBLAM or COHEPP, low-grade lymphoma patients either COP, CAP, NoSte or fludarabine. Solid tumor patients were receiving either high-dose polychemotherapy or low-dose palliative chemotherapy.

Definition of Therapy Response in AML

Cytoreduction was assessed by microscopic evaluation of marrow aspirates on day 14 and before the second course. According to the Cancer and Leukemia Group B [13], patients were grouped as responders (< 5% residual blasts), partial responders (5–25% blasts) or non-responders (> 25% blasts). Remission was defined as (a) complete remission, when patients achieved normalization of peripheral blood (no blasts, > 3000/µl granulocytes, 100 000/µl platelets) or (b) partial remission (< 5% blasts, > 1000/µl granulocytes, > 50 000/µl platelets).

Urine Processing

Early morning urine was collected two or three times per week during the first 28 days of therapy. After centrifugation, the samples were stored at − 20 °C until use. Thawed samples were again centrifuged at 8000 g for 10 min and supernatants concentrated 2–10-fold using Centrisart tubes according to the creatinine value to correct for differences in protein contents as described [14].

Assay of α_1-AT^{41}

Urinary proteins were boiled for 5 min and mixed 1:1 with sample buffer including 2% SDS, 0.15 M Tris-HCl and 5% β-mercaptoethanol and run in an ultrathin 4–22% polyacrylamide gel electrophoresis system with a maximum current of 1200 V, a power of 50 mA and 30 W for 3 h at 5°C. Separated proteins were transferred onto a polyvinylidene difluoride membrane (Immobilon P) by Western blotting with 10 V, 150 mA, 5 W at 20°C for 32 min in a semidry buffer system [15]. α1-AT and its fragments were specifically detected with a monoclonal antibody prepared against the proteolyzed urinary inhibitor as described [8] and detected by a second biotin-labeled anti-mouse antibody and streptavidin-conjugated peroxidase and the reaction visualized by 3,3′ diaminobenzidine plus nickel-cobalt enhancement [16].

After drying, the protein bands on the blot membrane were subjected to computer-assisted laser scanning densitometry by integration of the area under the peaks. Quantitation was obtained by comparison with a serial dilution of purified α_1-AT^{41}, yielding a standard curve as described [8].

Statistics

Statistical analysis was performed using the BMDP software package (BMDP Project, Academic Computing and Network Services, Northwestern University, Evanston, Ill) on a CDC Cyber NOS/VE computer. Differences in α_1-AT^{41} levels among the patient groups were analyzed by either the Mann-Whitney U test or the Kruskal-Wallis test at a significance level of $p < 0.05$. Cumulative time to reach remission, relapse-free survival and overall survival, as well as the best cut-off values, were calculated by the actuarial method of Kaplan and Meier [17]. The statistical significance of the obtained differences was tested wtih the Log rank test [18].

Results

Of the 27 AML patients, 20 (74%) were found to excrete the 41 kDa inhibitor fragment in their urines. Mean peak excretion (the highest value during the collection period) was 6.7 μg/mg creatinine (cr), with a range from 1.1 to 41 μg/mg. One out of ten ALL and three out of 13 NHL patients also had detectable amounts in their urines. In all other investigated patients, including those with nephrotic syndrome, who exhibited marked proteinuria, the protein could not be detected, at least within the detection limit of the assay (1 μg/mg cr). Within the AML patients, 11 of the 12 responders had measurable amounts of the fragment, with a median peak value of 9.5 μg/mg cr. In contrast, 4 of 7 non-responders excreted the protein, with a median concentration of 1.5 μg/mg cr. Partial responders had intermediate values (5.0 μg/mg). When responders and partial responders were taken together and compared with the non-responders, the difference is statistically significant ($p < 0.05$, Mann-Whitney U test). In a second step, the excretion of α_1-AT^{41} was correlated with time to reach remission. 19 evaluable AML patients receiving TAD as the induction protocol were separated into two groups, i.e. those with and those without detectable amounts of α_1-AT^{41}, and the cumulative time to reach remission compared. The analysis showed that those patients excreting the fragment achieved remission in a significantly shorter time than the non-excreters (median 40 vs 100 days, $p < 0.05$, log rank test).

Next, the follow-up data of remission duration and survival were analyzed and the α_1-AT^{41} values searched for a cut-off point to separate different groups. Figure 1 shows the result for relapse-free survival (RFS) when a cut-off of 3 μg/mg cr is used. Although the difference is not statistically significant, a trend can be observed, i.e. the patients excreting more than 3 μg/mg cr have a longer RFS. In the group excreting < 3 μg/mg cr, RFS is zero after 9 months, whereas in the higher excretion group a plateau is reached at 20% after 3 years. Figure 2 compares the two groups with the same cut-off in respect

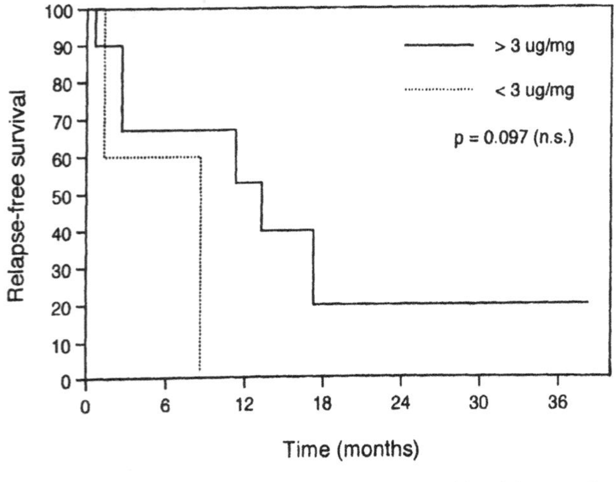

Fig. 1. Cumulative probability of relapse-free survival (RFS) in 19 AML patients treated according to the German AMLCG separated by a cut-off of 3 μg/mg creatinine α_1-AT^{41} peak excretion

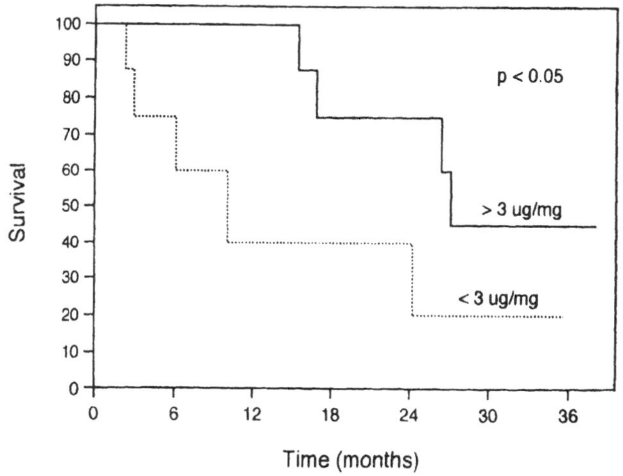

Fig. 2. Overall survival of 19 AML patients separated into two groups by a cut-off of 3 μg/mg creatinine α_1-AT^{41} peak excretion

to overall survival. It is evident that the patients in the group with > 3 μg/mg cr live significantly longer than those in the group below this value ($P < 0.05$, log rank test).

Discussion

We have recently reported that a fragment of α_1-AT can be observed in the urine of AML patients during remission induction chemotherapy [8]. At present, we believe that the inhibitor is truncated in plasma by proteinases released from the myeloid blast cells. By using an immunoenzymatic assay, the amounts of this protein were correlated with cytoreduction and an association was found in that adequate blast cell clearance is accompanied by higher values of α_1-AT^{41} than partial or non-response [9].

The results presented here indicate that this marker could be valuable for the discrimination of prognostically different subgroups of patients. However, the data stem from a small number of patients and should therefore be interpreted with caution until results of a larger trial, which is currently planned, become available.

In addition, some aspects of the assay and the mode of detection have to be improved. First, the densitometric scanning of immunoreactive protein bands, although reported as quantitative and comparable to standard radioimmunoassays [19], is in our opinion a rather semiquantitative technique. Thus, our aim is to generate an antibody specific for α_1-AT^{41} and unreactive with the native 53 kDa inhibitor, which would enable us to establish a sandwich type enzyme linked immunosorbent assay. Second, the timing of sample collection appears to be crucial; daily urine collection and integration of the whole excretion of the protein is rather laborious, but an estimation of a single sample probably does not reflect quantitative excretion of the fragment. Although we observed that the values of day 14 roughly reflect the integrated total excretion, the correlation was not statistically significant. Thus, the excretion of α_1-AT^{41} during the induction period has to be studied in more detail in more patients to find the best time for sample collection.

In conclusion, we present evidence that a fragment of α_1-AT found in the urine of AML patients during the induction period is associated with cytoreduction, time to reach remission and survival, and might thus contribute to the search for prognostic markers in this disease.

Acknowledgment. This work was supported by the Wilhelm Sander-Stiftung, grant 90.006.2.

References

1. Schiffer C.A., E.J. Lee, T. Tomiyasu, P.H. Wiernik, J.R. Testa (1989) Prognostic impact of cytogenetic

abnormalities in patients with de novo acute nonlymphocytic leukemia, Blood 73, 263–270.
2. Büchner Th., W. Hiddemann, B. Wörmann, A. Heinecke, M.C. Sauerland, D. R. Fonatsch, Beacher, D. Hosfeld, J. Goasguen, H. Löffler, U.W. Schäfer for the German AML Cooperative Group (1993) Factors determining outcome in patients with AML (Abstract), Blood 82 (Suppl.), 1929.
3. Löwenberg B. (1995) Post-remission treatment of acute myelogenous leukemia, N. Engl. J. Med. 332, 260–262.
4. Ellison R.R. (1982) Acute myelocytic leukemia, In: Holland J.F. and Frei E. (Eds.), Cancer Medicine, pp. 1407–1446, Philadelphia, Lea & Febiger.
5. Heinecke A., M.C. Sauerland, and Büchner Th. (1990) Predictive models for achievement of complete remission and duration of first remission in adult myeloid leukemia, In: Büchner Th., Schellong G., Hiddemann W., and Ritter J. (Eds.), Acute Leukemias II, Haematology and Blood Transfusion, 33, pp. 285–289, Berlin, Springer.
6. Maubach P.A., B. Emmerich, A. Willer, A. Ogilvie, and J. Rastetter (1984) Urinary glycoproteins in acute leukemia: a 41000 Da glycoprotein follows the kinetics of cytoreduction, Blut 48, 243–245.
7. Ogilvie, A., Eger G., Dengler R., Lottspeich F., Maubach P.A., and Emmerich B. (1990) The response-related urinary 41 kDa glycoprotein is a fragment of α_1-proteinase inhibitor (Abstract) Blood 76, 305.
8. Dengler R., G. Eger, F. Lottspeich, A. Plewan, A. Ogilvie, and B. Emmerich (1992) Proteolytic inactivation of α_1-proteinase inhibitor in vivo: detection, characterization and quantitation of the main fragment excreted in the urine of leukemia patients, Biol. Chem. Hoppe-Seyler 373, 581–588.
9. Dengler R., A. Plewan, U. Münstermann, R. Busch, G. Eger, and B. Emmerich (1995) Urinary excretion of proteolyzed α_1-antitrypsin: specificity, quantitation, and relation to therapy response in patients with acute myeloid leukemia, Clin. Cancer Res. 1, 199–205.
10. Büchner Th., D. Urbanit, W. Hiddemann, et al. (1985) Intensified induction and consolidation with or without maintenance chemotherapy for acute myeloid leukemia (AML): two multicenter studies of the German AML Cooperative Group, J. Clin. Oncol. 3, 1583–1590.
11. Kurrle E., G. Ehninger, M. Freund, et al. (1988) A multicenter study on intensive induction and consolidation therapy in acute myelogenous leukemia, Blut 56, 233–240.
12. Hölzer D., E. Thiel, H. Löffler, et al. (1988) Prognostic factors in a multicenter study for treatment of acute lymphoblastic leukemias in adults, Blood 71, 123–131.
13. Yates J., O. Glidewell, P. Wiernik, et al. (1982) Cytosine arabinoside with daunorubicin or adriamycin for therapy of acute myelocytic leukemia: a CALGB study, Blood 60, 454–462.
14. Lemann J., and B.T. Dumas (1987) Proteinuria in health and disease assessed by measuring the urinary protein/creatinine ratio, Clin, Chem. 33, 297–304.
15. Kyhse-Andersen J. (1984) Electroblotting of multiple gels: a simple apparatus without buffer tank for rapid transfer of proteins from polyacrylamide to nitrocellulose, J. Biochem. Biophys. Meth. 10, 203–214.
16. DeBlas A.L., and H. Cherwinski (1983) Detection of antigens on nitrocellulose paper immunoblots with monoclonal antibodies, Anal. Biochem. 133, 214–222.
17. Kaplan E.L., and P. Meier (1958) Non-parametric estimation from incomplete observations, J. Am. Stat. Assoc. 53, 457–481.
18. Lee E.T. (1980) Statistical methods for survival data analysis, pp. 324–335, Belmont, Wadsworth.
19. Howe J. and J.W.B. Hershey (1981) A sensitive immunoblotting method for measuring protein synthesis initiation factor levels in lysates of Escherichia coli, J. Biol. Chem. 256, 12836–12839.

Acute Leukemias V
Experimental Approaches
and Management of Refractory Diseases
Hiddemann et al. (Eds.)

Studies on Plasma Coagulation in Children with ALL Undergoing Therapy Using the COALL-05-92 Protocol

S. Eckhof-Donovan, R. Kirschke, I. Michelmann, D. Körholz, D. Schwamborn, and U. Göbel

Abstract. A survey conducted in 1993 in patients undergoing treatment using the COALL protocol revealed that not only the use of venous catheters, but also the induction phase as well as the administration of asparginase, represented risk factors for thrombosis. In order to better understand plasma coagulation activity during these phases of treatment, detailed coagulation activity during these phases of treatment, detailed coagulation analysis was performed. Eleven girls and 10 boys suffering from ALL, whose age at the time of diagnosis ranged from 1.4 to 13.1 years and whose leuocyte count at diagnosis between 1,100 and 1,258,000/µl, 11 were treated; according to the high-risk (HR) and 10 according to the low risk (LR) protocol of COALL 05-92. *Coagulation activation parameters:* thrombin-antithrombin-III complex (TAT), modified antithrombin III (ATM), prothrombin fragment (F1+2); *anticoagulatory parameters:* antithrombin (AT III), protein C (PC); *parameters of fibrinolytic capacity:* plasminogen activator inhibitor (PAI), plasminogen (Plmg), antiplasmin (AP). Evaluation of the available data shows coagulatory activity is increased in both the HR and LR groups (higher median values for TAT, ATM and F1+2). Median values for AT III remained within the reference values. PC values were low, particularly following ASP administration. The median values for PAI were within the normal range in both groups in all phases of treatment, and all other measured fibrinolytic parameters were also unremarkable. Not only at the time of diagnosis, but also during therapy, children with ALL have been shown to have increased coagulation activity which does not cause serious derangement of fibrinolytic capacity. Protein C would appear to be a more inconsistent parameter than AT III.

Introduction

Coagulation disturbances and thrombotic complications in the treatment of acute lymphoblastic leukemia in childhood are a frequently discussed issue. There are several different protocols that can be used for therapy of ALL in childhood. Our interest was to document experiences with the COALL-protocol, which was designed by the German Society for Pediatric Oncology and Hematology [1,2]. In 1993, a questionnaire was sent to all participating centers to see whether the clinical manifestation of thrombotic events or hemorrhagic infarctions appears to be a relevant problem [3]. In 286 patients the overall thromboses frequency was 2.1% (6/286). In 1.4% (4/286) patients a continous venous catheter, for example a Broviac catheter, could be regarded as thrombotic risk factor. Two patients (0.6%) developed thrombotic events without a contributing risk factor–so called idiopathic thromboses. Only one patient developed intracranial thrombosis, namely a sinus sagittalis superior thrombosis. He survived, but suffered from severe neurological complications. With regard to the time of thrombotic events during therapy, induction

University Children's Hospital Düsseldorf, Clinic for Pediatric Hematology and Oncology, Moorenstr. 5, 40225 Düsseldorf, Germany

therapy and application of asparaginase seemed to enhance thromboses [3].

To find out whether there are thrombogenic risk phases during treatment using the COALL-05-92 protocol, we planned detailed coagulation studies during therapy.

Material and Methods

Therapy Protocol

The COALL-05-92 protocol consists of a "high-risk" and a "low-risk" version. High and low-risk criteria include age, WBC and immunological type of ALL. Basic elements of the protocol are pre-induction, induction, intensive, CNS, reinduction and maintenance therapy. The main difference between "low-risk" and "high-risk" therapy is that each element of intensive therapy is repeated in the high-risk group. In addition, cyclophosphamide is added to the first element of intensive therapy. We summarize the combination chemotherapy and dosages in Table 1. Unless explicitly mentioned, *E.coli* asparaginase (medac, Germany) was used for treatment.

Patients Characteristics

Twenty-one patients from the University Children's Hospital Düsseldorf took part in our study. Characteristics at the time of diagnosis: sex, 11 female and 10 male; median age, 3.8 years (range 1.4–13.10 years); median WBC, 20, 150/µl (range 1,100/µl–1,258,000/µl); 10 low-risk patients, 11 high-risk patients.

None of our patients developed a thrombotic event during the study period.

Samples

Samples were taken during pre-induction therapy, induction and intensive therapy, since those periods seemed to be most interesting with regard to our basic question. As therapy is still running, the number of samples is not always complete in the single investigated period. During pre-induction and induction, therapy samples were taken by direct venous puncture or with the help of a peripheral venous line. During intensive therapy, most patients had a Broviac catheter as a continuous central venous catheter. Samples were diluted 1:10 with sodium citrate, centrifuged at 620 g for 10 min and stored at −70°C.

Laboratory Analysis

All coagulation studies were performed using commercially available reagents and methods. Routine coagulation analysis consisted of PTT, PT, TT, fibrinogen, F.II, F.V, and F.VII, and will not be discussed further.

Antithrombin III (Chromogenix, Sweden) and protein C (Chromogenix) were measured as coagulation inhibitors. Coagulation activation was investigated with the help of thrombin-antithrombin-III complex TAT (Behring, Germany), modified antithrombin III ATM (STAGO, France) and prothrombin fragment F1+2 (Behring). Plasminogen activator inhibitor PAI (Chromogenix), plasminogen (Chromogenix) and antiplasmin (Chromogenix) are participants of the fibrinolytic system and were investigated to get information about possible involvement.

Table 1. Combination chemotherapy for patients on the COALL-05-92 high-risk protocol during the investigated periods DNR, daunorubicin; VCR, vincristine; CYC, cyclophosphamide; MTX, methotrexate; ASP, asparaginase 6 MP, 6 mercaptopurine; VM 26, teniposide; ARA-C, adriamycine; 6 TG, 6 thioguanine; d, daily

Pre-induction Day -7	Induction 1,8,15,22	Int. 1a 30,31,33	Int. 1b 45,46,48	Int. 2a 57,59	Int. 2b 69,71	Int. 3a 86,87,89	Int. 3b 105,106,108
DNR	VCR	CYC	CYC	MTX	MTX	ARA-C	ARA-C
36 mg/m²	1.5 mg/m²	900 mg/m²	900 mg/m²	1 g/m²	1 g/m²	3 g/m²	3 g/m²
	DNR	MTX	MTX	VM 26	VM 26	ASP	ASP
	36 mg/m²	1 g/m²	1 g/m²	165 mg/m²	165 mg/m²	45,000/m²	45,000/m²
		ASP	ASP	ARA-C	ARA-C		
		45,000 U/m²	45,000 /m²	300 mg/m²	300 mg/m²		
	Prednisone p.o		6 MP p.o	6MP p.o	6 TG p.o		
	60 mg/m²d		100 mg/m²/d	100mg/m²/d	100 mg/m²/d		
MTX i.th		MTX i.th.	MTX i.th.	MTX i.th.	MTX i.th.		

Results During Pre-induction Therapy and Mode of Interpretation

Reference values for each parameter were confirmed by a pool of 20 healthy adults. All values of one patient during one therapy period were summarized as median value. In the following description we speak of "elevated" values when the median is above the reference values, and of "lowered" values when the median is below.

As the very first observations of coagulation studies during therapy might be most influenced by the disease as such, we chose the pre-induction period to demonstrate that we could not find significant differences between the two groups with regard to the investigated parameters. Therefore we did not differentiate between the two risk groups in the following presentation. Pathological values during pre-induction therapy are only found within the coagulation activation, and low-risk patients show even more coagulation activation than high-risk patients.

Median Values of Low-Risk Patients

As can be seen in Table 2, coagulation activation can be found in nearly all investigated periods. Particularly pre-induction, induction and the first part of intensive therapy seem to be involved. Another striking result is the lowering of Int. 3) in combination with lowering of plasminogen (Int. 1)

Median Values of High-Risk Patients

The results are quite similar, but plasminogen levels remain low even longer (Int. 1a, 1b, 2a), combined with low antiplasmin (Int. 1b) and elevation of plasminogen-activator-inhibitor levels (Int. 2a). The decrease in protein C seems to be connected with application of asparaginase (Int. 1a, 1b, 3a, 3b) (Table 3).

Median Values Under Asparaginase Therapy

In order to obtain more information on *E.coli* asparaginase (ASP) therapy, blood sampling was intensified as follows: 1 day before ASP (day – 1), shortly before ASP (day 0), 1 day after first application of ASP (day +1), shortly before second application (day +2), 1 day after second application (day +2), 2 days after second application (day +3), 3 days after second application (day +4). As ASP application is similar in both versions, we did not differentiate between high and low risk. We did not include results from the *Erwinia*-ASP-treatment (last intensive therapy element of low risk). More data are needed in order to compare the two forms of ASP with regard to the investigated side effects.

Table 2. Results during the low-risk protocol TAT; (thrombin-antithrombin-III complex; ATM, modified AT III; F1+2, prothrombin fragment; PC, protein C; AT III antithrombin III; PAI, PLGN-activator-inhibitor; PLGN plasminogen; AP,antiplasmin

Parameter (reference)	Pre-Induction median (range)	Induction median (range)	Int. 1 median (range)	Int. 2 median (range)	Int. 3 median (range)	Int. 4 median (range)
TAT (1.0–4.1ng/1)	44.6 (8.5–60.0)	4.8 (1.8–25–1)	4.7 (2.5–24.7)	6.9 (0.5–16.7)	4.8 (2.3–6.8)	4.0 (2.5–60.0)
ATM (<20µg/m1)	37 (10–49)	27 (23–39)	14 (4–26)	30 (23–76)	18 (3–47)	20 (8–104)
F1+2 (< 1.1 mmol/1)	5.0 (1.9–9.4)	1.5 (0.8–5.4)	1.7 (0.9–4.4)	1.7 (0.7–3.6)	1.1 (0.8–1.8)	1.2 (0.7–7.5)
PC (70–100%)	99 (69–100)	100 (90–100)	60 (30–100)	94 (49–100)	60 (43–85)	74 (58–100)
AT III (> 70%)	128 (92–190)	148 (126–194)	79 (38–140)	99 (70–140)	91 (56–116)	96 (60–134)
PAI (< 24 U/m1)	11 (7–37)	13 (2–28)	20.5 (4–30)	16 (14–38)	11 (4–15)	14 (2–23)
PLGN (70–135%)	108 (98–125)	102 (85–133)	53 (9–101)	94 (62–108)	70 (11–98)	78 (38–125)
AP (> 70%)	101 (77–136)	105 (90–136)	83 (53–126)	92 (40–110)	75 (51–110)	88 (51–127)

Table 3. Results during the high-risk protocol

Parameter (reference)	Pre-Induction median (range)	Induction median (range)	Int. 1a median (range)	Int. 1b median (range)	Int. 2a median (range)	Int. 2b median (range)	Int. 3a median (range)	Int. 3b median (range)
TAT	3.7	4.4	4.2	3.5	6.8	5.6	3.2	3.2
(1.0–4.1 ng/1)	(3.4–15.2)	(1.0–25.0)	(1.0–9.3)	(1.1–11.7)	(2.4–18.0)	(0.6–12.7)	(1.0–25.0)	(1.0–9.8)
ATM	40	97	19	25	45	33	18	17
(< 20 μg/ml)	(37–48)	(39–105)	(0–40)	(15–64)	(31–71)	(29–41)	(17–25)	(11–33)
F1+2	1.5	1.5	1.2	1.2	3.6	1.6	1.6	0.9
(< 1.1 mmol/1)	(1.5–3.2)	(0.5–5.8)	(0.7–2.0)	(0.7–1.8)	(1.8–6.9)	(1.0–1.8)	(0.9–6.2)	(0.8–1.6)
PC	98	100	55	55	80	92	70	66
(70–100%)	(83–100)	(93–100)	(25–100)	(27–100)	(61–105)	(67–100)	(32–100)	(41–124)
AT III	122	146	83	77	95	110	96	95
(> 70%)	(90–130)	(100–200)	(60–154)	(45–112)	(83–128)	(87–122)	(67–128)	(70–146)
PAI	6	17	18	14	25	10	13	16
(< 24 U/ml)	(1–8)	(5–37)	(2–26)	(4–34)	(5–40)	(4–15)	(3–34)	(8–37)
PLGN	92	94	51	44	69	91	83	72
(75–135%)	(72–100)	(86–123)	(35–169)	(26–83)	(53–91)	(48–120)	(51–101)	(51–103)
AP	91	104	97	60	98	99	102	94
(> 70%)	(79–103)	(68–131)	(42–133)	(28–106)	(79–105)	(90–113)	(55–119)	(68–105)

One of the most striking results is that even before ASP application coagulation activation can be shown with the same parameters as explained before. During therapy, a reduction of plasminogen and protein C levels appears. The ASP-dependent deficiency is demonstrated in Fig. 1.

The AT III median remained within reference values as before. The lowest value for AT III was 38% in a patient who reacted very sensitively to ASP with all parameters. She received subsitution therapy with AT III concentrate on day +2. Otherwise no substitution therapy was necessary in the presented patients, even though there were individual patients with AT III values below reference limits.

Discussion

The described data show that the antileukemic treatment using the COALL-05-92 protocol is associated with coagulation activation during the investigated periods of treatment. As we

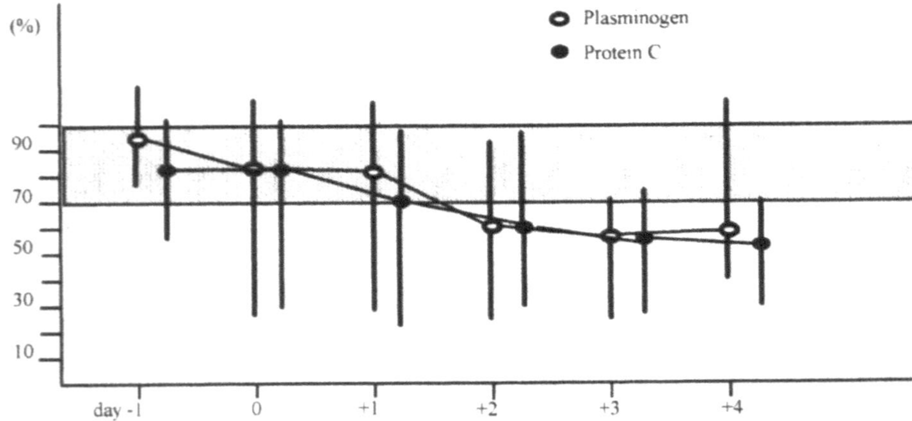

Fig. 1. Median values and ranges of protein C and plasminogen during *E.coli*-ASP treatment: 1 day before ASP (day – 1) shortly before ASP (0) 1 day after first ASP (+1), shortly before second ASP (+2), 1 day after second ASP (+3), 2 days after second ASP (+4)

could show earlier, patients with ALL show activated coagulation even before chemotherapy [4]. We could not show a clear enhancement of this finding during ASP therapy. Mitchell et al. [5] described similar results: at presentation, three of four plasma markers of in vivo thrombin activity (e.g. TAT and F1 +2) were increased in children with ALL. This increased thrombin generation was also documented throughout treatment. In our studies there was a remarkable reduction of the coagulation inhibitor protein C, and sometimes plasminogen as well. AT III appeared much more dependable. These findings are confirmed by earlier studies under a different therapy protocol [6,7]. Risseeuw-Appel et al. [8] investigated 20 children under a Dutch chemotherapy protocol that was based upon the BFM 86 study. They found that asparaginase only had minimal effect on the coagulation system. The overall effect is described as a slight imbalance towards thrombosis mainly because of gradual decrease of protein C activity.

Our data confirm this statement. In contrast to the above mentioned protocol, the COALL-05-92 protocol does not include asparaginase during induction therapy. This appears as an advantage, as prednisone and the destruction of leukemic cell mass themselves attribute to thrombogenic risk. Previously published investigations have supported the separation of induction therapy and ASP application [9,10].

In our study, AT III median values were within reference values, but we know from other studies that AT III levels may be reduced as well [6,11]. As mentioned before, some individual patients in our study group developed AT III deficiency.

As protein C seems to react most sensitively to ASP therapy, a procoagulable state can be assumed during this period of treatment. Protein C takes part in coagulation inhibition as well as in activation of fibrinolysis [12]. Impairment of fibrinolysis caused by protein C deficiency is therefore also possible.

Manifestation of thrombosis is a frequently discussed issue when dealing with ALL treatment in children. Combination of potentially thrombogenic drugs is a possible reason [11,13]. Asparaginase causes a depletion of l-asparagin. Besides selective leukemic cell killing, other organ systems suffer from a temporary impaired protein sysnthesis. This can mean acquired deficiency of coagulation factors and their inhibitors. But probably this effect is only part of a complex thrombogenic situation.

Referring to our initial question of whether we can find a connection between the clinical manifestation of thrombotic events described in a large group of patients [3] and plasma coagulation investigated in our study group, we think that reduced protein C and probably AT III levels on the basis of activated coagulation predispose to thrombotic events during ASP therapy. Any additional risk factor, for example a central venous catheter or combination with other thrombogenic drug such as prednisone, enhances the development of thrombotic complications.

Acknowledgments. This work was supported by the Elterninitiative Kinderkrebsklinik, Düsseldorf. We thank our medical assistants, E. Oellers and G. Göbel, for their vital help.

References

1. Janka-Schaub G.E., Winkler U., Göbel U., Graubner U., Gutjahr P., Haas RJ., Jürgens H., Spaar J. for the COALL Study Group. Rapidly Rotating Chemotherapy in Childhood Acute Lymphoblastic Leukemia: Preliminary Results of a Randomized Comparison with Conventional Therapy. Leukemia (1988) 2; 73–78
2. Winkler K., Beron G., Erttmann R., Jürgens H., Göbel U., Gutjahr P., Kabisch H., Kuhn N., Spaar H.J., J. Drescher, P., Thomas, G. Landbeck COALL-80-Studie zur Behandlung der akuten lymphoblastischen Leukämie (ALL) im Kindealter-ein Zwischenbericht Klin Pädiatr. (1983) 195, 161–167
3. Eckhof-Donovan S., Schwamborn D., Körholz D., Michelmann I., von Kries R., Nürnberger W., Göbel U. Thrombosen bei Kindern mit akuter lymphoblastischer Leukämie unter dem COALL-Protokoll Klin. Pädiatr. (1994) 206, 327–330
4. Eckhof-Donovan S., Ohlenbusch A., vom Orde A., von Kries R., Nürnberger W., Michelmann I. Activation of Coagulation in Children with ALL at the Time of Diagnosis. Klin Padiätr (1993) 205, abstract no. 303
5. Mitchell L., Hoogendoorn H., Giles A.R., Vegh P., Andrew M. Increased Endogenous Thrombin Generation in Children With Acute Lymphoblastic Leukemia: Risk of Thrombotic Complications in L-Asparaginase-Induced Antithrombin III Deficiency. Blood (1994) 83; 386–391
6. Priest J.R., Ramsay N.K.C., Bennett A.J., Krivit W., Edson J.R. The Effect of L-asparaginase of Antithrombin, Plasminogen, and Plasma Coagulation during Therapy for Acute Lymphoblastic Leukemia. J Pediatrics (1982) 100, 990–995

7. Priest J.R., Ramsay N.K.C., Steinherz P.G., Tubergen D.G., Cairo M.S., Sitarz A.L., Bishop A.J., White M.B., White B.S., Trigg M.E., Levitt C.J., Cich J.A., Coccia P.F. A Syndrome of Thrombosis and Hemorraghe complicating L-Asparaginase Therapy for Childhood Acute Lymphoblastic Leukemia. J Pediatrics (1982) 100, 984–989
8. Risseeuw-Appel I.M., Dekker I., Hop W.C.J., Hählen K. (1994) Minimal Effects of E.coli and Erwinia Asparaginase on the Coagulation System in Childhood Acute Lymphoblastic Leukemia: A Randomized Study. Medical and Pediatric Oncology (1994) 23, 335–343
9. Just C., Jürgens H., von Kries R., Wahn V., Göbel U. Immediate and long-term Alterations of Haemostasis due to Asparaginase. in: Wenzel E., Hellstern P., Morgenstern E., Köhler M., von Blohn G. (editors) Rational diagnosis and treatment of hemorrhagic diatheses and thromboembolic disorders, Schattauer Verlag (1986) 5.18–5.21
10. Schieffer M., Schwamborn D., von Kries R.,Göbel U. Structure and Concentration of Fibronectin in Children with Acute Lymphoblastic Leukemia in: Wenzel E., Hellstern P., Morgenstern E., Köhler M., von Blohn G. (editors) Rational diagnosis and treatment of hemorrhagic diatheses and thromboembolic disorders, Schattauer Verlag (1986) 5.13–7.17
11. Sutor A.H., Niemeyer C., Sauter S., Witt I., KaufmehlK., Rombach A.,. Brandis M, Riehm H. Changes in blood coagulation in treatment with ALL-BFM-90 and NHL-BFM-90 protocols. Klin Pädiatr (1992) 204, 264–273
12. Clouse L.H., Comp P.C. The Regulation of Hemostasis: the protein C System New Engl J Med (1986) 314, 1298–1304
13. Rodeghiero F, Castamann G., Dini E. Fibrinopeptide A changes during remission induction treatment with L-asparaginase in acute lymphoblastic leukemia: evidence for activation of blood coagulation Thromb Res (1990) 57, 31–38

Residual Leukemia

Acute Leukemias VI
Prognostic Factors
and Treatment Strategies
Büchner et al. (eds)

Methods for Detection of Minimal Residual Disease

J.F. San Miguel[1] and J.J.M. van Dongen[2]

General Considerations

The available treatment strategies for patients with leukemia results in a high complete remission rate, defined as < 5% detectable neoplastic cells by light-microscopic examination. However, many patients will eventually relapse due to persistence of low numbers of malignant cells that are undetectable by conventional cytomorphological techniques whose detection limit is 1–5 leukemic cells among 100 normal cells. The leukemic cell load under this level is called "minimal residual disease" (MRD). Owing to this patients are indiscriminately subjected to post-remission treatment to eliminate MRD, with the risk of certain cases being either under- and over-treated. Therefore, more sensitive techniques for detection of lower frequencies of leukemic cells are needed [1, 2]. These will allow us to evaluate the effectiveness of treatment through a more precise assessment of the tumor mass in order to predict impending relapses prior to clinical manifestations. The final goal of these studies is to establish a base for the design of patient-adapted post-remission treatments which would reduce the risk of both relapse and over-treatment. In addition, these studies will help to achieve a better assessment of the quality of bone marrow or peripheral blood stem cells scheduled for autologous transplantation and to tackle the important question of whether complete eradication of neoplastic cells is really mandatory for the cure of patients.

Techniques for MRD can be classified depending on the cellular structure identified [1]: (a) overall characteristics of the neoplastic cells, such as the morphology and the in vitro colony growth; (b) cytogenetic characteristics, evaluated either by conventional chromosomal analysis or fluorescence in situ hybridization (FISH); (c) the antigenic immunophenotype of blast cells assessed by multiparametric flow cytometry; (d) DNA content aneuploidy detected by flow cytometry; and (e) DNA sequences, analyzed either by Southern blot or polymerase chain reaction (PCR).

The general strategy in MRD detection is based on the identification at diagnosis of singular leukemic cell characteristics that permits one to distinguish them from residual normal cells. According to these characteristics (cytogenetics, immunophenotypic, or molecular), a custom-built probe will be established at diagnosis for the identification of possible residual leukemic cells during follow up. The efficacy of the different techniques available for the detection of MRD are based on : (a) specificity (to discriminate malignant from normal cells, without false-negative and positive results); (b) sensitivity (detection limit); and (c) reproducibility and applicability(easy standardization and speed in collecting results for the clinical application) (Table 1); (Fig. 1).

Morphology

The sensitivity of morphological analysis is low since, as mentioned above, it ranges between 1: 20 and 1: 100, which is equivalent to a residual

[1]Servicio de Hematologia, Hospital Universitario de Salamanca, Spain
[2]Department of Immunology, Erasmus University, Rotterdam, The Netherlands

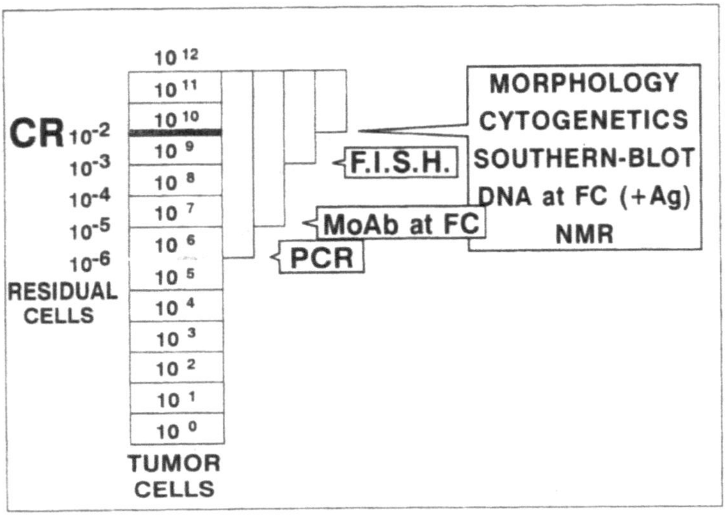

Fig. 1. Detection limits of MRD techniques

Table 1. Applicability of MRD techniques

	Immuno-Phenotype (%)	PCR Analysis (%)
B-ALL	90	100
T-ALL	90	100
AML	80	30–40
B-Cr. LPD B-NHL	?	100
CML	-	100

The percentages indicate the possibility for MRD detection within each group of AL.

cell mass of 10^{10}–10^{11} malignant cells. Moreover, special difficulties emerge to distinguish regenerative bone marrow from MRD [3].

Cytogenetics and FISH

Cytogenetics has the advantage that chromosome aberrations are specific leukemic markers. In addition, it permits the identification of many chromosomal changes within a sample. However, the sensitivity lies within the range of morphology since it only permits the detection of one leukemic cell among 20 normal cells. It should also be taken into account that the cytogenetic aberration may persist for a long time after complete remission has been achieved, and that a clonal selection could be induced when cells are being cultured in order to obtain cell mitosis [4].

Fluorescence in situ hybridization (FISH) is a rapid technique for detection of chromosomal abnormalities not only in metaphase cells but also in cell nuclei in interphase. Although probes for all recurring abnormalities are not yet available, the number is rapidly expanding. This technique is particularly advantageous for studying clonal chromosomal markers in slowly dividing cells such as multiple myeloma and other chronic lymphoproliferative disorders [5]. The sensitivity of centromeric probes for detection of trisomies is 1%, while in monosomies, due to possible artifacts, it is even lower (10%). Nevertheless, when two or three trisomies coexist, the signal points within a single cell become multiplied and thus the error chances decrease, leading to a sensitivity of 10^{-4} [6]. An additional attractive possibility of the FISH technique is the detection of chromosomal translocations by means of specific genomic probes. Several groups, including our own, are currently using this strategy to identify the t(9; 22)(BCR-ABL) [7] and probably soon molecular targets for t(8; 14), t(4; 11), t(8; 21), t(9; 11), etc. will become available. The combined analysis at single cell level of FISH, immunophenotype, and morphology represent an elegant approach for a comprehensive characterization of individual cells, with a high degree of sensitivity and specificity since leukemic cells are identified by a triple marker: chromosome/antigen/morphology [8]; nevertheless, this is a rather complex and time-consuming approach for routine MRD studies.

Cell Cultures

Cell culture techniques have also been used for the investigation of MRD [9–11]. Clonogenic leukemic cells (Colony-forming units lymphoid CFU-L), sharing the same chromosomal abnormality as the leukemic blast cell at diagnosis, have been detected in patients in morphological complete remission [11]. Moreover, the CFU-L are more sensitive for MRD detection than uncultured bone marrow cells since it has been shown the former displayed gene rearrangements that were undetectable in the fresh bone marrow cells [10, 11]. These findings support the clinical observation that patients in complete remission with a high number of CFU-L have a higher incidence of relapse [10]. However, it should be mentioned that CFU-L may persist in some patients that remain in full complete remission for many years and who are theoretically cured [12]. Thus, these would correspond to false-positive results unless these CFU-L were really not the clonogenic cells responsible for disease progression. A different approach to exploit cell cultures for detection of MRD could be based on the alteration in the normal growth pattern of CFU—granulocyte macrophage (CFU-GM) due to the persistence of leukemic hemopoiesis [13]. We have recently observed that the sequential investigation of the CFU-GM growth pattern may be helpful to predict acute myeloblastic leukemia (AML) relapse. In our experience, the proliferation pattern does frequently change during evolution. All patients that switched from an abnormal to a normal growth pattern remain in continous complete remission, while three out of five patients that showed the opposite switch (normal to abnormal) have relapsed. Thus, for the assessment of the real value of these analyses, sequential follow-up studies are mandatory, while single-point studies are not of value.

DNA Aneuploidy

Another alternative for MRD investigations is a DNA content study that permits the detection of an aneuploid peak by flow cytometry. The sensitivity of this technique is low since it requires the presence of a difference of DNA content of at least 5%. Nevertheless, the use of simultaneous staining for DNA content and precise antigens that identify the malignant clone may increase the sensitivity to 10^{-3} [14].

Immunophenotype

Immunophenotypic analysis is theoretically an optimal method for MRD investigation due to its speed and simplicity with a sensitivity ranging from 10^{-3} to 10^{-5}. However, it has the disadvantage of a lack of leukemic-specific antigens with the exception of some proteins resulting from gene fusions such as BCR-ABL or EZA-PBX1, but monoclonal antibodies (MAbs) for these latter markers are not yet available. In general, single immunologic marker analysis is not suitable for distinguishing leukemic cells from their normal counterpart because, as mentioned above, antigens found on leukemic cells are also expressed by normal hematopoietic cells [15–19]. One exception is the use of antibodies to terminal deoxynucleotidil transferase (TdT) to study meningeal infiltration in TdT+ cases of leukemia and lymphoma because TdT+ cells are normally absent from the cerebrospinal fluid [20]. The use of large panels of MAbs in double and triple combinations, analysed at flow cytometry, has shown that leukemic cells frequently display aberrant phenotypic characteristics that allow the distinction of leukemic from normal cells [14, 15, 17, 18, 22–24]. The three most important types of phenotypic aberrations are: lineage infidelity (i.e. expression of lymphoid-associated antigens in myeloid blast cells or vice-versa); maturational asynchronous antigen expression (i.e, CD34/CD20 or CD34/CD56) and increased intensity of antigen expression over-expression [1, 14–16]. In our experience, 73% of AML patients display an aberrant phenotype at diagnosis [23], and the incidence of aberrancies in B-lineage acute lymphoblastic leukemia (B-ALL) and T-ALL patients is 72% and 100%, respectively [24]. With the use of the specific combinations, optimal reagents, and appropriate flow-cytometric strategies, this approach enables the detection of one leukemic cell among 10^5 normal cells. Two possible pitfalls of this technique are the presence of more than one leukemic subpopulation at diagnosis and phenotypic switches at relapse. If several immunophenotypic different subpopulations are detected, it will be necessary to investigate all of them during follow up since perhaps a minor one may be the resistant subclone responsible for relapse. In 85% of our AML patients, two or more cell subpopulations were detected at diagnosis, and frequently these included small subclones represented by < 10% blast cells [25]. Phenotypic switches may occur and their incidence has not been clearly established in either AML or ALL. Although phenotypic changes are apparently common, they do not usually affect the criteria used for defining a phenotype as aberrant [15, 22]. In our experience, only 16% of AML patients, 22% of T-ALL, and 19% of B-ALL displayed changes in the aberrant phenotypes.

Molecular Biology

Finally, probably the most promising tool for detection of MRD is the investigation at molecular level of two types of tumor-specific markers: (a) clone-specific junctional regions generated physiologically through immunoglobulin (Ig) and T cell receptor (TCR) gene rearrangements or by illegitimate V(D)J recombinase activity (e.g., SIL-TAL1); and (b) disease-specific fusion regions of oncogenes involved in chromosomal translocations (e.g., PML/RAR)[17, 21, 26, 27]. These leukemia specific molecular targets can be analyzed by Southern blot or PCR. The first has a low sensitivity $1{:}10^2$, while PCR allows the detection of up to one leukemic cell among 1 million malignant cells; thus the latter is the molecular technique of choice for MRD detection [17, 26]. The strategy for the study of rearranged Ig and TCR includes the PCR analysis of the junctional region and the direct sequencing of the PCR products using oligonucleotide primers. Based on the obtained nucleotide sequence, junctional region-specific oligonucleotide probes are designed for detection of residual leukemic cells [17, 27–30]. This strategy may be used not only for ALL but also for some AML patients [10%–30%] that display inappropiate rearrangements of Ig and TCR genes [17, 31]. The study by PCR of fusion regions of genes involved in chromosomal translocations requires that the breakpoint should occur at a constant region of small size (< 2 b). The variability in translocation breakpoints precludes in many cases their study at the DNA level. However, these translocations frequently produce leukemiaspecific fusion mRNAs which can be used as PCR targets after reverse transcription into cDNA (RT-PCR) [17, 26]. The clinical value of these studies is still controversial. In B-ALL it has been shown that, at the end of therapy, a negative PCR result of Ig rearrangements does not exclude eventual relapse [32]. By contrast, it has been postulated [33] that in patients with acute promyelocytic leukemia, the persistence of positivity for RT-PCR to detect the PML/RAR fusion gene correlates highly with subsequent relapse, while the presence of serial negative results is associated with good prognosis. Some other chromosomal abnormalities may persist of long time, making therapeutic decisions especially complicated. Thus, the AML1/ETO fusion gene resulting from the t(8; 21) in M_2 leukemias can be detected in patients in continuous complete remission for > 5 years [26].

In these studies it is also very important to be aware of the limitations and pitfalls of PCR techniques: (a) false-positive results can be caused by amplification of sequences of normal cells or leukemic debris. Positive and negative controls must be included in all assays. In order to prevent cross-contamination, particularly with techniques based on RNA targets, the separation of laboratory space for DNA and RNA is important; special care must be taken following amplification, and those samples should be handled in a hood; (b) false-negative results may originate from samples of poor quality, control for DNA/RNA degradation is mandatory in these cases. In addition, Ig and TCR rearrangements may display oligoclonality at diagnosis and clonal evolution at relapse which can cause false-negative results if these gene junctional regions used for MRD detection [29, 30].

Although the real value of MRD studies remains controversial, and a definitive answer will not be reached until longitudinal prospective studies enrolling large number of patients are carried out, some consensus has already emerged based on the available data:

1. Sequential studies are mandatory in MRD investigations.

2. Single-point results have a very low value, especially during the early phase of treatment.
3. In some maligganancies it could take several years to eradicate all malignant cells (or the molecular abnormalities, e.g., AML1/ETO).
4. The switch from negative to positive results (two consecutive samples) predicts impending relapse.
5. The number of residual cells at the end of induction treatment has prognostic implifications.
6. The predictive value of these tests may vary among diseases. Independent evaluation of each neoplasia is necessary.

The data emerging from some on-going European and American cooperative studies will contribute to a final confirmation of whether or not MRD detection can really be used to adapt future treatment strategies in order to prevent both under-and over-treatment in patients with leukemia and lymphoma.

Acknowledgment. This work is part of a concerted action partially supported by the European Union's Biomedical and Health Research Biomed 1 Programme.

References

1. San Miguel JF, C. Bartram, D. Campana, M. Andreeff. Minimal residual disease in hematological malignancies. Rev. Inv. Clin (Suppl) 1994; 147-152.
2. Worman B, S. Konemans, M. Safford, et al. Immunophenotypic heterogeneity of leukemic cell in AML at diagnosis and after chemotherapy. Blood 1990; 76: 377a.
3. Bennett JM. Detection of relapse in acute leukemia: should we discontinue routine bone marrow serveillance?. Leukemia 1992;6: 1099-1110.
4. Dewald GW, M.A. Morris, V.C. Lilla. Chromosome studies in neoplastic hematological disorders. In: Clinical Laboratory Medicine, KD McClatchey, ed. Williams & Wilkins, Baltimore (1993).
5. Criel A, I. Wlodarska, P. Meeus, M. Stul, A. Louwagie, V. Hoof, M. Hudajat, C. Mecucci, H. Van den Berghe. Trisomy 12 is uncommon in typical chronic lymphocytic leukaemias. Br. J. Haematol. 1994; 87: 523-528.
6. Kibbelaar RE, F. Kok, E.J. Dreef, J.K. Kleiverda, C.J. Cornelisse, A.K. Kaap, PhM. Kluin. Statistical methods in interphase cytogenetics: an experimental approach. Cytometry 1993; 14: 716-724.
7. Tkachuk CD, C.A. Westbrook, M. Andreeff, et al. Detection of bcr-abl fusion in chronic myelogenous leukemia by in-situ hybridization. Science 1990; 250: 559-562.
8. Kibbelaar, R.E. H. van Camp. D.J. Dreef, et al. Combined immunophenotyping and DNA in situ hybridization study lineage involvement in patients with myelodysplastic syndromes. Blood 1992; 79: 1823-1828.
9. Uckun FM, J.H. Kersey, R. Haake, et al. Pretransplantation burden of leukemic progenitor cells as a predictor of relapse after bone marrow transplantation for acute lymphoblastic leukemia. N.Engl.J.Med. 1993; 329: 1296-1301.
10. Gerhartz MM, H. Schmetzer. Detection of minimal residual disease in acute myeloid leukemia. Leukemia 1990; 4: 508-516.
11. Miller CB. B.A. Zehnbaner. S. Piantadosi. S.D. Rowley. and R.J. Jones. Correlation of occult clonogenic leukemia drug sensitivity with relapse after autologous bone marrow transplantation. Blood 1991; 78: 1125-1131.
12. Estrov Z, T. Gunberger, I.D. Dube, Y-P. Wang, M.H. Freedman: Detection of residual acute lymphoblastic leukemia cells in cultures of bone marrow obtained in remission. N.Engl.J.Med. 1986; 315: 386-389.
13. Aul C, N. Gutterman, W. Schneider: Comparison of in vitro growth characteristics of blast cell progenitors (CFU-L) in patients with myelodysplastic syndromes and acute leukemia. Blood 1992; 80: 625-633.
14. Orfao A, J. Ciudad, M.C. López-Berges, A. López Borrasca, B. Vidriales, M.D. Caballero, B. Valverde, M. Gonzalez, J.F. San Miguel. Acute lymphoblastic leukemia (ALL): detection of minimal residual disease (MRD) at flow cytometry. Leukemia & Lymphoma 1994; 1: 87-90.
15. Campana D,E. Coustan-Smith, G. Janossy. The immunological detection of minimal residual disease in acute leukemia. Blood 1990; 76: 163-169.
16. Campana D, E. Coustan-Smith, F.G. Behm. The definition of remission in acute leukemia with immunologic techniques. B.M.T. 1991; 8: 429-437.
17. Van Dongen JJM, T.M. Breit, H.J. Adriaansen, A. Beishuizen, H. Hooijkaas. Detection of minimal residual disease in acute leukemia by immunological marker analysis and polymerase chain reaction. Leukemia 1992; 6: 47-59.
18. Worman B. Implications of detection of minimal residual disease. Current Opinion in Oncology 1993; 5: 3-12.
19. Adriaansen HJ, B.C. Jacobs, M.C. Kappers-Klunne, K. Hanle, H. Hooijkaas, J.J.M. van Dongen. Detection of residual disease in AML patients by use of double immunological marker analysis for terminal deoxynucleotidyl transferase and myeloid markers. Leukemia 1993; 7: 472-481.
20. Hooijkaas H, K. Hahlen, H.J. Adriaansen, I. Dekker, G.E. van Zanen, J.J.M. van Dongen. Terminal deoxynucleotidyl transferase (TdT)-positive cells in the cerebrospinal fluid and development of overt CNS leukemia: a 5-year follow-up study in 113 children with a TdT-positive leukemia or non-Hodgkin's lymphoma. Blood 1989; 74: 416-422.

21. Campana D, S. Yokota, E. Coustant-Smith, T.E. Hansen-Hagge, G. Janossy, C.R. Bartram. The detection of residual acute lymphoblastic leukemia cells with immunologic methods and polymerase chain reaction: a compartive study. Leukemia 1990; 9: 609–614.
22. Coustant-Smith E, F.G. Behm, C.A. Hurwitz, G.K.J. Rivera, D. Campana. N-CAM (CD56) expression by CD34+ malignant myeloblasts has implications for minimal residual disease detection in acute myeloid leukemia. Leukemia 1993; 7: 853–858.
23. Macedo A, A. Orfao, M.B. Vidriales, M.C. López-Berges, B. Valverde, M. Gonzalez, M.D. Caballero, F. Ramos, M. Martinez, J.F. San Miguel. Characterization of aberrant fenotypes in acute myeloid leukemia. Ann.Hematol. 1995; 70: 189–194.
24. Macedo A, A. Orfao, A. Martinez, B. Vidriales, M.C. López-Berges, J.F. San Miguel. Immunophenotype of C-kit cells in normal human bone marrow: implications for the detection of minimal residual disease. Br.J.Haematol. 1995; 89: 338–341.
25. Macedo A, Orfao A, M. Gonzalez, B. Vidriales, M.C. López-Berges, A. Martinez, J.F. San Miguel. Immunological detection of blast cell subpopulations in acute myeloblastic leukemia at diagnosis: implications for minimal residual disease studies. Leukemia (In press).
26. Bartram CR. Detection of minimal residualleukemia by the polymerase chain reaction: potential implications for therapy. Clin.Chim.Acta 1993; 217: 75–83.
27. Potter MN, N.C.P. Cross, J.J.M. van Dongen, G. Saglio, A. Oakhill, C.R. Bartram, J.M. Goldman. Molecular evidence of minimal residual disease after treatment for leukaemia and lymphoma: an updated meeting report and review. Leukemia 1993; 7: 1302–1314.
28. Ito Y, R. Wasserman, N. Galili, B.A. Reichard, S. Shane, B. Lange, G. Rovera Molecular residual disease status at the end of chemotherapy fails to predict subsequent relapse in children with B-lineage acute lymphoblastic leukemia. J.Clin.Oncol.1993; 11: 546–553.
29. Beishuizen A, M.A.J. Verhoeven, E.R. van Wering, K. Hahlen, H. Hoojikaas, J.J.M. van Dongen. Analysis of Ig and T-cell receptor genes in 40 childhood acute lymphoblastic leukemias at diagnosis and subsequent relapse: implications for the detection of minimal residual disease by polymerase chain reaction analysis. Blood 1994; 83: 2238–2247.
30. Kitchingman GR. Residual disease detection in multiple follow-up samples in children with acute lymphoblastic leukemia 1994; 8: 395–401.
31. Sanchez I. J.F. San Miguel. Corral et al. Gene rearrangement in acute non-lymphoblastic leukemia. Correlation with morphological and immunophenotypic characteristics of blast cells. Br.J.Haematol. 1995; 89: 104–109.
32. Lion T, T. Henn, A. Gaiger, P. Kahis, H. Dagner. Early detection of relapse after bone marrow transplantation in patients with chronic myelogenous leukaemia. Lancet 1993; 341: 275–276.
33. Lococo F, D. Diversio, P.D. Paudolfi et al.: Molecular evaluation of residual disease as predictor of relapse in acute promyelocytic leukemia. Lancet 1992; 340: 1437–1438.

Acute Leukemias VI
Prognostic Factors
and Treatment Strategies
Büchner et al. (eds)

Molecular Biological Detection of Minimal Residual Disease in Acute Lymphoblastic Leukemia

C.R. Bartram[1], T. Seriu[1], T.E. Hansen-Hagge[1], J.W.G. Janssen[1], and W.-D. Ludwig[2]

Introduction

During the last two decades substantial improvement has been made in the treatment of children with acute lymphoblastic leukemia (ALL). Chemotherapy alone induces complete clinical and hematologic remission in almost every patient and achieves cure rates of 75% [1, 2]. Progress in the treatment of adult ALL patients is less pronounced with long-term remissions in about 30% of cases [3]. This inferior outcome is at least partly explained by differences in the incidence of biologically defined leukemia subentities between both age groups [4]. In particular, BCR-ABL-positive ALL, the most aggressive ALL subtype, is observed in a third of the adults, but only in 4% of childhood ALL [5]. One major challenge of today's oncology is therefore to guarantee a timely diagnosis of prognostically relevant entities and to design more efficient treatment strategies for respective patients, the latter being undoubtedly the more difficult task.

Since most relapses originate from neoplastic cells escaping therapeutic intervention, sensitive methods are required in order to detect impending recurrences prior to clinical manifestation or to determine the quality of a morrow scheduled for autologous transplantation. On the other hand, an insufficiently characterized group of eventually cured ALL patients, particularly children, may in fact receive over-treatment and face adverse long-term effects. In this context, the introduction of polymerase chain reaction (PCR) techniques [6] has set new standards for the monitoring of leukemia patients by permitting the detection of as few as one leukemia cell within 10^4–10^6 normal cells in more than 90% of ALL cases. In the following, we will briefly discuss PCR studies which are hoped to ultimately provide a rationale for the design of patient-adapted treatment protocols.

Molecular Marker Categories

In principle, two marker systems can be used for PCR analyses in ALL patients. Probably the more important one is based on the unique patten of immunoglobulin (Ig) or T cell receptor (TCR) gene recombinations characterizing every ALL patient [7, 8]. Since the three landmark reports from 1989 on PCR strategies utilizing rearranged IgH [9], TCRγ [10], or TCRδ [11] loci, respectively, various techniques have been proposed for the generation of clonospecific junctional probes and their consecutive application to detect minimal residual disease (MRD). It is possible to design consensus primers which recognize the majority of V or J elements of a given Ig or TCR locus or, alternatively, to synthesize specific amplifiers that hybridize to individual V or J segments. The amplification product may then be isolated and directly used as a probe or, following sequence analysis, a junction-specific oligomer can be prepared. Yet

[1]Selection of Molecular Biology, Department of Pediatrics II, University of Ulm, Helmholtzstrasse 10, 89081 Ulm, Germany
[2]Department of Medical Oncology and Applied Molecular Biology, Robert-Rössle Cancer Center, Free University of Berlin, Germany

other approaches comprise the usage of a single-sided oligonucleotide primer or PCR-mediated RNAse protection analysis (for a review see [12, 13]). Recent modifications include the introduction of selection steps by usage of biotinylated PCR products in order to reduce unspecific background signals or the application of synthetic oligomers representing Ig or TCR junctions as clonospecific primers for consecutive rounds of amplification rather than as clonospecific probes [14–16]. Such adaptations improve and facilitate significantly the detection of MRD in ALL patients (Fig. 1). Extensive analyses of the IgH, TCRγ, and TCRδ loci from ALL patients, namely by the group of van Dongen [7, 8, 17–19], paved the way for the monitoring of MRD in principally all T-ALL cases and more than 90% of B-lineage ALLs. A limited set of restriction enzymes, well characterized probes and oligomers allow the initial identification of suitable Ig/TCR marker loci by Southern blotting and the consecutive amplification and sequencing of junctional regions.

However, since more than 50% of ALL patients show changes in Ig and TCR recombination patterns between diagnosis and subsequent relapse that may prevent the detection of leukemia cells if affecting the junctional region represented by the clonospecific probe [20], it appears mandatory to use at least two independent markers in order to confirm results derived from the application of a single PCR approach. False-negative results may also be caused by the focal persistence of residual leukemia cells [12]. This pitfall is of course associated with any type of MRD diagnostic and can probably not be avoided.

Illegitimate V(D)J recombinase activity at the TCRδ/α gene cluster mediates a 90-kb deletion on chromosome 1p32 that results in the fusion of the TAL1 and SIL genes in approximately 15% of T-ALL patients [21]. Since SIL-TAL fusion regions become similarly modified as Ig or TCR junctions, they represent attractive targets for the generation of clonospecific probes [22].

In contrast to the loci mentioned above, the second, steadily increasing marker category comprises disease-specific rather than patient-(clone-)specific gene recombinations. Table 1, probably already outdated when published, summarizes oncogene recombinations based on chromosomal abnormalities that are accessible to molecular genetic diagnosis [23, 24]. However, only a minority of them appear relevant for PCR studies aimed at the detection of MRD since most of these genetic lesions are very rare (< 1% of ALLs). From a practical point of view, four entities appear noteworthy. As mentioned above, the BCR-ABL recombination is the most common genetic abnormality in adult ALL with a particularly high incidence (50%) in B-precursor leukemias [5]. BCR-ABL transcripts can be used as a marker for leukemia cells in

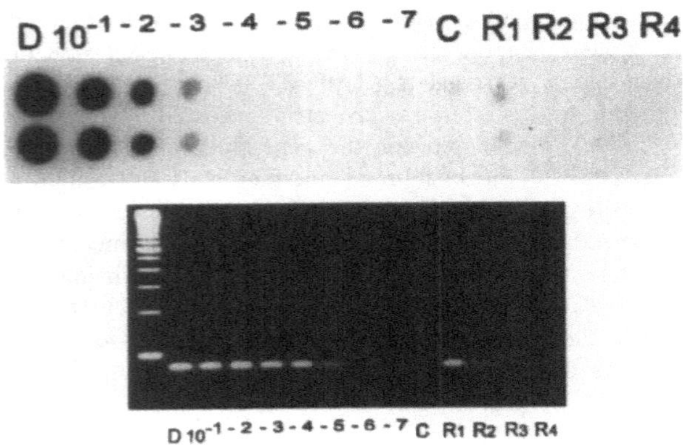

Fig. 1. Application of clonospecific TCRγ sequences either as a probe (*upper panel*) or as 5′ primer (allele-specific oligomer, ASO, *lower panel*). Leukemia cell DNA obtained from a patient with common ALL (*D*) was serially diluted into peripheral blood cell DNA of healthy individulas (*C*) at 10^{-1}–10^{-7}; 5 μl amplification products were dotted and hybridized with the clonospecific probe. Alternatively, DNA fragments obtained by ASO-PCR were run in a 3% agarose gel. Remission samples were obtained 1, 3, 6, and 9 months after initial diagnosis (*R1-R4*). Note a 100-fold increase in sensitivity and the detection of residual disease in sample R2 by ASO-PCR as compared to the usage of a clonospecific oligonucleotide probe

Table 1. Gene rearrangements in acute lymphoblastic leukemia

Chromosome defect	Genes involved	Cell lineage
1p32*	SIL-TAL1[b]	T
t(1; 7)(p32; q34)	TAL1-TCRβ	T
t(1; 7)(p34; q34)	LCK-TCRβ	T
t(1; 14)(p32; q11)	TAL1-TCRδ	T
t(1; 19)(q23; q13)	PBX1[c]-E2A	B
t(2; 8)(q12; q24)	Igk-MYC	B
t(4; 11)(q21; q23)	AF4[d]-ALL1[e]	B
t(5; 14)(q31; q32)	IL3-IgH	B
t(6; 11)(q27; q23)	AF6-ALL1	B
t(7; 9)(q34; q34)	TCRβ-TANr	T
t(7; 19)(q34; q24)	TCRβ-HOX11[F]	T
t(7; 19)(q34; q13)	TCRβ-LYL1	T
t(8; 14)(q24; q11)	MYC-TCRα	T
t(8; 14)(q24; q32)	MYC-IgH	B
t(8; 22)(q24; q11)	MYC-Igλ	B
9q34[a]	SET-CAN	B
t(9; 11)(p21; q23)	AF9-ALL1	B
t(9; 12)(q34; p13)	ABL-TEL	B
t(9; 22)(q34; q11)	ABL-BCR	B
t(10; 14)(q24; q11)	HOX11-TCRδ	T
t(11; 14)(q13; q11)	TTG2-TCRδ	T
t(11; 14)(p15; q11)	TTG1-TCRδ	T
t(11; 19)(p23; q13)	ALL1-ENL1[i],	B, T
t(11; X)(q23; q13)	ALL1-AFX	T
t(17; 19)(q22; q13)	HLF-E2A	B
t(X; 14)(q28; q11)	MTCP1-TCRδ	T

[a]submicroscopic deletion. Alternative designations: [b]SCL, TCL5; [c]PRL, [d]FEL, MLLT2; [e]MLL; HRX; [f]TAL2; [g]TCL3; [h]rhombotin; [i]LTG 19, MLLT1.

about a third of adult ALL patients and 4% of pediatric cases. The PBX1-E2A fusion of t(1; 19) represents the most common oncogene recombination in childhood ALL (6%) with a frequency of 25% in pre-B-ALL [23]. Translocations involving chromosome region 11q23 occur in about 7% of ALL with an exceptionally high incidence of 75% in infants (25–27). The spectrum of recombination partners comprises more than 20 different loci with a predominance of t(4; 11) and t(11; 19) in ALL [28]. An ALL1-AF4 rearrangement, the molecular hallmark of t(4; 11), is observed in 35% of children and adults with pre-pre-B-ALL [29] and can be used to monitor residual disease in about 5% of all ALL patients. Finally, HOX11 recombinations as a consequence of the t(4; 10), are observed in 7% of T-ALL. In summary, these genetic lesions constitute useful complementary tools for the detection of MRD by PCR in approximately 15% of children and 45% of adults with ALL. The fact that some of these genetic defects define biologically/prognostically distinct ALL subtypes is a specific advantage of this marker category.

Since the breakpoints of chromosomal translocations are often spread over large distances at the genomic level, hybrid mRNAs after reverse transcription into cDNA have to be used as amplification targets. Starting at the RNA level, however, requires specific care in handling cell samples and makes it necessary to establish scrupulous precautions to minimize the danger of false-positive results caused by contamination [30]. Moreover, quantification of residual disease at the transcript level (as compared to DNA-based PCR targets) poses problems which can only be overcome by the application of relatively complex competitive PCR analyses [31].

Note that the methods as discussed above are far from routine practice and require the expertise of specialized molecular genetic laboratories.

Preliminary Lessons from Retrospective Studies

Only very few PCR studies have thus far addressed the MRD status of ALL patients by targetting recombined oncogene sequences. Although the technical principles to monitor BCR-ABL-positive ALL were already introduced in 1988 [32], applications of this marker remain infrequent. This may be due to the short remission durations associated with this very aggressive ALL subtype. The few available data indicate that intensified chemotherapy or bone marrow transplantation may eradicate leukemia and thus constitute reasonable options for some patients [12, 33–36]. However, new treatment modalities (which, for example, correct altered signal transduction pathways triggered by the BCR-ABL product) are definitely required to cure the majority of respective patients. Apart from the Ph translocation, the t(4; 11) has been associated for a long time with a very poor prognosis. This high-risk group, however, has definitely improved following the introduction of intensified protocols [1]. Along this line, all bone marrow samples obtained from ALL1-AF4-positive ALL patients in continuous complete remission lacked evidence of MRD in recent studies [29, 37]. PCR analyses utilizing TAL1 [38, 39], E2A [40–42], or HOX11 [43] recombinations as PCR targets remain thus far anecdotal.

Much more insight into the remission status of ALL patients has been gained through the application of clonospecific Ig or TCR probes. More than 300 ALL cases have been studied by PCR (for a review until 1992 see [12, 13] and refererences herein). These investigations, however, are compromised by many shortcomings associated with retrospective analyses, namely case selection. Moreover, these studies frequently included different age groups, did not balance for biologically distinct ALL entities, and were based on various chemotherapeutic trials. Nevertheless, it appears appropriate to draw some general conclusions from the published data: (a) longitudinal analyses disclosed marked individual differences in the intervals between achievement of clinical remission and eradication of leukemic cells below the detection level of PCR—these dynamic disparities in reduction of malignant cells do not necessarily correlate with known risk factors and may define independent components of the individual response to chemotherapy; (b) the majority of ALL patients remain PCR positive at the end of remission induction, and residual leukemia cells show self-renewing capability [44]—it generally takes several months of consolidation or even maintenance therapy to convert into a PCR-negative status; (c) a constantly high level of leukemia burden several months after remission induction or a steady increase of blasts predicts relapse and can be diagnosed up to several months prior to clinical manifestaion; (d) the application of independent markers per patient appears important for a balanced interpretation of the remission status.

The possibility that residual disease at the end of induction therapy predicts long-term out-come i.e., relapse, is particularly intriguing [45, 46]. If this observation can be confirmed in controlled prospective trials, it would represent an important parameter for the future design of patient-adapted protocols. A related question concerns the relevance of PCR negativity at the end of chemotherapy. If the absence of MRD at the end of treatment is not sufficient to assure that a patient is cured [47], later relapses may escape timely detection unless off-therapy marrows are taken serially, which may not be practicable. As an aside, it will become interesting to evaluate systematically the predictive value of marrow analyses in patients with "isolated" extra-medullary relapses [48, 49].

The tools to tackle these issues are available and should be applied without further delay. We emphasize, however, that PCR analyses to monitor residual disease should currently be restricted to investigational studies in the frame work of therapeutic trials, they are not yet recommended for community practice.

Prospective Trials: The Next Crucial Step

Results from prospective PCR studies are still scanty, but in line with experiences from retrospective analyses [50, 51]. However, data from prospective trials enrolling large numbers of patients have to be awaited before case-adapted treatment protocols can be seriously considered. Since the diagnosis "ALL" comprises a variety of biologically/genetically defined subentities, respective parameters have to be taken into account. It appears, for example, less informative to determine the remission status of adult ALL patients without knowledge of their BCR-ABL status. Moreover, results emerging form PCR studies based on different treatment modalities may vary substantially.

To overcome some of these shortcomings, the European BFM Study Group has opened a prospective PCR trial after a series of intensive discussions, particularly taking ethical aspects into account. Approximately 500 children with ALL were recruited between 1992 and 1994 and will be monitored according to a fixed schedule of 10 marrow aspirates to be taken over a 3-year-period after diagnosis. The responsible molecular laboratories in Austria (R.E. Panzer-Grümayer), Germany (C.R. Bartram), Italy (A. Biondi), and The Netherlands (J.J.M. van Dongen) are using identical techniques, probes, and primers. Obligatory PCR targets constitute rearranged TCRγ, TCRδ, and SIL-TAL loci, other markers are optional. An advantage of this PCR study is the fact that the molecular data can be interpreted in the context of morphological, immunophenotypic, and cytogenetic parameters that are likewise determined according to standardized criteria [52]. It is reasonable to assume that a first set of informative data will be available by 1996, although final conclusions cannot be expected before the end of the study in 1997.

Our laboratory has recently started with the evaluation of a first series of 108 consecutive patients enrolled in the BFM trial from whom remission samples were taken over a period of 18 months after diagnosis. With a set of only two digests and four probes, suitable TCRγ and TCRδ recombinations were identified in 17/17 T-ALL and 80/91 precursor B-ALL, i.e., in 90% of cases under investigation. One T-ALL showed a SIL-TAL recombination. Taking into account the four TCRδ and α alleles that might rearrange in a leukemia cell clone, we determined two, three, or four junctions suitable for PCR analyses in 29%, 20%, and 9% of the cases, respectively. For 50% of the patients clonospecific TCRγ as well as TCRδ probes could be generated. This means that at least two independent markers were available in about 60% of the ALL cases. Since we also plan to include clonospecific IgH junctional probes, it appears feasible to generate multiple independent probes for almost every ALL patient. Owing to modifications of PCR protocols, as mentioned above, our analyses reached a detection level of 10^{-4}–10^{-6} in all cases. Remission samples have thus far been analyzed in 39 cases. In accordance with data from our retrospective studies, the majority of patients were still PCR positive at the end of remission induction. However, all patients who are in continuous complete remission became PCR negative within 9 months after diagnosis, most of them already during the first 3 months of treatment. Five of the 39 patients (three precursor B-ALL, two T-ALL) relapsed and died. In all cases this event could be predicted by PCR. One patient initially became PCR negative, but showed a steady increase of leukemia cells 3 months before clinical manifestation (12 months after diagnosis). Remarkably, four patients exhibited constantly high amounts ($>10^{-3}$) of residual blasts (Fig. 2). These patients relapsed on maintenance therapy 6–11 months after diagnosis.

Prospective trials such as the one of the European BFM Study Group will have to determine during the next few years the possible place of PCR analyses in the monitoring of ALL patients. Important questions remain to be answered. Do serial PCR analyses yield a benefit to individual patients (or at least to distinct ALL subtypes)? Is it possible to predict the long-term outcome at an early stage of treatment? Can a timely diagnosis of leukemia relapse be achieved for patients under or post treatment (and do effective therapeutic alternatives exist for these patients)? However, even if the ongoing prospective PCR trials indeed come up with promising data, the ultimate value of PCR-guided protocol adaptations will have to be further evaluated in consecutive randomized trials stratified according to molecular parameters. Thus, it might take another decade untill individualized ALL protocols eventually become reality.

Acknowledgments. We thank D.H.R. Erz for expert technical assistance, H. Barro for help with the

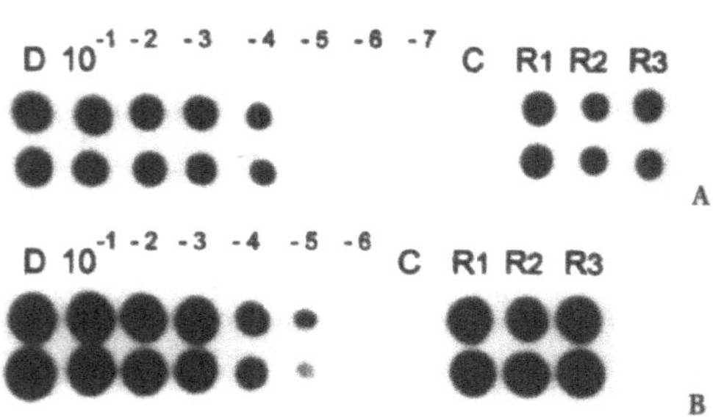

Fig. 2A, B. PCR analysis of the remission status with clonospecific TCRδ probes in two patients with T-ALL (**A**) and cALL (**B**). Note the constantly high amount of residual leukemia cells in remission samples R1 through R3 (obtained 1, 3, and 6 months after diagnosis). Both patients relapsed clinically 8 and 10 months after diagnosis, respectively

preparation of the manuscript, the participants in the multicenter ALL Trials for children (BFM) and Adults (BMFT) for continuous support, and the members of the BIOMED-1 Concerted Action on Minimal Residual Disease in Acute Leukemia, namely Professor J.J.M. van Dongen(Rotterdam) for fruitful cooperation. This work was supported by grants from the Deutsche Krebshilfe, Bundesministerium für Forschung und Technologie, the European Union, and Fördeskreis tumor-und leukämiekranke Kinder Ulm e.v.

References

1. Rivera GK, Raimondi SC, Hancock ML, Behm FG, Pui CH, Abromowitch M, Mirro Jr J, Ochs JS, Look AT, Williams DL, Murphy SB, Dahl GV, Kalwinsky DK, Evans WE, Kun LE, Simone JV, Crist WM (1991): Improved outcome in childhood acute lymphoblastic leukemia with reinforced early treatment and rotational combination chemotherapy. Lancet 337: 61–66
2. Reiter A, Schrappe M, Ludwig WD, Hiddemann W, Sauer S, Henze G, Zimmermann M, Lampert F, Havers MW, Niethammer D, Odenwald E, Ritter J, Mann G, Welte K, Gadner H, Riehm H (1994): Chemotherapy in 998 unselected childhood acute lymphoblastics leukemia patients. Results and conclusions of the multi-center trial ALL-BFM 86. Blood 84: 3122–3133
3. Hoelzer D (1994): Treatment of acute lymphoblastic leukemia. Sem. Hematol. 31: 1–15
4. Hoelzer D (1993): Acute lymphoblastic leukemia—progress in children, less in adults. N. Engl. J. Med. 329: 1343–1344
5. Maurer J, Janssen JWG, Thiel E, van Denderen J, Ludwig WD, Aydemir Ü, Heinze B, Fonatsch C, Harbott J, Reiter A, Riehm H, Hoelzer D, Bartram CR (1991): Detection of chimeric BCR-ABL genes in acute lymphoblastic leukaemia by the polymerase chain reaction. Lancet 337: 1055–1058
6. Saiki RK, Gelfand DH, Stoffel S, Scharf SJ, Higuchi R, Horn GT, Mullis KB, Erlich HA (1988): Primer-directed enzymatic amplification of DNA with a Thermostable DNA polymerase. Science 239: 487–491
7. van Dongen JJM, Wolvers-Tettero ILM (1991): Analysis of immunoglobulin and T-cell receptor genes: I Basic and technical aspects. Clin. Chim. Acta 198: 1–91
8. van Dongen JJM, Wolvers-Tettero ILM (1991): Analyses of immunoglobulin and T-cell receptor genes: II Possibilities and limitations in the diagnosis and management of lymphoproliferative disease and related disorders. Clin. Chim. Acta 198: 93–174
9. Yamada M, Hudson S, Tournay D, Bittenbender S, Shane SS, Lange B, Tsujimoto Y, Caton AJ, Rovera G (1989): Detection of minimal disease in hematopoietic malignancies of the B-cell lineage by using third-complementary-determining region (CDR-III)-specific probes. Proc. Natl. Acad. Sci. USA 86: 5123–5127
10. D'Auriol L, Macintyre E, Galibert F, Sigaux F (1989): In vitro amplification of T cell γ gene rearrangements: a new tool for the assessment of minimal residual disease in acute lymphoblastic leukemias. Leukemia 3: 155–158
11. Hansen-Hagge TE, Yokota S, Bartram CR (1989): Detection of minimal residual disease in acute lymphoblastic leukemia by in vitro amplification of rearranged T-cell receptor chain sequences. Blood 74: 1762–1767
12. Bartram CR (1993): Detection of minimal residual leukemia by the polymerase chain reaction: potential implifications for therapy. Clin. Chim. Acta 217: 75–83
13. Potter MN, Cross NCP, van Dongen JJM, Saglio G, Oakhill A, Bartram CR, Goldman JM (1993): Molecular evidence of minimal residual disease after treatment for leukaemia and lymphoma: an updated meeting report and review. Leukemia 7: 1302–1314
14. Seriu T, Hansen-Hagge TE, Erz DHR, Bartram CR (1995): Improved detection of minimal residual leukemia through modifications of polymerase chain reaction analyses based on clonospecific T-cell receptor junctions. Leukemia 9: in press
15. Brisco MJ, Tan LW, Orsborn AM, Morley AA (1990): Development of a highly sensitive assay, based on the polymerase chain reaction, for rare B-lymphocyte clones in a polyclonal population. Br. J. Haematol. 75: 163–167
16. Billadeau D, Blackstadt M, Greipp P, Kyle RA, Oken MM, Kay N, van Ness B (1991): Analysis of B-lymphoid maligancies using allele-specific polymerase chain reaction: a technique for sequential qualification of residual disease. Blood 78: 3021–3029
17. Breit TM, Wolvers-Tettero ILM, Hählen K, van Wering ER, van Dongen JJM (1991): Extensive junctional diversity of γ T-cell receptors expressed by T-cell acute lymphoblastic leukemias: implications for the detection of minimal residual disease. Leukemia 5: 1076–1086
18. Beishuizen A, Verhoeven MAJ, Mol EJ, Breit TM, Wolvers-Tettero ILM, van Dongen JJM (1993): Detection of immunoglobulin heavy-chain gene rearrangementsw by Southern blot analysis: recommendations for optimal results. Leukemia 7: 2045–2053
19. Breit TM, Wolvers-Tettero ILM, Beishuizen A, Verhoven MAJ, van Wering ER, van Dongen JJM (1993): Southern blot patterns, frequencies, and junctional diversity of T-cell receptor-δ gene rearrangements in acute lymphoblastic leukemia. Blood 82: 3063–3074
20. Beishuizen A, Verhoven MAJ, van Wering ER, Hählen K, Hooijkaas H, van Dongen JJM (1994): Analysis of Ig and T-cell receptor genes in 40 childhood acute lymphoblastics leukemias at diag-

nosis and subsequent relapse: implications for the detection of minimal residual disease by polymerase chain reaction analysis. Blood 83: 2238–2247
21. Breit TM, Mol EJ, Wolvers-Tettero ILM, Ludwig WD, van Wering ER, van Dongen JJM (1993): Site-specific deletions involving the tal-1 and sil genes are restricted to cells of the T cell receptor α/β lineage: T cell receptor δ gene deletion mechanism affects multiple genes. J. Exp. Med. 177: 965–977
22. Breit TM, Beishuizen A, Ludwig WD, Mol EJ, Adriaansen HJ, van Wering ER, van Dongen JJM (1993): Tal-1 deletions in T-cell acute lymphoblastics leukemia as PCR target for detection of minimal residual disease. Leukemia 7: 2004–2011
23. Raimondi SC (1993): Current status of cytogenetic research in childhood acute lymphoblastics leukemia. Blood 81: 2237–2251
24. Rabbitts TH (1994): Chromosomal translocations in human cancer. Nature 372: 143-149
25. Chen CS, Sorensen PHB, Domer PH, Reaman GH, Korsmeyer SJ, Heerema NA, Hammond GD, Kersey JH (1993): Molecular rearrangements on chromsome 11q23 predominate in infant acute lymphoblastics leukemia and are associate with specific biologic variables and poor outcome. Blood 81: 2386–2393
26. Cimino G, Lo Coco F, Biondi A, Elia L, Luciano A, Croce CM, Masera G, Mandelli F, Canaani E (1993): ALL-1 gene at chromosome 11q23 is consistently altered in acute leukemia of early infancy. Blood 82: 544–546
27. Heerema NA, Arthur DC, Sather H, Albo V, Feusner J, Lange BJ, Steinherz PG, Zeltzer P, Hammond D, Reaman GH (1994): Cytogenetic features of infants less than 12 months of age at diagnosis of acute lymphoblastics leukemia: impact of the 11q23 breakpoint on outdome: a report of the Children's Cancer Group. Blood 83: 2274–2284
28. Thirman MJ, Gill HJ, Burnett RC, Mbangkollo D, McCabe NR, Kobayashi H, Ziemin-van der Poel S, Kaneko Y, Morgan R, Sandberg AA, Chaganti RSK, Larson RA, Le Beau MM, Diaz MO, Rowley JD (1993): Rearrangements of the MLL gene in acute lymphoblastics and acute myeloid leukemias with 11q23 chromosomal translocations. N. Engl. J. Med. 329: 909–914
29. Janssen JWG, Ludwig WD, Borkhardt A, Spadinger U, Rieder H, Fonatasch C, Hossfeld DK, Harbott J, Schulz AS, Repp R, Sykora KW, Hoelzer D, Bartram CR (1994): Pre-pre-B acute lymphoblastics leukemia: high frequency of alternatively spliced ALL1-AF4 transcripts and absence of minimal residual disease during complete remission. Blood 84: 3835–3842
30. Kwok S, Higuchi R (1989): Avoiding false positives with PCR. Nature 339: 327–328
31. Lion T, Henn T, Gaiger A, Kahls P, Gadner H (1993): Early detection of relapse after bone marrow transplantation in patients with chronic myelogenous leukaemia. Lancet 341: 275–276
32. Kawasaki ES, Clark SS, Coyne MY, Smith SD, Champlin R, Witte ON, McCormick FP (1988): Diagnosis of chronic myeloid and acute lymphoblastic leukemias by detection of leukemia-specific mRNA sequences amplified in vitro. Proc. Natl. Acad. Sci. USA 85: 5698–5702
33. Roberts WM, Rivera GK, Raimondi SC, Santana VM, Sandlund JT, Crist WM, Pui CH (1994): Intensive chemotherapy for philadelphia-chromosome-positive acute lymphoblastic leukemia. Lancet 343: 331–332
34. Gekly GB, Bryant EM, Lee AM, Kidd PG, Thomas ED (1991): Chimeric BCR-abl messenger RNA as a marker for minimal residual disease in patients transplanted for Philadelphia chromosome-positive acute lymphoblastic leukemia. Blood 78: 458–465
35. Miyamura K, Tamimoto M, Morishima Y, Horibe K, Yamamoto K, Akatsuka M, Kodera Y, Kojima S, Matsuyama K, Hirabayashi N, Yazaki M, Imai K, Onozawa Y, Kanamura A, Mizutani S, Saito H (1992): Detection of Philadelphide chromosome-positive acute lymphoblastic leukemia by polymerase chain reaction: possible eradication of minimal residual disease by marrow transplantation. Blood 79: 1366–1370
36. Martin H, Atta J, Bruecher J, Elsner S, Stadler M, von Melchner H, Hoelzer D (1994): In patients with BCR-ABL-positive ALL in CR peripheral blood contains less residual disease than bone marrow: implications for autologous BMT. Ann. Hematol. 68: 85–87
37. Biondi A, Rambaldi A, Rossi V, Elia L, Caslini C, Basso G, Battista R, Barbui T, Mandelli F, Masera G, Croce C, Canaani E, Cimino G (1993): Detection of ALL1/AF4 fusion transcript by reverse transcription—polymerase chain reaction for diagnosis and monitoring of acute leukemias with the t(4; 11) translocation. Blood 82: 2943–2947
38. Jonsson OG, Kitchens RL, Baer RJ, Buchanan GR, Smith RG (1991): Rearrangements of the tal-1 locus as clonal markers for T cell acute lymphoblastic leukemia. J. Clin. Invest. 87: 2029–2035
39. Janssen JWG, Ludwig WD, Sterry W, Bartram CR (1993): SIL-TAL1 deletion in T-cell acute lymphoblastic leukemia. Leukemia 7: 1204–1210
40. Hunger SP, Galili N, Carroll AJ, Crist WM, Link MP, Clearly ML (1991): The t(1; 19)(q23; p13) results in consistent fusion of E2A and PBX1 coding sequences in acute lymphoblastics leukemias. Blood 77: 687–693
41. Izraeli S, Janssen JWG, Haas OA, Harbott J, Brok-Simoni F, Walther JU, Kovar H, Henn T, Ludwig WD, Reiter A, Rechavi G, Bartram CR, Gadner H, Lion T (1993): Detection and clinical relevance of genetic abnormalities in pediatric acute lymphoblastic leukemia: a comparison between cytogenetic and polymerase chain reaction analyses. Leukemia 7: 671–678
42. Devaraj PE, Foroni L, Sekhar M, Butler T, Wright F, Mehta A, Samson D, Prentice HG, Hoffbrandt AV, Secker-Walker LM (1994): E2A/HLF fusion cDNAs and the use of RT-PCR for the detection of minimal residual disease in t(17; 19)(q22; p13) acute lymphoblastic leukemia. Leukemia 8: 1131–1138

43. Kagan J, Finger LR, Besa E, Croce CM (1990): Detection of minimal residual disease in leukemic patients with the t(10; 14)(q24; q11) chromosmal translocation. Cancer Res. 50: 5240–5244
44. Estrov Z, Ouspenskaia MV, Felix EA, McClain KL, Lee MS, Harris D, Pinkel DP, Zipf TF (1994): Persistence of self-renewing leukemia progenitors during remission in children with B-precursor acute lymphoblastic leukaemia. Leukemia 8: 46–52
45. Wassermann R, Galili N, Ito Y, Silber JH, Reichard BA, Shane S, Womer RB, Lange B, Rovera G (1992): Residual disease at the end of inducation therapy as a predictor of relapse during therapy in childhood B-lineage acute lymphoblastic leukemia. J. Clin. Oncol. 10: 1879–1888
46. Brisco MJ, Condon J, Hughes E, Neoh SH, Sykes PJ, Seshardi R, Toogood I, Waters K, Tauro G, Ekert H, Morley AA (1994): Outcome prediction in childhood acute lymphoblastic leukaemia by molecular quantification of residual disease at the end of induction. Lancet 343: 196–200
47. Ito Y, Wasserman R, Galili N, Reiard BA, Shane S, Lange B, Rovera G (1993): Molecular residual disease status at the end of chemotherapy fails to predict subsequent relapse in children with B-lineage acute lymphoblastic leukemia. J. Clin. Oncol. 11: 546–553
48. Goulden N, Langlands K, Steward C, Katz F, Potter M, Chessels J, Oakhill A (1993): PCR assessment of bone marrow status in "isolated" extramedullary relapse of childhood B-precursor acute lymphoblastic leukemia. Br. J. Haematol. 87: 282–285
49. Neale GAM, Pui CH, Mahmoud HH, Mirro Jr J, Crist WM, Rivera GK, Goorha RM (1994): Molecular evidence for minimal residual bone marrow disease in children with "isolated" extramedullary relapse of T-cell acute lymphoblastic leukemia. Leukemia 8: 768–775
50. Nizet Y, van Daele S, Lewalle P, Vaerman JL, Philippe M, Vermylen C, Cornu G, Farrant A, Michaux JL, Martiat P (1993): Long-term follow-up of residual disease in acute lymphoblastics leukemia patients in complete remission using clonogenic IgH probes and the polymerase chain reaction. Blood 82: 1618–1625
51. Seriu T, Yokota S, Nakao M, Misawa S, Takaue Y, Koizumi S, Kawai S, Fujimoto T (1995): Prospective monitoring of residual disease during the course of chemotherapy in patients with acute lymphoblastic leukemia, and detection of contaminating tumor cells in peripheral blood stem cells for autotransplantation. Leukemia 9: in press
52. van der Does-van den Berg A, Bartram CR, Basso G, Benoit YCM, Biondi A, Debatin KM, Haas OA, Harbott J, Kamps WA, Köller U, Lampert F, Ludwig WD, Niemeyer CM, van Wering ER (1992): Minimal requirements for the diagnosis, classification, and evaluation of the treatment of childhood acute lymphoblastic leukemia (ALL) in the "BFM Family" Cooperative Group. Med. Pediatr. Oncol. 20: 497–505

Acute Leukemias VI
Prognostic Factors
and Treatment Strategies
Büchner et al. (eds)

Immunophenotypic Detection of Minimal Residual Disease in Acute Lymphoblastic Leukemia

J. Ciudad[1], J.F. San Miguel[2], M.C. Lopez-Berges[2], B. Valverde[1], B. Vidriales[2], A.M.A. Loperz[1], M. Gonzalez[2], R. Garcia-Sanz[2], and A. Orfao

Abstract. The aims of the present study were: (a) to analyze the incidence of leukemia-associated phenotypes within patients with acute lymphoblastic leukemia; (b) to determine the frequency and the causes of phenotypic changes in relapse samples, and (c) to analyze the clinical impact of the immunophenotypic detection of minimal residual disease in acute lymphoblastic leukemia (ALL). A total of 72 ALL cases (T lineage: 16, B lineage: 56 patients) were included in the study and a total of 323 complete remission follow-up bone marrow samples were analyzed; 78% of the cases displayed leukemia-associated phenotypes at diagnosis (T-lineage ALL: 100%, and B-lineage ALL: 72%). The overall distribution of the different types of leukemia-associated phenotypes was: lineage "infidelity" 56%, asynchronous antigen expression 23%, antigen over-expression 18%, tissue-restricted phenotypes 15%, and "rate" phenotypes 5%. The incidence of DNA aneuploidy was 15%, most of the cases corresponding to B-lineage leukemias. From these patients 75% displayed more than one aberrant phenotype. The presence of more than one blast cell population was detected in 28% of the cases.

Follow-up studies have shown that upon considering individually each of the immunological markers analyzed, phenotypic changes are relatively rare (6.4%), although they might be detected in a high proportion of patients (37%). However, an aberrant criterion was involved in the phenotypic changes in only 20% of these patients. Moreover, in all cases, at least one of the aberrations detected at diagnosis remained constant at relapse. Phenotypic changes were frequently related to technical artefacts (27%) and to the existence of minor blast cell populations at diagnosis (27%).

Regarding clinical outcome, on most occasions (84%) relapses were predicted by an increase in the proportion of bone marrow cells displaying leukemia-associated phenotypes. In addition, when an increase in the proportion of cells displaying a leukemia-associated phenotype was detected in two consecutive complete remission bone marrow samples, the patient tended to relapse (70% of the cases).

Introduction

At present, chemotherapeutic regimes used for the treatment of acute lymphoblastic leukemia (ALL) lead to the achievement of complete remission in a high proportion of patients. However, a relatively high percentage of these patients relapse due to the persistence of low numbers of leukemic cells that remain undetectable by conventional morphology and cytochemistry. This is known as minimal residual disease (MRD) [1–8]. It has been suggested that several methodological approaches could be of help for the detection of MRD in acute leukemias [9]. In order to be suitable for being used in MRD detection, each method should fulfill four criteria: they should be specific, sensitive, rapid, and reproducible. From the different approaches that have been tested up until now, the immunological detection of MRD represents

[1]Unit of Cytometry, University of Salamanca, Spain
[2]Department of Hematology, University Hospital of Salamanca, Spain

one of the most attractive methods [7, 9, 10]. However, for a long time two major disadvantages have been related to the use of immunological methods for the detection of MRD. First, with a few exceptions such as the proteins resulting from the fusion of translocated genes [11, 12], no leukemia specific antigens have been found [2, 13, 14]. Secondly, several reports have suggested the existence of phenotypic changes that may affect the blast cells at relapse [14–16], increasing the difficulty of following the leukemic cells in samples of morphological complete remission. However, the combined use of flow cytometry and multiple combinations of monoclonal antibodies have allowed for the identification of leukemia-associated phenotypes that are either absent or extremely rare in normal bone marrow (BM) samples [2, 6, 8, 18–23].

In the present paper, the contribution of flow cytometry to the detection of MRD in 72 consecutive patients suffering from ALL is explored. The aims of this study were to analyze the incidence of leukemia-associated phenotypes, to determine the frequency and the causes of phenotypic changes detected at relapse, and, finally, to analyze the clinical impact of monitoring the detection of cells with leukemia-associated phenotypes in complete remission BM samples.

Material and Methods

Patients

A total of 72 patients (33 children and 39 adults, ages ranging from 2 to 66 years) diagnosed as suffering from ALL according to morphological, cytochemical, and immunological criteria [24, 25] were included in the present study. All cases were treated according to the protocols of the Spanish PETHEMA Cooperative Group which included vincristine, prednisone, l-asparaginase and daunorubicin in the induction phase. The duration of chemotherapy treatment ranged between 24 and 30 months; two patients underwent alogeneic BM transplantation. Patients were followed for a mean period of 35 ± 28 months, ranging from 12 to 100 months. During this period 323 complete remission follow-up BM samples were analyzed. At present, 25 out of the 72 patients have relapsed (total number of relapses: 30) and the remaining patients remain in continuous morphological complete remission.

Immunological Studies at Diagnosis and Relapse

The immunophenotype of the ALL blast cells was analyzed in all cases at diagnosis by means of multiparametric flow cytometry, using multiple-staining combinations of monoclonal antibodies (MAbs), on erythrocyte-lysed (FACS lysing solution, Becton/Dickinson, San José, CA, USA) whole BM samples. The reactivity of the leukemic cells for the CD7, CD10, CD13, CD16, CD19, CD20, CD22, CD33, CD34, HLADR, and TDT was analyzed in all cases. In addition, the expression of the CD1, CD2, sCD3, cCD3, CD4, CD5, CD8, CD38, CD71 and TCR-alpha-beta antigens was also assessed in T-lineage ALL cases. The reactivity for the CD13 and CD33 myeloid-associated markers was analyzed using the leuM7 and leuM9 (Becton/Dickinson) MAbs conjugated with phycoerythrin, the most sensitive fluorochrome for flow cytometers equipped with a 488-nm argon ion laser. In all cases, the reactivity for both myeloid markers was assessed in either CD19 + (B-lineage ALL) or CD7 + (T-lineage ALL) blast cells. In order to analyze the incidence and the causes of the phenotypic changes at relapse, the 30 relapse samples were also analyzed using the same methodological approach.

Data acquisition and analysis were performed on a FACScan flow cytometer (Becton/ Dickinson) by means of the LYSYS II (Becton/ Dickinson) and PAINT-A-GATE PLUS (Becton/ Dickinson) software programs, respectively. For each tube combination, a minimum of 10 000 events were collected and analyzed. The analysis process was performed according to previously reported methods. From the 72 patients analyzed, 56 corresponded to B-lineage ALL and the remaining 16 to T-lineage ALL. The following criteria were used for the definition of leukemia-associated phenotypes: (a) lineage infidelity (co-expression of the CD13 and/or CD33 myeloid-related markers on the surface of the lymphoid blast cells); (b) asynchronous expression of differentiation markers; (c) antigen over-expression; and (d) abnormal localization in the BM of phenotypes restricted to other tissues. Phenotypes detected at a frequency lower than one cell in 10^5 leukocytes in normal human BM were also considered to be aberrant when detected at a higher frequency.

DNA Ploidy Studies at Diagnosis

The analysis of the DNA ploidy status of the ALL blast cells was performed using the Vindelov et al. technique [26, 27]. Briefly, between 5 and 10×10^5 leukocytes from ammonium chloride-lysed whole BM were washed in 1.5 m citrate buffer. Upon discharging the supernatant, the cell pellet was resuspended in 200 µ citrate buffer. Immediately after resuspending the cell pellet, 1.8 m solution A containing trypsin was added and the cells were incubated for 10 min at room temperature. Once this incubation period was complete, another 1.5 m solution B containing RNAse and a trypsin inhibitor were added and another 10-min incubation was performed at room temperature. Afterwards, 1.5 m solution C containing propidium iodide was added and a third incubation for at least 10 min (room temperature) in the dark was carried out. The measurement of DNA/propidium iodide fluorescence intensity was performed in a FACScan flow cytometer using the CellFit software program (Becton/Dickinson). In those cases in which the percentage of blast cells in the sample was higher than 90%, a second tube containing a mixture (2: 1) of the patient's sample and a sex-matched normal peripheral blood was prepared, acquired, and analyzed [27]. DNA aneuploidy was considered to exist when two different G0/G1 cell populations were detected in the DNA histogram according to the recommendations of the DNA Cytometry Consensus Conference [28].

Analysis of Minimal Residual Disease

For the investigation of MRD, different MAb combinations of the above-mentioned markers were used. These MAb combinations were adapted in each patient according to the phenotype of the blast cells observed at diagnosis. In addition, the CD10/CD20/CD19 MAb combination was explored in all complete remission BM samples analyzed. Data acquisition was performed on a FACScan flow cytometer using a two-step procedure. (a) 20,000 cells/test of the total samples were acquired; and (b) a second acquisition of either CD19 + (B-lineage ALL) or CD7+ (T-lineage ALL) cells was made through either a SSC/CD19 or a SSC/CD7 live gate, respectively. The sensitivity of this approach was at least 1×10^{-5}.

For the follow up of cases displaying DNA aneuploidy, a DNA/antigen double-staining method was performed using previously reported techniques [29]. Briefly, complete remission BM samples were stained with the appropriate MAbs fluorescein isothiacynate (FITC)-conjugated for 10 min at room temperature. Afterwards, erythrocytes were lysed using ammonium chloride; then the leukocytes were treated with RNAse and their DNA stained with propidium iodide.

Results

Incidence of Leukemia-Associated Phenotypes

From the 72 patients analyzed at diagnosis, 56 (78%) displayed leukemia-associated phenotypes: 16 out of 16 T-lineage ALL (100%) and 40 out of 56 B-lineage ALL cases (72%). The presence of lineage infidelity was the most commonly detected leukemia-associated phenotype (56% of the cases), with a similar incidence in T- and B-lineage ALL: 50% and 57%, respectively. The frequency of antigen over-expression, asynchronous antigen expression and phenotypes restricted to other tissues was 18%, 23%, and 15%, respectively. Other phenotypes absent or extremely rare in normal BM were detected in 5% of the cases. It should be mentioned that while antigen over-expression was restricted to B-lineage ALL (21% versus 0%), the presence of phenotypes restricted to tissues other than BM was characteristic of T-lineage ALL patients (69% versus 0%). Tables 1 and 2 show the distribution of the different aberrant phenotypes detected in T-and B-lineage ALL patients, respectively. It can be seen that the number of aberrations is much higher than the number of cases displaying leukemia-associated phenotypes, pointing to the fact that in a high proportion of the ALL cases analyzed the blast cells displayed more than one aberration. Actually,

Table 1. T-lineage ALL: incidence of leukemia-associated phenotype ($n = 16$)

	T-lineage ALL (n)
Lineage infidelity	13
Tissue-Restricted phenotypes	9
Asynchronous Antigen expression	5
Increase of rare phenotypes	10
DNA Aneuploidy	1

Table 2. B-lineage ALL: incidence of leukemia-associated pehnotypes ($n = 56$)

	B-lineage ALL (n)
Lineage infidelity	43
Asynchronous antigen expression	15
Antigen over-expression	12
DNA Aneuploidy	10

75% of the patients displaying leukemia-associated phenotypes showed only one aberrant criterion while in the remaining cases two, three, or even four different aberrations were detected. The overall incidence of DNA aneuploidy was 15%, most of the cases (10 out of 11) corresponding to B-lineage leukemias.

A detailed analysis of the blast cells of the patients included in the present study confirmed that they are heterogeneous since differences were detected not only among different patients but even within the same patient. In this sense, the presence of more than one population of leukemic cells was detected in 28% of the patients (46% of the T-lineage ALL and 24% of the B-lineage ALL patients).

Incidence and Causes of Phenotypic Changes at Relapse

Eleven out of the 30 relapse samples (37%) analyzed in the present study showed phenotypic changes in which at least one of the markers investigated was involved. Despite this apparently high incidence, the frequency of phenotypic changes affecting one marker as regards to the total number of tests performed was very low (6.4%) and it was slightly lower in T-lineage (4%) than in B-lineage (8%) ALL patients. Phenotypic changes involving leukemia-associated phenotypes were observed in six relapses (20%). However, it should be mentioned that in all these six relapse samples there were other leukemia-associated phenotypes detected at diagnosis, and, at least one of them remained constant in the blast cells of the relapse sample.

Upon analyzing the causes of the phenotypic changes detected at relapse, it was observed that in a relatively high proportion of cases they were associated with either technical questions, such as the use of different MAbs and the use of the same MAb conjugated with different fluorochromes (27% of the cases), or to the existence of more than one blast cell subset that changed its proportion between the diagnosis and the relapse (27% of the patients). From the remaining phenotypic changes 9% were associated with the analysis of samples from other tissues, while in the remaining 37% of patients the cause of the phenotypic changes is unknown.

Clinical Impact of MRD Detection

From the 56 patients that displayed a leukemia-associated phenotype at diagnosis, 30 cases (eight T- and 22 B-lineage ALL) displayed an increase in the percentage of cells with leukemia-associated phenotypes in two consecutive studies, while in the remaining 26 patients (eight T- and 18 B-lineage ALL) the proportion of BM cells displaying leukemia-associated phenotypes, progressively decreased from the diagnosis and either became undetectable or remained stable without displaying an increase. From the former group, 21 patients (70%) have relapsed. The mean follow up between the detection of the increase in the proportion of blast cells and the relapse ranged from 4 weeks to 20 months. Interestingly, the incidence of false positives (cases with an increase in the proportion of cells displaying leukemia-associated phenotypes, without relapsing) was higher for the B-lineage ALL (36%) than for the T-lineage acute leukemias (13%). Nevertheless, most false positives without a relapse were observed during the last follow-up studies.

Only four out of the 26 patients (15%) from those who had not displayed an increase in the proportion of cells with leukemia-associated phenotypes have relapsed, the incidence of false negatives (non predicted relapses) being similar in T-and B-lineage ALL: 13% and 17%, respectively.

Discussion

The clinical utility of the immunological methods for the detection of MRD in ALL greatly depends on the incidence of leukemia-associated phenotypes, their stability at relapse, and the sensitivity of these methods to detect leukemic cells which are present at low frequencies in complete remission samples. In the present study it is shown that most of the ALL cases display leukemia-associated phenotypes at diagnosis, with more than one aberrant criterion usually present in the ALL patient's blast cells. During the past decade, an increasing number of studies have been reported on the incidence of expression of myeloid-associated markers in ALL [1, 8, 23, 30–32], while the information on the incidence of other types of leukemia-associated phenotypes is still scanty [1, 23, 32, 33]. A careful analysis of the results reported shows a high degree of variability [31]. As an example, the incidence of CD13 and/or CD33 expression in ALL patients ranges from 5% to 46%. This great variability is probably related to methodological questions. Accordingly, the use of different fluorochromes and systems for the immunological detection of cell antigens as well as the variability of the criteria used to consider a case as being positive, clearly influences the final results. In the present study, the definition of leukemia-associated phenotypes was based on the analysis of the normal human BM. In addition, standardized procedures were used for the investigation of these phenotypes. For example, the expression of the pan myeloid-related markers CD13 and CD33 was always performed with the most sensitive fluorochrome, phycoerythrin. The expression of myeloid-associated markers was the most common aberration detected. The incidence of other types of aberration was similar.

Regarding antigen over-expression, which was restricted in our series to B-lineage ALL, the abnormally high levels of CD10 per cell was the most frequent leukemia-associated phenotype observed, in accordance to previous reports [33]. In contrast, the presence of tissue-restricted phenotypes, although absent in B-lineage ALL, was a common finding in T-lineage ALL due to the detection of phenotypes restricted to the thymus [34, 35]. Finally, it can be concluded from our data that the simultaneous assessment of antigens associated with early and late differentiation stages such as CD34 and CD20 is of great help in the identification of leukemia-associated phenotypes due to asynchronous antigen expression.

Several reports have suggested the existence of phenotypic changes in ALL [15–17]. Our results confirm that in fact they do exist and that, by using a large panel of MAbs, they can even be detected in a relatively high proportion of cases. However, in the context of all the tests performed they are relatively rare. Moreover, technical artefacts such as the use of different clones of MAbs as well as distinct fluorochromes may be associated with these changes. Interestingly, our results show that in a similar way to acute myeloblastic leukemia [18], a relatively high proportion of ALL cases (especially T-lineage patients) display more than one blast cell subset whose proportions frequently change during relapse. This also contributes to the detection of "false" phenotypic changes. These results point to the need for a careful analysis of the ALL blast cells at diagnosis to identify and characterize all the blast cell populations in order to be able to monitor each of them during the follow-up studies. Our results also indicate that further studies on this matter are still necessary since the cause of a high proportion of the phenotypic changes detected remains unknown.

Preliminary reports have indicated that the use of immunological methods for the detection of residual leukemic cells in ALL have an important clinical impact [2, 4, 6, 8, 10, 23, 32]. Accordingly, our results show that the observation of an increase in the percentage of BM cells displaying leukemia-associated phenotypes predicts, with a high sensitivity, the occurrence of relapse. Moreover, this approach also appears to be highly specific since most of the cases in which an increase in the percentage of BM cells with leukemia-associated phenotypes was detected, relapsed; from those who did not relapse, most had a short follow-up period after this increase was observed. These results support the notion that an adequate immunological monitoring of cells with a leukemia-associated phenotype in complete remission BM samples from ALL patients would allow for an early diagnosis of relapse.

In summary, our results show that the great majority of ALL patients display leukemia-associated phenotypes and that at least one of these aberrations remains constant at relapse. In addition, it is shown that MRD detection using the approach presented here would allow for the early diagnosis of relapse with both high sensitivity and specificity.

References

1. Campana D, E. Coustan-Smith, F.G. Behm. The definition of remission in acute leukemia with immunologic techniques. Bone Marrow Transpl 1991; 8: 429–37.
2. van Dongen JJM, T.M. Briet, H.J. Adriaasen, A. Beishuizen, H. Hooijkaas. Detection of minimal

residual disease in acute leukemia by immunological marker analysis and polymerase chain reaction. Leukemia 1992; 6(suppl 1): 47-59.
3. Lange BJ, G. Rovera. Detection of minimal residual leukemia in acute lymphoblastic leukemia. Hematol/Oncol Clin Am 1990; 4: 895-914.
4. Hooijkaas H, K. Hahlen, H.J. Adraasen, I. Dekker, G.E. van Zaden, J.J.M. van Dongen (1989) Terminal deoxynucleotidyl transferase positive cells in cerebrospinal fluid and development of overt CNS leukemia: a 5-year follow-up study in 113 children with Tdt positive leukemia or non-Hodgkin's lymphoma. Blood, 74, 416-21.
5. Hagenbeek A, A.C.M. Maertens. Minimal residual disease in acute leukemia: preclinical studies in a relevant rat model (BNML). Bailliere's Clin Hematol 1991; 4: 609-635.
6. Campana D, R. Otubo-Freitas, E. Coustan-Smith. Detection of residual leukemia with immunological methods. Technical developments and clinical implications. Leuk Lymph 1994; 13 (suppl 1): 31-34.
7. van Dongen JJM, H. Hooijkaas, H.J. Adraasen, K. Hahlen, G.E. van Zanen. Detection of minimal residual disease acute lymphoblastic leukemia by immunological marker analysis: possibilities and limitations. In: Minimal residual disease in acute leukemia edited by Lowenberg P and Hagenbeeck J. Martius Nijhoff Publishers, The Hague, 1986, pp 113-133
8. Campana D, E. Coustan-Smith, G. Janossy. The immunologic detection of minimal residual disease in acute leukemia. Blood 1990; 76: 163-171.
9. San Miguel JF, A. Macedo, J. Ciudad, M. Gonzalez, A. Orfao. Enfermedad minima residual. In: "Temas de Medicina Interna. Leucemias agudas". Ramiro Hernandez M and Kamiro S (eds). Interamericana McGraw-Hill, Mexico, 1993; 161-186.
10. Campana D. Applications of flow cytometry to study acute leukemia: in vitro determination of drug sensitivity and detection of minimal residual disease. Cytometry (Communications in Clinical Cytometry) 1994; 18: 68-74.
11. van Denderen J, A. Hermans, T. Meeuwsen. Antibody recognition of the tumor-specific bcr-abl joining region of the chronic myeloid leukemia. J Exp Med 1989; 169: 87-98.
12. Kamps MP, C. Murre, X.H. Sun, D.A. Baltimore new homeobow gene contributes the DNA binding domain of the t(1; 19) translocation protein in pre-B ALL. Cell 1990; 60: 547-556.
13. Janossy G, F.J. Bollum, K.F. Bradstock, J. Ashley. Cellular phenotypes of normal and leukemic hemopoietic cells determined by analysis with selected antibody combinations. Blood 1980; 56: 430-441.
14. Foon KA, R.F. Todd III. Immunologic classification of leukemia and lymphoma. Blood 1986; 68: 1-31.
15. Gomez E, J.F. San Miguel, M. Gonzalez, A. Orfao, M.C. Cañizo, J. Ciudad, A. Lopez Borrasca. Cambios fenotipicos de las leucemias agudas linfoblàsticas en recaida y resistentes. Sangre 1991; 36: 201-204.
16. Pui CH, S.C. Raimondi, F.G. Behem. Shifts in blast cell phenotype and karyotype at relapse of childhood lymphoblastic leukemia. Blood 1986; 68: 1306-1312.
17. Raghavacher A, W.D. Ludwig, C.R. Bartram. Clonal variation in childhood acute lymphoblastic leukemia at early and late relapse detected by analysis of phenotype and genotype. Eur J Pediatr 1988; 147: 503-507.
18. Macedo A, A. Orfao, M. Gonzalez, M.B. Vidriales, M.C. Lopez-Berges, A. Martinez, J.F. San Miguel. Immunological detection of blast cell subpopulations in acute myeloblastic leukemia at diagnosis: implications for minimal residual disease studies. Leukemia 1995 (in press).
19. Loken MR, V.O. Shah, K.L. Dattilio, C. Civin. Flow cytometric analysis of human bone marrow: II. Normal B-lymphocyte development. Blood 1987; 70: 1316-1324.
20. Campana D, G. Janossy, M. Bofill, L.K. Trejdosiewicz, M.A.D. Hoffbrand A.V. Human B-cell development: I. Phenotypic differences of B-lymphocytes in the bone marrow and peripheral blood tissue. J Immunol 1985; 134: 1524-1530.
21. Ryan DH, C. Chapple, S.A. Kossover, A.A. Sandberg, H.J. Cohen. Phenotypic similarities and differences between CALLA-positive acute lymphoblastic leukemia cells and normal marrow CALLA-positive B cell precursors. Blood 1987; 70: 814-819.
22. Hurwitz CA, M.R. Loken, M.I. Graham, J.E. Karp, M.J. Borowitz, D.J. Pullen. Asynchronous antigen expression in B lineage acute lymphoblastic leukemia. Blood 1988; 72: 229-307.
23. Orfao A, J. Ciudad, M.C. Lopez Berges, J.F. San Miguel. Acute lymphoblastic leukemia (ALL): detection of minimal residual disease (MRD) at flow cytometry. Leuk Lymph 1994; 13 (suppl 1): 87-90.
24. Bennett JH, D. Catovsky, M.T. Daniel, G. Flandrin, D.A.G. Galton, H.R. Gralnick. Proposals for the classification of the acute leukaemias. Br J Haematol 1976; 33: 451-458.
25. Bene MC, G. Castoldi, W. Knapp, W.D. Ludwig, E. Matutes, A. Orfao, M.B. van't Veer. Proposals for the immunological classification of acute leukemias. Leukemia, 1995 (in press).
26. Vindelov LL, I.b.J. Christensen, G. Jensen, N.I. Nissen: Limits of detection of nuclear DNA abnormalities by flow cytometric DNA analysis. Results obtained by a set of methods for sample-storage, staining and internal standardization. Cytometry 1983; 3: 332-338.
27. Vidriales MB, A. Orfao, M.C. Lopez-Berges, M. Gonzalez, A. Lopez-Macedo, J. Ciudad, A. Lopez, M.C. Cañizo, M.A. Garcia, J.F. San Miguel: DNA aneuploidy in acute myeloblastic leukemia is associated with a high expression of lymphoid markers. Cytometry (Communications in Clinical Cytometry) 1995; 22: (in press).
28. Shankey TV, P.S. Rabinovitch, B. Bagwell, K.D. Bauer, R.E. Duque, D.W. Hedley, B.H. Mayall, L.

Wheless: Guidelines for implementation of clinical DNA cytometry. Cytometry 1993; 14: 472–477.

29. Orfao A, R. Garcia-Sanz, M.C. Lopez-Berges, M.B. Vidriales, M. Gonzalez, M.D. Caballero, J.F. San Miguel: A new method for the analysis of plasma cell DNA content in multiple myeloma samples using a CD38/propidium iodide double staining technique. Cytometry 1994; 17: 332–339.
30. Bradstock KF, J. Kird, P.G. Grimsley, A. Kabral, W.G. Hughes. Unusual immunophenotypes in acute leukemias: incidence and clinical correlations. Br J Haematol 1989; 72: 512–518.
31. Drexler Hg, E. Thiel, W.D. Ludwig. Review of the incidence and clinical relevance of myeloid antigen-positive acute lymphoblastic leukemia. Leukemia 1991; 5: 637–645.
32. Drach J, D. Drach, H. Glassl, C. Gattringer, H. Huber. Flow cytoometric determination of atypical antigen expression in acute leukemia for the study of minimal residual disease. Cytometry 1992; 13: 893–901.
33. Lavabre-Bertrand T, G. Janossy, K. Ivory, R. Peters, L. Secker-Walker, A. Porwit-MacDonald. Leukemia-associated changes identified by quantitative flow cytometry: I. CD10 expression. Cytometry (Communications in Clinical Cytometry) 1994; 18: 209–217.
34. Reinherz EC, P.C. Kung, G. Goldstein, R.H. Levey, S.F. Schlosman. Discrete stages of human intrathymic differentiation. Analysis of normal and leukemic lymphoblasts of T-cell lineage. Proc Natl Acad Sci USA 1980; 77: 1588–1592.
35. Janossy G, N. Tidman, E.S. Papageorgiou, P.C. Kung, G. Goldstein. Distribution of T-lymphocyte subsets in the human bone marrow and thymus: an analysis with monoclonal antibodies. J Immunol 1981; 126: 1608–1613.
36. Bradstock KF, G. Janossy, N. Tidman, E.S. Papageorgiou, H.G. Prentice, M. Willoughby. Immunological monitoring of minimal residual disease in treated thymic acute lymphoblastic leukemia. Leuk Res 1981; 5: 301–309.

Acute Leukemias VI
Prognostic Factors
and Treatment Strategies
Büchner et al. (eds)

Molecular Biological Detection of Minimal Residual Disease in Acute Myeloid Leukemia

A. Biondi[1], D. Diverio[2], A. Luciano[1], R. Riccioni[2], and F. Lo Coco[2]

Abstract. The role of molecular detection of minimal residual disease (MRD) in different forms of acute myeloid leukemia (AML) is currently being explored by polymerase chain reaction (PCR) methods that can amplify a unique nucleotide sequence from 1 in 10^5 cells can detect MRD with a sensitivity that far exceeds standard light microscopy and routine cytogenetics.

In acute promyelocytic leukemia (APL) appropriate oligo primers complementary to PML and RAR-α sequences near the DNA breakpoints have been successfully used in PCR experiments to amplify the PML/RAR-α hybrid gene and sensitively detect MRD. Retrospective analysis of APL patients in different series has indicated the prognostic relevance of PCR evaluation of the PML/RARα rearrangement as a predictor of impeding relapse in APL. Moreover, in APL patients during long-term remission (4–5 years), RT-PCR analysis revealed the absence of PML/RAR-a fusion transcripts. Data of RT-PCR monitoring analysis of APL patients in a large longitudinal prospective Italian study are presented. By comparison, the recent findings on the persistence of the t(8; 21) translocation in patients with AML in long-term remission are discussed for the different implications of the detection of translocation-carrying cells in AML.

Introduction

The current treatment of acute myeloid leukemia (AML) patients leads to complete remission in 60%–70% of cases [1]. Despite the high remission rate, a significant proportion of AML patients develop a relapse within 1–3 years [2]. Apparently, low numbers of leukemic cells persist although they are undetectable by conventional cytomorphological techniques. These methods have a detection limit of 1%–5%, therefore more sensitive techniques are needed to evaluate the effectiveness of treatment, i.e., the reduction of tumor mass. More recently, immunological and molecular approaches that are able to detect small numbers of leukemic cells, below 10^{-4}–10^{-5}, have been developed [3]. The polymerase chain reaction (PCR) techniques for the detection of minimal residual disease (MRD) can be applied in AML patients whose blasts carry specific well-defined chromosome aberrations or cross-lineage rearrangements of immunoglobulin (Ig) and/or T-cell receptor (TCR) genes [3]. As shown in Table 1, the most frequent chromosomal translocations occurring in AML have been molecularly characterized and the chimeric genes have provided an important target for PCR-based detection at diagnosis and during the course of treatment [4].

We will discuss here the use of RT-PCR in the monitoring of the acute promyelocytic leukemia (APL) clone, together with the clinical relevance of the evaluation of residual disease in APL as compared to other AML subtypes.

Clinica Pediatrica, Università, Milano, H. S. Gerardo, Monza Italy Ematologia, Dipt. Biopatologia, Università "La Sapienza", Roma, Italy

Table 1. Chromosomal translocation breakpoints and genes in AML (modified from [4])

Type	Affected gene	Protein domain	Fusion protein
t(15; 17)(q21-q11-22)	PML (15q21) RARα (17q21)	Zinc-finger Retinoic acid receptor-alfa	Zinc-finger+RAR DNA and ligand binding
t(11; 17)(q23; q21.1)	PLZF (11q23) RARα (17q21)	Zinc-finger Retinoic acid receptor-alfa	Zinc-finger+RAR DNA and ligand binding
t(9; 11)(q21; q23)	MLL (11q23) AF9/MLL T3(9p22)	A-T hook/Zn-finger Ser-Pro rich	A-T hook+(Ser-Pro)
t(11; 19)(q23; p13)	MLL (11q23) ENL(19p13)	A-T hook/Zn-finger Ser-Pro rich	A-T hook+(Ser-Pro)
t(11; 17)(q23; q21)	MLL(11q23) AF17(17q21)	A-T hook/Zn-finger Cys-rich/leucine zipper	A-T hook + leucine zipper
t(8; 21)(q22; q22)	AML1/CBF α (21q22) ETO/MTG8 (8q22)	DNA binding/runt homology Zn-finger	DNA binding + Zn-fingers
t(16; 21)(p11; q22)	FUS (16p11)	Gin-Ser-Tyr/Gly-rich/RNA binding	Gin Ser-Tyr+DNA binding
t(6; 9)(p23; q34)	DEK (6p23) CAN (9q34)	? ZIP	?+ZIP
inv(16)(p13; q22)	Myosin MYH11 (16p13) CBF-beta (16q22)		DNA binding?

Molecular Detection of the t(15;17) Translocation by RT-PCR

Acute promyelocytic leukemia is characterized by a reciprocal translocation that involves chromosomes 15 and 17 (reviewed in [5]). The chromosome break sites were isolated by four groups [6–9] and shown to involve PML, a previously unknown gene coding for a putative novel transcription factor mapped on chromosome 15 and the gene for the retinoic acid receptor-α (RARα) on chromosome 17.

The chromosome 17 breakpoints are localized within a 16-kb DNA fragment of the RARα intron 2. By contrast, the chromosome 15 breakpoints are variably located in three regions of the PML locus. In 90%–92% of case, it is equally distributed between intron 6 (breakpoint cluster region 1; bcr 1) and intron 3 (bcr 3). In the remaining 8%-10% of cases, it is located within exon 6 (bcr 2).

Regardless of the extreme variability of the PML break site, PML/RARα genes that have the potential to encode for a fusion PML/RARα are consistently selected by the leukemic phenotype. In bcr 1 or bcr 3 cases, the 5' portion of PML intron 6 or 3, respectively, fuses with the 3' portion of RARα intron 2 [5]. During assemblage of the PML/RARα junction in the fusion transcript, the chimeric intron is spliced out and the longest PML and RARα open reading frames (ORFs) become aligned. The operative mechanism of bcr 2 is more complex: a cryptic donor site of the retained portion of PML exon 6 and the RAR intron 2 physiologic acceptor site take part in the assemblage [10].

While the PML/RARα is transcribed into mRNA in 100% of cases, the reciprocal RARα/PML has been found in only 70% of APL patients [11]. Therefore, amplification of the PML/RARα junction should be preferred for both diagnositc and monitoring studies [12–15]. Following reverse transcription to obtain the hybrid CDNA, oligomers derived from PML exons 3 and 5 and from RARα exon 3 are used to detect the chimeric fusion genes, as shown in Fig. 1.

Even by using a two-step reaction with nested primers, the sensitivity of the RT-PCR analysis of PML/RARα hybrid gene seemed to be lower if compared to the RT-PCR amplifcation of other fusion genes. In similar experiments, different groups, including ours, were able to detect as low as 50 pg total RNA, but only one out of 10^{-4}–10^{-5} PML/RARα-positive cells. Overall this means that the reported assay is approximately 1–2 log less sensitive than the RT-PCR applied to different chimeric genes, such as the bcr/abl in the t(9; 22) (16) or the AML1/ETO in the t(8; 21) [17–19]. In addition to the abovementioned limits, the availability of good quality RNA from leukemic blasts (more difficult in APL than in other hematological malignancies) and the choice of an appropriate source of sam-

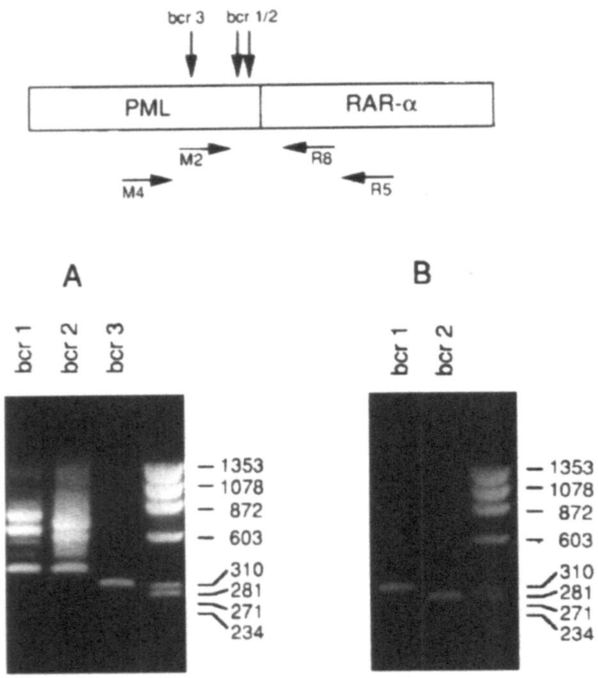

Fig. 1. Amplification of the differnt PML/RARα junctions by RT-PCR in t(15; 17)-positive APL patients at diagnosis. Primer M4, derived from PML exon 3, and primer R5 were used as a first cycle of PCR; then a second round of amplification was performed by using R8 as a nested primer. To obtain a better resolution of the PML/RARα junction corresponding to ber 1 and ber 2, a primer derived from PML exon 5 was used [15]

pling, should be considered in order to obtain proper results.

Clinical Relevance of RT-PDCR Analysis

The identification of the PML/RARα fusion gene has been proposed not only as a diagnostic tool but also for monitoring the APL clone. In a preliminary report, we found [20] that PCR positivity detected after consolidation was significantly correlated with clinical relapse, whereas a PCR-negative result was almost invariably associated with prolonged disease-free survivial. Several independent studies, [21, 22] have subsequently confirmed the predictive value of PCR positivity as an indicator of impending relapse. Based on these data obtained in retrospective APL series, the molecular monitoring of the APL clone has been included in the new on-going study for the treatment of newly diagnosed APL (AIDA) of the Italian cooperative adult and pediatric groups (GIMEMA and AIEOP) [23]. The protocol includes an initial course of all-trans retinoic acid (ATRA) (45 mg per m^2 per day orally for a minimum of 30 and a maximum of 90 days) and idarubicin given i.v. on day 2,4,6, and 8 at the dosage of 12 mg/m^2). Once complete remission is achieved, patients receive three courses of consolidation chemotherapy treatment without ATRA. Patients still PCR positive for the PML/RARα gene at the end of the consolidation phase, undergo bone marrow transplantation (either allogeneic or autologous) or are randomized in four different arms including no treatment or with methotrexate + 6-mercaptopurine alternated to ATRA. The preliminary results of the prospective molecular monitoring of APL patients enrolled in the AIDA protocol showed that approximately 30% of cases available for PCR monitoring at the end of induction (after the ATRA and idarubicin courses) persisted positive for the presence of PML/RARα. By contrast, virtually all cases analyzed so far have been PCR negative at the end of the third consolidation course. It is of course too early to draw any conclusions as to the predictive value of PCR positivity detected at the end of induction treatment, with respect to final outcome. In order to evaluate whether the PCR positivity detected at the end of induction treatment, reflects the persistence of bone-marrow progenitor cells expressing the PML/RARα gene, we have analyzed single hemopoietic colonies grown on semi-solid agar [24]. In three cases, a total of 36 colony-forming units—granulocyte macrophage (CFU-GM)colonies individually examined were negative for the presence of the fusion PML/RARα mRNA. The results are in line with the hypothesis that PCR positivity might reflect the persistence of differentiating cells in the bone marrow of APL patients still positive at the end of induction.

MRD Evaluation in APL vs Other Leukemias

The clinical significance of PCR monitoring in hematological malignancies is still a controversial issue. Chronic myelogenous leukemia (CML) patients in long-term remission have frequently been reported to remain PCR positive [25–28]. Similarly, in M2-type AML patients carrying the t(8,21) translocation, t(8; 21)-positive cells have been found several years after remission with no apparent correlation with subsequent relapse [17–19]. These findings are in marked contrast to those observed in APL. PCR positivity after consolidation is almost invariably associated with impending relapse, and by contrast, long-term survivors do not show PCR-detectable residual cells, suggesting that cure of the disease is accompanied by elimination of cells carrying the PML/RARα fusion gene [29]. We hypothesize that such discrepancies may be explained considering the biologic diversity of the different leukemia subtypes. The expression of the chimeric protein could play a different role with respect to clonal proliferation and aggressiveness, and the affected clone would require additional mutations to express the transformed phenotype. Alternatively, it is possible, as in the case of t(8; 21) cells, that the cell proliferation is repressed by a unknown mechanism. Overall, these findings further reinforce the need for large prospective studies in order to gain the appropriate perspective as the clinical relevance of molecular monitoring within each different AML subtype.

Acknowledgments. This work is partially supported by the Fondazione Tettamanti and by grants from the Associazione Italiana Ricerca sul Cancro (AIRC) and the Consiglio Nazionale delle Ricerche (PF ACRO, No. 92.02140).

References

1. Warrel RP Jr, de Thé H, Wang Z-Y, Degos L: Acute promyelocytic leukemia: N. Engl. J. Med. 329: 177, 1993
2. Food KA, Gale RP: Therapy of acute myelogenous leukemia: Blood Rev 6: 15, 1992.
3. Van Dongen JJM, Breit TM, Adriaansen HJ, Beishuizen A, Hooijkaas H: Leukemia 6: 47, 1992.
4. Rabbitts TH: Chromosomal translocations in human cancer: Nature 372: 143, 1994
5. Grignani F, Fagioli M, Alcalay M, Longo L, Pandolifi PP, Dontil E, Biondi A, Lo Coco F, Grignani F, Pelicci PG: Acute promyelocytic leukemia: from genetics to treatment. Blood, 83: 10, 1994
6. Borrow J, Goddard AD, Sheer D, Solomon E: Molecular analysis of acute promyelocytic leukemia breakpoint cluster region on chromosome 17. Science 249: 1577, 1990
7. de Thé H, Chomienne C, Lanotte M, Degos L, Dejean A: The t(15; 17) translocation of acute promyelocytic leukaemia fuses the retinoic acid receptor α gene to a novel transcribed locus. Nature 347: 558, 1990
8. Alcalay M, Zangrilli D, Pandolif PP. Long L, Mencarelli A, Giacomucci A, Rocchi M, Biondi A, Rambaldi A, Lo Coco F, Diverio D, Donti E, Grignani F, Pelicci PG: Translocation breakpoint of acute promyelocytic leukemia lies within retinoid acid receptor α locus. Proc Natl Acad Sci USA 88: 1977, 1991.
9. Lemons RS, Eilender D, Waldmann RA, Rebentisch M, Frej AK, Ledbetter DM, Willmann C, McConnel T, O'Connel P: Cloning and characterization of the t(15; 17) translocation breakpoint region in acute promyelocytic leukemia. Genes Chromosom Cancer 2: 79, 1990
10. Pandolfi PP, Alcalay M, Fagioli M, Zangrilli D, Mencarelli A, Diverio D, Bionid A, Lo Coco F, Rambaldi A, Grignani F, Rochette-Egly C, Gaube MP, Chambon P, Pelicci PG: Genomic variability and alternative splicing generate multiple PML/RARα transcripts that encode aberrant PML proteins and PML/RARα isoforms in acute promyelocytic leukemia. EMBO J 1: 1397, 1992
11. Alcalay M, Zangrilli D, Fagioli M, Pandolfi PP, Mencarelli A, Lo Coco F, Biondi A, Grignani F, Pelicci PG: Expression pattern of the RARα-PML fusion gene in acute promyelocytic leukemia. Proc. Natl Acada Sci USA 89: 4840, 1992.
12. Chang KS, Lu J, Wang G, Trujillo JM, Estey E, Cork A, Chu DT, Freireich EJ, Stass SA: The t(15; 17) breakpoint in acute promyelocytic leukemia cluster within two different sites of the myl gene: targets for the detection of minimal residual disease by polymerase chain reaction. Blood 79: 554, 1992
13. Castaigne S, Balitrand N, de Thé H, Dejean A, Degos L, Chomienne C: A PML-retinoic acid receptor alpha fusion transcript is constantly detected by RNA-based polymerase chain reaction in acute promyelocytic leukemia. Blood 79: 3110, 1992

14. Chen S-J, Chen Z, Chen A, Tong J-H, Dong S, Wang Z-Y, Waxman S, Zelent A: Occurrence of distinct PML-RARα isoforms in pateints with acute promyelocytic leukemia detected by reverse transcriptase/polymerase chain reaction. Oncogene 7: 1223, 1992.
15. Biondi A, Rambalid A, Pandolfi PP, Rossi V, Giudici G, Alcalay M, Lo Coco F, Diverio D, Pogliani EM, Lanzi EM, Mandelli F, Masera G, Barbui T, Pelicci PG: Molecular monitoring of the myl/RAR-α fusion gene in acute promyelocytic leukemia by polymerase chain reaction. Blood 80: 492, 1992
16. Kawasaki ES, Clark SS, Coyne MY, Smith SD, Champlin R, Witte DN, McCromick FP: Diagnosis of chronic myeloid and acute lymphocytic leukemia by detection of leukemia-specific mRNA sequence amplified in vitro. Proc. Natl Acad Sci USA 85: 5698, 1988.
17. Nucifora G, Larson RA, Rowley JD: Persistence of the 8; 21 translocation in patients with acute myeloid leukemia type M2 in long-term remission. Blood 82: 712, 1993.
18. Maruyama F, Stass SS, Estey EH, Cork A, Hirano M, Ino T, Freireich EJ, Yang P, Chang K-S: Detection of AML1/ETO fusion transcript as a tool for diagnosing t(8; 21) positive acute myelogenous leukemia. Leukemia 8: 40, 1994.
19. Kusek R, Laczika K, Knöbl P, Friedl J, Greinix H, Kahls P, Linkesch W, Schwarzinger I, Mitterbauer G, Purtscher B, Haas OA, Lechner K, Jaeger U: AML1/ETO fusion mRNA can be detected in remission blood samples of all patients with t(8; 21) acute myeloid leukemia after chemotherapy or autologous bone marrow transplantation. Leukemia 8: 735, 1994.
20. Lo Coco F, Diverio D, Pandolif PP, Bionid A, Rossi V, Avvisati G, Rambaldi A, Arcese W, Petti MC, Meloni G, Mandelli F, Grignani F, Masera T, Barbui T, Pelicci PG: PCR evaluation of residual disease as a predictor of cure or relapse in acute promyelocytic leukemia. Lancet, 340: 1437, 1992
21. Miller WH Jr, Kakizuka A, Frankel SR, Warrel RP Jr, De Blasio A, Levine K, Evans RM, Dimitrovski E. Reverse transcription polymerase chain reaction for the rearranged retinoic acid receptor alpha clarifies diagnosis and detects minimal residual disease in acute promyelocytic leukemia. Proc. Natl Acad Sci USA 89: 2694, 1992
22. Huang W, Sun G-L, Li X-S, Cao Q, Lu Y, Jang G-S, Zhang F-Q, Chai J-R, Wang Z-Y, Waxman S, Chen Z, Chen S-J: Acute promyelocytic leukemia: clinical relevance of two major PML/RARα isoforms and detection of minimal residual disease by retrotranscriptase polymerase chain reaction to predict relapse. Blood 82: 1264, 1993
23. Avvisati G, Baccarani M, Ferrara F, Lazzarino M, Resegotti L, Mandelli F (for the GIMEMA): AIDA protocol (ALL-trans retinoic acid+idarubicin) in the treatment of newly diagnosed acute promyelocytic leukemia (APL): a pilot study of the Italian cooperative group GIMEMA. Blood 84: 380(a), 1994.
24. Hernandez A, Osterholz J, Price CM, Wiedemann LM, Gordon MY, Goldman JM, Morgan GJ, Detection of the hybrid BCR/ABL messenger RNA in single CFU-GM colonies using the polymerase chain reaction. Exp. Hematology 18: 1142, 1990.
25. Pignon JM, Henni T, Amselem S, Vidaud M, Dugquesnoy P, Vernant JP, Kuents M, Cordonnier C, Rochant H, Goossens M: Frequent detection of minimal residual disease by use of the polymerase chain reaction in long-term survivors after bone marrow transplantation for chronic myeloid leukemia. Leukemia 4: 83, 1990
26. DEfau M-H. Kerckaert J-P, d'Hooghe MC, Fenaux P, Lai J-L, Jouet JP, Grandchamp B, Detection of minimal residual disease in chronic myeloid leukemia patients after bone marrow transplantation by polymerase chain reaction. Leukemia 4: 1, 1990.
27. Hughes T, Morgan GJ, Martiat P, Goldman JM: Detection of residual leukemia after bone marrow transplantation for chronic myeloid leukemia: role of polymerase chain reaction in predicting relapse. Blood 77:874, 1991.
28. Lee M-S, Kantarjian H, Talpaz M, Freireich EJ, Deisseroth A, Trujillo JM, Stass SA: Detection of minimal residual disease by polymerase chain reaction in Philadelphia chromosome-positive chronic myelogenous leukemia following interferon therapy. Blood 79: 1920, 1992
29. Diverio D, Pandilfi PP, Biondi A, Avvisati G, Petti MC, Mandelli F, Pelicci PG, Loco F. Absence of RT-PCR detectable residual disease in patients with acute promyelocytic leukemia in long-term remission. Blood, 82: 3556, 1993

Acute Leukemias VI
Prognostic Factors
and Treatment Strategies
Büchner et al. (eds)

Detection of Minimal Residual Disease in Cytogenetically Defined Prognostic Subgroups of AML

B. Wörmann[1], S. Könemann[1], D. Grove[1], D. Haase[1], C. Fonatsch[2], T. Büchner[3], L.W.M.M. Terstappen[4], and W. Hiddemann[1]

Introduction

The structure of chemotherapy in patients with newly diagnosed acute myeloid leukemia (AML) has become highly standardized. It consists of one or two courses of induction chemotherapy, consolidation, maintenance or intensified consolidation with or without stem cell support [3]. Intensification of consolidation therapy increases the number of patients in long-term disease-free survival [9]. The most efficient prevention of relapse can be achieved through myeloablative therapy with subsequent bone marrow transplantation from HLA-matched donors [1]. However, intensification of postremission therapy leads to a significant increase of deaths in complete remission [4, 9].

Potential future approaches may reserve high-risk therapy to AML patients with an unfavorable prognosis. Currently, the most widely accepted prognostic variables are age above 60, secondary leukemia, and cytogenetic features. Unfavorable karyotypes include −5/5q−, −7/7q−, and complex karyotypic abnormalities [2]. The long-term disease-free survival of these patients is only about 10%. In contrast, the prognosis for patients with t(8; 21), t(15; 17) and inv 16 is significantly above average, with a chance of long-term disease-free survival for about 50% of all patients [1]. Identification of these pre-therapeutic risk factors is based on patient history, morphology, and cytogenetic and molecular biological analysis.

Another option for stratification of postremission therapy is based on detection of minimal residual disease. Hematological complete remission has been defined as regeneration of normal hematopoiesis, absence of extramedullay disease, and a blast count $\leq 5\%$ in bone marrow aspirates [6]. Several methods are capable of detecting leukemia-associated markers with a significantly higher sensitivity. The most frequently used methods are the flow cytometric detection of cells with a leukemia-associated immunophenotype and polymerase chain reaction (PCR) of fusion genes or clone-specific gene rearrangements. The sensitivity of these methods for detection of persistent leukemic cells is 1×10^{-3} to 1×10^{-5} [5, 12]. Recent data on the detection of leukemia-associated markers in hematological remission are inconclusive. While rtPCR for PML/RARα has frequently disappeared in patients with acute promyelocytic leukemia in long-term complete remission (CR) [7], transcripts of AML1/ETO have been detected several years after achievement of hematological CR, without clinical evidence of relapse [8, 10].

The likely hypothesis is that risk factors defined before treatment and the chance of detection of minimal residual disease (MRD) in remission are not unrelated. In a continuing prospective study on the clinical significance of

[1]Department of Internal Medicine, Division of Hematology/Oncology, Robert-Koch-Str. 40, 37075 Göttingen, Germany
[2]Institute of Medical Biology, University of Vienna, Währinger-Str. 10, 1090 Vienna, Austria
[3]Department of Internal Medicine A, Domagkstr. 3, 48129 Münster, Germany
[4]Immunicon Corporation, 1313 Masons Mill 2, Huntingdon Valley, PA 19006, USA

persistent cells with the leukemia-associated phenotype (LAP), we have analyzed bone marrow aspirates from 15 patients with favorable prognositc factors and from 9 patients with unfavorable features.

Material and Methods

Patients

Twenty-four patients with newly diagnosed AML were enrolled in the study. All patients were treated at the Departments of Internal Medicine of the Universities of Münster and Göttingen between April 1989 and May 1994. Diagnosis was based on light microscopic evaluation of Pappenheim-stained slides by two independent hematocytologists. Classification was according to the criteria of the FAB group and included evaluation of cytochemical reactions with PAS, esterase, and peroxidase. All patients were treated according to the protocol of the German AML Cooperative Group [3]. Patients under the age of 60 received double induction chemotherapy with TAD9 and high-dose Ara-C and mitoxantrone, followed by one course of consolidation with TAD9 and 3-year maintenance therapy. Patients above the age of 60 received a second course of induction chemotherapy only if the blast count on day 16 was above 5%. Patients treated after 1990 were included in a randomized study comparing placebo versus granulocyte-macrophase colony-stimulating factor given 24 h prior to start of chemotherapy as a priming agent, with continuous daily administration of the drug until neutrophil recovery was achieved [11].

Bone marrow aspirates were taken from all patients prior to therapy and at recovery of platelets and neutrophil after induction chemotherapy.

Cell Preparation

Bone marrow aspirates were prepared for flow cytometric analysis by lysing erythrocytes. One volume of bone marrow was diluted with 14 volumes of the lysing solution [10^{-4} mol EDTA, 10^{-3} mol $KHCO_3$, 0.17 mol NH_4Cl in H_2O (pH 7.3)] and gently mixed. After lysis for 3–5 min at room temperature, the cells were centrifuged at 200 *g* for 5 min at room temperature. The pellet was resuspended in a volume of RPMI 1640 14 times larger than the original bone marrow volume, and centrifuged at 200 *g* for 5 min at 4°C. Following two washing steps the cells were finally resuspended in PBS containing 1% BSA and 20 mmol HEPES (pH 7.3). Cell concentration was 2×10^5 to 1×10^6 cells/ml. Monoclonal antibodies were added at a concentration of 5–20 µl/sample, adjusted to pretitering on normal bone marrow. After 30 min on ice, the cells were washed once with 2 ml PBS at 4°C. The pellet was resuspended in 1 ml 0.5% paraformaldehyde in PBS. Control cells were incubated with fluorescence-labeled isotype controls.

Flow Cytometry

Flow cytometric analysis was performed on a FACScan (BDIS, San Jose, CA, USA) using FACScan research software. The instrument was set up using T lymphocytes as reference by gating on CD3-positive lymphocytes in the FITC channel followed by adjustment of the light scatter detectors to locate the CD3-positive lymphocytes in a standard position of forward light scatter and orthogonal light scatter. Scatter and fluorescence signals were determined for each cell and data of 20,000 events were stored in list mode datafiles.

Data Analysis

The analysis of the five dimensional data was performed with the Paint-a-Gate Plus software (BDIS). This program transforms orthogonal light scatter according to a polynomial function and increases the resolution between cell populations in orthogonal light scatter.

Statistical Analysis

Treatment response was defined according to the guidelines of the NCI consensus report [6]. CR was defined by the presence of less than 5% leukemic blasts in the bone marrow aspirates, ⩾1500 neutrophils/mm^3, ⩾100 000 platelets/mm^3, and by absence of extramedullary disease. Remission duration was calculated from achievment of CR to relapse. The last timepoint of observation was February 15, 1996. Patients who died in CR were classified as in continous CR Lifetable analysis was calculated according to kaplan and Meier, and significances were determined by the logrank test, using the SPSS program system.

Results

Identification of Prognostic Factors at Diagnosis

Data from the 24 patients are summarized in Tables 1 and 2. Five patients had t(8; 21). By morphology, three patients were classified as having AML M2, two as AML M4. Three patients were diagnosed as having AML M3. In two of them the morphological diagnosis was confirmed by the cytogenetic presence of t(15; 17). This was not found in one patient (UPN 17), although local and central evaluation of the bone marrow slides unanimously classified the leukemia as M3. The largest group of these patients with favorable prognostic karyotypes comprised seven patients with AML M4 Eo and inv 16. All patients were treated according to the protocol except one patient, who was mentally retarded (UPN 121). She achieved CR after only one course of TAD9, and later received a second course of TAD9 as consolidation. Maintenance therapy was not initiated.

Nine patients had secondary acute leukemia. In six of them, a myelodysplastic syndrome was diagnosed as antecedent hematological disorder. Two further patients had a previous history of breast cancer which had been treated with radio- and adjuvant chemotherapy. The last patient was diagnosed with low-grade non-Hodgkin lymphoma 11 years prior to diagnosis of AML. He had been treated with COP.

Table 1. Characteristics of patients with favorable prognostic factors

UPN	Age (years)	Sex	FAB group	Minimal residual disease	Remission duration (months)
17	36	w	M3	–	65 +
94	22	w	M3	–	53 +
105	64	w	M4Eo	–	53 +
116	33	m	M4	–	6 +
121	52	w	M2	–	6
129	34	m	M2	+	4
166	48	m	M4Eo	–	12
169	56	w	M4	+	4
204	21	w	M4Eo	–	35+
210	60	w	M2	–	17
214	66	m	M4Eo	–	32 +
1004	37	m	M4Eo	–	25 +
1143	36	w	M4Eo	–	21 +
1311	29	w	M3	+	15 +
1564	81	m	M4Eo	+	4

–, absent; +, present

Table 2. Characteristics of patients with unfavorable prognostic factors

UPN	Age (years)	Sex	FAB group	Minimal residual disease	Remission duration (months)
51	57	m	M4	+	10
65	72	m	M6	+	7
70	58	m	M	+	15
81	61	m	M1	+	10
90	47	m	M	+	1
109	78	w	M2	+	3
114	49	w	M2	+	51+
142	66	w	M5	+	2
1128	51	m	M	+	12

Detection of Cells with the Leukemia-Associated Phenotype in CR

The leukemia-associated phenotype was analyzed using multiparameter flow cytometry in the bone marrow aspirates of all 24 patients prior to therapy. An informative combination of antibodies was defined for each patient and was used for follow-up analysis. The persistence of cells with the leukemia-associated phenotype was determined in all 24 patients at achievement of hematological CR. Leukemic cells were identified in 4 of the 15 with favorable prognostic factors, and in 9 of the 9 patients with unfavorable prognostic factors. Data are summarized in Tables 1 and2.

Correlation of MRD Results to Clinical Outcome

Lifetables according to Kaplan-Meier analysis are presented in Fig. 1 and 2. The group of patients with favorable factors had an excellent prognosis. The projected percentage of patients without relapse is 71% for patients without residual leukemic cells and 50% for patients with residual leukemic cells. Patients with unfavorable prognostic factors had a very poor prognosis. Only one patient stayed in continuous CR, now at 61 months. At later follow-up analysis this patient had no residual leukemic cells after consolidation therapy. All other patients relapsed, with a median remission duration of 7 months.

Discussion

During the past 20 years the prognosis of patients with newly diagnosed AML has significantly improved. Together with progress in suppority care this has mainly been achieved through intensification of chemotherapy in the induction, consolidation, and maintenance phases. Large multicenter trials have also allowed the identification of prognositc factors. Currently, individualized risk-adapted therapy is intensively debated on two competing principles: the first uses pretherapeutic parameters, the strongest risk factors being etiology of the leukemia, age, cytogenetic subgroup, and LDH; the second is based on detection of minimal residual disease in hematological CR.

Our study shows that these two principles are not competing, but rather are complimentary. As part of an ongoing multicenter trial on the clinical significance of the detection of persisting cells with a leukemia-associated phenotype, we analyzed 24 patients with cytogenetic or morphologically defined prognostic features. All 24 patients had an informative immunophenotype. This very high rate may either be due to the small number of patients or to the selection

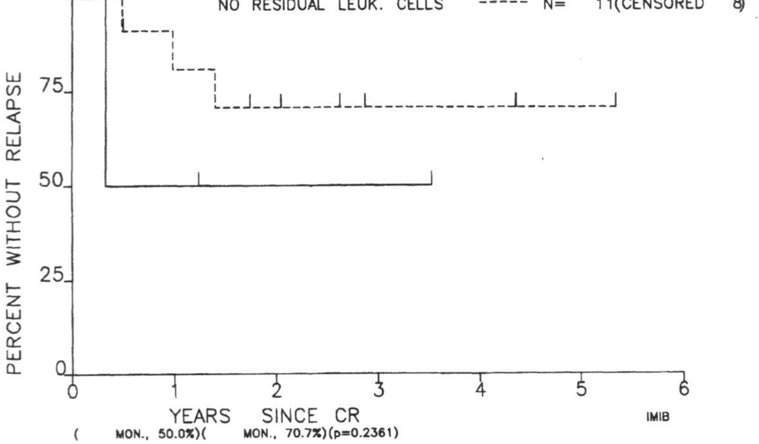

Fig. 1. Relapse-free survival of patients in cytogenetically favorable prognostic subgroups in relation to presence or absence of residual leukemic cells

of patients involved. It has previously been reported that patients with AML M2 and t(8; 21) have a high rate of aberrant antigen expression involving CP19 and CD56. Expression of lymphoid lineage-associated antigens has also been described in patients with AML M3 and AML M4E. Comparable data have not yet been published on patients with secondary leukemia. The complex genetic abnormalities in these patients, however, may also indicate that surface antigen expression may deviate from that in normal hematopoiesis.

At achievement of CR only 4 of 15 patients with favorable karyotypes had detectable leukemic cells. Due to the small patient group, the difference in therapy outcome in patients with and those without residual leukemic cells was not significantly different. It is conceivable that patients with persistent leukemic cells in CR even in prognostically favorable subgroups are those that will eventually relapse. This has to be tested in larger patient populations. In these three cytogenetic entities, multiparameter flow cytometry competes with the molecular biological detection of fusion transcripts for detection of 2MRD. Persistence or reappearacne of PML/RARα transcripts in patients with acute promyelocytic leukemia is associated with an unfavorable prognosis [7]. The results are not as clear as in patients with t(8; 21). AML1/ETO transcripts are consistently found in hematological CR [8, 10]. Multiparameter flow cytometry may have lower sensitivity but higher specificity.

All nine patients with secondary acute leukemia had persistent leukemic cells at achievement of CR. This is not an unexpected finding, but it supports the validity of detection of residual disease using multiparameter flow cytometry. The majority of these patients only had a short remission duration on standard chemotherapy with consolidation and maintenance. Higher cure rates in these patients [4]. require new experimental approaches. Even myeloablative therapy with allogeneic bone marrow transplantation leads to long-term disease-free survival in only 20%–30% of patients Analysis of MRD in these patients does not provide additional information for the overall prognosis

Our data further clarify the potential significance of detection of minimal residual disease by multiparameter flow cytometry in patients with newly diagnosed AML in hematological CR. We underline the interdependence of prognostic factors at different time points of treatment follow-up and the necessity to perform these studies as part of large multicenter trials with standardized chemotherapy

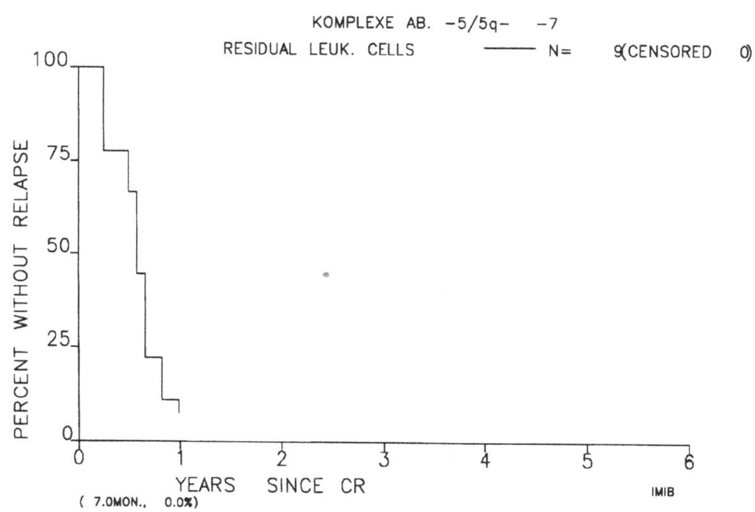

Fig. 2. Relapse-free survival of patients with cytogenetically unfavorable prognostic factors

References

1. Appelbaum F. R, Downing J., Willman C. (1995). The biology and therapy of acute myelogeneous leukemia. Hematology 1995. Education Program. Am. Soc. Hematol 23-35
2. Arthur D.C., Berger R., Golomb H.M., Swansbury G.J., Reeves B. R., Alimena G., van den Berghe H., Bloomfield C.D., de la Chapelle A., Dewalt G.W., Garson O.M., Hagemeijer A., Kaneko Y., Mitelman F., Pierre K.V., Ruutu T., Sakurai M., Lawler S.D., Rowley J.D. (1989) The clinical significance of Karyotype in acute myelogenous leukemia. Cancer Genet Cytogenet 40: 203
3. Büchner T., Hiddemann W. (1990) Treatment strategies in acute myeloid leukemia (AML). A. First-line chemotherapy. Blut 60: 61
4. Burnett A.K., Goldstone A.H., Stevens R., Hann I., Rees J.K., Wheatley K (1995) Biological characterisitcs of disease determine the outcome of allogeneic or autologous BMT in AML CR1. Blood 86 (10) [suppl.1] 616a (2452)
5. Campana D., Pui C.H. (1995) Detection of minimal residual disease in acute leukemia: Methodologic advances and clinical significance. Blood 85: 1416–1434
6. Cheson B.D., Cassileth P.A., Head D.R., Schiffer C.A., Bennett J.M., Bloomfield C.D., Brunning R., Gale R.P., Grever M. R., Keating M.J., Sawitsky A, Stass S., Weinstein H., Woods W.G. (1990) Report of the National Cancer Institute-sponsored workshop on definitions of diagnosis and response in acute myeloid leukemia. J. Clin Onc of 8: 813–818
7. Diverio D., Pandolfi P.P., Rossi V., et al. (1994) Monitoring of treatment outcome in acute promyelocytic leukemia by RT-PCR. Leukemia 8: 1105
8. Kusec R., Lackzika K., Knobl P., Friedl J., Greinix H., Kahls P., Linkesch W., Schwarzinger I., Mitterbauer G., Purtscher B. et al (1990) AML1/ETO fusion mRNA can be detected in remission blood samples of all patients with t(8; 21) acute myeloid leukemia after chemotherapy or autologous bone marrow transplantation. Leukemia 8: 735–739
9. Mayer R.J., Davis R.B., Schiffer C.A. et al (1994) Intensive postremission chemotherapy in adults with acute myeloid leukemia. N. Engl. J. Med. 331: 896–903
10. Nucifora G., Larson R.A., and Rowley J.D (1993). Persistence of the 8; 21 translocation in patients with acute myeloid leukemia type M2 in long-term remission. Blood 82: 712–715
11. Wörmann B., Hiddemann W., Frisch J., Zühlsdorf M., Rottmann R., Boeckmann A., Reuter C., Freire E.A., Innig G., Schulz G., Büchner Th (1991): In vitro and in vivo effects of rh GM-CSF in acute myeloid leukemia (AML). Behring Inst. Mitt. 90: 28–38
12. Wörmann B., Safford M., Könemann S., Büchner T., Hiddemann W., Terstappen L.W. (1993) Detection of aberrant antigen expression in acute myeloid leukemia by multiparameter flow cytometry. Recent Result Cancer Res 131: 185.

New Strategies: Nucleoside Analogs

Acute Leukemias VI
Prognostic Factors
and Treatment Strategies
Büchner et al. (eds)

Current Approaches in the Treatment of Chronic Lymphocytic Leukemia

E. Montserrat, F. Bosch, and C. Rozman

Abstract. In the last 2 decades, important advances have been made in the understanding of the biology, natural history, and prognosis of chronic lymphocytic leukemia (CLL). In addition, treatment possibilities in patients with CLL have changed as a result of the availability of new drugs and treatment strategies. Patients in early clinical stage (Binet A; Rai 0) with non-diffuse bone marrow histopathology, and low stable blood lymphocyte levels have a long survival and should not be treated unless the disease progresses. In contrast, patients with poor prognostic features, such as advanced clinical stage (Binet B, C; Rai III, IV), diffuse bone marrow infiltration or high and rapidly increasing blood lymphocyte levels have a median survival inferior to 5 years and need therapy. Chloroambucil has been the mainstay for CLL treatment, but new agents, particularly the purine analogs, offer great promise. Among these, fludarabine is the treatment of choice for patients failing standard therapies, and its role as frontline therapy is being investigated. Whatever the treatment used, however, cure is rarely achieved. A number of situations (e.g., autoimmune cytopenias, hypersplenism) require special treatment approaches (e.g., corticosteroids, splenectomy). Transplants of progenitor hemopoeitic cells are also increasingly performed and deserve further investigation.

Introduction

Chronic lymphocytic leukemia (CLL) is the most frequent form of leukemia in Western countries. Clinical features of CLL are due to the progressive accumulation of immuno-incompetent B lymphocytes in bone marrow and lymphoid organs and the immune disturbances that accompany the disease [1, 2]. The prognosis of patients with CLL is variable. In the last 2 decades significant advances have been made in the therapy of CLL [3–5]. This review focuses on when and how to treat patients with CLL.

When to Treat

Treatment decisions in CLL should not be made without taking into consideration the following items: (a) disease diagnosis; (b) patient characteristics; (c) symptoms; (d) prognosis; and (e) pace of the disease.

Diagnosis

Since CLL may be confounded with other chronic lymphoproliferative disorders, criteria to diagnose CLL have been proposed [6,7] (Table 1). Although, in the past, an absolute lymphocyte count of $15 \times 10^9/l$ was considered as the threshold for defining CLL, a diagnosis of CLL can be made whenever there is an absolute increase in the number of lymphocytes in blood and their morphology and immunophenotype (i.e., low density SmIg, CD5+, CD19+, CD20+, CD23+) are consistent with the diagnosis. The French-America-British (FAB) Group [8] has divided CLL into different morphological vari-

Postgraduate School of Hematology "Farreras Valenti", Department of Medicine, University of Barcelona, Barcelona Hospital Clinic, Villarroel, 170-08036 Barcelona, Spain

ants on the basis of the proportion of atypical lymphoid cells in peripheral blood (Table 1). This subclassification should be reanalyzed in light of the recent identification of lymphomas (e.g., splenic lymphoma with villous lymphocytes, mantle cell lymphoma) that can mimic CLL morphologically or immunophenotypically.

Patient Characteristics

The median age of patients with CLL at diagnosis is 65 years, with only 10%–15% of them being under 50 years of age. In addition, these patients may have associated diseases, thus excluding them from intensive treatment approaches. In younger patients, age by itself should not be considered as criterion to initiate therapy. In these patients, however, the goal of treatment, once indicated, should be to eradicate the disease.

Disease Symptoms

A number of symptoms that justify therapy in CLL are usually recognized [5, 6].

General Symptoms. These are B symptoms: weight loss, fever without infection, night sweats, weakness, or easy fatigability). However, systemic symptoms in uncomplicated CLL are infrequent. Therefore, infections or the transformation of CLL to a more aggressive lymphoproliferative disorder such as large-cell lymphoma (Richter syndrome) should be discarded before assuming that general symptoms reflect disease activity.

Compressive Problems. Bulky lymphadenopathy and/or splenomegaly can cause compressive problems.

Increased Susceptibility to Bacterial Infections with Hypogammaglobulinemia. Infection susceptibility usually correlates with low immunoglobulin levels and advanced disease, with the latter being the major reason to initiate therapy.

Prognosis

The median survival of patients with CLL has increased from about 5 years in the early 1970s to about 8 years; this is due to the larger proportion of patients currently diagnosed when asymptomatic. Clinical stages [9, 10], bone marrow histopathology [11, 12], blood lymphocyte levels [13, 14], lymphocyte doubling time [15, 16], lymphocyte morphology [17, 18], and cytogenetic abnormalities [19, 20] are reliable predictors of survival (Tables 2–4). These prognostic factors apply to all patients with CLL regardless of their age [21].

Clinical staging systems are the most useful prognostic parameters. Nevertheless, other variables may add discriminant power to clinical stages. For example, among patients in early stage, those with a diffuse bone marrow histopathologic pattern and/or rapidly increasing lymphocyte counts are likely to progress, whereas in those with non-diffuse bone marrow involvement and low, stable blood lymphocyte levels the disease tends to have an indolent and non-progressive (Smoldering) course [22, 23].

Pace of Disease

After diagnosis, patients should be observed without treatment for several weeks to accurately establish the stage of the disease, to calculate doubling time, and to assess the pace of the dis-

Table 1. Chronic lymphocytic leukemia; diagnostic criteria [6–8]

1. Absolute lymphocytosis in peripheral blood
   $> 5 \times 10^9$/l (National Cances Institute/Working Group)
   $> 5 \times 10^9$/l (International Workshop on CLL)
2. The majority of lymphocytes should be small and mature in appearance
   Morphologic subtypes (FAB Group)
   - 2.1 Typical or classic CLL ($\leqslant$ 10 % atypical lymphocytes)
   - 2.2 Atypical or mixed CLL/PL (prolymphocytes in blood between 11% and 54%)
   - 2.3 Atypical or mixed: variable proportion of atypical lymphocytes in blood with $<$ 10% prolymphocytes
3. Characteristic immunophenotype
   SmIg +/−, CD5 +, CD19 +, CD20 +, CD23 +, FMC7 −/ +, CD22 +/−
4. Bone marrow infiltration
   > 30% lymphocytes in bone marrow aspirate, or consistent pattern in bone marrow biopsy

Table 2. Chronic lymphocytic leukemia; Rai staging system

Risk	Stage	Characteristics	Median survival (years)
Low	0	Lymphocytosis alone	> 15
Intermediate	I	Lymphocytosis Lymphadenopathy	9
	II	Lymphocytosis Spleen and/or liver enlargement	5
High	III	Lymphocytosis Anemia (Hb < 11 g/dl)	2
	IV	Lymphocytosis Platelets $< 100 \times 10^9$/l	2

Table 3. Chronic lymphocytic leukemia; Binet staging system

Stage	Characteristics	Median survuval (years)
A	No anemia, no thrombocytopenia, fewes than 3 lymphoid areas[a] enlarged	12
B	No anemia, no thrombocytopenia, three or more areas enlarged	5
C	Anemia (Hb < 10 g/dl) and/or platelets $< 100 \times 10^9$/l	2

[a]Lymphoid areas considered are: cervical, axillary, and inguinal lymphadenopathies (whether uni- or bilateral), spleen, and liver.

ease and its severity. This may be of value in patients in whom the decision regarding the need for therapy is not clear enough.

In summary, patients with no risk factors (i.e., those in early clinical stage with a non-diffuse bone marrow pattern, and low and stable blood lymphocyte levels) have a very long survival and should not be treated unless the disease progresses. In contrast, patients with poor prognostic features (i.e., those with advanced clinical stage, diffuse bone marrow histopathology, high and/or rapidly increasing blood lymphocyte counts) have a median survival of less than 5 years and require therapy.

Table 4. Chronic lymphocytic leukemia: other prognostic factors

Parameter	Median survival (years)
Bone marrow histopathologic pattern	
Non-diffuse	10
Diffuse	3–5
Number of lymphocytes in blood	
$\leqslant 50 \times 10^9$/l	6
$> 50 \times 10^9$/l	3–4
Doubling time	
> 12 months	10
⩽ 12 months	5
Lymphocyte morphology in peripheral blood	
⩽ 5% prolymphocytes	5–6
> 5% prolymphocytes	3–4
Cytogenetic abnormalities	
Normal Karyotype	> 10
Multiple and complex abnormalities	5–6

N.B. The number of lymphocytes and prolymphocytes in blood as well as doubling time behave as continuous variables: the higher the number of cells or the shorter the doubling time, the poorer the prognosis. In most instances, these poor risk factors are not found in isolation but accompanying advanced disease.

How to Treat

Patients with Early and Stable Disease. Treatment of patients in an early stage (Binet A; Rai 0) has resulted in a delay in the rate of progression of the disease but no survival benefit [24–27]; in one study, patients treated from diagnosis with continuous chlorambucil had a higher incidence of second neoplasms [25]. Therefore, the current notion is that patients with early and stable disease should not be treated unless the disease progresses. Whether patients with early stage but unfavorable features (e.g., diffuse bone marrow biopsy, high and/or rapidly increasing blood lymphocyte counts) could gain benefit from being treated before they actually progress has not been addressed in clinical trials.

Patients with Advanced Clinical Stage Due to High Tumor Burden and Bone Marrow Failure. Over the last 2 decades, chlorambucil (e.g., 0.4–0.8 mg/kg orally every 2 weeks) has been the treatment of choice for the majority of these patients. Although patients treated with cyclophosphamide, doxorubicin, vincristine, and prednisone, (CHOP) achieve a higher response rate, this does not translate into longer survival [28–31]. Nevertheless, front-line treatment with CHOP might be indicated in the rare tumoral forms of the disease with compressive problems, a setting in which a rapid response is desirable; in such cases, local radiotherapy may also be useful. Patients failing frontline therapy should be treated with combination chemotherapy or fludarabine [5, 32–36]. Preliminary results of ongoing trials in which fludarabine is being compared to CHOP and cyclophosphamide, doxorubicin, and prednisone (CAP) show a higher response rate for fludarabine; whether this will translate into a longer survival remains to be seen, with more follow up being necessary [35,36]. At present, frontline therapy with fludarabine or other purine analogues should only be considered if forming part of clinical trials.

Patients with Cytopenias Due to Immune Mechanism. These patients, i.e., stage C (III, IV) (immune), should be initially treated with corticosteroids (e.g., prednisone 40 mg/m^2 daily given orally), with cytotoxic agents (e.g., cyclophosphamide 50–100 mg orally per day) only being added in case of no response after 4–6 weeks of treatment. In patients with autoimmune hemolytic anemia not responding to or difficult to control with corticosteroids plus cytotoxic agents, high-dose immunoglobulin or cyclosporine may be tried. A proportion of these patients, however, eventually require splenectomy or low-dose spleen radiation [5].

Another form of apparently advanced CLL not due to bone marrow infiltration is pure red-cell aplasia (PRCA) which may be occasionally, associated with CLL. Excellent treatment results have been reported with cyclosporine with or without prednisone [5, 37].

Patients with Hypersplenism. There are cases of CLL in which the anemia and/or the thrombocytopenia are entirely or partially due to hypersplenism. In such cases, splenectomy or low-dose radiotherapy over the spleen may be more effective than chemotherapy [5].

Therapy of Systemic Complications. Hypogammaglobulinemia is frequent in CLL and is the major cause of infections which are the major cause of death. In a placebo-controlled randomized study, 400 mg/kg immunoglobulin given intravenously at intervals of 3 weeks for 1 year was found to be effective and well tolerated (38). Prophylactic immunoglobulin, however, had no impact on survival and cost/benefit considerations make the routine use of immunoglobulin in all patients with hypogammaglobulinemia debatable [39]. Relatively lower doses of immunoglobulin (10 g every 3 weeks; 250 mg/kg every 4 weeks) might be as effective as higher doses, with this having important practical and economic derivations [40, 41]. The role of oral antibiotics as prophylaxis has not been formally investigated. As in other settings, recombinant hemopoietic growth factors may overcome neutropenia related to treatment [42]. Finally, erythropoietin may be useful to treat anemia unresponsive to other measures [43].

New Treatment Approaches

Purine Analogues. Deoxycoformycin (DCF), fludarabine, and 2-Chlorodeoxyadenosine (2-CDA) are related purine analogues which have demonstrated high activity in CLL. All these agents inhibit DNA synthesis in replicating cells, but their mechanisms of action in lymphoid malignancies are largely unknown. DCF is a potent inhibitor of adenosine deaminase; 2-CDA may induce DNA strand breaks. Both fludarabine and 2-CDA appear to activate in vitro cellular apoptosis [5, 34]. Unfortunately, there are no studies comparing the relative merits of purine analogues in CLL therapy. Results reported with these drugs are summarized in Table 5, and are presented in detail elsewhere in this volume.

Biotherapy. New approaches to treat CLL include monoclonal antibodies (MAbs), interferon (IFN), and cytokines. [MAbs], either alone (e.g., Campath) or conjugated with toxins (B4-blocked ricin), cytotoxic agents or radioisotopes

Table 5. Chronic lymphocytic leukemia: summary of treatment results with purine analogues

Agent	Trials[a] (n)	Patients (n)	Previous therapy	Response		
				CR (%)	PR (%)	CI (%)
Deoxycoformycin	6	152	Yes	0–4	16–35	16–65
Fludarabine	12	1159	Yes	0–38[b]	14–68	0–68
	3	138	No	25–74[b]	6–75	
2-Chlorodeoxyade-	6	179	Yes	0–39	2–60	16–20
nosine	1	20	No	25	60	

[a]Not including patients treated in randomized studies [35, 36].
[b]Including some patients in complete remission but with persistent lymphoid nodules or aggregates in bone marrow biopsy (for complete list of reference see [5]).
CR. complete remission;
PR. partial remission;
CI. clinical improvement.

(I131) are being actively investigated; the response is usually partial and transient. MAbs might be useful to eliminate residual disease in patients achieving good response after chemotherapy [44–47]. (IFN) has no effect in patients with advances and heavily pretreated disease. In contrast, IFN is more effective in patients with early disease and no prior therapy, although no complete remission is obtained [48–50]. IFN might further improve responses achieved with chemotherapy [51,52]. The combined use of IFN and cytotoxic agents deserves investigation in large clinical trials [48]. Interleukins (e.g., IL-2, IL-4, IL-6) are also under study. IL-2 has proven to have limited clinical activity with considerable toxicity [53–55].

Allogeneic Bone Marrow Transplantation. Experience with allogeneic bone marrow transplantation in CLL is increasing [56–58] (Table 6). The European and International Bone Marrow Transplant Registries have collected 54 patients who received an allogeneic bone marrow transplant because of CLL. Of these 38 patients (70%) achieved hematologic remission, 24 (44%) are alive at a median of 27 months (range 5–80 months) post-transplant; 3-year survival probability was 46%. Cytofluorometry and/or molecular biology techniques have shown some of the remissions achieved after transplant to be molecular, with no evidence of residual disease. Relapses, sometimes as late as 4 years after transplant, may be observed [58].

Table 6. Chronic lymphocytic leukemia: summary of treatment results with transplants

Study	Patients (n)	Age Median (years)	Range (years)	CR	CCR Follow up (n)	(months)	BMT-related deaths (n)
Rabinowe et al. 1993 [56]							
Allogeneic	8	40	31–34	6	6	6–18	
Autologous	12	45	27–54	10	10	6–31	1
Khouri et al. 1994 (57)							
Allogeneic [a]	11	42	25–55	7	7	6–36	1
Autologous	11	59	37–66	6	3	4–29	1
EMBT 1994 [58]							
Autologous	11	50	41–59	NR	8	3–24	1
IBMTR/EBMT 1995 [59]							
Allogeneic	54	41	21–57	38	24	5–80	25

[a]One syngeneic transplant (alive in continuous complete remission at 19 months after transplantation).
CCR, continous complete remission;
BMT, bone marrow transplant;
NR, not reported.

Autotransplants. There are several reports on autotransplants in CLL [56–58] (Table 6). All patients had advanced disease before transplantation and received cyclophosphamide and total body irradiation (TBI) as the conditioning regimen. In about half of the cases the bone marrow graft was purged with MAbs against B cells. A meaningful analysis of these cases is precluded by a short median follow up (i.e., less than 2 years).

The role of transplants in CLL treatment has not yet been completely defined and should be considered as experimental. Nevertheless, the possibility of performing an allogeneic bone marrow transplant should be considered in any young patient with CLL for whom an HLA-histocompatible donor is available. However, the potential benefits from a transplant (i.e., cure?) should be balanced with its risks (i.e., high mortality rate related to the procedure). Patients with poor prognostic factors are reasonable candidates. In contrast, transplants are not indicated in persons with CLL and no poor-risk factors. Under some circumstances (e.g., non-availability of an HLA-histocompatible donor, advanced age) and, provided a complete clonal remission has been achieved with standard therapy, autografts may be an alternative to allografts. Nevertheless, experience with autografts in CLL is still more preliminary than that with allografts and should also be considered as an experimental procedure.

Treatment Goals

As in any other malignancy, the prolongation of survival is the most important aim in CLL therapy. However, there are subjects with CLL in whom the disease does not affect, or only modestly affects, survival. Therefore, treatment should not be decided without taking risk factors into consideration.

For patients requiring therapy, considerable data indicate that response to treatment is associated with increased survival, and that survival correlates with the degree of response. Nevertheless, the disease is rarely, if ever, cured. Therefore, in most patients with CLL needing treatment, the most reasonable aim is to obtain the highest response with acceptable toxicity. In contrast, in young patients with poor-risk factors, experimental approaches are warranted in an attempt to achieve a cure.

Acknowledgments. This work has been performed thanks in part to grants 91/213, 93/0303, and 95/257 from Fondo de Investigaciones Sanitaries de la Seguridad Social (FISS), SAL 89/963 from Comision Interministerial de Cienciay Tecnologia (Spain), and the Jose Carreras International Foundation 93/P-CR.

References

1. Galton DAG: The pathogenesis of chronic lymphocytic leukemia. Can Med Assoc J 1966; 94: 1005–1010
2. Dameshek W: Chronic lymphocytic leukemia—an accumulative disease of immunologically incompetent lymphocytes. Blood 1967; 29: 566–584
3. Foon KA, Rai KR, Gale RP: Chronic lymphocytic leukemia: new insights into biology and therapy. Ann Int Med 1990; 113: 525–539
4. Dighiero G, Travade Ph, Chevret S et al.: (French Cooperative Group on CLL): B-cell chronic lymphocytic leukemia: present status and future directions. Blood 1991; 78: 1901–1914
5. Montserrat E, Rozman C: Chronic lymphocytic leukemia: present status. Ann Oncol 1995; in press.
6. Cheson BD, Bennet JM, Rai KR et al.: Guidelines for clinical protocols for chronic lymphocytic leukemia: recommendations of the National Cancer Institute-Sponsored Working Group. Am J Hematol 1988; 29: 152–163
7. International Workshop on CLL: Chronic lymphocytic leukemia: recommendations for diagnosis, staging, and response criteria. Ann Int Med 1989; 110: 236–238
8. Bennet JM, Catovsky D, Daniel MT et al.: Proposals for the classification of chronic (mature) B and T lymphoid leukemias. J Clin Pathol 1989; 42: 567–584
9. Rai KR, Sawitsky A, Cronkite EP et al: Clinical staging of chronic lymphocytic leukemia. Blood 1975, 46: 219–234
10. Binet JL, Auqier A, G. Dighiero et al.: A new prognostic classification of chronic lymphocytic leukemia derived from a multivariate survival analysis. Cancer 1981; 48: 198–206
11. Rozman C, Montserrat E, Rodriguez-Fernandez JM et al: Bone marrow histologic pattern—the best single prognostic parameter in chronic lymphocytic leukemia: a multivariate survival analysis of 329 cases. Blood 1984, 64: 642–648
12. Geisler C, Ralfkiaer E, Hansen MM et al.: The bone marrow histological pattern has independent prognostic value in early stage chronic lymphocytic leukemia. Br J Haematol 1986; 62: 47–54
13. Rozman C, Montserrat E, Feliu E et al.: Prognosis of chronic lymphocytic leukemia: a multivariate survival analysis of 150 cases. Blood 1982; 59: 1001–1005
14. Baccarani M, Cavo M, Gobbi M et al.: Staging of chronic lymphocytic leukemia. Blood 1982; 59: 1191–1196.

15. Montserrat E, Sanchez-Bisono J, Vinolas N et al.: Lymphocyte doubling time in chronic lymphocytic leukaemia: analysis of its prognostic significance. Br J Haematol 1986; 62: 567–575
16. Molica S, Alberti A: Prognostic value of lymphocyte doubling time in chronic lymphocytic leukemia. Cancer 1987; 60: 2712–2716
17. Melo JV, Catovsky D, Galton DAG: The relationship between chronic lymphocytic leukaemia and prolymphocytic leukaemia: I. Clinical and laboratory features of 300 patients and characterization of an intermediate group. Br J Haematol 1986; 63: 377–387.
18. Vallespi T, Montserrat E, Sanz MA: Chronic lymphocytic leukaemia: prognostic value of lymphocyte morphological subtypes. A multivariate analysis in 146 patients. Br J Haematol 1991; 77: 478–485
19. Juliusson G, Oscier DG, Fitchett M et al: Prognostic subgroups in chronic lymphocytic leukemia defined by specific chromosomal abnormalities. N Engl J Med 1990; 323: 720–724
20. Juliusson G, Gahrton G: Cytogenetics in CLL and related disorders. Bailliere's Clin Haematol 1993; 6: 821–848
21. Montserrat E, Gomis F, Vallespi T et al: Presenting features and prognosis of chronic lymphocytic leukemia in younger adults. Blood 1991; 78: 1545–1551
22. Montserrat E, Vinolas N, Reverter JC et al.: Natural history of chronic lymphocytic leukemia: on the progression and prognosis of early clinical stages. N Rev Franc Hematol 1988; 30: 359–361
23. Montserrat E, Vinolas N, Reverter JC et al.: "Smouldering" chronic lymphocytic leukaemia. Leuk Lymphoma 1991; 5 (suppl): 183–187
24. Shustik C, Mick R, Silver R et al.: Treatment of early chronic lymphocytic leukemia: intermittent chlorambucil versus observation. Hematol Oncol 1988; 6: 7–12
25. French Cooperative Group on Chronic Lymphocytic Leukemia: Effects of Chlorambucil and therapeutic decision in initial forms of chronic lymphocytic leukemia (stage A): results of a randomized clinical trial on 612 patients. Blood 1990; 75: 1414–1421
26. French Cooperative Group on Chronic Lymphocytic Leukaemia: Natural history of stage A chronic lymphocytic leukaemia in untreated patients. Br J Haematol 1990, 76: 45–57
27. Catovsky D, Richards S, Fooks J et al.: (MRC Working Party on leukaemia in Adults): CLL trials in the United Kingdom. Leuk Lymphoma 1991: 5 (suppl): 105–112
28. French Cooperative Group on Chronic Lymphocytic Leukaemia: Effectiveness of "CHOP" regimen in advanced chronic lymphocytic leukaemia. Lancet 1986; 1: 1346–1349
29. Hansen MM, Andersen E, Birgens H et al.: CHOP versus chloranbucil plus prednisolone in chronic lymphocytic leukemia. Leuk Lymphoma 1991; 5 (suppl): 97–100
30. Kimby E, Mellstedt H: Chlorambucil/prednisone versus CHOP in symptomatic chronic lymphocytic leukemias of B-cell type. A randomized trial. Leuk Lymphoma 1991; 5 (suppl): 93–96
31. Spanish Cooperative Group on CLL: Treatment of chronic lymphocytic leukemia: a preliminary report of Spanish (PETHEMA) trials. Leuk Lymphoma 1991; 5 (suppl): 89–91
32. O'Brien S, Kantarjian H, Beran M et al.: Results of fludarabine and prednisone therapy in 264 patients with chronic lymphocytic leukemia with multivariate analysis-derived prognostic model for response to treatment. Blood 1993; 82: 1695–1670
33. Keating MJ, O'Brien S, Kantarjian H et al.: Long-term follow-up of patients with chronic lymphocytic leukemia treated with fludarabine as a single agent. Blood 1993; 81: 2878–2884
34. Keating MJ, McLaughlin P, Plunkett W et al.: Fludarabine: present status and future development in chronic lymphocytic leukemia and lymphoma. Ann Oncol 1994; 5 (suppl 2): 79–83
35. Hiddemann W, Johnson S, smith A et al.: (Multinational CLL Cooperative Group): Fludarabine versus cyclophosphamide, adriamycin, prednisone (CAP) for the treatment of chronic lymphocytic leukemia: results of a multinational prospective randomized trials (abstract) Blood 1994; 84 (suppl 1): 461a.
36. French Cooperative Group on CLL: Comparison of fludarabine (FDB), CAP and CHOP in previously untreated stage B and C chronic lymphocytic leukemia: first interim results of a randomized clinical trial in 247 patients (abstract). Blood 1994; 84; (suppl 1): 461a
37. Chikappa G, Pasquale D, Zarrabi MH et al.: Cyclosporine and prednisone therapy for pure red cell aplasia in patients with chronic lymphocytic leukemia. Am J Hematol 1992; 41: 5–12
38. Cooperative Group for the Study of Immunoglobulin in Chronic Lymphocytic Leukemia: Intravenous immunoglobulin for the prevention of infection in chronic lymphocytic leukemia. A randomized controlled clinical trial. N Engl J Med 1988; 319: 902–907
39. Weeks JC, Tierney MR, Weinstein MC: Cost effectiveness of prophylactic intravenous immune globulin in chronic lymphocytic leukemia. N Engl J Med 1991; 325: 81–86
40. Chapel H, Dicato M, Gamm H et al.: Immunoglobulin replacement in patients with chronic lymphocytic leukaemia: a comparison of two dose regimes. Br J Haematol 1994; 88: 209–212
41. Jurlander J, Hartmann Geisler C, Hansen MM: Treatment of hypogammaglobulinaemia in chronic lymphocytic leukaemia by low-dose intravenous gammaglobulin. Eur J Haematol 1994; 53: 114–118
42. Hollander AAMJ, Kluin-Nelemans HC, Haak HR et al.: Correction of neutropenia associated with chronic lymphocytic leukemia following treatment with granulocyte-macrophage colonystimulating factor. Ann Hematol 1991; 62: 32–34
43. Pozlopoulos Ch, Panayiotidis P, Angelpoulos MK et al.: Treatment of anaemia in B-chronic lymphocytic leukaemia (B-CLL) with recombinant human

erythropoietin (r-HuEPO) (abstract) Br J Haematol 1994; 87 (suppl 1): 232
44. Stickney DR, Foon KA: Biologic response modifiers: therapeutic approaches to lymphoproliferative diseases. Current Opin Oncol 1992; 4: 847–855
45. Grossbard ML, Press OW, Appelbaum FR et al.: Monoclonal antibody-based therapies for leukemia and lymphoma: Blood 1992; 80: 863–878
46. Rabinowe SN, Grossbard ML, Nadler LM: Innovative treatment strategies for chronic lymphocytic leukemia: monoclonal antibodies, immunoconjugates, and bone marrow transplantation. In: Chronic Lymphocytic Leukemia: Scientific Advances and Clinical Developments. Cheson BD (editor). Marcel Dekker Inc. New York, 1993; p: 337–367
47. Levy R: Idiotype/granulocyte-macrophage colony-stimulating factor fusion protein as a vaccine for B-cell lymphoma. Nature 1993; 362: 755–758.
48. Montserrat E, Villamor N, Urbano-Ispizua A et al.: Alpha interferon in chronic lymphocytic leukemia. Eur J Cancer 1991; 27 (suppl 4): 74–77
49. Rozman C, Montserrat E, Vinolas N et al.: Recombinant alpha-2 interferon in the treatment of B-chronic lymphocytic leukemia in early stages. Blood 1988; 71: 1295–1298
50. Ziegler-Heitbrock HWL, Schlag R, Flieger D et al.: Favorable response of early stage B CLL patients to treatment with IFN-alpha-2. Blood 1989; 73: 1426–1430
51. Montserrat E, Villamor N, Urbano-Ispizua A et al.: Treatment of early stage B-chronic lymphocytic leukemia with alpha-2b interferon after chlorambucil reduction of the tumoral mass. Ann Hematol 1991; 63: 15–19
52. Ferrara F, Rametta V, Mele G et al.: Recombinant interferon alpha-2A as maintenance treatment of patients with advanced stage chronic lymphocytic leukemia responding to chemotherapy. Am J Hematol 1992; 41: 45–49
53. LeMaistre CF, Meneghetti C, Rosenblum M et al.: Phase I trial of an interleukin-2 (Il-2) fusion toxin (DAB_{486}IL-2) in hematologic malignancies expressing the IL-2 receptor. Blood 1992; 79: 2547–2554
54. Kay NE, Oken MM, Mazza JJ et al.: Evidence for tumore reduction in refractory or relapsed B CLL patients with infusional interleukin 2. N Rev Franc Hematol 1988; 30: 475–478
55. LeMaistre CF, Rosenblum MG, Reuben JM et al.: Therapeutic effects of generically engineered toxin (DAB_{486}IL-2) in patient with chronic lymphocytic leukaemia. Lancet 1991; 337: 1124–1125
56. Rabinowe SN, Soiffer RJ, Gribben JG et al.: Autologous and allogeneic bone marrow transplantation for poor prognostic patients with B-cell chronic lymphocytic leukemia. Blood 1993; 82: 1366–1376
57. Khouri IF, Keating MJ, Vriesendorp HM et al.: Autologous and allogeneic bone marrow transplantation for chronic lymphocytic leukemia: Preliminary results. J Clin Oncol 1994; 12: 748–758
58. Michallet M, Archimbaud E, Juliusson G et al: Autologous transplants in chronic lymphocytic leukemia. Report of 11 cases (abstract). Br J Haematol 1994; 87 (suppl 1): 172
59. Michallet M, Archimbaud E, Rowlings PA et al.: HLA-identical sibling bone marrow transplants for chronic lymphocytic leukemia (submitted for publication).

Prognostic Factors
and Treatment Strategies
Büchner et al. (eds)

Fludarabine for the Treatment of Advanced Chronic Lymphocytic Leukemia: Results of a Prospective Randomized Comparison with Cyclophosphamide, Doxorubicin and Prednisone

W. Hiddemann[1], S. Johnson[2], A. Smith[3], M. Björkholm[4], Löffler[5], B. Emmerich[6], P.J. Wyld[7], and J. Binet[8]
for the French Cooperative Group on CLL

Abstract. The current study was initiated to compare the efficacy and side effects of single agent fludarabine treatment with cyclophosphamide, doxorubiein, and prednisone (CAP) in previously untreated and pretreated patients with advanced-stage chronic lymphocytic leukemia (CLL) by way of a prospective randomized clinical trial. Patients with (a) previously untreated B-CLL of Binet stages B or C, or (b) relapsed B-CLL pretreated with non-anthracycline-containing regimens for more than 6 months but less than 3 years were randomly assigned to either fludarabine given at a dose of 25 mg/m^2 per day over 5 consecutive days or CAP comprising cyclophosphamide 750 mg/m^2 per day and doxorubicin 50 mg/m^2 on day 1 and prednisone 40 mg/m^2 per day on days 1-5. Both regimens were repeated every 28 days for a total of six courses.

A total of 196 patients were entered into the trial of whom 100 were previously untreated, while 96 patients had received prior therapy. Remission rates were significantly higher in fludarabine-than CAP-treated patients, with overall response rates of 60% vs. 44%, respectively ($p = 0.023$). Further analysis indicated a higher response to fludarabine in both untreated and pretreated cases which was statistically significant, however, in pretreated cases only (48% vs. 27%, $p = 0.036$). Patients achieving complete or partial remission after fludarabine experienced a significantly longer event-free interval than the comparable CAP-treated group, with a median response duration of 796 days for fludarabine and 270 days for CAP ($p = 0.002$). This difference translated into a tendency towards a longer survival for fludarabine-treated patients which was not statistically significant, however, at the time of evaluation (1302 days vs. 999, $p = 0.40$).

Treatment-associated side effects consisted predominantly in myelosuppression and granulocytopenia occuring after 19% of courses with fludarabine and after 22% CAP treatment cycles. CAP-treated patients, however, experienced a higher frequency and severity of nausea and vomiting (25% vs. 5%, $p < 0.001$) as well as of hair loss and allopecia (65% vs. 2%, $p < 0.001$)

The current data demonstrate a significantly higher activity of fludarabine in patients with advanced-stage CLL which is most pronounced in previously treated patients. In relapsed CLL fludarabine, therefore, represents the current treatment of first choice.

Introduction

After years of stagnation and lack of therapeutic progress, new perspectives have recently arisen in the treatment of chronic lymphocytic leukemia (CLL) through the introduction of

[1]Department of Hematology and Oncology, University of Göttingen, Germany
[2]Taunton Somerset Hospital, Taunton, UK
[3]Department of Hematology, Royal United Hospital, Bath, UK
[4]Department of Medicine, Karolinska Hospital, Stockholm, Sweden
[5]Department of Hematology and Oncology, University of Kiel, Germany
[6]Department of Internal Medicine, University of München, Germany
[7]Inversk Clinical Research Ltd., Edinburgh, UK
[8]Department of Hematology, Group Hospitalier Pitié-Salpétriére, Paris, France

purine analogues and fludarabine in particular. Fludarabine was extensively investigated in patients failing on or relapsing after conventional therapy and was thus approved for second-line treatment by the respective authorities in several countries. Based on these promising results, fludarabine is also being applied in previously untreated patients and combined with additional agents to further improve its activity [1–9]. Side effects such as the prolonged suppression of CD4 lymphocytes and the associated increased risk of infections [5, 10–12] caution its widespread application outside controlled clinical trials at the present time and warrant a prospective comparison with standard therapies. The current study was intiated to compare the efficacy and side effects of fludarabine with one of the most effective and broadly used combination regimens comprising cyclophosphamide, doxorubicin and prednisone (CAP) [13–15] in previously untreated and pretreated patients with advanced-stage CLL by way of a prospective randomized clinical trial.

Patients, Materials, and Protocols

Patients of either sex with B-CLL as defined by the National Cancer Institute (NCI) Working Group [16] at ages older than 18 years were considered for entry into the study if they presented with either [a] previously untreated B-CLL of Binet stages B or C; or (b) relapsed B-CLL pretreated with chlorambucil or similar non-anthracycline or anthrachinone-containing regimens for more than 6 months but less than 3 years. All patients had to be in need of therapy as defined by an impairment of normal hematopoiesis, presence of B symptoms or progressive disease. Patients with poor performance status (World Health Organization WHO, scale 4) were excluded, as were cases with abnormal renal or liver function, uncontrolled autoimmune hemolytic anemia or thrombocytopenia, HIV-related disease, T-CLL or prolymphocytic leukemia and Richter's syndrome.

The initial diagnostic work-up included the assessment of history and physical examination, the determination of complete blood counts and immunoglobulin levels, liver and renal function, as well as bone marrow aspiration and biopsy for morphology and immunophenotyping, respectively.

Randomization and Protocols

Eligible patients underwent a central randomization procedure for the assignment to either fludarabine or CAP therapy by telephone or fax using preformed randomization lists. Randomization was balanced for each participating institution and stratified for prior or no prior therapy, stage B or C according to Binet, and age below or above 70 years.

Fludarabine was given at a dose of 25 mg/m^2 per day over 5 consecutive days by 30-min infusion. CAP comprised cyclophosphamide 750 mg/m^2 per day and doxorubicin 50 mg/m^2 per day both given by intravenous infusion on day 1, and orally administered prednisone 40 mg/m^2 per day on days 1–5. Both regimens were repeated every 28 days for a total of six courses. In case of incomplete but continuing therapeutic response at that time, up to four further cycles were allowed to be given.

Response was assessed according to NCI Working Group criteria [16]. Complete remission (CR) was defined by the disappearance of all palpable disease and the normalization of blood counts with granulocyte counts greater than 1 500/mm^3, thrombocyte counts greater than 100 000/mm^3, and hemoglobin greater than 11.0 g/dl as well as bone marrow lymphocyte percentage less than 30% in both aspiration and biopsy material. A partial remission (PR) required a greater than 50% reduction of measurable disease manifestations and a more than 50% improvement of all abnormal blood counts. Progressive disease was defined as a greater than 10 000/mm^3 lymphocyte count and a more than 25% increase above remission values or a greater than 50% increase in marrow infiltration or a corresponding enlargement of lymph nodes, liver, or spleen.

Treatment related toxicity was evaluated according to WHO criteria. Survival was calculated from the 1st day of treatment to death or last follow up progression-free interval comprised the period from the end of therapy to disease progression or death.

Evaluation Procedures and Statistics

Fludarabine and CAP therapy were primarily compared for their respective response rates after the completion of the six initial treatment courses. Patients terminating therapy prior to this end point were classified as treatment failures unless the reason for early withdrawal was achievement of CR or PR. Response rates in both treatment groups were compared using the Mantel-Haenszel test.

Treatment-associated side effects were assessed by the modified Student's test. Survival curves and progression-free intervals were determined according to Kaplan and Meier, and the log rank test was applied for comparison.

Study Conduct

The study was performed under regulatory approval from the participating countries, Germany, France, Sweden, and the United Kingdom. It was conducted in accordance with the updated declaration of Helsinki and approved by the ethics committees at the participating institutions. Prior to study entry, all patients gave their informed consent after having been informed about the aim and investigational nature of the trial.

Results

Patient Characteristics

During the study enrolment period from May 1990 until July 1992, 208 patients were entered from 40 participating institutions in France, Germany, Sweden, and the United Kingdom. Institutions and responsible investigators are listed in Appendix 1. A total of 102 patients were randomized for CAP and 106 patients were assigned to fludarabine therapy. Six patients in each group were subsequently excluded because of non-adherence to entry criteria or protocol violation. Of the remaining 196 patients 100 were previously untreated while 96 had received prior therapy with one to three different regimens; 105 patients presented with stage B disease according to Binet, 89 had stage C, and two previously pretreated cases were at stage a. Patient characteristics are summarized in Table 1.

Table 1. Fludarabine vs. CAP in chronic lymphocytic leukemia: patient characteristics

	Fludarabine	CAP
n	100	96
Age 1/m Range (years)	39–79	43–78
Median (years)	63	62
Male (n)	74	63
Female (n)	26	33
Binet stage A (n)	1	1
Binet stage B (n)	54	51
Binet stage C (n)	45	44
No prior therapy (n)	52	48
Prior therapy	48	48

Treatment Response and Side Effects

From the 196 evaluable patients a total of 102 (52%) responded with 29 (15%) patients achieving CR and 73 (37%) obtaining PR. Remission rates were significantly higher in fludarabine than in CAP-treated patients, with overall response rates of 60% for fludarabine and 44% for CAP ($p = 0.023$). Correspondingly, more CRS were observed after fludarabin than after CAP (18% vs. 11%, $p = 0.20$). Further analysis according to prior therapy or no preceding treatment indicated a higher response to fludarabine in both patient groups, which was statistically significant only in pretreated cases, Table 2.

A total of 68 (35%) patients did not complete the scheduled number of six treatment courses; 35 received fludarabine while 35 were on CAP treatment. Reasons for early withdrawals are given in Table 3 and indicate a higher rate of progressive disease, including progressive disease-associated deaths, during CAP as compared to fludarabine (21%, 12%, $p = 0.065$). Twelve patients died during therapy, nine on fludarabine and three on CAP. Of the nine deaths during fludarabine treatment, three were due to progressive disease and four due to severe infections. One patient each died from myocardial infarction and intracerebral hemorrhage related

Table 2. Fludarabine vs. CAP in chronic lymphocytic leukemia: Response

	Fludarabine		CAP		
	n	CR+PR *n*(%)	*n*	CR+PR (*n*)%	(*p*)
All patients	100	60 (60)	96	42 (44)	0.023
Untreated	52	37 (71)	48	29 (60)	0.26
Pretreated	48	23 (48)	48	13 (27)	0.036

Table 3. Fludarabine vs. CAP in chronic lymphocytic leukemia: patients not completing six treatment cycles

	Fludarabine (*n*)	CAP (*n*)
Progressive disease	9	21
Death from		
Infection	4	3
Progression	3	–
Other causes	2	–
Intercurrent illness		
Infection	5	3
Other causes	10	7
Partial remission	–	1
	33	35

to severe thrombocytopenia. All three deaths during CAP were caused by infections. Excluding the progressive disease-associated deaths, mortality rates were similar in both regimens.

Intercurrent illness prompted the cessation of therapy in 25 (13%) patients, 15 (15%) of the 100 being on fludarabine and 10 (10%) of the 96 patients on CAP. Of the ten patients terminating fludarabine early because of non-infectious complications, five revealed newly occurring autoimmune phenomena including autoimmune hemolytic anemia ($n=2$), autoimmune thrombocytopenia ($n=2$), or pure red cell aplasia ($n=1$). The latter case has been reported previously [17]. Similar events were not observed during CAP treatment.

Treatment—associated side effects are summarized in Table 4. Myelosuppression and granulocytopenia in particular comprised the predominant toxicity after both regimens but were mostly mild to moderate. Granulocytopenia of WHO grade III or IV was experienced after 19% of fludarabine treatment courses and after 22% of CAP cycles, respectively. CAP was however, associated with a significantly higher rate, and severity of nausea and vomiting (25%, 5%, $p<0.001$), as well as of hair loss and complete alopecia (65%, 2%, $p<0.001$).

Response Duration and Survival

The assessment of response duration and survival is based on a median observation time of 31 months (range 1–52 months).

Patients achieving CR or PR after fludarabine experienced a significantly longer progression-free interval than the comparable CAP group. The median duration of response was 796 days for fludarabine and 270 days for CAP ($p=0.002$) (Fig. 1). This difference translated into a tendency towards a longer survival for fludarabine-treated patients which was, however, not statistically significant at the time of evaluation. The median survival was 1302 days after fludarabine and 999 days after CAP ($p=0.40$)

Discussion

Following the first promising reports by Grever et al. [2] and Keating et al. [3] about the high activity of fludarabine in advanced, CLL evidence has been accumulated by subsequent studies that fludarabine represents the most active currently available single agent in the treatment of CLL and may thus provide a new perspective in the management of this disorder. A prospective comparative evaluation with stan-

Table 4. Fludarabine vs. CAP in chronic lymphocytic leukemia: cumulative side effects-all Patients

	Fludarabine WHO I/II (*n*)	(%)	WHO III/IV (*n*)	(%)	CAP WHO I/II (*n*)	(%)	WHO III/IV (*n*)	(%)
Granulocytopenia	130	(27)	91	(19)	90	(20)	98	(22)
Thrombocytopenia	90	(18)	68	(14)	87	(19)	58	(13)
Anemia	137	(28)	35	(7)	155	(34)	35	(8)
Infection	98	(19)	21	(4)	74	(16)	12	(3)
Hepatic	35	(7)	4	(1)	28	(7)	2	(0.5)
Renal	33	(7)	–	–	22	(5)	–	
Diarrhea	20	(4)	2	(0.5)	8	(2)	–	
Nausea/vomiting	23	(5)	2	(0.5)	96	(21)	17	(4)
CNS	16	(3)	1	(0.2)	3	(0.5)	–	
Peripheral neuropathy	7	(2)	2	(0.5)	2	(0.5)	–	
Hair loss	8	(2)	1	(0.2)	210	(46)	86	(19)

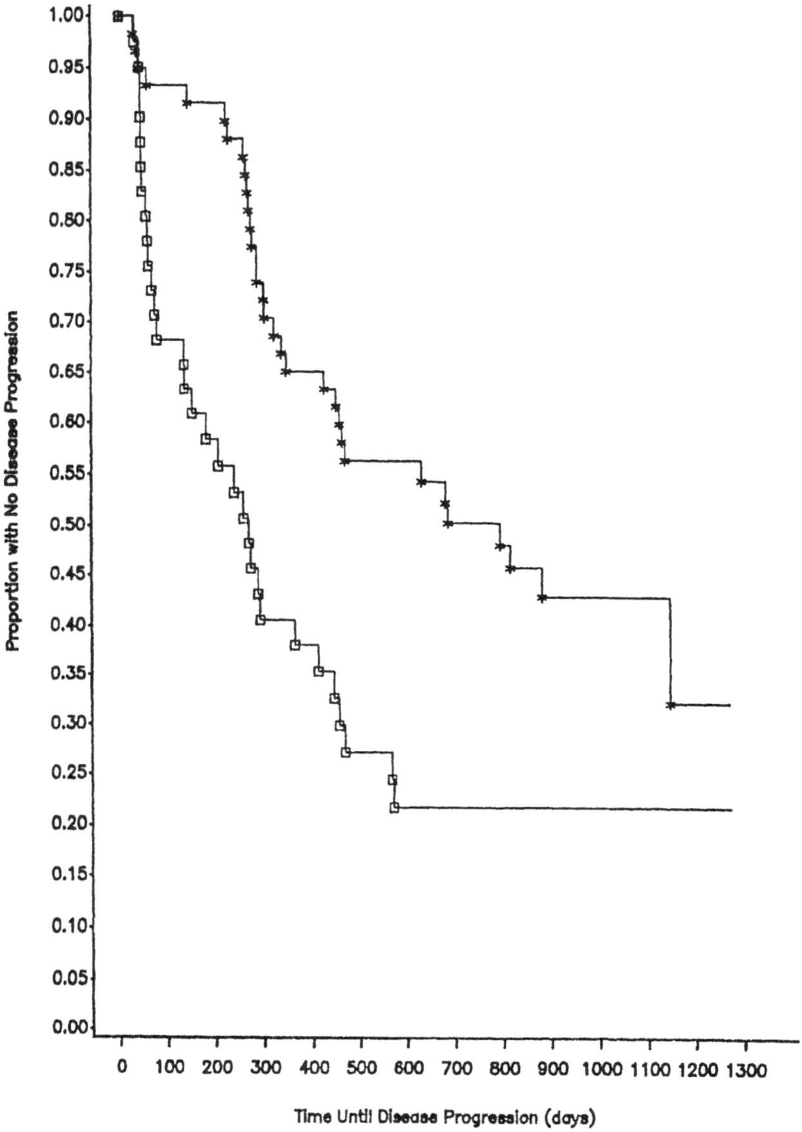

Fig. 1. Progression-free intervals for patients with complete or partial remission after fludarabine (asterisks) or CAP therapy (squares) The median response duration was 796 days after fludarabine and 270 days after CAP ($p = 0.002$)

dard therapies was lacking, however, and precluded a more definite judgement.

The data obtained in the current study clearly demonstrate a significantly higher response rate after fludarabine than CAP with overall remission rates of 60%, 44%, respectively ($p = 0.023$). Further analysis of previously untreated and pretreated cases revealed that 71% of previously untreated patients achieved CR or PR by first-line therapy with fludarabine as compared to a 60% response rate after CAP ($p = 0.26$). In previously treated patients the difference was even more pronounced with 48% remissions after fludarabine and 27% responses after CAP ($p = 0.036$). These data are in accordance with preceding phase II studies demonstrating responses to fludarabine in 38%–57% of previously treated patients and in up to 79% in patients without prior therapy (2–5, 7, 18]. They also confirm the comparatively low efficacy of conventional salvage regimes in relapsed CLL including the anthracycline-containing combinations such as CAP and cyclophosphamide, doxorubicin, vincristine, and prednisone [13].

In the current trial fludarabine not only proved more effective in terms of inital response, but was also associated with fewer side effects. While myelosuppression and granulocytopenia in particular comprised the predominant toxicity after both regimens and occurred in 19% of courses with fludarabine and in 22% of CAP cycles, CAP-treated patients experienced a higher frequency and severity of nausea and vomiting (25% vs, 5%, $p < 0.001$), as well as of alopecia and complete hair loss (65% vs. 2%, $p < 0.001$). These differences appear especially relevant in view of the fact that both regimens are primarily applied for palliation and that good tolerance facilitates the acceptance and performance of therapy.

In contrast to other investigations, no increase in infections events was observed during or after fludarabine therapy. This complication has been associated with the sustained reduction of lymphocyte counts and of CD 4 helper cells in particular [10–12, 19]. In addition, an impairment of antibody activiy and even granulocyte function has been reported [20–21]. However, in accordance with the current results, the most mature study on this issue recently published by O'Brien and coworkers [5] did not reveal a higher incidence of infections among 264 CLL patients treated with fludarabine except for patients receiving fludarabine in combination with prednisone. Antimicrobial prophylaxis as advocated by several investigators already seems, therefore, not generally required during fludarabine therapy.

These data warrant further exploration and emphasize the need for prospective analyses which are also required to evaluate the impact of treatment on disease-free and overall survival. At the time of evaluation, the higher response rate achieved by fludarabine in the present trial did not translate into a statistically significant improvement of overall survival either in untreated or in pretreated patients. However, the median progression-free interval was significantly longer in patients responding to fludarabine.

References

1. Chun HG, Leyland-Jones B, Cheson BD: Fludarabine phosphate—a synthetic purine antimetabolite with significant activity against lymphoid malignancies. J. Clin Oncol 9: 175–188, 1991
2. Grever MR, Kopecky KJ, Coltman CA et al.: Fludarabine monophosphate—a potentially useful agent in chronic lymphocytic leukemia. Nouv Res Fr Hematol 30: 457–459, 1988
3. Keating MJ, Kantarjian H, Talpaz M et al.: Fludarabine—a new agent with major activity against chronic lymphocytic leukemia. Blood 74: 19–25, 1989
4. Hiddemann W, Rottmann R, Wörmann B et al.: Treatment of advanced chronic lymphocytic leukemia by fludarabine—results of a clinical phase-II study. Ann Hematol 63: 1–4, 1991
5. O'Brien S, Kantarjian H, Beran M et al.: Results of fludarabine and prednisone therapy in 264 patients with chronic lymphocytic leukemia with multivariate analysis-derived prognostic model for response to treatment. Blood 82: 1695–1700, 1993
6. Keating MJ, Estey E, O'Brien S et al.: Clinical experience with fludarabine in leukemia. Drugs 47, Suppl 6: 39–49, 1994
7. Keating MJ, O'Brien S, Kantarjian H et al.: Long-term follow-up of patients with chronic lymphocytic leukemia treated with fludarabine as a single agent. Blood 81: 2878–2884, 1993
8. Robertson LE, O'Brien S, Kantarjian H et al.: Fludarabine plus doxorubicin in previously treated chronic lymphocytic leukemia. Blood 82, Suppl. 1, 140a, 1993
9. Elias L, Stock-Novack D, Head DR et al.: A Phase I trial: combination fludarabine monophsphate and chlorambucil in chronic lymphocytic leukemia: Southwest Oncology Group Study. Leukemia 7: 361–365, 1993
10. Wijermans PW, van der Linden JSM, Gerrits WBJ, Haak HL: Severe immuno deficiency and opportunistic infections seen in patients treated with fludarabine monophosphate. Blood 80, Suppl 1, 46a, 1992
11. Bergmann, Fenchel K, Jahn B, Mitrou PS, Hoelzer D: Immunosuppressive effects and clinical response of fludarabine in refractory chronic lymphocytic leukemia. Ann Oncol 4: 371–375, 1993
12. Byrd JC, Hargis JB, Kester K, Hospenthal DR, Weidner S, Diehl L: Fludarabine therapy for lymphoid malignancies is associated with a high number of opportunistic pulmonary infections. Blood 82, Suppl 1, 538a, 1993
13. Keating MJ, Scouras M, Murphy S et al.: Multiple agent chemotherapy (POACH) in previously treated and untreated patients with chronic lymphocytic leukemia. Leukemia 2: 157–164, 1988
14. Keating MJ, Hester JP, McCredie KB et al.: Long-term results of CAP therapy in chronic lymphocytic leukemia. Leuk Lymph 2: 391–397, 1990
15. French Cooperative Group of CLL: Comparison of fludarabine (FDB), CAP and ChOP in previously

untreated stage B and C chronic lymphocytic leukemia (CLL). First interim results of a randomized clinical trial in 247 patients. Blood 83, Suppl. 1: 461a, 1994
16. Cheson BD, Bennett JM, Rai KR et al.: Guidelines for clinical protocols for chronic lymphocytic leukemia. Recommendations of the National Cancer Institute Sponsored Working Group. Am J Hematol 29: 152–163, 1989
17. Leporrier M, Reman O, Troussard X: Pure red-cell aplasia with fludarabine for chronic lymphocytic leukaemia. Lancet i.: 555, 1993
18. Sorensen JM, Vena Dm Fallavollita A, Cheson BD: Treatment of refractory chronic lymphocytic leukemia (CLL) with fludarabine monophosphate (FAMP) under the group C protocol. Proc. Am Soc Clin Oncol 11: 264, 1992
19. Seymour JF, Kurzrock R, Freireich EJ Estey EH, Anderson MD: Prolonged CD4+ lymphocytopenia is the cost of durable responses to 2-chlorodeoxyadenosine (2-CdA) in patients (PTS) with hairy cell leukemia (HCL). Blood 82, Suppl. 1: 142a, 1993
20. Priebe T, Kandil O, Nakic M, Pan BF, Nelson JA: Selective modulation of antibody response and natural killer cell activity by purine nucleoside analogs. Cancer Res 48: 4799–4803, 1988
21. Priebe T, Ruiz L, Nelson JA: Adenosine receptors and modulation of natural killer cell activity by purine nucleosides and their analogs. Cell Immunol 130: 513–519, 1990
22. Schäfer C, Brochmann C, Büchner Th, Hiddemann W, Wörmann B: In vivo effects of fludarabine on immunocompetent cells in patients with chronic lymphocytic leukemia and low grade non-Hodgkin lymphoma. Ann Hematol 67, Suppl.: 412, 1993

Appendix

Participating institutions and responsible investigators in order of the number of patients entered.

The French Cooperative Group on CLL:

Dr. P. Fenaux
Service de Maladies du Sang
Hôpital Huriez
59037 Lille
France

Prof. Dr. J.L. Binet
Department d'Hematologie
La Pitie Salpetriere
47 Boulevard de l'Hôpital
Paris 75651
France

Prof. Dr. M. Leporrier
Sce d'Hematologie
CHRU de Caen
Avenue Georges Clemenceau
14033 Caen
France

Dr. P. Travade Service Saint-Vincent
Hotel Dieu
63000 Clermont-Ferrand
France

Prof. Dr. H. Piguet
Sce d'Hematologie
Centre Henri Becquerel
Rue d'Amiens
766038 Rouen
France

Dr. C. Linassier
Sce D'Oncologie Medicale
Hôpital Bretonneau
2 Boulevard Tonnele
37000 Tours
France

Dr. B. Desablens
Sce d'Hematologie
Hôpital Sud BP 3009
80030 Amiens
France

Dr. B. Dreyfus
Dept. d'Hematologie
Hôpital de la Miletrie
Pavillon de Blaye-BP 577
86021 Poitiers
France

Prof. Dr. C.P. Brizard
Dept. d'Hematologie
Hôpital Nord
Avenue Albert Raymond
42277 St. Priest en Jarez
France

Dr. B. Murgue
Dr. T. Russet
Sce d'Hematologie
Hôpital Lapeyronie
Route de Ganages
34059 Montpellier
France

Dr. P. Souteyrand
Service d'Hematologie

Centre Hospitalier d'Avignon
Hôpital de la Durance
305 Rue Raoul Follereau
84025 Avignon
France

Dr. S. Johnson
Dr. M.J. Phillips
Musgrove Park Hospital
Taunton
Somerset TA1 5DA
England

Prof. Dr. W. Hiddemann
University of Göttingen
Dept. of Hematology/Oncology
Robert-Koch-Str. 40
37075 Göttingen
Germany

Dr. A Smith
Dr. S. Roath
Dept. of Hematology
Royal South Hants Hospital
Brunton's Terrace
Off St. Mary's Road
Southampton SO9 4XY
England

Prof. Dr. H. Löffler
Städtisches Krankenhaus
II. Medizinische Klinik and Poliklinik
Chemnitzstraße 33
24116 Kiel
Germany

Dr. M. Björkholm
Dr. E. Ösby
Dept. of Medicine
Karolinska Hospital
10401 Stockholm
Sweden

Prof. Dr. B. Emmerich
University of München
Medizinische Klinik Innenstadt
Ziemssenstr. 1
80336 München
Germany

Prof. B. Coiffier
Hopital Lyon-Sud
Head Department of Hematology
Chemin du Grand Revoyet
69310 Pierre-Bénite
France

Prof. Dr. E. Thiel
Dr. W. Knauf
University of Berlin/Steglitz
Hindenburgdamm 30
12203 Berlin
Germany

Dr. G. Juliusson
Karolinska Institute
Huddings
14186 Stockholm
Sweden

Dr. R. Marcus
Dept. of Hematology
Addenbrookes Hospital
Hills Road
Cambridge CB2 2QQ
England

Dr. A.G. Prentice
Dr. J.A. Copplestone
Dept. of Haematology
Derriford Hospital
Plymouth
Devon PL6 8DH
England

Prof. Dr. M. Freund
University of Hannover
Konstanty-Gutschow-Str. 8
30625 Hannover
Germany

Dr. P.W. Milligan
Dept. of Clinical Haematology
Pathology Unit
East Birmingham Hospital
Bordesley Green East
Birmingham B9 5ST
England

Dr. D. Winfield
Dept. of Haematology
Royal Hallamshire Hospital
Glossop Hospital
Glossop Road
Sheffield S10 2JF
England

Dr. J. Yin
Dept. of Haematology
Manchester Royal Infirmary
Manchester M13 9WL
England

Prof. Dr. K.P. Hellriegel
Dept. of Internal Medicine
Hospital Moabit
Turmstr. 21
10559 Berlin
Germany

Prof. Dr. D.K. Hossfeld
University of Hamburg/Eppendorf
Dept. of Medicine
Martinistr. 52
20251 Hamburg
Germany

Dr. E. Kimby
Dept. of Medicine
Danderyds Hospital
182 788 Danderyd
Sweden

Prof. A.K. Burnett
College of Medicine
University of Wales
Department of Hematology
Heath Park
Cardiff CF4 4XN
England

Prof. T.A. Lister
Dept. of Medical Oncology
St. Bartholomew's Hospital
West Smithfield
London EC1A 7BA
Englnad

Dr. N. Lucie
Dept. of Haematology
Western Infirmary
Glasgow G11 6NT
Scotland

PD Dr. L. Kanz
University of Freiburg
Hugstetter Str. 55
79106 Freiburg
Germany

Dr. R. Lerner
Dept. of Medicine
Sodersjukhuset
10064 Stockholm
Sweden

Dr. C. Lindemalm
Dept. of Oncology
Radiumhemmet, Karolinska Hospital
10401 Stockholm
Sweden

Dr. A. Child
Dept. of Haematology
Leeds General Infirmary
Great George Street
Leeds LS1 3EX
England

Prof. T. Hamblin
Dr. D. Oscier
Dept. of Haematology
Bournemouth General Hospital
Castle Lane East
Bournemouth BM7 7DW
England

Dr. J.G. Smith
Dr. R.J. Singer
Royal United Hospital
Combe Park
Bath BA1 3NG
England

Dr. A. Parker
Dept. of Haematology
Royal Infirmary
Edinburgh EH3 9YW
Scotland

Dr. J. Whittaker
Dept. of Haematology
University Hospital of Wales
The Health
Cardiff CF4 4XN
Great Britain

Dr. P. Wyld
Inveresk Clinical Research Ltd.
Deputy Medical Director
Research Park, Riccarton
Edinburgh EH14 4AP
Scotland

Acute Leukemias VI
Prognostic Factors
and Treatment Strategies
Büchner et al. (eds)

Potential Immunological Action of Purine Nucleoside Analogs

G. Dighiero

Abstract. Purine nucleoside analogs are a new class of drugs with activity against nondividing lymphocytes; thus, they should play a major role in the treatment of low-grade lymphoid malignancies.

These drugs have been shown to have strong effect in DNA systhesis on actively dividing cells, through interference with DNA polymerases and ribonucleotide reductase, and for some of them through inhibition of DNA primase and DNA ligase. However, the cell cycle kinetics of low-grade lymphocytic lymphomas is characterized by the presence of very low-growth fractions. Hence, the action of these drugs in slowly progressing lymphoid malignancies cannot be accounted for by the same mechanism observed in actively proliferating tumors and needs to be explained through activity against quiescent resting lymphocytes. Recent work has stressed the role of purine analogs in inducing programmed cell death of quiescent lymphocytes, which could be explained through the induction of accelerated DNA strand breaks. This process leads to consumption of NAD for poly(ADP-ribose) synthesis, which could induce critical depletion of adenosine-5′-triphosphate (ATP).

In addition, as their action extends to normal resting lymphocytes, deleterious effects related to their immunosuppressive action are also observed, i.e., prolonged lymphopenia predominating in T cells and especially in the CD4 subset and an increased frequency of opportunistic infections. Nevertheless, beneficial effects of this immunosuppressive action have also been reported for 2-chlorodeoxyadenosine (2CDA) in the case of autoimmune hemolytic anemia associated with chronic lymphocytic leukemia (CLL). These last results could offer some promise for these drugs in the field of immunosuppression.

To substantiate this possibility, a considerable amount of work needs to be carried out in order to better define the mechanisms of action of these drugs, as well as their potential activity on different immunological effectors. Also, studies in animal models of autoimmune disease should be undertaken.

Introduction

The introduction of nucleoside analogs constituted an important progress in the treatment of low-grade lymphoid malignancies. The initial success of the pyrimidine nucleoside cytarabine in the treatment of acute leukemia prompted the search for purine nucleoside analogs. Among these, deoxycoformycin (DCF), an inhibitor of adenosine deaminase (ADA), fludarabine monophosphate (FLU), a fluorinated analog of adenine that is relatively resistant to ADA and 2-chloro-2'-deoxyadenosine (2-CDA), a drug also resistant to ADA through the introduction of a choro at the carbon 2, have been shown as the most promising drugs. All three drugs have displayed impressive activity in the treatment of chronic lymphocytic leukemia (CLL), low-grade lymphoma, and hairy-cell leukemia (Plunkett

Unité d'Immunohématologie et d'Immunopathologie, Institut Pasteur, 28 rue du Docteur Roux, 74724 Paris Cedex 15, France

and Saunders, 1993, O'Dwyer et al., 1988, Chun et al., 1991 and Piro et al., 1988).

These drugs have been shown to have a strong effect in DNA synthesis on actively dividing cells through interference with DNA polymerases and ribonucleotide reductase, and for some of them through inhibition of DNA primase and DNA ligase (reviewed by Plunkett et al. 1993 and Plunkett and Saunders (in press)). However, the cell cycle kinetics of low-grade lymphocytic lymphomas is characterized by the presence of very low-growth fractions. Hence, the action of these drugs in slowly progressing lymphoid malignancies cannot be accounted for by the same mechanism observed in actively proliferating tumors and needs to be explained through activity against quiescent resting lymphocytes. In addition, as their action extends to normal resting lymphocytes, deleterious effects related to their immunosuppressive action are also observed, i.e., prolonged lymphopenia predominating in T cells and especially in the CD4 subset and an increased frequency of opportunistic infections (Byrd et al., 1993 and Seymour et al., 1993). Nevertheless, beneficial effects of this immunosuppressive action have also been reported for 2-CDA in the case of autoimmune hemolytic anemia associated with CLL (Piro et al., 1988). These last results could offer some promise for these drugs in the field of immunosuppression.

In this work, we shall review the putative mechanisms involved in the immunosuppression induced by purine analogs and discuss the experiments that should be devised to substantiate this question.

Are Purine Analogs Mimicking Adenosine Deaminase Deficiency?

In humans, a genetic deficiency of ADA causes severe combined immunodeficiency. This disease is characterized by a selective lymphopenia of both T and B cells resulting in reduced cellular and humoral immune capacity, which may be attributed to the toxic effect of deoxyadenosine accumulation. (Giblett et al. 1972, Martin and Gelfand, 1981 and Hirschhorn and Ratech, 1983).

It was reasonable to assume that analogs of deoxyadenosine resistant to cellular deamination might mimic the ADA-deficient state and have a potential therapeutic activity on resting lymphocytes without damaging other cell types (Carson et al. 1977, 1978, 1980 and 1982). Initial work demonstrated that when T lymphoblasts were exposed to the strong ADA inhibitor deoxycoformycin (DCF), there was a preferential accumulation of deoxyadenosine-5′-triphosphate (dATP) (O'Dwyer et al., 1988). The metabolic effect of deoxyadenosine in nondividing human lymphocytes is the consequence of the progressive accumulation of strand breaks in DNA. In addition, it has been shown that repair of DNA breaks is associated with the synthesis of poly(ADP-ribose). This polymer is produced from NAD in a reaction catalyzed by the chromatin-associated poly(ADP-ribose) synthetase, which results in a depletion of the NAD content of the cell. This depletion induces a profound alteration of the cellular reducing power that results in programmed cell death (PCD). Hence, it appears that nucleoside analogs can act on quiescent lymphocytes via an apoptotic process (Brox et al. 1984, Seto et al., 1985, Carson et al., 1986, O'Dwyer et al, 1988 and Plunkett et al., 1993). As this is a central point to understand the effect of nucleoside analogs, we shall briefly review this point.

What Is the Role of Apoptosis in the Immunosuppression Induced by Nucleoside Analogs?

The term "programmed cell death" was initially used by developmental biologists to describe the loss of specific cells which occurs in a temporal and spatial manner and corresponds to a physiological process during development. PCD was initially thought to differ from death induced by the classical necrotic process in that it requires new gene expression which is necessary to activate the process. More recently, immunologists extended the concept of PCD to any cell death, dependent on de novo gene expression (reviewed by Arends et al. 1990 and Schwartz and Osborne, 1993). However, not all cells dying in a programmed fashion display the stereotypic changes associated with apoptosis, and suppression of apoptosis by inhibitors or RNA and/or protein synthesis does not appear to be universal.

In most cases, apoptosis has been reported to be abrogated by inhibitors of macromolecular synthesis like cycloheximide, actinomycin D, puromycin and emetine (Schwartz and Osborne 1993). An exception to this rule is the cytotoxic T lymphocyte (CTL)-induced apoptosis in target cells, where DNA fragmentation occurs within 20 min, excluding the possibility that protein synthesis could occur. In addition, apoptosis induced by glyotoxin in HL-60 cells following treatment by calcium ionophore and that induced by mild hyperthermia have not been shown to depend on protein synthesis (Collins et al., 1991).

As regards purine nucleoside analogs, work by Carson et al. (1983) demonstrated that 2-CDA could selectively harm resting normal human lymphocytes. This effect appeared to be very selective for this purine analog when compared to other clinically useful anticancer agents affecting purine and pyrimidine metabolism (cytarabine, 6-thioguanine, 5-fluouracil, and hydroxyurea). To explain this action, it was speculated that there was a relstionship between DNA strand breaks, NAD metabolism, and PCD (Berger et al., 1979 and 1985, Seto et al. 1985 and Carson et al. 1986) Under normal conditions, resting lymphocytes are continuously breaking and rejoining DNA. When this physiological process is accelerated, it leads to consumption of NAD for poly(ADP-ribose synthesis), which could induce lethal ADP and ATP depletion. This hypothesis was substantiated by the fact that supplementation of the medium with the NAD precursor nicotinamide or 3-aminobenzamide, an inhibitor of poly(ADP-ribose) synthetase, prevented NAD depletion and prevented 2-CDA toxicity. Although attractive, this hypothesis needs to be further substantiated since there is controversy as to whether resting quiescent lymphocytes contain a sizable amount of preexistent single-strand breaks (Jostes et al. 1989 and Boerrigter, 1991). In addition, the activation of poly(ADP-ribose) polymerase by a DNA-damaging agent is not necessarily indicative of a role for polyADP-rybosylation in DNA repair (Boerrigter, 1991).

Similar depletion in both NAD and ATP, which could be prevented by addition of either nicotinamide or 3-aminobenzamide, were observed by Brager and Grever (1986) when normal lymphocytes were incubated with 10 μM FLU. In addition, rat thymocytes incubated with FLU were shown to undergo PCD. Recent work by Robertson et al. (1993) succeeded in demonstrating that 24–72-h incubation of CLL lymphocytes with either 2-CDA or FLU clearly accelerated the spontaneous process of PCD observed when these cells are cultured in usual conditions; 2-CDA appeared to determine more DNA cleavage than FLU. In addition, this effect was not observed in all CLL cases studied. Previously untreated patients displaying spontaneous DNA fragmentation after short-term culture exhibited the higher levels of in vitro DNA fragmentation after exposure to purine nucleoside analogs, and this correlated well with a favorable response to chemotherapy. On the contrary, relative resistance to spontaneous or nucleoside analog-induced PCD correlated with a poor response to chemotherapy. Interestingly, nucleoside analog-induced PCD did not appear to be inhibited by inhibition of protein synthesis and by depletion of extracellular calcium, whereas the intracellular chelator BAPTA-AM completely inhibited DNA fragmentation. In a previous report, Collins et al. (1991) also showed that spontaneous PCD in CLL lymphocytes does not require protein synthesis.

What Are the Mechanisms Involved in Nucleoside Analog-Induced Immunosuppression?

Available evidence concerning the mechanisms involved in nucleoside analog-induced immunosuppression is scarce. Clinical studies in low-grade lymphoid malignancies have shown that treatment with these drugs is frequently associated to long-lasting T cell lymphopenias predominating in CD4 cells and with the appearance of opportunistic infections (Byrd et al., 1993 and Seymour et al., 1993). ADA levels have been found to be tenfold greater in T cells than in B cells and to predominate in immature thymocytes when compared to mature ones (Huang et al., 1981 and Barton et al., 1979). In addition, since T cells display greater ATP accumulation (Carson et al., 1970 and 1981 and Wortmann et al., 1979), it has been shown that ADA inhibition affects more T than B cells (Carson et al., 1978 and Fox et al. 1981). ADA inhibition also results in impairment of E-rosette formation (Ballet et al., 1976, Lum et al., 1978) and mitogenic response (Carson and Seegmiller, 1976 and Hovi et al., 1976). On the other hand, contradictory results have been obtained when antibody production and natural killer (NK) function were explored. Priebe et al. (1988, 1990a and 1990b) showed that the nucleoside analog tubercidin reduced NK activity whereas FLU stimulated NK cell activity. On the contrary, enhances antibody production, through decrease of NK activity whereas FLU decreases antibody activity.

Conclusion

Available evidence indicates that nucleoside analogs are new drugs with strong activity against nondividing lymphocytes and should thus play a major role in the treatment of low-grade lymphoid malignancies. As these drugs are active against resting lymphocytes, harmful effects related to this action were expected and have been reported. However, this harmful effect observed during the treatment of lymphoid malignancies could hold some promise when dealing with autoimmune diseases.

To substantiate that possibility, a considerable amount of work should be carried out to better define the mechanism of activity of these drugs as well as their action on the different immunological populations. Also, studies in animal models of autoimmune disease should be designed.

The hypothesis that nucleoside analogs act through the increase of single-strand DNA breaks has been advanced. The DNA repair process that ensues will determine an increase in poly(ADP-ribose) which depletes the cell content in NAD and ATP content, leading lymphocytes to PCD. This hypothesis is supported by considerable experimental work. However, the possibility that quiescent lymphocytes in normal conditions contain a sizable amount of single-strand DNA breaks and the obligatory role of polyADP-ribosylation in DNA repair remain controversial issues. Although there is evidence indicating that nucleoside analogs exert at least part of their action on quiescent lymphocytes through an induced apoptosis process, the fact that this activity is not dependent on protein synthesis remains puzzling.

The evidence concerning functional impairment of T,B, and NK cells was obtained during the 1970s and the early 1980s and needs to be updated. All the experimental work was performed on PBL cells using the functional tests available at that time. A functional study taking into account the different immunological subsets and the progresses accomplished in studying the cytokine cascade are needed to further define the putative immunosuppressive action of these drugs. For instance, can the potential immunosuppression induced by these drugs be accounted for only through the induction of PCD? Do these drugs preferentially affect one special subset of T cells (TH1, TH2, suppressor cells, etc)? What is their action on the secretion of the different cytokines? Since both CD4 and CD8 subsets derive from a common double-positive cell, why does the long-lasting lymphopenia observed after treatment with these drugs predominate in CD4 subset? These are some of the main questions that need to be answered in order to seriously consider these drugs as potential immunosuppressive agents.

Finally, trials in animal models of autoimmune disease should be planned to better define the action of these drugs. The NZB mouse model, characterized by a polyclonal stimulation of B cells and Coombs-positive autoimmune hemolytic anemia, may constitute a suitable model to explore the action of nucleoside analogs in suppressing antibody responses, and this could substantiate initial observations in humans indicating that 2-CDA may have a beneficial effect in autoimmune hemolytic anemia associated with CLL. MRL-lpr/lpr mice have a rapidly progressive illness characterized by massive lymphadenopathy, arthritis and membranoproliferative glomerulonephritis associated with the production of anti-DNA and rheumatoid factor autoantibodies. This mouse model associating lymphoproliferation and autoimmune manifestations could also constitute a privilegiate model to study purine nucleoside analogs. Interestingly, it has recently been shown that these mice display a mutation in the APO-1/fas gene whose expression is known to induce apoptosis (Wu et al., 1993 and Chu et al., 1993). The abnormal expression of this molecule could result in inappropriate cell survival and could explain the accumulation of lymphocytes in the peripheral organs observed in these mice. MRL-lpr/lpr mice could thus constitute a suitable model for the study of apoptosis induced by purine analogs.

Finally, if the immunosuppressive action of purine analogs is substantiated, they could play a role in the treatment of graft-versus-host disease, and this can also be investigated in animal models.

References

Arends WJ, Morris RG, and Wyllie AH. Apoptosis. The role of the endonuclease. American Journal of Pathology 136: 593–608, 1990

Ballet JJ, Insel R, Merler E, Rosen FS. Inhibition of maturation of human precursor lymphocytes by conformycin, an inhibitor of the enzyme adenosine deaminase. J Exp Med 143: 1271–6, 1976

Barton R, Martiniuk F, Hirschhorn R, Goldschneider I. The distribution of adenosine deaminase among lymphocyte populations in the rat. J Immunol 122: 216–20, 1979

Berger NA, Sikorski W, Petzold SJ, and Kurohara KK. Association of poly(adenosine diphosphoribose) synthesis with DNA damage and repair in normal human lymphocytes. J Clin Invest 63: 1164–1171, 1979

Berger NA, Berger SJ, Catino DM, Petzold SJ, and Robins RK. Modulation of nicotinamide adenine dinucleotide and poly(adenosine diphosphoribose) metabolism by the synthetic "C" nucleoside analogs, tiazofurin and selenazofurin. J Clin Invest 75: 702–709, 1985

Boerrigter METI. DNA strand break metabolism in human lymphocytes: a reevaluation. Exp Cell Res 196: 1–5, 1991

Boldt DH, Von Hoff DD, Kuhn J, and Hersh M. Effects on human peripheral lymphocytes in vivo administration of 9-β-D-arabinofuranosyl-2-fluoroadenine-5'-monophosphate (NSC 312887), a new purine antimetabolite. Cancer Research 44: 4661–4666, 1984

Brager PM, and Grever MR. 9-β-D-arabinofuranosyl-2-fluoroadeniine reduces NDA in normal lymphocytes and neoplastic cells in CLL. Pro American Ass Cancer Research 27: 21–□, 1986

Brockman RW, Schabel FM Jr, and Montgomery JA. Biologic activity of 9-β-D-arabinofuranosyl-2-fluoroadenine, a metabolically stable analog of 9-β-D-arabinofuranosyladenine. Biochem Pharmacology 26: 2193–2196, 1977

Brox L, Ng A, Pollock E, and Belch A. DNA strand breaks induced in human T-lymphocytes by the combination of deoxyadenosine and deoxycoformycin. Cancer Res 44: 934–937, 1984

Carrera CJ, Terai C, Piro LD, Saven A, Beutler E, and Carson DA. 2-Chlorodeoxyadenosine chemotherapy triggers programmed cell death in normal and malignant lymphocytes. International Journal Purine Pyrimidine Research 2 (Suppl. 1): 39–□, 1991

Carson DA, Seegmiller JE. Effect of adenosine deaminase inhibition upon human lymphocyte blastogenesis. J Clin Invest 57: 274–82, 1976

Carson DA, Kaye J, and Seegmiller JE. Lymphospecific toxicity in adenosine deaminase deficiency and purine nucleoside phosphorylase deficiency: possible role of nucleoside kinase (s . Proc Natl Acad Sci USA 74: 5677–5681, 1977

Carson DA, Kaye J, and Seegmiller JE. Differential sensitivity of human leukemic T cell lines and B cell lines to growth inhibition by deoxyadenosine. J Immunol 121: 1726–1731, 1978

Carson DA, Kaye J, Matsumoto S, Seegmiller JE, Thompson L. Biochemical basis for the enhanced toxicity of deoxyribonucleosides toward malignant human T cells lines. Proc Natl Acad Sci USA 76: 2430–3, 1979

Carson DA, Wasson DB, Kaye J, Ullman B, Martin DW Jr, Robins RK, and Montgomery JA. Deoxycytidine kinase-mediated toxicity of deoxyadenosine analogs toward human lymphoblasts in vitro and toward murine L12110 leukemia in vivo. Proc Nat Acad Sci USA 77: 6865–6869, 1980

Carson DA, Kaye J, Matsumoto S, Seegmiller JE, Thompson L. Biochemical basis for the enhanced toxicity of deoxyribonucleosides toward malignant human T-cells lines. J Immunol 126: 348–352, 1981

Carson DA, Wasson DB, Lakow E, and Kamatani N. Possible metabolic basis for the different immunodeficient states associated with genetic deficiencies of adenosine deaminase and purine nucleoside phophorylase. Proc National Academic Science USA 79: 3848–3852, 1982

Carson DA, Wasson DB, Taetle R, and Yu A. Specific toxicity of 2-clorodeoxyadenosine toward resting and proliferating human lymphocytes. Blood 62: 737–743, 1983

Carson DA, Wasson DB, and Beutler E. Antileukemic and immunosuppressive activity of 2-chloro-2'-deoxyadenosine. Proc Natl Acad Sci USA 81: 2232–2236, 1984

Carson DA, Seto S, Wasson DB, and Carrera CJ. DNA strand breaks, NAD metabolism and programmed cell death. Experimental Cell Research 164: 273–281, 1986

Carson DA, Carrera CJ, Wasson DB, and Yamanaka H. Programmed cell death and adenine nucleotide metabolism in human lymphocytes. Adv Enzyme Reg 27: 395–404, 1987

Chun HG, Leyland-Jones B, and Cheson B. Fludarabine phosphate: a synthetic purine antimetabolite with significant activity against lymphoid malignancies. Journal of Clinical Oncology 9: 175–188, 1991

Cohen A, Hirschhorn R, Horowitz D, Rubinstein A, Polmar SH, Hong R, and Martin DW Jr. Deoxyadenosine triphosphate as a potentially toxic metabolite in adenosine deaminase deficiency. Proc Natl Acad Sci USA 75: 472–476, 1978

Coleman M, Donofrio SJ, Hutto JJ, Hahn L, Daoud A, Lampkin B, and Dyminski J. Identification and quantitation of adenine deoxynucleotides in erythrocytes of a patient with adenosine deaminase deficiency and severe combined immunodeficiency. J Biol Chem 253: 1619–1626, 1978

Collins JM, Greishaber CK, and Chabner BA. Pharmacologically guided phase I clinical trials based upon preclinical drug development. J Natn Cancer Inst 82: 1321–1326, 1990

Creissen D, and Shall S. Regulation of DNA ligase activity by poly(ADP-ribose). Nature (Lond) 296: 271–272, 1982

Donofrio J, Coleman Ms, Hutton JJ, Daoud A, Lampkin B, and Dyminski J. Overproduction of

adenine deoxynucleosides and deoxynucleotides in adenosine deaminase deficiency with severe combined immunodeficiency disease. J Clin Invest 62: 884–887, 1978
Durkacz BW, Omidiji O, Gray DA, and Shall S. (ADP-ribosen) participates in DNA excision repair. Nature (Lond) 283: 593–596, 1980
Fox RM, Piddington SK, Tripp EH, Tattersall MH. Ecto-adenosine triphosphate deficiency in cultured human T and null leukemia lymphocytes. A biochemical basis for thymidine sensitivity. J Clin Invest 68: 544–52, 1981
Gandhi V, Nowak B, Keating MJ, and Plunkett W. Modulation of arabinosylcytosine metabolism by arabinosyl-2-fluoroadenine in lymphocytes from patients with chronic lymphocytic leukemia: implications for combination therapy. Blood 74: 2070–2075, 1989
Gandhi V, Kemena A, Keating MJ, and Plunkett W. Fludarabine infusion potentiates arabinosylcytosine metabolism in lymphocytes of patients with chronic lymphocytic leukemia. Cancer Research 52: 897–903, 1992b
Giblett ER, Anderson JE, Cohen B, Pollara B, and Meuwissen HJ. Adenosine-deaminase deficiency in two patients with severely impaired cellular immunity. Lancet 1067: 1069–1972,
Grever MR, Leiby J, Kraut E, Metz E, Neidhart J, Balcerzak S, and Maslepis L. A comprehensive phase I and II clinical investigation of fludarabine. Sem Oncol 17 (Suppl 8): 39–48, 1990
Griffig J, Koob T, and Blakley RL. Mechanisms of inhibition of DNA synthetis by 2-chlorodeoxyadenosine in human lymphoblastic cells. Cancer Research 49: 6923–6928, 1989
Hershfield Ms, Fetter JE, Small MC, Bagnara AS, Williams SR, Ullman B, Martin DW Jr, Wasson DB, and Carson DA. Effects of mutational loss of adenosine kinase and deoxycytidine kinase on deoxy ATP accumulation and deoxyadenosine toxicity in cultured CEM human T-lymphoblastoid cells. J Biol Chem 257: 6380–6386, 1982
Hirota Y, Yoshioka A, Tanaka S, Watanabe K, Otani T, Minowada J, Matuda A, Ueda T, and Wataya Y. Imbalance of deoxyribonucleoside triphosphates, DNA double-strand breaks and cell death cause by 2-chlorodeoxyadenosine in mouse FM3A cells. Cancer Research 49: 915–919, 1989
Hirschhorn R, and Ratech H. Genetic deficiencies of adenosine deaminase and purine nucleoside phosphorylase and their implications for therapy of leukemias. Curr Top Hematol 4: 1–35, 1983
Hovi T, Smyth JF, Allison AC, Williams, SC. Role of adenosine deaminase in lymphocyte proliferation. Clin Exp Immunol 23: 395–403, 1976
Huang P, and Plunkett W. Action of 9-β-D-arabinofuranosyl-2-fluoroadenine on RNA metabolism. Molec Pharmacology 39: 449–455, 1991
Huang AT, Logue LG, Engelbrecht GL. Two biochemical markers in lymphocyte populations. Br J Haematol 34: 631–8,1981
Huang P, Chubb S, and Plunkett W. Incorporation of 9-β-D-arabinofuranosyl-2-fluoroadenine into DNA and its chain termination effect on DNA synthesis. J Biol Chem 265: 16617–16625, 1990
Jostes R, Reese JA, Cleaver JE, Molero M, and Morgan WF. Quiescent human lymphocytes do not contain DNA strand breaks detectable by alkaline elution. Exp Cell Res 182: 513–520, 1989
Kantarjian HM, Alexanian R, Koller CA, Kurzrock R, and Keating MJ. Fludarabine therapy in macroglobulinemic lymphoma. Blood 75: 1928–1931, 1990
Keating M, Kantarjian H, Talpaz M, Redman J, Koller C, Barlogie B, Velasquez W, Plunkett W, Freireich EJ, and McCredie KB. Fludarabine: a new agent with major activity against chronic lymphocytic leukemia. Blood 74: 19–25, 1989
Kefford RF, and Fox RM. Deoxycoformycin-induced response in chronic lymphocytic leukemia: deoxyadenosine toxicity in non-replicating lymphocytes. Br J Haematol 50: 627–636, 1982
Kefford RF, and Fox RM. Purine deoxynucleoside toxicity in non-dividing human lymphoid cells. Cancer Res 42: 324–330, 1982
Kester K, Hospenthal DR, Weidner S., and Diehl L. Fludarabine therapy for lymphoid malignancies is associated with a high number of opportunistic pulmonary infections. Blood 82: 138 a–, 1993
Leiby JM, Snider KM, Kraut EH, Metz EN, Malspeis L, and Grever MR. Phase II trial of 9-β-D-arabinofuranosyl-2-fluoroadenine 5′-monophosphate in non-Hodgkin's lymphoma: prospective comparison of response with deoxycytidine kinase activity. Cancer Research 47: 2719–2722, 1987
Lum CT, Schmidtke JR, Sutherland DE, Najarian JS. Inhibition of human T-cell rosette formation by the adenosine deaminase inhibitor erythro-9-(2-hydroxyl-3-nonyl) adenine hydrochloride (EHNA). Clin Immunol Immunopathol 10: 258–61, 1978
Martin DW Jr, and Gelfand EW. Biochemistry of diseases of immunodevelopment. Annu Rev Biochem 50: 845–877, 1981
Matsumoto SS, Yu J, and Yu AL. Inhibition of RNA synthesis by deoxyadenosine plus deoxycoformycin in resting lymphocytes. J Immunol 131: 2762–2766, 1983
Mitchell BS, Mijias E, Daddona PE, and Kelley WN. Purinogenic immunodeficiency diseases: selective toxicity of deoxyribonucleosides for T cells. Proc Natl Acad Sci USA 75: 5011–5014, 1978
O'Dwyer PJ, Wagner B, Leyland-Jones B, Wittes RE, Cheson BD, and Hoth DF. 2'-Deoxycoformycin (Pentostatin) for lymphoid malignancies. Rational development of an active new drug. Ann International Medicine 108: 733–743, 1988
Parker WB, Bapat AR, Shen J-X, Towsend AJ, and Cheng Y-C. Interaction of 2-halogenated dATP analogs (F, Cl and Br) with human DNA polymerases, DNA primase and ribonucleotide reductase. Molec Pharmacology 34: 485–491, 1988
Piro LD, Carrera CJ, Beutler E, and Carson DA. 2-Chlorodeoxyadenosine: an effective new agent for the treatment of chronic lymphocytic leukemia. Blood 72: 1069–1073, 1989

Plunkett W, and Chubb S. Toxicity, metabolism and incorporation into DNA and RNA of arabinosyl-2-fluoroadenine (F-ara-A). Proc Am Ass Cancer Research 26: 19–□, 1985

Plunkett W, Huang P, and Gandhi, V. Metabolism and action of fludarabine phosphate. Sem Oncology 17 (Suppl 8): 3–17, 1990

Priere T, Kandil O, Nakic M, Pan BF, and Nelson JA Selective modulation of antibody response and natural killer cell activity by purine nucleoside analogs. Cancer Research. 48 4799: 4803–1988,

Priere T, Platsoucas CD, and Nelson JA. Adenosine receptors and modulation of natural killer cell activity by purine nucleosides. Cancer Research 50: 4328–4331, 1990a

Priere T, Ruiz L, and Nelson JA. Role of natural killer cells in the modulation of primary antibody production by purine nucleosides and their analogs. Cell Immunology 130: 513–519, 1990b

Redman J, Cabanillas F, McLaughlin P, Hagemeister F, Velasquez W, Swan F, Rodriguez M, Plunkett W, and Keating M. Fludarabine phosphate: a new agent with major activity in low grade lymphoma. Proc Am Ass Cancer Research 29: 221–□,1988

Robertson Le, Chubb S, Hittelman WN, Sandoval A, and Plunkett W. Programmed death (apoptosis) in chronic lymphocytic leukemia cells after fludarabine and chlorodeoxyadenosine. Blood 78: 172a–□, 1991b

Robertson LE, Chubb S, Meyn RE, Story M, Ford R, Hittelman WN, and Plunkett W. Induction of apoptotic cell death in chronic lymphocytic leukemia by 2-chloro-2'- deoxyadenosine and 9-β-D-arabinosyl-2-fluoroadenine. Blood 81: 143–150, 1993

Seto S, Carrera CJ, Kubota M, Wasson DB, and Carson DA. Mechanism of deoxyadenosine and 2-chlorodeoxyadenosine toxicity to nondividing human lymphocytes. Journal of Clinical Invest 75: 377–383, 1985

Seymour JF, Kurzrock R, Freireich EJ, Estey EH, Anderson MD. Prolonged CD4+ lymphocytopenia, is the cost of durable responses TO2-chlorodeoxyadenosine (2-CdA) in patients (PTS) with hairy cell leukemia (HCL). Blood 82: 142 a–, 1993

Siaw MFE, Mitchel BS, Koller A, Coleman MS, and Hutton JJ. ATP depletion as a consequence of adenosine deaminase inhibition in man. Proc Natl Acad Sci USA 77: 6157–6161, 1980

Snyder RD, Van Houten B, and Regan JD. The inhibition of ultraviolet radiation-induced DNA repair in human diploid fibroblasts by arabinofuranosyl nucleosides. Chem Bio Interact 50: 1–14, 1984

Spriggs D, Robbins G, Mitchell T, and Kufe D. Incorporation of 9-β-D-arabinofuranosyl-2-fluoroadenine into HL-60 cellular RNA and DNA. Biochem Pharmacology 35: 247–252, 1986

Thelander L, and Reichard P. Reduction of ribonucleotides. Annu Rev Biochem 48: 133–158, 1979

Tseng WC, Derse D, Cheng YC, Brockman RW, and Bennett LL Jr. In vitro activity of 9-β-D-arabinofuranosyl-2-fluoroadenine and the biochemical actions of its triphosphate on DNA polymerases and ribonucleotide reductase from HeLa cells. Molec Pharmac 21: 474–477, 1982

Ullman B, Gudas LJ, Cohen A, and Martin DW Jr. Deoxyadenosine metabolism and cytotoxicity in cultured mouse T lymphoma cells: a model for immunodeficiency disease. Cell 14: 365–375, 1978

Wortmann RL, Mitchell BS, Edwards NL, Fox IH. Biochemical basis for differential deoxyadenosine toxicity to T and B lymphoblasts: role for 5'-nucleotidase. Proc Natl Acad Sci USA 76: 2434–7, 1979

Bibliography

Arends WJ, Morris RG, and Wyllie AH. Apoptosis. The role of the endonuclease. American Journal of Pathology 136: 593–608, 1990

Berger NA, Sikorski W, Petzold SJ, and Kurohara KK. Association of poly(adenosine diphosphoribose) synthesis with DNA damage and repair in normal human lymphocytes. J Clin Invest 63: 1164–1171, 1979

Berger NA, Berger SJ, Catino DM, Petzold SJ, and Robins RK. Modulation of nicotinamide adenine dinucleotide and poly(adenosine diphosphoribose) metabolism by the synthetic "C" nucleoside analogs, tiazofurin and selenazofurin. J Clin Invest 75: 702–709,1985

Boerrigter METI. DNA strand break metabolism in human lymphocytes: a reevaluation, Exp Cell Res 196: 1–5, 1991

Boldt DH, von Hoff DD, Kuhn J, and Hersh M. Effects on human peripheral lymphocytes in vivo administration of 9-β-D-arabinofuranosyl-2-fluoroadenine-5'-monophosphate (NSC 312887), a new purine antimetabolite. Cancer Research 44: 4661–4666, 1984

Brager PM, and Grever MR. 9-β-D-Arabinofuranosyl-2-fluoroadeniine reduces NDA in normal lymphocytes and neoplastic cells in CLL. Pro American Ass Cancer Research 27: 21–□, 1986

Brockman RW, Schabel FM Jr, and Moontgomery JA. Biologic activity of 9-β-D-arabinofuranosyl-2-fluoroadenine, a metabolically stable analog of 9-β-D-harabinofuranosyladenine. Biochem Pharmacology 26: 2193–2196, 1977

Brox L, Ng A, Pollock E, and Belch A. DNA strand breaks induced in human T-lymphocytes by the combination of deoxyadenosine and deoxycoformycin. Cancer Res 44: 934–937, 1984

Carrera CJ, Terai C, Piro LD, Saven A, Beutler E, and Carson DA. 2-Chlorodeoxyadenosine chemotherapy triggers programmed cell death in normal and malignant lymphocytes. International Journal Purine Pyrimidine Research 2 (Suppl. 1): 39–□, 1991

Carson DA, Kaye J, and Seegmiller JE. Lymphospecific toxicity in adenosine deaminase deficiency and purine nucleoside phosphorylase deficiency: possible role of nucleoside kinase(s). Proc Natl Acad Sci USA 74: 5677–5681, 1977

Carson DA, Kaye J, and Seegmiller JE. Differential sensitivity of human leukemic T cell lines and B cell

lines to growth inhibition by deoxyadenosine. J Immunol 121: 1726–1731, 1978
Carson DA, Wasson DB, Kaye J, Ullman B, Martin DW Jr, Robins RK, and Montgomery JA. Deoxycytidine kinase-mediated toxicity of deoxyadenosine analogs toward human lymphoblasts in vitro and toward murine L12110 leukemia in vivo. Proc Nat Acad Sci USA 77: 6865–6869, 1980
Carson DA, Wasson DB, Lakow E, and Kamatani N. Possible metabolic basis for the different immunodeficient states associated with genetic deficiencies of adenosine deaminase and purine nucleoside phosphorylase. Proc Natl Acad Sci USA 79: 3848–3852, 1982
Carson DA, Wasson DB, Lakow E, and Kamatani N. Possible metabolic basis for the different immunodeficient states associated with genetic deficiencies of adenosine deaminase and purine nucleoside phosphorylase. Proc National Academic Science USA 79: 3848–3852, 1982
Carson DA, Wasson DB, Taetle R, and Yu A. Specific toxicity of 2-clorodeoxyadenosine toward resting and proliferating human lymphocytes. Blood 62: 737–743, 1983
Carson DA, Wasson DB, and Beutler E. Antileukemic and immunosuppressive activity of 2-chloro-2' -deoxyadenosine. Proc Natl Acad Sci USA 81: 2232–2236, 1984
Carson DA, Seto S, Wasson DB, and Carrera CJ. DNA strand breaks, NAD metabolism and programmed cell death. Experimental Cell Research 164: 273–281, 1986
Carson DA, Carrera CJ, Wasson DB, and Yamanaka H. Programmed cell death and adenine nucleotide metabolism in human lymphocytes. Adv Enzyme Reg 27: 395–404, 1987
Chun HG, Leyland-Jones B, and Cheson B. Fludarabine Phosphate: a synthetic purine antimetabolite with significant activity against lymphoid malignancies. Journal of Clinical Oncology 9: 175–188, 1991
Cohen A, Hirschhorn R, Horowitz D, Rubinstein A, Polmer SH, Hong R, and Martin DW Jr. Deoxyadenosine triphosphate as a potentially toxic metabolite in adenosine deaminase deficiency. Proc Natl Acad Sci USA 75: 472–476, 1978
Coleman M, Donofrio SJ, Hutto JJ, Hahn L, Daoud A, Lampkin B, and Dyminski J. Identification and quantitation of adenine deoxynucleotides in erythrocytes of a patient with adenosine deaminase deficiency and severe combined immunodeficiency. J. Biol Chem 253: 1619–1626, 1978
Collins JM, Greishaber CK, and Chabner BA. Pharmacologically guided phase I clinical trials based upon preclinical drug development. J Natn Cancer Inst 82: 1321–1326, 1990
Creissen D, and Shall S, Regulation of DNA ligase activity by poly(ADP-ribose). Nature (Lond) 296: 271–272, 1982
Donofrio J, Coleman MS, Hutton JJ, Daoud A, Lampkin B, and Dyminski J. Overproduction of adenine deoxynucleosides and deoxynucleotides in adenosine deaminase deficiency with severe combined immunodeficiency disease. J. Clin Invest 62: 884–887, 1978
Durkacz BW, Omidiji O, Gray DA, and Shall S. (ADP-ribose)$_n$ participates in DNA excision repair. Nature (Lond) 283: 593–596, 1980
Gandhi V, Nowak B, Keating MJ, and Plunkett W. Modulation of arabinosylcytosine metabolism by arabinosyl-2-fluoroadenine in lymphocytes from patients with chronic lymphocytic leukemia: implications for combination therapy. Blood 74: 2070–2075, 1989
Gandhi V, Kemena A, Keating MJ, and Plunkett W. Fludarabine infusion potentiates arabinosylcytosine metabolism in lymphocytes of patients with chronic lymphocytic leukemia. Cancer Research 52: 897–903. 1992b
Giblett ER, Anderson JE, Cohen B, Pollara B, and Meuwissen HJ. Adenosine-deaminase deficiency in two patients with severely impaired cellular immunity. Lancet 1067: 1069–1972
Grever MR, Leiby J, Kraut E, Metz E, Neidhart J, Balcerzak S, and Maslepis L. A comprehensive phase I and II clinical investigation of fludarabine. Sem Oncol 177 (Suppl 8): 39–48, 1990
Griffig J, Koob T, and Blakley RL. Mechanisms of inhibition of DNA synthetis by 2-chlorodeoxyadenosine in human lymphoblastic cells. Cancer Research 49: 6923–6928, 1989
Hershfield MS, Fetter JE, Small MC, Bagnara AS, Williams SR, Ullman B, Martin DW Jr, Wasson DB, and Carson DA. Effects of mutational loss of adenosine kinase and deoxycytidine kinase on deoxy ATP accumulation and deoxyadenosine toxicity in cultured CEM human T-lymphoblastoid cells. J Biol Chem 257: 6380–6386, 1982
Hirota Y, Yoshioka A, Tanaka S, Watanabe K, Otani T, Minowada J, Matuda A, Ueda T, and Wataya Y. Imbalance of deoxyribonucleoside triphosphates, DNA double-strand breaks and cell death cause by 2-chlorodeoxyadenosine in mouse FM3A cells. Cancer Research 49: 915–919, 1989
Hirschhorn R, and Ratech H. Genetic deficiencies of adenosine deaminase and purine nucleoside phosphorylase and their implications for therapy of leukemias. Curr Top Hematol 4: 1–35, 1983
Huang P, and Plunkett W. Action of 9-β-D-arabinofuranosyl-2-fluoroadenine on RNA metabolism. Molec Pharmacology 39: 449–455, 1991
Huang P, Chubb S, and Plunkett W. Incorporation of 9-β-D-arabinofuranosyl-2-fluoroadenine into DNA and its chain termination effect on DNA synthesis. J Biol Chem 265: 16617–16625, 1990
Jostes R, Reese JA, Cleaver JE, Molero M, and Morgan WF. Quiescent human lymphocytes do not contain DNA strand breaks detectable by alkaline elution. Exp Cell Res 182: 513–520, 1989
Kantarjian HM, Alexanian R, Koller CA, Kurzrock R, and Keating MJ. Fludarabine therapy in macroglobulinemic lymphoma. Blood 75: 1928–1931, 1990
Keating M, Kantarjian H, Talpaz M, Redman J, Koller C, Barlogie B, Velasquez W, Plunkett W, Freireich EJ, and McCredie KB. Fludarabine: a new agent with

major activity against chronic lymphocytic leukemia. Blood 74: 19–25, 1989
Kefford RF, and Fox RM. Purine deoxynucleoside toxicity in non-dividing human lymphoid cells. Cancer Res 42: 324–330, 1982
Kefford RF, and Fox RM. Deoxycoformycin-induced response in chronic lymphocytic leukemia: deoxyadenosine toxicity in non-replicating lymphocytes. Br J Haematol 50: 627–636, 1982
Leiby JM, Snider KM, Kraut EH, Metz EN, Malspeis L, and Grever MR. Phase II trial of 9-β-D-arabinofuranosyl-2-fluoroadenine 5'-monophosphate in non-Hodgkin's lymphoma: prospective comparison of response with deoxycytidine kinase activity. Cancer Research 47: 2719–2722, 1987
Martin DW Jr, and Gelfand EW. Biochemistry of diseases of immunodevelopment. Annu Rev Biochem 50: 845–877, 1981
Matsumoto SS, Yu J, and Yu AL. Inhibition of RNA synthesis by deoxyadenosine plus deoxycoformycin in resting lymphocytes. J Immunol 131: 2762–2766, 1983
Mitchell BS, Mijias E, Daddona PE, and Kelley WN. Purinogenic immunodeficiency diseases: selective toxicity of deoxyribonucleosides for T cells. Proc Natl Acad Sci USA 75: 5011–5014, 1978
O'Dwyer PJ, Wagner B, Leyland-Jones B, Wittes RE, Cheson BD, and Hoth DF. 2'-Deoxycoformycin (Pentostatin) for lymphoid malignancies. Rational development of an active new drug. Ann International Medicine 108: 733–743, 1988
Parker WB, Bapat AR, Shen J-X, Towsend AJ, and Cheng Y-C. Interaction of 2-halogenated dATP analogs (F, Cl and Br) with human DNA polymerases, DNA primase and ribonucleotide reductase. Molec Pharmacology 34: 485–491, 1988
Piro LD, Carrera CJ, Beutler E, and Carson DA. 2-Chlorodeoxyadenosine: an effective new agent for the treatment of chronic lymphocytic leukemia. Blood 72: 1069–1073, 1989
Plunkett W, and Chubb S. Toxicity, metabolism and incorporation into DNA and RNA of arabinosyl-2-fluoroadenine (F-ara-A). Proc Am Ass Cancer Research 26: 19–□, 1985
Plunkett W, Huang, P and Gandhi, V. Metabolism and action of fludarabine phosphate. Sem Oncology 17 (Suppl 8): 3–17, 1990
Priere T, Kandil O, Nakic M, Pan BF, and Nelson JA Selective modulation of antibody response and natural killer cell activity by purine nucleoside analogs. Cancer Research. 48 4799: 4803–1988
Priere T, Platsoucas CD, and Nelson JA. Adenosine receptors and modulation of natural killer cell activity by purine nucleosides. Cancer Research 50: 4328–4331, 1990a
Priere T, Ruiz L, and Nelson JA. Role of natural killer cells in the modulation of primary antibody production by purine nuucleosides and their analogs. Cell Immunology 130: 513–519, 1990b
Redman J, Cabanillas F, McLaughlin P, Hagemeister F, Velasquez W, Swan F, Rodriguez M, Plunkett W, and Keating M. Fludarabine phosphate: a new agent with major activity in low grade lymphoma. Proc Am Ass Cancer Research 29: 221–□, 1988
Robertson LE, Chubb S, Hittelman WN, Sandoval A, and Plunkett W. Programmed death (apoptosis) in chronic lymphocytic leukemia cells after fludarabine and chlorodeoxyadenosine. Blood 78: 173a–□, 1991b
Robertson LE, Chubb S, Meyn RE, Story M, Ford R, Hittelman WN, and Plunkett W. Induction of apoptotic cell death in chronic lymphocytic leukemia by 2-chloro-2'-deoxydenosine and 9-β-D-arabinosyl-2-fluoroadenine. Blood 81: 143–150, 1993
Seto S, Carrera CJ, Kubota M, Wasson DB, and Carson DA. Mechanism of deoxyadenosine and 2-chlorodeoxyadenosine toxicity to nondividing human lymphocytes. Journal of Clinical Invest 75: 377–383, 1985
Siaw MFE, Mitchel BS, Koller A, Coleman MS, and Hutton JJ. ATP depletion as a consequence of adenosine deaminase inhibition in man. Proc Natl Acad Sci USA 777: 615–6161, 1980
Snyder RD, Van Houten B, and Regan JD. The inhibition of ultraviolet radiation-induced DNA repair in human diploid fibroblasts by arabinofuranosyl nucleosides. Chem Bio Interact 50: 1–14, 1984
Spriggs D, Robbins G, Mitchell T, and Kufe D. Incorporation of 9-β-D-arabinofuranosyl-2-fluoroadenine into HL-60 cellular RNA and DNA. Biochem Pharmacology 35: 247–252, 1986
Thelander L, and Reichard P. Reduction of ribonucleotides. Annu Rev Biochem 48: 133–158, 1979
Tseng WC, Derse D, Cheng YC, Brockman RW, and Bennett LL Jr. In vivo activity of 9-β-D-arabinofuranosyl-2-fluoroadenine and the biochemical actions of its triphosphate on DNA polymerases and ribonucleotide reductase from HeLa cells. Molec Pharmac 21: 474–477, 1982
Ullman B, Gudas LJ, Cohen A, and Martin DW Jr. Deoxyadenosine metabolism and cytotoxicity in cultured mouse T lymphoma cells: a model for immunodeficiency disease. Cell 14: 365–375, 1978

Acute Leukemias VI
Prognostic Factors
and Treatment Strategies
Büchner et al. (eds)

Fludarabine and Fludarabine, Mitoxantrone, Dexamethasone in the Management of Low-Grade Non-Hodgkin Lymphomas

C. Pott-Hoeck[1], M. Unterhalt, D.S. Sandford, H. Markert, M. Freund, A. Engert, W. Gassmann, W. Holtkamp, M. Seufert, K. Hellriegel, B. Knauf, R. Nieberding, B. Emmerich, P. Koch, B. Wörmann, and W. Hiddemann

Abstract. Low-grade non-Hodgkin lymphomas (NHL) comprise a heterogeneous group of disorders both in terms of their cellular origin and composition and in terms of their clinical course. Their common characteristics are low to moderate proliferative activity and a slowly progressive clinical course with median survival times ranging from approximately 3 to 8 years for the different histologic subtypes. Although a wide array of therapies, comprising single agent and combination chemotherapy or combined modality approaches including radiotherapy, have been available during the last years, most patients succumb to their disease. In the early stages I and II and selected cases of stage III disease, radiotherapy has curative potential. Initial chemotherapy for patients with advanced stage III and IV disease produces remission rates of more than 60–80% without any curative potential. The impact of interferon alpha (IFN) in addition to or after cytoreductive chemotherapy on remission duration and survival was investigated in different studies, and preliminary results of the German Low-Grade NHL Study Group and others reveal a favorable effect of IFN maintenance therapy on disease-free survival. Treatment at relapse remains an important feature in management of NHL, and several new treatment strategies including myeloablative radio-chemotherapy protocols with subsequent retransfusion autologous or allogeneic hematopoietic stem cells are under investigation. With the development of the structurally related purine analogs fludarabine phosphate, 2-deoycoformycine and 2-chlorodeoxyadensoine, new perspectives in the therapy of low-grade NHL were provided. Fludarabine has proved effective in the treatment of chronic lymphocytic leukemia (CLL) and low-grade NHL, predominantly of the follicular subtype. In a consecutive multicenter phase II study the German Low-Grade NHL Study Group investigated fludarabine in combination with mitoxantrone and dexamethasone (FMD) in 39 patients with refractory or relapsed low-grade NHL and achieved a response rate of 39%, with 6 (21%) complete and 5 (18%) partial remission. All patients were heavily pretreated and had 6 (21%) complete and 5 (18%) partial remissions. All patients were heavily pretreated and had received two to five preceding regimens (median 2). Histologic subtypes included 14 centroblasticcentrocytic NHL, 10 centrocytic NHL, 13 lymphoplasmocytoid immunocytoma, one T-chronic lymphocytic leukemia and one monocytoid B-cell lymphoma. Treatment-associated toxicity was moderate, with myelosuppression comprising the major side effect.

Introduction

The differences in histology, biology and clinical course of non-Hodgkin lymphomas (NHL) served as the basis for several classification systems, among which the Working Formulation and the Kiel classification are nowadays mostly applied. The natural history of lymphomas and their response to therapy under i.e. the working formulation, the most popular classification

[1] Department of Hematology and Oncology, University of Göttingen, Germany for the German Low-Grade Non-Hodgkin's Lymphoma Study Group

currently used in the United States, which discriminates between low-grade, intermediate-grade and high-grade lymphomas (1). A different, more biologically oriented approach was taken by the Kiel classification, which attempts to group the non-Hodgkin lymphomas according to their normal cellular counterparts and the physiologic stages of lymphopoesis from which the malignant clone may have emerged (2). Increasing insights into the biology and physiologic development of the lymphatic system, provided by novel immunologic and molecular techniques, make this approach most attractive and are the basis for the most recently proposed Revised European American Lymphoma (REAL) classification [3], developed by an International Lymphoma Study Group of pathologists. Although the clinical impact of this proposal is still under debate, it attempts to incorporate the current knowledge of lympnoma biology and promises to become a widely accepted classification system that will facilitate the international comparability of studies and clinical data.

Treatment Options

Low-grade NHL are characterized by a long clinical course with median survival times ranging from approximately 3 years for centrocytic (CC) or mantle-cell lymphomas (MCL) to 5–8 years for centroblastic-centrocytic (CB-CC) or follicular lymphomas (FL). Therapy of low-grade lymphomas depends mainly on the extent of the disease. In the early stages I and II, at which approximately only 15–20% of low-grade NHL are diagnosed, as well as selected cases of stage III disease, radiotherapy may be applied with curative intent (6–8). Patients with stage I and II disease experience long-lasting disease-free survival and may even be cured by extended field or total nodal irradiation using doses of around 30 Gy [6]. However, in the majority of cases the lymphoma has spread to stages III and IV at the time of diagnosis due to the indolent course of the disease. The long-term perspectives in the advanced stages III and IV are dismal, and current conventional regimens offer no chance for disease eradication and cure. Therapeutic management is, therefore, mainly directed towards palliation and cytostatic therapy is usually withheld until the occurrence of disease-associated symptoms or lymphoma progression [9]. Frequently used regimens are of mild to moderate intensity and comprise chlorambucil with or without prednisone; cyclophosphamide, vincristine, prednisone (COP); or prednimustine and mitoxantrone (PmM), as recently reported by the German Low-Grade Lymphoma Study Group [10]. The application of anthracyclines or more intensive multi-agent combinations did not prove advantageous for response rate, response duration or survival and hence cannot be recommended outside controlled clinical trials [11].

Some hope may be gained, however, from the administration of interferon alpha (IFN) together with or after successful cytoreductive chemotherapy. Recent data indicate that IFN may prolong the disease-free and possibly also the overal survival, especially in patients with follicular lymphomas [12–16]. Similarly to high-grade lymphomas, early intensification by myeloablative radio-chemotherapy with subseuqent retransfusion of autologous or allogeneic hematopoietic stem cells may offer a certain potential for cure but will also rely on a preceding reduction of the lymphoma cell mass by effective anti-lymphoma chemotherapy [17–21].

With the development of the structurally related purine analogs fludarabine phosphate, 2-deoxycoformycine and 2-chlorodeoxyadensoine, new perspectives in the therapy of low-grade lymphoid malignancies were provided. A number of phase I and II studies have shown a significant activity of fludarabine in the treatment of chronic lymphocytic leukemia (CLL) and relapsed or refractory low-grade NHL [22–26], predominantly of the follicular subtype. On the basis of synergistic effects of fludarabine and mitoxantrone in the treatment of NHL [27], the German Cooperative NHL Study Group initiated a multicenter phase II study for the treatment of relapsed low-grade NHL to investigate the anti-lymphoma activity and toxicity of fludarabine in combination with mitoxantrone and dexamethasone (FMD) in the treatment of patients with relapsed or refractory low-grade NHL.

Patients and Methods

Patient Population

Patients were primarily recruited from the multicenter trial of the German Cooperative NHL Study Group with a randomized comparison of two different induction regimens (COP versus

tion only [10]. Beside these we included all patients who were refractory or relapsed after a conventional oral or intreavanous chemotherapy regimen. Criteria for the evaluation of FMD were the rate of complete and partial remission and the duration of a subsequent event`free interval as well as the incidence and severity of treatment-related side effects.

We included patients with recurrent or refractory NHL who had progressive or bulky disease and required therapy as defined by the presence of B-symptoms and/or signs of impairment of the hematopoetic system. The following histologic subtypes were represented 14 centroblastic-centrocytic NHL, 10 centrocytic NHL, 13 lymphoplasmocytoid immunocytoma, one T-chronic lymphocytic leukemia and one monocytoid B-cell lymphoma.

All patients were required to have adequate marrow function except in the presence of lymphoma infiltration of the bone marrow, with granulocytes $>1500/\mu l$ and platelets $>100{,}000/\mu l$, as well as adequate liver function (bilirubin <2.0 mg/dl), renal function (creatinine <1.5 mg/dl) and sufficient cardiac function. Dose reduction was assigned in case of treatment-associated myelosuppression not related to bone marrow involvement.

Patients were excluded from the study if there was any possibility of primary potentially curative radiotherapy or if they were older than 75 years.

Tumor response and toxicity were evaluated and graded according to WHO criteria. Complete remission (CR) was defined as absence of all signs of disease for more than 4 weeks, including normalization of peripheral blood counts, with granulocytes $>1500/mm^3$, Hb >12 g/dl and platelet $>100{,}000/mm^3$. Partial remission (PR) was defined as more than 50% decrease of all measurable lymphoma manifestations for at least 4 weeks and normalization of peripheral blood counts. Remission duration was the time from documentation of remission until relapse. As survival we defined the period from first day of therapy until death.

Treatment Plan

Preceding initial therapy, diagnostic staging procedures, including physical examination, chest X-ray, abdominal sonography, bone marrow aspirate and biopsy and computed tomography of involved sites of disease were done after every two cycles. Fludarabine was administered at a dose of 25 $mg/m^2/day$ by a 30-min infusion on days 1–3 together with mitoxantrone 10 $mg/m^2/day$ on day 1 as a 30-min infusion and dexamethasone 20 mg/day on days 1–5 orally. Cycles were repeated every 28 days for an initial series of 4 courses. Further treatment was adapted to response as follows: Patients achieving a complete remission after 4 cycles received 2 further courses of therapy as consolidation and no further treatment subsequently. Patients with CR or PR after 6 cycles also received 2 further courses of therapy until a maximum of 8 courses, regardless of whether CR or PR was achieved. Patients with minor response or stable disease after 4 cycles were excluded from the study, as were patients with progressive NHL at any stage.

Results

Thirty-nine patients from 8 participating centers entered the study and received 167 cycles of therapy with the combination FMD. Histologic subtypes included 14 centroblastic-centrocytic (CB-CC) NHL, 10 centrocytic (CC) NHL, 13 lymphoplasmocytoid immunocytoma (LP-IC), one T-chronic lymphocytic leukemia and one monocytoid B-cell lymphoma. All patients were heavily pretreated and had received 2–5 preceding regimens (median 2). In accordance with to the normal age distribution observed in patients with low-grade NHL, the patients in our study were mainly elderly, with the majority being older than 50 years.

In a previous phase II trial for the treatment of relapsed low-grade NHL [27] with fludarabine as single agent, our group could show an overall response rate of 32% including 5 CR (13.5%) and 7 PR (18.9%), corresponding to response rates found in the literature. A comparison of the treatment results of fludarabine monotherapy with the combination therapy FMD is shown in Fig. 1.

Patients treated with the combination FMD achieved not only a higher overall remission rate of 39%, including 5 (18%), but also a higher rate of CR (6 patients, 21%), than fludarabine monotherapy. Furthermore, response to treatment seems to be more rapidly achieved by patients treated with FMD, where 4 CR were obtained after only 4 treatment cycles.

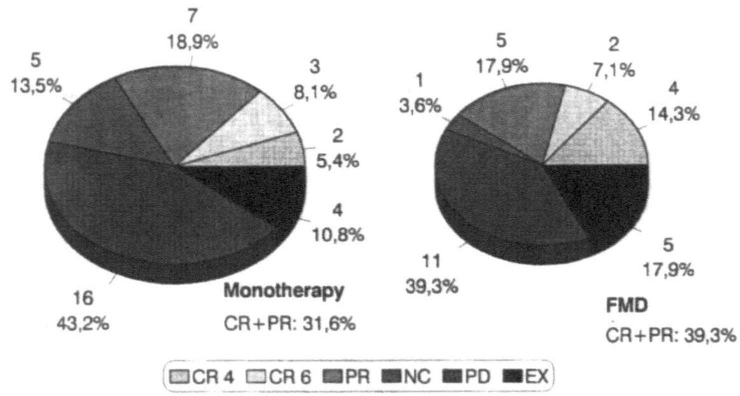

Fig. 1. Fludarabine monotherapy vs FMD after induction therapy

Five patients (17.9%) died during treatment with FMD; 1 patient died from myocardial infarction, the other 4 succumbed to disease progression or infection. There was no significant difference from the death rate with fludarabine monotherapy.

Despite the higher overall remission rate with FMD in the treatment of low-grade NHL, there was no difference between the event-free interval (Fig. 2) and the time to relapse or death (Fig. 3) in the two treatment groups.

Compared to fludarabine as single-agent therapy, the treatment with FMD does not provide any advantage with respect to overall survival, as shown in Fig. 4. However, analysis of the patient subgroups in the survival curves reveals that patients responding with a CR or PR to treatment with FMD have a significantly higher probability of survival, with a median survival time of 10.3 months compared to 8.3 months in non-responder Similar results were achieved by fludarabine monotherapy, where patients achieving a remission had a median survival time of 20 months, compared to 5.8 months in the non-responder group.

Analysis of the side effects shows that acute toxicity of FMD was mild. Only a few cases of nausea and vomiting occurred, as seen in previous studies [23]. The main treatment-associated side effects of FMD consisted in hematotoxicity. Forty-eight percent of the patients presented with a WHO grade 3–4 myelosuppression, which led in 7 cases (18.4%) to WHO grade 3–4 infections.

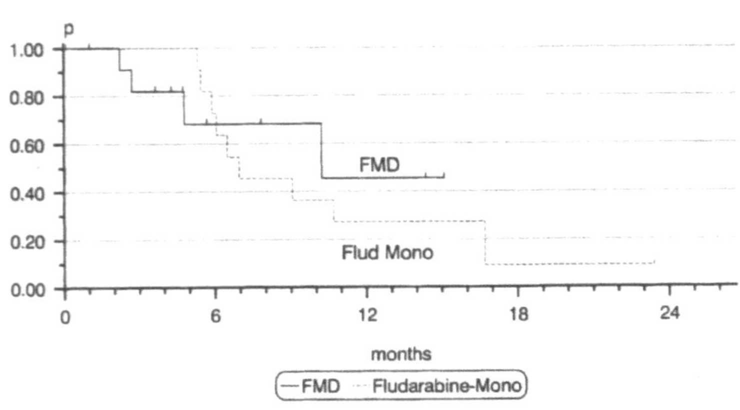

Fig. 2. Event-free interval after FMD and fludarabine monotherapy (all patients with CR or PR after induction therapy)

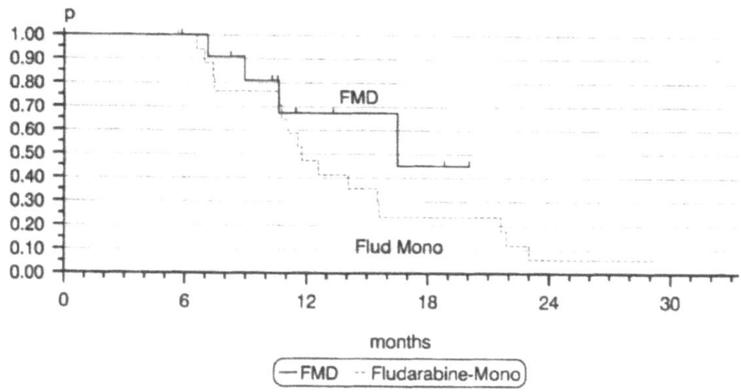

Fig. 3. Time to relapse or death after start of therapy with FMD and fludarabine monotherapy (all patients with CR, PR, MR or SD)

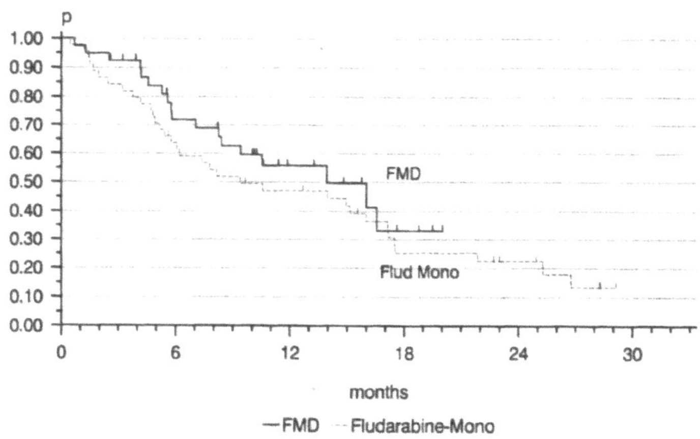

Fig. 4. Survival after start therapy with FMD and fludarabine monotherapy

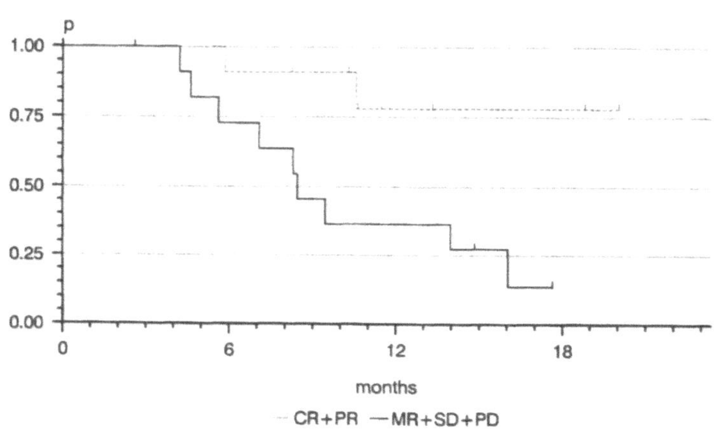

Fig. 5. Survival after start of therapy with FMD

Platelets were affected in 29% of patients having grade 3–4 toxicity, but only a few moderate bleeding complications resulted. WHO grade 3–4 hematotoxicity was the reason for dose reduction in 10% of the cases treated with FMD.

A comparison of hematotoxicity of FMD with the monotherapy (Fig. 6) indicates only marginal differences in the extent of hematotoxicity, with a tendency towards a higher incidence of WHO grade 3–4 granulocytopenia in patients treated with FMD.

Discussion

The development of new strategies in NHL treatmentin currently a highly attractive field of research. Treatment options for advanced disease include strategies with IFN maintenance or even myeloablative chemo-radiotherapy followed by autologous bone marrow or peripheral stem-cell transplantation.

The introduction of purine analogs in the treatment of lymphoid malignancies has had a substantial impact on the management of lymphoid malignancies and may allow exploration of novel treatment strategies with curative potential which have not been available so far. The current study of the German Cooperative NHL Study Group clearly demonstrates that FMD is effective in a heavily pretreated patient group with relapsed or refractory NHL. In a previous phase II trial for the treatment of relapsed low-grade NHL [26] our group showed that an overall response rate of 31% is achieved with fludarabine as single agent, corresponding to response rates found in the literature. The results of the consecutive phase II study indicate that the combination therapy with FMD appears to be more effective, with an overall response rate of 39%. However, analysis of the survival after treatment with fludarabine as single agent or FMD have shown that patients achieving a remission have a significantly higher probability of survival than patients with minimal or no response. A comparison of the survival curves of all patients in the two different studies reveals no advantage in survival for the patients treated with FMD.

Undoubted fludarabine has immunosuppressive effects through a depletion of T-cell subsets [28]. Different investigators found a decrease in the absolute CD4+ and CD8+ counts associated with fludarabine therapy, and an increased incidence of opportunistic infections has been discussed [29, 30]. On the other hand, long-term follow-up of patients in remission after single-agent therapy with fludarabine revealed no increased incidence of opportunistic infections despite diminished CD4+ counts [31]. Hence, the persistent suppression of CD4+ lymphocytes may not only facilitate the emergence of opportunistic infections but also enhance the risk of secondary malignancies.

These results encourage participation in prospective studies which are currently under way and will help to define the appropriate indication and timing of these promisng new agents.

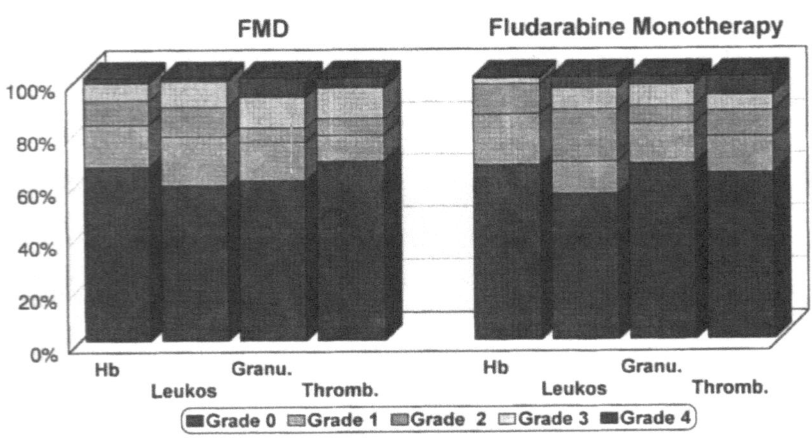

Fig. 6. Hematelogic toxicity in patient with Low-grade NHL

References

1. The Non-Hodgkin's Lymphoma Pathologic Classification Project: National Cancer Institute sponsored study of classifications of non-Hodgkin's lymphomas. Summary and description of a working formulation for clinical usage. Cancer 1982; 49: 2112–35.
2. Stansfeld AG, J. Diebold, Y. Kanci et al. Updated Kiel classification for lymphomas. Lancet 1988; 603 I: 292–293.
3. Harris NL, E.S. Jaffe, H. Stein et al. A proposal for an international consensus on the classification of lymphoid neoplasms. Blood 1994; 84: 1381–92.
4. Brittinger G, P. Meusers, M. Engelhard. Strategien der Behandlung von Non-Hodgkin-Lymphomen. Internist 1986; 27: 485–97.
5. Horning SJ, S.A. Rosenberg. The natural history of initially untreated low-grate non-Hodgkin's lymphomas. N Engl J Med 1984; 31: 1471–75.
6. Epelbaum R, A. Kuten, N.M. Coachman et al. Stage I-II low-grade non-Hodgkin's lymphoma: prognostic factors and treatment results. Strahlenth Onkol 1992; 168 (2): 66–72.
7. Armitage JO. Treatment of non-Hodgkin's lymphoma. N Eng J Med 1992; 328: 1023–30.
8. Sack H. V. Budach, M. Stuschke et al.: Non-Hodgkin lymphomas (NHL)—early stages. Interim results of a multicentre trial. Cancer Res Clin Oncol 1992, 118 (suppl.): R 115.
9. Young RC, D.L. Longo, Glastein et al. The treatment of indolent lymphomas: watchful waiting v. aggressive combined modality treatment. Semin Hematol 1988; 25 (suppl. 2) 11–16.
10. Hiddemann W, M. Unterhalt, P. Koch et al. New aspects in the treatment of advanced low-grade non-Hodgkin's lymphomas: prednimustine/mitoxantrone (PmM) vs. cyclophosphamide/vincristine/prednisone (COP) followed by interferon vs. observation only—a preliminary update of the German low-grade Lymphoma Study Group. Sem Oncol 1994, in press.
11. Kimby E, M. Björkholm, G. Gahrton et al.: Chlorambucilprednisone vs. CHOP in symptomatic low-grade non-Hodgkin's lymphomas: randomized trial from the Lymphoma Group of Central Sweden. Ann Oncol 1994 5, Suppl. 2: 67–71.
12. Hagenbeek A, P. Carde, R. Somers et al. Maintenance of remission with human recombinant alpha-2 interferon (Roferon-A) in patients with stages III and IV low-grade malignant non-Hodgkin's lymphoma. Results from a prospective, randomised phase III clinical trial in 331 patients. Blood (suppl. 1) 1992; 80: 74a.
13. Chisesi T, M. Congiu, A. Contu et al. Randomized study of chlorambucil (CB) compared to interferon (alfa-2b) combined with CB in low-grade non-Hodgkin's lymphoma: an interim report of a randomized study. J Eur J Cancer 1991; 27 (suppl 4): 31–33.
14. Price CGA, A.Z.S. Rohatiner, W. Steward et al. Interferon 2b in the treatment of follicular lymphoma: preliminary results of a trial in progress. Ann Oncol 1991; 2 (suppl 2): 141–45.
15. Peterson BA, G. Petroni, M.M. Oken et al. Cyclophosphamide versus cyclophosphamide plus interferon alfa-2b in follicular low-grade lymphomas: a preliminary report of an intergroup trial (CALGB 8691 and EST 7486). Proc Am Soc Clin Oncol 1993; 12: 366.
16. Smalley RV, J.W. Andersen, M.J. Hawkins et al.: Interferon alfa combined with cytotoxic chemotherapy for patients with non-Hodgkin's lymphoma. N Engl J Med 1992; 19: 1336–41.
17. Horning SJ: Treatment approaches to the low-grade lymphomas. Blood 1994 83: 881–84.
18. Schouten HC, P. Colombat, L.F. Verdonck, N.C. Gorin, B. Björkstrand, G. Taghipour, A.H. Goldstone. Autologous bone marrow transplantation for low-grade Non-Hodgkin's lymphoma: The European Bone Marrow Transplant Group Experience.Ann Oncol 1994; 5 (suppl.2): 147–49.
19. Rohatiner AZS, A. Freedman, L. Nadler, J. Lim, T.A. Lister. Myeloablative therapy with autologous bone marrow transplantation as consolidation therapy for follicular lymphoma.Ann Oncol 1994; 5 (suppl.2): 143–46.
20. Freedman A, J. Gribben, S. Rabinowe et al. Autologous bone marrow transplantation in advanced low-grade B-cell non-Hodgkin's lymphoma in first remission. Blood 1993; 82 (suppl. 1): 332a.
21. Vose JM, C. Peterson, P.J. Bierman et al. Comparison of high-dose therapy and autologous bone marrow transplantation for T-cell and B-cell non-Hodgkin's lymphomas. Blood 1990; 76: 424–31.
22. Keating MR, H. Kantarjian, S. O'Brien et al. Fludarabine: a new agent with marked cytoreductive activity in untreated CLL. J Clin Oncol 1991; 9: 44–49.
23. Hiddemann W, R. Rottmann, B. Wörmann et al. Treatment of advanced CLL by fludarabine: results of a clinical phase II study. Annals Hematol 1991; 63: 1–4.
24. Leiby JM, K.M. Snider, E.H. Kraut et al. Phase II trial of 9-ß-D-arabinofuranosyl-2-fluoroadenine-5'-monophosphate in non-Hodgkin's lymphoma: prospective comparison of response with deoxycytidine kinase activity. Cancer Res 1987; 47: 2719–22.
25. Redman JR, F. Cabanilas, W.S. Velasques et al. Phase II trial of fludarabine phosphate in lymphoma: an effective agent in low-grade lymphoma. J Clin Oncol 1992; 10: 790–94.
26. Hiddemann W, M. Unterhalt, C. Pott et al. Fludarabine single agent therapy for relapsed low grade non-Hodgkin's lymphomas: a phase II study of the german low-grade non-Hodgkin's lymphoma study group. Sem Oncol 1993; 20 (suppl.7): 28–31.
27. McLaughlin P, F. Swan, F. Hagemeister et al. Phase I study of the combination of fludarabine, mitoxantrone and dexamethasone in low-grade lymphoma. J Clin Oncol 1994; 12: 575–79.
28. Boldt DH, Von Hoff DD, Kuhn, et al. Effects on-human peripheral lymphocytes of in vivo adminis-

tration of 9-β-D-arabinofuranosyl-2-fluoroadenine-5'-monophosphate (NSC 312887), a new purine antimetabolite. Cancer Res 1984; 44: 4661–66.

29. O'Brien S, Kantarjian H.M. Beran et al. Results of fludarabine and prednisone therapy in 264 patients with chronic lymphocytic leukemia with multivariate analysis—derived prognostic model for response to treatment. Blood 1993; 82, 1695–1700.

30. Bergmann L, K. Fenchel, B. Jahn et al. Immunosuppressive effects and clinical response of fludarabine in refractory CLL. Ann Oncol 1993; 4: 371–73.

31. Keating M, S. O'Brien, H. Kantarjian, W. Plunkett, E. Estey, C. Koller, N. Beran, E. Freireich. Longterm follow up of patients with CLL treated with fludarabine as a single agent. Blood 1993; 81: 2878–84.

Acute Leukemias VI
Prognostic Factors
and Treatment Strategies
Büchner et al. (eds)

Fludarabine in Low-Grade Lymphoma: St. Bartholomew's Hospital Experience

A.Z.S. Rohatiner[1], E. Tirovola[1], E.A. Pigaditou[1], J.S. Whelan[1], P.M.W. Johnson[1], A.J. Norton[2], J.A.L. Amess[3], J. Matthews[1], and T.A. Lister[1]

Abstract. Between February 1989 and February 1995, 122 patients with low-grade non-Hodgkin's lymphoma received fludarabine: 25 mg/m^2 daily for 5 days, repeated every 3-4 weeks, to a maximum of eight cycles. Eighty patients received fludarabine at first or subsequent recurrence, or when the disease was deemed resistant to conventional therapy, 26 patients were treated in the context of minimal residual disease (MRD) in the bone marrow and/or lymph nodes in the hope of eventually proceeding to myeloablative therapy with autologous bone marrow transplantation. A further 16 newly diagnosed patients received fludarabine as initial therapy.

A total of 118 patients are evaluable for response. The response rate (complete remission, CR,+ partial remission, PR) in previously treated patients was 45/102 (45%) overall: 31/76 (41%) in patients with recurrent or resistant disease and 14/26 (54%) in patients with MRD. The response rate was somewhat higher in newly diagnosed patients, i.e. 11/16 (69%).

The predominant toxicity was myelosuppression, 55% and 31% of previously treated and newly diagnosed patients, respectively, requiring admission to hospital for treatment of infection. There were six treatment-related deaths (from infection), all in patients with unresponsive disease. Five patients developed unusual neurological symptoms possibly ascribable to treatment with fludarabine; four subsequently recovered fully.

These results confirm the efficacy of fludarabine in inducing regression of low-grade lymphoma and its potential toxicity.

Introduction

Within the morphological and immunological diversity of lowg-rade non-Hodgkin's lymphomas, one overriding factor remains constant: except in rare circumstances, these diseases are demonstrably incurable with current treatment. Characteristically, the clinical course is one of repeated remissions and recurrences with a median survivial between 5 and 10 years [1-4]. The inexorable pattern of recurrence means that, almost always, death occurs as a consequence of the disease, with or without transformation to high-grade histology [1-5]. An experimental approach is therefore justified.

The rationale for using fludarabine in lymphoid malignancies is based on pre-clinical studies which showed activity against L1210 and P388 leukaemia [6] and against lymphoma in a human tumour-cloning system [7]. Several clinical studies subsequently demonstrated fludarabine to be effective in chronic lymphocytic leukaemia and, more recently, in low-grade lymphoma[8-15].

The experience in patients with low-grade non-Hodgkin's lymphoma treated at St. Bartholomew's Hospital (SBH) over a 6-year period forms the basis of this analysis and includes patients previously reported as part of a collabo-

[1]ICRF Department of Medical Oncology, St. Bartholomew's Hospital, London ECIA 7BE, UK
[2]Department of Histopathology, St. Bartholomew's Hospital, London, ECIA 7BE, UK
[3]Department of Haematology, St. Bartholomew's Hospital, London ECIA 7BE, UK

rative trial [10] and a phase II study which is currently in progress at SBH [15].

Patients and Methods

Patients

A total of 122 patients comprise three groups:

1. Eighty who received fludarabine at first or subsequent recurrence (43 patients) or when the disease was deemed resistant to conventional treatment (37 patients). Virtually all of the latter group had received an adriamycin-containing treatment and, when this was not effective, were treated with fludarabine.
2. Twenty-six patients were treated following therapy with chlorambucil and/or an adriamycin-containing treatment. A good response had been achieved, but MRD was present in the bone marrow and/or lymph nodes. Fludarabine was therefore used in an attempt to induce CR, with a view to then proceeding to myelo-ablative therapy with autologous bone marrow transplantation (ABMT). Clinical characteristics for groups (1) and (2) are shown in Table 1.
3. Sixteen newly diagnosed patients (Table 2) received fludarabine as initial therapy.

Treatment

Fludarabine was reconstituted in 10 ml sterile water and given intravenously over 10 min, at a dose of 25 mg/m^2 for 5 days, repeated every 21–28 days depending on the peripheral blood count and the clinical situation. The aim was to administer two cycles of treatment beyond the point of maximum response, as measured by clinical examination, radiological findings and evaluation of the bone marrow. If, after two cycles of treatment, there was no evidence of response, no further fludarabine was administered. Patients were admitted to hospital when they became febrile or had other symptoms and signs of infection in the context of neutropenia. Antibiotics and blood products were given as appropriate.

Table 1. Clinical characteristics of evaluable patients with recurrent/resistant disease

Gender M: F (*n*)		63: 43
Age Median—(years)		49
—Range (years)		26–79
Histology (*n*)		
	Lymphocytic	4
	Centroblastic centrocytic follicular	53
	Centroblastic/ centrocytic diffuse	1
	Low-grade B-cell unclassified	11
	Mantle cell	5
	Peripheral T-cell	2
		76

Table 2. Clinical characteristics of newly diagnosed patients

Gender	M: F (*n*)	12: 4
Age Median—(years)		52
	— Range (years)	(40–77)
Histology (*n*)		
	Lymphoplasmacytoid	10
	Centroblastic/centrocytic diffuse	1
	T zone	3
	Peripheral T cell	1
	Low-grade unclassified	1
Stage (*n*)		
	IE (GI tract)	1
	II	1
	III	1
	IV	13

Definitions

Complete remission was defined as the disappearance of all measurable disease. *Partial remission* was defined as a greater than 50% reduction in measurable disease as evidenced by clinical examination, CT scan findings and a bone marrow aspirate and trephine biopsy. The treatment was deemed to have *failed* when the response was anything less than PR. Death from infection occurring during a cycle of treatment was considered to be a *treatment-related death. Recurrent disease* signifies first or subsequent recurrence. *Resistant disease* was defined as failure or progression following conventional treatment. *Minimal residual disease* was defined as lymph nodes less than 2 cm in diameter, or an equivocal CT scan, ± less than 20% bone marrow infiltration on a trephine biopsy.

Results

Response to Treatment

Table 3 shows details of the overall response to treatment.

Previously Treated Patients. A Total of 102 patients are evaluable for response, 76 with recurrent/resistant disease, 26 with MRD. Overall, the response rate (CR+PR) was 45/102 (45%); 17/41 (41%) and 14/35 (40%) for patients with recurrent and resistant disease, respectively. Thirty-seven patients in whom a response was achieved subsequently received myelo-ablative therapy with ABMT, 27 immediately and ten following alternative, additional treatment to try and improve on the response to fludarabine. Response according to histological subtype is shown in Table 4. There was no evidence of response in 51 patients, fludarabine was therefore stopped. There were six treatment-related deaths (see below). For the 26 evaluable patients treated in the context of MRD, the response rate was 14/26 (52%), 18 of the latter 26 patients actually received myelo-ablative therapy with ABMT.

Table 3. Response to therapy

	(*n*)	(%)
Previously treated patients		
Response (CR+PR)	45/102	45
Recurrent disease	17/41	41
Resistant disease	14/35	40
MRD	14/26	52
Treatment failed	51/102	49
Treatment-related deaths		
Newly diagnosed Patients		
Response (CR)	11/16 (6 CR)	69
Treatment failed	5/16	31

Newly Diagnosed Patients. The response rate was higher in the 16 newly diagnosed patients (11/16, 69%) with CR being achieved in six patients.

Toxicity

Treatment was given on an out-patient basis with minimal clinical toxicity. Myelosuppression was the predominant toxicity, 51% of previously treated and 31% of newly diagnosed patients requiring admission to hospital for neutropenic fever. There were six deaths from infection, five in patients with recurrent/resistant disease who were not responding to fludarabine at the time.

Five patients developed unusual neurological symptoms whilst receiving fludarabine: four recovered spontaneously and one died. Details of the symptoms and findings are shown in Table 5 and have been described in full in a previous report [16].

Discussion

These results confirm the activity of fludarabine in low-grade lymphoma [8–15]. Significant activity in extensively pre-treated patients was

Table 4. Response to therapy according to histological subtype (patients with recurrent/resistant disease)

Histology	Patients (*n*)	Response (CR+PR) (*n*)	treatment failed (*n*)	Treatment related death (*n*)
Lymphocytic	2	2/2	–	–
Lymphoplasmacytoid	26	10/26	11	5
Centroblastic/centrocytic	32	14/32	18	–
Mantle cell	4	1/4	3	–
Peripheral T cell	2	0/2	2	–
Low-grade unclassified	10	4/10	5	1
Total	76	31/76	39	6

Table 5. Neurological symptoms and signs in five patients receiving fludarabine

	Histological subtype	Clinical details
1	Follicular	Headaches and right-sided hemiparesis. At autopsy, no cerebral lymphoma, but histology showed vascular intimal hyperplasia
2	T cell	Headaches and right-sided hemiparesis Complete recovery
3	Follicular	Previous Cerebrovascular attack Left-sided weakness, Complete recovery
4	T cell	Generalised weakness CSF protein elevated conduction studies suggestive of demyelination Gradual spontaneous improvement
5	CLL	Tremor and unsteadiness of gait Generalised weakness and areflexia Conduction studies—slowing of motor conduction Velocity suggestive of a demyelinating peripheral neuropathy Complete recovery

observed. It appears to be particularly active in lymphoplasmacytoid lymphoma which is perhaps not surprising in view of the activity in chronic lymphocytic leukaemia (CLL). In general, clinical toxicity was not a major problem although the drug is clearly myelosuppressive, an appreciable number of patients requiring admission to hospital for treatment of infection.

Neurological toxicity is a potential concern. Whilst it is not possible to be sure as to whether the neurological symptoms observed in the five patients described above were necessarily attributable to treatment with fludarabine, four patients recovered spontaneously when fludarabine was stopped.

Thus, fludarabine represents a useful addition to the treatment options currently available for patients with low-grade lymphoma. A number of studies are currently in progress which will hopefully further define its role as initial treatment, either alone or in combination.

References

1. Anderson T, De Vita VT, Simon RM et al. Malignant lymphoma: II. Prognostic factors and response to treatment of 473 patients at the National Cancer Institute. Cancer, 1982; 50: 2708–2721
2. Brittinger G, Bartels H, Common H et al. Clinical and prognostic relevance of the Kiel Classification of non-Hodgkin's lymphoma. Results of a prospective multi-centre study by the Kiel Lymphoma Group. Hematol Oncol, 1984; 2: 269
3. Gallagher CJ, Gregory WM, Jones AE, Stansfeld AG, Richards M, Dhaliwal HS, Malpas JS & Lister TA. Follicular lymphoma: prognostic factors for response and survival. J Clin Oncol, 1986; 4: 1470–1480
4. Richards MA, Hall PA, Gregory WM, Dhaliwal HS, Stansfeld AG, Amess JA & Lister TA. Lymphoplasmacytoid and small cell centrocytic non-Hodgkin's lymphoma—a retrospective analysis from St Bartholomew's Hospital 1972–1986. Hematol Oncol, 1989; 7: 19–35
5. Jones SE, Fuks Z, Bull M et al. Non Hodgkin's lymphoma: IV. Clinicopathologic correlation in 405 cases. Cancer, 1973; 31: 806–823
6. Tavoussi M & Avramis VI. Pharmacodynamics of fludarabine phosphate (F-ara-AMP) in P388 leukaemia-bearing mice after toxic and non-toxic regimens. Proc ASCO, 1986; 5: 45
7. Lathan B & Diehl V, Clark GM, et al. Cytotoxic activity of 9-β-D-arabinofuranosyl-2-fluoroadenine 5-monophosphate (fludarabine, NSC 312887) in a human tumor cloning system. Eur J Cancer Clin Oncol 1988, 24: 1891–1895.
8. Leiby JM, Snider KM, Kraut EH et al. Phase II trial of 9-β-D-arabinofuranosyl-2-fluoroadenine 5'-monophosphate in non-Hodgkin's lymphoma: prospective comparison of response with deoxycytidine kinase activity. Cancer Research 1987, 47: 2719–2722.
9. Hochster H & Cassileth P. Fludarabine phosphate therapy of non-Hodgkin's lymphoma. Semin Oncol, 1990; 17: 63

10. Whelan JS, Davis CL, Rule S, Ranson M, Smith OP, Mehta AB, Catovsky D, Rohatiner AZ, Lister TA. Fludarabine phosphate for the treatment of low grade lymphoid malignancy. Br J Cancer 1991; 64(1): 120.
11. Hochster HS, Kim KM, Green MD, et al. Activity of fludarabine in previously treated non-Hodgkin's low-grade lymphoma: results of an Eastern Co-operative Oncology Group study. J Clin Oncol 1992, 10: 28–32
12 Redman JR, Cabanillas F, Velasquez WS, et al. Phase II trial of fludarabine phosphate in lymphoma: an effective new agent in low-grade lymphoma. J Clin Oncol 1992, 10: 790–794
13. Hiddeman W, Unterhalt M, Pott C, et al. Fludarabine single-agent therapy for relapsed low-grade non-Hodgkin's lymphomas—a phase II study of the German low-grade non-Hodgkin's Lymphoma Study Group. Semin Oncol 1993, 20, (suppl 7), 28–31
14. Zinzani PL, Lauria F, Rondelli D, et al. Fludarabine—an active agent in the treatment of previously treated and untreated low-grade non-Hodgkin's lymphoma. Ann Oncol 1993; 4: 575–578
15. Pigaditou A, Rohatiner AZS, Whelan JS, et al. Fludarabine in low-grade lymphoma. Semin Oncol 1993, 20 (suppl 7): 24–27
16. Johnson et al. Neurological problems related to fludarabine. Br J Cancer (1994) 70, 966–968

Acute Leukemias VI
Prognostic Factors
and Treatment Strategies
Büchner et al. (eds)

Future Role of Purine Analogues in Oncology

M.J. Keating

Abstract. The purine analogues fludarabine monophosphate and 2-chlorodeoxyadenosine (2-CDA) have emerged as major new drugs in the management of hematologic malignancies. The initial activity of these drugs was noted in indolent lymphoid malignancies, and 2-CDA has emerged as the treatment of choice in hairy cell leukemia (HCL) and fludarabine as the most active single agent studied in chronic lymphocytic leukemia (CLL). Numerous effects of these drugs on the activities of enzymes important in DNA synthesis and repair have been identified, and a key role in induction of apoptosis has been noted. Fludarabine and 2-CDA both enhance the formation of cytosine arabinoside triphosphate (ara-C) in leukemic cells and have been demonstrated to inhibit repair of DNA damage caused by radiation, cisplatinum, and mitoxantrone. This activity presumably extends to other drugs. Fludarabine has the highest documented complete (CR) and partial (PR) remission rate in both previously treated and untreated patients with CLL. Comparative studies against salvage and frontline regimens have demonstrated superiority in response rate. Combinations of fludarabine with anthracyclines, alkylating agents, and mitoxantrone are being actively explored in CLL. The activity of fludarabine and 2-CDA in low-grade lymphoma has led to combinations of these agents with mitoxantrone and corticosteroids. The addition of corticosteroids appears to enhance the probability of opportunistic infections. The activity of fludarabine in enhancing ara-CTP formation in acute leukemia, myelodysplastic syndrome (MDS) has led to exploration of this combination alone, fludarabine + ara-C (FA), or together with GCSF (FLAG), and with idarubicin (FLAG/Ida). All three regimens are very active in poor and better prognosis patients with acute myelogenous leukemia (AML) and MDS and are well tolerated. The effect of fludarabine in inhibiting repair of DNA damage has led to protocols and solid tumor clinical trials with cisplatinum in ovarian cancer. Trials with cisplatinum or radiation in head and neck cancer are being initiated. Purine analogues as single agents in the indolent lymphoproliferative diseases are likely to be used for many years. The extended role will be in combinations both in hematologic malignancies and solid tumors. The immunosuppressive effect of the purine analogues is likely to lead to increased use of these drugs in preparative regimens for bone marrow transplantation and perhaps use in enhancing cytotoxicity in association with preparative regimens in autologous and allogeneic bone marrow transplants.

Introduction

Discovery of the activity of purine analogues fludarabine and 2-chlorodeoxyadenosine (2-CDA) in lymphoproliferative disorders has been an observation of major clinical significance [1–6]. The role of these drugs in the future, however, will depend on exploitation of the multiple effects that these agents have on activity of a variety of enzymes active in DNA replication

Division of Medicine, University of Texas, M.D. Anderson Cancer Centre, Houston, Texas 77030, USA

and repair [7]. Fludarabine was demonstrated in phase I clinical trials to be active in chronic lymphocytic leukemia (CLL) and low-grade lymphoma [1, 3] and to have a dramatic effect in decreasing T cell subpopulations in patients with solid tumors [8]; 2-CDA, on the other hand, was demonstrated to have striking clinical activity in hairy cell leukemia (HCL) [4] and has been more recently explored in CLL [5] and low-grade lymphoma [6]. The present discussion will omit 2-deoxycoformycin, an agent which has a different mechanism of action to fludarabine and 2-CDA, being a potent inhibitor of adenosine deaminase, an enzyme which tends to degrade fludarabine and 2-CDA. Both fludarabine and 2-CDA have a muliplicity of effects in inhibiting DNA polymerase, ribonucleotide reductase and they are incorporated into DNA as triphosphate forms [7]. The incorporation into DNA correlates well with cytotoxicity. Fludarabine is the only purine analogue which is incorporated into RNA as the triphosphate.

This presentation will review some of the clinical activity of fludarabine in combinations predominantly studied at the M.D. Anderson Cancer Centre (MDACC). Many of the conclusions drawn will be applicable to 2-CDA.

Fludarabine in CLL

The activity of fludarabine in CLL was demonstrated in early studies by Grever and his colleagues [1]. Activity of an agent with so many possible effects on DNA synthesis in low-grade lymphoproliferative disorders was somewhat unexpected. In particular, because of the effect of fludarabine in decreasing normal T cell subsets in preference to B cell subsets, it was anticipated than fludarabine may be more active in T cell malignancies than to B cell malignancies [8]. Following these observations a phase I/II clinical trial was conducted with fludarabine as a single agent in CLL at the MDACC [2]. Seventy-eight patients were eventually entered on this clinical trial and more than half of the patients obtained a complete (CR) or partial response (PR). Using National Cancer Institute Working Group (NCIWG) criteria for response [9], two thirds of the responders achieved CR. However, two thirds of these CR patients had persistent lymphoid nodules which may or may not have been malignant. It is thought, at the present time, that these patients indeed have residual malignant lymphocyte clusters and should be considered as partial responders.

The next study which was undertaken in previously treated patients with CLL was the co-administration of fludarabine at 30 mg/m^2 per day with prednisone 30 mg/m^2 per day [10]. As shown in Table 1, there is no difference in overall response rate, CR rate, and as shown in Fig. 1, there is no difference in survival. An observation which was made is that patients with the addition of corticosteroids begin to exhibit a propensity to develop infections with *Pneumocystis carinii* pneumonia and *Listeria* monocytogenes [10, 11]. This, associated with other side effects of corticosteroids in elderly patients, argues against the use of corticosteroids in conjunction with purine analogues as there is no demonstrated benefit of this approach clinically.

Based on the elegant pharmacodynamic studies of Plunkett and colleagues which demonstrated that F-ara-ATP, the triphosphate form of fludarabine, persists in CLL cells for prolonged periods, a study was set up to explore the ability to administer the drug on a weekly basis [7, 12]. The postulate was that the long-lasting effect of F-ara-ATP in CLL cells would allow persistent activity of the drug while myelosuppression may be spared. The outcome of this study, however, demonstrated a decrease in the response rate by a factor of two with only one patient in four achieving a response with a low CR rate [12]. No survival advantage or disadvantage to this approach was noted, presumably because a number of these patients then went on to salvage therapy with more intensive fludarabine regimens. No improvement in probability of developing myelosuppression or infectious complications was noted in this study.

As a prelude to possible combination therapy approaches with fludarabine and other myelosuppressive agents, a 3-day schedule was evaluated [13]. Fludarabine was given at 30 mg/m^2 per day for 3 days every 4 weeks. The schedule has 60% of the dose intensity of the fludarabine and fludarabine plus prednisone 5-day regimens. The response rate dropped down to 46% with a decrease in the CR rate. However, there was a halving of the infectious complications and the survival of this group of patients, if anything, was slightly superior to the survival that was noted for the 5-day regimens (Fig. 1). The study also illustrated that, as opposed to the 5-day regimens where there is a prompt fall of

Table 1. Response (complet+partial response) of 373 previously treated patients with CLL receiving fludarabine regimens by prognostic factors (MDACC trials)

Prognostic factor	Response total		Significance
	(*n*)	(%)	
Overall	181/373	49	
Rai stage			
0	14/17	82	
I-II	99/153	65	$p<.001$
III-IV	82/220	37	
Binet stage			
A	60/89	67	
B	58/103	56	$p<.001$
C	63/181	35	
Age (years)			
<70	158/306	52	$p=.01$
70	23/67	34	
Refractory	120/272	4	$p=.005$
Non-refractory	61/101	60	
Prior treatment regimens			
1	53/86	62	
2–3	102/211	48	$p<.001$
>3	26/76	34	
Regimens			
Fludarabine (5-day)	45/78	57	
Fludarabine (5-day) + prednisone	88/169	52[a]	
Weekly fludarabine	11/46	24	$p<.05$
Fludarabine (3-day)	37/80	46	

[a]Compared with each of the other regimens.

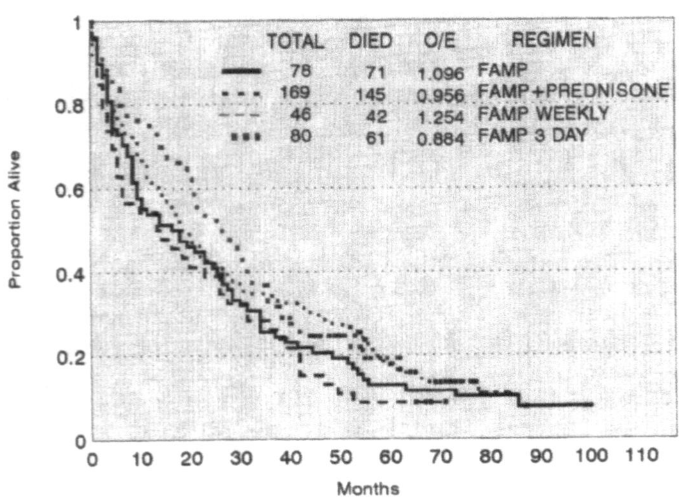

Fig. 1. Survival CLL (PRIOR treatment) by fludarabine regimen

CD4 and CD8 T lymphocyte miosing subpopulations to an average value of approximately 200/µl after three courses, the level of CD4 counts at 3 months of the 3-day regimens was still a median of >500/µl and the level fell to approximately 200/µl only after six courses.

This was associated with a decrease in the episodes of fever and infection. Myelosuppression was also less prominent in the 3-day schedule than in the 5-day schedule.

This series of studies illustrates that dose intensity and schedule of administration of fludarabine still requires further exploration. In particular, subsets of patients more likely to suffer complications of myelosuppression and infectious morbidity may benefit from a less intensive approach to therapy using a 3-day schedule rather than the 5-day schedule. Comparative studies of these two approaches would be useful in the future to answer this question.

After completing the 3-day fludarabine schedule, fludarabine was combined with doxorubicin and initially with prednisone in the FLAP regimen [14]. After the effect of corticosteroids to increase opportunistic infections was noted, corticosteroids were discontinued. The study demonstrated that fludarabine could be given at a dose of 30 mg/m^2 per day for 4 days with the addition of doxorubicin 50 mg/m^2 on day 1. Whether this is the optimal schedule for co-administration of fludarabine plus doxorubicin is not known at this time. The response rate was similar to fludarabine as a single agent, but a number of patients who were resistant to fludarabine responded to the combination. As doxorubicin is obviously active in low-grade and intermediate-grade lymphoma, possible interaction between the purine analogue and doxorubicin in such patient subsets would be of interest.

In low-grade lymphoma, fludarabine/mitoxanrone/dexamethasone is a well-tolerated effective regimen. Subsequently a combination study of fludarabine 30 mg/m^2 per day for 3 days with mitoxantrone 12 mg/m^2 on day 1 was conducted in CLL. The early results of this study do not suggest that there is an improvement in the response rate in the combination over fludarabine as a single agent administered for 5 days (unpublished data).

The overall results from these series of studies illustrate that in previously treated patients the response to fludarabine therapy alone or in combinations is of the order of 50% (Table 1). The response rate is lower in patients that have myelosuppression, in particular anemia, and is correlated strongly with a number of prior treatment regimens which the patient receives [2, 10, 12]. The albumin level is another major factor in predicting probability of response. Patients with low serum albumin have much lower probability of response and a higher likelihood of developing infectious complications, in particular, fatal complications. A prognostic factor analysis of risk factors for response and early death has illustrated that a combination of the hemoglobin level, number of prior treatments, and albumin is able to predict patients who have probabilities of achieving a remission varying from 13% to 74% [15]. Questions are still present as to whether the addtion of other agents to fludarabine is likely to be a benefit. The combination of fludarabine plus chlorambucil has not proven to be easily administered [16]. An intergroup study in the United States comparing fludarabine with chlorambucil and the combination of these two drugs led to early discontinuation of the combination arms because of excessive toxicity.

The results of 2-CDA in patients with CLL demonstrate that there is a similar overall response rate to that noted with fludarabine but that the CR rate appears to be less (Table 2) [18–20]. This may be related to presistent thrombocytopenia as a complication of the 2-CDA. Continued studies of this drug at lower dose levels may be of interest.

Untreated CLL

The activity of fludarabine as a single agent in previously untreated patients with CLL is striking, with approximately 80% of the patients responding and 60%–70% of these patients achieving CR [17]. However, as in the previously treated patients, the CR patients had persistent lymphoid nodules in approximately 50% of the patients so that the true CR rate is more of the order of 30%–35%. The addition of corticosteroids in similar fashion to the previously treated patients led to the same overall response rate with a somewhat lower CR rate [10]. These was no survival advantage to the addition of corticosteroids (Fig. 2), and the same conclusion can be drawn for untreated patients as previously treated, namely that corticosteroids do not add to the response rate, survival, or time-to-progression of patients with CLL and possibly increase the risk of opportunistic infections. Corticosteroid use, therefore, should be restricted to the management of the immunologic complications such as autoimmune hemolytic

Table 2. Comparison of response rates for previously treated CLL patients receiving fludarabine or 2-CDA (MDACC)

Regimen	Patients (*n*)	CR (%)	PR (%)	CR+PR (%)
Fludarabine				
Fludarabine (5-day) [2]	78	29	28	57
Fludarabine (5-day) + prednisone [10]	169	37	15	52
Weekly fludarabine [12]	46	15	9	24
Fludarabine (3-day) [13]	80	25	21	46
2-CDA				
2-CDA [18]	90	4	40	44
2-CDA [19]	18	39	28	67
2-CDA [20]	26	0	31	31

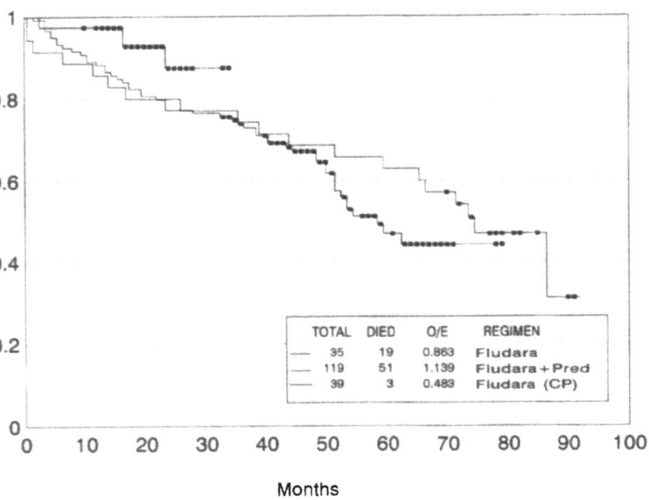

Fig. 2. Survival untreated CLL by fludarabine regimens

anemia and immunologic thrombocytopenia. Early trials of the combination of fludarabine plus mitoxantrone in previously untreated patients with CLL suggest that there is no advantage to the combination over the single-agent fludarabine results (unpublished data).

Low-Grade Lymphoma

A number of investigators have noted that fludarabine is active in low-grade lymphoma (LGL) [21–25]. This is also being found with 2-CDA [6]. The overall response rate for fludarabine in patients with previously treated relapsed or refractory LGL has demonstrated a response rate of approximately 60% with 15%–20% of patients able to achieve CR [21]. The activity of fludarabine in LGL has led to a combination program at MDACC of Fludarabine, mitoxantrone, and dexamethasone (FMD). In the phase I study the recommended dose was fludarabine 25 mg/m^2 per day for 3 days, mitoxantrone 12 mg/m^2 on day 1, and dexamethasone 40 mg per day for 5 days [26]. This combination is now being evaluated in previously untreated patients with LGL and the overall response rate is 95% in 51 previously treated patients [27]. The regimen is well tolerated. A number of patients have developed *Pneumocystis carinii* infections and Bactrim prophylaxis is now recommended if corticosteroids are to be administered. The response rate appears to be similar across all the low-grade morphologies. This study has now led to a randomized comparative trial of FMD with a series of alternating regimens (alternating triple therapy, ATT) in LGL at our institution being monitored by polymerase chain reaction (PCR) to detect residual cells with abnormalities in bcl-2. Studies such as this should lead to an evaluation of the activity of FMD in frontline or relapsed management of LGL. No reports are available of the activity of fludarabine combined with doxorubicin in LGL. The Eastern Cooperative Group has conducted a study of fludarabine plus cyclophosphamide in previously untreated patients with LGL and the results have been published in abstract form [28]. A very high response rate has been noted and the regimen appears to be well tolerated. The presumed mechanism for combinations such as this is the inhibition of repair of DNA damage caused by mitoxantrone, doxorubicin, and alkylating agents. This may lead to a synergistic cytotoxicity and a higher CR rate.

Cytosine Arabinoside in Acute Myelogenous Leukemia and Myelodysplastic Syndrome

Gandhi and colleagues [7, 29] have demonstrated that pretreatment of cell lines leads to a consistent increase in formation of the triphosphate form of cytosine arabinoside (ara-CTP). Studies in patients confirm that in almost every patient studied there will be approximately a twofold increase in formation of ara-CTP as a result of pre-administration of fludarabine [7, 29]. Two mechanisms are proposed for this effect. First, inhibition of ribonucleotide reductase leads to a decrease in deoxynucleotide pools to compete for ara-C uptake in formation. However, the major effect which has been demonstrated has been a direct stimulation of the enzyme deoxycytidine kinase by F-ara-ATP. F-ara-A and ara-C compete for deoxycytidine kinase so that the scheduling of the administration of fludarabine 4 h prior to the administration of ara-C appears to be important.

Based on these studies, a regimen combining fludarabine 30 mg/m^2 with ara-C 1–2g/m^2 given over 2–4 h as a couplet administered on 5 consecutive days has been developed [30]. The encouraging results with this regimen in poor-prognosis patients with acute myelogenous leukemia (AML) and myelodysplastic syndrome (MDS) has led to the combination of these drugs with granulocyte colony-stimulating factor (G-CSF) [31]. G-CSF has been administered 1 day prior to the chemotherapy and during the entire course of chemotherapy until patients achieve remission. This regimen (FLAG) has slightly increased the overall response rate but not to a statistically significant degree. The response rate in patients with AML and MDS is slightly superior in the FLAG-treated patients compared to the FA patients [31]. More recently idarubicin has been combined with FLAG and the overall response rate is slightly lower compared to the FLAG regimen. The subset of AML patients who were treated with these regimens are those with adverse cytogenetics and/or a myelodysplastic onset of AML. Patients with favorable karyotypes namely inv 16, t(8; 21), and t(15; 17) or diploid patients are excluded from this study. The results with this combination appear superior to our historical controls but further follow up of this approach is necessary and comparative studies need to be conducted. Similar results are noted for MDS patients.

Other Possibilities

Fludarabine has been demonstrated to be synergistic with radiation in a variety of animal model systems [32]. In addition, fludarabine inhibits the repair of DNA damage associated with alkylating agents and inhibits excision of DNA adducts formed with platinum analogues [33]. All these activities suggest that fludarabine may be used in the future in a modulatory fashion combined with a variety of chemotherapeutic agents, anthracyclines, anthraquinones, alkylating agents, irradiation, and platinum analogues. Whether these activities will translate into a higher response rate in patients with solid tumors being treated with such combinations is uncertain at the present time.

Immunosuppression

Another observation which is of interest is the consistent T cell immunosuppression associated with fludarabine and 2-CDA[34–36]. After two to three courses of treatment, the CD4 and CD8 lymphocyte subpopulations decreased to approximately 200/μl and after discontinuation of treatment there is a very slow, modest return towards normal levels in patients who have been off treatment for 12–24 months. This effect on T cell subsets without other organ toxicities suggests that purine analogues may be very effective drugs when administred as immunosuppressive agents. It has been noted that, in patients who have received purine analogues before allogeneic bone marrow transplant at our institution, there is a remarkably low incidence of graft-versus-host disease [37]. Whether this activity will be more widely applicable in other transplantation areas remains to be investigated. The oral bioavailability of fludarabine [38]and 2-CDA [39] suggest that chronic low-dose administration schedules can be explored in the future which may lead to a difference in response in hematologic malignancies and would lead to a more acceptable methodology for immunosuppressive regimens.

A combination study of fludarabine radiation has been initiated at MDACC in patients with bulky head and neck cancer who have not had CR to 5 weeks of radiation therapy. A 2-week boost of fludarabine plus radiation will be given directly to residual tumor to see if the tumor shrinks in size.

Conclusions

Purine analogues have a wide variety of biochemical and biologic activities. Not all of these are well understood at the present time. The interactions between other drugs suggest that in the future, rather than as a single agent, fludarabine will be used in a variety of combination studies. The immunosuppressive potential of the purine analogues in autoimmune disorders should be further evaluated.

References

1. Grever MR, Kopecky KJ, Coltman CA, et al.: Fludarabine monophosphate: a potentially useful agent in chronic lymphocytic leukemia. Nouv Rev Fr Hematol 30: 457–459, 1988.
2. Keating MJ, Kantarjian H, Talpaz M, et al.: Fludarabine: a new agent with major activity against chronic lymphocytic leukemia. Blood 74: 19–25, 1989.
3. Von Hoff DD: Phase I clinical trials with fludarabine phosphate. Sem Oncol 17: 33–38, 1990.
4. Piro LD, Carrera CJ, Carson DA, et al.: Lasting remissions in hairy-cell leukemia induced by a single infusion of 2-chlorodeoxyadenosine. N Engl J Med 322: 1117–1121, 1990.
5. Piro LD, Carrera CJ, Beutler E, et al.: 2-Chlorodeoxyadenosine: an effective new agent for the treatment of chronic lymphocytic leukemia. Blood 72: 1069–1073, 1988.
6. Saven A, Emanuele S, Kosty M, et al.: 2-Chlorodeoxyadenosine activity in patients with untreated, indolent non-Hodgkin's lymphoma. Blood 86: 1710–1716, 1995.
7. Plunkett W, Huang P, Gandhi V: Metabolism and action of fludarabine phosphate. Sem Oncol 17: 3–17, 1990.
8. Boldt DH, Von Hoff DD, Kuhn JG, et al.: Effects on human peripheral lymphocytes of in vivo adminstration of 9-β-D-arabinofuranosyl-2-fluoroadenine-5′-monophosphate (NSC 312887), a new purine antimetabolite. Cancer Res 44: 4661-4666, 1984.
9. Cheson BD, Bennett JM, Rai KR, et al.: Guidelines for clinical protocols for chronic lymphocytic leukemia: recommendations of the National Cancer Institute-Sponsored Working Group. Am J Hematol 29: 152–163, 1988.
10. O'Brien S, Kantarjian H, Beran M, et al.: Results of fludarabine and prednisone therapy in 264 patients with chronic lymphocytic leukemia with multivariate analysis-derived prognostic model for response in treatment. Blood 82: 1695–1700,1993.
11. Anaissie E, Kontoyiannis DP, Kantarjian H, et al.: Listeriosis in patients with chronic lymphocytic leukemia who were treated with fludarabine and prednisone. Am J Med 117: 466–469, 1992.
12. Kemena A, O'Brien S, Kantarjian H, et al.: Phase II clinical trial of fludarabine in chronic lymphocytic leukemia on a weekly low-dose schedule. Leuk Lymph 10: 187–193, 1993.
13. Robertson LE, O'Brien S, Koller C, et al.: A phase II evaluation of a three day schedule of fludarabine in chronic lymphocytic leukemia with comparison to other schedules. Leukemia, in press.
14. Robertson LE, O'Brien S, Kantarjian H, et al.: Fludarabine plus doxorubicin in previously treated chronic lymphocytic leukemia. Leukemia 9: 943–945, 1995.
15. Keating MJ, Smith TL, Lerner S, et al.: Prediction of prognosis following fludarabine therapy as secondary therapy for chronic lymphocytic leukemia. Leuk Lymph, in press.
16. Weiss M, Spiess T, Berman E, et al.: Concomitant administration of chlorambucil limits dose intensity of fludarabine in previously treated patients with chronic lymphocytic leukemia. Leukemia 8: 1290–1293, 1994.
17. Keating MJ, O'Brien S, Kantarjian H, et al.: Long-term follow-up of patients with chronic lymphocytic leukemia treated with fludarabine as a single agent. Blood 81: 2878–2884, 1993.
18. Saven A, Carrera CJ, Carson DA, et al.: 2-Chlorodeoxyadenosine treatment of refractory chronic lymphocytic leukemia. Leuk Lymph 5: 133–138, 1991.

19. Juliusson G, Liliemark J: High complete remission rate from 2'-chlor-2'-deoxyadenosine in previously treated patients with B-cell chronic lymphocytic leukemia: response predicted by rapid decrease of blood lymphocyte count. J Clin Oncol 11: 679-689, 1993.
20. Tallman MS, Hakimian D, Zanzig C, et al.: Cladribine in the treatment of relapsed or refractory chronic lymphocytic leukemia. J Clin Oncol 13: 983-988, 1995.
21. Hochster HS, Kim K, Green MD, et al.: Activity of fludarabine in previously treated non-Hodgkin's low-grade lymphoma: results of an Eastern Cooperative Oncology Group Study. J Clin Oncol 10: 28-32, 1992.
22. Redman JR, Cabanillas F, Velasquez W, et al.: Phase II trial of fludarabine phosphate in lymphoma: an effective new agent in low-grade lymphoma. J Clin Oncol 10: 790-794, 1992.
23. Whelan JS, Davis CL, Rule S, et al.: Fludarabine phosphate for the treatment of low grade lymphoid malignancy. Brit J Cancer 64: 120-123, 1991.
24. Zinzani PL, Lauria F, Rondelli D, et al.: Fludarabine: an active agent in the treatment of previously treated and untreated low-grade non-Hodgkin's lymphoma. Ann Oncol 4: 575, 1993.
25. Hiddemann W, Pott-Hoeck C: Fludarabine in the management of malignant lymphomas. Drugs 47: 50-56,1994.
26. McLaughlin P, Hagemeister FB, Swan Jr F, et al.: Phase I study of the combination of fludarabine, mitoxantrone, and dexamethasone in low-grade lymphoma. J Clin Oncol 12: 575-579, 1994.
27. McLaughlin P, Hagemeister FB, Romaguera J, et al.: Fludarabine, mitoxantrone, and dexamethasone (FMD): an effective new regimen for low grade lymphoma. J Clin Oncol, in press.
28. Hochster H, Oken M, Bennett J, et al.: Efficacy of cyclophosphamide and fludarabine as first line therapy of low-grade non-Hodgkin's lymphoma-ECOG 1491. 36th Annual Meeting of the American Society of Hematology, Nashville, TN, Dec 2-6, 1994.
29. Gandhi V, Estey E, Keating MJ, et al.: Fludarabine potentiates metabolism of cytarabine in patients with acute myelogenous leukemia during therapy. J Clin Oncol 11: 116-124, 1993.
30. Estey E, Plunkett W, Gandhi V, et al.: Fludarabine and arabinosylcytosine therapy of refractory and relapsed acute myelogenous leukemia. Leuk Lymph 9: 343-350, 1993.
31. Estey E, Thall P, Andreeff M, et al.: Use of granulocyte colony-stimulating factor before, during, and after fludarabine plus cytarabine induction therapy of newly diagnosed acute myelogenous leukemia or myelodysplastic syndromes: comparison with fludarabine plus cytarabine without granulocyte colony-stimulating factor. J Clin Oncol 12: 671-678, 1994.
32. Plunkett W, Gandhi V, Huang P, et al.: Fludarabine: pharmacokinetics, mechanisms of action, and rationales for combination therapies. Semin Oncol 20: 2-12, 1993.
33. Yang LY, Li L, Trujillo JM, et al.: Fludarabine synergizes cisplatin cytotoxicity in LoVo human colon carcinoma cells by inhibiting repair of cisplatin-induced DNA damage. Proc Amer Assoc Cancer Res 34: 347, 1993 (abstract).
34. Keating MJ: Immunosuppression with purine analogues-the flip side of the gold coin. Ann Oncol 4: 347-348, 1993.
35. Seymour JF, Kurzrock R, Freireich EJ, et al.: 2-Chlorodeoxyadenosine induces durable remissions with prolonged suppression of CD4+lymphocyte counts in patients with hairy cell leukemia. Blood 83: 2906-2911, 1994.
36. Bergmann L, Fenchel K, Jahn B, et al.: Immunosuppressive effects and clinical response of fludarabine in refractory chronic lymphocytic leukemia. Annals Oncol 4: 371-375, 1993.
37. Khouri IF, Keating MJ, Vriesendorp HM, et al.: Autologous and allogeneic bone marrow transplantation for chronic lymphocytic leukemia: preliminary results. J Clin Oncol 12: 748-758, 1994.
38. Kemena A, Keating M, Plunkett W: Oral bioavailability of plasma fludarabine and fludarabine triphosphate (F-ara-ATP) in peripheral CLL cells. Onkologie 14: 83-?, 1991b.
39. Liliemark J, Juliusson G: Cellular pharmacokinetics of 2-chloro-2'-deoxyadenosine nucleotides: comparison of intermittent and continuous intravenous and subcutaneous and oral administration in leukemia patients. Clin Cancer Res 1: 385-390, 1995.

New Strategies: Idarubicin

Acute Leukemias VI
Prognostic Factors
and Treatment Strategies
Büchner et al. (eds)

Intracellular Effects of Anthracyclines: Distribution, DNA-Binding and Genotoxicity

F. Gieseler, S. Valsamas, J. Kunze, C. Zernak, and M. Clark

Abstract. Anthracyclines are widely used in cancer therapy, but their mode of action is still not completely unveiled. These drugs have a number of intracellular effects such as direct membrane toxicity, liberation of free oxygen radicals, DNA intercalation and induction of DNA strand breaks via inhibition of topoisomerase II. In therapeutically relevant concentrations, the latter seems to be the cytotoxic principle, although neither inhibition of topoisomerase II alpha, nor the induction of strand breaks alone is sufficient for cell death. Anthracyclines are highly lipophilic and tend to accumulate several thousand -fold in leukemia cells. Even at IC_{50} concentrations, the intranuclear amount of idarubicin in HL-60 cells was well above the possible DNA intercalation sites. Within 20 min after treatment of the cell with idarubicin, the DNA was saturated. the number of DNA strand breaks increased until 3 h after treatment and was then repaired until 24 h after treatment. After treatment of the cells with idarubicin at the IC_{50} concentration the maximal amount of apoptotic cells (50%) was reached 70 h after treatment. From the experiments it can be concluded that the cellular reaction upon DNA binding and genotoxicity induced by anthracyclines plays a major role in apoptotic cell death after treatment with these drugs.

Introduction

A number of intracellular effects of anthracyclines are known, amongst them direct membrane toxicity, liberation of free oxygen radicals and genotoxicity due to inhibition of topoisomerase II. The direct membrane toxicity and the liberation of free oxygen radicals are dose-dependent effects which are thought to be responsible for side effects of chemotherapy, namely cardiotoxicity. Anthracyclines are highly lipophilic substances which accumulate in cell membranes. Especially with high plasma concentration peaks, there is a risk of acute cardiotoxcity. A number of experimental data indicate, that free oxygen radicals are responsible for the delayed cardiotoxicity [2]. Although this has been described for doxorubicin, there is no reason to believe that there are principle differences between the anthracyclines. Oxygen radicals are produced by electron transport between flavin-dehydrogenases or iron-bearing proteins, catalysed by the anthracyclines' chinolon ring system. Repetitive reduction and oxidation of anthrachinones produce oxygen radicals, especially when this happens near the sarcoplasmatic reticulum or the mitochondrial oxygen chain. The amount of free oxygen radicals in these experiments was high enough to induce tissue damage which resembles anthracycline-induced cardiotoxicity in many characteristics [2]. Myocardial cells are rich in mitochondria and, in contrast to liver or lung cells, they have poor protection against free oxygen radicals, as their peroxide-reducing capacity is solely dependent on the glutathion/glutathion-peroxidase cycle [1].

It is widely accepted that, in therapeutical concentrations, the induction of DNA strand

Medizinische Poliklinik der Universität, Klinikstr. 8, 97070 Würzburg, Germany breaks via inhibition of topoisomerase II is the cytotoxic priniciple in chemotherapy with anthracyclines. Anthracyclines intercept the topoismerase II action after induction of DNA double strand breaks [6]. One of the prerequisites for this interaction is the intercalation of the anthracycline molecules into the DNA double strands. The induced DNA strand breaks might be recognized by the cell and repaired. The interrelations between intranuclear drug concentration, DNA binding, the induction of DNA strandbreaks and cell death are the subject of the investigations described here.

Material and Methods

All used materials are commercially available. CCRF-CEM cells and HL-60 cells are from ATCC, Bethesda, Maryland. Examination of anthracycline cellular uptake and DNA binding have been described before [4]. The amount of anthracyclines in whole cells and nuclei has been determined by fluorescense analysis after extraction by HCL/isopropanole of cells or nuclei. The wavelength was 480 nm for excitation and 560–590 nm for emission. The fluorescense quenching of the AT-binder Hoechst 33342 (fluorescense resonance energy transfer, mercury lamp ex. 300–600 nm, 435 nm excitation filter) was used to examine the DNA binding of anthracyclines.

Viability of cells was determined by the use of the alamar blue substrate which alters fluorescence emission when reduced by viable cells in the same way as the widely used MTT assay. The comet assay was performed as described in the literature with the alteration that for chromatin observation no electrophoresis was applied [5]. Photographic images were scanned using an Apple One Scanner and processed using the program NIH Image on a Powerbook 180.

Results

In order to intercalate into DNA and inhibit topoisomerase II, anthracyclines have to cross the outer cell membrane, the cytoplasma, the nuclear membrane and the nucleosome. The time course of the intracellular distribution and the saturation time for the different compartments are shown in Table 1. Owing to their highly lipophilic nature, the anthracyclines could be detected in the nucleus within 10 min. after the incubation. This was also true for idarubicin, idarubicinol, as well as for daunorubicin in normal lymphocytes, promyelocytic HL-60 cells and T-lymphoblastic CCRF-CEM cells. As shown in Table 1, 33% of the intracellular idarubicin could be extracted from the nuclei of HL-60 cells.

The fluorescense energy resonance transfer between the DNA-bound Hoechst dye 33342 and the anthracycline molecule results in a shift of the fluorescence wavelength and was used to determine the DNA binding of anthracyclines. Because the DNA binding of H33342 is different in each living cell, only the relative amount of quenching by anthracyclines can be estimated using this method. The saturation time of DNA binding sites as described in Table 1 is the time in which the plateau of DNA binding is reached. Although nuclear idarubicin saturation is reached within 8 min. in HL-60 cells, 20 min. are needed to achieve the plateau of DNA binding. For daunorubicin, the DNA binding time was even 45 min.

The topoisomerase II action is inhibited by anthracyclines after the induction of a DNA double strand break. This results in the formation of the "cleavable complex" which consists of the DNA, the bound topoisomerase II and the drug [6]. After stabilization of this complex by SDS treatment and proteolytic treatment of the cells, the DNA strand breaks can be quantified

Table 1. Intracellular pharmacodynamics of idarubicin, HL-60 cells were treated with idarubicin 1,873 μM (= 1 μg/ml) which is the IC 50. The saturation amount reached in whole cells or nuclei is calculated for 10^6 cells

	Membranes and cytoplasma	Nucleus	DNA
Saturation time (min)	5	8	20
Saturation amount ($\mu M/10^6$ cells)	5124	4259	–
Distribution	77	33	–

by using the comet assay as described under Material and Methods. The assay shown in Fig. 1 demonstrated the genotoxicity induced by idarubicin under different reaction conditions.

Inspection of the nuclei without electrophoresis allows the detection of alterations in the chromatin structure, experiments of this kind are shown on the left. In panel A, the nuclei are seen directly after treatment. There is chromatin structure and a small corona can be detected; these nuclei look the same as nuclei from untreated cells. In panel C, a nucleus shown 3 h after treatment. The chromatin is compacted and a corona can be seen. This corona is thought to represent the opened chromatin loops (due to strand breaks) which are still fixed to the nuclear matrix [5]. In panel E, 48 h after treatment, an apoptotic nuclear body is shown in the uppper part and an unaltered nucleus is shown in the lower part. Remember, the cells have been treated with idarubicin, IC_{50}.

In the right column, the nuclei can be seen after electrophoresis Panel B, directly after treatment, shows a small triangled shaped tail. In

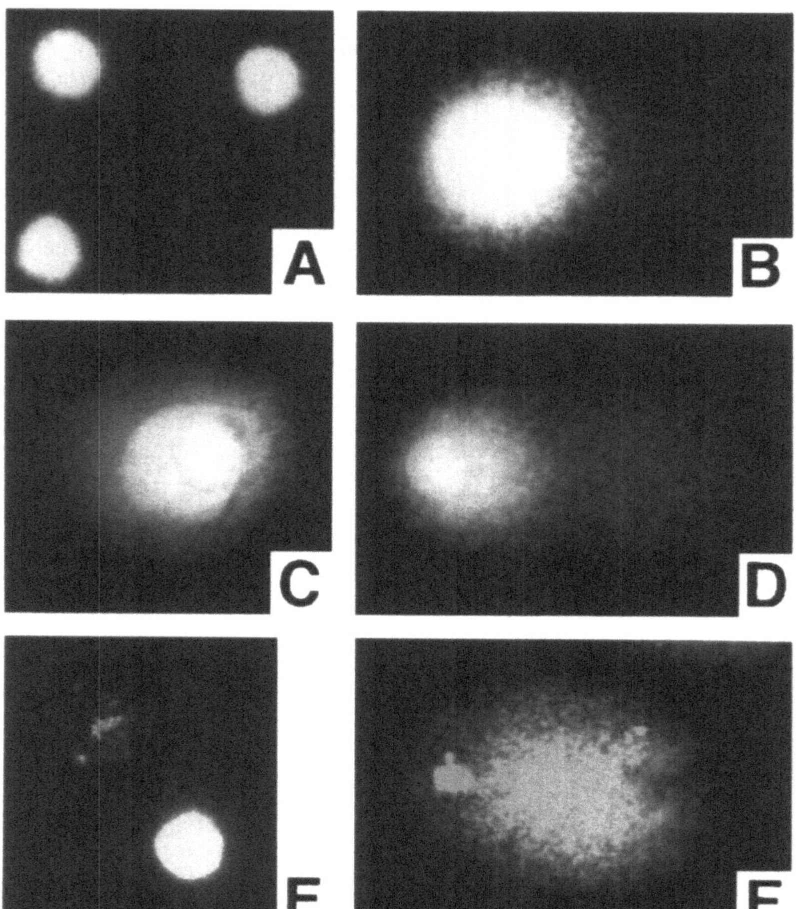

Fig. 1A–F. Comet assays of CCRF-CEM cells after treatment with idarubicin (IC_{50}, 1 µg/ml, 90 min). *Left column*, without electrophoresis; *right column*, with electrophoresis. **A, B** directly after treatment; **C** and **D**, 3 h after treatment. The experiment without electrophoresis (*left*) was performed to examine chromatin alterations upon treatment. The first alteration is chromatin condensation, approx 3 h after treatment (**C**). At this timepoint a high number of DNA strand breaks produce a long comet after electrophoresis of the nuclei (**D**)

cells treated with daunorubicin instead of idarubicin no strand breaks can be detected directly after treatment (not shown). Three hours after treatment, the highest amount of strand breaks can be detected, the comet tail is shown in panel D. A bulk of DNA can be extracted from apoptotic nuclei, as shown in panel F. At this stage, the length of the comet tail is not in good correlation with the amount of strand breaks, but the fluorescense intensity must be taken into account, e.g. with the use of the "tail moment" (length of comet X% of fluorescense in the tail) [5].

The DNA strand breaks (comet length) and the index of non-viable cells are shown in Fig. 2. The amount of non-viable cells and the comet length are displayed in relation to the untreated control. Therefore 1 means that the number of non-viable cells or the comet length is the same as in the control. Although a high number of DNA strand breaks can be observed 3 h after treatment, the viability of the cells was not altered until 12 h after treatment. Most of the early strand breaks (3 h) are repaired by the cells within 24 h. At this time point, the amount of death increases to reach a plateau at 50 h with the concentration of anthracycline used in these experiments (IC_{50}).

Discussion

Anthracyclines are highly lipophilic and these substances are gathered in high intracellular concentrations. Table 1 shows, the accumulation of idarubicin in HL60 cells. The drug has been found in the nucleus of the cells within 10 min. Obviously, the outer cell membrane, the cytoplasma and the nuclear membrane are crossed within minutes. The intracellular and even the intranuclear drug concentrations were several 1000 fold higher than the extracellular concentration was. The intranuclear drug concentration after incubation of the cells with idarubicin 1.873 μM (which represents the IC_{50}) was even higher than the theoretically existing anthracycline binding sites of a human cell: the number of DNA base pairs is about 4×10^9. The highest density of intercalated anthracyclines is one anthrycycline per ten base pairs. After multiplication with Loschmidt's number (6.02×10^{23} molecules = 1 Mol), maximally 6.7×10^{-9} *M* anthracyclines in 10^6 cells might bind to the DNA. In living cells, the number must be below this because anthracyclines can only bind where no histones cover the DNA. From these experiments it can be concluded that even at the IC_{50} concentration of idarubicin, enough drug

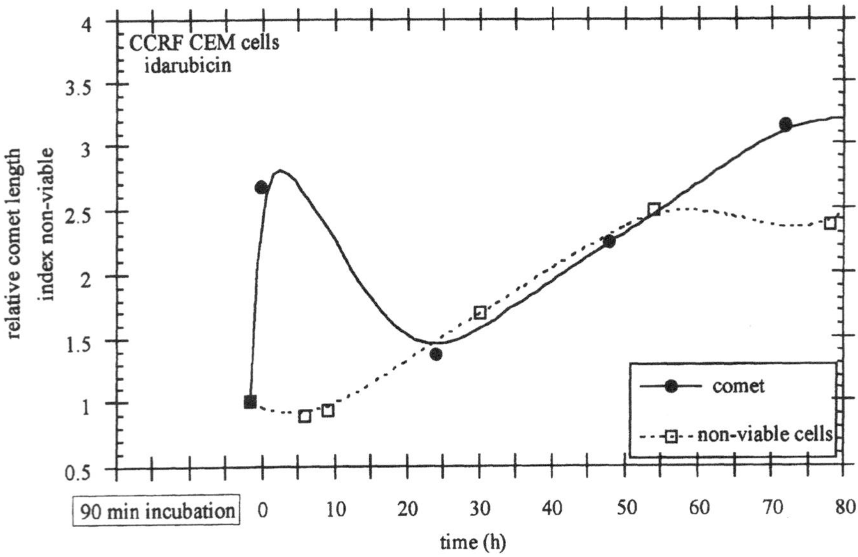

Fig. 2. DNA strand breaks and cell death after treatment with idarubicin (same conditions as in Fig. 1). Although the number of DNA strand breaks is high three h after treatment, the number of dead cells starts to increase 12 h after treatment

Table 2. Pharmacodynamic phases in the treatment of cells with anthracyclines which can be discriminated after treatment

Hour	Event	Endpoint
0-1.5	Intracellular distribution	DNA binding
1.5-3	Chromatin condensation, formation of the cleavable complex	DNA breaks
3-24	DNA repair	DNA excision
24-96	Chromatin fragmentation	DNA loss, apoptotic cell death

arrives in the nucleus to cover all possible DNA binding sites. This makes differences of the intracellular or intranuclear drug concentration as a factor for cellular sensitivity unlikely.

From the pharmaco-dynamic aspect, three different phases can be distinguished in the treatment of hematopoetic cells with anthracyclines (Table 2). After binding of the anthracyclines to the DNA, a ternary complex consisting of topoisomerase II, DNA and the drug, is formed. This complex has been called the cleavable complex (CC) because, after treatment with SDS, DNA strand breaks can be seen [3, 6]. Within this complex, the topoisomerase II is trapped after inducing DNA double or single-strand breaks, therefore not able to religate the DNA strands. Obviously the formation of the complex is not directly cytotoxic as no increase of non-viable cells can be observed before 12 h after treatment and the plateau of cell killing is not achieved before 50 h after treatment (Fig. 2).

Once the cells have recognized the DNA damage, they react in a complex manner. This reaction, under the unphysiological condition of inhibited topoisomerase II, is the final event resulting in apoptosis. The alteration of chromatin structure and induction of DNA strand breaks are shown in Fig.1. The left column shows the nuclei without electrophoresis; and the right column shows the nuclei with electrophoresis; 1-3 h after treatment, the chromatin condenses (Fig. 1C). Beginning at 24 h after treatment, chromatin fragmentation and apoptotic bodies can be observed (Fig. 1E) The amount of DNA breaks in correlation with cell death is shown in Fig. 2. Although the initial DNA strand breaks are high 3 h after treatment, virtually no loss of viability can be observed at this time point. However, in the experiments we performed with CCRF-CEM cells, the amount of strand breaks after 3 h is in good correlation with the cell killing after 72 h. Table 2 shows the time course of a treatment with anthracyclines. About 1.5 h after treatment of the cells, the intracellular distribution ends with DNA binding of the drugs. The first morphological alterations of the cells (chromatin condensation) and DNA strand breaks could be observed 1.5–3 h after treatment. Most of the DNA breaks were repaired within the first 24 h. After this time, the number of apoptotic cells increases until 70 h after treatment. Investigations of the factors which are crutial for successful treatment with anthracyclines might help to optimize chemotherapy.

References

1. Dorshow JH, Akman S, F.F.C, Esworthy S. Role of gluthatione—gluthatione peroxidase cycle in the cytotoxicity of anticancer quinones. Pharmmacol Ther 1990; 47: 359–370
2. Dorshow JH, Locker GY, Meaers CE. Enzymatic defenses in the mouse heart against reactive oxygen metabolites: alterations produced by doxorubicin. J Clin Invest 1980; 65: 128–135
3. Gale KC, Osheroff N. Uncoupling the DNA cleavage and religation activities of topoisomerase II with a single-stranded nucleic acid substrate: evidence for an active enzyme cleaved DNA intermediate. Biochemistry 1990; 29: 9538–9545
4. Gieseler F, Biersack H, Brieden T, Manderscheid J, Nüßler V. Cytotoxicity of anthracyclines: correlation with cellular uptake, intracellular distribution and DNA-binding. Ann. Hematol. 1994; 69 (Suppl. 1): S13–S17
5. McKelvey-Martin VJ, Green MH, Schnezer P, Pool-Zobel BL, De Meo MP, Collins A. The single gel electrophoresis assay (comet assay): a European review. Mut Res 1993; 288: 47–63
6. Robinson MJ, Corbett AH, Osheroff N. Effects of topoisomerase II-targeted drugs on enzyme-mediated DNA cleavage and ATP hydrolysis: evidence for distinct drug interaction domains on topoisomerase II. Biochemistry 1993; 32: 3638–43

Acute Leukemias VI
Prognostic Factors
and Treatment Strategies
Büchner et al. (eds)

Specific Role of Idarubicin During Induction Therapy of Childhood Acute Myeloblastic Leukemia

J. Ritter, U. Creutzig, and M. Zimmermann for the Cooperative Childhood AML-BFM Study Group[a]

Abstract. The combination of an anthracycline and cytosine arabinoside (ara-C) is considered standard therapy for remission induction in acute myeloblastic leukemia (AML). Recently, (4-demethoxydaunorubicin idarubicin, IDA) has been found to be active in AML in adults. Furthermore, the therapeutic index of IDA may be higher than that of daunorubicin (DNR) regarding cardiotoxicity—a major problem, especially in children. Thus, one aim of study AML-BFM-93 was to compare IDA with DNR during induction treatment of childhood AML in a randomized trial. From January 1, 1993 to May 31, 1994, 51 children with newly diagnosed AML received 3 × 12 mg/m^2 IDA together with ara-C and etoposide (AIE) for remission induction treatment. All children received further intensification/consolidation chemotherapy followed by cranial irradiation and maintenance chemotherapy for a total treatment duration of 18 months.

51 evaluable children 38 developed fever during bone marrow aplasia. No severe liver or kidney toxicity (WHO grade > II) was found in 51 evaluable children. The median time to recovery of the neutrophil count in 23 evaluable children was 26 days. Thirty-seven children achieved a complete remission (CR rate 73%)

These preliminary data of the ongoing study show that IDA can be used for remission induction treatment in childhood AML. So far, no significant differences have been found between the IDA and the DNR groups concerning toxic deaths, non response, and remission rate. However, further follow up of this study is necessary.

Introduction

Results of treatment of childhood acute myeloblastic leukemia (AML) have shown significant improvement during the last 20 years. Recently, the administration of intensive induction, consolidation, intensification, and maintenance therapy together with an appropriate CNS-directed treatment and with appropriate supportive care have resulted in remission rates of 70%–80% and produced significant cure rates of more than 50% of all children coming in complete remission (CR) [1].

Intensive remission induction treatment in children as in adults, consists of a combination

University Children's Hospital, Albert-Schweitzer-Str. 33, 48129 Münster, Germany
[a]Participating Members:
R. Mertens (Aachen); A. Gnekow (Augsburg); R. Dickerhoff (St. Augustin); G.F. Wündisch (Bayreuth); G.Henze (Berlin); U. Bode (Bonn); H.-J. Spaar/T Lieber (Bremen); W. Eberl (Braunschweig); I. Meyer (Datteln); U. Göbel (Düsseldorf); J.D. Beck (Erlangen); B. Kornhuber (Frankfurt); M. Lakomek (Göttingen); F. Lampert/R. Blütters-Sawatzki (Gieβen); H. Winkler/G. Janka-Schaub (Hamburg); K. Debatin/B. Selle (Heidelberg); H. Riehm/P. Weinel (Hannover); N. Graf/M. Müller (Homburg/Saar); G. Nessler (Karlsruhe); T. Wehinger (Kassel); M. Rister (Koblenz); F. Berthold (Koln-Univ.); W. Sternschulte (Köln); R. Schneppenheim (Kiel); P. Bucsky (Lübeck); O. Sauer (Mannheim); P. Gutjahr (Mainz); R. Eschenbach (Marburg); W. Müller (Mönchengladbach); R.J. Haas (München); St. Müller-Weihrich (München-Schwabing); C. Bender-Götze (München-Univ.); P. Klose (Müchen-Harlaching); A. Jobke (Nürnberg-Cnopfsche); U. Schwarzer (Nürnberg/Städt.-Kinderklinik); J. Treuner (Stuttgart); D. Niethammer/H. Scheel-Walter (Tübingen); W. Hartmann† (Ulm); J. Kühl (Würzburg).

of an anthracycline together with cytosine arabinoside (ara-C) and a third drug—mainly 6-thioguanine or etoposide.

Idarubicin, an anthracycline derived from daunorubicin, was synthesized in an attempt to find new analogs with an improved spectrum of activity and diminished acute or chronic toxicity, as compared to daunorubicin [2]. Recently, idarubicin has been found to be at least as effective as daunorubicin as an induction regimen in newly diagnosed AML in adults [3–5]. Furthermore, the therapeutic index of idarubicin may be higher than that of daunorubicin regarding cardiotoxicity—a major problem especially in children [6]. Thus, one aim of study AML-BFM-93 was to compare idarubicin with daunorubicin during induction treatment of childhood AML in a randomized trial. The preliminary results of children treated with idarubicin of this ongoing trial are presented.

Patients and Methods

From January 1, 1993 until May 31, 1994, a total of 51 consecutive, previously untreated patients < 17 years of age were enrolled in the idarubicin arm of the cooperative study AML-BFM-93.

Patient characteristics and disribution to the different French-American-British Group (FAB) subtypes are shown in Table 1.

The treatment protocol of study AML-BFM-93 evolved from studies AML-BFM-83 and -87[7], the outline of this protocol is shown in Fig. 1. All patients were initially, randomized to receive either ADE ara-C 100 mg/m^2 per day continuous infusion for 2 days followed by 30 min infusion every 12 h on days 3–8, daunorubicin 30 mg/m^2 30 min, infusion every 12 h on dcsyd 3,4,5 and VP-16 150 mg/m^2 60 min infusion on days 6,7,8) or AIE (idarubicin 12 mg/m^2 30 min infusion every 24 h on days 3,4,5 instead of daunorubicine). Further treatment consisted of consolidation therapy with seven drugs and intensification with high-dose ara-C together with VP-16 in standard-risk patients, whereas high-risk patients were randomized to receive

Table 1. Patient characteristics—AML-BFM-93 —AIE induction (diagnosed January 1993 - June 1994)

Total (*n*)		51
Boys (*n*)		24
Girls (*n*)		27
Age (range)		3 months–16 years
Median (years)		7
White blood cell count - Range		1.600–438.000/µl
Median		23.650/µl
FAB	MO	4
	M1	4
	M2	14
	M3	2
	M4	9
	M5	13
	M6	1
	M7	4

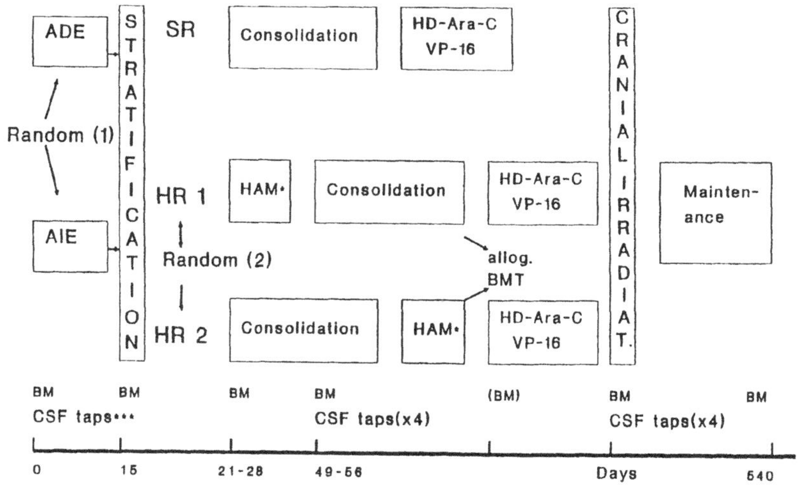

Fig. 1. Treatment plan of study AML-BFM-93 (*HAM*, HD-draC/mitoxantrone)

either high-dose ara-C together with mintoxantrone, followed by consolidation and intensification (HR1) or consolidation followed by high-dose ara-C together with mintoxantrone and intensification with HD-ara-C plus VP-16 (HR2). All children in remission received cranial irradiation together with 4 intrathecal doses of ara-C followed by maintenance treatment of a total duration of 18 months.

Results

The outcome of remission induction therapy of the first 51 children in the AIE branch are shown in Table 2. Three children died within the first 6 weeks in bone marrow aplasia. Eleven children were nonresponders. Of the 51 children 37 (73%) attained CR. So far, six children have relapsed on treatment, whereas 31 children are still in continuous CR, four of them after allogeneic bone marrow transplantation.

Toxicity after AIE induction is shown in Table 3. No severe liver or kidney toxicity (WHO grade > II) was found in 49 evaluable children. One child developed severe cardiotoxicity (WHO grade III) on day 21 with *Streptococcus viridans* septicemia, which was reversible after treatment with digoxin, steroids, and diuretica. This child is still in remission after 18 months of further treatment with complete recovery of cardiac function. A total of 38 children developed fever during bone marrow aplasia, eight of them with clinical and radiological signs of penumonia. The median time to recovery of the neutrophil count in 31 evaluable children was 26 days (range 13–34 days). In 42 evaluable patients, bone marrow blasts on day 15 after the beginning of AIE were ≤5% in 32 children and > 5% in ten children.

Table 2. Preliminary treatment results—AML-BFM-93 AIE induction (diagnosed 1993 - 1994)

Patients	(*n*)51
Early deaths	3
Nonresponders	11
CR	37
Relapses	6
In continuous CR	31[a]

[a] (Four after allogeneic bone marrow transplantation)

Table 3. Toxicity after AIE induction

Patients	(*n*) 51
Liver	0
Renal	0
Cardiotoxicity	1 (WHO III)
Skin reaction	1 (WHO III)
Infection	38

Discussion

Three previous studies in adults with newly diagnosed ANL showed superior CR rates in idarubicin-containing regimens as compared to daunorubicin, Berman et al. [3] described a CR rate of 48 of 60 (80%) adults in the idarubicin-containing arm compared to 35 of 60 (58%) patients, $p = .005$, in the daunorubicin-containing arm. Wiernik et al.[5] described a CR in 68/97 (70%) patients in the idarubicin-containing arm, as compared to 65/111 (59%; $p = .08$) in the daunorubicin-containing arm. The difference in CR rates was significant in patients aged 18–50 years ($p = .035$). Vogler et al.[4] described CR rates in 75 of 105 (71%) on the idarubicin arm compared to 65 of 113 (58%; p=.03) in the daunorubicin arm.

Experiences with idarubicin with AML are scarce. Sackman-Mauriel et al.[8] used idarubicin instead of daunorubicin in the induction phase in a clinical trial similar to protocol AML-BFM-87[9]. Thirth-six patients under the age of 21 were treated at seven cancer centers. Of the 36 33 (91.7%) patients in this noncomparative study went in to CR after a mean duration of treatment of 33.6 days (range 22–63 days).

The preliminary data of the ongoing study of AML-BFM-93 show that idarubicin can be used for remission induction treatment in childhood AML. The main toxicity was fever in severe bone marrow aplasia. So far, no severe liver or kidney toxicity has been observed in the first 51 children. One child developed severe cardiotoxicity 21 days after induction during septicemia in bone marrow aplasia, which was completely reversible. So far, no significant differences have been found between the idarubicin-and the daunorubicin-containing arms concerning toxic death, nonresponders and remission rate in this ongoing study. Further patient accrual and longer follow up are obviously required to evaluate the specific role of idarubicin during induction therapy in childhoold AML.

Acknowledgment. This work was supported by the Deutsche Krebshilfe.

References

1. Hurwitz CA, Mounce KG, Grier HE (1995) Treatment of patients with acute myelogenous leukemia: review of clinical trials of the past decade. J Pediatr Hematol Oncol, 17: 185–197.
2. Arcamone F, Bernardi L, Giardini P, et al. (1976) Synthesis and antitumor activity of 4-demethoxyc-daunorubicin, 4-demethoxy-7-9-diepidaunorubicin and their anomers. Cancer Res 60: 829–834.
3. Berman E, Heller G, Santorsa J, et al. (1991) Results of a randomized trial comparing idarubicin and cytosine arabinoside with daunorubicin and cytosine arabinoside in adult patients with newly diagnosed acute myelogenous leukemia. Blood 77: 1666–1674.
4. Vogler WR, Velez-Gracia E, Weiner RS, Flaum MA, Bartolucci AA, Omura GA, Gerber MC, Banks PLC (1992) A phase III trial comparing idarubicin and daunorubicin in combination with cytarabine in Acute myelogenous leukemia: a Southeastern Cancer Study Group. JCO 10:1103–1111
Ref ID : 828
5. Wiernik PH, Banks PLC, Case DC, Jr., Arlin ZA, Perlman PO, Todd MB, Ritch PS, Enck RE, Weitberg AB (1992) Cytarabine plus idarubicin or daunorubicin as induction and consolidation therapy for previously untreated adult patients with acute myeloid leukemia. Blood 79: 313–319.
6. Ganzina F, Pacciarini MA, De Pietro N (1986) Idarubicin (4-demethoxydaunorubicin). A preliminary review of preclinical and clinical studies. Invest New Drugs 4: 85–105.
7. Ritter J, Creutzig U, Schellong G (1992) Treatment results of three consecutive German childhood AML trials: BFM-78, -83, and -87. Leukemia 6: 59–62.
8. Sackmann-Muriel F, Fernandez-Barbieri MA, Santarelli MT, Matus-Ridley M, Rosso A, Negri-Aranguren P, Cerutti I, Gomel M, Kvicala R (1993) Results of treatment with an intensive combination induction regimen containing idarubicinin children with acute myeloblastic leukemia: preliminary report of the Argentine Group for treatment of acute leukemia. Semin Oncol 20: 34–38.
9. Creutzig U, Ritter J, Zimmermann M, Schellong G, for the AML-BFM Study Group (1993) Does cranial irradiation reduce the risk for bone marrow relapse in acute myelogenous leukemia (AML): unexpected results of the childhood AML Study BFM-87. J Clin Oncol 11: 279–286.

Acute Leukemias VI
Prognostic Factors
and Treatment Strategies
Büchner et al. (eds)

Overview of Current Treatment for Acute Myeloid Leukemia

P.H. Wiernik

Abstract. Idarubicin is a more active anthracycline than daunorubicin for induction therapy of acute myeloid leukemia (AML). A cytarabine-based postremission regimen, bone marrow transplantation, or a combination of the two approaches improve disease-free survival and enhances the cure rate in this disease. Combinations of all-trans-retinoic acid and induction chemotherapy and superior to either approach alone in acute promyelocytic leukemia (APL). Yeast-derived rhGM-CSF given during induction theraphy improves the safety of that therapy and enhances outcome in elderly patients with AML.

Introduction

The purpose of this paper is to provide an overview of certain aspects acute myeloid leukemia (AML) therapy and to draw conclusions of a general nature whenever possible.

Materials and Methods

Published literature on induction and postremission therapy of AML were reviewed and, whenever possible, reported results were updated by personal communication.

Results

Induction Therapy

One of the most interesting recent studies of induction therapy for AML was published by the Australian Leukemia Study Group approximately 5 years ago [1]. That study compared induction therapy with a standard dose and schedule of cytarabine and daunorubicin with an identical regimen to which etoposide was added. The complete response rate was similar after the two treatments but the triple-drug regimen yielded a significantly longer disease-free and overall survival in patients under the age of 55 years and those differences have persisted (J.F. Bishop, personal communication, 1995). No significant differences in outcome were observed in older patients. The study is important for two reasons. First, it demonstrates clearly that a manipulation during induction therapy can favorably affect remission duration and survival. It further suggests that, as more effective treatments are developed, cure may be obtained with induction therapy alone without postremission treatment. The lack of efficacy of postremission therapy has been clearly demonstrated in other hematologic malignancies for which substantially effective induction theraphy has been developed, such as advanced Hodgkin's disease and diffuse large-cell lymphoma. Secondly, the Australian study demonstrates the difficulty in making meaningful therapeutic observations in elderly patients which can be readily observed in younger patients. This latter point should not be interpreted to mean that older patients should not be studied, but the study of a therapeutic intervention in elderly patients alone may not allow for the observation of a modest step forward presumably because of the myriad of comorbidities that plague the elderly in most cases.

Albert Einstein Cancer Center and Montefiore Medical Center, Bronx, New York, USA

The late Zalmen Arlin compared a standard cytarabine and daunorubicin regimen with a similar regimen in which daunorubicin was replaced by mitoxantrone [2]. There were no significant differences in outcome between the two induction regimens, wich argues for the equivalency of daunorubicin and mitoxantrone. More recently, Pavlovsky et al. [3] conducted a study of identical design and reported virtually identical results. There are no published comparisons of idarubicin and mitoxantrone combined with cytarabine for induction therapy of newly diagnosed patients with AML. However, the Eastern Cooperative Oncology Group (ECOG) has recently embarked on a study (E3993) in which elderly AML patients are randomized to receive induction therapy with cytarabine and daunorubicin, mitoxantrone, or idarubicin along with a growth factor or a placebo. No results are available from that study at this date.

The combination of cytarabine, mitoxantrone, and etoposide has been a popular induction therapy for relapsed or refractory patients with AML, especially in Europe [4]. Unfortunately, there are no prospective comparative trials from wich one could assess the merits of this regimen relative to others. The situation is reminiscent of the previous acceptance on anecdotal grounds of the superiority of high-dose cytarabine plus amsacrine [5] until a prospective comparative study by the Southwest Oncology Group (SWOG) demonstrated no advantage for the addition of amsacrine to high-dose cytarabine [6].

There are a number of randomized induction therapy trials in which a combination of cytarabine and daunorubicin (A+D) was compared with cytarabine and idarubicin (A+I), and all have shown an advantage for the latter combination over the former. Berman et al. [7], in a single-institution study for patients with AML under the age of 60 years, reported a significantly greater complete response rate, remission duration, and survival in patients treated with A+I compared with those treated with A+D, and a recent unpublished update of that study demonstrates that those significant differences continue to be observed (E.Berman, personal communication, 1995). In a multicenter study of similar design [8] those same differences in outcome were observed in younger patients (under the age of 60 years) but not in older patients. A recent unpublished update of that study also demonstrates that those outcome differences have been maintained (Fig. 1).

In a Southeast Oncology Group study (SEG) of similar induction therapy design [9], the complete response rate with A+I was significantly greater than that with A+D. The postremission protocol in that study incorporated a test of late intensification with A+I or A+D, depending upon the patient's initial induction therapy. A recent update of the study demonstrates no difference in disease-free or overall survival with respect to induction therapy. However, remission duration is significantly longer in patients who received late intensification compared with patients who did not, and those patients who were given A+I during induction and late inten-

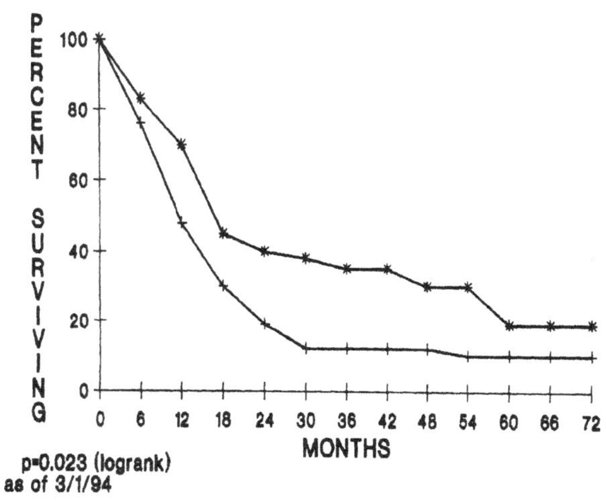

Fig. 1. Updated overall survival data (age 60 or less) from the study by Wiernik et al. [8] Asterisks, A+1; crosses, D+A

sification phases of the protocol had significantly longer disease-free (and overall) survival than any other group of patients (E. Velez-Garcia, personal communication, 1995). Finally, the GIMEMA group studied A+I vs. A+D as induction therapy in elderly patients [10]. There was no difference in response rate or duration, or overall survival between the two treatment groups, as might be expected from the results obtained in elderly patients by Bishop et al. [1] and in the multicenter study described above [8], but a significantly greater number of patients achieved a complete response with one course of A+I than with one A+D course in the GIMEMA study. This observation was also made in the Berman [7] and multicenter study [8] but not in the SEG study [9].

These studies all demonstrate the superiority of idarubicin over daunorubicin in combination with cytarabine as induction therapy for AML, especially in patients under the age of 60 years, and this clinical observation is supported by a number of laboratory investigations that demonstrate more favorable pharmacokinetics for idarubicin than daunorubicin [11] and less interference of *p*-glycoprotein with idarubicin activity than with that of daunorubicin [12–14]. The presence of *p*-glycoprotein on the surface of leukemic cells from patients with de novo AML has repeatedly been demonstrated to impair response to A+D [15–17].

Turning now to acute promyelocytic leukemia (APL), there is general agreement that a major limitation on the effectiveness of all-trans-retinoic acid in this leukemia is the clinical pharmacokinetics of the agent. Trans-retinoic acid induces its own catabolism, presumably by a cytochrome P-450 mechanism [18]. Schwartz et al. [19] have demonstrated that fluconazole, an inhibitor of P-450, inhibits the in vitro catabolism of all-trans-retinoic acid have recently demonstrated the same in patients with APL. However, whether fluconazole inhibition of all-trans-retinoic acid catabolism can translate into more effective antileukemic activity remains to be studied. At the present time, optimal therapy for APL appears to be initial therapy with all-trans-retinoic acid followed by chemotherapy with an anthracycline plus cytarabine, as first demonstrated by Fenaux et al. [18], who reported a 96% complete response rate and a substantial fraction of durable remissions with this approach. Although the French used daunorubicin in these studies, idarubicin may be a better choice, since Berman [21] demonstrated that the latter is significantly more active than the former in APL, as it is in AML in general.

Postremission Therapy

There is considerable debate about the most effective post remission therapy for patients with AML. A number of studies suggest equivalent long-term survival for patients undergoing bone marrow transplantation or chemotherapy alone. However, none of those studies analyzes outcome with respect to major prognostic factors such as karyotype and immunophenotype. A current intergroup study conducted by ECOG (EST 3489) will provide information on the relative merits of autologous and allogeneic bone marrow transplantation, and chemotherapy alone in patients who have been characterized by immunophenotype and karyotype. The results of that study may provide a basis for selection of one option over another for a specific AML patient in the future.

It is possible to draw broad conclusions about the relative merits of a number of programs employing chemotherapy alone as post`remission therapy for AML and, in my view, no clearly superior treatment has emerged. Figure 2 includes a number of curves that represent the best-published results with certain regimens that have recently attracted interest. The Cancer and Leukemia Group B (CALGB) curve represents that group's data on high-dose Cytosine arabinoside (ara-C), 3 gm/m^2 every 12 h for 6 days for patients under the age of 45 years, followed by daunorubicin and standard-dose

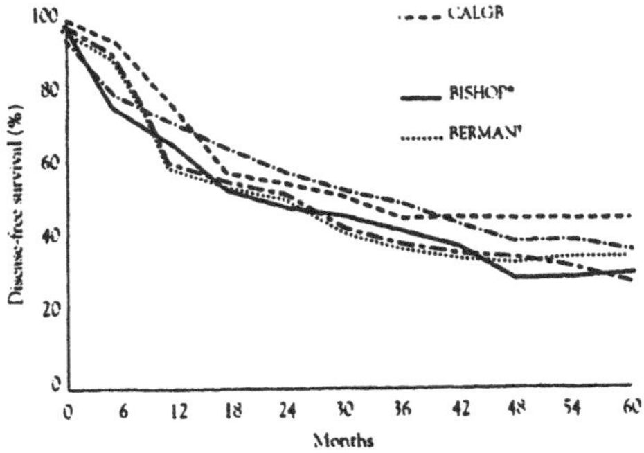

Fig. 2. A comparison of selected published postremission treatments for adults with AML. See text for details

cytarabine [22]. The Schiller curve represents a similar approach with high-dose cytarabine alone [23]. The Bishop curve represents the Australian results in patients up to the age of 55 years in whom cytarabine, daunorubicin, and etoposide were given as induction therapy, and followed by less intensive but more prolonged postremission therapy than the studies represented in the first two curves [1]. Ther Berman curve represents the Memorial study of induction therapy with cytarabine and idarubicin, followed by short-term administration of truncated induction courses after remission in a group of adult patients 60 years old or younger [7]. The Wiernik curve represents a study begun in 1978 at the National Cancer Institute Baltimore Cancer Research Center in which patients with a median age of 47 years and a range in age of 14–72 years were induced with cytarabine and daunorubicin and then treated with cytarabine and thioguanine in short intensive courses every 3 months for 3 years [24, 25]. This curve represents the oldest patients with the longest follow up in this figure. A reasonable interpretation of these curves is that they are not different one from another. They cannot be statistically analyzed, however, because they do not represent a prospective, randomized comparison. The figure suggests that there are several options available that will achieve what would currently be accepted as optimal long-term results: a) improve induction therapy (Bishop and Berman curves); b) provide short-term, intensive post-remission therapy (CALGB and Schiller curves); or c) provide long-term less intensive postremission therapy (Wiernik curve). Options a. and c. are available to patients of all ages, while option b. is too toxic for patients beyond middle age. There is no evidence from other studies that combining options improves outcome.

Second Remission Therapy

There is little doubt that bone marrow transplantation can offer long-term disease-free survival to patients in second remission [26]. However, for a variety of reasons [27], these procedures are not available to a large number of patients who might benefit from them. Therefore, it is appropriate to study other methods of potential cure for patients in second remission. The ECOG study randomized patients in second remission to receive low-dose cytarabine or no treatment, and the treatment arm was associated with a significantly longer second remission duration [28]. That study proved that chemotherapy during second remission was beneficial. biological response modifiers have recently been studied in second remission alone or in conjuction with other modalities. Some small studies of interleukin-2 (IL-2), for instance, given either alone [29, 30] or in conjuction with autologous bone marrow transplantation [31] have given results that were provocative enough to lead to prospective intergroup studies that are nearing implementation.

Supportive Care

Two recently completed studies asked whether granulocyte-macrophage colony-stimulating factor (GM-CSF) given soon after the completion of induction therapy for AML in elderly patients would improve hematologic recovery to a clinically significant degree. The ECOG study utilized yeast-derived GM-CSF and CALGB studied *Escherichia coli*-derived GM-CSF. In both studies the growth factor was compared with a placebo. Both studies have been published only in abstract form to date [32, 33]. There was no evidence from either study that the administration of GM-CSF was detrimental in the setting in which it was studied, which is important because of the concern in some quarters that such a growth factor might stimulate the leukemic clone. In the ECOG study, patients receiving the growth factor had significantly more rapid recovery of the peripheral granulocyte count and significantly fewer infections. However, in the CALGB study the outcome with growth factor or placebo was similar. possible explanations for these dissimilar results are the different sources of the recombinant growth factor, different chemotherapy doses in the two studies, and the somewhat different age groups studied. Further study will clearly be necessary to resolve the true role, if any, for GM-CSF in this setting.

Discussion

Much progress has been made in the treatment of adults with AML. Complete remission is obtained in at least 75% of all patients, and a fraction of responders, perhaps as large as 30%, is apparently cured with currently available methodology. The induction regimen of idarubicin and cytarabine has proven superior to daunorubicin and cytarabine regimens in all prospective, randomized studies. Studies in which mitoxantrone and daunorubicin in combination with cytarabine were compared have yielded equivalent results for those treatments. Combination of all-trans-retinoic acid and standard chemotherapy appear to be optimal induction therapy for APL. Whether cytarabine adds to the activity of anthracylines in APL as it does in other French-American-British Group (FAB) types is debatable. Yeast-derived rhGM-CSF, given after marrow hypoplasia is obtained during induction therapy, facilitates therapy and improves outcome in elderly patients with AML. Postremission regimens based on cytarabine clearly improve disease-free survival, although the optimal dose of that agent has not yet been determined. The relative merits of bone marrow transplantation and chemotherapy alone for postremission treatment continue to be debated, but currently ongoing trials are likely to identify the best available approach to various AML subtypes. Certain immunologic agents, such as IL-2, are under evaluation in patients in second remission, and early reports suggest that they may have activity in that setting. Although studies designed to optimize treatment with currently available agents are important, the most likely future accomplishments to significantly further improve results in AML are discoveries of new active agents against the disease.

References

1. Bishop JF, Lowenthal RM, Joshua D, et al.: Etoposide inacute nonlymphocytic leukemia. Blood 75: 27-32, 1990.
2. Arlin Z, Case Jr DC, Moore J, et al.: Randomized-multicenter trial of cytosine arabinoside with mitoxantrone or daunorubicin in previously untreated adult patients with acute nonlymphocytic leukemia (ANLL). Leukemia 4: 177-183, 1990.
3. Pavlovsky S, Gonzalez Llaven J, Garcia Martinez MA, et al.: A randomized study of mitoxantrone-plus cytarabine versus daunomycin plus cytarabine in the treatment of previously untreated adult patients with acute nonlymphocytic leukemia. Ann Hematol 69: 11-15, 1994.
4. Archimbaud E, Fenaux P, Reiffers J, et al.: Granulocyte-macrophage colony-stimulating factor inassociation totimed-sequential chemotherapy with mitoxantrone, etoposide, and cytarabine for refractory acute myelogenous leukemia. Leukemia 7: 372-377, 1993.
5. Arlin ZA, Ahmed T, Mittelman A, et al.: A new regimen of amsacrine with high-dose cytarabine is safe and effective therapy for acute leukemia. J Clin Oncol 5: 371-375, 1987.
6. Karanes C, Kopecky KJ, Durie BGM, et al.: Increasedrisk of earlydeathwith high dose ara-C (HDAC) and m-AMSA compared to HDAC alone or HDAC and mitoxantrone in high risknonlymphocytic leukemia. Proc Am Soc Clin Oncol 8: 201, 1989.
7. Berman E, Heller G, Santorsa J, et al.: Results of a randomized trial comparing idarubicin and cytosine arabinoside with daunorubicin and cytosine arabinoside in adult patients with newly diagnosed acute myelogenous leukemia. Blood 77: 1666-1674, 1991.
8. Wiernik PH, Banks PLC, Case Jr DC, et al.: Cytarabine plus idarubicin or daunorubicin as induction and consolidation therapy for previously untreated patients with acute myeloid leukemia. Blood 79: 313-319, 1992.
9. Vogler WR, Velez-Garcia E, Weiner RS, et al.: A phase III trial comparing idarubicin and daunorubicin in combination with cytarabine in acute myelogenous leukemia: a Southeastern Cancer Study Group study. J Clin Oncol 10: 1-9, 1992.
10. Mandelli F, Petti MC, Ardia A, et al.: A randomised clinical trial comparing idarubicin and cytarabine to daunorubicin and cytarabine in the treatment of acute non-lymphoid leukaemia. Eur J Cancer 27: 750-755, 1991.
11. Robert J, Rigal-Huguet F, Hurteloup P: Comparative pharmacokinetic study of idarubicin and daunorubicin in leukemia patients. Hematol Oncol 10: 111-116, 1992.
12. Berman E, McBride M: Comparative cellular pharmacology of daunorubicin and idarubicin-in human multi-drugresistant cells. Blood 79: 3267-3273, 1992.
13. Muller MR, Lennartz K, Boogen C, et al.: Cytotoxicity of adriamycin, idarubicin, and vincristine in acute myeloid leukemia: chemosensitization by verapamil in relation to P-glycoprotein expression. Ann Hematol 65: 206-212, 1992.
14. Petrini M, Mattii L, Valentini P, et al.: Idarubicin is active on mdr cells: evaluation of DNA synthesis inhibition on P388 cell lines. Ann Hematol 67: 227-230, 1993.
15. Zhou D-C, Marie J-P, Suberville A-M: Relevance of mdrlgene expression in acute myeloid leukemia and comparison ofdifferent diagnostic methods. Leukemia 6: 879-885, 1992.
16. Gsur A, Zochbauer S, Gotzl M, et al.: MDRI RNA expression as a prognostic factor in acute myeloid leukemia: an update. Leukemia & Lymphoma 12: 91-94, 1993.
17. Miwa H, Kita K, Nishii K, et al.: Expression of mdrl gene in acute leukemia cells: association with CD7+acute myeloblastic leukemia/acute lymphoblastic leukemia. Blood 82: 3445-3451, 1993.
18. Muindi JRF, Frankel SR, Huselton C, et al.: Clinical pharmacology of oral all-trans retinoic acid in patients with acute promyelocytic leukemia. Cancer Res 52: 2138-2142, 1992.

19. Schwartz EL, Hallam S, Gallagher RE, et al: Inhibition of all-trans retinoic acid metabolism by fluconazole in vitro and in a patient with acute promyelocytic leukemia. Proc Am Soc Clin Oncol, in press, 1995.
20. Fenaux P, Castaigne S, Dombret H, et al.: All-transretinoic acid followed by intensive chemotherapy gives a high complete remission rate and may prolong remissions in newly diagnosed acute promyelocytic leukemia: a pilot study on 26 cases. Blood 80: 2176–2181, 1992.
21. Berman E: A review of idarubicin in acute leukemia.Oncology 7: 91–107, 1993.
22. Mayer RJ, Davis RB, Schiffer CA, et al.: Intensive postremission chemotherapy in adults with acute myeloid leukemia. N Engl J Med 331: 896–903, 1994.
23. Schiller G, Gajewski J, Territo M, et al: Long-term outcome of high-dose cytarabine-based consolidation chemotherapy for adults with acute myelogenous leukemia. Blood 80: 2977–2982, 1992.
24. Dutcher JP, Wiernik PH, Markus S, et al.: Intensive maintenance therapy improves survival in adult acute nonlymphocytic leukemia: an eight-year follow-up. Leukemia 2: 413–419, 1988.
25. Dutcher JP, Wiernik PH, Markus S, et al.: Fifteen-year follow-up of adult patients with acute myeloid leukemia(AML): study BCRC 7802. Proc XXV Cong Intl Soc Hematol, 1994 (abstract no.48)
26. Spinolo JA, Dicke KA, Horwitz LJ, et al.: High-dose chemotherapy and unpurged autologous bone-marrow transplantation for acute leukemia in second or subsequent remission. Cancer 66: 619–626, 1990.
27. Berman E, Little C, Gee T, et al.: Reasons that patients with acute myelogenous leukemia do not undergo allogeneic bone marrow transplantation. N Engl J Med 326: 156–160, 1992.
28. Oken MM, Kim K, Mazza JJ, et al.: Maintenance low-dose ara-C improves complete remission duration from salvage induction therapy for relapsed and refractory acute myeloid leukemia. Proc Am Soc Clin Oncol 10: 220, 1991.
29. Wiernik PH, Dutcher JP, Todd M, et al.: Polyethylene glycolated interleukin-2 as maintenance therapy for acute myelogenous leukemia in second remission. Am J Hematol 47: 41–44, 1994.
30. Bergmann L, Heil G, Kolbe K, et al.: Interleukin-2 bolus infusion as late consolidation therapy in 2nd remission of acute myeloblastic leukemia. Leukemia & Lymphoma 16: 271–280, 1995.
31. Benyunes M, Higuchi C, Lindgren C, et al.: IL-2 +LAK cell therapy after autologous BMT (ABMT) for hematologic malignancies. Blood 78 (suppl 1): 246a, 1991.
32. Rowe JM, Andersen J, Mazza JJ, et al.: PhaseIII randomized place bo-controlled study of granulocyte-macrophage colony stimulating factor (GM-CSF) in adult patients (55–70 years) with acute myelogenous leukemia (AML). A study of the Eastern Cooperative Oncology Group (ECOG). Blood 82 (suppl 1): 329a, 1993.
33. Stone R, George S, Berg D, et al.: GM-CSF `v' placebo during remission induction for patients > – 60 years old with denovo acute myeloid leukemia: CALGB study # 8923. Proc Am Soc Clin Oncol 13: 304, 1994.

Acute Leukemias VI
Prognostic Factors
and Treatment Strategies
Büchner et al. (eds)

Chemotherapy for Acute Myeloid Leukemia: the State of the Art and the Contribution of Idarubicin

T. Büchner

The trends in modern chemotherapy for AML are best exemplified by the multicenter randomized trials listed in Table 1. In these trials a total of 7554 patients have been treated. The overall complete remission rate is 63% and the 5-year relapse-free survival rate is 21%. A certain chronological trend can be seen in that 5-year remission rates in excess of 25% are found only in publications from the 1990. The same, however, is true for mortality in remission of 10% and more, indicating the limits of the generally increasing treatment intensity. The table shows the trials or treatment arms within trials in order of the intensity of chemotherapy in the induction, consolidation and maintenance phases. Intensification appears as a determinant of outcome in that 5-year remission rates of 30% and over are produced only by intensified consolidation or induction regimens [9, 13–15]. The role of maintenance as a determinant of outcome is underlined in that reduced maintenance [6, 8, 10] or no maintenance after standard consolidation [3] resulted in low 5-year remission rates. On the other hand, the effect of maintenance may be replaced by that of intensified consolidation [9, 10, 15].

The results of an inter-study comparative analysis can only be an approximation, since different trials used different selection criteria regarding age and exclusion of patients in remission.

The trials cited randomly compared different drugs or strategies, and significant differences between alternatives compared were found in seven trials. Thus, differences in the CR rate were in favor of aclarupicin vs (dounorubicin) as part of induction treatment [9]. idarubicin(IDR) vs DNR [12], and DNR full dose vs half dose [13]. Differences in CR duration were in favor of cytosine arabinoside (AraC) infusion vs bolus in induction [1], AraC s.c. vs i.v. maintenance[1], chemotherapy vs Bacillus Calmette Guerain (BCG) in maintenance [2], maintenance vs no maintenance [3], and AraC high dose vs standard dose in postremission therapy (14). Improved cure rates of 35%–40% in younger patients resulted from regimens using high-dose AraC in induction [13] or postremission treatment [9,14].

IDR has been compared with DNR in three multicenter trials [3,8,9] and a single-center trial [17]. IDR has produced superior CR rates in three trials (Table 2), with no long-term results published so far (Table 3).

In conclusion Among anthracyclines different drugs and dosages may affect the CR rate, with advantages for IDR over intermediate-dose DNR. For cure, high-dose AraC appears to play a leading role.

References

1. Rai RR, J.F. Holland, O.J. Glidewell et al.: Treatment of acute myelocytic leukemia: a study by Cancer and Leukemia Group B. Blood 58 (1981) 1203–1212
2. Vogler WR, E.F. Winton, D.S. Gordon et al.: A randomized comparison of postremission therapy in acute myelogenous leukemia: a Southeastern Cancer Study Group trial. Blood 63 (1984) 1039–1045

University of Münster, Germany

Table 1. Chemotherapy intensity and outcome in multicenter randomized trials

Study	Ref. no.	Therapy intensity			Complete remission	Five years disease-free survival	Mortality in remission	Positive selection	
		Induction	Consolidation	Maintenance				Age (years)	exclusions in remission
CALGB 87	6	++		+	56%	12%	9%		
CALGB 91	8	++		+	61%	10%	3%		
ECOG 92	10	++		+	68%	16%	0	15–65	Yes
CALGB 81	1	++		++	53%	22%	?	0–83	Yes
AMLCG 85	3	++	++		59%	6%	2%		Yes
SECSG 84	2	++	++	+	66%	10%	3%		Yes
EORTC 86	5	++	++	+	64%	17%	?	10–65	Yes
DSHSG 91	9	++	+++		58%	35%	10%	17–65	
ECOG 92	10	++	+++		68%	27%	21%	15–65	Yes
EORTC 95	15	++	+++		66%	30%	22%	11–59	Yes
AMLCG 85	3	++	++	++	59%	25%	5%		Yes
BMRC 86	4	++	++	++	67%	18%	?	0–83	
GIMEMA 92	11	++	++	++	68%	24%	10%	15–55	
SECSG 92	12	++	++	++	71%	19%	23%		
CALGB 94	14	++	++	++	64%	22%	3%		Yes
EORTC 89	7	++	++	+++	67%	23%	4%	10–65	Yes
AMLCG 92	13	+++	++	++	62%	30%	6%		
CAIGB 94	14	++	+++	++	64%	37%	5%		Yes

+ Reduced intensity; ++ intensity as in standard treatment; +++ intensive chemotherapy

Table 2. Effects of idarubicin versus daunorubicin on response to induction treatment

Source	Induction	Dosage (mg/m²)	Age (years)	No. of Patients	CR rate	*P*
Berman		IDR 12			80	
et al. 791 [17]	5+3	IDR 50	16–60	120	58%	0.005
Mandelli		IDR 12			40%	
et al. 791 [15]	7+3	DNR 45	58–78	249	39%	
Wiernik		IDR 13			70%	
et al. 792 [16]	7+3	DNR 45	18→60	208	59%	0.08
Vogler		IDR 12			71%	
et al. 792 [12]	7+3	DNR 45	15→60	218	58%	0.3

Table 3. Effects of idarubicin versus daunorubicin on long-term results

Source	Remission therapy	Arm	Age (years)	Relapse-free Survivial median 2-3 years	
				months	
Berman		IDR			
et al. 791 [17]	5+3 × 2	DNR	16–60	–	–
Mandelli		IDR		12	22%
et al. 791 [15]	5+5+2 × 4,5+5 × 6	DNR	58–78	12	22%
Wiernik		IDR		9	35%
et al. 792 [16]	5+3 × 2	DNR	18→60	8	6%
Vogler		IDR		14	22%
et al. 792 [12]	5+1 × 3,4+2 × 4	DNR	15→60	11	15%

3. Büchner T, D. Urbanitz, W. Hiddemann et al: Intensified induction and consolidation with or without maintenance chemotherapy for acute myeloid leukemia (AML): two multicenter studies of the German AML Cooperative Group. J Clin Oncol 3 (1985) 1583–1589
4. Rees JKH, R.G. Gray, D. Swirsky et al: Principal results of the Medical Research Council's 8th acute myeloid leukaemia trial. The Lancet 29 (1986) 1236–1241
5. Hayat M, U. Jehn, R. Willemze et al: A randomized comparison of maintenance treatment with androgens, immunotherapy, and chemotherapy in adult acute myelogenous leukemia. Cancer 58 (1986) 617–623
6. Preisler H, R.B. Davis, J. Kirshner et al: Comparison of three remission induction regimens and two postinduction strategies for the treatment of acute nonlymphocytic leukemia: a Cancer and Leukemia Group B study. Blood 69 (1987) 1441–1449
7. Zittoun R, U. Jehn, D. Fiere et al: Alternating v repeated postremission treatment in adult acute myelogenous leukemia: a randomized phase III study (AML6) of the EORTC Leukemia Cooperative Group. Blood 73 (1989) 896–906
8. Dillmann RO, R.B. Davis, M.R. Green et al: A comparitive study of two different doses of cytarabine for acute myeloid leukemia: a phase III trial of Cancer and Leukemia Group B. Blood 78 (1991) 2520–2526
9. Hansen OP, J. Pedersen-Bjergaard, J. Ellegaard et al: Aclarubicin plus cytosine arabinoside versus daunorubicin plus cytosine arabinoside in previously untreated patients with acute myeloid leukemia: a Danish national phase III trial. Leukemia 5 (1991) 510–516
10. Cassileth PA, E. Lynch, J.D. Hines et al: Varying intensity of postremission therapy in acute myeloid leukemia. Blood 79 (1992) 1924–1930
11. Mandelli F, M.L. Vegna, G. Avvisati et al: A randomized study of the efficacy of postconsolidation therapy in adult acute nonlymphocytic leukemia: a report of the Italian Cooperative Group GIMEMA. Ann Hematol 64 (1992) 166–172
12. Vogler WR, E. Velez-Garcia, R.S. Weiner et al: A phase III trial comparing idarubicin and daunorubicin in combination with cytarabine in acute myelogenous leukemia: a Southeastern Cancer Study Group study. J Clin Oncol 10 (1992) 1103–1111
13. Büchner T, W. Hiddemann, G. Löffler et al: Improved cure rate by very early intensification combined with prolonged maintenance chemotherapy in patients with acute myeloid leukemia: Data from the AML Cooperative Group. Sem Hematol 28 (1991) 76–69
14. Mayer R.J, R.S. Davis, C.A. Schiffer et al: Intensive postremission chemotherapy in adults with

acute myeloid leukemia. N Engl J Med 6 (1994) 896–942
15. Mandelli F, M.C. Petti, E. Arida et al: A randomised clinical trial comparing idarubicin und cytarabine to daunorubicin and cytarabine in the treatment of acute nonlymphoid leukaemia. Eur J Cancer 27 (1991) 750–755
16. Wiernik PH, P.L.C. Banks, D.C. Case et al: Cytarabine plus idarubicin or daunorubicin as induction and consolidation therapy for previously untreated adult patients with acute myeloid leukemia. Blood 79 (1992) 313-319
17. Berman C, G. Heller, J.A. Santorsa et al: Results of a randomized trial comparing idarubicin and cytosine arabinoside with daunorubicin and cytosine arabinoside in adult patients with newly diagnosed acute myelogenous leukemia. Blood 77 (1991) 1666–1674

Acute Leukemias VI
Prognostic Factors
and Treatment Strategies
Büchner et al. (eds)

Phase II Trial of Idarubicin, Fludarabine, Cytosine Arabinoside and Filgrastim (G-CSF) for Treatment of Refractory, Relapsed, and Secondary Acute Myeloid Leukemia

H.T. Steinmetz[1], M. Schwonzen[1], A. Glasmacher[2], P. Staib[1], I. Katay[1], A. Neufang[1], A. Schulz[1], V. Diehl[1], and P.D. Wickramanayake[1]

Abstract. The combination of fludarabine and cytosine arabinoside (ara-C) with a simultaneous infusion of granulocyte colony-stimulating factor (G-CSF; FLAG) is an effective chemotherapy to induce remission in poor-prognosis acute myeloid leukemia (AML) [5]. We started a phase II trial adding idarubicin to FLAG (Ida-FLAG) in order to improve the response rate and its duration. Patients refractory to or with first relapse after standard chemotherapy and patients with secondary AML, a history of myelodysplasia or signs of trillineage dysplasia at diagnosis (MDS-AML) were included. Ida-FLAG consisted of idarubicin 8 mg/m^2 on days 1,3,5; fludarabine 25 mg/m^2 1 h i.v. on days1–5; ara-C 1000 mg/m^2 1 h i.v. every 12h on days 1–5; and Filgrastim 400 $\mu g/m^2$ continuous infusion from day O until recovery of absolute neutrophil count (ANC) > 1000/µl.

A total of 35 patients were included within the first 12 months of study. Nine patients (seven male, two female) with refractory AML had a median age of 48 years (range 22–68 years), eight patients (three male, five female) with AML in first relapse had a median age of 59 years (range 30–75 years) and 18 patients (12 male and six female) with secondary AML or MDS-AML had a median age of 56 years (range 45–67 years). Thirty-four patients were evaluable for response after a first course of ida-FLAG. Complete remission (CR) was achieved in 21 patients (62%) overall, in one of nine patients (11%) with refractory AML, in seven of eight patients (87%) with relapsed AML, and in 13 of 17 patients (76%) with MDS-AML. Seven patients (21%) died within 28 days from severe infection. Toxicity was evaluated in 27 patients surviving the first course of ida-FLAG. The median of the duration of G-CSF infusion was 24.5 days (range 17-66 days), of white blood cell count (WBC) < 3000/µl 20 days (range 11–44 days), of WBC < 500/µl 17 days (range 6–31 days), of ANC < 1500/µl 20 days (range 11–37 days), of ANC < 500/µl 18 days (range 9–31 days), of platelets < 50 000/µl 24 days (range 13–68 days) and, of days with fever > 38 °C 4 days (range 1–33 days).

Idarubicin-FLAG is a well-tolerated chemotherapy which induces a high rate of CR in patients with relapsed or secondary AML. It is too early to comment on the duration of response and surivival. The toxicity should be monitored carefully especially in the second cycle. It may be warranted and worthwhile to compare the efficacy of ida-FLAG with other protocols for secondary or relapsed AML.

Introduction

Recently it has been demonstrated that a treatment of acute myeloid leukemia (AML) blasts with fludarabine followed by cytarabine (ara-C) enhances the intracellular concentration of ara-C triphosphate (ara-CTP) resulting in an improved ara-C cytotoxicity [6]. The active triphosphate of fludarabine could be increased by preincubation of blasts with granulocyte colony-stimulating factor(G-CSF) [5]. In addition, G-CSF given prior to chemotherapy possi-

[1]First Department of Internal Medicine, University Hospital, 50924 Köln, Germany
[2]First Department of Internal Medicine, University Hospital, Bonn, Germany

bly recruits blasts into the cell cycle [1, 4]. This "priming" may enhance cytotoxicity too. G-CSF given after chemotherapy reduces the time of granulocytopenia and the rate of infections [9]. Based on this in vitro evidence and clinical studies, the fludarabine ara-C-G-CSF (FLAG) regimen has been given to patients with high-risk AML and has been proven to be effective [5, 12].

Idarubicin has shown some evidence for a more potent activity against AML than other anthracyclines [2,11,13]. Moreover, there are some experimental data demonstrating a synergistic efficialy of idarubicin and G-CSF by enhanced expression of DNA topoisomerase II in leukemic cells [10].

In order to improve the effectivity of the FLAG regimen we added idarubicin (Ida-FLAG) and started a phase II study in patients with high-risk AML to evaluate the response rate, duration of response, and toxicity of Ida-FLAG.

Patients and Methods

The AML was diagnosed from bone marrow smears by cytomorphological and cytochemical criteria. The subgroup of AML were classified according to the French-American-British Group (FAB) classification. Patients refractory to (REF-AML) or with a first relapse (1R-AML) after standard induction therapy were eligible. Standard therapy for patients with age <60 years was TAD-HAM chemotherapy according to the study of the AML Cooperative Group (AMLCG, Prof. Büchner, Münster, Germany) and for patients >60 years a combination of aclarubicine mg/m^2 on days 1–4, etoposide (VP-16, 100 mg/m^2 on days 1–3), and cytarabine (100 mg/m^2 every 12 h on days 1–7 (AVA-7).

Patients with an AML secondary to a myeloproliferative disorder and patients with a history of a myelodysplasia according to the FAB classification or with a trilineage myelodysplasia (TMD) at initial diagnosis of AML (MDS-AML) were included as a third group. The age of patients had to be > 18 years. Written informed consent had to be obtained. Exclusion criteria were a history of an allergic reaction to one of the study drugs or a severe concomitant disease, judged as contraindication against any intensive chemotherapy.

From January 1994 until January 1995 35 patients with AML entered the study: 13 female and 22 male with a medium age of 56 years range 22–75 years.Characterisitcs of patients and subgroups of AML according to the FAB classification are given in Table 1. Ida-FLAG therapy consisted of idarubicin 8 mg/m^2 on days 1,3,5; fludarabine 25 mg/m^2 1h-v-i.v on days 1–5; ara-C 1000 mg/m^2 every 12 h 1 h iv on days 1–5; and filgrastim 400 µg/m^2 continuous infusion on day 0 until recovery of ANC > 1000/µl. All patients received selective oral antibiotic prophylaxis and in case of fever an antibiotic thera-

Table 1. Characteristics of 35 patients included from January 15th 1994 to January 15th 1995

	Refractory AML (n = 9)		Frist relapse AML (n = 8)		MDS-AML (n = 18)		Total (n = 35)
Sex							
Male (n)	7		3		12		22
Female (n)	2		5		6		13
Age							
Median (years)	48		59		56		56
Range (years)	22–68		30–75		32–71		22–75
FAB classification	M0	2	M1	1	MDS	9	
	M2	2	M2	4	TMD	5	
	M4	1	M4	2	Sec. AML	4	
	M5	1	M6	1			
	M7	2					
	MDS	1					
Karyogram							
Normal	–		1		5		6
Aberration	6		2		7		15
Not determined	3		5		6		14

MDS, history of MDS at diagnosis of AML; TMD, trilineage myelodysplasia at diagnosis, sec. AML, history of myeloproliferative disease at diagnosis.

py according to the criteria of the PEG-II trial [8]. Bone marrow aspiration was performed between days 9–11 and after recovery of hematopoiesis but at least between days 28 and 35.

In case of a complete remission (CR) a second-cycle Ida-FLAG was recommended after a rest of 2–4 weeks. In case of a partial response (PR, significant reduction of blasts in bone marrow, but more than 5%) a second cycle Ida-FLAG could be given. An allogeneic bone marrow transplantation with a related or unrelated donor was recommended if possible for all patients with CR or PR.

Results

Response. After the first 12 months of study 34/35 patients were evaluable for response after the first cycle of Ida-FLAG. CR was achieved in 21 patients (62%) overall. Three patients had a significant reduction of blasts, three had a persistence of blasts in bone marrow and seven patients (21%) died within the first 28 days. Cause of death was a severe infection in all cases. The response after the first cycle with regard to the subgroups is shown in Table 2. Thirteen patients (one with IR-AML, 12 with MDS-AML) received a second cycle of Ida-FLAG for consolidation.

Survival and Duration of Response. One patient with refractory disease after TAD-HAM who achieved a CR after Ida-FLAG is in continuous CR (cCR) after 20 weeks without further therapy. Another refractory patient with a history of chronic myelomonocytemic leukemia (MDS-CMMoL), treated without success with AVA-7 and TAD-9 before, achieved a significant reduction of blasts. After 22 weeks AML relapsed. He was treated again with Ida-FLAG off study and achieved a nearly complete reduction of blasts once more. From the seven CR patients with 1R AML, one is in cCR after 35 weeks (duration of first remission after TAD-HAM =10 months). The other six patients had a relapse (duration of remission: 32, 29, 24, 13, 13, 6 weeks). One 30-year-old lady refractory to TAD-HAM achieved a 10-month lasting first CR with FLAG; 6 weeks after achieving the second CR with Ida-FLAG she relapsed and was successfully transplanted with the bone marrow of an unrelated donor. Thirteen patients with MDS-AML achieved CR, of whom 12 received a second cycle Ida-FLAg. Three patients died due to infectious complications within 28 days after consolidation therapy. Four patients are in cCR (29+, 27+, 26+, 24+ weeks). Two patients died with signs of myelodysplasia but without evidence for a relapse of AML. Three patients are receiving consolidation therapy now. General survival from beginning of Ida-FLAG therapy, the event-free survival, and the duration of remission are shown in Table 3.

Toxicity. Alopecia was common, nausea and vomiting could be sufficiently controlled, and relevant mucositis was a rare event. Hematological toxicity was comparable to other high-dose therapies. The median of the duration of G-CSF infusion was 24.5 days (range 17–66 days) in 27 survivors of the first cycle. The duration of leukocytopenia, a white blood cell count (WBC) <500/μl or <3000/μl, was a median 17 days range 6–31 days and 20 days range 17–66 days respectively. Granulocytopenia, ANC< 500/μl or <1500/μl, was a median 18 days range 9–31 days and 20 days range 11–37 days respectively. Hematological toxicity with regard to the subgroups is shown in Table 4. The MDS-AML patients, who received Ida-FLAG as a first high-dose chemotherapy, had a shorter duration of aplasis than the pretreated patients with refractory or relapsed AML. All patients had a fever > 38 °C mostly classified as fever of unknown origin (with negative culture results and without evidence for a focus)) (Table 5). Until now the rate of atypical infections has not increased. In

Table 2. Efficacy of the first cycle of Ida-FLAG

	Refractory AML ($n=9$)		First relapse AML ($n=8$)		MDS-AML ($n=17$)		Total ($n=34$)	
	(n)	(%)	(n)	(%)	(n)	(%)	(n)	(%)
CR	1	11	7	87	13	76	21	62
No remission	5	56	-		1	6	6	17
Early death	3	33	1	12	3	18	7	21

Table 3. Response to Ida-FLAG, survival, event-free survival, and duration of remission. Evaluation after 12 months of study

	No.	Response to first cycle	Ida-FLAB for olidation	Survival from Ist day of therapy (weeks)	Event free survival[a] (weeks)	Duration of complete remission (weeks)	Comments
REF-	1	PR	–	54+	6		
-AML	2	ED	–	3	3	–	
	3	ED	–	4	4	–	
	4	PD	–	30	5	–	
	5	ED	–	4	4	–	
	6	PD	–	24+	4	–	
	7	PD	–	5	4	–	
	8	CR	–	20+	20+	16+	
	9	PD	–	11	5	–	
IR-	1	CR	–	51+	37	32	
-AML	2	CR	+	50+	29	24	
	3	CR	–	–	–	13	
	4	ED	–	3	3	–	
	5	CR	–	48+	9	5	
	6	CR	–	36+	9	6	Allogencic BMT, week 11
	7	CR	–	35+	35+	29+	
	8	CR	–	17	1	13	
MDS-	1	CR	+	36	23	18	Death in bone marrow aplasia, no blasts
-AML	2	CR	+	34	22	18	
	3	CR	+	33+	33+	29+	
	4	CR	+	32+	32+	27+	
	5	CR	+	13	13	9	Septic death during second cycle
	6	CR	+	30+	30+	26+	
	7	CR	–	29+	29+	25+	
	8	CR	+	28+	28+	24+	
	9	CR	+	11	11	6	Septic death during second cycle
	10	ED	–	4	4	–	
	11	PR	–	–	–	-	Lost to follow up
	12	CR	+	9	9	5	Septic death during second cycle
	13	ED	–	3	3	–	
	14	ED	–	3	3	–	Blastycrisis of CML
	15	CR	+	11+	10	5	Relapse with start of second cycle
	16	CR	+	9+	9+	3+	
	17	CR	+	5+	5+	1+	
	18	n.d.	–	4+	4+	–	

[a]Events: no remission, relapse, death.

general Ida-FLAG was well tolerated in this group of high-risk patients. In the second cycle of Ida-FLAG the median duration of G-CSF infusion was 27.5 days (range 21–33 days), of WBC $< 500/\mu l$ 21 days (range 11–29 days), and of ANC $< 500/\mu l$ 21 days (range 12–31 days). In four of seven evaluable patients who surivived the second cycle the time until recovery of hematopoiesis was longer than in the first course, in three it was shorter.

Discussion

This is a very preliminary evaluation of a phase II trial in high-risk patients with AML. However,

Table 4. Hematological toxicity in survivors of the first cycle Ida-FLAG

	Refractory AML ($n=6$)		First relapse AML ($n=7$)		MDS-AML ($n=14$)		Total ($n=27$)	
	Median days	Range days	Median days	Range days	Median days	Range days	Median days	Range days
G-CSF infusion	27	23–30	29	17–66	22.5	18–39	24.5	17–66
WBC								
< 500/µl	18.5	12–22	19	6–31	14.5	12.24	17	6–31
< 3000/µl	24	15–28	24	11–44	18	15–35	20	11–44
ANC								
< 500/µl	21.5	12–25	19	9–31	16	12–26	18	9–31
< 1500/µl	24	14–25	22	1–37	17.5	14.34	20	11–37
Platelets								
< 50000/µl	25.5	21.38	30	13–68	22.5	17–42	24	13–68
Transfusion								
Erythrocytes	9	2–20	6	0–22	8	4–18	8	0–22
Platelets	8	1–13	5	2–19	6	3–12	6	1–19

Table 5. Days with fever, i.v. antibiotics, and hospitalization in survivors of the first cycle Ida-FLAG

	Refractory AML ($n=6$)		First relapse AML ($n=7$)		MDS-AML ($n=14$)		Total ($n=27$)	
	Median days	Range days	Median days	Range days	Median days	Range days	Median days	Range days
Temp. > 38 °C	9	2–15	4	1–33	4	1–12	4	1–33
Antibiotics (i.v.)	25.5	21–29	21	9–39	12.5	7.25	15	7–39
In hospital[a]	31	30–39	36.5	19–68	26.5	21–42	29	19–68

[a] Until discharge in patients with CR or evidence of persistence of leukemia (end of study) in non-responders.

the Ida-FLAG regimen seems to be a very effective combination to induce a CR in patients with relapsed or secondary AML. As a consequence of the different subgroups of patients with different risks of death of relapse the number of patients will be enlarged for the final assessment of effectivity.

It is very early to comment on the preliminary evaluation of survival and remission duration. Neverthless, it is our impression that it may be warranted and worthwhile to compare the efficacy of Ida-FLAG with other protocols for relapsed AML, in particular since there is no gold standard of second line therapy for relapsed patients. Patients with secondary or MDS-AML have a specialty high risk for relapse after conventional induction [3,7]. Therefore, new strategies such as Ida-FLAG may be beneficial and should be compared to standard induction. Despite some benefits in the group of refractory patients, the rescue therapy in this group remains an unsolved problem.

The toxicity of one-cycle Ida-FLAG is moderate and the subjective tolerance very good. Until now there is no evidence for an increase of atypical infections. However with regard to three septic deaths in 13 patients treated with a second cycle, the infectious toxicity and immunological deficiencies should be monitored in detail. The impairment of the lymphatic system by fludarabine possibly induces a higher incidence of severe and rapidly fatal infections. The relative importance of each single drug in the Ida-FLAG regimen is only supported by experimental data and has not been proven by clinical evidence until now. Therefore, the repeated application of Ida-FLAG and the value of each drug should be tested in comparative studies.

References

1. Baer M, Bernstein SH, Brunetto VI, Mindermann H, Rustum Y, Block AW, Mrocek K, Bloomfield CD, Herzig CD (1993) In vivo recombinant human G-CSF priming in previously untreated acute myeloid leukemia. Blood, 22(10): 328a, Abstract
2. Berman E, Heller G, Santorsa JA, McKenzie S, Gee T, Kempin S, Gulati S, Andreeff M, Kolitz J, Gabrilove J, Reich L, Mayer K, Keefe D, Trainor, Schluger A, Pennenberg D, Raymond V, O'Reilly R, Jhanwar S, Young C, Clarkson B (1991) Results of a randomized trial comparing idarubicin and cytosine arabinoside with daunorubicin and cytosine arabinoside in adult patients with newly diagnosed acute myelogenous leukemia. Blood 77(8): 1666ff
3. Büchner T, Hiddemann W, Wörmann B, Heinecke A, Sauerland MC, Fonatsch C, Becher R, Hossfeld D, Goasguen J, Löffler H, Schaefer UW (1993) Factors determining therapeutic outcome in patients with AML. Blood 22(10):192a, Abstract 754
4. Drach J. Pereira-Leahy JM, Sanchez-Williams G, Dunne C, Zhao S, Liu Y, Estey E, Andreeff M (1992) Treatment with G-CSF, fludarabine and aRA-C (FLAG) of poor prognosis AML and MDS: biological effects and response. Blood 80 Suppl.1:448a Abstract 1782
5. Estey E, Gandi V, Keating M, Plunkett W (1993) G-CSF potentiates clinical and pharmakcokinetic responses to fludarabine and aRA-C in AML and MDS. Proc ASCO 12:301, Abstract 986
6. Gandhi V, Estey E, Keating MJ, Plunkett W (1993) Fludarabine potentiates metabolism of cytarabine in patients with acute myelogenous leukemia during therapy. J Clin Oncol 11: 116–124
7. Kuriyama K. Tomonaga M, Matsuko T, Kobayashi T, Miwa H, Shirakawa S, Tanimoto M, Adachi K, Emi N, et al. (1994) Poor response to intensive chemotherapy in de novo acute myeloid leukaemia with trillineage myelodysplasia. Br J Haematol 86: 767–773
8. Meyer P, Adam D, Hiddemann W, Link H, Maschmeyer G, Helmerking M (1992) Interventionstherapie von Infektionen und Fieber unklarer Genese bei neutropenischen Patienten mit malignen hämatologischen Grunderkrankungen. Zeitschrift für antimikrobielle antineoplastische Chemotherapie 10: 1–27
9. Ohno R., et al. (1990) Effect of G-CSF after intensive induction therapy in relapsed or refractory acute leukemia. N Eng J Med 323(13): 871–877
10. Towatari M, Ito Y, Morishita Y, Tanimota M, Kawashima K, Morishima Y, Andoh T, Saito H (1990) Enhanced expression of DNA topoisomerase II by recombinant human G-CSF in human leukemia cells. Cancer Res 50: 7198–7202
11. Vogler W, Velz-Garcia E, Weiner RS, Flaum MA, Bartolucci AA, Omura GA, Gerber MC, Banks PLC (1992) A phase III trial comparing idarubicin and daunorubicin in combination with cytarabine in acute myelogenous leukemia: Southeastern Cancer Study Group study. J Clin Oncol 10(7): 1103ff
12. Wickramanayake PD, Rumpsfeld M, Karayl I, Sieg K, Rüffer U, Schulz A, Steinmetz T, Diehl V (1994) Treatment with filgratsim (G-CSF), fludarabine and ara-C (FLAG) is effective to induce remission in AML refractory or relapsed to TAD-HAM induction. Ann Hematol 68: A33, Abstract 130
13. Wiernik O, Banks PLC, Case Dc, Arlin ZA, Periman PO, Todd MB, Ritch PS, Enck RE, Weitberg AB (1992) Cytarabine plus idarubicin or daunorubicin as induction and consolidation therapy for previously untreated adult patients with acute myeloid leukemia. Blood 79(2): 313f

New Strategies Using Growth Factors: G-CSF

Acute Leukemias VI
Prognostic Factors
and Treatment Strategies
Büchner et al. (eds)

Mechanisms of Regulated Drug Sensitivity

E.A. McCulloch

Abstract. Regulated drug sensitivity (RDS) is defined as the influence of growth regulators on the drug sensitivity of cancer cells measured in culture. The blast stem cells of acute myeloblastic leukemia (AML) provide a suitable model system. Myelopoietic growth factors, all-trans-retinoic acid (ATRA) and hydrocortisone (HC) have been found to alter some drug dose-response curves, with degree and direction of effect often schedule dependent. GM-CSF and HC were found to protect AML blasts against cytosine arabinoside (ara-C) killing; G-CSF increased sensitivity. ATRA regularly increased sensitivity only if given after the drug. Regulator-mediated change in cell cycle parameters was a potential mechanism for RDS. Measurements using high specific activity tritiated thymidine (^{3}HTdR) to identify stem cells in the S phase provided evidence against this attractive hypothesis. We compared RDS using different drugs. Unlike ara-C, anthracycline sensitivity was changed by ATRA or HC but not by growth factors. Thus, a single mechanism is unlikely to explain RDS. We asked if the protooncogene bcl-2, known to influence apoptosis, was part of the RDS mechanism. We found that bcl-2 was down-regulated by retinoic acid. Bcl-2 has an anti-oxidant effect. Exogenous H_2O_2 is metabolized to produce free radicals; we asked if sensitivity to H_2O_2 was regulated. We found that ATRA after H_2O_2 increased killing, while HC before H_2O_2 was protective. We asked whether N-acetylcysteine (NAC), a potent radical scavenger, would alter drug sensitivity. We found that NAC before agent provided partial protection against the lethal effects of both ara-C and H_2O_2. We concluded that ara-C, in addition to direct killing following incorporation into DNA, causes the production of toxic free radicals. ATRA may sensitize and HC protect through mechanisms that influence the outcome of damage by free radicals. The control network that regulates intracellular redox is complex and includes members of the bcl-2 family and cytochromes; the network provides many targets, permitting drug sensitivity to be regulated by more than one mechanism.

Introduction

Chemotherapy is the major treatment available for patients with disseminated malignancies. Leukemia is a valuable example since the disease is widespread when first diagnosed and often responds to treatment with drugs. Unfortunately, in adults, the disease usually recurs and then is less responsive to therapy. These features of leukemia make it a suitable site in which to seek for mechanisms of drug response and resistance. Further, malignant leukemic cells can easily and safely be obtained as single-cell suspensions for laboratory studies. The development of cell culture methods, now often combined with molecular techniques, makes it possible to evaluate the biological characteristics of leukemic cells; interactions with drugs can also be examined in some detail.

This paper contains an account of studies in which the blast cells from the peripheral blood

The Ontario Cancer Institute/Princess Margaret Hospital, 500 Sherbourne St., Toronto, Canada M4X 1K9

of patients with acute myeloblastic leukemia (AML) were examined in cell culture in order to observe interactions between regulatory molecules and chemotherapeutic drugs. It is necessary to review briefly some characteristics that drug responses have in common, regardless of cell or agent. Features of AML are reviewed as essential background for the work. Then a description is provided of observations showing that the responses of AML blast cells to cytosine arabinoside (ara-C), cisplatin and the anthracycline daunourubcin (DNR) can be influenced by myeloid growth factors and ligands for the steroid superfamily of intracellular receptors. Putative mechanisms of this regulated drug sensitivity (RDS) are then introduced as the major thrust of the paper.

Proximal and Distal Cellular Responses to Drugs

Dose-Response Curves

When drug and cell interact, the result may either be proliferative death or survival either because of repair or because injury was escaped. It is these two alternative fates that provide the basis of standard dose-response curves, where survival or death are plotted as a function of drug concentration. For many drugs, including are-C [1], the anthracyclines DNR or idarubicin (IDA) [2] and cisplatinum (cisplatin) [3], we have found it convenient to construct semi-longarithmic plots, with survival on the vertical logarithmic axis and drug concentration on the linear horizontal axis. Drug dose—cell survival relationships plotted in this way may show an initial shoulder followed by exponential decline with increasing dose and may be characterized by two parameters: Dq, the dose required to reach exponential decline; and Do, the slope of the exponential curve, given as dose required to reduce survival to 37%. This style of data presentation is derived from radiation biology, where the shoulder is attributed to repair of sublethal damage and the exponential decline is considered a reflection of the random nature of radiation interactions with matter [4,5].

It is now appreciated that the binary outcome of "death" or "survival" is strongly influenced not only by the inherent toxicity of the drug but also by many cellular events. Unlike drug-specific toxicity, cell-mediated contributions are likely to contribute to the outcome of exposure to many different drugs; hence they are collectively termed "multiple-drug resistance" or MDR mechanisms [6]. These are attractive for study because of their potential to explain heterogeneity of response to drug and because they may be manipulated to improve efficacy. Cellular contributions to the outcome of drug exposure may usefully be divided into two classes: first, using a nomenclature proposed by Dr. Mark Minden, Cellular mechanisms that act from the time of exposure to drug until interaction with an important target may be considered "proximal"; second, responses by the cell following injury may be considered "distal."

Proximal Resistance

Perhaps the best known of proximal MDR mechanisms is that mediated through the action of *p*-glycoprotein (Pgp); Pgp is a complex molecule imbedded in the cell membrane were it acts as a pump, moving toxic molecules, including many drugs, from the cytoplasm to the extra cellular space. In this way, effective exposure to drug is reduced and with it cytotoxicity [7]. A Pgp-mediated mechanism may, in contrast, be favorable for treatment; recently it has been shown the Pgp is expressed strongly in very primitive normal stem cells; it may act in such cells to increase efficacy by protecting stem cells against lethal damage from drugs [8]. A second proximal mechanism links cell function to drug action. Many chemotherapeutic agents are analogues of normal DNA precursors; for example, ara-C is a nucleoside analogue. Such drugs must usually be incorporated into DNA to be toxic; thus, cells not in the synthetic (S) phase of the cycle are protected. This mechanism is particularily important for normal stem cells since these are often out of cycle in a Go state [9].

Distal Resistance

Distal mechanisms have long been known to protect cells against injury from ionizing or ultraviolet irradiation by repairing damaged DNA. Genes for many enzymes responsible for DNA repair have now been cloned, often using cells from patients with genetically determined disorders, such as xeroderma pigmentosa [10]; their importance in preserving genomes from degradation by toxins was recognized when the magazine *Science* honored the family of repair enzymes as the Molecule of the Year (*Science*, December 23, 1994). The family's general importance is emphasized by studies showing that DNA repair and DNA transcription have many common features [11]. Repair of drug-damaged DNA is recognized as a mechanism for drug resistance [12]. An example of direct repair is the removal of O^6 alkylguanine from DNA of nitrosourea-treated cells by alkyltransferase [13]. Excision repair is a more general mechanism for removing bulky adducts [14, 15] and is important in survival of cells treated with many DNA-damaging chemotherapeutic drugs.

The induction of repair genes is but one part of the multifaceted response of mammalian cells to injury. Genes that are not themselves repair genes mediate such important responses as G1 arrest of the cell cycle and apoptosis [16] providing further instances of how response to injury shares mechanisms with normal cellular functions. A prominent example is the tumor-suppressor gene encoding p53. The wild-type protein is a potent inhibitor of cell proliferation, acting, at least in part, through a G1 block in the cell cycle. Cells exposed to chemotherapeutic agents that cause breaks in DNA (but not to drugs that kill by other mechanisms) show striking increases in their nuclear p53 protien; the increase requires protein synthesis but appears to result from enhanced p53 stability rather than increased transcription [17]. Further p53 is required for apoptosis of E1A-transformed mouse embryo fibroblasts. Cells expressing p53 are more sensitive to irradiation or drugs than p53-negative cells, when viability is assessed by fluorescein isothiocyanate (FITC) uptake [18]. Nelson and Kastan [19] has proposed a model that envisages DNA breaks followed by up-regulation of p53 resulting either in G1 arrest or in apoptosis. The model includes the participation of other genes, particularly GADD45, a member of a family of growth arrest and DNA inducible genes. The model does not specify whether G1 arrest protects from apoptosis.

The proto-oncogene bcl-2 is the first of a family of genes that are important regulators of apoptosis [20]. Bcl-2, first identified from breakpoint analysis of a 14; 18 translocation, plays a role in lymphoid development where it inhibits apoptosis; bcl-2 is now known to be active in the development of other body systems, including the nervous system. Bcl-2 also promotes survival of factor-dependent cell lines when deprived of factor. Bcl-x, a bcl-2-related gene, was first isolated from chicken lymphoid cells. In human cells two cDNAs, a long (bcl-xl) and a short (bcl-xs) form are transcribed from the same gene by alternate splicing. Bcl-xl acts like bcl-2 to prevent apoptosis following factor deprivation, while the short form inhibits over-expression of bcl-2[21]. Another family member, Bax was discovered because its product co-precipitated with Bcl-2. Bax forms inhibitory heterodimers with bcl-2; it has been proposed that the balance between bcl-2 and Bax proteins in heterodimers is an important mechanism in the regulation of apoptosis [22]; regardless, it seems that a complex controlling network is in place. The network may be of importance in chemotherapy because, in model systems, bcl-2 has been shown to protect against damage by ionizing radiation and drugs [23].

It is now known how the bcl-2 gene product protects cells; an attractive possibility is that the protein acts as an antioxidant [24]. Hydroxyl radicals (HO), the most powerful of oxygen radicals are produced in water by ionizing radiation and are probably the mechanism by which radiation causes DNA breaks; breaks in DNA are also seen after drug treatment [25] and it is this form of damage that induces repair enzymes. Bcl-2 is localized, although not exclusively, in mitochondria, principle sites of radical production. Evidence that radicals are important in apoptosis was obtained by showing that treatment with the scavenger N-acetylcysteine protects interleukin-3 (IL-3)- requiring cells when deprived of factor. Evidence for interaction of bcl-2 and free radicals has been found in experiments showing that over-expression of bcl-2 protects against damage with H202 which is converted in cells to hydroxyl radicals. Finally, interaction with redox systems would influence many cell types, since changes in redox potential affects many regulatory pathways [26–28]; thus redox is a plausible target for mechanisms of multiple drug resisitance and sensitization.

AML as a Model

Biology

Acute myeloblastic leukemia is an attractive model for studying drug-cell interactions. It is a clonal hemopathy [29]; genetic evidence is available that the disease begins in a very early hemopoietic stem cell, although there remains controversy as to whether the cell of origin is always pluripotent or may sometimes be committed to granulopoiesis [30, 31]. Production of apparently normal myeloid cells continues after transformation; indeed clinical remissions may be based on differentiation from leukemic stem cells [30–34]. The dominant and diagnostic population consists of morphologically undifferentiated blast cells. Immunophenotypic studies of AML blast show that these express a variety of differentiation markers; however these are often present as in appropriate combinations of early and late markers (asynchrony) or antigens normally restricted to myelopoiesis or lymphopoiesis are found together on single blasts (lineage infidelity or mixed lineage leukemia) [35–40]. These data have been interpreted to mean that differentiation continues in AML blasts but is aberrant; the finding of immunoglobulin gene re-arrangements in AML blasts provides molecular support for this view [41,42].

Cell Culture

Acute myeloblastic leukemia blasts can readily be obtained as >90% pure single-cell suspensions [43]. Cell culture studies of blasts are consistent with the view that the hierarchical cell structure of normal hemopoiesis is maintained in AML. When blasts are plated in growth medium made viscid by methylcellulose, colony formation is observed, provided myelopoietic growth factors are included. Plating efficiency in methylcellulose (PEmc) is usually low, indicating that a minority of blasts are clonogenic [44]. Cells can be recovered from methylcellulose and replated; a secondary plating efficiency (PE2) is obtained, indicating that clonogenic blasts have the stem cell property of self-renewal, although the low values of PE2 (usually <1%) indicate the renewal rarely occurs in methylcellulose cultures [45]. Blasts may also be cultured in suspension; changes in clonogenic cell number can be measured as a function of time by plating from suspension into methylcellulose [46]. Increase in clonogenic cell number is considered a measure of self-renewal; however, the doubling time of clonogenic cells is suspension is usually 2–3 days, longer than their 8–12 h generation time [47]. Thus, in suspension, new clonogenic cells are added by self-renewal, but their number decreases as some pass through determination and initiate terminal divisions.

The hierarchical model of blast cells has implications for therapy. Since the malignant population is maintained by stem cells, these are the appropriate targets for treatment. Control requires that stem cells, rather than the whole population, must be eliminated or greatly reduced in number. It is probable that the success of cytotoxic chemotherapy with doses that permit return of normal marrow function is achieved because only the significant stem cell subpopulation, not all leukemic cells, must be eliminated or reduced significantly. Culture methods may be valuable because plating in methylcellulose and changes in clonogenic cell recovery after suspension may be used together to measure stem cell numbers and behavior. Several investigators have reported significant associations between low stem cell renewal, measured in culture, and clinical outcome [48–52]. The culture methods can be used to measure drug dose-response curves. The technique has the advantage of great flexibility since culture conditions can be altered, permitting cells to be exposed to drugs under defined physiological conditions. Most importantly the method is selective; that is, by using colony formation as an endpoint, the observed dose-response curve is that of the crucial blast stem cell population.

Regulated Drug Sensitivity

Myelopoietic Growth Factors

The observation of RDS is an example of the power of the culture methods to demonstrate the influence of cellular processes on drug response. Blast stem cells in culture respond to many of the regulator that govern normal hemopoiesis. Blast cells usually depend for proliferation and survival on the myelopoietic growth factors IL-3 granulocyte-macrophage colony-stimulating factor (GM-CSF), G-CSF CSF-1 [53–58]and the ligand for the receptor encoded by c-KIT (kit ligand, KL) [58, 59] striking synergism is often seen when two or more factors are combined. The response to factor varies greatly among blast populations in terms of active factor or combinations and in the extent of stimulation. IL-3, GM-CSF, and KL act preferentially on normal early stem cells with multilineage potential, while the normal targets for G-CSF and CSF-1 are lineage-restricted, committed progenitors. An equivalent lineage or stage specificity is not seen when blast cells are treated with growth factors; rather, the mitogenic effects dominate but usually include support of both self-renewal and terminal divisions.

Ligands for Steroid Receptors

Blast stem cells, like normal progenitors respond to the ligands that bind intracellular steroid recepotors [60–62]. All-trans-retinoic acid (ATRA) is an important example. Normal progenitors are often stimulated by ATRA, although recently inhibition of early erythropoietic cells has been reported [63–65]. ATRA was observed to induce differentiation in promyelocytic leukemic populations (APL) [66], and recent success in the treatment of it is an important precedent for the value of biological therapy. Retinoic acid receptors are expressed regularly in AML cell lines. In suspension, clonogenic cell renewal is usually inhibited; however, when fresh cells are examined, both inhibition and stimulation have been observed [67,68].

Features of RDS

The reponses of blast cells to regulators provided evidence that their growth patterns were responsive to external control. Since cell physiology may influence drug response, we tested the sensitivity of blast cells to drugs under a variety of conditions. Regularly, blasts were found to be more ara-C or cisplatinum sensitive in G-CSF than in IL-3 or GM-CSF [3,69–71]. Figure 1 is an example; it shows survival curves for OCI/AML-1 cells exposed to increasing doses of ara-C for 6 days in suspension culture, then harvested,washed, and plated in methylcellulose to determine clonogenic cell recovery. The survival curves for cells in IL-3 or GM-CSF were not different; but both were significantly ($p < 0.001$) less sensitive than aliquots of the same cell line exposed to ara-C in the presence of G-CSF. Steroid ligands also influenced sensitivity. HC was found to be protective[72], while ATRA increased or decreased sensitivity depending on target cell and schedule[73,74]. These phenomena were grouped together under the term regulated drug sensitivity.

Proximal Mechanisms Considered

Regulated drug sensitivity might best make a contribution to understanding leukemia or to improving care if its mechanism were understood. We began to test candidate proximal mechanisms.

Proliferative and Cycle State

Using cell culture methods, it had been possible to estimate the balance between self-renewal and terminal divisions that characterized the growth pattern of each blast population under specified growth factor stimulation. It was attractive to

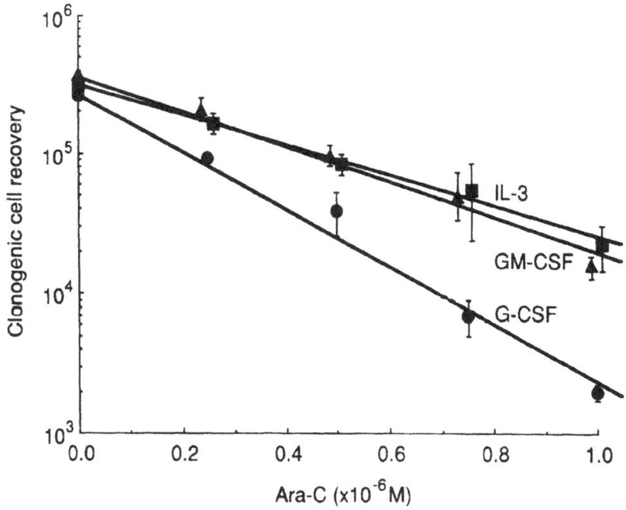

Fig. 1. Ara-C dose-response curves for OCI/AML-1 cells exposed to drug in the presense of one of IL-3, GM-CSF, or G-CSF. For description see text. (From [70]) leukemia blast cells from ara-C. By Koistinen et al, Leukemia 5: 789–795 1991

expect that the factor manipulations that set growth patterns and drug sensitivity might use the same cell processes as the basis for both phenotypes. That is, self-renewing cells might have a different sensitivity from terminal dividing cells. The early data [69] supported this hypothesis but, as the number of observations increased, it became clear that the effect of growth factors on ara-C sensitivity was a function of the factor not the physiological state of the cells[70].

Many of our experiments used ara-C, chosen because of its importance in the treatment of AML. It is widely accepted that ara-C must be incorporated into DNA to be lethal[75]; thus, ara-C sensitivity might be regulated by mechanisms that altered the proportion of cells in the S phase of the cycle. Many clinical investigators found this mechanism attractive; it was proposed that growth factors be employed in the treatment of AML to "recruit" cells into S phase, where they would be susceptible to attack by ara-C; in the laboratory measurements associated with this hypothesis, blast cells from patients were cultured with or without added factor and then the toxicity of ara-C determined. Usually increased sensitivity was observed[76–78]. This experimental design has an important drawback. The underlying assumption, well supported by data, is that AML blasts are factor sensitive. It follows that blast cells maintained without factor may well be entering apoptosis; since cellular machinery may be generally impaired in apoptotic cells, the apparent resistance of such cells to ara-C may be an artifact.

The growth factor experiments that demonstrated RDS were designed to compare cells in comparable growth states; that is, the drug dose-responses of cells exposed to two different factors or factor combinations were measured. Although these conditions would be expected to maintain the S phase fraction in each population, the possibility remained that the S phase fraction was affected by the culture conditions. The capacity of high specific activity tritiated thymindine (^{3}HTdR) to destroy clonogenicity following incoporation into DNA— "thymidine suicide," was used to measure the percentage of cells in the S phase under various conditions. An experimental design was developed in which blast cells were pulsed with either ^{3}HTdR at increasing specific activity or ara-C at increasing drug concentration; the cells were washed and than plated in methylcellulose to determine survival of clonogenic cells. When this design was applied to cells cultured with G-CSF, as expected, the ^{3}HTdR response curve was characterized by an initial decrease in survival to about 50% as cells in the S phase were inactivated, followed by a plateau as cells in G2-M-G1 were spared. The curve for cells pulsed with ara-C was similar, as expected if the drug kills when incorporated into S phase cells. In contrast, however, when blast cells were cultured in GM-CSF or IL-3, the usual form of the ^{3}HTdR curve was maintained, but little or no killing was seen in cultures pulsed with ara-C[70]. Thus, the effect of ara-C was dependent on the growth factors present during exposure and independent of the fraction of cells in the S phase of the cycle.

Regulated drug sensitivity mediated by ATRA or HC was also tested for a cell cycle-mediated mechanism. Since ATRA and HC are not required for cell proliferation, an experimental design was feasible where controls and cells exposed to agent could be tested under the same growth conditions. The protocol used to study the protective effect of HC is an example. Blast cells were pulsed with either ^{3}HTdR or ara-C, as in the growth factor experiments described above, and for each cycle-specific agent, controls were compared to cells exposed to HC. Results obtained for the factor-dependent cell line OCI/AML-1, grown in medium conditioned by 5637 cells, and the factor-independent line OCI/AML-2 are shownin Fig. 2. Cells exposed to ^{3}HTdR as controls or after HC, and ara-C-treated control cells gave very similar dose-reponse curves, characteristic of selective killing of S-phase cells; in contrast, for both cell lines, HC protected against ara-C toxicity. Thus, as in the growth factor experiments, HC influenced survival following ara-C even for cells shown to be in the S phase of the cycle by reason of susceptibility to killing by ^{3}HTdR. These and other experiments of similar design make it very unlikely that RDS is mediated by regulator-induced changes in cell cycle parameters.

Transport and Metabolism

Transport mechanisms mediated by Pgp are potential contributors to RDS. Neither ara-C nor cisplatinum are among the many drugs whose sensitivity is influenced by Pgp; and RDS can be seen readily in AML populations that are negative for Pgp expression. We considered that drug metabolism was a more probable proximal RDS mechanism. Two approaches were used to

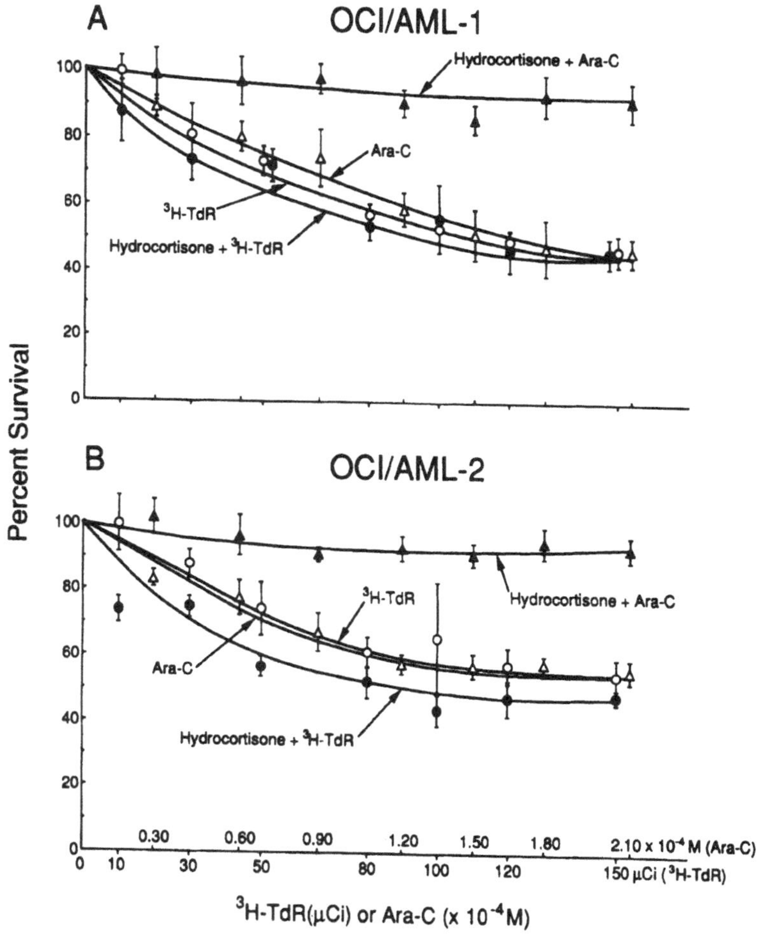

Fig. 2. Dose-response curves for OCI/AML-1 and OCI/AML-2 cells exposed for 20 min to increasing specific activity ^{3}HTdR or increasing concentration of ara-C; experimental groups were treated with hydrocortisone before agent; controls were treated only with agent. For description see text. (From[7])

test the metabolic hypothesis. First, we asked if HC protects blast cells from ara-C toxicity by decreasing incorporation into DNA. We compared the incorporation of ^{3}HTdR and ^{3}Hara-C into OCI/AML-2 cells as controls or after treatment with HC; while the measurements were made on the bulk population, we considered that the results might be relevant to the clonogenic population since the plating efficiency of OCI/AML-2 cells apporaches 20%. The results are given in Table 1. While more ^{3}HTdR was incorporated than ^{3}Hara-C, treatment with HC did not affect the extent of incorporation by either labelled precursor. Thus, support was not obtained for HC protection based on decreased incorporation of ara-C into DNA. We based a second test for metabolic mechanisms on the specificity of drug cytotoxicity; we argued that, if drugs with different requirements for killing

Table 1. Incorporation of ^{3}HTdR or ^{3}Hara-C in DNA of OCI/AML-2 cells (counts in DNA).(Rediafted from [72])

Hydrocortisone	Time 0	Incubated (2 h)
^{3}Hara-C		
Control	2.2×10^3	1.7×10^4
Present	2.4×10^3	2.1×10^4
^{3}HTdR		
Control	1.1×10^4	3.7×10^5
Present	1.7×10^4	4.0×10^5

were regulated in a similar fashion, it was unlikely that regulators were changing response by affecting metabolism. Accordingly, cisplatin and ara-C sensitivites were tested in the presence of either G-CSF, GM-CSF or combinations. Regularly dose-response curves for both drugs were altered in the same direction in response to the culture milieu[3], a result that did not support a metabolic explanation of RDS. Thus, an extensive search failed to uncover a plausible proximal mechanism of RDS.

Distal Mechanisms Preferred

Two strategies were used in a search for distal mechanisms of RDS. The first was a study of events immediately after drug injury. The purpose was to see if changes following injury indicated repair and if such changes could be influenced by regulators. The second strategy was a search for changes in gene following exposure to regulators where the observations were consistent with RDS. For both strategies we used established cell lines whose drug sensitivity was increased when ATRA was given after drug and where protection was observed when HC was given before drug.

Kinetics of Appearance and Loss of Nicks in DNA Following Drug Treatment

We choose to use a modification of the nick translation assay of Masuck et al. [25] because this method permits kinetic measurements of early events [79, 80]. The method is limited because it does not select for blast stem cells. Accordingly, the clonogenic assay was used in parallel to control systematic differences between the bulk population and stem cells. This comparison showed that the dose-response curves for both ara-C and DNR were similar for both methods. Kinetics were determined by exposing cells to drug in suspension, washing, assaying for nicks in DNA and clonogenic cell recovery, then reculturing; after 24 h the cultures were again harvested, the assays and reculture procedures repeated. At each subculture, the cell number was re-adjusted to the original starting value. For both drugs the proportion of cells with damaged DNA increased with time after drug and then recovered. We interpreted the data as showing that sublethal damage in DNA became lethal with time and evident as nicks in DNA. There was a striking kinetic difference between ara-C and DNR. For the former the maximum damage was seen 2 days after drug, while for the latter nicked DNA continued to increase for 6–7 days.

If, as postulated, the observed kinetics reflect responses to injury, the experimental system is suitable to ask whether the mechanism of RDS is distal. Blast cells were exposed to HC before drug and to ATRA after drug; then kinetics were measured and compared with controls exposed to drug only. At the earliest time point, little or no difference was seen between controls and cells exposed to regulators. As expected, damage became evident with time in the controls. For cells treated with HC before drug, many fewer cells with nicks in DNA appeared; ATRA after drug markedly increased evidence of damage. These changes were particularly evident in cells treated with DNR since, following this drug, evidence of damage in controls continued to grow for about week. Thus, the studies with the nick translation assay disclosed events that are not readily detected with the clonogenic assay because of the time in culture required for colony formation. These events may represent sublethal damage becoming lethal or being repaired. The effects of ATRA and HC are highly consistent with distal mechanisms that either favor or inhibit repair.

A further mechanistic point emerged from these experiments: anthracycline toxicity is regulated by ATRA and HC. In previous work, no evidence was found of anthracycline regulation by growth factors; indeed, anthracycline curves were used as controls against nonspecific culture artifacts as explanations for changes seen when cells were exposed to ara-C under different conditions. It follows that the mechanism of regulation by ATRA and HC may be different than those that subserve the growth factor effects.

Proposed Distal Mechanism

As discussed earlier [2, 3], distal mechanisms are both multiple and complex. The studies with the nick translation assay allowed us to conclude that post-injury events were probable targets for RDS. With this information, it became reasonable to seek specific genetic mechanisms. As criteria, we asked that a potential gene of interest would have an expression response pattern that was compatible with the RDS. Bcl-2 was an attractive candidate because of its known effects on apoptosis. We found it expressed in many but not all AML blast populations; we tested bcl-2 expression AML cell lines following exposure to either ATRA, ara-C, or both. A striking down-regulation of bcl-2 expression was seen in cells treated with ATRA; when both ATRA and ara-C were given, the down-regulation was reduced or prevented [81]. These expression responses supported the possibility that bcl-2 was involved. The literature provided many other reasons for investigating bcl-2, including an association between bcl-2 and outcome in AML[82]and evidence that increased bcl-2 expression resulted in drug resistance [23].

It has been proposed that bcl-2 has an antioxidant effect and that this contributes to its capacity to suppress apoptosis. H_2O_2 can be added to cultures where it is metabolized in cells to yield the free radical HO. We prepared dose-response curves for AML blasts exposed for 8 h to H_2O_2; the curves were characterized by an initial shoulder followed by a rapid exponential decline. We then sought an association between bcl-2 expression and H_2O_2 sensitivity; the test used three cell lines; Northern analysis readily demonstrates bcl-2 expression in OCI/AML-2 and OCI/AML-5 cells, while expression can only be shown in OCI/AML-1 cells using Polymerase chain reaction(PCR). We found that OCI/AML-1 cells were about 100 fold more sensitive to H_2O_2 than either of the bcl-2-expressing lines.

The next requirment was to link the observations the H_2O_2 to those with drugs. Ara-C was metabolized to the triphosphate and incorporated into DNA, where it acts as a chain terminator [83, 84]. We asked if, in addition to chain termination, ara-C in cells might lead to the production of toxic free radicals. We used a known radical scavenger, *N*-acetylcysteine (NAC), to test this hypotesis. We found that treatment of blast cells with NAC before ara-C markedly reduced drug toxicity. The protection was entirely schedule dependent; NAC with ara-C or after drug was without effect. This result provided indirect but strong evidence for a role for free radicals in ara-C toxicity [81].

If radical production following ara-C exposure is important in RDS, it would be expected that damage by free radicals would be subject to RDS. We tested this possibility using three OCI/AML cell lines. The cells were treated with HC before H_2O_2 and with ATRA after peroxide; each treatment had its own control because the time relations of exposure were not indentical. The results are shown as H_2O_2 survival curves Fig. 3. For OCI/AML-2 and OCI/AML-5 cells, HC clearly protected while ATRA sensitized. Only the HC protection was demonstrated for OCI/AML-1 cells since these do not express the retinoic acid receptor. However, examination of the H_2O_2 dose scales for the survival curves shows the 100-fold difference in sensitivity mentioned earlier.

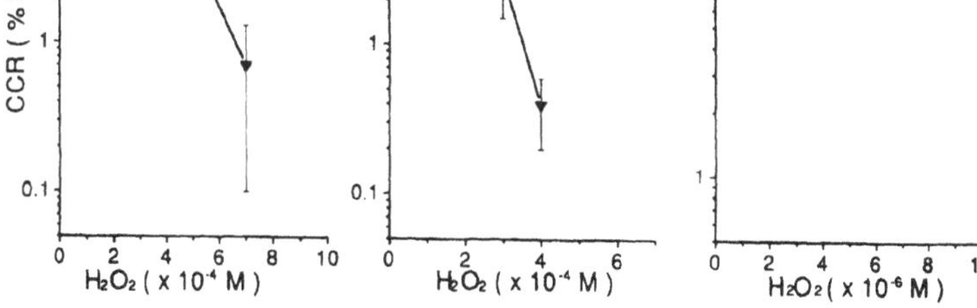

Fig. 3A–C. Hydrogen peroxide dose-response curves for three OCI/AML cell lines: **A** OCI/AML-S; **B** OCI/AML-2; **C** OCI/AML-1. Control survival curves are compared to cells treated with hydrocortisone before drug or with retinoic acid after drug. For description see text. *Squares*,HC control; *circles*, HC(+); *triangles*. ATRA control; *inverted triangles*, ATRA (+). (From[81])

In summary, we suggest the following hypothesis. Ara-C kills cells in at least two ways: by terminating DNA chain elongation and by inducing the formation of free redicals. Bcl-2 protein directly or indirectly decreases toxicity resulting from free radicals. Ara-C toxicity is regulated by ATRA by its action on bcl-2 expression. This proposal is a specific example of a distal mechanism of RDS.

How Many Mechanisms?

The observation that anthracycline sensitivity is regulated by ATRA and HC but not by growth factors made it necessary to postulate two mechaninsms of RDS, one for factors, one for steroids. The mechanism described for regulation by ATRA may not include regulation by HC; although HC protects against H_2O_2 sensitivity, treatment of bcl-2-postitive AML blast cells does not alter HC expression; an effect of HC on Bax is an obvious thought, but, as yet, support for it has not been found experimentally. It is possible, of course, that each example of RDS is mechanistically unique. Alternatively, the regulatory network that is actived following cell injury presents many places where regulators could make changes; the results of changes in different places might have quite similar consequences for drug response. If this latter view is supported, many mechanisms of RDS may coexist within a single system of cell defense against injury.

Conclusion

Therapy of cancer is now limited by the intractable nature of disseminated disease. A systemic treatment is clearly needed; yet many malignant cell populations are resistant to available chemotherapeutic drugs. Leukemia is a useful model because both sensitivity and resistance can be demonstrated in blast cells. In this paper, an attempt is made to illustrate the extensive systems that govern what happens when cell meets drug and how the response to drug is modulated by cellular mechanisms. RDS provides examples of how crucial cell systems may be manipulated by external forces. If mechanisms were well understood, drugs might be combined with biologicals so that resistance can be minimized. Clinical trial might then be proposed to see if such manipulation is useful in patient care.

Acknowledgment. The work described in this paper was supported by the National Cancer Institute of Canada and the Medical Research Council of Canada

References

1. Niho Y, Till JE, McCulloch EA: Effect of arabinosyl cytosine on granulopoietic colony formation by marrow cells from leukemic and non-leukemic patients. Exp. Hematol. 1976; 4: 63–69.
2. Curtis JE, Minden MD, Minkin S, McCulloch EA: Sensitivities of AML blast stem cells to idarubicin and daunorubicin: a comparison with normal hematopoietic progenitors. Leukemia 1994; in press.
3. Wang Y-F, Kelleher CA, Minkin S, McCulloch EA: The effects of rGM-CSF and rG-CSF on the cisplatinum sensitivity of the blast cells of acute myeloblastic leukemia. Leukemia 1991; 5: 239–248.
4. Whitmore GF, Till JE: Quantitation of cellular radiobiological responses. Ann.Rev. Nucl.Sci.1964; 14: 347–374.
5. Bump EA, Brown JM: Role of glutathione in the radiation response of mammalian cells in vitro and in vivo. Pharmac. Ther. 1990; 47: 117–136.
6. Simon SM, Schindler M: Cell biological mechanisms of multidrug resistance in tumors. Proc.Natl.Academ.Sci (USA) 1994; 91: 3497–3504.
7. Gerlach JH, Kartner N, Bell DR, Ling V : Multidrug resistance. Cancer Surveys 1986; 5: 25–46.
8. Chaudhary PM, Roninson IG: Expression and activity of p-glycoprotein, a multidrug efflux pump, in human hematopoietic stem cells. Cell 1991; 66: 85–94.
9. Bruce WR, Valeriote FA: Normal and malignant stem cells and chemotherapy. In: The proliferation and spread of neoplastic cells. M.D. Anerson symposium on fundamental cancer research 1967; 21: 409–420
10. Hoeijmakers JHJ, Bootsma D: Molecular genetics of eukaryotic DNA excision repair. Cancer Cells 1990; 2: 311–320.
11. Hanawalt PC: Transcription-coupled repair and human disease. Science 1994; 266: 1957–1958.
12. Link CJ,Jr, Burt RK, Bohr VA : Gene-specific repair of DNA damage induced by UV irradiation and cancer chemotherapeutics. Cancer Cells 1991; 3: 427–436.
13. Gerson SL, Trey JE, Miller K: Potentiation of nitrosourea cytotoxicity in human leukemic cells by inactivation of O^6-alkylgluanine-DNA alkyltransferase. Cancer Research 1988; 48: 1521–1527.
14. Wood RD, Coverley D: DNA excision repair in mammalian cell extracts. BioEssays 1991; 13: 447–453.
15. Sancar A: Mechanisms of DNA excision repair. Science 1994; 266: 1954–1956.
16. Koury MJ: Programmed cell death (apoptosis) in hemopoiesis. Exp. Hematol. 1992; 20: 391–394.

nuclear accumulation of the tumor suppressor protein p53 by DNA-damaging agents. Oncogene 1993; 8: 307–318.
18. Lowe SW, Ruley HE, Jacks T, Houseman DE: p53-dependent apoptosis modulates the cytotoxicty of anticance agents. Cell 1993; 74: 957–967.
19. Nelson WG,Kastan MB: DNA strand breaks: the DNA template alterations that trigger p53-dependent DNA damage response pathways. Mol. and Cell Biol. 1994; 14: 1815–1823.
20. Korsmeyer SJ: Bcl-2 initiates a new category of oncogenes: regulators of cell death. Blood 1992; 80: 879–886.
21. Boise LH, Gonzales-Garcia M, Postema CE, Ding L, Lindsten T, Turka LA, Mao X, Nunez G, Thompson, CB : Bcl-x, a bcl-2-related gene that functions as a dominant regulator of apoptotic cell death. Cell 1993; 74: 597–608.
22. Oitval ZN, Milliman CL, Korsmeyer SJ: Bcl-2 heterodimerizes in vivo with a conserved homolog, Bax, the accelerated programmed cell death. Cell 1993; 74: 60–619.
23. Miyashita T, Reed JC, Sabido O, Oriol, P, Roubi N, Vasselon C, Archimbaud E, Magaud J-P, Guyotat D: Bcl-2 oncoprotein blocks chemotherapy-induced apoptosis in a human leukemia cell line. Blood 1993; 81: 151–157.
24. Hockenbery DM, Oltval ZN, Yin M-X, Millman CL, Korsmeyer SJ : Bcl-2 functions in an antioxidant pathway to prevent apoptosis. Cell 1993; 75: 241–251.
25. Masuck TM, Taylor AR, Lough J: Arabinosylcytosine-induced accumulation of DNA links in mytotube nuclei detected by in situ nick translation. J. Cell. Physiol. 1990; 144: 12–17.
26. Hayashi T, Ueno Y, Okamoto T: Oxidoreductive regulation of nuclear factor kappa B: involvement of a cellular reducing catalyst thioredoxin. J. Biol. Chem. 1993; 268: 11380–11388.
27. Bauskin AR, Alkalay I, Ben-Heriah Y: Redox regulation of a protein tyrosine kinase in the endoplasmic reticulum. Cell 1991; 66: 685–696.
28. Pognonec P, Kato H, Roeder RG: The helix-loop-helix/leucine repeat transcription factor can be functionally regulated in a redox-dependent manner. J. Biol. Chem. 1992; 267: 24563–24567.
29. McCulloch EA, Till JE: Stem cells in normal early haemopoiesis and certain clonal haemopathies. In: Recent advances in haematology 1977 (A. V.Hoffbrandt, M.C. Brain, and J. Hirsch eds) ppage 85–110, Churchill-Livingston, Londan New York.
30. Fearon ER, Burke PJ, Schiffer CA, Zehnbauer BA, Vogelstein B: Differntiation of leukemic cells to polymorphonuclear leukocytes in patients with acute nonlymphocytic leukemia. New Engl. j. Med 1986; 315: 15–24.
31. Fialkow PJ, Singer JW, Adamson JW, Vaidya K, Dow LW, Ochs J, Moohr JW: Acute nonlymphocytic leukemia: heterogeneity of stem cell origin. Blood 1981; 57: 1068–1073.
32. Jacobson RJ, Temple MJ, Singer JW, Powell J, Fialkow PJ: A clonal complete remission in a ing in a multipotent stem cell. New Engl J Med 1984; 310: 1513–1517.
33. Fialkow PJ, Singer JW, Raskind WH, Adamson JW, Jacobson RJ, Berstein DI, Dow LD, Najfeld, V, Veith R: Clonal development, stem-cell differntiation and clinical remissions in acute nonlymphocytic leukemia. N Engl J Med 1987; 317: 468–473.
34. Najifeld V, Zucker-Franklin D, Adamson J, Sainger J, Troy K, Fialkow PJ : Evidence for clonal development and stem cell origin of M7 megakaryocytic leukemia. Leukemia 1988; 2: 351–357.
35. Smith LJ, Curtis JE, Messner HA, Senn JS, Furthmayr H, McCulloch EA : Lineage infidelity in acute leukemia. Blood 1983; 61: 1138–1145.
36. Lantham GR, Bollum FW, Williams DL, Stass SA : Simultaneous occurrence of terminal deoxynucleotidyl transferase and myeloperoxidase in individual leukemic blasts. Blood 1984; 64: 318.
37. Neame PB, Soamboonsrup P, Browman G, Barr, RD, Saeed N, chan, BB, Berger A, Wilso, WEC, Walker IR, McBride JA : Simultaneous sequential expression of lymphoid and myeloid phenotypes in acute leukemia. Blood 1985; 65: 142–148.
38. Vaughn WP, Civin CI, Weisenburger DD, Karp JE, Graham ML, Sanger WG, Grierrson HL, Joshi SS, Burke,PJ: Acute leukemia expressing the normal hematopoietic stem cell membrane glycoprotein CD34 (My10). Leukemia 1988; 2: 661–666.
39. Kurtzberg J, Waldmann TA, Davey MP, Bigner SH, Moore JO, Hershfield MS, Haynes BF: CD7+, CD4−, CD8− acute leukemia: a syndrome of malignant pluripotent lymphohematopoietic cells. Blood 1989; 73: 381–390.
40. Hurwitz CA, Loken MR, Graham ML, Karp JE, Borowitz MJ, Pullen DJ, Civin CI: Asynchronous antigen expression in B lineage acute lymphoblastic leukemia. Blood 1988; 72: 299–307.
41. Cheng GYM, Minden MD, Toyonaga B, Mak TW,McCulloch EA : T-cell receptor and immunoglobulin gene rearrangements in acute myeloblastic leukemia. J.Exper. Med 1986; 65: 894–901.
42. Foa R, Casorati G, Giubellino MC, Basso G, Schiro, R, Pizzolo G, Lauria F, LeFranc, MP, Rabbitts TH, Migone N: Rearrangements of immunoglobulin and T cell receptor beta and gamma genes are associated with terminal deoxyncleotidyl transferase expression in acute myeloid leulemia. J. Exper. Med. 1987; 165: 879–890.
43. Minden MD, Buick RN, McCulloch EA : Separation of blast cell and T-lymphocyte progenitors in the blood of patients with acute myeloblastic leukemia. Blood 1979; 54: 186–195.
44. Buick RN, Till JE, McCulloch EA : Colony assay for proliferative blast cells circulating in myeloblastic leukaemia. Lancet 1977; 1: 862–863.
45. Buick RN, Minden MD, McCulloch EA : Self-renewal in culture of proliferative blast progenitor cells in acute myeloblastic leukemia. Blood 1979; 54: 95–104.
46. Nara N, McCulloch EA : The proliferation in suspension of the progenitors of the blast cells in acute myeloblastic leukemia. Blood 1985; 65: 1484–1493.

47. Minden MD, Major P, Wu A, Kufe DW: Generation time of leukemic blast progenitor cells. Cell Tissue Kinet. 1981; 16: 577–582.
48. Curtis JE, Messner HA, Minden MD, Minkin S, McCulloch EA : High dose cytosine arabinoside in the treatment of acute myeloblastic leukemia: contributions to outcome of clinical and laboratory attributes. J. Clin.Oncol. 1987; 5: 532–543.
49. McCulloch EA, Curtis JE, Messner HA, Senn JS, Germanson TP : The contribution of blast cell properties to outcome variation in acute myeloblastic leukemia (AML). Blood 1982; 59: 601–608.
50. McCullocha EA, Buick RN, Curtis JE, Messner HA. The heritable nature of clonal characteristics in actue myeloblastic leukemia. Blood, 1981; 58: 105–109.
51. Nara N: Association between secondary colony-plating efficiency of blast progenitors and the remission induction outcome of acute myeloblastic leukemia patients. Acta Haematol. JPN. 1988; 51: 1624–1629.
52. Delmer A, Marie J-P, Thevenin D, Cadiou M, Viguie F, Zittoun R : Multivariate analysis of prognostic factors in acute myeloid leukemia: value of clonogenic leukemic cell properties. J. Clin. Oncol. 1989; 7: 738–746.
53. Kelleher C, Miyauchi J, Wong G, Clark S, Minden MD, McCulloch EA : Synergism between recombinant growth factors, GM-CSF and G-CSF, acting on the blast cells of acute myeloblastic leukemia. Blood 1987; 69: 1498–1503.
54. Young DC, Wagner K, Griffin JD: Constitutive expression of the granuocyte-macrophage colony-stimulating factor gene in acute myeloblastic leukemia. J Clin. Invest 1987; 79: 100–106.
55. Nara N, Murohashi I, Suzuki T, Yamashita Y, Maruyama Y, Aoki, N, Tanikawa S: Effects of recombinant human granulocyte colony-stimulating factor (G-CSF) on blast progenitors from acute myeloblastic leukaemia patients. Br. J.Cancer 1987; 56: 49–51.
56. Motoji T, Takanashi M, Fuchinoue M, Masuda M, Oshimi K, Mizoguchi H : Effect of recombinant GM-CSF and recombinant G-CSF on colony formation of blast progenitors in acute myeloblastic leukemia. Exper. Hemat. 1989; 17: 56–60.
57. Rodgriguez-Cimadevilla JC, Beauchemin V, Villeneuve L, Letendre F, Shaw A, Hoang T: Coordinate secretion of interleukin-1-ß and granulocyte-macrophage colonystimulating factor by the blast cells of acute myeloblastic leukemia: role of interleukin-1 as an endogenous inducer. Blood 1990; 76: 1481–1489.
58. Wang C, Koistinen P, Yang GS, Williams DE, Lyman SD, Minden MD, McCulloch EA : Mast cell growth factor, a ligand for the receptor endcoded by c-kit, effects the growth in culture of the blast cells of acute myeloblastic leukemia. Leukemia 1991; 5: 493–499.
59. Witte ON: Steel locus defines new multipotent growth factor. Cell 1990; 63: 5–6.
60. Beato M: Gene regulation by steroid hormones. Cell 1989; 56: 335–344.
61. Evans RM: The steroid and thyroid hormone receptor superfamily. Science 1988; 240: 889–895.
62. Fuller PJ : The steroid receptor superfamily: mechanisms of diversity. FASEB J 1991; 5: 3092–3099. 63. Douer D, Koeffler HP: Retinoid enhances colony-stimulating factor-induced growth of normal human myeloid progenitor cell in vitro. Exp. Cell Res. 1982; 138: 193–198.
64. Douer D, Koeffler HP: Retinoic acid enhances growth of human early erythroid progenitor cells in vitro. J. Clin. Invest. 1982; 69: 1039–1041.
65. Gratas C, Menot ML, Dresch C, Chomienne C: Retinoic acid supports granulocytic but not erythroid differentiation of myeloid progenitors in normal bone marrow cells. Leukemia 1993; 7: 1156–1162.
66. Breitman TR, Collins SJ, Keene BR: Terminal differentiation of human promyelocytic leukemia cells in primary culture in response to retinoic acid. Blood 1981; 57: 1000–1004.
67. Wang C, Curtis JE, Minden MD, McCulloch EA: Expression of a retinoic acid receptor gene in myeloid leukemia cells. Leukemia 1989; 3: 264–269.
68. Gallagher RE, Said F, Papenhausen PR, Paietta E, WierniK PH: Expression of retinoic acid receptor-α mRNA in human leukemia cells with variable responsiveness to retinoic acid. Leukemia 1989; 3: 789–795.
69. Miyauchi J, Kelleher CA, Wang C, Minkin S, McCulloch EA: Growth factors influence the sensitivity of leukemic stem cells to cytosine arabinoside in culture. Blood 1989; 73: 1272–1278.
70. Koistinen P, Wang C, Curtis JE, McCulloch EA : Granulocyte-macrophage colony-stimulating factor and interleukin-3 protect leukemic blast cells from ara-C toxicity. Leukemia 1991; 5: 789–795.
71. Koistinen P, Wang C, Yang GS, Wang Y-F, Williams DE, Lyman SD, Minden MD, McCulloch EA : OCI/AML-4, an acute myeloblastic leukemia cell line: regulation and response to cytosine arabinoside. Leukemia 1991; 5: 704–711.
72. Yang GS, Wang C, Minkin S, Minden MD, McCulloch EA : Hydrocortisone in culture protects the blast cells of actue myeloblastic leukemia from the lethal effects of cytosine arabinoside. J.Cell Physiol. 1991; 148: 60–67.
73. Lishner M, Curtis JE, Minkin S, McCulloch EA : Interaction between retinoic acid and cytosine arabinoside affecting the blast cells of acute myeloblastic leukemia. Leukemia 1989; 3: 784–788.
74. Yang GS, Minden MD, McCulloch EA : Influence of schedule on regulated sensitivity of AML blasts to cytosine arabinoside. Leukemia 1993; 7: 1012–1019.
75. Kufe DW, Major PP, Egan M, Beardsley GP : Correlation of cytotoxicity with incorporation of ara-C into DNA. Journal of Biological Chemistry 1980; 255: 8997–9000.
76. Cannistra SA, Groshek P, Griffin JD : Granulocyte-macrophage colony-stimulating factor enhances the cytotoxic effects of cytosine arabinoside in acute myeloblastic leukemia and in the myeloid blast crisis phase of chronic myeloid leukemia. Leukemia 1989; 3: 328–334.

77. Carrington PA, Hill RJ, Stenberg PE, Levin J, Corash L, Schreurs J, Baker G, Levin FC: Multiple in vivo effects of interleukin-3 and interleukin-6 on murine megakaryocytopoiesis. Blood 1991; 77: 34–41.
78. Cannistra SA, DiCarlo J, Groshek P, Kanakura Y, Berg D, Mayer RJ, Griffin JD: Simultaneous administration of granulocyte-macrophage colony-stimulating factor and cytosine arabinoside for the treatment of relapsed acute myeloid leukemia. Leukemia 1991; 5: 230–238.
79. Yang GS, Wang C, Mincen MD, McCulloch EA: Fluorescence labelling of nicks in DNA from leukemic blasts cells as a measure of demage following cytosine arabinoside; application to the study of regulated drug sensitivity. Leukemia 1994; 8: 2052–2059.
80. Yang GS, Minden MD, McCulloch EA: Regulation by retinoic acid and hydrocortisone of the anthracycline sensitivity of blast cells of acute myeloblastic leukemia. Leukemia 1994; 8: 2065–2075.
81. Hu Z, Yang GS, Li M, Miyamoto N, Minden MD, McCulloch EA: Mechanism of cytosine arabinoside toxicity to the blast cells of acute myeloblastic leukemia: involvment of free radicals. Leukemia 1995; in press.
82. Campos L, Rouault J-P, Sabido O, Oriol P, Roubi, N, Vasselon C, Archimbaud E, Magaud J-P, Guyotat D: High expression of bcl-2 protein in acute myeloid leukemia cells is associated with poor response to chemotherapy. Blood 1993; 81: 3091–3096.
83. Kufe DW, Spriggs DR: Biochemical and cellular pharmacology of cytosine arabinoside. Seminars in Oncology 1985; 12: 34–48.
84. Mikita T, Beardsley GP: Functional consequences of arabinosylcytosine structural lesions in DNA. Biochemistry: 1988 27: 4698–4705

Acute Leukemias VI
Prognostic Factors
and Treatment Strategies
Büchner et al. (eds)

Current Status of Granulocyte Colony-Stimulating Factor and Granulocyte-Macrophage Colony-Stimulating Factor in the Management of Acute Lymphoblastic Leukemia

O.G. Ottmann and D. Hoelzer

Introduction

In recent years, intensification of remission induction and consolidation chemotherapies have considerably improved treatment results in childhood and adult acute lymphoblastic leukemia (ALL), with 70%–90% of adult patients initially achieving a complete remission 9CR) [2, 10]. The probability of long-term disease-free survial and cure in adult patients (20%–35%) remains unsatisfactory, however, due primarily to high relapse rates in both high and standard -risk groups, indicating that currently employed treatment intensities are frequently insufficient [9, 23]. Nevertheless, myelosuppression is the dose-limiting toxicity with current treatment regimens, in which infectious complications are the major cause of morbidity and are largely responsible for age-related mortality rates of 3%–20% during induction therapy [3, 8, 28]. Myelosuppression also necessitates frequent treatment delays which prolong hospitalization and decrease the planned dose intensity of cytotoxic agents, which may adversely affect overall treatment outcome.

The rationale for using hematopoietic growth factors as adjuncts to chemotherapy for ALL is based on numerous clinical trials in patients with solid tumors, lymphomas and following bone marrow transplantation, which show that granulocyte colony-stimulating factor (G-CSF) and granulocyte-macrophage CSF (GM-CSF) are able to mitigate neutropenia, reduce the incidence of febrile and infectious episodes, and in some studies allow dose intensification of chemotherapy [4, 16, 18, 22, 25–27]. The following overview will summarize and critically assess the clinical values of G-CSF and GM-CSF in ALL as far as can presently be ascertained on the basis of published clinical trials.

G-CSF and GM-CSF Post-Chemotherapy for ALL

The potential value of prophylactic administration of G-CSF or GM-CSF following induction or early postremission chemotherapy has been examined in both adult and pediatric patients with ALL, with the majority of clinical studies investigating G-CSF.

Encouraging results were reported in an early nonrandomized study by Kantarjian et al. [12], in which 14 patients with newly diagnosed ALL in CRI after induction therapy received postremission intensification with a 3 day course of high-dose cytosine arasinoside ara-C, mitoxantrone, and vincristine followed by G-CSF (5 μg/kg s.c. starting day 4 until neutrophil regeneration). Compared with a historical control group, the duration of neutropenia $<500/\mu l$ in the G-CSF-treated patients was reduced by 4 days (14 days vs. 18 days, $p<0.001$). In this small number of patients and with few events, there was a statistically non-significant trend towards a lower incidence of febrile episodes, severe infections, and early death.

Impressive, though still preliminary, support for the efficacy and safety of prophylactic G-CSF in ALL comes from a randomized, open-label

Zentrum der Inneren Medizin, Universitätsklinikun, Theodor-Stern-Kai 7, 60590 Frankfurt, Germany

trial in children with high-risk ALL treated in the ALL-BFM-90 study [30]. Forty-two patients were randomized to receive either successive 6 days cycles of multi-agent chemotherapy alone or followed by G-CSF given s.c. at 5 μg/kg per day starting on day 7. An interim analysis based on 13 patients in the G-CSF group and 15 patients in the control group who received a total of 92 and 119 chemotherapy cycles, respectively, showed that neutropenic episodes occurred less frequently in the G-CSF group with 47 episodes (median duration 19 days) as opposed to 114 episodes (median duration 72 days) in the control arm (Table 1). The median duration of febrile neutropenia was reduced from 24 days to 9 days, and there were fewer infectious episodes requiring i.v. antibiotics with G-CSF than in the controls (25 episodes vs. 10 episodes).

In a randomized, placebo-controlled study of 184 patients with newly diagnosed ALL conducted by the Cancer and leukemig Group B CALGB, (protocol 9111), G-CSF (5 μg/kg/ per day s.c.) was administered starting 1 day after the end of induction therapy until neutrophil recovery (Table 2) (Larson et al., 1994). The duration of granulocytopenia ($<1000/\mu l$) was shortened significantly in the G-CSF arm compared with the controls ($p<0.001$), both in the patients <60 years (15 days with G-CSF vs. 21 days with placebo) and in the older (>60 years) patients (16 days vs. 29 days). The incidence of severe infections and death during induction was slightly lower in the G-CSF arm, although this was not statistically significant (Table 2). Overall, elderly patients appeared to benefit particularly from the adjuvant administration of G-CSF.

The utility of GM-CSF in ALL has so far been tested only sporadically. In an early non-randomized trial by Kantarjian et al. [11], 34 refractory adult ALL patients treated with high-dose cytarabine and mitoxantrone over 3 days followed by GM-CSF (125 $\mu g/m^2$ i.v., starting on day 4) were compared with an identically treated historical control group ($n=29$) that had received no growth factor support. Recovery of granulocyte counts above 500/μl occurred 8 days earlier in the GM-CSF-treated patients compared with historical controls (25 days vs. 33 days, $p<0.01$), with an albeit non significant trend towards lower induction mortality in the GM-CSF group (6% vs. 28%). GM-CSF reduced neither the incidence of febrile episodes nor of documented infections, and CR rates were identical in both groups. while survival was prolonged in the GM-CSF-treated patients (31 vs. 20 weeks, $p=0.05$), this was not clinically relevant.

Concurrent Administration of Chemotherapy and G-CSF or GM-CSF

In contrast to the aforementioned studies in which GM-CSF or GM-CSF was administered after completion of chemotherapy, the sequential application of cytotoxic agents and growth factor support is not feasible in BFM-based induction regimens, in which cytotoxic agents are scheduled daily over prolonged time periods. With these widely employed protocols, e.g., that of the German multicenter study of intensified treatment in adult ALL (GMALL), chemotherapy and growth factors have to be given simultaneously, a setting in which the stimulation of normal progenitor cells could conceivably aggravate instead of ameliorate therapy-induced myelosupression.

The feasibility of administering G-CSF concomitantly with induction therapy for newly diagnosed adult ALL was first tested in two independent pilot studies by the GMALL study group [20] and by the Vienna group [24] using a nearly identical chemotherapy protocol. These two trials differed in that G-CSF was given throughout the whole 8 weeks of intensive induction treatment by the Vienna group, whereas the GMALL pilor study restricted G-CSF administration to weeks 5–8 of induction in patients who had achieved a CR or partial remission following weeks 1–4. Both studies indicated that the concomitant administration of G-CSF and this specific induction chemotherapy is safe, with a trend towards reduced neutropenia compared with historical controls. This was confirmed in a subsequent randomized open-label study by the GMALL, which prospectively addressed two unique aspects of hemopoietic growth factor support in the treatment of ALL: (a) the *simultaneous* administration of G-CSF and chemotherapy; and (b) the combination of G-CSF with parallel prophylactic CNS and (in T-lineage ALL) mediastinal irradiation. Seventy-six adult patients with ALL were randomly assigned to receive either G-CSF ($n=37$) or no growth factor ($n=39$) parallel to induction chemotherapy and prophylactic cranial irradiation. The median duration of neutropenia

Table 1. Clinical Trails of G-CSF or GM-CSF in pediatric ALL

Author	Patients	Chemotherapy	Growth factor	(*n*)	Neutyropenia		Incidence of infections	Relapse rate (%)	Follow-up	
					Episodes % (therapy cycles)	Duration (days)			Median (Months)	Range (Months)
Welte 1993 [30]	High risk	Consolidatin (All--BFM 90): V,I,P,E,ADR MP,TG, Hd-araC, HdMTX L-asp i. th.	G-CSF	15	51% of 92 cycles		40	20	n.g.	5–26
			Control	13	95% of 119 cycles		80	15	n.g.	7–22
Calderwood 1994 [1]	High risk CRI	Consolidation C, araC, MP, i. th, CNS-rad	GM-CSF	20		6[a]/11.5[b]	81	10	18.2	3–37
			Placebo	20		7[a]/12[b]	79	0		
Dibenedetto 1995 [5]	CRI, intermediate risk	AIEOP-consolidation C,araC, MP, triple i. th.	G-CSF	14		16[c]	14	n.g.	n.g.	
			Control	18		19	11	n.g.	n.g	

[a] <500/μl.
[b] <1000/μl.
[c] <200/μl.
C, cyclophosphamide; V, vincristine; E, etoposide; P, prednisone; HdMTX, high-dose methotrexare; Hd-araC high-dose cytarabine; MP, 6-mercaptopurine; TG, thioguanine, L-asp: asparaginase; ADR, doxorubicin; rad, prophylactic cranial irradation; i.th, intrathecal therapy; n.g., not given.

Table 2. Randomized Clinical Trials of G-CSF or GM-CSF in adult ALL

Author	Patients	Chemotherapy	Growth factor	(*n*)	Days until ANC>500/μl	Significance (%)	Incidence of infections (%)	Early deaths (%)	CR rate (%)
Geissler 1994 [7]	Untreated ALL	GMALL-induction: VCDP, L-asp,MP araC, rad, i th	G-CSF	12	21		8[a]	0	100
			Control	12	30	$p<004$	42[a]	2	67
Larson 1994 [15]	Untreated ALL (>60years)	CALGB 9111-induction VCDP L-asp	G-CSF	n.g.	15/16		53	4	91
			Placebo	n.g.	21/29	$p<0.001$	66	11	80
Ottmann 1995 [21]	PR/CRI	GMALL-induction phase II (C.araC, MP, rad, i,th.)	G-CSF	37	8		43	0	n.a.
			Control	39	12.5		56	3	n.a.

[a] Denotes incidence of febrile neutropenia.
C, cyclophosphamide; V, vincristine; p, prednisone; MP, 6-mercaptopurine, L-asp, asparaginase; D, daunorubicin; rad, prophylactic cranical irradation; i.th, intrathecal therapy, n.g. not given; n.a. not applicable.
Patients include AML (n = 67), CML-blast crisis ($n = 9$) and AL ($n = 30$). No subgroup analysis performed.

(< 1 × 109/1) *during* chemotherapy was 8 days in patients receiving G-CSF compared with 12.5 days in the control group. A similar reduction from 11.5 to 7 days was observed in patients with T-ALL receiving additional mediastinal irradiation. The incidence of nonviral infections was reduced by 50%, from 32 episodes in the control arm to 16 episodes in the G-CSF arm. Prolonged interruptions of chemotherapy administration were less frequent, with delays of 2 weeks or more occurring in only 24% of patients receiving G-CSF as opposed to 46% in the control arm. Accordingly, chemotherapy was completed significantly earlier with the use of G-CSf (39, 44 days, $p = 0.008$). The probability of disease-free survival was not significantly different between the two groups.

These findings are supported by preliminary results from a randomized, open-label study using essentially the same chemotherapy protocol, in which G-CSF is started on day 2 of induction and given throughout the 8-week period of induction chemotherapy (Table 2) [7]. An interim analysis based on 24 randomized patients showed a 100% CR rate in the G-CSF arm as compared to 67% in the control arm. Recovery from neutropenia occurred more rapidly, and adherence to the intended treatment schedule was improved with G-CSF. Febrile neutropenia occurred in five of 12 patients and fatal infectious complications in two of 12 patients in the control arm, compared with no deaths and one episode of febrile neutropenia with G-CSF.

These findings differ from those of a randomized, placebo-controlled trial utilizing GM-CSF during an induction regimen for high-risk childhood ALL [1]. In this study, concurrent GM-CSF did not ameliorate the degree or duration of chemotherapy-induced myelosuppression and did not influence the incidence of fever, number of hospital days, days on i.v. antibiotics, or the number and severity infectious complications (Table 1).

Possible reasons for this discrepancy are the use of GM-CSF instead of G-CSF, the different patient populations studied (childhood vs. adult ALL), and the GM-CSF administration schedule, in which GM-CSF was not administered daily throughout induction treatment until neutrophil recovery, but was given in two 7-day courses separated by a GM-CSF-free interval of 1 week duration.

In another randomized, open-label study in pediatric patients with intermediate-risk ALL in first CR, 14 patients received G-CSF (10 µg/kg per day s.c.) and 18 patients no growth factor during weeks 5–8 (phase II) of a BFM-based induction regimen [5]. The media duration of therapy was 37 days in the G-CSF group 36 days in the control group, only one patient in the G-CSF arm (7%) and two patients in the control arm (14%) completed phase II according to schedule (Table 1). Similarly, the two groups did not differ in terms of duration of granulocytopenia (< 200/µl), frequency of febrile episodes, and documented infections or duration of hospitalization.

Discussion

Several recent controlled studies support the safety of administering G-CSF or GM-CSF in conjunction with induction and consolidation chemotherapy in lymphoid acute leukemias in adult and pediatric patients. A clear majority of these studies also demonstrates that prophylactic administration of G-CSF after chemotherapy significantly accelerates neutrophil recovery, and most studies show a reduced rate of febrile episodes and infections. If is of substantial interest that not only the conventional sequential but also the parallel administration of hematopoietic growth factors with combined chemoradiotherapy is possible without aggravating myelotoxicity, at least in conjunction with the examined therapeutic regimens. As shown by two randomized studies in adult ALL, this mode of application even facilitates a better adherence to the scheduled chemotherapy and thus more rapid completion of therapy. These results should not be uncritically extrapolated to other chemotherapy combinations, however, as indicated by the enhanced myelotoxicity observed in patients with colorectal tumors receiving G-CSF simultaneously with 5-fluouracil plus leukovorin [17].

Theoretical concerns that G-CSF or GM-CSF could stimulate leukemic cell proliferation are not supported by the results obtained in the clinical trials to date. Despite the observed expression of G-CSF or GM-CSF receptors on blast cells in occasional patients with ALL [6, 13, 29] or lymphomas [14] there has been no clinical evidence for stimulation of leukemic cell growth or acceleration of relapses by either of the investigated growth factors.

The well-established safety of G-CSF or GM-CSF administration contrast with partially divergent results regarding their clinical efficacy in ALL. In contrast to G-CSF, which has been shown to be beneficial in terms of shortened neutropenia, fewer febrile and infectious episodes, and fewer chemotherapy delays [7, 15, 21, 30], a potential clinical benefit of GM-CSF is at present supported by only one study showing a reduction of neutropenia duration compared with a historical control group. A randomized, double-blind study of GM-CSF in children with high-risk ALL, on the other hand, fails to show an advantage of GM-CSF compared with placebo. It appears unlikely that this lack of effect was due to the study of pediatric patients, since substantial benefits of growth factor (G-CSF) administration in this age have been reported by Welte et al. [30]. A more likely explanation is the scheduling of GM-CSF in the study by Calderwood et al. in which an interruption of 1 week's duration may have abrogated the stimulatory effect of GM-CSF on hematopoietic recovery. Irrespective of these theoretical considerations, there has as yet been no clear demonstration of the clinical efficacy of GM-CSF as hemopoietic support in the treatment of ALL.

Despite the encouraging and reproducible beneficial effects of G-CSF regarding rapidity of hematopoietic recovery and decreased infectious morbidity, it remains to be established whether G-CSF improves either remission rates or overall treatment outcome. The consistently more rapid hematologic recovery facilitated by G-CSF in adult as well as childhood ALL has resulted in an increased dose intensity by improving adherence to the scheduled protocol or allowing the application of more chemotherapy cycles in a given time period [7, 21, 30]. While it is questionable whether the relatively small increments that were achieved will have a major impact on treatment response, it should be noted that these studies were not designed to maximize dose intensity.

Owing to the small number of fatal complications in the published studies, an apparent trend towards a lower mortality with G-CSF is currently not amenable to statistical analysis. Conceivably, lowering mortality during induction and/or postremission intensification may affect long-term treatment results. It is anticipated that ongoing and future prospective, controlled trials will clarify these important issues.

References

1. Calderwood, S., Romeyer, F., Blanchette, V., Chan, H., Doyle, J., Greenberg, M., Lorenzana, A., Malkin, D., Saunders, F., Weitzman, S., Zipursky A., Freedman M.H. Concurrent RhGM-CSF does not offset myelosuppression from intensive chemotherapy: randomized placebo-controlled study in childhood acute lymphoblastic leukemia: Am. J. Hematol 47: 27–32 (1994)
2. Champlin R, Gale RP. Acute lymphoblastic leukemia: recent advances in biology and therapy. Blood 73: 2051 (1989)
3. Copelan EA, McGuire EA. The biology and treatment of acute lymphoblastic leukemia in adults. Blood 85: 1151–1168 (1995)
4. Crawford J, Ozer H, Stoller R, Johnson D, Lyman G, Tabbara I, Kris M, Grous J, Picozzi V, Rausch G, Smith R, Gradishar W, Yahanda A, Vincent M, Stewart M, Glaspy J: Reduction by granulocyte colony-stimulating factor of fever and neutropenia induced by chemotherapy in patients with small-cell lung cancer. N Engl J Med 325: 164–170 (1991)
5. Dibendetto, SP, Ragusa, R, Ippolito, A.M., LoNigro, L, DiCataldo, A., D'Amico, S., Miraglia, V.. Assessment of the value of treatment with granulocyte colony-stimulating factor in children with acute lymphoblastic leukemia: a randomized clinical trial. Eur. J. Haematol. 55: 93–96 (1995)
6. Freedman, M.H., Grunberger, T., Correa, P., Axelrad, A.A., Dube, I.D., Cohen, A. Autocrine and paracrine growth control by granulocyte-monocyte colony-stimulating factor of acute lymphoblastic leukemia cells. Blood 81: 3068–3075 (1993)
7. Geissler K, Koller E, Hinterberger W, Niederwieser D, Knöbl P, Pabinger I, Werner D, Scherrer R, Schwarzinger I, Friedl J, Jaeger U, Lechner K. Concomitant administration of granulocyte colony-stimulating factor (G-CSF) and induction chemotherapy of adult acute lymphoblastic leukemia (ALL)-first results of a multicenter, open-label, phase III study in randomized parallel groups. Blood 84: (Suppl. 1) 911 (abstr)(1994)
8. Hoelzer D: Which factors influence the different outcome of therapy in adults and children with ALL? Bone Marrow Transplant 4 Suppl 1: 98 (1989)
9. Hoelzer D. Therapy of the newly diagnosed adult with acute lymphoblastic leukemia. Hematol Oncol Clin North Am 7: 139–160 (1993)
10. Hoelzer D. Treatment of acute lymphoblastic leukemia. Semin Oncol 31: 1 (1994)
11. Kantarijan, H.M., Estey, E.H., OBrian, S., Anaissie, E., Beran, M., Rios, M.B., Keating M.J., Gutterman, J. Intensive chemotherapy with mitoxantrone and high-dose cytosine arabinoside followed by granulocyte macrophage colony-stimulating factor in the treatment of patients with acute lymphocytic leukemia. Blood 79: 876–881 (1992)

12. Kantarijan, H.M., Estey, E.H., O'Brian, S., Anaissie, E., Beran, M., Pierce, S., Robertson, L., Keating, M.J. Granulocyte colony-stimulating supportive treatment following intensive chemotherapy in acute lymphocytic leukemia in first remission. Cancer 72: 2950–2955 (1993)
13. Kita K; Nishii K; Ohishi K; Morita N; Takakura N; Kawakami K; Miwa H'; Shirakawa S. Frequent gene expression of granulocyte colony-stimulating factor (G-CSF) receptor in CD7+ surface CD3-acute lymphoblastic leukaemia. Leukemia 7: 1184–1190 (1993)
14. Kondo S, Okamura S, Niho Y, Gondo H, Hayashi S: Human granulocyte colony-stimulating factor receptor expressed on T-cell malignant lymphoma cells. Blood 1: 1630 (1992)
15. Larson RA, Linker CA, Dodge RK, George SL, Davey FR, Frankel SR, Powell BL, Schiffer CA: Granulocyte colony-stimulating factor (Filgrastim: G-CSF) reduces the time to neutrophil recovery in adults with acute lymphoblastic leukemia receiving intensive remission induction chemotherapy: Cancer and Leukemia Group B study 9111. Proc of ASCO 13: 305 (1994)[abstr.]
16. Maher D.W., Lieschke, G.J., Green, M., Bishop, J., Stuart-Harris, R., Wolf, M., Sheridan, W.P., Kefford, R.F., Cebon, J., Olver, I., McKendrick, J., Toner, G., Bradstock, K., Lieschke, M., Cruickshank, S., Tomita, D.K., Hoffmann, E.W., Fox, R.M., Morstyn, G. Filgrastim in patients with chemotherapy-induced febrile neutropenia. Annual Int Med 121: 492–501 (1994)
17. Meropol NJ, Miller LL, Korn EL, Braitman LE, MacDermott ML, Schuchter LM: Severe myelosuppression resulting from concurrent administration of granulocyte colony-stimulating factor and cytotoxic chemotherapy. JNCI 84: 1201–1203 (1992)
18. Neidhart J, Mangalik A, Kohler W, Stidley C, Saiki J, Duncan P, Souza L, Downing M: Granulocyte colony-stimulating factor stimulates recovery of granulocytes in patients receiving dose-intensive chemotherapy without bone marrow transplantation. J. Clin Oncol 7: 1685 (1989)
19. Ohno R, Tomonaga M, Kobayashi T, Kanamaru A, Shirakawa S, Masaoka T, Omine M, Oh H, Nomura T, Sakai Y, Hirano M, Yokomaku S, Nakayama S, Yoshida Y, Miura AB, Morishima Y, Dohy H, Niho Y, Hamajima N, Takaku F: Effect of granulocyte colony-stimulating factor after intensive induction therapy in relapsed or refractory acute leukemia. N Engl J Med 323: 871–877 (1990)
20. Ottmann, O.G., Ganser, A., Freund, M., Heil, G., Hiddemann, W., Heit, W., Gracien, E., and Hoelzer, D. Simultaneous administration of granulocyte colony-stimulating factor (Filgrastim) and induction chemotherapy in acute lymphoblastic leukemia—a pilot study. Ann. Hematol. 67: 161–167 (1993)
21. Ottmann OG, Hoelzer D, Gracien E, Ganser A., Kelly K, Reutzel R, Lipp T, Busch FW, Schwonzen M, Heil G, Wandt H., Koch P, Kolbe K, Heyll A, Bentz M, Peters S, Diedrich H, Dethling J., Meyer P., Nowrousian, M.R., Löffler, B., Weiss, A., Kneba M., Föller, A., Graf M., Hecht, Th. Concomitant granulocyte colony-stimulating factor and induction chemoradiotherapy in adult acute lymphoblastic leukemia: a randomized phase III trial. Blood 86: 444 (1995)
22. Pettengell R, Gurney H, Radford JA, Deakin DP, James R, Wilkinson PM, Kane K, Bertley J, Crowther D: Granulocyte colony-stimulating factor to prevent dose-limiting neutropenia in non-Hodgkin's lymphoma: a randomized controlled trial. Blood 80: 1430 (1992)
23. Preti A and Kantarjian HM. Management of adult acute lymphoblastic leukemia: present issues and key challenges. J. Clin Oncol 12: 1312–1322 (1994)
24. Scherrer, R., Geissler, K., Kyrle, P.A., Gisslinger, H., Jäger, U., Bettelheim, P., Laczika, K., Locker, G., Scholten, C., Sillaber, C., Schwarzinger, I., Thalhammer, F., and Lechner, K. Granulocyte colony-stimulating factor (G-CSF) as an adjunct to induction chemotherapy of adult acute lymphoblastic leukemia (ALL). Ann. Hematol. 66: 283–289 (1993)
25. Sheridan WP, Morstyn G, Wolf M, Dodds A, Lusk J, Maher D, Layton JE, Green MD, Souza L., Fox RM: Granulocyte colony-stimulating factor and neutrophil recovery after high-dose chemotherapy and autologous bone marrow transplantation. Lancet 2: 891 (1989)
26. Schriber UJR; Negrin RS; Chao NJ; Long GD; Horning SJ; Blume KG: The efficacy of granulocyte colony-stimulating factor following autologous bone marrow transplantation for non-Hodgkin's lymphoma with monoclonal antibody purged bone marrow. Leukemia 7: 1491 (1993)
27. Taylor KM, Jagannath S, Spitzer G, Spinolo JA, Tucker SL, Fogel B, Cabanillas FF, Hagemeister FB, Souza LM: Recombinant human granulocyte colony-stimulating factor hastens recovery after high-dose chemotherapy and autologous bone marrow transplantation in Hodgkin's disease. J Clin Oncol 7: 1791 (1990)
28. Telford MW, Kempin S, Kritz A, Sogoloff H, Gee T, Berman E, Scheinberg D, Little C, Gaynor J, Belanger C, Bertino J, Andreeff M, McKenzie S, Clarkson B: Severe toxicity limits intensification of induction therapy for acute lymphoblastic leukemia. Leukemia 7: 832 (1993)
29. Tsuchiya H., Adachi N., Asou N., Takatsuki K., Matsuda I., Kawano F., Murakami T., Mizutani S., Watanabe M. Responses to granulocyte colony-stimulating factor (G-CSF) and granlocytemacrophage CSF in Ph1-positive acute lymphoblastic leukemia with myeloid surface markers. Blood 77: 411 (1991)
30. Welte, K., Mempel, K., Reiter, A., Yakisan, E., Odenwald, E., Pfetsch, M., Zwingers, T., Schwab, G., and Riehm, H. A randomised phase III study of recombinant human granulocyte colony-stimulating factor (r-metHuG-CSF) in childhood high risk acute lymphoblastic leukemia. Blood 82: 194a, (1993) (Abstract)

Acute Leukemias VI
Prognostic Factors
and Treatment Strategies
Büchner et al. (eds)

Peripheral Blood Stem Cell Transplantation in Acute Myeloid Leukemia

J. Reiffers, J.-M. Boiron, P. Cony-Makhoul, G. Marit, F.-X. Mahon, and A. Broustet

Introduction

Autologous peripheral blood stem cell (PBSC) transplantation was first successfully performed in patients with acute myelogenous leukemia (AML) during the mid 1980s. Since these reports [1–3], the number of patients undergoing PBPSC transplantation has increased, as the use of PBSC rather than bone marrow offers many advantages which can be summarized as follows: hematopoietic recovery following PBSC transplantation is significantly quicker than that usually observed after unpurged or purged bone marrow transplantation (BMT), and this can lead to a decrease in the morbidity and mortality of the transplant procedure [4]; PBSC are very easy to collect by means of leukapheresis, thus avoiding the need for patients to have general anesthesia; PBSC could be less contaminated by residual leukemic cells, which could lead to a decrease in the relapse risk following transplantation. However, the latter question is still unanswered as their are no clinical or biological data that can either confirm or refute this hypothesis [5]. Moreover, there is no clinical evidence that PBSC transplantation can produce a higher proportion of long-term survivors.

In this review, we focus our attention on the use of PBSC transplantation in AML. Before analyzing the clinical resuslts, we summarize the problems of mobilization and collection and the main data concerning hematopoietic recovery.

PBSC Mobilization and Collection

It is obvious that the numbers of PBSC collected (usually assessed by the colony forming unit—granulocyte macrophage CFU-GM assay and more recently by CD34-positive cell evaluation) depend on the concentration of blood progenitor cells at the time of collection.

During the steady state, the CFU-GM concentration is usually very low (about 50–100/ml) and the number of leukaphereses that would be necessary to collect 10×10^4/kg CFU-GM could be close to 30 procedures (about 0.3×10^4/kg CFU-GM per collection). We and others have reported that a 10–50-fold increase in the CFU-GM blood concentration could be obtained during the regenerative period following intensive chemotherapy [6, 7]. Leukaphereses performed during this "recirculation phase" (which lasts about 5–10 days) make it possible to collect high numbers of CFU-GM [4] (Table 1). In leukemic patients, as well as in other hematological malignancies or solid tumors, several factors can influence the rate of PBSC recirculation. These include the dose of chemotherapy used for mobilization (the higher the dose, the higher the recirculation) and the type of chemotherapy used, as some drugs which cause long-lasting damage to hematopoietic progenitors cannot be successfully used to mobilize PBSC. However, the rate of PBSC recirculation is mainly influenced by the number of courses of chemotherapy administered to patients before PBSC collection since the hematopoietic reserves may

Bone Marrow Transplant Unit, CHR Bordeaux, 33064 Pessac France and URA CNRS 1456, University of Bordeaux II, 33076 Bordeaux, France

Table 1. Recirculation and collection of CFU-GM in patients with AML according to different types of mobilization

Type of mobilization	Recirculation (/ml)	(Highest recorded peak level	Collection (x10[4])
Induction chemotherapy (de novo AML)	2274	(1133-3796)	627
Induction chemotherapy (AML in relapse)	not done		182
Consolidation chemotherapy	1286	(240-2279)	147
Consolidation chemotherapy and G-CSF	not done		213

have been depressed by successive myelotoxic treatments. This is illustrated in Table 1 which shows that PBSC recirculation and collection is significantly greater in AML patients after induction chemotherapy than after either consolidation treatment or chemotherapy administered for leukemic relapse (for the latter patients, many courses of chemotherapy have been used to induce and maintain the first complete remission).

More recently, it has been clearly shown that hematopoietic growth factors (HGF) can be used either alone or in combination with chemotherapy to increase PBSC recirculation. Granulocyte colony-stimulating factor G-CSF) or granulocyte-macrophage CSF (GM-CSF) have been reported (and more recently some other HGF) mainly in patients treated for solid tumors or lymphoid malignancies such as multiple myeloma, non-Hodgkin lymphomas or Hodgkin's disease [8-10]. In patients with AML, HGF are not routinely used to decrease the duration of marrow aplasia and thus to increase PBSC mobilization. However, when combined with chemotherapy to induce PBSC mobilization, G-CSF seems to be able to increase the yield of CFU-GM collected (personal data, Table 1).

Hematopoietic Recovery

As previously mentioned, the main advantage of PBSC transplantation over BMT is the short duration of marrow aplasia. We have reported that leukemic patients undergoing chemotherapy-mobilized PBSC transplantation achieve granulocytic and platelet recovery after a median number of 14.5 (range 9–20) days and 24 (range 10–35) days, respectively [6]. This latter hematopoietic recovery is quicker than that usually observed after unpurged or purged BMT [4, 11]. However, particularly in AML, some patients have a delayed platelet engraftment which is seen when the number of CFU-GM transplanted is lower than $15–25 \times 10^4$/kg [12, 13]. In some other cases, there may be a double wave of engraftment which is characterized by a rapid hematopoietic recovery (within 3 weeks) followed by a drop in the white blood cell (WBC) and platelet counts (≈6 weeks–3 months) before the patients recover a stable and trilineage engraftment [11, 12].

The differences observed in the hematopoietic recovery after either chemotherapy-mobilized PBSC transplantation or BMT have been reported in numerous series of patients. In the retrospective analysis of the European Bone Marrow Transplant (EBMT) Registry, the median number of days to achieve 500 polymorphonuclear cells/mm^3 was 15.5 days (range 9–60) and was significantly lower than the observed after BMT (27 days range 9–389) ($p<0.001$). However, there were no statistical difference for platelet recovery [14]. In the prospective study conducted by the BGMT group comparing BMT and PBSC transplantation for AML in first remission (CRI), we also found a statistical difference for granulocytic ($p<0.001$) but not for platelet engraftment [15]. The shorter period of granulocytopenia was accompanied by a significant reduction in the number of days of hospitalization or of amphotericin B administration, but not in the number of days with fever or intravenous antibiotic administration. Using PBSC mobilized with both chemotherapy and G-CSF, we recently observed that the duration of thrombocytopenia was significantly reduced as compared to that seen after chemotherapy- mobilized PBSC transplantation or BMT (Table 2).

Clinical Results in AML

In 1984, the patients who were transplanted with PBSC had AML in relapse. In most cases, following the myeloablative therapy (cyclophos-

Table 2. Hematopoietic recovery in AML patients undergoing PBSC transplantation

Reference	PMN[a]		Platelets[b]	
	Median	Range	Median	Range
EBMT study [11]	15.5	9–60	27	9–389
Korbling et al. [166]	14	–	30	–
Reiffers et al. [15]	13	11–20	87	55–120
Mobilization with chemotherapy+G-CSF	15	11–17	14	10–31

[a]PMN number of days to reach 500 polymorphonuclear cells/mm^3.
[b]Platelets, number of days to reach 50,000 platelets/mm^3.

phamide and total body irradiation TBI), a complete remission (CR) was achieved but its duration was usually very short, not exceeding 6 months, [1, 2]. Similar results were observed in patients undergoing autologous BMT for AML in relapse.

The number of patients who have been transplanted in second CR is very low. We recently reviewed our own cases and found that the 3-year disease-free survival was 20%–35%, similar to that reported with autologous BMT.

Most AML patients have been transplanted in first CR. Körbling et al. [16] reported the results obtained in 20 patients transplanted with PBSC collected following induction or consolidation chemotherapy. Although the patients were given a very intensive preparatory regimen (200 mg/kg cyclophosphamide and 14.4 Gy TBI), most had a leukemic relapse (14/20), so the 2 year disease-free survival was only 35%. These results were inferior (although the difference was not statistically significant) to those observed in an historical series of 23 patients who underwent autologous (purged) BMT in the same institution using the same conditioning regimen. Similar results were also reported by six collaborating centers in Australia: 36 patients were transplanted after the Bu-Cy2 conditioning regimen and the 2 year disease-free was 38% [17]. More recently, Sanz et al. [18] reported on a series of patients who underwent autologous PBSC transplantation. They also used the combination of busulfan and cyclophosphamide as a preparatory regimen and obtained results comparable to those of patients undergoing BMT.

To compare the results of PBSC versus BMT for AML in first CR, we retrospectively reviewed the data of patients reported to the EBMT Registry. For the 886 patients undergoing BMT, the 3-year disease-free survival and the actuarial risk of relapse were 42%±30% and 5%±3% respectively. These results were statistically different from those observed in the 63 patients transplanted PBSC alone, as the disease-free survival and risk of relapse were 33%±6% and 64%±7%, respectively (p<0.01 and p<0.0007). However, using multivariate analysis, there was no statistical difference between PBSC transplantation and BMT. More recently, we compared the results obtained in 57 patients undergoing PBSC transplantation in Europe with those of 114 patients who were matched for age, interval diagnosis-transplantation, and conditioning regime and who received BMT. No statistical differences were seen among the latter groups for disease-free survival, risk of relapse, and transplant-related mortality (unpublished data).

To analyze better the possible differences between BMT and PBSC transplantation, we undertook a prospective study comparing these two modalities of transplantation (BGMT Study). All patients received the same conditioning regimen (busulfan and melphalan). After a median follow up of 36 months, we were unable to detect any differences between the two groups (Fig. 1) [15].

Conclusion

Thus, there are no convincing data showing that the relapse risk could be lesser or greater than that observed after autologous BMT. This is in agreement with the biological study performed by To et al. [5] who could not detect any differences in the rate of residual leukemic cells between PBSC transplantation and BMT [5]. However, prospective studies enrolling a larger

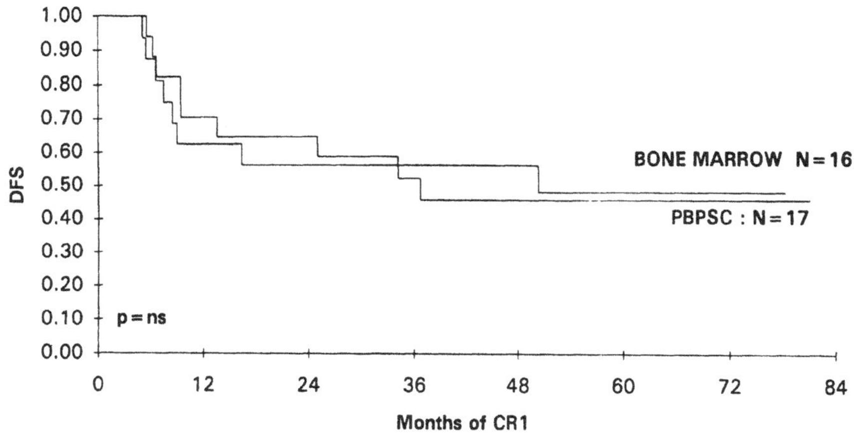

Fig. 1. BGMT-87 study. Comparison of PBPSC transplantation and BMT. transplantation for AML in first CR (age < 55 years). DFS, disease-free survival

number of patients than that of the BGMT study are needed to compare PBSC transplantation and BMT. A lower risk of relapse observed after PBSC transplantation could signify either a lower contamination by leukemic cells in PBSC than in bone marrow or other mechanisms such as a higher content of cytotoxic lymphoid cells in the PBSC samples as compared to bone marrow.

References

1. J. Reiffers, Ph. Bernard, B. David et al. (1986) Successful autologous transplantation with peripheral blood hemopoietic cells in a patient with acute leukemia. Exp. Hematol. 14: 312–315
2. C.A. Juttner, L.B. To, D.N. Haylock, A. Brandford et al (1985) Circulating autologous stem cells collected in very early remission from acute non-lymphoblastic leukaemia produce prompt but incomplete haemopoietic reconstitution after high-dose melphalan or supralethal chemotherapy. Br. J. Haematol, 61: 739–746
3. S. Castaigne, F. Calvo, L. Douay et al. (1986) Successful haematopoietic reconstitution using autologous peripheral blood mononucleated cells in a patient with acute promyelocytic leukaemia. Br. J. Haematol. 63: 209–211
4. J. Reiffers, G. Marit., G. Vezon, P. Cony-Makhoul, J.M. Boiron, M. Monrastruc, A. Rice, A. Broustet (1992) Autologous blood stem cell grafting in hematological malignancies. Present status and future directions. Transf. Sc. 13: 399–405
5. L.B. To, J. Russell, S. Moore & C.A. Juttner (1987) Residual leukaemia cannot be detected in very early remission peripheral blood stem cell collections in acute non-lymphoblastic leukaemia. Leuk. Res., 11: 327–330
6. J. Reiffers, G. Vezon, Ph Bernard et al. (1988) Stem cell apheresis in patients with acute non-lymphocytic leukemia. Plasma Ther. Transfus. Technol. 9: 115–118
7. L.B. To, D.N. Haylock, R.J. Kimber & C.A. Juttner (1984) High levels of circulating haemapoietic stem cells in very early remission from acute non-lymphoblastic leukaemia and their collection and cryopreservation. Br. J. Haematol., 58: 399–410
8. W.P. Dheridan, C.G. Begley, C.A. Juttner et al. (1992) Effect of peripheral blood progenitor cells mobilised by filgrastim (g-CSF) on platelet recovery after high-dose chemotherapy. The Lancet 1: 640–642
9. J.M. Boiron, G. Marit, C. Faberes et al. (1993) Collection of peripheral blood stem cells in multiple myeloma following single high-dose cyclosphosphamide with and without recombinant human granulocyte-macrophage colony-stimulating factor (rhGM-CSF). Bone Marrow Transplant. 12: 49–55
10. S. Siena, M. Bregni, B. Brando, F. Ravagnani et al. (1989) Circulation of CD 34+ hematopoietic stem cells in the peripheral blood of high dose cyclophosphamidetreated patients: enhancement by intravenous recombinant human granulocyte-macrophage colony stimulating factor. Blood, 74: 1095–1911
11. J. Reiffers, G. Leverger, G. Marit et al. (1989) Hematopoietic reconstitution after autologous blood stem cell transplantation. In Bone Marrow Transplantation: Current controversies»: Gale RP, Champlin RE (eds) Alan Liss, New-York, p 313–320
12. J. Reiffers (1991) Purged autologous bone marrow: better and worse than circulating stem cells? In «Advances in Haemapheresis»: CT Smith Sebinga and L. Kater (eds), Kluwer Academic Publishers, Dordrecht, p 103–112

13. C.A. Juttner, L.B. To, D.N. Haylock et al. (1991) Granulocyte macrophage progenitor numbers in peripheral blood stem cell autotransplantation. In «Advances in Haemapheresis»: CT Smit Sebinga and L. Kater (eds), Kluwer Academic Publishers, Dordrecht, p 91–102
14. J. Reiffers, M. Korbling, M. Labopin et al. (1992) Autologous blood stem cell transplantation versus autologous bone marrow transplantation for acute myeloid leukemia in first complete remission. Int. J. Cell Clon. 10 (Supp) 111–113
15. J. Reiffers, A.M. Stoppa, M. Attal, M. Michallet (1994) Is there a place for blood stem cell transplantation for the younger adult patient with acute myelogenous leukemia. J. Clin. Oncol. 12: 1100–1101
16. M. Korbling, T.M. Fliedner, R. Holle et al. (1991) Autologous blood stem cell (ABSCT) versus purged bone marrow transplantation (pABMT) in standard risk AML: influence of source and cell composition of the autograft on hemopoietic reconstitution and disease-free survival. Bone Marrow Transplant. 7: 343–349
17. J. Szer, C.A. Juttner, L.B. To et al. (1992) Post-remission therapy for acute myeloid leukemia with blood-derived stem cell transplantation. Results of a collaborative phase II trial Int. J. Cell Cloning 10: 114–117
18. M.A. Sanz, J. De LA Rubia, G.F. Sanz, G. Martin, J. Martinez et al. (1993) Busulfan plus cyclophosphamide followed by autologous blood stem cell transplantation for patients with acute myeloblastic leukemia in first complete remission: a report from a single institution. J. Clin. Oncol. 11: 1661–1667

New Strategies Using Growth Factors: GM-CSF, PIXY 321

Acute Leukemias VI
Prognostic Factors
and Treatment Strategies
Büchner et al. (eds)

Growth Factors in AML: Updates

T. Büchner, W. Hiddemann, B. Wörmann, M. Zühlsdorf, R. Rottmann, G. Innig, G. Maschmeier, W.-D. Ludwig, M.-C. Sauerland, and A. Heinecke for the AMLCG

Abstract. Hematopoietic growth factors (GF) are administered in patients with acute myeloid leukemia (AML) in order to overcome two limitations of chemotherapy: (1) its myelotoxicity and (2) the chemoresistance of minimal residual disease. GF have been used after chemotherapy in 11 clinical studies, eight of them on older or otherwise high-risk AML patients. The GF used were GM-CSF in seven, G-CSF in three and M-CSF in one of the studies. Beneficial effects of GF could be shown on the duration of neutropenia in eight studies, frequency of infections or fever in four studies, mortality or survival in two studies and remission rate in one study. The benefits in remissions and survival were all seen in high-risk patients. One leukemic regrowth or disease-free survival in the other studies. GF priming strategies are based upon their stimulation of AML blasts in vitro, their modulation of cellular AraC metabolism and enhancement of clonogenic cell kill by AraC. Protective effects of GF against clonogenic cell kill or apoptosis were also described. There are data from ten clinical studies using GF, also prior to or simultaneously with chemotherapy. One study showed significance and two studies a tendency to longer disease-free survival, two other studies a trend to more remissions. A disadvantage in the remission rate and survival was found in one study, and prolonged thrombocytopenia in two studies. Nine of ten studies found no evidence for an adverse effect of GF priming on the course of the disease. In most studies GF priming was only adminstered in one or two chemotherapy courses. One study giving 4–5 courses with GF priming found a reduction in relapses during the first half-year. In conclusion, supportive use of GF in the treatment of AML may have its place in high-risk rather than standard-risk situations. GF priming approaches may not have been adequately investigated so far, and an extension of this strategy to more treatment courses now appears justified and more promising. From clinical data available so far, all administration of GF in AML has to be regarded as investigational.

Introduction

Among human leukemias, acute myeloid leukemia has been a particular challenge for the administration of hematopoietic growth factors (GF) ever since their introduction during the late 1980s. Since AML blasts belong to the target cells of GF there was serious concern about adverse affects on the progression of the diesease. On the other hand it appeared to have potential to overcome the limitations in the treatment of AML represented by the high treatment-related mortality due to myelosuppression and by the chemoresistant minimal residual disease that produces recurrence of leukemia in the majority of patients.

Use of GF for Supportive Care in AML

The supportive use of GF in AML has now been investigated in the 11 major studies summarized in Table 1.

University of Münster, Germany

Table 1. Supportive use of growth factors in AML: synopsis of clinical studies

Study Reference	Special risk	Product	Growth factor Daily dose	Start	Control	Chemotherapy Dose	No. of patients	GF benefit	No difference	GF worse
German [1–3]	Early/multiple relapse or age 65+	GM-CSF (yeast)	250 μg/m²	Day 4 after chemo.	Historic	Relapses high dose, Age 65+ standard	112	Neutropenia ($p = 0.02$), mortality ($p = 0.009$)	Disease-free survival, leukemic regrowth	
ECOG [4]	Age 55–70	GM-CSF (yeast)	250 μg/m²	Day 4 after chemo.	Placebo	Standard	124	Neutropenia ($p = 0.001$), grade 4/5 infections ($p = 0.002$), survival (p=0.048)	Disease-free survival	
Houston [5]	Poor prognosis	GM-CSF (*E. coli*)	120 μg/m²	Day 1 after chemo.	Historic	Standard	12 GM-CSF		Neutropenia outcome	
CALGB [6]	Age 60+	GM-CSF (*E. coli*)	5 μg/kg	Day 1 after chemo.	Placebo	Standard	388	Neutropenia ($p = 0.02$),	Mortality remissions, leukemic regrowth survival, hospitalization	
GOELAM/ [7]	Age 55–75	GM-CSF (*E. coli*)	5 μg/kg	With start of chemo.	Placebo	Standard	209	Neutropenia ($p = 0.002$) disease-free survival ($p = 0.024$)	Mortality, remissions, infections, survival, hospitalization	
EORTC/ GIMEMA [8]	Age 15–60	GM-CSF (*E. coli*)	5 μg/kg	Day 1 after chemo.	Random	Standard	102		Infections, hospitalization	Remissions ($p = 0.008$), event-free-survival ($p = 0.01$)
EORTC/ HOVON [9]	Age 60+	GM-CSF (*E.coli*)	5 μg/kg	Day 1 before chemo.	Random	Standard	326	Neutropenia ($p = 0.001$)	Remission, infections, survival, disease-free-survival	Fever, fluid retention
Japan [10]	Relapsed/refractory acute leukemias	G-CSF	200 μg/m²	Day 2 after chemo.	Random	Standard or intensified	108	Neutropenia ($p < 0.01$), doc. infections ($p = 0.028$)	Fever, leukemic regrowth, relapses	

France, Italy Belgium [11]	Age 65+	G-CSF	5 µg/kg	Day 2 after chemo.	Placebo	Standard	172	Neutropenia ($p < 0.001$), remissions ($p = 0.002$)	Mortality at 8 weeks infections, leukemic regrowth, survival
Europe, Australia [12]		G-CSF	5 µg/kg	Day 1 after chemo.	Placebo	Standard	521	Neutropenia ($p = 0.0001$), fever ($p = 0.009$), antibiotics ($p = 0.0001$), hospitalization ($p = 0.0001$)	Remissions, disease-free survival, survival
Japan [13]		M-CSF	8×10^6U	Day 1 after chemo., three courses	Placebo	Intensive consolidation	198	Febrile neutropenia ($p = 0.003$), days required for 3 courses ($p = 0.005$), antimicrobial agents ($p = 0.018$), platelet transfusions ($p = 0.026$)	

The first clinical study using GM-CSF in patients with AML started in 1987 and was restricted to patients with a high risk of treatment-related mortality, such as patients 65 years of age or older and patients with an early first relapse or a second relapse [1, 2]. Yeast-derived GM-CSF, 250 μg/m^2/day continuous. i.v. infusion, was started on day 4 after chemotherapy provided that the blasts in bone marrow were reduced to less than 5%. Infusion of GM-CSF continued until the blood neutrophils reached 2000/mm^3. Thirty-six patients entered the study: 25 older patients with newly diagnosed AML and 11 patients with relapses. The results were historically compared with those from 56 patients receiving the same chemotherapy without GM-CSF. Under GM-CSF the neutrophil recovery time could indeed be reduced by a median of 1 week when compared with that in the control patients, and there was a reduction in early deaths from 39% to 14% ($p = 0.009$) in the entire study group and from 44% to 12% in the older patients ($p = 0.007$)[3].

The original dosage and schedule of yeast-derived GM-CSF for high-risk AML [3] was tested in a randomized placebo-controlled trial conducted by the ECOG in elderly patients with newly diagnosed AML. One hundred and twenty-four patients 55–70 years of age were involved, and the median neutrophil recovery time to 1000/mm^3 was reduced by 7 days ($p = 0.001$). This effect also translated into a reduction in the overall treatment-related toxicity ($p = 0.049$) and in grade 4/5 infections ($p = 0.002$) and a superior median survival in the GM-CSF arm (10.6 vs 4.8 months, $p = 0.048$) [4].

In contrast, a pilot study at M.D. Anderson Cancer Center in Houston could not confirm an acceleration of neutrophil recovery or improved outcome in 12 patients with newly diagnosed AML and a poor prognosis [5]. In this study a comparatively low daily dose of 120 μg/m^2/day *E. coli*-derived GM-CSF was used.

In a large randomized placebo-controlled trial involving 388 patients, the CALGB addressed the effect of GM-CSF after chemotherapy in patients 60 years of age and older with newly diagnosed AML. *E. coli*-derived GM-CSF, 5 μg/kg/day by 6-h i.v. infusion, was started 1 day after the first induction course and continued until the blood neutrophils recovered to 1000/mm^3. The median neutrophil recovery time was 2 days shorter in the GM-CSF group ($p = 0.02$), whereas no significant difference was found in complete remissions, mortality, persistent leukemia, leukemic regrowth and total survival [6]. In this trial GM-CSF was discontinued in 32% of patients—34% in the GM-CSF arm and 31% in the placebo arm—for reasons of side effects attributed by physicians to GM-CSF. Thus, the data from one-third of the patients could not contribute to the issue of GM-CSF effects, although this group, with side effects most likely related to infections rather than to GM-CSF and with a much lower response rate, might have especially benefitted from GM-CSF support.

Most recently the GOELAM group in France reported the results of GM-CSF vs placebo in patients 55–75 years of age. *E. coli*-derived GM-CSF, 5 μg/kg/day 6-h i.v. infusion, was given during induction by standard dose cytosine arabinoside (AraC) and idarubicin and was continued until neutrophils recovered. The duration of neutropenia was 4 days shorter in the GM-CSF arm ($p = 0.002$), but the incidence of febrile episodes and bacteremias and the duration of hospitalization were similar in both arms. GM-CSF was prematurely stopped for reasons of toxicity in 14% of GM-CSF patients and 3% of placebo patients [7].

In a European study of EORTC/GIMEMA, 102 patients 15–60 years of age received *E. coli*-derived GM-CSF randomly at various timings. Those with the GF after induction chemotherapy actually had a disadvantage in their remission rate and event-free survival [8].

An other European study by EORTC/HOVON randomized 326 patients over age 60 to receive *E.coli*-derived GM-CSF from 1 day before chemotherapy until neutrophil recovery or chemotherapy alone. There was a significant reduction in the neutrophil recovery time but no benefit in clinical outcome. GM-CSF showed significant toxicity manifested by more frequent fever and fluid retention [9].

Like GM-CSF, G-CSF was first investigated in a mixed population of patients with relapsed or refractory acute leukemias, including AML, ALL, CML blast crisis and AML after myelodysplasia. One hundred and eight patients were randomized to receive either chemotherapy followed by G-CSF or chemotherapy alone. G-CSF reduced neutropenia by 1 week ($p < 0.01$) and lowered the incidence of infections ($p = 0.028$) [10].

An AML Cooperative Study Group in France, Italy and Belgium treated 172 patients 65 years of age and older with G-CSF after standard induction treatment. When compared with placebo the duration of neutorpenia was reduced by 6 days ($p < 0.001$) and the complete remission rate was increased (70 vs 47%, $p = 0.002$), but the induction mortality and overall survival were not improved [11].

The largest study on GF or placebo support in AML has recently been conducted at 31 centers in Europe and Australia. G-CSF 5 μg /kg/day or placebo was started 1 day after each induction and consolidation chemotherapy course and continued until neutrophil recovery. In the patients with G-CSF the neutrophils recovered 5–7 days earlier ($p = 0.0001$), which translated into reductions in days with fever ($p = 0.009$), days with antibiotics ($p = 0.0001$) and days in hospital ($p = 0.0001$), while the remission rate and survival were not influenced by G-CSF [12]. The use of human natural M-CSF following chemotherapy has been investigated in a study in 198 patients randomized to receive three consolidation courses with M-CSF or placebo following each course. M-CSF significantly reduced the incidence of febrile neutropenia, the requirement for antimicrobial agents and platelet support, and the number of days required to give the three consolidation courses [13].

Importantly, no major adverse effects of GF after chemotherapy on the course of AML have been observed so far. The first study revealed leukemic regrowth in 2 of 30 patients under GM-CSF [3], and the CALGB reported 2% leukemic regrowth in each arm, GM-CSF and placebo [6]. In one patient the regrowth was completely reversible after cessation of GM-CSF [3, 14], but the regrowth continued uninfluenced in 1 patient [3] and 5 patients [6] and thus appeared GM-CSF independent. Furthermore, the duration of response was not significantly affected by GM-CSF [3, 6]. In the three studies on G-CSF [10–12] and the one study on M-CSF [13] after chemotherapy, there was again no evidence of stimulating leukemic regrowth.

In summary, GF for supportive use has proved safe and effective in reducing neutropenia in the vast majority of studies. Additional clinical benefits were achieved in some studies, preferentially in high-risk situations, where GF support may have its place.

GF Priming in AML

Other approaches with GF aim at enchancement of the antileukemic effect of chemotherapy by recruitment of chemoresistant resting leukemic cells into sensitive phases of the cell cycle. Even in vitro, a kind of recruitment can be observed when AML blasts are stimulated by GF to multiply and produce colonies [15–18]. The GM-CSF-induced increase in leukemic S phase cells also increased the leukemic clonogenic cell kill by AraC in vitro [19]. In 18 patients with newly diagnosed AML recruitment could then be demonstrated in vivo after a 24- to 48-h infusion of *E. coli*-derived GM-CSF, 250 μg/m^2/day continuous i.v. infusion prior to chemotherapy. There was a shift of leukemic blasts from G_0 with low RAN and DNA content to higher RNA and DNA content, corresponding to the G_1 and S phases, and also an increase in S phase cells incorporating BrdU, which was found in the majority of patients. GM-CSF continued during and after chemotherapy until neutrophil recovery, and 83% of patients achieved a complete remission [20].

GM-CSF priming strategies as used in the above study may also benefit from a modulation of the cellular metabolism of antileukemic drugs. Thus, we could show that the incorporation of AraC into DNA in leukemic blasts in vitro was increased 1.5- to 8.5-fold (median twofold) by 48 h preincubation and simultaneous incubation together with GM-CSF, an effect found in 23 out of 28 cases [21].

GF preexposure and presence also significantly increased the clonogenic cell kill by AraC in colony essays using semi-solid medium. The effect observed in leukemic blasts from AML patients was not observed in normal hematopoietic precursors (CFU-GM) [22]. The enhancement of the AraC antileukemic cytotoxicity by GF in vitro was related to their growth simulatory effect and varied among patients [23]. Contradicting the priming concept using GM-CSF, others discussed a protection of AML cells against antileukemic agents by this GF. Thus, AML blasts in vitro showed a substantial clonogenic cell kill after a 20-min pulse of AraC only if cultured in G-CSF, not in GM-CSF or IL-3. However, if the exposure to AraC was extended to 6 days, there was substantial cell kill with all three growth factors, though most marked with G-CSF, and mixing G-CSf and GM-CSf together brought the result close to that of G-CSF [24]. These data suggest an enhancement of cytotoxicity by these growth factors rather than leukemic cell protection, at least when AraC was present for an adequate time.

In a clinical setting, 56 patients with newly diagnosed AML received *E.coli*-derived GM-CSF at either 20 or 125 μg/m² once daily subcutaneously during a period varying between 0 and 8 days prior to chemotherapy. This inhomegenous population showed the lowest complete remission rate and shortest survival when compared with two historical control groups. The authors postulated that leukemic cell resistance was induced by GM-CSF [25].

Apoptosis, or programmed cell death, is one of the effects of antileukemic chemotherapy. In a murine leukemic cell line, nuclear condensation and fragmentation and internucleosomal DNA fragmentation, typical features of apoptosis, were found to be induced by TGFβ and were prevented by GM-CSF and G-CSF. GM-CSF and G-CSF also inhibited apoptosis induced by AraC, while the overall clonogenic cell reduction was not reduced. The authors proposed that apoptosis may be regulated independently from other mechanisms of cell kill [26]. In human AML cell lines, apoptosis induced by AraC was enhanced by a preexposure to PIXY 321, a GM-CSF/IL-3 fusion protein. This effect also occurred with an apoptosis-specific induction of the c-jun gene and a reduction of bcl 2 gene expression [27].

Thus, in the therapeutic in vivo situation different effects of GM-CSF may interfere with and even antagonize each other. In addition, potential recruitment effects on early leukemic stem cells in vivo may not be detectable in vitro and may only be reflected by an improved long-term outcome of patients from chemotherapy. Therefore, a recent German multicenter randomized trial in patients with newly diagnosed AML on GM-CSF priming and long-term administration in five consecutive chemotherapy cycles compared with identical chemotherapy alone [28–30] may give some answers. Yeast-derived GM-CSF, 250 μg/m² by once daily s.c. injection, was started 24 h before chemotherapy and continued until neutrophil recovery in both induction courses, in the consolidation course and in the first two maintenance courses. Chemotherapy was standard dose TAD [31] for induction and consolidation and reduced TAD courses for monthly maintenanace, given until 3 years of remission were completed. The second induction course was high-dose AraC with mitoxantrone [32] and was given to patients of 60 years and older if the bone marrow after the first course contained 5% or more residual blasts, and to all patients under 60 years. In addition, the AraC dose was 3 g/m² × 6 in the younger and 1g/m² × 6 in the older patients. A total of 114 patients with a median age of 51 (17–75) years entered the study. Some 79% of the GM-CSF patients and 84% of the controls went into remission, and persistent leukemia was observed in 4% and 18% of patients. Patients under 60 years of age achieved complete remissions in 82% and 73% of case and show a continuous remission rate after 4 years of 51% and 44%, while during the first half year there was a tendency of fewer relapses in the GM-CSF arm (3% vs 22%) [33]. Figure 1 shows an update of event-free survival.

Table 2 summarizes the data available from 10 clinical studies on GF priming.

In a South German placebo controlled study, 80 patients with newly diagnosed AML received standard dose induction and consolidation chemotherapy and a late consolidation of AraC 3 g/m² × 12 with daunorubicin 30 mg/m² × 3. *E. Coli*-derived GM-CSF 250 μg/m²/day s.c. injection or placebo was started 48 h prior to chemotherapy and continued until neutrophil recovered and was administered in the second induction course and in the two consolidations. There were no differences in the response to induction between the randomized groups. Disease-free survival after 41 months in patients under age 50 was 65% in the GM-CSF and 58% in the placebo group ($p = 0.03$), but in patients over age 50 disease-free survival was 20% vs 31% ($p = 0.28$) [34].

In the GOELAM study mentioned above [7] GM-CSF or placebo was administered concomitantly with chemotherapy and thereafter in patients over age 55. The disease-free survival at 2 years was 44% vs 19% in favor of GM-CSF ($p = 0.024$).

Different schedules of *E.coli*-derived GM-CSF were investigated in 102 patients, aged 15–60 years, by the EORTC/GIMEMA Leukemia Cooperative Group. GM-CSF 5 μg/kg/day was given randomly (1) from 24 h prior to the start of a standard-dose AraC/idarubicin course and continued until the end of this course, from the end of the course until day 28 or neutrophil recovery, or (3) as in 1 plus 2 or (4) chemotherapy was given alone. A significantly negative impact on the CR rate and event-free survival was found from GM-CSF given after chemotherapy, while results from GM-CSF before and during chemotherapy were similar to those of

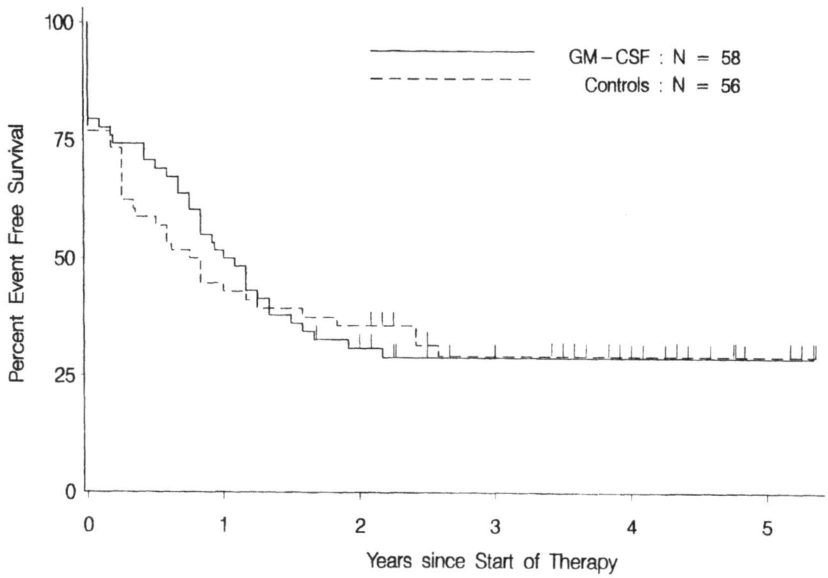

Fig. 1. Randomized study of multiple-course GM-CSF priming and long-term administration in primary AML. Event-free survival of all patients entering comparing GM-CSF patients and control patients without GM-CSF. Age is 16–75 years and events are non-achievement of remission, death in remission and relapse. Tick marks represent patients alive in remission. The 4-year event-free survival rate is 29% in both arms. In the 88 patients unter age 60 the 4-year event-free survival rate is 38% in the GM-CSF and 32% in the control arm ($p = 0.3$), and the corresponding disease-free interval is 53% vs 45% ($p = 0.3$)

controls [8]. Disease-free survival was not reported.

GM-CSF priming was also an attempt of the large European study in 326 older patients [9]. Again, no benefit in outcome could be demonstrated. Instead of GM-CSF, three studies used G-CSF for their priming strategies. Given for 3 days before chemotherapy, G-CSF has no adverse effect on the recovery of neutrophils and platelets [35]. Accelerated neutrophil recovery was found after G-CSF, preceding by 1 day a fludarabine high-dose AraC chemotherapy for unfavorable AML or myelodysplasis [36] and by 2 days standard chemotherapy for refractory AML [37]. In both studies [36, 37] G-CSF was continued until the recovery of neutrophils.

Besides some general side effects typical for cytokines there was no major specific toxicity from GF priming regimens. In particular, the data on blast clearance, persistent leukemia and disease-free survival gave no evidence for a chemoresistance induced by GF priming. In both German studies, however, the recovery of platelets showed a significant delay in the GM-CSF arm [30, 34] suggesting an impairment of early hematopoietic progenitor cells by GF priming. This effect did not cause major clinical problems. On the contrary, it permits speculation that early leukemic progenitors may be affected similarly.

In summary, GF priming remains an interesting therapeutic approach in AML. Negative effects on the course of the disease have rarely been observed, while there seems to be an advantage in disease-free survival. The priming strategy may be more effective in a multiple course design.

References

1. Büchner Th, Hiddemann W, Koenigsmann M et al. Human recombinant granulocyte-macrophage colony-stimulating factor (GM-CSF) treatment of patients with acute leukemias in aplasis and at high risk of early death. Behring Inst Mitt 83: 308, 1988.
2. Büchner T, Hiddemann W, Koenigsmann M, et al. Recombinant human GM-CSF following chemotherapy in high-risk AML. Bone Marrow Transplantation 6: 131–134, 1990.
3. Büchner Th, Hiddemann W, Koenigsmann M et al. Recombinant human granulocyte-macrophage

Table 2. Growth factor priming in AML: synopsis of clinical studies

Study References	Special Risk	Product	Growth factor Daily dose	Start	Controls	Chemotherapy dose	No. of patients	No. of courses chemo. plus GF	GF Benefit	No difference	GF worse
Vienna/NY [20]	Age 25–77	GM-CSF (*E. coli*)	250 μg/m²	1–2 days before chemo.	Historic	Standard	18 GM-CSF 39 controls	1–2	Complete neutropenia ($p < 0.05$)	remissions 85%	
Houston [25]	Adults	GM-CSF (*E. coli*)	20 or 120 μm/m²	0–8 days before chemo.	Historic	intermediate or high dose	56 GM-CSF 176 controls	3–4			Remissions (p=0.01), survival ($p < 0.034$)
AML CG [28–30]	Age 16–75	GM-CSF (yeast)	250 μg/m²	1 day before chemo.	Random	Standard (3–4 courses), high dose (1 course)	114	4–5	Disease-free-survival age < 60 (n.s.)	Remissions, persistent leukemia, blast clearance, neutropenia, survival	Thrombo-penia ($p < 0.05$)
South German [34]	Age 17–73	GM-CSF (*E. coli*)	250 μg/m²	2 days before chemo.	Placebo	Standard (2 courses), high dose (1 course)	80	3	Disease-free-survival age < 60 (n.s)	Remissions, neutropenia, survival	Thrombo-penia ($p < 0.05$)
GOELAM [7]	Age 55–75	GM-CSF (*E. coli*)	5 μg/kg	With start of chemo.	Placebo	Standard	209	1–2	Disease-free survival (p=0.024), neutropenia (p=0.002)	Remissions, survival	
EORTC/ GIMEMA [8]	Age 15–60	GM-CSF (*E. coli*)	5 μg/kg	1 day before chemo.	Random	Standard	102	1–		Remissions, resistance, mortality	
EORTC/ HOVON [9]	Age 60+	GM-CSF (*E. coli*)	5 μg/kg	1 day before chemo.	Randosm	Standard	321	1	Neutropenia (p=0.001)	Remissions infections, disease-free survival,	Fever, fluid retention
Buffalo [35]	Primary and secondary AML	G-CSF	10 μg/kg	3 days before chemo. then stop	Unprimed controls	High dose	17 G-CSF	1		neutropenia, thrombopenia	

Houston [36]	AML rather unfavorable karyotypes, and myelodysplasias	G-CSF	500 µg/m2	1 day before or at start of chemo.	Historic	High dose	112	1	Neutropenia (p=0.001)	Remissions, infections, survival
Japan [37]	Relapsed or refractory	G-CSF	200 µg/m2	2 days before chemo.	Placebo	standard	58	1	Neutropenia ($p < 0.001$) remissions (n.s.)	Fever, infections. AML cell growth, AML regrowth, event-free survival, diaease-free survival

colony-stimulating factor after chemotherapy in patients with acute myeloid leukemia at higher age or after relapse. Blood 78: 1190–1197, 1991.
4. Rowe JM, Andersen J, Mazza JJ et al. A randomized placebo-controlled Phase III study of granulocyte-macrophage colony stimulating factor (GM-CSF) in adult patients (>55–70 years) with acute myelogenous leukemia (AML). A study of the Eastern Cooperative Oncology Group (E1490). Blood: 86: 457, 1995.
5. Estey EH, Dixon D, Kantarjian HM et al. Treatment of poor-prognosis, newly diagnosed acute myeloid leukemia with Ara-C and recombinant human granulocyte-macrophage colony stimulating factor. Blood 75: 1766–1769, 1990.
6. Stone RM, Berg DT, George SL et al. Granulocyte-macrophage colony-stimulating factor after initial chemotherapy for elderly patients with primary acute myelogenous leukemia. New Engl J Med 332: 1671–1677, 1995.
7. Witz F, Harousseau JL, Cahn JY et al. CM-CSF during and after remission induction treatment for elderly patients with acute myeloid leukemia (AML). Ann Hematol 70 (Suppl II): 163: A135, 1995.
8. Zittoun R, Mandelli F, de Witte T et al., Recombinant human granuocyte-macrophage colony-stimulating factor (GM-CSF) during induction treatment of acute myelogenous leukemia (AML). A randomized trial from EORTC/GIMEMA leukemia cooperative groups. Blood 84 Suppl 1: 231 a, 1994
9. Löwenberg B, Suciu S, Zittoun R et al. GM-CSF during as well as after induction chemotherapy (CT) in elderly patients with acute myeloid leukemia (AML). The EORTC/ HOVON Phase III trial (AML 11). Blood 86 Suppl 1: 433 a, 1995
10. Ohno R, Tomonaga M, Kobayashi T et al. Effect of granulocyte colony-stimulating factor after intensive induction therapy in relapsed or refractory acute leukemia. N Engl J Med 323: 871–877, 1990
11. Dombret H, Chastang C, Fenaux P et al. A controlled study of recombinant human granulocyte colony-stimulating factor in elderly patients after treatment for acute myelogenous Leukemia. N Engl J Med 22: 1678–1683, 1995
12. Heil G, Hoelzer D, Sanz MA et al. Results of a randomized double-blind placebo controlled phase III study of filgrastim remission induction and early consolidation therapy for adults with de-novo acute myeloid leukemia. Blood 86 Suppl 1: 267 a, 1995
13. Ohno R, Miyawaki S, Hatake K et al. Macrophage-colony stimulating factor (M-CSF) reduces the incidence and duration of febrile neutropenia and shortens the period required to finish three courses of intensive consolidation therapy in acute myeloid leukemia (AML): a double-blind controlled study. Blood 86 Suppl 1: 266a, 1995
14. Koenigsmann M, Hiddemann W, Büchner Th, Reversible leukaemic regrowth under GM-CSF treatment after chemotherapy for AML. Leukemia Research 15: 37–41, 1991.
15. Griffin JD, Young D, Herrmann F et al. Effects of recombinant human GM-CSF on proliferation of clonogenic cells in acute myeloblastic leukemia. Blood 67: 1448–1453, 1986.
16. Kelleher C, Miyauchi J, Wong G et al. Synergism between recombinant growth factors GM-CSF and G-CSF, acting on the blast cells of acute myeloblastic leukemia. Blood 69: 1498–1503, 1987.
17. Miyauchi J, Kelleher CA, Yang YC et al. The effect of three recombinant growth factors, IL-3, GM-CSF, and G-CSF, on the blast cells of acute myeloblastic leukemia maintained in shortterm suspension culture. Blood 70: 657–663, 1987.
18. Vellenga E, Young DC, Wagner K et al. The effect of GM-CSF and G-CSF in promoting growth of clonogenic cells in acute myeloblastic leukemia. Blood 69: 1771–1776, 1987.
19. Cannistra SA, Groshek P, Griffin JD. Granulocyte-macrophage colony-stimulating factor enhances the cytotoxic effects of cytosine arabinoside in acute myeloblastic leukemia and in the myeloid blast crisis phase of chronic myeloid leukemia. Leukemia 3: 328–334, 1989.
20. Bettelheim P, Valent P, Andreeff M et al. Recombinant human granulocyte-macrophage colony-stimulating factor in de novo acute myeloid leukemia. Blood 77: 700–711, 1991.
21. Reuter C, Auf der Landwehr U, Schleyer E et al. Modulation of intracellular metabolism of cytosine arabinoside in acute myeloid leukemia by granulocyte macrophage colony stimulating factor. Leukemia 8: 217–225, 1994.
22. Zühlsdorf M, Busemann C, Weißpfennig S et al. Priming with rhGM-CSF or rh-IL-3 for AML progenitors versus CFU-GM in vivo and in vitro: Significant increase in therapeutic ratio for cytosine arabinoside. Proc AACR 85: 211, 1994.
23. Van Der Lely N, De Witte T, Wessels J et al. In vitro response of blasts to IL-3, GM-CSF, and G-CSF is different for individual AML patients: factors that stimulate leukemic clonogenic cells also enhance Ara-C cytotoxicity. Ann Hematol 68: 225–232, 1994.
24. Koistinen P, Wang C, Curtis JE et al. Granulocyte-macrophage colony-stimulating factor and interleukin-3 protect leukemic blast cells from Ara-C toxicity. Leukemia 5: 789–795, 1991.
25. Estey E, Hall PT, Kantarjian H et al. Treatment of newly diagnosed acute myelogenous leukemia with granulocyte-macrophage colony-stimulating factor (GM-CSF) before and during continuousinfusion high-dose Ara-C + daunorubicin: comparison to patients treated without GM-CSF: Blood 79: 2246–2255, 1992.
26. Lotem J, Sachs L. Hematopoietic cytokines inhibit apoptosis induced by transforming growth factor ß1 and cancer chemotherapy compounds in myeloid leukemic cells. Blood 80: 1750–1778, 1992.
27. Bhalla K, Tang C, Ibrado AM et al. Granulocyte-macrophage colony-stimulating factor/interleukin-3 fusion protein (pIXY 321) enhances high-dose Ara-C induced programmed cell death

or apoptosis in human myeloid leukemia cells. Blood 80: 2883–2890, 1992.
28. Büchner Th, Hiddemann W, Rottmann R et al. Multiple course chemotherapy with or without GM-CSF priming and longterm administration for newly diagnosed AML. Proc ASCO 29: 301, 1993.
29. Büchner T, Hiddemann W, Wörmann B et al. The role of GM-CSF in the treatment of acute myeloid leukemia. Leukemia and Lymphoma 11; 21–24, 1993.
30. Büchner T. Hematopoietic growth factors in cancer treatment. Stem Cells 12: 241–252, 1994.
31. Büchner T, Urbanitz D, Hiddemann W, et al. Intensified induction and consolidation with or without maintenance chemotherapy for acute myeloid leukemia (AML): two multicenter studies of the German AML Cooperative Group. J Clin Oncol 12: 1583–1589, 1985.
32. Hiddemann W, Kreutzmann H, Straif K et al. High-dose cytosine-arabinoside and mitoxantrone: A highly effective regimen in refractory acute myeloid leukemia. Blood 69: 744, 1987.
33. Büchner Th, Hiddemann W, Wörmann B et al. for the AML Cooperative Group. Hematopoidic growth factors in acute myeloid leukemia. Hematology and Blood Transfusion 1996 (in press).
34. Heil G, Chadid L, Hoelzer D et al. GM-CSF in a double-blind randomized, placebo controlled trials on therapy of adult patients with de novo acute myeloid Leukemia (AML). Leukemia 9: 3–9, 1995.
35. Baer M.R., Bernstein SH, Brunetto VL et al. In vivo revombinant human G-CSF priming in previously untreated acute myeloid leukemia. Blood 26 Suppl 1: 328a, 1993.
36. Estey E, Thall P, Andreeff M et al. Use of granulocyte colony stimulating factor before, during and after fludarabine plus cytarabine induction therapy of newly diagnosed acute myelogenous leukemia or myelodysplastic syndromes: Comparison with fludarabine plus cytarabine without granulocyte colony-stimulating factor. J Clin Oncol 12: 671–678, 1994.
37. Ohno R. Naoe T, Kanamaru A et al. A double-blind study of granulocyte colony-stimulating factor started two days before induction chemotherapy in refractory acute myeloid leukemia. Blood 83: 2086–2092, 1994

Acute Leukemias VI
Prognostic Factors
and Treatment Strategies
Büchner et al. (eds)

Granulocyte-Macrophage Colony-Stimulating Factor-Based Priming Concepts in Acute Myeloid Leukemia

J.J. Wielenga

Introduction

The majority of patients with acute myeloid leukemia (AML) achieve a complete remission (CR) following modern chemotherapy. Unfortunately, most of them will relapse sooner or later as a consequence of residual AML cells which survived chemotherapy. Attempts to overcome this minimal residual disease by bone marrow transplantation (BMT) or other intensive treatment modalities are not always possible or successful. Eventually, the most frequent cause of treatment failure is resistance to chemotherapy that may develop as a result of a variety of mechanisms. One of these mechanisms may be related to the observation that a large fraction of clonogenic AML cells is not in S phase during cytosine arabinoside ara-C exposure [1]. Recruitment of AML cells into S phase in vivo following stimulation with hemopoietic growth factors (HGFs) may contribute to overcome this kinetic resistance of quiescent AML cells to ara-C. In addition, metabolic activation following exposure to HGFs may increase the intrinsic sensitivity of the AML cells to chemotherapy. This concept, called priming, has been tested in vitro as well as in several clinical studies. Butturini [2] demonstrated that an increase in cell cycle activity by HGFs parallels an increase in ara-C inhibition. Andreef [3] observed an increased in vitro ara-C toxicity if hemopoietic growth factor addition resulted in a six fold increase of cells in S phase. Ara-C efficacy was not increased in cases in which a smaller effect of growth factors on cytokinetics was observed. Similar data have been reported by other groups [4–8]. Other, not all cycle-related mechanisms may also play a role [9–11].

Materials and Methods

Clinical Studies

Published data on clinical studies are summarized and interpreted for the efficacy of the priming concept. Furthermore, preliminary data from 460 patients, treated in a study on granulocyte-macrophage colony-stimulating factor (GM-CSF)-based priming were analyzed. This study was recently performed by the Dutch, Swiss, and Belgian co-operative HOVON-SAKK centers. Inclusion criteria were: previously untreated AML, age 15–60 years, WHO performance 2 or less, and informed consent. Chemotherapy was conventional dose ara-C and daunomycin in cycle 1, intermediate dose ara-C and am-sacrine in cycle 2, and mitoxantrone etoposide in cycle 3. GM-CSF administration (5 μg/kg per day continuously i.v.) was according to randomization in arm la GM-CSF was started 24 h before chemotherapy and continued until the end of chemotherapy: in arm 1 b GM-CSF was started 24 h before chemotherapy and continued until granulocytes were above $0.5 \times 10^9/l$ or until day 28. In arm 2a GM-CSF was not given and in arm 2b GM-CSF was started after chemotherapy and continued until granulocytes were above $0.5 \times 10^9/l$ or until day 28. This study has

Department of Hematology, Academic Hospital Rotterdam, Dr. Molewaterplein 40, 3015 GD Rotterdam, The Netherlands

a factorial design: for the analysis the pooled data of arms 1a and b will be compared with the pooled data of arms 2a and b to analyze the priming effect, while the pooled data of arm 1a and 2a will be compared with the pooled data of arm 1b and 2b to analyze the effect of GM-CSF after chemotherapy.

Comparison of In Vitro and In Vivo Growth Factor Response of AML

To examine potential differences between in vivo and in vitro response of human AML to hemopoietic growth factors, mice with severe combined immuno deficiency (SCID) were transplanted with human AML cells as described [12]. Briefly, female specific pathogen-free CB17 scid/scid mice (5–8 weeks of age) were obtained from Harlan CPB Austerlitz, The Netherlands. They were housed under pathogen-free conditions and supplied with sterile food and acidified drinking water with 100 mg/l ciprofloxacin (Bayer AG, Leverkusen, Germany). Prior to transplantation, mice were irradiated with 3.5 Gy TBI, delivered by a ^{137}Cs source. AML cell suspensions were injected into a lateral tail vein. On day 35 after transplantation, mice were sacrificed by CO_2 inhalation followed by cervical dislocation. Cell suspensions obtained from the bone marrow (BM) were labelled with phycoerythrin conjugated monoclonal antibodies against CD33/CD45 and analyzed by FACSCAN.

Results

Clinical Studies

Several clinical studies on GM-CSF have been published over the last 5 years. Some of these studies only concern the administration of GM-CSF following chemotherapy for mitigation of pancytopenia [13–14]. Other studies were also aimed at the priming concept [7–8, 15–22] These studies are summarized in Table 1. In these studies the efficacy of GM-CSF based priming was evaluated by comparison of the complete remission (CR) rate following remission induction chemotherapy with and without GM-CSF. In most studies, a significant difference between GM-CSF- treated groups and controls was not found for CR rate, except for the study by Estey [15], in which the CR rate in the historical control group without GM-CSF was significantly higher as compared to the study group primed with GM-CSF. Preliminary data of the study performed by the Dutch, Swiss, and Belgian co-operative HOVON-SAKK centers are shown in Table 2. Significant differences for CR rate were not found.

Granulocyte-macrophage colony-stimulating Factor was not always given according to the protocol. A delay was sometimes necessary if the number of peripheral blasts was high, sometimes there was a temporary interruption, often for suspected drug fever, and in approximately 30 % of the patients GM-CSF was stopped prematurely. Reasons for early discontinuation were presumed side effects in approximately 45 of these patients. It is difficult to evaluate side effects in the context of toxic and intensive chemotherapy. Side effects observed more frequently in the GM-CSF-treated groups were fluid retention and hypotension. Side effects such as fluid retention, fever, hypotension, and allergic skin reactions were reasons for premature discontinuation in 45 out of 244 patients. Other side effects were less common and not clearly related to GM-CSF.

Table 1. Effects of GM-CSF-Based priming in AML

GM-CSF + Chemotherapy		Chemotherapy		Reference
(*n*)	CR (%)	(*n*)	CR (%)	
18	83	39	100	[7]
56	48	110/66	65/74	[15]
10	70	27	66	[19]
20	30	38	43	[16]
20	85	30	na	[18]
41	81	39	79	[20]
na	75	na	84	[21]
49	59	53	62	[22]

Table 2. Preliminary results of HOVON 4A study

	GM-CSF priming		GM-CSF post chemotherapy	
	Yes (n)	No (%)	Yes (n) (%)	No (n) (%)
CR	95 79	84 76	88 75	91 81
No CR	25 21	26 24	29 25	22 19
	120	110	117	113

Comparison of In Vitro and In Vivo Growth Factor Response of AML

The in vitro proliferation of AML measured by tritiated thymidin incorporation was compared to in vivo proliferation, as measured by massive BM infiltration 35 days after xenogenic transplantation. In Table 3 the results of four AML cases are shown. In case 1 in vivo and in vitro proliferation was observed in the presence as well in the absence of interleukin 3 (IL-3). In case 2, in vivo and in vitro proliferation was observed in the presence of IL-3 only. In cases 3 and 4, stimulation of in vivo AML proliferation by IL-3 was not predicated by in vitro stimulation as measured by tritiated thymidin incorporation: in case 3, in vitro proliferation was observed in the presence of IL-3 only, while in vivo proliferation was IL-3 independent. In case 4 spontaneous proliferation of AML was observed in vitro, while IL-3 was required to obtain in vivo growth.

Discussion

The concept of GM-CSF-based priming is theoretically interesting, and in vitro data suggest that it might work. However, so far the clinical data do not support this. If we look at the number of blast cells in the peripheral blood before and after GM-CSF, we see a heterogeneic response: in most patients, the number of blast cells rose, in some patients it remained unchanged, and in one patient it went down. Also, in in vitro response to GM-CSF, there is variability among patients. Therefore, it is possible that some patients may benefit from GM-CSF-based priming while other patients do not.

In vitro response to a growth factor is not always predictable for the situation in vivo as demonstrated in a preclinical model using SCID mice.

If we compare the potential favorable and unfavorable effects of GM-CSF-based priming, the influence on cell cycle kinetics, and the effects on ara-C metabolism counterbalance the risk to stimulate AML growth and to interfere with the cytotoxic effects of the treatment. This balance between favorable and unfavorable effects may be variable among patients. A higher dose of GM-CSF or a different priming schedule might be more effective. Another HGF or a combination of different HGFs might be more appropriate.

In conclusion, many questions on GM-CSF-based priming remain unanswered. Most of these questions cannot be answered in clinical studies. Therefore, we recently started preclinical studies in SCID mice aimed at these questions. The answers could be the basis for future clinical studies with GM-CSF or other hemopoietic growth factors.

Table 3. Comparison of in vivo and in vitro stimulation of AML by IL-3

AML Case no.	In vitro proliferation		In vivo proliferation	
	+IL-3	−IL-3	+IL-3	−IL-3
1	+	+	+	+
2	+	−	+	−
3	+	−	+	+
4	+	+	+	−

References

1. Minden MD, Till JE, McCulloch EA: Proliferative state of blast cell progenitors in acute myeloblastic leukemia (AML). Blood 52: 592–600, 1978.
2. Butturini A, Santucci MA, Gale RP, Perocco P, Tura S: GM-CSF incubation prior to treatment with cytarabine or doxorubicin enhances drug activity against AML cells in vitro: a model for leukemia chemotherapy. Leukemia Research 14: 743–749, 1990.
3. Andreeff M, Tafuri A, Hegewisch-Becker S: Colony-stimulating factors (rhG-CSF, rhGM-CSF, rhIL-3, and BCGF) recruit myeloblastic and lymphoblastic leukemic cells and enhance the cytotoxic effects of cytosine-arabinoside. Hamatol Bluttransfus 33: 747–762, 1990.
4. Lista P, Porcu P, Avanzi GC, Pegorano L: Interleukin-3 enhances the cytotoxic activity of 1-β-D-arabinofuranosylcytosin (ara-C) on acute myeloblastic leukemia (AML) cells. Br J Hematol 69: 121–123, 1988.
5. Tafuri A, Andreeff M: Kinetic rationale for cytokine induced recruitment of myeloblastic leukemia followed by cycle-specific chemotherapy in vitro. Leukemia 4: 826–834, 1990.
6. Cannistra SA, Groshek P, Griffin JD: Granulocyte-macrophagecolony-stimulating factor enhances the cytotoxic effects of cytosine arabinoside in acute myeloblastic leukemia and the myeloid blastic crisis of chronic myeloid leukemias. Leukemia 8: 328–334, 1989.
7. Bettelheim P, Volent P, Andreef M, Tafuri A, Haimi J, Gorischek C, Muhm M, Sillaber CH, Haas O, Vieder L, Maurer D, Scholz G, Speiser W, Geissler K, Kier P, Hinterberger W, Lechner K: Recombinant human granulocyte-macrophage colony-stimulating factor in combination with standard induction chemotherapy in de novo acute myeloid leukemia. Blood 77: 700–711, 1991.
8. Cannistra SA, DiCarlo J, Groshek P, Kanakura Y, Berg D, Mayer RJ, Griffin JD: Simultaneous administration of granulocyte-macrophage colony-stimulating factor and cytosine arabinoside for the treatment of relapsed acute myeloid leukemia. Leukemia 5: 230, 1991
9. Wormann B, Reuter C, Zuhlsdorf M, Buchner T, Hiddemann W: Experimental basis for the use of recombinant human granulocyte-macrophage colony-stimulating factor in patients with acute myeloid leukemia. Semin Oncol 21 (6 Suppl 16): 39–43, 1994.
10. te Boekhorst PA, Lowenberg B, Vlastuin M, Sonneveld P: Enhanced chemosensitivity of clonogenic blasts from patients with acute myeloid leukemia by G-CSF, IL-3 or GM-CSF stimulation. Leukemia 7: 1191–1198, 1993.
11. Yang GS, Minden MD, McCulloch EA: Influence of schedule or regulated sensitivity of AML blasts to cytosine arabinoside. Leukemia 7: 1012–1019, 1993.
12. Terpstra W, Prins A, Visser T, Wognum B, Wagemaker G, Löwenberg B, Wielenga JJ: Conditions for engraftment of human acute myeloid leukemia (AML) in SCID mice. Leukemia, in press.
13. Estey EH, Dixon D Katarjian HM, Keating MJ, McCredie K, Bodey GP, Kurzrock R, Talpaz M Freireich EJ, Deisseroth AB: Treatment of poor prognosis, newly diagnosed acute myeloid leukemia with ara-C and recombinant granulocyte-macrophage colony-stimulating-factor. Blood 75: 1766–1769, 1990.
14. Estrov Z, Estey EH, Andreef M, Talpaz M, Kurzrock R, Reading CL, Deisseroth AB, Gutterman JU: Comparison of in vivo and in vitro effects of granulocyte-macrophage colony stimulating factor (GM-CSF) in patients with acute myeloid leukemia. Exp Hematol 20: 558–564, 1992.
15. Estey E, Thall PF, Kantarjian, H, O'Brien S, Koller CA, Beran M, Gutterman J, Deisseroth A, Keating M: Treatment of newly diagnosed acute myelogenous leukemia with granulocye-macrophage colony-stimulating factor (GM-CSF) before and during continuous-infusion of high dose ara-C + daunorubicin: comparison to patients treated without GM-CSF. Blood 79: 2246–2255, 1992.
16. Archimbaud E, Fenaux P, Reiffers J, Cordonnier C, Leblond V, Travade P, Troussard X, Tilly H, Auzanneau G, Marie JP: Granulocyte-macrophage colony-stimulating factor in association to timed-sequential chemotherapy with mitoxantrone, etoposide, and cytarabine for refractory aute myelogenous leukemia. Leukemia 7: 372–377, 1993.
17. Buchner T, Hiddemann W, Koenigsmann M, Zuhlsdorf M, Wormann B, Boeckmann A, Freire EA, Innig G, Maschmeyer G, Ludwig WD: Recombinant human granulocyte-macrophage colony-stimulating factor after chemotherapy in patients with acute myeloid leukemia at higher age or after relapse. Blood 78: 1190–1197, 1991.
18. Valent P, Sillaber C, Geissler K, Andreeff M, Tafuri A, Vieder L, Schulz G, Lechner K, Bettelheim P: Treatment of de novo acute myelogenous leukemia with recombinant granulocyte macrophage-colony-stimulating factor in combination with standard induction chemotherapy: effect of granulocyte macrophage-colony-stimulating factor on white blood cell counts. Med Pediatr Oncol Suppl 2: 18–22, 1992.
19. Puntous M, Lacombe F, Dumain P, Marit G, Cony-Makhoul P, Belloc F, Boiron JM, Laurent G, Bernard P, Reiffers J: Treatment of relapsed acute myeloid leukemia using GM-CSF before intensive chemotherapy. Leuk Lymphoma 12: 95–102, 1993.
20. Heil G, Chadid L, Hoelzer D, Seipelt G, Mitrou P, Huber C, Kolbe K, Mertelsmann R, Lindemann A, Frisch J; GM-CSF in a double-blind randomized, placebo controlled trial in therapy of adult patients with de novo acute myeloid leukemia (AML). Leukemia 9: 3–9, 1995.
21. Buchner T, Hiddemann W, Wormann B, Rottmann R, Maschmeyer G, Ludwig WD, Zuhlsdorf M, Buntkirchen K, Sander A, Aswald J: The role of GM-CSF in the treatment of acute

myeloid leukemia. Leuk Lymphoma 11 Suppl 2: 21–24, 1993.
22. Zittoun R, Mandelli F, de Witte T, Willemze R, Thaler J, Hayat M, Stryckmans P, Peetermans M, Dardenne M, Solbu G, Suciu S: Recombinant human granulocyte-macrophage colony-stimulating factor (GM-CSF) during induction treatment of acute myelogenous leukemia (AML). A randomized trial from EORTC-GIMEMA leukemia cooperative groups. Blood 82 suppl: 231a, 1994.

Acute Leukemias VI
Prognostic Factors
and Treatment Strategies
Büchner et al. (eds)

Cancer and Leukemia Group B Studies with Hematopoietic Growth Factors in Patients with Acute Myeloid Leukemia

C.A. Schiffer[1], R. Stone[2], J. Moore[3], and B. Peterson[4] for the CALGB, (Lebanon, NH)

Abstract. The Cancer and Leukemia Group B (*CALGB*) has evaluated the use of hematopoietic growth factors in patients with acute myeloid leukemia (AML) using a number of different strategies. *CALGB protocol 8923* was a prospectively randomized, double-blind trial in patients with de novo AML > than 60 years of age receiving initial induction chemotherapy. There was no benefit in terms of improvement in complete remission (CR) rate, survival, or infectious morbidity from granulocyte-macrophage colony-stimulating factor (GM-CSF) begun the day after completion of chemotherapy and administered until neutrophil recovery. *CALGB protocol 9022* was a pilot study evaluating the feasibility of administering sequential courses of intensive consolidation treatment to patients with AML < than 60 years of age in first complete remission. Patients receiving diaziquone and mitoxantrone as their third course of consolidation experienced profound, sustained neutropenia. Subsequent cohorts received the same doses followed by G-CSF, which produced a statistically and clinically significant reduction in the duration of neutropenia < than 500/µl. *CALGB protocol 9021* is an ongoing randomized study evaluating the effect of GM-CSF "priming" as a means of increasing responsiveness to therapy with high-dose cytosine arabinoside ara-C in patients with refractory or relapsed AML. The CALGB is awaiting the results of other trials in progress prior to focusing on further investigations with hematopoietic growth factors in patients with AML.

Although prolonged disease-free survival can be achieved in approximately 20% of adults with de novo acute myeloid leukemia (AML), death from infectious complications and drug resistance limit the success of treatment in the majority of patients. Hematopoietic growth factors are being evaluated by a number of investigators as a means of decreasing the duration of neutropenia, there by potentially attenuating the impact of infections, as well as a means of enhancing sensitivity to S-phase-specific chemotherapeutic agents by increasing the number of cells in cell cycle. The CALGB has conducted studies addressing each of these questions and the results of these studies will be briefly summarized.

CALGB 8923 was a recently completed double-blind trial in which patients with de novo AML > than 60 years of age were randomized to receive either granulocyte-macrophage colony-stimulating factor (GM-CSF) (Schering Corporation 5 µg/kg per day administered intravenously over 6 h) or a placebo infusion [1]. The GM-CSF/placebo was begun the day after completion of a standard regimen of daunorubicin (3 days) and ARA-C (7 days). A total of 379 evaluable patients were randomized; pretreatment demographic characteristics were the same in both groups with an overall median age of 68 years. There were no clinically important

[1]Division of Hematologic Malignancies, University of Maryland Cancer Center, Division of Hematology/Medical Oncology, University of Maryland School of Medicine, Baltimore, Maryland 21201, USA
[2]Dana Farber Cancer Institute, Boston MA, USA
[3]Duke University School of Medicine, Durham NC, USA
[4]University of Minnesota School of Medicine, Minneapolis MN, USA

differences between the GM-CSF and placebo recipients in complete response (CR) rate [52% vs 54%, respectively], duration of neutropenia < than 500/μl (15 vs 17 days, $p=0.2$), duration of hospitalization (27 days vs 30 days, $p=.06$), overall survival or CR duration. Approximately one third of patients in *both* arms did not complete the scheduled duration of infusion, almost always because of the perception by the treating physician that toxicities were due to the study infusion. There was no difference between the GM-CSF and placebo recipients when only the subgroup of patients who completed the scheduled infusion as per protocol were considered. Only 2% of patients were removed from study because of the concern that the infusion may have stimulated leukemic cell growth; the incidence of treatment failure due to apparent chemotherapy-resistant leukemia was the same in both arms. Lastly, an identical fraction of patients in both arms were able to go on to receive post-remission consolidation therapy.

Comment. Although there was a small but statistically significant reduction in the duration of neutropenia in patients receiving the GM-CSF infusion, this did not result in any improvement in clinically relevant measurements of outcome. In general, the results of this very large trial are consistent with most smaller trials of similar design using GM-CSF although some analogous studies using G-CSF have not yet been completed or reported. It is not necessarily surprising that there was no important reduction in the incidence of severe infections. A significant fraction of patients with AML either present with fever and infection or develop fevers requiring antibiotic therapy within the first 1–2 weeks of admission to the hospital. Hematopoietic growth factors cannot be expected to entirely eliminate the prolonged nadir blood counts resulting from intensive induction chemotherapy, particularly in patients with primary marrow disorders and, thus, most patients are profoundly neutropenic at the time infections become manifest. At best, the growth factors might be able to accelerate neutrophil recovery in responding patients after the period of aplasia. This has the potential for decreasing the duration of therapy with antibiotics or amphotericin B, possibly limiting longer-term side effects, thereby perhaps enhancing the ability to deliver intensive post-remission chemotherapy. Although we were unable to demonstrate such a favorable effect using GM-CSF in our study, trials underway or under analysis should evaluate these possible end points. Based on our results, the CALGB is not currently planning studies utilizing growth factors as a means of decreasing infections morbidity so as to increase response rates following induction chemotherapy.

CALGB 9022 was a pilot study evaluating the feasibility of administering three courses of intensive post-remission chemotherapy to patients with de novo AML < than 60 years of age who achieved remission following induction therapy with daunorubicin and ARA-C [2]. Patients were scheduled to receive one course of high-dose cytosine arabinoside ara-C, followed by high-dose cyclophosphamide and etoposide with the last course consisting of diaziquone (AZQ) and mitoxantrone. Doses were derived from prior CALGB phase I/II studies in patients with either de novo or relapsed AML [3–5]. The high-dose ara-C, administered as six doses over a 5-day period, and the cyclophosphamide/etoposide regimens were relatively well tolerated. In contrast, severe myelosuppression was noted when mitoxantrone (12 mg/m^2 × three daily doses) was combined with AZQ 28 mg/m2 or AZQ 24 mg/m^2 per day × 3 days by continuous infusion. Two subsequent cohorts of sequentially treated patients received G-CSF 5 μg/kg per day beginning on day 4 until neutrophil recovery. The median duration of neutropenia (less than 500/μl) in the two groups not receiving G-CSF was 35 and 30 days respectively which was decreased significantly ($p<.001$) in the cohorts of patients receiving AZQ 24 mg/m^2 (median 20 days neutropenia) or 28 mg/m^2 (median 23 days) along with the same dose of mitoxantrone and G-CSF. There was also a suggestion of a decrease in the duration of severe thrombocytopenia in the third cohort of patients ($p=.12$). There was no difference in the duration of CR when the 61 patients treated without G-CSF were compared to the 59 patients receiving G-CSF, suggesting no apparent stimulation of residual leukemic cells in these patients. The CALGB is currently comparing the effect of three courses of post-remission high-dose aRA-C and the regimen piloted in protocol 9022, with the third course consisting of AZQ administered at 28 mg/m^2 per day for 3 days in combination with mitoxantrone and G-CSF. This ongoing study is designed to determine whether outcome can be improved by using a sequence of agents, all of which have been identified as having substantial activity in patients with AML in relapse, as compared with the use of single-agent ara-C alone.

Comment. This study evaluating sequential cohorts of younger patients with AML demonstrated a marked shortening of the duration of neutropenia with G-CSF following the administration of intensely myelosuppressive post-remission consolidation. This effect was less apparent in studies reported by the Eastern Cooperative Oncology Group (ECOG) [6] and German Leukemia groups [7]. Although the results of our pilot study are suggestive that hematopoietic growth factors may permit safer delivery of intensive post-remission therapy, these results should be confirmed in a randomized trial. Of note is that there was no adverse effect on relapse rate in patients receiving the growth factors in these CALGB trials. This is consistent with the results of most other randomized trials using these agents after the administration of chemotherapy for AML.

CALGB 9021 evaluates the effect of GM-CSF administered intravenously by continuous infusion for a maximum of 5 days prior to the administration of 12 doses of high-dose ara-C (2 gm/m^2 per dose) for patients with AML refractory to induction therapy or in first relapse. The GM-CSF is continued until 24 h after the completion of the chemotherapy. This study will complete accrual shortly; approximately 170 patients have been randomized to date. Twenty percent of patients were refractory to induction therapy while 47% had short initial complete responses of less than 6 months. The overall CR rate of 43% is quite reasonable in this group of relatively refractory patients. The results in the two treatment arms remain coded. In general, the infusion of GM-CSF has been well tolerated, and most patients have completed the infusion prior to the need to initiate chemotherapy.

Comment. This study evaluates the important concept of "recruitment" of leukemic cells to enhance cytotoxicity of ara-C. There is considerable in vitro and some in vivo evidence, suggesting increased ara-C cytotoxicity after incubation with growth factors [8–10]. It remains to be seen in clinical trials, however, whether sufficient numbers of clonogenic leukemic cells can be recruited from the resting state allowing increased cytotoxicity with both higher CR rates and longer durations of response. Studies from other groups are in progress evaluating this concept both as primary treatment and in patients in relapse. It is likely that there will be considerable interpatient variability in the degree of proliferation induced by different cytokines. Similarly, there is also heterogeneity within the blast population from an individual patient in the responsiveness to growth factors. Thus, even with large clinical trials, it may be possible to "miss" important beneficial (or harmful) effect in subgroups of patients. The development of in vitro assays more predictive of an effect in individual patients are critical in this regard but have been hampered by difficulties in reproducibly growing and characterizing subpopulations of clonogenic leukemic cells.

Summary. Overall, the results from multiple groups evaluating various sequences of chemotherapy and growth factors have been relatively disappointing. The CALGB is awaiting the maturation of other trials either in progress or recently completed prior to considering new studies incorporating growth factors in patients with AML. Based on the available data, it would appear that there is as yet no proven role for the addition of hematopoietic growth factors to standard chemotherapeutic approaches.

References

1. Stone R, George S, Berg D, Pacuicci P, Schiffer CA. GM-CSF vs placebo during induction therapy for patients > 60 years old with de novo acute myeloid leukemia: CALGB study #8923. ASCO Proc 13: 304, 1994.
2. Moore JO, Schiffer CA, Amrein PC, Dodge RK, George SL, Silver R, Blanton B. G-CSF reduces the duration of both granulocytopenia and thrombocytopenia after AZQ/mitoxantrone consolidation in acute myelogenous leukemia—CALGB 9022. Blood 80(suppl 1): 291a, 1992.
3. Lee EJ, Paciucci A, Amrein P, Schulman P, Davis R, Schiffer CA. A randomized phase II trial of 3 regimens in the treatment of relapsed or refractory acute myeloid leukemia (AML) in adults: a CALGB study. Blood 76: 294a, 1990.
4. Amrein PC, Davis RB, Mayer RJ, Schiffer CA. Treatment of relapsed and refractory acute myeloid leukemia with diaziquone and mitoxantrone: a CALGB phase I study. Am J Hematol 35: 80–83, 1990.
5. Mayer RJ, Davis RB, Schiffer CA, Berg DT, Powell BL, Schulman P, Omura GA, Moore JO, Mcintyre

OR, Frei E, for the Cancer and Leukemia Group B. Intensive postremission chemotherapy in adults with acute myeloid leukemia. N Engl J of Med 331: 896–903, 1994.
6. Rowe JM, Andersen J, Mazza JJ, Paietta E, Bennett JM, Hayes A, Oette D, Wiernik PH. Phase III randomized placebo-controlled study of granulocyte-macrophage colony stimulating factor (GM-CSF) in adult patients (55-70 years) with acute myelogenous leukemia (AML). A study of the Eastern Cooperative Oncology Group (ECOG). Blood 82 (suppl): 329a, 1993.
7. Büchner Th, Hiddemann W, Rottmann R, Wormann B, Maschmeyer G, Ludwig W-D, Sauerland MC, Frisch J, Schultz G. Multiple course chemotherapy with or without GM-CSF priming and longterm administration for newly diagnosed AML. Proc ASCO 12: 301, 1993.
8. Bhalla K, Birkhofer M, Arlin A, Grant S, Lutzky J, Graham G. Effect of recombinant GM-CSF on the metabolism of cytosine arabinoside in normal and leukemic human bone marrow cells. Leukemia 2: 810–813, 1988.
9. Cannistra SA, Groshek P, Griffin JD. Granulocyte-macrophage colony-stimulating factor enhances the cytotoxic effects of cytosine arabinoside in acute myeloblastic leukemia and in the myeloid blast crisis phase of chronic myeloid leukemia. Leukemia 3: 328–334, 1989.
10. Reutler C, Auf der Landwehr U, Schleyer E, Zuhlsdorf M, Ameling C, Rolf C, Wormann B, Buchner T, Hiddemann W. Modulation of intracellular metabolism of cytosine arabinoside in acute myeloid leukemia by granulocyte-macrophage colony-stimulating factor. Leukemia 8: 217–225, 1994.

Acute Leukemias VI
Prognostic Factors
and Treatment Strategies
Büchner et al. (eds)

Preclinical Evaluation of Granulocyte-Macrophage Colony-Stimulating Factor/Interleukin 3 Fusion Protein (PIXY 321) in Acute Myeloid Leukemic Cells

A. Tafuri, M.T. Petrucci, M.G. Mascolo, C. Ciliberti, M.R. Ricciardi, and L. De Felice

Abstract. Hemopoietic growth factors (GFs) can stimulate proliferation of leukemia cells, such effect furnished a rationale for acute myeloid leukemia (AML) treatment based on priming of quiescent blasts into cell cycle. Cell kinetic in vitro studies have suggested that GFs may enhance cytosine arabinoside (ara-C) cytotoxicity. While clinical trials based on this approach are progressing with discordant results, new cytokines are now entering into clinical use. PIXY 321 is a novel fusion protein of recombinant human granulocyte-macrophage colony-stimulating factor (GM-CSF) and interleukin-3 (IL-3), that exhibits biologic effects of both its parent cytokines. To assess the in vitro role of this cytokine in the GF/chemotherapy strategy, we have exposed 20 AML samples to several GFs including PIXY 321, stem cell factor, (SCF) IL-3, GM-CSF, and G-CSF, used alone and in combination. Cell kinetic effects of cytokines were evaluated by the flow-cytometric acridine orange (AO) technique, thereafter cells were exposed to the S-phase specific agent ara-C. Clonogenic growth of leukemic colonies colony-forming units—lymphoid, in methylcellulose was then evaluated to detect proliferative and cytotoxic effects on AML samples. We report that AML cells can be effectively recruited into cell cycle by PIXY 321, as demonstrated by a significant G_0 decrease ($p = 0.001$) and S phase increase ($p = 0.0001$). Clonogenic cell growth analysis showed a significant increase in CFU-L in 62.5% of the samples exposed to PIXY 321. These effects resulted in ara-C sensitization as demonstrated by an increase of CFU-L inhibition (75.9% vs 51.4% in presence f ara-C alone). compared to other cytokines, SCF, induced the lowed mean effects on ara-C sensitization that in some cases was even lower than the cytotoxicity achieved by ara-C alone. We conclude that PIXY 321 may be useful in combination with cycle-specific agents to prime quiescent blasts into cell cycle and to potentially enhance the cytotoxic effects of chemotherapy.

Introduction

Human recombinant hematopoietic growth factors (GFs), including interleukin-3 (IL-3) and granulocyte-macrophage colony-stimulating factor (GM-CSF), regulate proliferation and differentiation of normal and leukemic progenitor cells [1-3] with overlapping but distinct hematopoietic effects. Preclinical studies have shown that these two molecules act synergistically in stimulating hematopoiesis. A novel fusion protein, PIXY 321, derived from these two GFs was constructed to combine their complimentary biologic effects. In vitro studies have shown that PIXY 321 binds to cells that express specific receptors for GM-CSF and IL-3, with similar affinities to the single cytokines. Another cytokine now undergoing clinical investigation, is the stem cell factor (SCF), a multipotent CSF, more active on primitive hematopoietic progenitor cells, that acts after binding to its specific surface receptor, the protein encoded by the protooncogene c-kit.

Several reports [4-9] have documented the IL-3 or GM-CSF can enhance cytosine arabi-

Hematology, Department of Human Biopathology, University La Sapienza of Rome, Via Benevento 6, 00161 Rome, Italy

noside (ara-C) cytotoxicity in acute myeloid leukemia (AML) in vitro. We have previously compared the effects of three hematopoietic growth factors, IL-3, GM-CSF, and G-CSF, alone and in combinations, on leukemic blasts treated with either cycle-specific and non-specific agents [10]. We demonstrated that IL-3 and especially cytokine combinations including IL-3 were the most effective in the mobilization of the G_0 pool and found a strong correlation between kinetic changes and enhancement of ara-C-induced cytotoxicity. Several mechanisms have been proposed to explain leukemic cell sensitization by GF priming. In addition to kinetic rationale, Bhalla et al. [11], evaluating PIXY 321 activities in human myeloid leukemic cell, lines, found that enhancement of ara-C cytotoxicity was promoted by an increase of oligonucleosomal DNA fragmentation. Pietsch et al. [12], studying effects of SCF on primary myeloid leukemic cells, found that combination of GFs including SCF induced a strong synergistic proliferative response, most likely helping quiescent stem cells to enter cell cycle.

Since cytokine/chemotherapy (GF/CT) combinations are now being investigated in patients with discordant results [13–15], we attempt in the present study to evaluate the priming effect of the novel cytokine PIXY 321 that is now entering clinical use [16]. Several GFs were tested alone and in combination in this study. Ara-c was chosen as the cell cycle-specific agents most widely used in the treatment of AML.

Material and Methods

Samples. Patient characteristics are listed in Table 1. The mean percentage of blasts was 80% (range 60%–98%). Peripheral blood and bone marrow samples were obtained after informed consent, according to institutional policy, from 20 AML patients. Mononuclear cells were separated by Ficoll-Hypaque density gradient centrifugation (Lymphoprep, Nycomed Pharma, Oslo, Norway). Diagnosis was based on the morphologic, cytochemical and immunologic surface marker profiles of the cells.

Biologic Reagents. PIXY 321 (GM-CSF/IL-3 fusion protein) and SCF were kindly provided by Immunex (Seattle, WA) and were used at a concentration of 10 ng/ml and 100 ng/ml, respectively. IL-3 was supplied by Sandoz Ltd. (Basel, Switzerland) and used at a concentration of 20 ng/ml, GM-CSF and G-CSF (from Schering and Roche, respectively) were both used at 500 U/ml. All cytokine concentrations had previously been found to be effective [17].

Table 1. Patient characteristics

Patient no	FAB	Tissue	Blast (%)	WBC[a]
1	M2	PB	70	62.2
2	M4Eo	PB	83	19
3	M2	BM	70	83.2
4	M5a	BM	95	275
5	M4Eo	BM	78	104
6	M4	BM	98	161
7	M5a	BM	74	1.5
8	M5a	PB	80	49
9	M3	PB	80	24.4
10	M0	PB	80	23.8
11	M1	BM	78	22.9
12	M5a	BM	91	144
13	M2	BM	84	8.1
14	M4	BM	81	130
15	M2	BM	80	4.6
16	M5a	BM	83	195
17	n.c.	BM	61	79.5
18	M4Eo	BM	60	9.4
19	M5	BM	90	143

[a]White blood cell count = 1×10^6/l.
nc, not classified; PB, peripheral blood; BM, bone marrow.

Suspension Cultures. According to cell availability, blast cells obtained after gradient separation were resuspended in RMPI 1640 medium, supplemented with 10% fetal calf serum (FCS), 1% L-glutamine and 1% penicillin streptomycin (all by Gibco, Milan). The cells numebr was adjusted to a starting concentration of 1.0×10^6 cells/ml. Cells were cultured for 48 h at 37°C in 5% CO_2 with and without (control culture) the above-reported cytokines used alone or in combination GM+IL-3 and SCF+PIXY 321. The culture period had previously been identified as optimal for recruitment into S phase [18]. Then, before drug exposure, cell number/viability was assessed by trypan blue exclusion and kinetic studies were performed.

Kinetic Studies. In order to evaluate cell cycle recruitment and proliferation the AO (Polysciences, Warrington, PA) flow cytometric technique was performed after 48 h of cytokine incubation. Cell cycle was determined by measuring cellular DNA and RNA content (percentage of cells in G_0, G_1, S, and G_2M, mean RNA content per cell in each phase of the cell cycle) as previously described [19]. Pretreatment with Triton X-100 makes the cells permeable to AO and at low pH nucleic acids remain insoluble. Subsequent staining with the dye, in the presence of a chelating agent (ethylene diaminetetra-acetic acid EDTA) which makes cellular RNA single stranded, results in metachromatic red staining of RNA, while the native DNA intercalates the dye and stains orthochromatically green. The RNA content of G_1 cells was expressed as RNA index (RNA-I G_1) determined as the ratio of the mean RNA content of the G_1 cells of the samples times ten, divided by the median RNA content of control lymphocytes [20]. G_0 cells were defined as cells with an RNA content equal or less than that of control lymphocytes.

Clonogenic Assay. Clonogenic cell growth was measured by clonogenic assay in methylcellulose, as previously reported [21]. Briefly, after 48 h of liquid coulture, 3×10^5 cells were resuspended and plated in 1 ml IMDM containing 30% FCS, betamercaptoethanol 5×10^{-5} *M* and 10% 5637 conditioned medium, and 0.8% methylcellulose to assess day 7 leukemic cluster/colony-forming units (CFU-L > 8 cells/ > 20 cells) growth, as previously described [10] and the results were expressed as number of CFU-L × 100 000 cells seeded.

Drug Exposure and Cytotoxicity. In vitro sensitization to ara-C was measured after 48 h of cytokine exposure by adding ara-C at a concentration of 1 μM for 24 h. In order to assess whether drug cytotoxicity was enhanced by cytokine priming, control samples treated only with ara-C were also established. cytotoxicity of ara-C was evaluated as the percentage of inhibition of CFU-L, as previously described [10].

Flow Cytometry Measurements and Analysis. A modified FACScan (Becton Dickinson, Mountainview, CA) was used to measure fluorescence upon excitation at 488 nm. for each analysis 5000–10 000 cells were measured at separate wavelength bands for green [F_{530}-DNA (AO)] and red [$F_{>620}$-RNA (AO)]. Samples were analyzed using a Hewlett Packard micro-computer (Moded 310) and Becton Dickinson software including Consort 30, FACScan Research, Lysis, and Paint-a-gate.

Statistical Analyses. Based on the percentage of G_0 and S phase, and on CFU-L number, proliferative changes were considered positive only when values increased >25%. Significance levels between different groups were determined by paired two-sided Student's test.

Result

Cell Kinetic Effects. Table 2 summarizes average results obtained comparing cytokine effects after 48 h of liquid culture. Exposure to GFs generally results in significant cell cycle changes (Fig. 1) for all cytokines tested (Table 2). PIXY 321, GM-CSF+IL-3, and the combination of SCF+PIXY 321 were the most effective in terms of mean (m) G_0 percentage decrease (from 50% to 33.1%, 31.4%, and 25.2%, respectively). The same results were obtained when effects were evaluated on S phase and on RNA index (Fig. 2). PIXY 321 increased the percentage of cells in DNA synthesis from a mean value of 6.8% to 17.3%, this result was almost comparable to that obtained by the combination of GM-CSF+IL-3 (m = 18.7%). The combination of SCF+PIXY induced the highest proliferative effect in terms of S phase (m = 22.9%). Among the single cytokines SCF resulted in a mean value of 15.8%.

When individual samples were analyzed separately, an increase in S phase higher than 25% was observed in the majority of cases. Thus, PIXY 321 induced significant proliferative changes in 89.4% of the samples, GM-CSF+IL-3 in 90%, and SCF+PIXY in 88.8% of the cases. Using SCF, alone 88.3% of the samples showed a significant increase in S phase.

Effects on Clonogenic Cell Growth. The clonogenic assay confirmed the ability of cytokines to promote CFU-L growth. All cytokines were capable of increaseing clonogenic leukemic growth more that two fold (Table 3). PIXY 321 induced an increase of CFU-L of 3.5-fold ($p = 0.03$), and the increase induced by GM-CSF+IL-3 was similar. The highest clonogenic proliferative chages were seen in the presence of SCF+PIXY 321 (6.7-fold increase), whereas SCF alone resulted in a 2.5-fold increase of CFU-L mean number.

Effects on Ara-C Cytotoxicity. When the S phase-specific agent ara-C was used at 1 uM, after cytokine exposure in liquid culture, a significant increase

Table 2. Cell cycle change

	G_0 (%)	G_1 (%)	S (%)	G_2M (%)	RNA-I GI
Control	50	39.81	6.8	1.16	16.3
G	41.3	42.14	14.6	1.8	19
p	0.005	0.97	0.001	0.015	0.0001
GM	39.6	43.26	14.9	1.85	19.3
p	0.004	0.61	0.0007	0.078	0.0007
IL 3	36.6	45.64	14.6	3	20
p	0.003	0.33	0.0005	0.000	0.0005
SCF	33.6	49.1	15.8	2.4	19.7
p	0.002	0.01	0.0002	0.025	0.0001
PIXY 321	33.1	47.44	17.3	2	19.8
p	0.001	0.00	0.0001	0.018	0.0004
GM+IL3	31.4	47.49	18.7	2.3	20.6
p	0.001	0.02	0.0001	0.007	0.0001
SCF+PIXY 321	25.2	48.22	22.9	3.9	22.6
p	0.001	0.03	0.0001	0.0002	0.0001

Cell cycle results are expressed as the percentage of cells in G_0 and S phase. Significance levels between different groups were determined by paired two-sided Student's t test. RNA-I G1 RNA index G1.

in CFU-L inhibition was found for all cytokines except SCF. Ara-C alone resulted in a CFU-L inhibition of 51.4%. The highest ara-C cytotoxic effect on clonogenic precursor inhibition was obtained using SCF+PIXY 321 (77%) and PIXY 321 alone (75.9%). GM-CSF+IL-3 and GM-CSF alone enhanced cytotoxicity, inhibiting CFU-L by 73.2%. Interestingly, SCF alone, compared to the other conditions, was the cytokine that induced the lowest mean value of CFU-L inhibition (66.1%). Thus, in 33% of the samples treated with SCF, the cytotoxic effects were lower than those induced by ara-C alone, suggesting protective effects of SCF on leukemic cell killing.

Discussion

In this study we investigated the in vitro proliferative effects induced by PIXY 321 on AML blast cells induced in order to evaluate whether priming of quiescent blasts by this cytokine may result in enhanced cytotoxicity of the cycle-specific agent ara-C. We demonstrated that the fusion protein of GM-CSF and IL-3 is capable of recruiting myeloid cells into cell cycle, resulting in enhanced leukemic cell killing. Under the experimental conditions tested, almost 80% of AML samples had a significant increase of S phase after exposure to PIXY 321. Clonogenic growth confirmed these data, although the proliferation increased in a lower percentage of cases (62.5%). Nevertheless, when cytokine-induced kinetic changes were determined by flow-cytometric methods, recruitment of the overall population correlated with proliferation measured by clonogenic assays in the majority of cases.

Our data suggest that PIXY 321 plus SCF is the more effective combination in terms of induction of proliferation an enhancement of ara-C cytotoxicity. SCF is rather ineffective in terms of blast sensitization if used in the absence of PIXY 321. The role of SCF in protection from apoptosis may be considered to explain these results since, in some AML samples, a lower leukemia cell killing was documented using ara-C after SCF priming, compared to this agent alone.

Results obtained in our study evaluating priming activity of PIXY 321 on AML blasts confirmed previous data [11] that showed enhanced ara-C-induced programmed cell death by PIXY 321 in human myeloid leukemic cells. This is one of the mechanisms that have been reported to explain the effectivenesss of the cytokine priming in AML blast cell sensitization. Other alternative mechanisms which may be involved are represented by a selective enhancement of

Fig. 1A–H. Cell cycle changes measured by AO technique in AML blasts treated with G-CSF (**B**), GM-CSF (**C**), IL-3 (**D**), SCF (**E**), PIXY 321 (F), GM-CSF+IL-3 (**G**), PIXY 321+SCF (**H**). Results were compared to control culture (**A**)

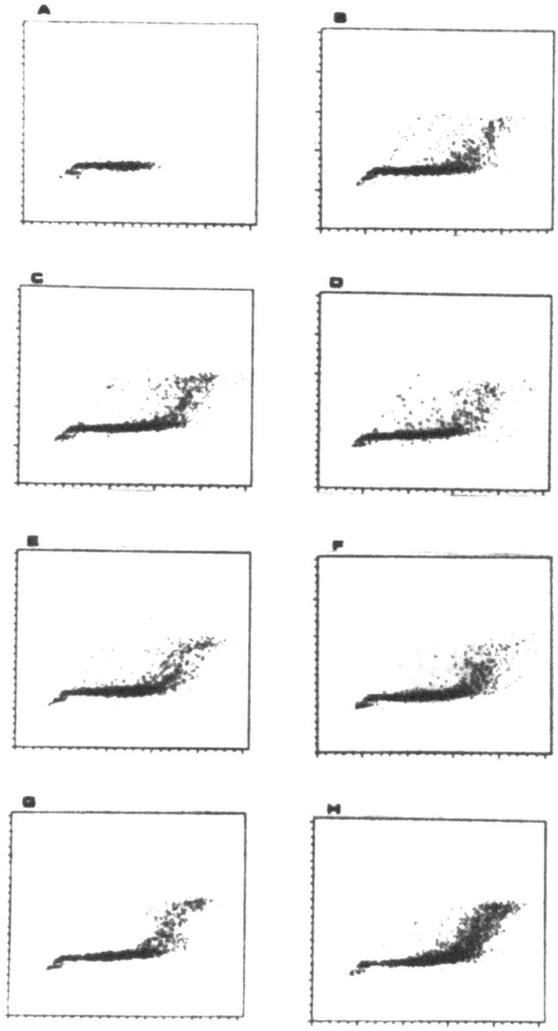

ara-CTP formation in leukemic cells [5]. In the future a better comprehension may help to explain the discordant results obtained in clinical trials. Although the proliferative response does not necessarily predict effective sensitization, none of the samples that failed to show recruitment had an increase in leukemic cell killing by ara-C. Ongoing clinical investigations need criteria to select patients who could potentially benefit from this approach: in vivo GM-CSF-induced recruitment only in de novo AML patients with low pretreatment S phase and proliferative response induced by GM-CSF was associated with achievement of complete remission [22]. In relapsed patients additional mechanisms of resistance to chemotherapy may confound the potential beneficial effects of GF/CT combinations.

In conclusion, with the present, study, we add in vitro evidence supporting the use of PIXY 321 in AML priming. We conclude that the combination of this cytokine with SCF may further enhance the benefical effects. These findings provide a rationale for clinical investigation based on a regimen containing PIXY 321 used as a priming cytokine.

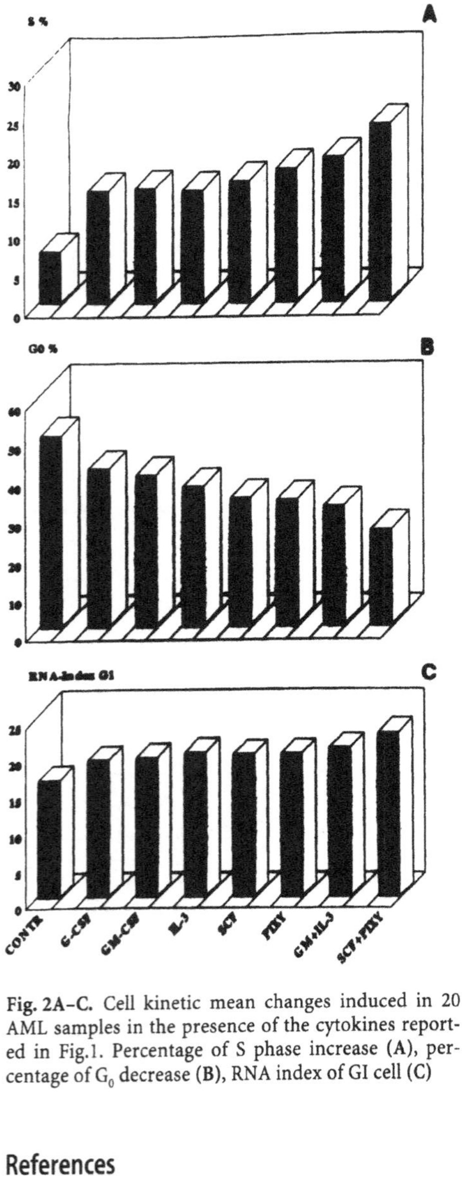

Fig. 2A–C. Cell kinetic mean changes induced in 20 AML samples in the presence of the cytokines reported in Fig.1. Percentage of S phase increase (**A**), percentage of G_0 decrease (**B**), RNA index of GI cell (**C**)

Table 3. Clonogenic growth

	CFU-L (*n*)	CFU-L (-fold increase)	CFU-L% inhibition Ara-C 1 u*M*
Control	798		51.46
G	879.5	2.11	67.94
p	n.s.	n.s.	0.034
GM	987.5	2.31	73.27
p	n.s.	n.s.	0.023
IL-3	1120	2.92	72.42
p	n.s.	n.s.	0.01
SCF	1779	2.51	66.18
p	n.s.	n.s.	n.s.
PIXY 321	1759	3.59	75.95
p	0.034	n.s.	0.005
GM+IL3	1804	3.53	73.27
p	0.039	n.s.	0.028
SCF+ PIXY 321	2880	6.72	77
p	n.s.	n.s.	0.002

References

1. Vellenga E, Ostapovica D, O'Rourke B, Griffin JD. Effects of recombinant IL-3, GM-CSF, and G-CSF on proliferation of leukemic clonogenic cells in short-term and long-term cultures. Leukemia 1987; 1: 584–589.
2. Strife A, Lambek C, Wisniewski D, Gulati S, Gasson JC, Golde DW, Welte K, Gabrilove JL, Clarkson B. Activities of four purified growth factors on highly enriched human hematopoietic progenitor cells. Blood 1987; 69: 1508–1523.
3. Kelleher C, Miyauchi J, Wong G, Clark S, Minden MD, McCulloch EA. Synergism between recombinant growth factors, GM-CSF and G-CSF, acting on the blast cells of acute myeloblastic leukemia. Blood 1987; 69: 1498–1503.
4. Lista P, Porcu P, Avanzi GC and Pegoraro L. Interleukin-3 enhances the cytotoxic activity of L-beta-d-arabinofuranosylcytosine (ara-C) on acute myeloblastic leukemia (AML) cells. British J Haematology 1988; 69: 121–123.
5. Bhalla K, Birkhofer M, Arlin Z, Grant S, Lutzky J, Graham G: Effect of recombinant GM-CSF on the metabolism of cytosine arabinoside in normal and leukemic human bone marrow cells. Leukemia 1988; 2: 810–813
6. Cannistra SA, Groshek P and Griffin JD. Granulocyte-macrophage colony-stimulating factor enhances the cytotoxic effects of cytosine arabinoside in acute myeloblastic leukemia and in the myeloid blast crisis phase of chronic myeloid leukemia. Leukemia 1989; 3: 328–334.
7. Miyauchi J, Kelleher CA, Wang C, Minikin S, McCulloch EA. Growth factors influence the sensitivity of leukemic stem cells to cytosine arabinoside in culture. Blood 1989; 73: 1272–1278
8. Brach B, Klein H, Platzer E, Mertelsmann R, Herrmann F: Effect interleukin-3 on cytosine arabinoside mediated cytoxicity of leukemic myeloblasts. Exp. Hematology 1990; 18: 748–753.
9. Santini V, Nooter K, Delwel R, Lowenberg B. Susceptibility of acute myeloid leukemia (AML) cells from clinically resistant and sensitive patients to daunomycin (DNR): assesment in vitro after simulation with colony stimulating factors (CSFs). Leukemia Research 1990; 14: 337–380.
10. Tafuri A, Lemoli RM, Chen R et al. Combination of hematopoietic growth factors containing IL-3 induced acute myeloid leukemia cell sensitization to cycle specific and cycle non specific drugs. Leukemia 1994; 8: 749–757.

11. Bhalla K, Tang C, Ibrado AM, Grant S, Tourkina E, Holladay C, Hughes M, Mahoney ME, Huang Y. Granulocyte-macrophage colony-stimulating factor interleukin-3 fusion protein (PIXY 321) enhances high-dose ara-C-induced programmed cell death or apoptosis in human myeloid leukemia cells. Blood 1992; 80: 2883–2890.
12. Pietsch T, Kyas U, Steffens U, Yakisan E, Hadam M, Ludwig WD, Zsebo K, Welte K. Effects of stem cell factor (c-kit ligand) on proliferation of myeloid leukemia cells: heterogeneity in response and synergy with other hematopoietic growth factors. Blood 1992; 80: 1199–1206.
13. Bettelheim P, Valent P, Andreeff M, Tafuri A, Haimi J, Gorischek C, Muhm M, Sillaber C, Haas O, vieder L, Maurer D, Schulz G, Speiser W, Geissler K, Kier P, Hinterberger W, Lechner K. Recombinant human granulocyte-macrophage colony stimulating factor in combination with standard induction chemotherapy in de novo acute myeloid leukemia. Blood 1991; 77: 700–711
14. Estey E, Thall PF, Kantarjian H, O'Brien S, Koller C, Beran M, Gutterman J, Deisseroth A, Keating M: Treatment of newly diagnosed acute myelogenous leukemia with granulocyte-macrophage colony-stimulating factor (GM-SCF) before and during continuous-infusion high-dose are-C + daunorubicin: comparison to patients treated without GM-CSF. Blood 1992; 79: 2246–2255.
15. Estey E, Kantarjian H, O'Brien S, Beran M, Feldman E, Freireich E, Keating M. Treatment of poor-prognosis myelodysplastic syndromes (MDS) with AML-type chemotherapy. Blood 1992; 80 suppl.1: 1783
16. Vadhan-Rai SV, Broxmeyer HE, Andreeff M et al. In vivo biologic effects of PIXY 321, a synthetic hybrid protein of recombinant human GM-CSF and IL-3 in cancer patients with normal hematopoiesis: a phase I study. Blood 1995; 86: 2098–2105
17. Tafuri A and Andreeff M. Kinetic rationale for cytosine-induced recruitment of myeloblastic leukemia followed by cycle-specific chemotherapy in vitro. Leukemia 1990; 12: 826–834
18. Tafuri A, Hegewisch S, Souza L, Andreeff M. Stimulation of leukemic blast cells in vitro by colony stimulating factors (G-CSF, GM-CSF) ad interleukin-3 (IL-3): evidence of recruitment and increased cell killing with cytosine arabinoside (ara-C). Blood 1988; 72: 105a.
19. Andreeff M, Darzynkiewicz Z, Sharpless TK, Clarkson BD, Melamed MR. Discrimination of human leukemia subtypes by flow cytometric analysis of cellular DNA and RNA. Blood 1980; 55: 282–293
20. Andreeff M, Assing G, Cirrincione C. Prognostic value of DNA/RNA flow cytometry in myeloblastic and lymphoblastic leukemia in adults: RNA content and S-phase predict remission duration and survival in multivariate analysis. Ann NY Acad Sci 1984; 468: 387–406
21. Buich B, Till JE, McCulloch EA: Colony assay for proliferative blast cells circulating in myeloblastic leukaemia. Lancet 1977; i: 862–863
22. Tafuri A, De Felice L, Petrucci MT, Mascolo MG, Valentini T, Fenu S, Petti MC, Andreeff M, Mandelli F. Kinetic changes and correlation to clinical response in AML patients treated with and without GM-CSF prior to therapy. Blood 1992; 80 suppl.1: 1143a

Acute Leukemias VI
Prognostic Factors
and Treatment Strategies
Büchner et al. (eds)

Initial Trial of PIXY 321 Following Autologous Bone Marrow Transplantation

J.M. Vose[1] and J.E. Anderson[2]

Introduction

The use of high-dose chemotherapy and autologous bone marrow transplantation (ABMT) for the treatment of relapsed or high-risk lymphoid malignancies has now been demonstrated to result in long-term disease-free survival in a number of patients [1–4]. However, severe and prolonged neutropenia can lead to infectious complications which can be fatal in a number of cases. The routine use of myeloid hematopoietic growth factors such as granulocyte-macrophage colony-stimulating factor (GM-CSF) and granulocyte colony-stimulating factor (GM-CSF) and granulocyte colony-stimulating factor (G-CSF) post ABMT have now been documented in several phase III trials to decrease the neutropenic period and number of infectious complications [5–8]. However, thrombocytopenia post ABMT remains a clinical problem with the administration of currently available GM-CSF or G-CSF not affecting the time to platelet transfusion independence.

PIXY 321 is a genetically engineered fusion molecule resulting from the linkage of interleukin-3 (IL-3) and GM-CSF by a flexible amino acid linker sequence that allows the binding domains of the ligands to fold into their native configurations [9,10]. The rationale for using PIXY 321 post ABMT was to try to enhance both neutrophil and platelet recovery following high-dose chemotherapy and ABMT. Since PIXY 321 has been shown to be a potent stimulator of both committed and multipotential progenitor cells and has been shown to enhance both neutrophil and platelet recovery in primates following whole body radiotherapy [11], it was felt this molecule could offer a possible potential for enhancement of engraftment in both cell lines post ABMT.

Materials and Methods

Patient Selection. Fifty patients with Hodgkin's disease and non-Hodgkin's lymphoma undergoing high-dose chemotherapy and ABMT were eligible for the study of PIXY 321 post ABMT in this phase I/II trial. Patients were enrolled at the University of Nebraska Medical Center and Fred Hutchinson Cancer Research Center from June 1992 to November 1993. Eligible patients included male and female patients aged 18–70 with a Karnofsky performance status of ≥ 70, a bilirubin 1.5 mg/dl, creatinine ≤ 1.5 mg/dl, and a MUGA ejection fraction $\geq 45\%$. All patients had autologous bone marrow harvested per standard techniques with a minimum of 1.0×10^8 nucleated cells/kg patients body weight collected.

Cytokine. The PIXY 321 used in this study was provided by Immunex (Seattle, Washington). After completion of the high-dose chemotherapy and infusion of autologous bone marrow, patients received one of the following doses of PIXY 321: 50 µg/m^2 ($n = 1$), 125 µg/m^2 ($n = 3$), 250 µg/m^2 ($n = 3$), 500 µg/m^2 ($n = 15$), 750 µg/m^2

[1] University of Nebraska Medical Center, Omaha, Nebraska 68198-3330, USA
[2] Fred Hutchinson Cancer Research Center, USA

($n=25$), or 1000 μg/m^2 ($n=3$). Initially there were three patients per dose level above 50 μg/m^2 with administration of the PIXY 321 evaluated. Subsequently, subcutaneous PIXY 321 was tested at the 500 μg/m^2 or 750 μg/m^2 dose levels either as a daily or twice-per-day dosing. The patients received a maximum number of 21 doses. Early discontinuation was done prior to the 21 doses if patients achieved an absolute neutrophil count (ANC) of $\geqslant$ 1500 cells/mm^3 for 2 consecutive days and a self-sustaining platelet count $\geqslant$ 20000 cells/mm^3 prior to the 21 doses.

Transfusion Criteria. When the patient had a hemoglobin $\leqslant$ 8. 0 gm/dl, or if the patient's condition otherwise demonstrated a need for transfusion, a two-unit irradiated packed red blood cell transfusion was administered. For a platelet count $\leqslant$ 20000 cells/mm^3, a single-donor irradiated platelet product or 6 units of random donor platelets were administered.

Statistical Analysis. Neutrophil engraftment was defined as the first of 2 consecutive days that the patient achieved an ANC $\geqslant$ 500 cells/mm^3 following the expected nadir. Platelet independence was defined as the first of 7 consecutive days following the expected nadir that the patient had a platelet count $\geqslant$ 20000 cells/mm^3 without transfusion. Time to event outcomes were evaluated using life table techniques by Kaplan-Meier estimates.

Results

A total of 50 patients were treated on this phase I/II trial with 16 patients undergoing high-dose chemotherapy and ABMT for Hodgkin's disease and 34 for non-Hodgkin's disease. Other characteristics are outlined in Table 1. The engraftment was analyzed by disease since there was a large difference in engraftment between the two subtypes.

Hodgkin's Disease Patients. The median day to engraft $\geqslant$ 500 ANC was 22 days (range 12–42) and the median days to platelet independence was 24 days (range 13–105+).

Non-Hodgkin's Disease Patients. The median days to engraft $\geqslant$ 500 ANC was 16 days (range 9–28) and the median days to platelet transfusion independence was 20 (range 10–39+).

Above 50 μg/m^2 there did not appear to be a dose-response effect. The effect of the route of administration was determined, at what was determined, based on several phase I/II studies, to be the optimum dose of 750 μg/m^2. Patients receiving 750 μg/m^2 by the i.v. route had a median time to reach an ANC of 500 cells/mm^3 of 19 days and a median time to platelet transfusion independence of 23 days. For patients receiving 750 μg/m^2 by daily subcutaneous dosing, the median time to reach an ANC of 500 cells/mm^3 was 15 days and the median time to platelet transfusion independence was 16 days. For patients receiving 750 μg/m^2 by twice-a-day subcutaneous dosing, the median time to reach an ANC of 500 cells/mm^3 was 13 days and the median time to platelet transfusion independence was 20 days (Table 2).

Safety and Tolerability. Adverse events that were grade 3 or 4 according to the National Cancer Institute (NCI) common toxicity criteria included fever (40%), nausea (8%), chills (8%), stomatitis (20%), rash (8%), edema (4%), pleural effusion (0%), and headache (4%). In the transplant population it is difficult to determine if an adverse event is related to the transplant regimen, underlying disease, medication used post transplant, or an infectious complication.

Table 1. Patient characteristics ($n=50$)

	Years	n	%
Median age (range)	43 (19–66)		
Sex			
Male		25	50
Female		25	50
Diagnosis			
Hodgkin's		16	32
Non-Hodgkin's		34	68

Table 2. Engraftment according to route of administration at 750 μg/m^2

Route	500 ANC (Median)	Platelet independance (days)
Intravenous	19	23
Subcutaneous daily	15	16
Subcutaneous twice a day	13	20

Discussion

The routine use of myeloid growth factors such as GM-CSF or G-CSF following high-dose chemotherapy and ABMT has now been demonstrated to enhance the engraftment of neutrophils post ABMT, as well as decreasing the number of documented infections. However, these factors do not enhance the other hematopoietic cell lineages.

Preliminary data with the use of IL-3 alone post ABMT as published by Nemunaitis et al. [12] demonstrated equivalent neutrophil engraftment to historical controls receiving GM-CSF; however, the platelet engraftment was not superior to the historical controls receiving GM-CSF. The sequential use of IL-3 followed by GM-CSF has also recently been reported by Fay et al. [13]. In this study, 37 patients undergoing ABMT for lymphoid malignancies received IL-3 at either 2.5 or 5.0 $\mu g/m^2$ per day for either 5 or 10 days, followed by GM-CSF at 250 $\mu g/m^2$ per day i.v. as a 2-h infusion. If all patients at the different dose levels were considered together, the median time to recover an ANC$\geqslant$500 cells/mm^3 was 14 days and the median time to platelet independence was 15 days. Compared to similar patients treated in the Nemunaitis randomized GM-CSF vs. placebo trial, the neutrophil and platelet engraftment were improved.

The engraftment data in the current phase I/II PIXY 321 trial overall demonstrate a time to 500 ANC of 18 days and platelet independence of 21 days. At the optimal dose of 750 $\mu g/m^2$per day by subcutaneous daily administration, the time to reach an ANC of $\geqslant$500 cells/mm^3 was 15 days and the time to platelet independence was 16 days. This engraftment is very similar to the engraftment obtained with the sequential IL-3/GM-CSF reported by Fay et al, [13].

Mobilized peripheral blood progenitors have now become a standard of care at many transplant centers. When compared to the patients at the optimum dose of PIXY 321 of 750 $\mu g/m^2$ subcutaneously in the current trial, the engraftment demonstrated in lymphoma patients using G-CSF or GM-CSF-mobilized peripheral blood progenitors is similar with respect to the platelet independence time. However, patients receiving G-CSF- or GM-CSF-mobilized peripheral blood progenitors have been reported to have a median time to engraft to an ANC of 500 cells/mm^3 of 10–18 days [14, 15].

Further evaluation comparing the types of autologous hematopoietic stem cell sources when stimulated with multilineage or earlier acting cytokines will be necessary for a complete comparison.

References

1. Philip T, Armitage JO, Spitzer G, et al. High-dose therapy and autologous bone marrow transplantation after failure of conventional chemotherapy in adults with intermediate-grade or high-grade non-Hodgkin's lymphoma. N Engl J Med 316: 1493–1498.
2. Petersen FB, Appelbaum FR, Hill R, et al. Autologous marrow transplantation for malignant lymphoma: a report of 101 cases from Seattle. J Clin Oncol 8: 638–647, 1990.
3. Vose JM, Anderson JR, Kessiger A, et al. High-dose chemotherapy and autologous hematopoietic stem-cell transplantation for aggressive non-Hodgkin's lymphoma. J Clin Oncol 11: 1846–1851, 1993.
4. Nademanee A, Schmidt GM, O-Donnell MR, et al. High-dose chemoradiotherapy followed by autologous bone marrow transplantation in adult patients with poor-risk aggressive lymphoma: a pilot study. Blood 5: 1130–1134, 1992.
5. Nemunaitis J, Rabinowe SN, Singer JW, et al. Recombinant granulocyte-macrophage colony-stimulating factor after autologous bone marrow transplantation for lymphoid cancer. N Engl J Med 324: 1773–1778, 1991.
6. Gorin NC, Coiffier B, Hayat M, et al. Recombinant human granulocyte-macrophage colony-stimulating factor after high-dose chemotherapy and autologous bone marrow transplantation with unpurged and purged marrow in non-Hodgkin's lymphoma: a double-blind placebo-controlled trial. Blood 80: 1149–1157, 1992.
7. Gulati SC and Bennett CL: Granulocyte-macrophage colony-stimulating factor (GM-CSF) as adjunct therapy in relapsed Hodgkin's disease. Ann Intern Med 116: 177–182, 1992.
8. Schmitz N, Dreger P, Zander A, et al. A randomized, controlled, multicentre study of granulocyte colony stimulating factor (filgrastim) in patients with Hodgkin's disease and non-Hodgkin's lymphoma undergoing autologous bone marrow transplantation. Blood 82: 568a, 1993.
9. Curtis BM, Williams DE, Broxmeyer He, et al. Enhanced hematopoietic activity of a human granulocyte-macrophage colony-stimulating factor/interleukin-3 fusion protein. Proc Natl Acad Sci USA 88: 5809–5813, 1991.
10. Williams DE, Park LS, Broxmeyer HE, et al. Hybrid cyokines as hematopoietic growth factors. Intl J Cell Clon 9: 542–547, 1991.

11. Williams DE, Dunn JT, Park LS, et al. In vivo effects of a GM-CSF/IL-3 fusion protein (PIXY 321) in sublethally irradiated monkeys. Biotechnol Therapeutics 4: 17–29, 1993.
12. Nemunaitis J, Appelbaum FR, Singer JW, et al. Phase I trial with recombinant human interleukin-3 in patients with lymphoma undergoing autologous bone marrow transplantation. Blood 82: 3273–3278, 1993.
13. Fay JW, Lazarus H, Herzig R, et al. Sequential administration of recombinant human interleukin-3 and granulocyte-macrophage colony-stimulating factor after autologous bone marrow transplantation for malignant lymphoma: a phase I/II multicenter study. Blood 84: 2151–2157, 1994.
14. Chao NJ, Schriber JR, Grimes K, et al. Granulocyte colony-stimulating factor "mobilized" peripheral blood progenitor cells accelerate granulocyte and platelet recovery after high-dose chemotherapy. Blood 81: 2031–2035, 1993.
15. Bishop MR, Anderson JR, Jackson JD, et al. High-dose therapy and peripheral blood progenitor cell transplantation: effects of recombinant human granulocyte-macrophage colony-stimulating factor on the autograft. Blood 83: 610–616, 1994.

New Strategies: Antifungal Treatment

Acute Leukemias VI
Prognostic Factors
and Treatment Strategies
Büchner et al. (eds)

Fluconazole Prophylaxis of Invasive Fungal Infections During Intensive Chemotherapy for Relapsed Acute Myeloid Leukemia: Interim Analysis of a Randomized Multicenter Trial

G. Behre[1], T. Büchner[2], A. Grote-Metke[3], M. Planker[4], U. Kubica[5], H. Eimermacher[6], D. Braumann[7], W. Gaßmann[8], P. Schönrock-Nabulsi[9], A. Großhans[10], J. Karow[11], C. Schadeck-Gressel[12], and W. Hiddemann[1], for the German AML Cooperative Group

Abstract. Invasive fungal infections are a major cause of death in neutropenic patients with hematologic malignancies. Fluconazole has broad-spectrum antifungal activity, excellent oral bioavailability, and few side effects. However, its efficacy for prevention of invasive fungal infections in neutropenic patients remains controversial. Therefore, an open prospective randomized multicenter trial was initiated to assess the impact of fluconazole prophylaxis on the incidence of invasive fungal infections and patients' outcome during intensive chemotherapy (sequential high-dose cytosine arabinoside (ara-C) and mitoxantrone plus granulocyte colony-stimulating factor) for relapsed or refractory acute myeloid leukemia. Patients were randomly assigned to either fluconazole 400 mg/day orally administered, in addition to standard antimicrobial prophylaxis with trimethoprim-sulfamethoxazole, colistin, and amphotericin B suspension, or to standard antimicrobal prophylaxis alone. The interim analysis of 33 patients indicates that fluconazole prophylaxis reduced the overall mortality (17% versus 47%) and infection-related mortality in particular (12% versus 29%). This reduction of mortality also led to a higher complete remission rate (61% versus 40%). However, fluconazole prophylaxis did not reduce th incidence of documented invasive fungal infections (11% versus 7%; all caused by *Candida* species), pneumonia (39% versus 27%), or the requirement for systemic amphotericin B therapy (76% versus 27%). One possible explanation for these results could be that, although fluconazole prophylaxis could not reduce the occurrence of invasive fungal infection, it could reduce their associated mortality. A completion of the ongoing trial is needed to substantiate these findings and to define the potential role of fluconazole prophylaxis in patients with acute myeloide leukemia.

Introduction

Invasive fungal infections are a major cause of infection-related mortality in patients with acute myeloid leukemia (AML) [1, 2], and therefore,

[1]Department of Hematology/Oncology, University of Göttingen, Robert-Koch-Str. 40, 37075 Göttingen, Germany
[2]Department of Hematology/Oncology, University of Münster, Albert-Schweitzer-Str. 33, 48149 Münster, Germany
[3]Ev. Hospital, Werler Str. 110, 59063 Hamm, Germany
[4]Städt. Krankenanstalten, Lutherplatz 40, 47805 Krefeld, Germany
[5]Central Hospital St. Jürgen, St. Jürgen Str. 1, 28205 Bremen, Germany
[6]St. Marien Hospital, Bergstr. 56, 58095 Hagen, Germany
[7]Department of Medicine II, General Hospital Altona, Paul-Ehrlich-Str. 1, 22763 Hamburg, Germany
[8]Department of Medicine II, University Hospital, Chemnitzstr. 33, 24116 Kiel, Germany
[9]Department of Hematology, Hospital, St. Georg, Lohmühlenstr. 2, 20099 Hamburg, Germany
[10]Städtisches Krankenhaus, 67653 Kaiserslautern, Germany
[11]Krankenanstalten Düren, Roonstr. 30, 52351 Düren, Germany
[12]St. Johannes Hospital, An der Abtei 11, 47166 Duisburg, Germany

new strategies for prevention and intervention are urgently needed.

Fluconazole is one of the most attractive agents for prevention of invasive fungal infections because it has broad-spectrum antifungal activity, excellent oral bioavailability and tissue penetration, and few side effects [3]. Fluconazole is highly recommended for the treatment of oropharyngeal or esophageal candidosis, as life-long maintenance therapy for AIDS patients with cryptococcal meningitis, as therapy for coccidioidal meningitis, and as therapy for candidemia in patients who are not neutropenic or otherwise immunosuppressed [4]. However, the efficacy of fluconazole for prevention of invasive fungal infections in neutropenic patients remains controversial [5–10]. Winston et al. [6] did not find a survival benefit or a decrease in invasive fungal infections among patients with acute leukemia who received prophylactic fluconazole while undergoing myelosuppressive chemotherapy. In contrast, in patients undergoing bone marrow transplantation, both systemic and superficial infections were reduced among fluconazole recipients [5].

Therefore, and open prospective randomized multicenter trial was initiated by the German AML Cooperative Group to assess the impact of fluconazole prophylaxis on the incidence of invasive fungal infections and patients' out come during intensive chemotherapy with sequential high-dose cytosine arabinoside (ara-C) and mitoxantrone plus granulocyte colony-stimulating factor for relapsed or refractory AML.

Materials and Methods

Patients

Patients fulfilling all of the following criteria were eligible for the study: (a) AML with bone marrow relapse (leukemic cells > 25%) or a persistent leukemic blast population after two induction courses; (b) age > 18 years; (c) written informed consent. Patients with one of the following criteria were excluded: (a) antecedent hematologic disorder and secondary leukemia; (b) preceding autologous or allogeneic bone marrow transplantation; (c) contraindications against intensive cytostatic therapy; (d) documented prior allergic reaction against study drugs.

Prior to the start of salvage therapy with sequential high-dose ara-C and mitoxantrone plus granulocyte colony-stimulating factor (S-HAM + G-CSF) patients were randomized to receive fluconazole in addition to standard antimicrobial prophylaxis with trimethoprim-sulfamethoxazole, colistin, and amphotericin B suspension versus standard antimicrobial prophylaxis alone. The study was initiated after approval by the ethics committees at the participating institutions and is in accordance with the declaration of Helsinki.

Interventions

Reinduction Therapy with S-HAM. Cytosine arabinoside is given as a 3-h infusion twice daily every 12 h on days 1, 2, 8, and 9. The dose of ara-C was adjusted to disease status and age: patients less than 60 years of age with refractory AML as defined by primary non-response to induction therapy, early relapse with remission duration of less than 6 months, and secondary and subsequent relapse were treated with 3.0 g/m^2 ara-C while older patients and patients with first relapse after more than 6 months, remission duration received 1.0 g/m^2 ara-C. All patients received mitoxantrone 10 mg/m^2 per day by a 30-min infusion on days 3, 4, 10, and 11.

Antimicrobial Prophylaxis and Therapy. Prior to cytostatic chemotherapy with S-HAM, patients were randomly assigned to either fluconazole 400 mg/day orally administered in addition to standard antimicrobial prophylaxis [11] with trimethoprim-sulfamethoxazole 160 mg/800 mg tid, colistin sulfate capsules 2 ml U po tid, and amphotericin B suspension 2400 mg po qd, or to standard antimicrobial prophylaxis alone. Upon the occurrence of fever or clinical signs of infection, systemic antimicrobial therapy was administered according to the interventional antimicrobial study II of the Paul Ehrlich Society for Chemotherapy [11].

Statistical Analysis

Patients are followed and evaluated until recovery of neutrophils > 1000/µl. The primary end point of the study is the incidence of invasive fungal infections and/or requirement of additional systemic antifungal therapy with amphotericin B. It is planned to enroll 168 patients into the study to detect a significant difference between the two treatment groups with a power of 80% ($\beta = 0.2$) at the $\alpha < 0.05$ level in χ^2 test by Mantel-Haenszel, assuming that the incidence of invasive fungal infections and/or the requirement of systemic amphotericin B therapy can be reduced from 50% in the control group to 30% in the fluconazole group.

Results

Patient Characteristics and Risk Factors. Patients' characteristics and risk factors such as age, given dose of ara-C, neutrophil recovery > 500/μl after start of chemotherapy, systemic antifungal therapy during preceding course of antineoplastic chemotherapy, infections at study entry, and compliance to standard antimicrobial prophylaxis were balanced between the groups with or without fluconazole prophylaxis (Table 1).

Patient Outcome. The overall mortality from reinduction therapy was 30%. There were 47% early deaths in the control group compared to only 17% in the fluconazole group. This reduction of mortality also translated into a higher complete remission rate (61% versus 40%) (Table 2).

Table 1. Patient characteristics and risk factors

	Fluconazole ($n = 18$)	Control ($n = 15$)
Age		
Median (years)	53	44.5
Range (years)	22–73	18–72
Antineoplastic chemotherapy		
3 g/m^2 ara-C: < 60 years + refractory AML (n)	3	3
(%)	17	20
1 g/m^2 ara-C: < 60 years + RD > 6 months (n)(%)	9	8
(%)	50	53
1 g/m^2 ara-C: > 60 years (n)	6	4
(%)	33	27
Neutrophil recovery > 500/μl (n)		
Day after start of chemotherapy—Median—	30.5	35
Range	25–57	28–44
Prior systemic antifungal therapy (n)	12	11
(%)	67	73
For invasive aspergillosis (n)	2	1
For invasive candidosis (n)	2	2
For suspected invasive fungal infection (n)	4	5
For FUO (n)	4	3
Infections at study entry (n)	5	2
(%)	28	13
Pneumonia (n)	1	
FUO (n)	4	1
Soft tissue infection (n)		1
Standard antimicrobial prophylaxis (n)	15	12
(%)	83	80

Table 2. Efficacy of antineoplastic chemotherapy

	Total ($n = 33$)		Fluconazole ($n = 18$)		Control ($n = 15$)	
	(n)	(%)	(n)	(%)	(n)	(%)
Complete remission	17	52	11	61	6	40
Partial remission	2	6	1	6	1	7
Persistent leukemia	4	12	3	17	1	7
Early death	10	30	3	17	7	47
In aplasia with blasts	1				1	
In aplasia without blasts		7	3		4	
Blast status not evaluable		2			2	

Incidence of Invasive Fungal Infections. Two microbiologically documented invasive fungal infections occured in the fluconazolegroup, one fungemia and sepsis caused by *Candida krusei*, and one fungemia and pneumonia caused by *Candida tropicalis* (Table 3). In the control group, there was one documented invasive fungal infection, a fungemia and sepsis by *Candida tropicalis*. The incidence of pneumonia was 39% in the fluconazole and 27% in the control group (Table 3). Of patients receiving fluconazole prophaylaxis, 76% subsequently required systemic antifungal therapy with intravenous amphotericin B, whereas only 27% of the control group were administered systemic amphotericin B therapy. An additional 27% of the control group received antifungal therapy with itraconazole or fluconazole (Table 4). However, the fluconazole group received a median of three consecutive regimens of antibacterial chemotherapy, whereas the control group only got 1.5 cycles of systemic intravenous antibacterial chemotherapy. The infection-related mortality was lower in the fluconazole than in the control group (12% versus 29%) (Table 4).

Discussion

The present interim analysis of the prospective randomized evaluation of fluconazole for the prevention of invasive fungal infections in patients undergoing intensive chemotherapy for relapsed or refractory AML indicates that fluconazole prophylaxis may reduce the overall mortality (17% versus 47%) and infection-related mortality (12% versus 29%) substantially. Futhermore, this reduction of mortality was also transferred into a higher complete remission rate (61% versus 40%). However, fluconazole prophylaxis could not be shown to reduce the incidence of documented invasive fungal infections (11% versus 7%; all caused by *Candida* species), pneumonia (39% versus 27%), or systemic amphotericin B therapy (76% versus 27%). One possible explanation for these results could be that, although fluconazole prophylaxis could not reduce the occurrence of invasive fungal infections, it could reduce their associated mortality.

The efficacy of fluconazole for prevention of invasive fungal infections in neutropenic patients remains controversial. In a multicenter trial by Goodman et al. [5], 400 mg fluconazole daily decreased the incidence of death due to invasive fungal infections in bone marrow transplant recipients (10 of 177 versus 1 of 179), most of whom had received allogeneic transplants. All the protection afforded seemed to be in invasive candidosis, not aspergillosis. However, fluconazole did not result in decreased use of empiric

Table 3. Incidence of infections

	Fluconazole (n = 18)		Control (n = 15)	
	(n)	(%)	(n)	(%)
No infection/FUO	1	6	1	7
FUO	11	61	8	53
Only clinically documented infection	6	33	6	40
Pneumonia	4	22	2	13
Sepsis			1	
Gastrointestinal infection	2		2	
Perineal infection			1	
Clinically and microbiologically documented infection	4	22	4	27
Fungemia and sepsis:				
Candida krusei	1			
Candida tropicalis			1	
Fungemia and pneumonia:				
Candida tropicalis	1			
Bacteremia and sepsis and pneumonia:				
Streptococcus viridans	1		1	
Pseudomonas aeruginosa	1		1	
Bacteremia:				
Proteus vulgaris			1	

Table 4. Efficacy of antimicrobial therapy

Patients with infection or FUO	Fluconazole ($n = 17$)	Control ($n = 14$)
Antifungal therapy (n)	13	8
(%)	76	57
Intravenous amphotericin B (n)	13	4
(%)	76	27
Itraconazole (n)		2
Fluconazole (n)		2
Antibacterial therapy		
regimens—Median	3	1.5
Range (n)	1–7	1–3
Efficacy		
Complete response (n)	14	9
Partial response (n)	1	1
Infection-related mortality (n)	2	4
(%)	12	29
Causes of death	Fungemia and sepsis (*Candida krusei*) Gastrointestinal infection	Fungemia and sepsis (*Candida tropicalis*) Pneumonia Sepsis Bacteremia and sepsis and pneumonia (*Strept. viridans*)

amphotericin B, nor has an effect of overall survival been demonstrated. By contrast, in patients with acute leukemia, the same dose of fluconazole did not decrease the incidence of invasive fungal infections, reduce the empiric use of amphotericin B, or decrease the death rate [6]. In most studies, fluconazole prophylaxis has decreased the incidence of mucocutaneous candidiasis, but this complication can also be diagnosed readily and treated when present.

Meanwhile, there is justifiable concern that widespread fluconazole prophylaxis and lengthy periods of use may promote the outgrowth of drug-resistant fungal pathogens [12]. Windgard et al. [13] reported that the incidence of *Candida krusei* infection among 84 patients treated with fluconazole was seven times higher than that among 335 patients without fluconazole prophylaxis. Also, *Candida glabrata* emerges as an important pathogen in patients receiving fluconazole prophylaxis [14]. In the present trial, one fatal fungemia and sepsis due to *Candida krusei*, and one fungemia and pneumonia caused by *Candida tropicalis* occured during fluconazole prophylaxis.

Controlled comparative trials in targeted patients groups are needed to determine the beneficial role, if any, of antifungal prophylaxis. Therefore, a completion of the ongoing trial is needed to define the potential role of fluconazole prophylaxis in patients with AML.

References

1. Pizzo PA. Management of fever in patients with cancer and treatment-induced neutropenia. N Engl J Med 1993; 328: 1323–32
2. Löwenberg B. Post-remission treatment of acute myelogenous leukemia. N Engl J Med 1995; 332: 260–2
3. Como JA, Dismukes WE. Oral azole drugs as systemic antifungal therapy. N Engl J Med 1994; 330: 263–272
4. Mangino JE, Moser SA, Waites KB. When to use fluconazole. Lancet 1995; 345: 6–7
5. Goodman JL, Winston DJ, Greenfield RA, Chandrasekar PH, Fox B, Kaizer H, Shadduck RK, Shea T, Stiff P, Friedman DJ, Powderly WG, Silber JL, Horowitz H, Lichtin A, Wolff SN, Nangan KF, Silver SM, WeisdorfD, Ho WG, Gilver G, Buell D. A controlled trial of fluconazole to prevent fungal infections in patients undergoing bone marrow transplantation. N Engl J Med 1992; 326: 845–51
6. Winston DJ. Chandrasekar PH, Lazarus HM, Goodman JL, Silber JL, Horowitz H, Shadduck RK, Rosenfeld CS, Ho WG, Islam MZ, Buell DN. Fluconazole prophylaxis of fungal infections in

patients with acute leukemia. Ann Intern Med 118: 1993; 495–503
7. Menichetti F, Del Favero A, Martino P, Bucaneve G, Micozzi A, D'Antonio D, Ricci P, Carotenuto M, Liso V, Nosari AM, Barbui T, Fasola G, Mandelli F, The GIMEMA Infection Program. Preventing fungal infection in neutropenic patients with acute leukemia: fluconazole compared with oral amphotericin B.Ann Intern Med 1994; 120: 913–8
8. Bodey GP, Anaissie EJ, Elting LS, Estey E, O'Brien S, Kantarjian H. Antifungal prophylaxis during remission induction therapy for acute leukemia fluconazole versus intravenous amphotericin B. Cancer 1994; 73: 2099–106
9. Walsh TJ, Lee JW. Prevention of invasive fungal infections in patients with neoplastic disease. Clin Infect Dis 1993; 17,Suppl. 2: 468–80
10. Working party of the British Society for Antimicrobial Chemotherapy. Chemoprophylaxis for candidosis and aspergillosis in neutropenia and transplantation: a review and recommendations. J Antimicrob Chemother 1993; 32: 5–21
11. Meyer P, Adam D, Hiddemann W, Link H, Maschmeyer G, Helmerking M für die Studiengruppe Infektionen in der Hämatologie/Onkologie der Paul-Ehrilich-Gesellschaft für Chemotherapie e. V.. Interventionstherapie von Infektionen und Fieber unklarer Genese bei neutropenischen Patienten mit malignen hämatologischen Grunderkrankungen — Studie II Zeitschrift für antimikrobielle antineoplastische Chemotherapie 1992; 10: 1–27
12. Rex JH, Rinaldi MG, Pfaller MA. Resistance of candida species of fluconazole. Antimicrob Agents Chemotherapy. 1995; 39: 1–8
13. Wingard JR. Merz WG, Rinaldi MG, Miller CB, Karp JE, Saral R. Association of Torulopsis glabrata infections with fluconazole prophylaxis in neutropenic bone marrow transplant patients. Antimicrob Agents Chemother 1993; 37: 1847–9
14. Wingard JR, Merz WG, Rinaldi MG, Johnson TR, Karp JE, Saral R. Increase in Candida krusei infection among patients with bone marrow transplantation and neutropenia treated prophylactically with fluconazole. J Engl J Med 1991; 325: 274–7.

Acute Leukemias VI
Prognostic Factors
and Treatment Strategies
Büchner et al. (eds)

Current Approaches in the Prevention of Invasive Aspergillosis

J. Beyer[1], S. Schwartz[2], G. Behre[3], K. Lenz[1], W.-D. Ludwig[4], W. Hiddemann[3], and W. Siegert[1]

Abstract. Apart from the use of high-efficacy particulate air (HEPA) filtration, no established strategy for the prevention of invasive aspergillosis (IA) exists to date, and several attempts with topical or systemic prophylaxis have failed. However, in animal studies as well as in early phase I/II trials in humans, prophylactic aerosol amphotericin B showed promising results. An ongoing open-label, randomized, multicenter trial is investigating the efficacy of this approach.

Introduction

Invasive aspergillosis (IA) is increasingly recongnized as a severe infection in patients with hematologic malignancies or after bone marrow transplantation [1]. Difficulties in the early clinical diagnosis [10] as well as the poor response of IA to antifungal treatment [4, 6] has prompted an intensive search for effective prophylactic strategies [3]. Laminar air flow facilities with high-efficacy particulate air (HEPA) filtration [12] can reduce the incidence of IA by elimination of aspergillus spores from ambient air, but these are expensive and unavailable in many centers. Prophylactic intravenous amphotericin B desoxycholate [18] was reported to prevent reactivation of IA during repetitive periods of neutropenia in patients with a history of previous disease. Unfortunately, a prophylactic effect of other less toxic strategies such as intranasal amphotericin B spary [7], low-dose intravenous amphotericin B [9], intravenous liposomal amphotericin B [13], or oral itraconazol [14] has not been demonstrated in randomized clinical trials so far. Prophylactic inhalations with amphotericin B aerosols, however, represent a novel approach, avoiding the systemic side effects of this drug, and results from animal studies as well as from initial phase I/II trials in humans have suggested prophylactic efficacy [2, 5, 11]. These preliminary data are under further investigation in an ongoing randomized multicenter trial.

Materials and Methods

From March 1993 until April 1994, 115 patients with hematologic malignancies or autologous bone marrow transplantation and an expected duration of neutropenia of $<500/\mu l$ for more than 10 days were randomized to receive prophylactic amphotericin B inhalations (group A) or no inhalation prophylaxix (group B). Patients with one of the following criteria were excluded: (a) proven or suspected invasive pulmonary aspergillosis during a preceding neutropenic episode; (b) treatment with itraconazol or intravenous amphotericin B during the last 3 months; (c) concomitant prophylaxis with itraconazol or intravenous amphotericin B; (d) laminar air flow units; (e) pulmonary infiltrate at time of randomization; (f) prior participation in the study.

[1]Universitätsklinikum Rudolf Virchow, Spandauer Damm 130, 14050 Berlin, Germany
[2]Universitätsklinikum Benjamin Franklin, Hindenburgdamm 30, 12200 Berlin, Germany
[3]Universitätsklinikum Gottingen, Robert-Koch-Strasse 40, 37075 Göttingen, Germany
[4]Robert Rössle Kilink, Lindenburger Weg 80, 13122 Berlin, Germany

Patients randomized to group A inhaled 10 mg aerosol amphotericin B twice daily. For each inhalation, 10 mg amphotericin B desoxycholate preparation for intravenous use (Bristol Myers Squibb, Munich, Germany) was diluted with sterile water to a total volume of 5 ml and nebulized with RespirGard II nebulizer (Marquest, Englewood, CO, USA) and the Lifetec jetair δ 10 (Salvia, Schwalbach, Germany) compressor at a flow rate of 8 ml/min, with the Pari boy or with the Pari I./S. II (Pari Werke, Starnberg, Germany). Each inhalation lasted for 15–20 min, and each nebulizer was used only twice to avoid bacterial contamination. Amphotericin B inhalations were initiated at the beginning of chemotherapy and stopped after recovery of neutrophils >1000/μl. In case of intravenous amphotericin B therapy, the continuation of amphotericin B inhalations was optional.

Invasive aspergillosis or systemic candidiasis was classified as possible, probable, or proven depending on whether there was clinical suspicion alone, or whether additional radiological, mycological, or histological confirmation could be obtained. Empiric intravenous amphotericin B was started in all study patients after 3–5 days of fever despite broad-spectrum antibiotics.

Results

A total of 115 patients from five institutions were include in this analysis; 65 patients randomized to group A and 50 patients to group B. Patient characteristics such as age, disease entity, conticosteroid comedication, treatment with hematopoietic growth factors, and median duration of neutropenia were balanced between the two groups (Table 1).

The incidence of possible, probable, or proven IA was 3/65 (5%) patients in group A who received aerosol amphotericin B prophylaxis as compared to 6/50 (12%) patients in group B in whom no aerosol amphotericin B was used. This difference was statistically not significant. No statistically signigificant differences were observed in the incidence of possible, probable, or proven systemic candidiasis or other fungal infections (Table 2), in the use of intravenous amphotericin B (26/65, 40%, patients in group A verus 19/50, 38%, patients in group B) or in the incidence of fever unresponsive to broad-spectrum antibacterial agents (22/65, 34%, patients in group A versus 18/50, 36%, patients in group B). The differences between the two study groups in the incidence

Table 1. Patient characteristics

	Inhalation ($n=65$)	No inhalation ($n=50$)
Age		
Median (years)	43	43
Range (years)	19–73	18–81
Underlying disease		
Acute myeloid leukemia (n)	38	29
(%)	58	58
Relapse of acute lymphoblastic leukemia/ high-grade non-Hodgkin's lymphoma (n)	5	8
(%)	8	12
High-dose chemotherapy with autologous stem cell rescue for solid tumors (n)	22	15
(%)	34	30
Leukocytopenia < 1000/μl		
Median (days)	17	15
Range (days)	0–48	0–47
Granulocytopenia < 500/μl		
Median (days)	18	18
Range (days)	4–50	0–50
Corticosteroid comedication	14	9
Therapy with hematopoetic growth factors (G-CSF/GM-CSF)	34	17

Differences between the two groups were not significant; p >0.05 test or Mann-Withney test).

Table 2. Effect of inhaled amphotericin B on the incidence of systemic fungal infections

	Inhalation ($n=65$)		No inhalation ($n=50$)	
	(n)	(%)	(n)	(%)
Invasive pulmonary aspergillosis	3	5	6	2
Proven	1		1	
Probable	2		4	
Possible	0		1	
Systemic candidiasis	9	14	4	8
Proven	1		0	
Probable	2		1	
Possible	6		3	
Possible systemic fungal infection	7	11	6	12

Differences between the two groups were not significant; $p > 0.05$, test.

of other infections, (classified as bacteremia/fungemia, pneumonia, other clinically documented infections, other clinically and microbiologically documented infections, fever of unknown origin, and no infection, was also statistically not significant.

The mortality was 11/65 (17%) in group A versus 9/50 (18%) in group B ($p > 0.05$) for an overall mortality of 20/115 (17%): 14 patients died from infections, three from progressive acute myeloid leukemia, two from cerebral bleeding, and one from toxic renal failure. Infective causes of death comprised pneumonias in seven patients (of these, two *Aspergillus*, one cytomegalovirus, one *Xanthomonas Maltophilia*, and three without microbiological confirmation), and sepsis in four patients (of these, three Gram negative, and one without microbiological confirmation). Adverse reactions consisted predominantly of coughing, bad taste, and nausea, which were reported by 35/65 (54%), 33/65 (51%), and 24/65 (37%) patients, respectively. Side effects resulted in the premature discontinuation of the inhalations in 15/65 (23%) patients. One patient who stopped the inhalations prematurely developed suspected IA after termination of the prophylaxis

Discussion

The occurrence of IA in patients with hematologic malignancies remains a life-threatening complication that may occur with an incidence of 10% or more in patients with prolonged neutropenia. Unfortunately, current approaches to prevent this condition have been largely unsuccessful. Laminar air flow is too expensive and unavailable for many patients for many patients at risk, and the general use of systemic prophylaxis with intravenous amphotericin B is limited by the toxicity of this drug. Despite preliminary reports of several non-randomized studies, no other prophylactic strategy could be established thus far.

This interim analysis of an ongoing prospective randomized trial of prophylactic aerosol amphotericin B administrations in neutropenic patients after myelosuppressive chemotherapy demonstrated a 5% incidence of possible, probable, or proven IA in patients receiving prophylaxis with aerosol amphotericin B, which compares to a 12% incidence in patients who recived no such prophylaxis. This reduction failed statistical significance. However, these results were expected and, were in accordance with data from animal experiments and statistical considerations.

Only a few patients have been included in this interim analysis which was performed primarily to be able to detect unexpected adverse events and to stop the trial early. A total of 380 patients will be required to detect a 9% reduction in the incidence of IA with prophylactic amphotericin B aerosol administrations as a realistic goal in the ongoing trial. Yet, the occurrance of possible, probable, as well as proven IA in patients receiving aerosol amphotericin B is worrisome and indicates that, even if this prophylaxis should reduce the incidence of IA, it will not be possible to completely prevent this condition in high-risk patients.

Most, but not all, of the previous trials investgating aerosol amphotericin B in humans reported a very low frequency of side effects from the inhalations. Manageable, but frequent side effects such as coughing, bad taste, and nausea were observed in the majority of patients in the present study, causing early discontinuation of the inhalation prophylaxis in 23%. However, as with any kind of prophylactic intervention, compliance of patients with the prophylaxis is crucial. This is underscored by the occurance of suspected IA in a patient with premature discontinuation of the inhalations prior to neutrophil recovery.

In conclusion, prophylactic aerosol amphotericin B might be promising for the prevention of IA in neutropenic patients. However, further recruitment of patients in the ongoing trial is required before more definite statements can be made. Because of the still undetermined efficacy of this intervention, the search for other approaches such as the application of hematologic growth factors or new antifungal drugs should continue.

References

1. Andriole VT (1993) Infections with Aspergillus species. Clin Insfect Dis 17 Suppl 2: 481–486
2. Beyer J, Barzen G,Risse G,Weyer C, Miksits K, Dullenkopf K, Huhn D, Siegert W (1993) Aerosol amphotericin B for prevention of invasive pulmonary aspergillosis. Antimicrob Agencs Chemother 37: 1367–1369
3. Beyer J, Schewartz S, Heinemann V, Siegert W (1994) Strategies in prevention of invasive pulmonary aspergillosis in immunosuppressed or neutropenic patients. Antimicrob Agents Chemother 38: 911–917
4. Büchner T, Roos N (1992) Antifungal treatment strategy in leukemia patients. Ann Hematol 65: 153–161
5. Conneally E, Cafferkey MT, Daly PA, Keane CT, McCann SR (1990) Nebulized amphotericin B as prophylaxis against invasive aspergillosis in granulocytopenic patients. Bone Marrow Transplant 5: 403–406
6. Denning DW, Stevens DA (1990) Antifungal and surgical treatment of invasive aspergillosis: review of 2,121 published cases. Rev Infects Dis 12: 1147–1201
7. Jeffery GM, Beard MEJ, Ikram RB, Chua J, Allen JR Heaton DC, Hart DNJ, Schousboe MI (1991) Intranasal amphotericin B reduces the frequency of invasive aspergillosis in neutropenic patients. Am J Med 90: 685–692
8. Karp JE, Burch PA, Merz WG (1988) An approach to intensive antileukemia therapy in patients with previous invasive aspergillosis. Am J Med 85: 203–206.
9. Perfect J, Klotman ME, Gilbert CC, Crawford DD, Rosner GL, Wright KA, Peters WP (1992) Prophylactic intravenous amphotericin B in neutropenic autologous bone marrow transplant recipients. J Infect Dis 165: 891–897.
10. Rüchel R (I993) Diagnoisis of invasive mycoses in severely immunospressed patients. Ann Hematol 67: 1–11
11. Schmitt HJ, Bernard EM, Häuser M, Armstrong D (1988). Aerosol amphotericn B is effective for prophylaxis and theraphy in a rat model of pulmonary aspergillosis. Antimicrob Angents Chemother 32: 1676–1679
12. Sherertz RJ, Belani A, Kramer BS, Elfenbein GJ, Weiner RS, ML Sullivan, RG Thomas, GP Samsa (1987) Impact of air filtration on nosocomial aspergillus infections.Am J Med 83: 709–718
13. Tollemar, J, Ringden O, Andersson S, Sundberg B, Ljungman P, Tyden G (1993) Randomized double-blind study of liposomal amphotericin B (amphotericin bisome) prophylaxis of invasive fungal infections in bone marrow transplant recipients. Bone Marrow Transplant 12: 577–582
14. Vreugdenhil G, van Dijke BJ, Donnelly P, Novakova IRO, Raemaekers JMM, Hoogkamp-Korstanje MAA, Koster M, de Pauw BE (1993) Efficacy of itraconazole in the prevention of fungal infections among neutropenic patients with hematological malignancies and intensive chemotherapy. A double blind, placebo controlled study. Leuk Lymphoma 11: 353–358.

Acute Leukemias VI
Prognostic Factors
and Treatment Strategies
Büchner et al. (eds)

Early Empiric Antifungal Treatment of Infections in Neutropenic Patients Comparing Fluconazole with Amphotericin B/5-Flucytosine

G. Silling[1], W. Fegeler[2], N. Roos[3], R. Schomaker[4], M. Essink[4], and T. Büchner[4]

Abstract. In order to improve outcome in neutropenic patients with hematological malignancies we administered i.v. antifungal agents early as part of an empiric antimicrobial regimen. Additionally, we compared the tolerability and efficacy of fluconazole (FCA) versus amphotericin B and 5-flucytosine (ABF) within a prospective randomized study. Antifungal treatment started on day 4 if fever of >38.5°C did not respond to i.v. antibiotics. In the case of additional pulmonary infiltrates or other evidence of invasive fungal infection, antifungal treatment started upfront together with the antibiotics. If fever or infiltrates persisted after 1 week, FCA was replaced by ABF. A total of 98 patients entered the study, 49 in each arm; all suffered from severe neutropenia with neutrophils <1000/µl.

A total of 42 FCA and 41 ABF patients suffered from fever of unknown origin; eight and seven respectively, had pulmonary infiltrates when fever occurred. Response to fever was achieved in 29/39 FCA and 37/49 ABF. This difference was statistically not significant. Fourteen of 20 nonresponders to FCA responded when ABF was given, so an overall response of 81.6% was achieved. In this high-risk population, 20 patients died, six in the FCA and 14 in ABF arm. Among those death six and eight were due to infections, four and five were fungal infections, and one and four patients died form aspergillosis.

We conclude that FCA and ABF seem to be equally effective in controlling microbiologically non-documented infections in neutropenic patients with hematological malignancies. Because of its lower toxicity, FCA may be preferred as a first-line empiric antifungal agent and—in the case of non-response-be replaced after 1 week.

Introduction

Neutropenic patients who suffer from hematological malignancies are at high risk to develop fungal infections [1, 2]. Although prevention procedures [3] like the introduction of laminar air flow or high-efficacy particulate air HEPA filters, protective isolation, selective gut decontamination or the use of growth factors [4] could reduce infectious complications, there still remains a high incidence due to prolongation of neutropenia and intensification of chemotherapy. At the same time, it is difficult to diagnose mycosis [5] and even the introduction of high-resolution computer tomography [6, 7] to recognize early suggestive pulmonary or hepatosplenic manifestations is often too late to initiate antifungal treatment. Therefore, empiric strategies have been established [8-12]. Additionally, pulmonary infiltrates have to be considered as a major problem because outcomes of those patients is worse and in prolonged neutropenia nearly one half of pneumonia infections where a pathogen could be identified were caused by fungi [12]. So not only the empiric antibiotic therapy seems to be reasonable but also the early empiric antifungal

[1]Dept. of Internal Medicine IV (Hematology/Oncology), University of Aachen, Germany
[2]Dept. of Microbiology, University of Münster, Germany
[3]Dept. of Radiology, University of Münster, Germany
[4]Dept. of Internal Medicine A (Hematology/Oncology), University of Münster, Germany

treatment. As amphotericin B—with or without 5-flycytosine (5-FC)-is still the standard antifungal agent, its use is limited by the associated side effects like fever, chills, and nephrotoxicity, although the intravenous infusion of saline and predosing of pethidine or paracetamol are able to mitigate these adverse reactions. Fluconazole (FCA) seems to be less toxic and also effective in fungal infections [13–18]. We therefore conducted a prospective randomized study to compare the toxicity and efficacy of FCA versus amphotericin B and 5-FC (ABF) in neutropenic patients for the empiric treatment of fever of unknown origin (FUO) or for the treatment of fungal infections.

Patients and Methods

Patients and Treatment Regimen. Patients qualified for this study when a prolonged neutropenia had to be expected. They suffered from hematological malignancies, predominantly from acute leukemias. They were included when they had first fever >38.5°C and neutrophils <1000/µl. Patients were stratified into two groups (Fig. 1) depending on whether they had pulmonary infiltrates, evidence of mycosis or not (FUO). The latter group received a combination of two antibiotics and, if there was no response after 4 days, the antibiotic regimen was changed and the antifungal regimen was randomly assigned. After 1 week of antifungal treatment, there was a second evaluation. In the case of non-response to FCA patients were changed to ABF, in the case of non-response to ABF, the physicians were free to choose any other agent.

If pulmonary infiltrates were seen on X-ray or any other evidence of mycosis occurred on the day of inclusion, the antifungal treatment was started together with the initial combination of antibiotics. If fever did not respond, antibiotics were changed on day 4 (first evaluation), efficacy of antifungals was evaluated after 1 week in order to have identical conditions in both groups. If patients responded to the antifungal regimen, it was continued for 4 weeks in patients with pulmonary infiltrates or for 1 week after temperature reached <37.5°C in FUO patients.

Dose. Amphotericin B was administered in a dose of 0.5 mg/kg (0.1+0.4) on day 1 and 0.75 mg/kg per day (max. 50 mg) on days 2–7; after day 7 it was given every other day except for those patients who had evidence of aspergillosis; they received a daily dose of 1.0 mg/kg. 5-Flucytosine was administered at a daily dose of 150mg/kg on days 1–14 and adapted when creatinine levels rose. On day 1 patients received a loading dose of 11.4 mg/kg (max. 800 mg) FCA and 5.7 mg/kg perday (max. 400 mg) on the following days.

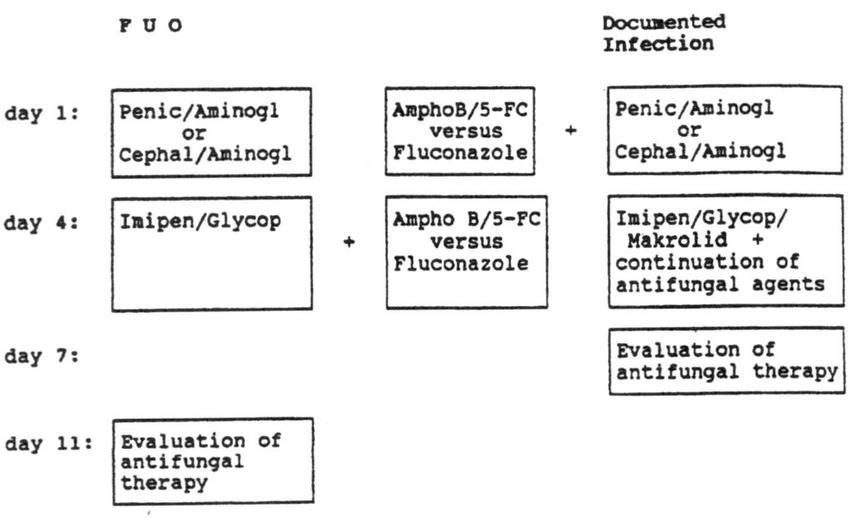

Fig. 1. Treatment regimen

Evaluation of Efficacy. In neutropenic patients fever is often the only symptom of infection, and in our study patients qualified for inclusion with the occurrence of fever. Therefore this was the main criterion of response. Response was evaluated when the antifungal agents were changed from FCA to ABF or another antifungal drug, or the antimycotic therapy was stopped because of cure or death. Response was achieved when temperature was <37.6°C. Additionally, other signs of fungal infection or microbiological documentation were monitored. Invasive fungal infections were diagnosed according to the following characteristics. Mycosis was proven only by biopsy or autopsy, it was highly suspected when there were positive blood cultures or typical lesions in high-resolution computer tomography (HR-CT) with the characteristic signs of *Candida* or *Aspergillus* [6, 7]. A rise in antigen or antibody titer or positive cultures from multiple body sites the reflecting extensive colonization made an invasive fungal infection suspected. Response of documented infections was defined as disappearance of radiological signs (X-ray and/or HR-CT) or negative cultures.

Results

Patients Characteristics. Ninety-eight patients entered the study, 49 in each arm. Predisposing factors to impair outcome such as age and underlying disease (Table 1) were well balanced, especially with regard to de novo diagnosis, or resistant or relapsed disease status. The median age was 47.9 years for the FCA patients and 45.6 years for the ABF patients, range 16–77 and 18–73, respectively.

Table 1. Hematological malignancies

	FCA (*n*)	ABF (*n*)
Acute myeloid leukemia(primary)	24	23
Acute myeloid leukemia(relapsed)	14	12
Myelodysplastic syndrome	1	3
Acute lymphoblastic leukemia (relapsed)	4	4
Lymphoma	6	6
Chronic myelogenous leukemia	0	1

Response to Fever. All 98 patients suffered from febrile neutropenia when they were randomized to the antifungal regimen. A total of 42 patients of the FCA group and 41 patients of the ABF group had FUO, whereas seven and eight patients also had primary pulmonary infiltrates. In both groups patients needed a mean of 5 days to respond to the randomized regimen. Response to fever was achieved in 29/49 (59.2%) FCA and 37/49 (75.5%) ABF patients (Table 2). At evaluation after 1 week, the results were 25 and 29 patients, respectively; 23 and 30 patients were still neutropenic when fever resolved. All these differences were not statistically significant. Another 14 patients responded when FCA was replaced by ABF, so the overall response for all patients initially randomized to FCA was 43/49 (87.7%).

Radiological Signs to Infection. Pulmonary infiltrates were seen at the beginning of antimicrobial therapy in seven FCA and eight ABF patients. A further 13 and 18 patients, respectively, developed pulmonary infiltrates during the treatment episode. In 5/20 FCA and 19/26 ABF patients these infiltrates resolved. This difference was

Table 2. Response to fever

	FCA		ABF		*p*
	(*n*)	(%)	(*n*)	(%)	
$n = 98$	49		49		
Defervescence	29	59.2	37	75.5	>0.05
Within 7 days	25		29		>0.05
While neutropenic	23		30		>0.05
Crossover	20				
Defervescence	14				
Non-response	6				
Overall response	43	87.7	37	75.5	>0.05

statistically significant, so the ABF regimen seems to be more effective in pneumonia. It has to be remembered that numbers are small.

Fungal Infections. Evidence of fungal infections occurred in ten FCA and 14 ABF patients. In four and seven patients respectively *Candida* were isolated, whereas *Aspergillus* was found in five and seven patiens. Response rates are shown in Table 3. With regard to the inhibitory concentrations of FCA, it could not be expected that it would be effective in aspergillosis and indeed nobody in our study in whom *Aspergillus* was detected responded to FCA. On the other hand, aspergillosis did not occur more often in the FCA group, so one can at least say that the use of FCA does not favor the occurrence of *Aspergillus*. Additionally, outcome of those patients was not worse when they received ABF as soon as there was any evidence of aspergillosis, as four of five patients responded after crossing over. One patient in the FCA group died as a consequence of invasive mycosis due to *Trichosporum beigelii* sepsis. The lung was the primary organ where mycosis could be diagnosed so fungal infections were associated with pneumonia in 9/10 in the FCA and in 9/14 in the ABF group.

Fatal Outcome. In this high-risk group, 20 patients died from infections or other causes. Six FCA and eight ABF patients died from infections, four and five of these were due to mycosis, and one and four were due to aspergillosis, respectively. In the ABF arm, seven patients died from other causes such as intracranial hemorrhage (three), cerebral infarction (one), cardiogenic shock (one), or progression of the underlying disease (two). One of these patients died as a consequence of cerebral hematoma and invasive pulmonary candidiasis that was resistant to therapy, and it was not possible to decide which was the leading cause of death.

Table 3. Fungal infections

	FCA (*n*)	ABF (*n*)
Mycosis	10	14
Candida	4	7
Response (after crossover)	1(+1)	5
Aspergillus	5	7
Response (after crossovern)	0(+4)	3
Trichosporum beigelii	1	
Response	0	

Toxicity. In general FCA was well tolerated and no major side effects occurred. The severity and symptoms of the underlying disease, side effects of cytostatic therapy or other necessary agents do not allow evaluation of minor side effects. In a few cases amphotericin B caused mild elevations (WHO 1 and 2) of serum creatinine, but these were reversible. Substitution of potassium is lower under the FCA regimen.

Discussion

In this prospective randomized study all patients suffered from fever and in most of them, 42 FCA and 41 ABF, the causes was not known. Seven and eight additionally had pulmonary infiltrates. In these patients, neither the overall response to fever nor the response within 7 days or while neutropenic differed significantly. As the groups were comparable with respect to risk factors such as age and underlying disease, both regimens are equally effective in the empiric treatment of neutropenic patients with hematological diseases. Additionally, treatment was successful in 14/20 FCA patients who received crossover therapy. So the overall response was 80/98 (81.6%).

Twenty FCA and 26 ABF patients developed pulmonary infiltrates, but regression was achieved less often in FCA patients. This difference was significant. Drawing the conclusion that the standard regimen seems to be much more effective has to be restricted considering that it look pulmonary infiltrates more than 1 week to disappear and in the case of nonresponse to FCA the antifungal regimen was changed on day 7, but ABF was continued because of a lack of better alternatives. It also has to be considered that pulmonary infiltrates may be caused by *Aspergillus*. Therefore, whether it is reasonable to change to amphotericin B whether with or without 5-FC remains an unanswered question.

Analysing the response rates of patients who had a proven invasive fungal infection, it is evident that this subgroup had the worst outcome. This does not depend on the inefficacy of the antifungal agent but on the method, as most of the proven fungal infections were diagnosed by autopsy, as biopsy was not possible because of the high risk of bleeding complications associated with thrombocytopenia. When mycosis was only suspected, response rates were better than in those patients where it was highly suspected. The explanation may be that mycosis is already advanced when diagnosis is possible. Consequently, treatment of the latter group is much more difficult and less successful than treating an emerging fungal infection. This again confirms the importance of early empiric treatment strategies leading to the conclusion that FCA and ABF seem to be equally effective in the early and empiric treatment of hematological patients who suffer from severe neutropenia. Therefore, the well-tolerated FCA should be administered in FUO patients but, in the case of refractoriness or evidence of aspergillosis or pneumonia with a high incidence of aspergillosis, it should be replaced by ABF.

References

1. Pfaffenbach B, Donhuijsen K, Pahnke J et al. (1994) Systemische Pilzinfektionen bei hämatologischen Neoplasien. Medizinische Klinik 89: 299-304
2. Bodey G, et al (1992) Fungal infections in cancer patients: an international autospy survey study. Eur J Clin Microbiol Infect Dis. 11: 99-109
3. Kibber CC, Prentice HG (1994) Infection control aspects of bone marrow transplantation. Current opinion in Infectious Diseases 7: 427-429
4. American Society of Clinical Oncology (1994) American Society of Clinical Oncology Recommendation for the use of hematopoetic colony-stimulating factors: evidence-based, clinical practice guidelines. Journal of Clinical Oncology 11: 2471-2508
5. Horn R, Wong B, Kiehn T et al. (1985) Fungemia in a cancer hospital: changing frequency, earlier onset, and results of therapy. Rev Infect Dis. 7: 646-655
6. RoosN, Vasallo P, Fahrenkamp A et al. (1990) Pulmonary aspergillosis and candidiasis: differentiation using CT. Radiology 177 (suppl.): 359
7. Kuhlmann JE, Fishman EK, Siegelmann SS (1985) Invasive pulmonary aspergillosis in acute leukemia: characteristics findings on CT, the CT halo sigh, and the role of CT in early diagnosis. Radiology, 157: 611-614
8. EORTC International Antimicrobial Therapy Cooperative Group (1989) Empiric antifungal therapy in febrile granulocytopenic patients. American Journal of Medicine 86: 668-672
9. Pizzo PA, Robichaud KJ, Gill FA, Witebsky FG (1982) Empiric antibiotic and antifungal therapy for cancer patients with prolonged fever and granulocytopenia. American Journal of Medicine 72: 101-111
10. Sugar AM (1990) Empiric treatment of fungal infections in the neutropenic host. Arch Inter Med 150: 2258-2264
11. Bodey GP (1986) Fungal infection and fever of unknown origin in neutropenic patients. The American Journal of Medicine 80 (Suppl 5C): 112-119
12. Maschmeyer G, Link H, Hiddemann W et al. (1994) Empirische antimikrobielle Therapie bei neutropenischen Patienten, Ergebnisse einer multizentrischen Studie der Arbeitsgruppe Infektionen in der Haematologie der Paul-Ehrlich-Gesellschaft. Medizinische Klinik 89(3): 114-123
13. Como JA, Dismukes WE (1994) Oral azole drugs as systemic antifungal therapy. New England Journal of Medicine 330: 263-271
14. Van't Wout JW, Mattie H, van Furth R (1988) A prospective study of the efficacy of fluconazole (UK-49858) against deep-seated fungal infections. J Antimicrob Chemoth 21: 665-672
15. Ikemoto H (1989) A clinical study of fluconazole for the treatment of deep mycosis. Diagn Microbiol Infect Dis12. 239 S
16. Anaissie E, Bodey GP, Kantarjian H et al. (1991) Fluconazole therapy for chronic disseminated candidiasis in patients with leukemia and prior amphotericin B therapy. The American Journal of Medicine 91: 142-150
17. Graninger W, Presteril E, Schneeweiss et al. (1993) Treatment of Candida albicans fungaemia with fluconazole. Journal of Infection 26: 133-146
18. Rex JH, Bennett JE, Sugar AM et al. (1994). A randomized trial comparing fluconazole with amphotericin B for the treatment of candidemia in patients without neutropenia. The New England Journal of Medicine 331: 1325-1332

Pharmacology

Acute Leukemias VI
Prognostic Factors
and Treatment Strategies
Büchner et al. (eds)

Dependence of Asparaginase-Induced Coagulopathy on Serum Asparaginase Activity: A Randomized Trial

U. Nowak-Göttl, J. Boos, G. Werber, E. Ahlke, and H. Jürgens

Abstract. Hypercoagulability and thrombosis are well-documented side effects of leukemia treatment with L-asparaginase (L-asp). To determine hemostatic alterations of different *Escherichia coli* asparaginase preparations, a randomized prospective study was carried out in 20 leukemic children (ALL-BFM 90): ten patients each received L-asp Crasnitin (Bayer AG) and Medac (originally purchased from Kyowa Hakko Kyogo, Japan). Blood samples for coagulation studies were obtained prior to and whilst on medication. L-asp activity was significantly ($p = 0.001$) higher in the Kyowa-treated patients, leading to prolonged asparagine depletion and longer inhibition of hepatic protein synthesis. Futhermore, alterations of hemostatic parameters were more pronounced in the Kyowa group. Clearly correlated with serum asparaginase activity, values of fibrinogen, antithrombin III, plasminogen, and α2-antiplasmin were significantly decreased and D-dimer formation was found to be markedly higher than in patients treated with *E. coli* asparaginase type A purchased from Bayer. A 13-year-old boy developed thrombosis and a 7-year-old girl acquired intermediate insulin-dependent hyperglycemia (both treated with Kyoma asparaginase).

Introduction

Alterations in hemostasis have frequently been observed in patients with leukemia, and thrombotic events are well documented in patients receiving L-asparaginase (L-asp) as a single agent or in combination with vincristine or prednisone, sometimes complemented by an anthracycline [1–7].

A wide range of circulating half-lives with the employment of different commercially available asparaginase preparations from *Eschericia coli* and *Erwinia chrysanthemi* has been reported [8–10]. The present study was designed to prospectively evaluate hemostatic parameters in leukemic children randomized to receive two different *E. coli* asparaginase preparation with different half-lives, and to relate changes of coagulations to serum asparaginase activity.

Methods

Twenty leukemic children diagnosed within a 9-month period and treated according to the ALL-BFM-90 study protocol 1 (part 1: prednisone 60 mg/m^2 on days 1–29; *E. coli* asparaginase 10 000 U/m^2 on days 12, 15, 18, 21, 24, 27, 30, 33; vincristine 1.5 mg/m^2 and daunorubicin 30 mg/m^2 on days 8, 15, 22, 29) were randomized to receive one of the two *E. coli* asparaginase preparations officially approved in Germany: L-asp Crasnitin (Bayer, Leverkusen, Germany) or Medac (Medac, Hamburg, Germany; originally purchased from Kyowa Hacco Kyogo, Japan). No patient had an individual or family history of bleeding or thrombophilia.

A total of 11 blood samples per patient were obtained at the onset of the disease, prior to the first and each subseequent dose of L-asp and 3 days after the last asparaginase adminstrations.

Department of Pediatric Hematology and Oncology, University Hospital Münster, Albert-Schweitzer-Str. 33, 48129 Münster, Germany

Blood samples were drawn into premarked 3-ml plastic tubes (citrate 3.8%/blood: 1: 10; Saarstedt), immediately placed on iced water and centrifuged at 4°C and 3000 *g* for 20 min. Fibrinogen was measured according to Clauss [11]. Antithrombin III, plasminogen, and α2-antiplasmin were measured by enzymatic procedure using chromogenic substrates S 2765, 2403, 2251 as described earlier [12]. D-Dimer formation was measured with EIA-D-Dimer micro (Behring Werke, Marburg, Germany [13].

Controls included calibration plasma, normal and abnormal control plasma (IL Test, Instrumentation Laboratory, Italy. Serum asparaginase activity [14] and asparagine levels [15] were simultaneously determined throughout the testing period.

Statistics

Calculations of medians and ranges and non-parametric statistics (Wilcoxon-Mann-Whitney: U test, Spearman rank) were performed using the Apple computer (Macintosh Performa 630) Stat view 4.02 program [16].

Results

Alterations of hemostatic parameters were more severe in those patients who received " Kyowa" asparaginase: decreased values of fibrinogen, antithrombin III, plasminogen, and α2antiplasmin were found (Figs 1, 2), along with significantly enhanced D-dimer formation (Fig. 3).

Furthermore, pharmcokinectic data (Fig. 3) of patients receiving Kyowa L-asp show signifi-

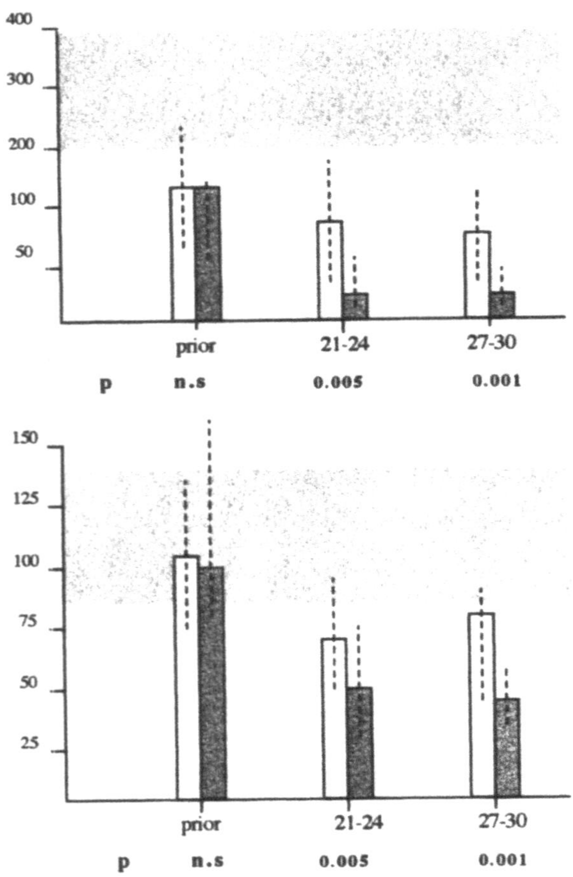

Fig. 1a,b. Fibrinogen (a, mg/dl) and antithrombin III (%) in 20 leukemic children prior to and after administration of different *E.coli* L-asparaginase preparations—(median, ranges, *p* values (Wilcoxon-Man-Whitney: Bayer asp, *open columns*; $n = 10$/Kyowa asp *shaded columns*; $n = 10$)

cantly ($p = 0.001$) enhanced L-asp activity compared to children treated with the Bayer type A preparation.

Table 1 shows a significant correlation between coagulation and serum asparaginase activity ρ and p values): the highest L-asp activity is clearly associated with the lowest values of fibrinogen, antithrombin III, plasminogen, and α2-antiplasmin, and with enhanced D-dimer formation.

Both groups of patients showed complete asparagine depletion, at a detection limit of 0.1 µm, during the course of asparaginase treatment (for further information see [18].

The children randomized to Kyowa l-asp, a 13-year-old boy and a 7-year-old girl, developed thrombosis on day 31 and intermediate insulin-dependent hyperglycemia, respectively. No patient treated with the Bayer prepartion showed evidence of these complications.

Discussion

L-Asparaginase is and enzyme that provides specific metabolic therapy for acute lymphoblastic leukemia (ALL) and non-Hodgkin lymphomas. This enzyme catalyses the conversion of the amino acid L-asp to aspartic acid and ammonia, which leads to rapid depletion of the circulating pool of asparagine and glutamine, and results in a decreased protein synthesis [8].

Data of this study show a significant decrease of fibrinogen, antithrombin III, plasminogen, and α2-antiplasmin, as well as significantly enhanced D-dimer formation, all clearly correlated to serum asparaginase activity.

In humans, circulating half-lives of asparaginase enzymes from *E.coli* and *E.chrysanthemi* vary within a wide range. Moreover, half-lives differ not only between *E.coli* strains type A and type B, but also among different commercial

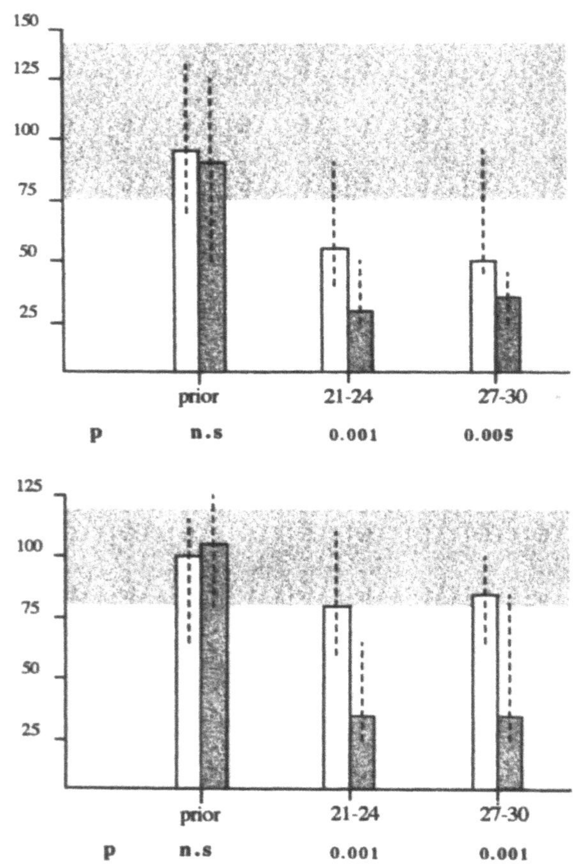

Fig. 2a,b. Plasminogen (%) and α2-antiplasmin (%) in 20 leukemic children prior to and after administration of different *E.coli* L-asparaginase preparations- (Median, ranges, p values (Wilcoxon-Man-Whitney: Bayer asp, *open columns*; $n = 10$/Kyowa asp, *shaded columns*; $n = 10$)

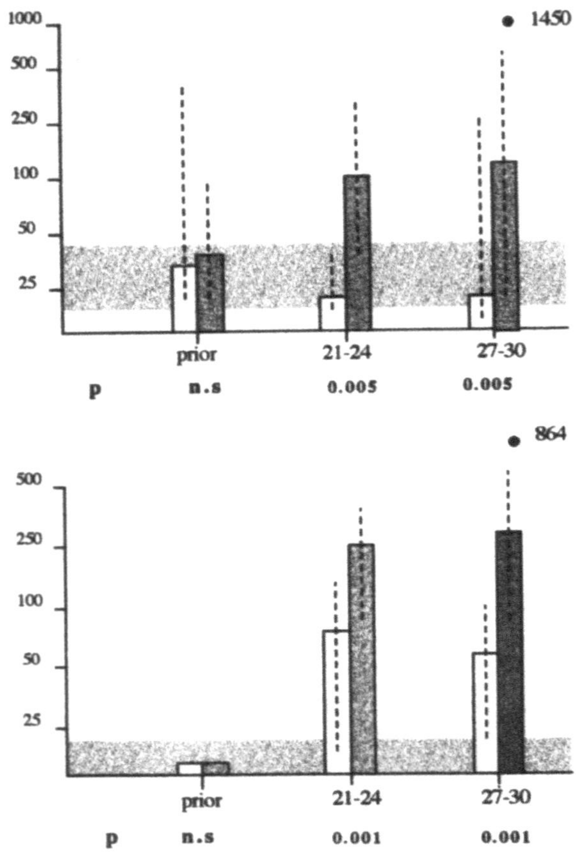

Fig. 3 a,b. D-Dimer (μg/l) formation and asparaginase activities (Iu/l) in 20 leukemic children prior to and after administration of different *E.coli* L-asparaginase preparations–(Median, ranges, *p* values (Wilcoxon-Man-Whitney: Bayer asp, *open columns*; $n = 10$/ Kyowa asp, *shaded columns* $n = 10$)

Table 1. Correlation (Spearman rank) between coagulation and fibrinolytic proteins and asparaginase activity *P* and *p* value) in leukemic children randomized to Bayer type A asparaginse ($n = 10$) and Kyowa asparaginase ($n = 10$)

Parameter	*P*	*p*-value
Fibrinogen	−0.487	0.023
Antithrombin III	−0.617	0.026
Plasminogen	−0.472	0.025
α2-Antimplasmin	−0.735	0.036
D-Dimer	0.581	0.05

E.coli preparations [8,-10,18]. One of the most obvious distinctions between the two *E.coli* asparaginase preparations administered in this study is the absence of cystine in the Kyowa L-asp, which also has a lower isoelectric point, a longer clearance time, and a longer half-life of 11–15 h as reported for the type A L-asp, a prolonged asparagine depletion with the Kyowa preparation is found. With respect to these observations, this may lead to longer inhibition of protein synthesis, which then may be the cause of a higher rate of side effects.

However, our results show not only a downregulation of coagulation proteins: the enhanced D-dimer formation along with decreased values for plasminogen and α2-antiplasmin signify an activated fibrinolytic system.

Along with studies on asparaginase pharmacokinetics and asparagine depletion, dose recommendations need to be tailored to the specific asparaginase preparation employed to assure optimal antineoplastic efficacy while minimizing the hazard of complications.

References

1. Semerano N, Montemurro P, Giordano P et al. Unbalanced coagulation—fibrinolysis potential during l-asparaginase therapy in children with acute lymphoblastic leukemia. Thromb Haemostas 1990; 64(1): 38–40
2. Leone G, Gugliotta L, Mazzucconi MG et al. Evidence of a hypercoagulable state in patients with acute lymphoblastic leukemia treated with low dose of E.coli asparaginase. A GIMEMA study. Thromb Haemostas 1993; 69(1): 12–15
3. Kucuk O, Kwaan HC, Gunnar W, Wasquez RM.Thromboembolic complicatins associated with L-asparaginase therapy. Cancer 1985;55: 702–6
4. Homans AC, Rybak ME, Baglini RL, Tiarks C, Steiner ME, Forman EN. Effect of L-asparaginase administration on coagulation and platelet function in children with leukemia. J Clin Oncol 1987; 5: 811–7
5. Pui CH, Jackson CW, Chesney CM, Abilgaard CF. Involvement of von Willebrand factor in thrombosis following asparaginase-prednisone-vincristine therapy for leukemia. Am J Hematol 1987; 25: 291–8
6. Mitchell L, Hoogendoorn H, Giles AR et al. Increased endogenous thrombin generation in children with acute lymphoblastic leukemia: risk of thrombotic complications on l-asparaginase-induced antithrombin III deficiency. Blood 1994; 83: 836–391
7. Nowak-Göttl U, Wolff J, Kuhn N et al. Enhanced thrombin generation, P-von Willebrand factor, P-fibrin, D-dinner and P-plasminogen activator inhibitor 1: predictive for venous thrombosis in asparaginase-treated children. Fibrinolysis 1994: 8(2): 63–65
8. Capizzi R, Holcenberg JS. l-Asparaginase. In Holland J, Frei E, eds. Cancer Medicine. Philadelphia. Lea & Frebiger 1992
9. Ohnuma T, Holland JF, Freemann A et al. Biochemical and pharmacological studies with asparaginse in man. Cancer Res 1979; 30: 2297–2305
10. Wriston JC, Yellin TO. l-Asparaginase: a review. Advanced Enzymol Relat Areas Mol Biol 1973; 39: 185–248
11. Clauss A. Gerinnungsphysiologische Schnellmethode zur Bestimmung des Fibrinogens. Acta haemat (Basel) 1957;237
12. Nowak-Göttl U, Funk M, Mosch G et al. Univariate tolerance regions for fibrinogen, antithrombin III, proteinC, protein S, plasminogen and α2-antiplasmin in children using the new automated coagulation laboratory (ACL) method. Klin Pädiatr 1994; 206: 437–439
13. Heaton DC, Billings JD, Hickton CM. Assessment of d-dimer assays for the diagnosis of deep vein thrombosis. J. Lab Clin Med 1987; 110: 588–91
14. Bergemeyer HU. Methoden der enzymatischen Analyse. l-Asparaginase.3. überarbeitete und erweiterte Auflage, Verlag, Chemie 1974; 464–46512
15. Lenda K, Svenneby G. Rapid high-performance liquid chromatographic determination of amino acids in synaptosomal abstracts. J Chrom 1980; 198: 516–519
16. Sachs L. Angewandte Statistik. Siebte Auflage, Springer Verlag, Berlin, Heidelberg New York. 1992: 380–391
17. Arens A, Rauenbusch E, Iron E, Wagner O, Bauer K, Kaufmann W. Z. Physiol Chem 1970; 351: 197
18. Boos J, Werber G, Ahlke E, Nowak-Göttl U, Verspohl E,Jürgens H. Significant differences in the pharmacokinetics of two L-asparaginse from Escherichia coli. In Büchner T, Hiddemann W, Wörnemann B, Ritter (Eds) Haematology and Blood Transfusion, Springer Verlag Berlin Heidelberg New York London Paris Hong Kong Barcelona Budapest, 1995: in press
19. Mashburn LT, Landin LM. In Grundmann E, Oettgen HF (Eds) Recent results in cancer research. Springer New York 1970; 33: 48

Acute Leukemias VI
Prognostic Factors
and Treatment Strategies
Büchner et al. (eds)

Significant Differences in the Pharmacokinetics of two L-Asparaginase Preparations from *Escherichia coli*

J. Boos[1], G. Werber[1,2], E. Ahlke[1], U. Nowak-Göttl[1], E.J. Verspohl[2], and H. Jürgens[1]

Abstract. Asparaginase (ASE) preparations from two biological sources (*Escherichia coli* and *Erwinia caratovora*) and companies are in clinical use. Current treatment protocols prescribe the dose and schedule but not the preparation to be used. As a rule, *E.coli* preparations are given (Asparaginase medac, Medac-GmbH, Germany; or Crasnitin, Bayer AG, Germany) unless allergic reactions occur.

We initiated a drug-monitoring project to measure asparaginase activity as well as serum amino acid levels in children on the acute lymphoblastic leukemia/non-Hodgkin lymphoma Berlin-Frankfurt-Münster study group 90 (ALL/NHL-BFM 90) treatment protocols. Samples were taken immediately prior to the application and additionally on the occasion of routine diagnostic punctures. In protocol 1, the dose administered was 10 000U/m^2 every 3 days (days 12–33).

Asparaginase activity was significantly higher in children treated with Asparaginase medac (162 samples/38 patients: median 441 U/1) than in children on Crasnitin (49 samples/10 patients: median 79 U/l).

The serum asparagine levels ranged around the detection limit (0.1 μ*M*) in both groups. While glutamine was similar (365/368 μ*M*), glutamic acid was elevated in the Asparaginase medac group (77 vs, 146 μ*M* median). The pharmacokinetic calculation of pooled data resulted in a $T_{1/2}$ of about 24 h for Asparaginase medac and about 15 h for Crasnitin.

There are significant differences between asparaginase preparations even when obtained from *E coli.* The relatively high activity observed with Asparaginase medac is not necessary to reach complete asparagine depletion. In the discussion about side effects of asparaginase, the preparation should, therefore, be specified in every study and the dosages should be defined taking pharmacokinetic differences into account.

Introduction

Asparaginase is an enzyme with notable activity against acute lymphoblastic leukemia (ALL)(for review see [1,2]). Depletion of asparagine in plasma (normal value ≈40–80 μ*M*) and cerebrospinal fluid (normally > 4 μ*M*) deprives leukemic cells of this amino acid which is essential for lymphoblastic blast cells.

Asparaginase preparations from two biological sources (*Escherichia coli* [3] and *Erwinia caratovora* [4] and several companies and with different chemical and immunological characteristics [5] are in clinical use. Current treatment protocols prescribe the dose and schedule but not the preparation to be used. As a rule, in our hospital *E coli* preparations are given (Asparaginase medac, Medac-GmbH, Germany; or Crasnitin, Bayer AG, Germany) unless allergic reactions occur. Eight asparaginase infusions of 10 000 units/m^2 are included in the induction protocol of the (ALL-Berlin-Frankfurt-Münster Study Group 90) trial Fig. 1.

An increasing number of adverse reactions, e.g., hyperglycemia, pancreatitis, bleeding com-

[1]Department of Pediatric Hematology/Oncology, University of Münster, 48149, Münster, Germany
[2]Institute of Pharmaceutical Chemistry, University of Münster, 48149 Münster, Germany

Fig. 1. Induction therapy of the ALL- and NHL-BFM trial. *PRED*, prednisone *VCR*, vincristine; *DNR*, daunorubium *L-ASP*, l-asparaginase, *CP*, cyclophosphamide; *ARA-C*, cytosine arabinoside; *6-TG*, 6-thioguanine; *MTX i.th.*, intrathecal methotrexate; *km*,bone marrow; *Tag*, day

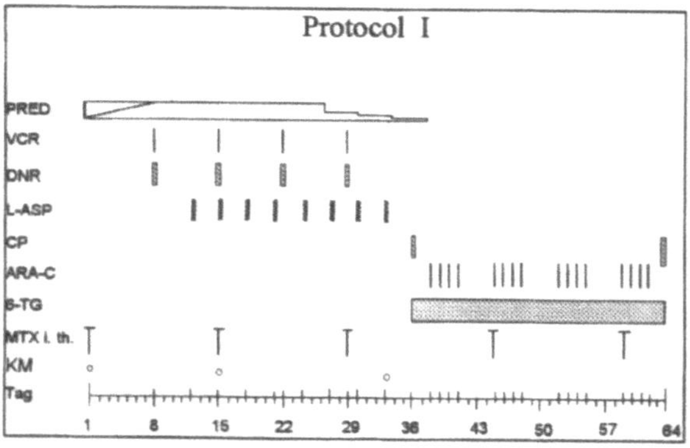

plications or thrombosis [6, 7], evoked renewed discussion about dosage, scheduling, and the overall value of asparaginase.

We therefore initiated a drug monitoring project to measure asparaginase activity as well as asparagine and other serum amino acid levels in children on the ALL/non-Hodgkin lymphoma-BFM 90 treatment protocols.

The main questions were: do the children reach asparagine depletion, is the dose of 10 000 U/m^2 adequate, and are different preparations equivalent?

Methods

Samples were taken from children on protocol 1 of the ALL/NHL-BFM trials before each application (see Fig. 1, day 3 after the previous application) and additionally on the occasion of routine diagnostic punctures. Informed consent was obtained from parents and patients as well.

The samples were put on ice and divided into two parts. One part was immediately centrifuged after withdrawal and deproteinized by the addition of sulfosalicylic acid 10%, then analyzed for amino acids. The other part was immediately frozen and analyzed for asparaginase activity (for details see [8]).

The sensitivity limit was 20 U/l for the asparaginase activity and 0.1 μM for asparagine.

Results

Asparaginase activity was significantly higher in children treated with Asparaginase medac. A total of 162 samples from 38 patients, taken 3 days after infusion of 10 000 Units/m^2 Asparaginase medac, showed a median of 441 U/l compared to a median of 79 U/l for those on Crasnitin (49 samples/10 patients). This difference was obvious on all days of protocol1 when trough levels were measured (Fig. 2).

The corresponding serum asparagine levels ranged around the detection limit (0.1 µM) in both groups. While glutamine was similar (366/361 µM), glutamic acid was elevated only in the Asparaginase medac group (145 vs 80 µM, median of 175/51 samples).

In addition to the trough levels, additional samples were collected and tested at varying intervals from the application in many children. The pharmacokinetic calculation of these pooled monitoring data yielded a $T_{1/2}$ of about 24 h for Asparaginase medac and about 15 h for Carsnitin (Fig. 3).

Discussion

Children with ALL have a very good chance, currently about 80%, for long-term survival. The incidence of thrombotic events varies between 0% and 15% but, irrespective of the incidence, such hazardous events are not acceptable in the treatment of children with such good prognosis. The current discussion focussed on variables such as additional treatment with vincristine or corticoids and the time schedule of asparaginase applications. In many publications the source of asparaginase (*E.coli* or *E.caratovora*) is given, but the trade names or preparations are not specified. It is a well-known phenomenon that *E.caratovora* asparaginase has a shorter half-life

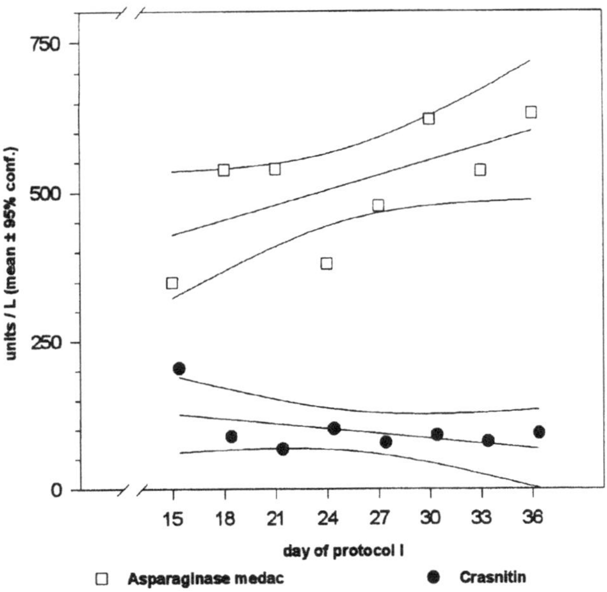

Fig. 2. Asparaginase activity prior to each application in protocol (4–27 observations/point: mean and 95% confidence interval). *Squares*, Asparaginase medac; *circles*, Crasnitin

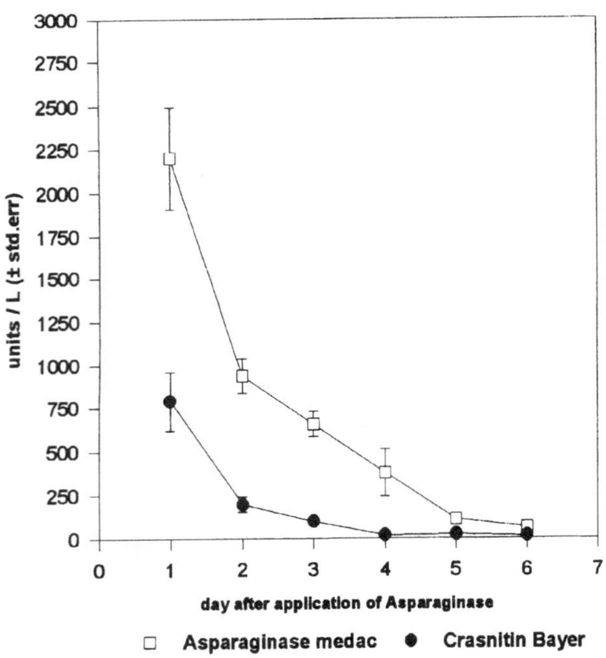

Fig. 3. Mean and standard deviation of all plasma activities taken 1-6 days after asparaginase application. *Squares*, Asparaginase medac; *circles*, Crasnitin

than *E.coli* asparaginase [9] and that this results in a different intensity of asparagine depletion [10,11].

In a current investigation, the treatment strategy of protocol 1 successfully depleted asparagine in children on *E.coli* asparaginase independent of the preparation used.

Focussing on the plasmatic activity of the enzyme, however, significant differences were observed even between different preparations from *E.coli*. Similar dosages of 10 000 U/m^2 Asparaginase medac resulted in significantly higher plasma levels and biological activity compared to Crasnitin. Such high plasmatic activity was not necessary to reach complete asparagine depletion, while it resulted in an increased turnover of glutamine and significantly higher levels of glutamic acid, an amino acid with potentially toxic effects, for example on endothelial cells.

The pharmacokinetic calculation, based on all monitoring data with reference to the time after application, showed that differences in plasma activity are a consequence of differences in pharmacokinetic parameters, e.g., a longer half-life of *E.coli* Asparaginase medac compared to Crasnitin (see Fig.3).

In the discussion regarding the antileukemic effects as well as side effects of asparaginase, the respective preparation, should therefore, be specified in every publication. Clinical trials should define dose schedules specifying the preparation and taking the pharmacokinetic differences into account. The BFM treatment schedules were developed decade ago when only the *E.coli* asparaginase from Bayer (Crasnitin) was available in Germany. Riccardi et al. [12] in a pharmacokinetic study, defined plasma levels of 100 U/l as optimal to deplete asparagine in plasma and cerebrospinal fluid.

Based on the present monitoring data, we propose that in children on Asparaginase medac the activity observed is higher than necessary and that complete asparagine depletion will be obtained with significantly lower dosages than with Crasnitin.

Acknowledgments. The research project reported in this paper was supported by funds from the Federal Department of Research and Technology, no. 01 EC 9401. The responsibility for the contents of this publication rests with the authors.

References

1. Wriston JC, Jr., Yellin TO. (1973) l-Asparaginase: a review. Adv Enzymol Relat Areas Mol Biol 39: 185–248.
2. Chabner BA, Collins JM. (1990) Enzyme therapy: l-asparaginase. In Cancer Chemotherapy: Principles and Practice. J.B. Lippincott Company, Philadelphia 397–407
3. Mashburn LT, Wriston JC, Jr.(1964) Tumor inhibition effect of l-asparaginase from Escherichia coli. Arch Biochem Biophys 105: 450–452.
4. Ohnuma T, Holland JF, Meyer P.(1972) Erwinia carotovora asparaginase in patients with prior anaphylaxis to asparaginase from E.coli. Cancer 30: 376–381.
5. Koerholz D, Brueck M, Nuernberger W, Juergens H, Goebel U, Wahn V.(1989) Chemical and immunological characteristics of four different l-asparaginase preparations. Eur J Haematol 42: 417–424
6. Mitchell L, Hoogendoorn H, Giles AR, Vegh P, Andrew M.(1994) Increased endogenous thrombin generation in children with acute lymphoblastic leukemia: risk of thrombotic complications in l-asparaginase-induced antithrombin III deficiency. Blood 83: 386–391
7. Sutor AH, Niemeyer C, Sauter S, Witt I, Kaufmehl K, Rombach A, Brandis M, Riehm H.(1992) Gerinnungsveränderungen bei Behandlung mit den Protokollen ALL-BFM-90 und NHL-BFM-90. Klin Pädiatr 204: 264–273
8. Werber G, Ahlke E, Nowak-Göttl U, Jürgens H, Verspohl E, Boos J.(1995) Asparaginase activities in vitro and highly sensitive to different buffer conditions. Haematology and Blood Transfusion 38, in press
9. Asselin BL, Whitin JC, Coppola DJ, Rupp IP, Sallan SE, Cohen HJ.(1993) Comparative pharmacokinetic studies of three asparaginase preparations. J Clin Oncol 11: 1780–1786.
10. Boos J, Werber G, Verspohl E, Nowak-Göttl U, Jürgens H.(1994) Asparagine levels in children on E.coli and Erwinia asparaginase therapy. Haematology and Blood Transfusion, 37: in press
11. Werber G, Boos J, Ahlke E, Nowak-Göttl U, Verspohl E, Jürgens H.(1995) Pharmacokinetic/pharmacodynamic monitoring of l-asparaginase in children. Haematology and Blood Transfusion 38: in press
12. Riccardi R, Holcenberg JS, Glaubiger DL, Wood JH, Poplack DG. (1981) l-Asparaginase pharmacokinetics and asparagine levels in cerebrospinal fluid of rhesus monkeys and humans. Cancer Res 41: 4554–8

Acute Leukemias VI
Prognostic Factors
and Treatment Strategies
Büchner et al. (eds)

Pharmacokinetic/Pharmacodynamic Monitoring of L-Asparaginase in Children

G. Werber[1,2], J. Boos[1], E. Ahlke[1], U. Nowak-Göttl[1], E.J. Verspohl[2], and H. Jürgens[1]

Abstract. Asparaginase preparations from different biological sources and companies are in clinical use. In the event of adverse reactions substitutions are common. The half-life of *Erwinia* asparaginase is significantly shorter compared to asparaginase obtained from *Escherichia coli.* Questions remain with respect to whether the pharmacodynamic effects are comparable. Therefore, we performed an asparaginase monitoring focussing on the comparability of asparaginase activity as well as asparagine serum levels.

Therapy according to protocol acute lymphoblastic leukemia non-Hodgkin lymphoma Berlin-Frankfurt-Münster Study Group 90 (ALL/NHL-BFM 90) was initiated with *E.coli* asparaginase (Asparaginase medac, Crasnitin Bayer, Germany), and in the case of allergic reactions continued with *Erwinia* asparaginase (Erwinase, Speywood, USA). All children underwent monitoring for asparaginase activity and serum asparagine levels; samples were taken immediately prior to the applications. The dose administered was 10000 U/m^2 every 3 or 4 days according to protocol II. Fifty protocol II patients, i.e., 26 children on Asparaginase medac, eight on Crasnitin, and 16 on Erwinase were compared. The asparaginase activity on day 3 (trough level) was higher in children receiving *E.coli* asparaginase (Asparaginase medac 528 U/l; Crasnitin 49 U/l median) than in those on Erwinase (< sensitivity limit).

The corresponding asparagine levels remained above the sensitivity limit of the analaysis (100 n*M*) in only six of 26 children on Asparaginase medac (all < 0.5 m*M*). On Crasnitin two of eight children were completely depleted, four were nearly depleted (> 0.1, < 0.5 m*M*), and two had normal asparagine levels. In the group switched to Erwinase only two of 16 children showed complete asparagine depletion and in two others asparagine levels were near the sensitivity limit of analysis. In 12 children, the levels covered the whole range up to normal concentrations.

Introduction

L-Asparaginase (L-Asparagine amidohydrolase, EC 3.5.1.1) is an enzyme that catalyzes the hydrolysis of the generally not essential amino acid L-asparagine to L-asparagine to L-aspartic acid and ammonia. Its antileukemic potency is due to the lack of L-asparagine synthetase in some tumor cells, most notably human lymphoblasts [1]. The depletion of L-asparagine within the cells inhibits protein synthesis causing cell death. Today, in clinical trials enzymes derived from *E.coli* and *Erwinia chrysanthemi* (former *carotovora*) are administered. Since *Erwinia* asparaginase does not share antigenic cross-reactivity with the *E.coli* asparaginase [2] substitutions in case of hypersensitive reactions are common [3–5]. Although *E.coli* and *Erwinia* preparations differ in their chemical and pharmacokinetic properties, they are generally administered in the same dose and schedule [6].

We studied patients with childhood acute lymphoblastic leukemia (ALL) on ALL-Berlin-

[1]Department of Pediatric Hematology/Oncology, University of Münster, 48129 Münster, Germany
[2]Institute of Pharmaceutical Chemistry, University of Münster, 48129 Münster, Germany

Frankfurt-Münster Study Group [BFM] 90 protocol II that uses i.v. L-asparaginase during consolidation therapy. Additional chemotherapy consisted of dexamethasone (daily), vincristine and adriamycin (once weekly). As part of the monitoring we measured L-asparaginase activity and L-asparagine in serum samples. This report describes the pharmacokinetic and pharmacodynamic effects of different enzyme preparations.

Patient Sample Collection

According to the protocol ALL/NHL-BFM 90, therapy was initiated with *E.coli* asparaginase (Asparaginase medac, Crasnitin, Bayer, Germany) and in the case of allergic reactions continued with *Erwinia* asparaginase (Erwinase, USA Speywood). The dose administered was 10,000 U/m^2 i.v. on days 8, 11, 15, and 18 according to protocol II. Samples were taken immediately prior to each application. A sample of 3 ml whole blood was drawn and allowed to clot on ice. Serum was separated, one part was frozen at −8°C for enzyme activity analysis, the other part was deproteinized immediately (400 µl serum + 100 µl sulfo-salicylic acid, SSA, 10%) and frozen at −8°C for amino acid analysis. Samples of 50 patients, i.e., 26 children on Asparaginase medac, eight on Crasnitin, and 16 on Erwinase, were collected.

Methods

L-Asparaginase Activity Assay. We determined the enzyme activity by photometric detection of the ammonia release after reaction with Nessler's reagent. Units of enzyme activity were defined as micromoles of ammonia released per minute at 37°C. A mixture of 100 µl serum and 400 µl 0.044 m*M* L-asparagine buffer solution was incubated at 37 °C for exactly 45 min. After addition of 250 µl trichloroacetic acid 24.5% (w/w) and centrifugation, 250 µl supernatant were added to Nessler's solution (2000 µl water plus 250 µl Nessler's reagent). The optical density at 450 nm was compared with an ammonium sulfate Nessler standard curve. The sensitivity limit of analysis was 20 U/l.

Amino Acid Analysis. Amino acid levels in serum were measured using an RP-HPLC technique following precolumn derivatization with *o*-phthaldialdehyde (OPA) and fluorescence detection according to Lenda and Svenneby [7]. The sensitivity limit of the anlaysis was 0.1 µ*M*.

Definition. The assessment of asparagine depletion under therapy with asparaginase is listed in Table 1.

Results

Our initial study focussed on the pharmacodynamics of L-Asparaginase by comparing the enzyme activity and asparagine depletion measured in patient sera following *E.coli* asparaginase (Asparaginase medac $n = 16$ and Crasnitin $n = 8$) or *Erwinia* asparaginase (Erwinase $n = 26$) administration. Fig. 1 shows the activities of the three groups prior to each application. The corresponding asparagine levels remained above the sensitivity limit (100 n*M*) in only six of 26 children on Asparaginase medac (all < 0.5 m*M*). Two of eight children on Crasnitin were completely depleted, four were nearly depleted (> 0.1 < 0.5 m*M*), and two had normal asparagine levels. In the group switched to Erwinase only two of 16 children showed complete

Table 1. Serum asparagine levels divided in to categories. Values are percentiles of all samples in one group (Asparaginase medac n=93; Crasnitin: $n = 24$; Erwinase: n = 51).

Category	Asparagine	Asparaginase Medac			Crasnitin			Erwinase		
	[µ*M*)	[%]	(s/p)[a]	p[b]	(%)	(s/p)[a]	p[b]	[%]	(s/p)[a]	p[b]
Complete depletion	⩽0.1	91.4	(85/26)	20	58.3	(14/6)	2	21.6	(11/7)	2
Nearly complete depletion	⩽0.5	8.6	(8/6)	6	16.7	(4/4)	4	27.5	(14/11)	2
Moderate reduction	⩽1.0							17.6	(9/7)	5
Slight to normal levels	⩽1.0				25.0	(6/2)	2	33.3	(17/7)	2
Variable asparagine levels										5

[a]Number = samples per patients, [b]Number of patients.

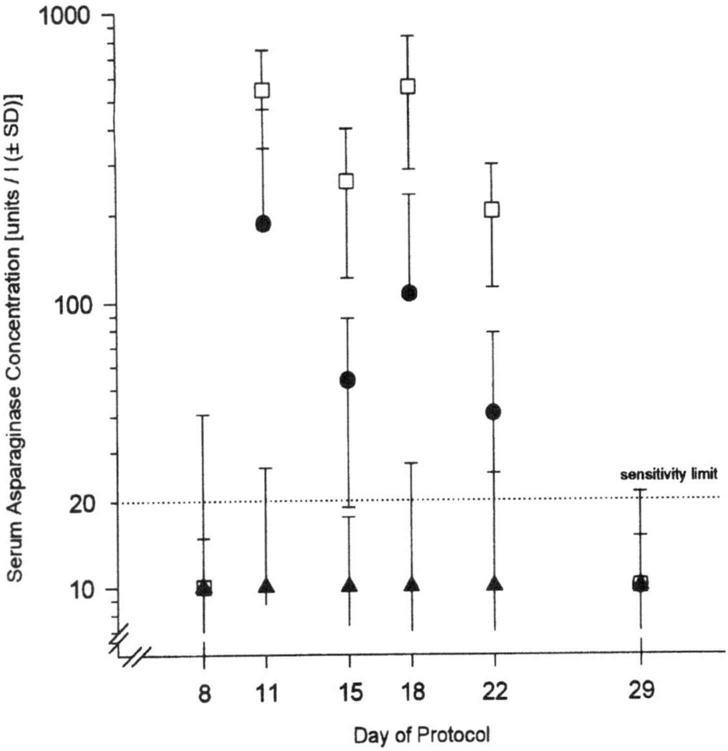

Fig. 1. Asparaginase activity in sera of patients treated with *E. coli* asparaginase (*squares*, Asparaginase medac®: n = 26 patients, *circles*, Crasnitin®: n = 8 patients), and *Erwinia* asparaginase (*triangles* Erwinase®: n = 16 patients) following the schedule of protocol II ALL-BFM 90. Values are mean ± SD

asparagine depletion and in two others asparagine levels were close to the sensitivity limit. In five children the asparagine levels were moderately reduced, and two children showed slightly reduced or normal asparagine levels. The other five children had variable asparagine levels (Fig. 2 and Table 1).

Table 1 lists the results of asparagine level distribution of all collected samples (last day in protocol is day 22). Most samples (91.4%) of patients treated with Asparaginase medac were completely and only 8.6% nearly completely depleted. In the Crasnitin group, 25% of all samples (two patients) showed normal asparagine levels, whereas 58.3% were completely and 14.7% nearly completely depleted. Patients treated with Erwinase in the case of allergic reaction to one of the *E.coli* asparaginases showed the whole range of asparagine levels. Of all samples 26% were completely depleted, 27.5% showed nearly complete depletion, 17.6% showed moderate reduction, and in 33.3% slight to normal levels of asparagine were measured.

The results of comparing the trough enzyme activity (3 days after asparaginase administration) of the three asparaginase preparations are shown in Fig. 3. Children receiving Asparaginase medac showed the highest activity (528 U/l median). Values were ten fold higher than those on Crasnitin (49 U/l median). Notably, serum activities of patients treated with Erwinase were not measurable (< sensitivity limit) (Fig. 3).

Discussion

Multiple clinical trials have demonstrated the importance of asparaginase as part of ALL chemotherapy [8–11]. *E.coli* as well as *Erwinia* preparations are commonly used at the same schedule and dose [6]. We observed marked differences in the depletion of L-asparagine between children treated with two *E.coli*

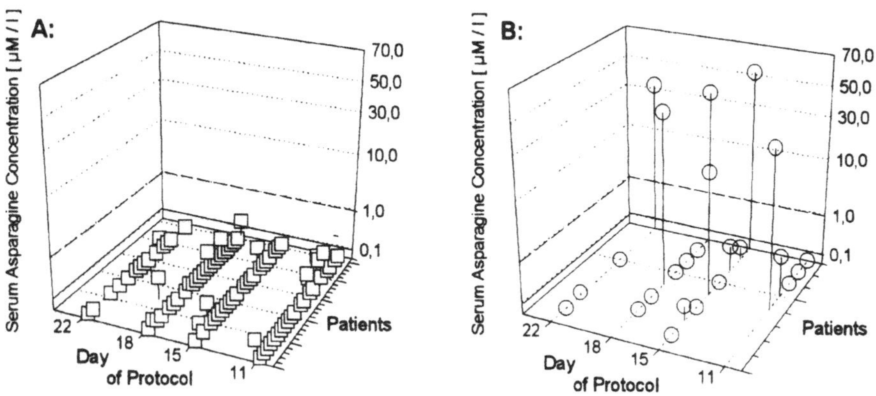

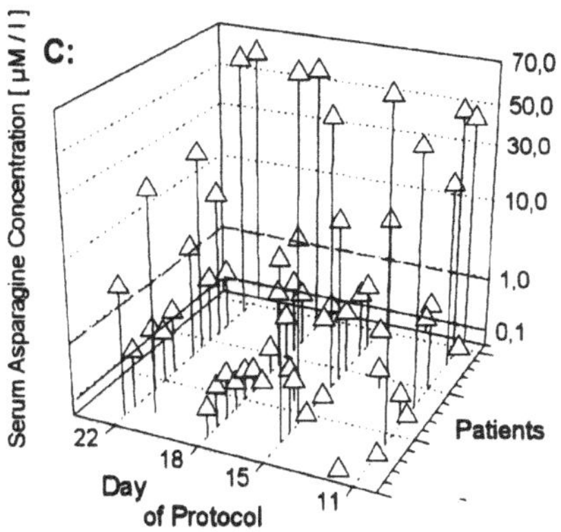

Fig. 2A–C. Serum asparagine concentrations in patients treated with **A** Asparaginase medac ($n=26$ patients), **B** Crasnitin ($n=$ eight patients, showed normal serum levels); or **C** Erwinase ($n=16$ patients, two were completely depleted, two showed normal serum concentrations). For every group all patients are listed. The serum asparagine levels are shown according to the day of protocol

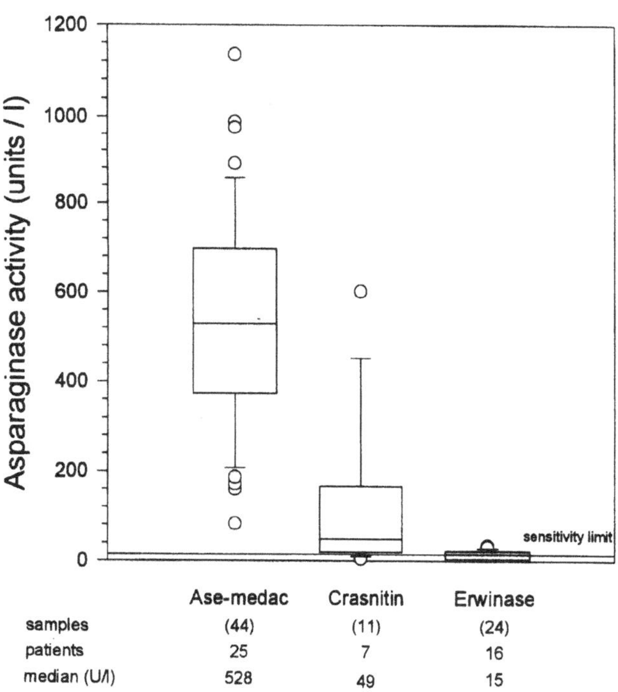

Fig. 3. Serum asparaginase activity 3 days after asparaginase application in patients treated following the schedule of protocol II ALL-BM 90

asparaginase and *Erwinia* asparaginase preparations. While the depletion was complete with Asparaginase medac and complete or nearly complete with Crasnitin (in two children the levels remained normal), there was a wide range of asparagine levels in children on *Erwinia* asparaginase.

It is known that *E.coli* asparaginase and *Erwinia* asparaginase differ in their chemical properties and pharmacokinetics [12]. Some investigators have determined the half-life of *E.coli* asparaginase in patients after i.v. (0.33–1.2 days) and i.m. (1.4–1.8 days) administration [13]. According to Asselin et al. [6] the biological half-life of *Erwinia* asparaginase is significantly shorter than that of *E.coli* asparaginase both for i.v. and i.m. administration. The insufficient and variable asparagine depletion in the *Erwinia* group could be explained by the short half-life of *Erwinia* asparaginase. Substitution of a drug with a half-life of 1.3 days by one with a half-life of 0.6 days requires changes in dose or frequency of application.

All children treated with *Erwinia* asparaginase had shown prior allergic reaction to *E.coli* asparaginase (11 to Asparaginase medac and five to Crasnitin, respectively) in the preceding induction therapy of the protocol. Another explanation for this observation is that cross-reacting antibodies might inactivate *Erwinia* asparaginase in children allergic to *E.coli* asparaginase. Strikingly, none of them showed clinical signs of adverse reactions during the monitored consolidation therapy.

During consolidation therapy like in protocol I [14] we again noticed a great difference of enzyme activity between the two *E.coli* asparaginases. Furthermore, two children on Crasnitin showed normal asparagine levels. Enzyme activities were undetectable after 3 days, whereas the other six patients on Crasnitin showed median levels of 109 U/l 3 days and 62 U/l 4 days after Crasnitin application. This could be due to neutralizing antibodies shorten the half-life of Crasnitin. Again, neither of the children showed any clinical signs of allergic reactions. In conclusion, substitution of different asparaginase preparations should take pharmacokinetic differences into account, and pharmacodynamic monitoring is warranted.

Acknowledgments. The research project reported in this paper was supported by funds from the Federal Department of Research and Technology (BMFT) and additional from the BMFT, no.01 EC 9401. The resposibility for the contents of this publications rests with the authors.

References

1. Broome JD. (1981) L-Asparaginase: discovery and development as a tumor-inhibitory agent. Cancer Treat. Rep.65: Suppl 4, 111–114.
2. Wade HE, Elsworth R, Herbert D, Keppie J, Sargeant K. (1968) A new L-asparaginase with antitumour activity? Lancet.2: 776–777.
3. Dellinger CT and Miale TD. (1976) Comparison of anaphylactic reactions to asparaginase derived from Escherichia coli and from *Erwinia* cultures. Cancer. 38: 1843–1846.
4. Ohnuma T, Holland JF, and Meyar P. (1972) *Erwinia* carotovora asparaginase in patients with prior anaphylaxis to asparaginase from E.coli. Cancer. 30: 376–381.
5. Evans WE, Tsiatis A, Rivera G, Murphy SB, Dahl GV, Denison M, Crom WR, Barker-LF, and Mauer AM. (1982) Anaphylactoid reactions to Escherichia coli and *Erwinia* asparaginase in children with leukemia and lymphoma. Cancer. 49: 1378–1383.
6. Asselin BL, Whitin JC, Coppola DJ, Rupp IP, Sallan SE, and Cohen HJ. (1993) Comparative pharmacokinetic studies of three asparaginase preparations J. Clin. Oncol. 11: 1780–1786.
7. Lenda K and Svenneby G. (1980) Rapid high-performance liquid chromatographic determination of amino acids in synaptosomal extracts. J.Chromatogr. 198: 516–519.
8. Tallal L, Tan C, Oettgen H, Wollner N, McCarthy M, Helson L, Burchenal J, Karnofsky- D, and Murphy ML. (1970) E.Coli l-asparaginase in the treatment of leukemia and solid tumors in 131 children. Cancer. 25: 306–320.
9. Sallan SE, Hitchcock Bryan S, Gelber R, Cassady JR, Frei E3, and Nathan DG. (1983) Influence of intensive asparaginase in the treatment of childhood non-T-cell acute lymphoblastic leukemia. Cancer Res. 43: 5601–5607.
10. Clavell LA, Gelber RD, Cohen HJ, Hitchcock Bryan S, Cassady JR, Tarbell NJ, Blattner SR, Tantravahi R, Leavitt P, and Sallan SE. (1986) Four-agent induction and intensive asparaginase therapy for treatment of childhood acute lymphoblastic leukeima. N. Engl. J.Med. 315: 657–663.
11. Ertel IJ, Nesbit ME, Hammond D, Weiner J, and Sather H. (1979) Effective dose of L-asparaginase for inducion of remission in previously treated children with acute lymphocytic leukemia: a report from children's Cancer Study Group. Cancer Res.39: 3893–3896.
12. Wriston JC, Jr. and Yellin TO. (1973) L-Asparaginase; a review. Adv. Enzymol. Relat. Areas. Mol. Biol. 39: 185–248.
13. Ho DH, Yap HY, Brown N, Benjamin RS, Friereich EJ, Blumenschein GR, and Bodey GP. (1981)

Clinical pharmacology of intramuscularly administered L-asparaginase. Clin. Pharmacol. 21: 72–78. J.
14. Boos J, Werber G, Ahlke E, Nowak-Göttl U, Verspohl EJ, Jürgens H. (1995) Significant differences in the pharmacokinetics of two L-Asparaginase preparations from Escherichia coli. Haematology and Blood Transfusion [In Press].

Acute Leukemias VI
Prognostic Factors
and Treatment Strategies
Büchner et al. (eds)

Asparaginase Activities In Vitro Are Highly Sensitive to Different Buffer Conditions

G. Werber[1,2], E. Ahlke[1], U. Nowak-Göttl[1], H. Jürgens[1], E.J. Verspohl[2], and J. Boos[1]

Abstract. Different asparaginase (Ase) preparations from various biological sources (*Escherichia coli* and *Erwinia carotovora*) are currently in use as potent antileukemic enzymes in the treatment of acute lymphoblastic leukemia (ALL) in children. According to the acute lymphoblastic leukemia/non-Hodgkin lymphoma Berlin-Frankfurt-Münster Study Group 90 (ALL/NHL-BFM-90) protocol, therapy is initiated with *E.coli*-Ase (Asparaginase Medac, Medac GmbH Germany, Crasnitin Bayer AG, Germany) and in the case of allergic reaction substituted by *Erwinia*-Ase (Erwinase, Porton, USA). There are, however, important questions concerning the comparability of these different preparations.

Therefore, we compared the enzyme activity of *E.coli*-Ase and *Erwinia*-Ase in vitro at different pH conditions (pH 7.0–8.5, each experiment five times) and various (eight) buffer conditions.

Physiological phosphate/buffered saline (PBS) buffer resulted in only 50%–65% and 80% –95% of the activity specified by the manufactures of *Erwinia*-Ase and *E.coli*-Ase, respectively.

The expected activity was detectable at pH 7.3 and pH 8.5. In saline solutions (0.9%) the activity decreased to 20% and 60%, respectively. Buffers containing boric acid (pH 8.5) or Tris (pH 7.3) and additional bovine serum albumin (BSA) resulted in a more reliable determination of enzyme activity with reference to the specifications on the vials (100% ± 10%). In all experiments, *E.coli*-Ase showed higher activity than *Erwinia*-Ase. In conclusion, the acitvity of asparaginase preparations depends on the conditions of the solution and *Erwinia*-Ase is more sensitive than *E.coli*-Ase.

Introduction

L-Asparaginase (Ase) (L-asparagine amidohydrolase, EC 3.5.1.1) is part of most chemotherapy protocols for childhood and adult acute lymphoblastic leukemia (ALL). The enzyme catalyzes the hydrolysis of the generally not essential amino acid L-asparagine to L-aspartic acid and ammonia. Its antileukemic potency is due to the lack of L-asparagine synthetase in some tumor cells [1, 2]. The discovery that Ase derived from *Escherichia coli* had antitumor activity allowed the enzyme to be produced in adequate amounts for clinical use [3]. Today, enzymes derived from *E.coli* and *Erwinia chrysanthemi* (former carotovora) are administered in clinical trials. According to the ALL/non-Hodgkin lymphoma Berlin Frankfurt-Münster Study Group 90 (ALL-NHL-BFM-90) protocol, therapy is initiated with *E.coli*-Ase (Asparaginase Medac Medac GmbH, Germany and Crasnitin Bayer AG, Germany) and in the case of allergic reaction substituted by *Erwinia*-Ase (Erwinase, Speywood, former Porton, USA). Although *E.coli* and *Erwinia* preparations differ in their chemical and pharmacokinetic properties, they are generally administered at the same dose and schedule [4]. There are important questions whether different preparations are comparable or even identical.

[1]Department of Pediatric Hematology/Oncology, University of Münster, 48149 Münster, Germany
[2]Institute of Pharmaceutical Chemistry, University of Münster, 48149 Münster, Germany

We studied the enzyme activity of two *E.coli*-Ase preparations and *Erwinia*-Ase in vitro under standard and modified buffer conditions and the different behaviour of each Ase to various pH values in a physiological buffer Phosphate-buffered saline, (PBS).

Methods

The enzyme activity was determined by photometric detection of the ammonia release after reaction with Nessler's reagent. Units of enzyme activity were defined as micromoles of ammonia released per minute at 37°C. A mixture of 100 µl sample and 400 µl 0.044 m*M* L-asparagine buffer solution was incubated at 37°C for exactly 45 min. After addition of 250 µl trichloroacetic acid 24.5 % w/w) and centrifugation, 250 µl supernatant were added to Nessler's solution (2000 µl water plus 250 µl Nesslers reagent). The optical density at 450 nm was compared with an ammonium sulfate Nessler standard curve. The sensitivity limit of detection was 20 U/l (Fig. 1).

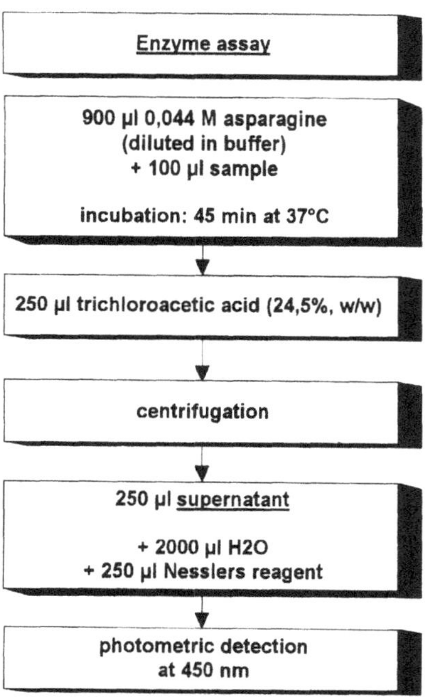

Fig. 1. Method to determine asparaginase activity

Results

First the enzyme activity of each L-Ase was studied in a physiological buffer (0.01 *M* phosphate buffer, pH 7.2), used to quantitatively determine the enzyme activity. Each manufcturer's specification claimed 10 000 U/vial. The *E.coli*-Ase activity was determined at a mean of 9395 (±1194) U/vial (±SD) for Asparaginase Medac and of 8897 (±2031) U/vial (±SD) for Crasnitin, and for *Erwinia*-Ase only of 5581 (±963) U/vial (±SD) (Fig. 2).

We measure the activity of all three Ases at different pH conditions in the buffer. The pH range tested was 7.0–8.5. The pH optimum of *E.coli*-Ases under these buffer conditions was in the physiological range pH 7.2 (Asparaginase Medac) and pH 7.4 (Crasnitin). Asparaginase Medac showed an additional activity optimum at pH 8.0. The highest activity of Erwinase was measured at pH 8.2 (Fig. 3).

The enzyme activity of *E.coli*-Ase (Asparaginase Medac) and *Erwinia*-Ase (Erwinase) was determined under different buffer conditions (Fig. 4.5). Table 1 lists the buffer used. All manufacutres determine the enzyme activity of their Ase at different buffer compositions. the expected activity was measured at pH 7.3 and 8.5. Buffers containing boric acid (pH 8.5) or Tris (pH 7.3) and additional bovine seium albumin (BSA) resulted in a more reliable determination of enzyme activity with reference to the specifications on the vial (100%±10%). In all experiments *E.coli*-Ase showed higher results than *Erwinia*-Ase. In saline solution (0.9%) the activity decreased to 60% and 20%, respectively.

Comparing the activity in NaCl (0.9%), NaCl (0.9%)+BSA, human albumin, and Tris (pH 7.3)+BSA, only 20%–35% were measured in pure NaCl. All showed higher activity after addition of BSA to NaCl. Activity of *E.coli*-Ases specified was measured in human albumin while the activity of *Erwinia*-Ase reached only about 60%. In Tris (pH 7.3) + BSA all Ases showed expected values.

Discussion

The aim of this study was the analysis of different behavior under various pH and buffer conditions of three Ase preparations, obtained from various biological sources, which differ in their

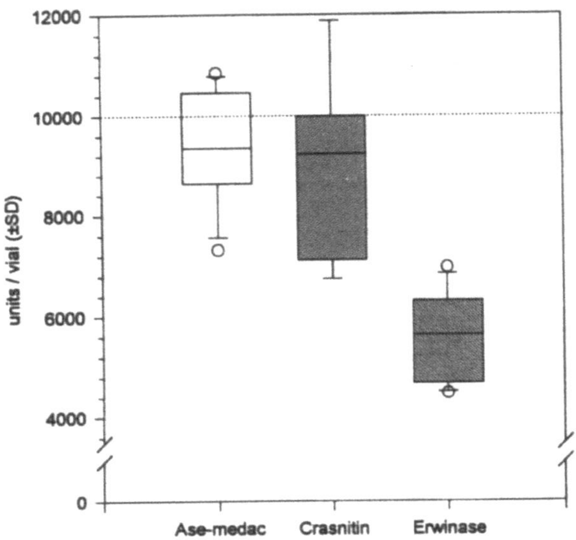

Fig. 2. Asparaginase activity of two *E. coli*-Ases (Asparaginase Medac and Crasnitin) and *Erwinia*-Ase (Erwinase) measured under physiological buffer conditions in 0.1 *M* phosphate buffer. The extends of the *box* indicate the 25th and 75th percentiles of the measured activity, the *line* inside marks the value of the 50th percentile. *Capped bars* indicate the 10th and 90th percentiles, and *symbols* mark all data outside the 10th and 90th percentile

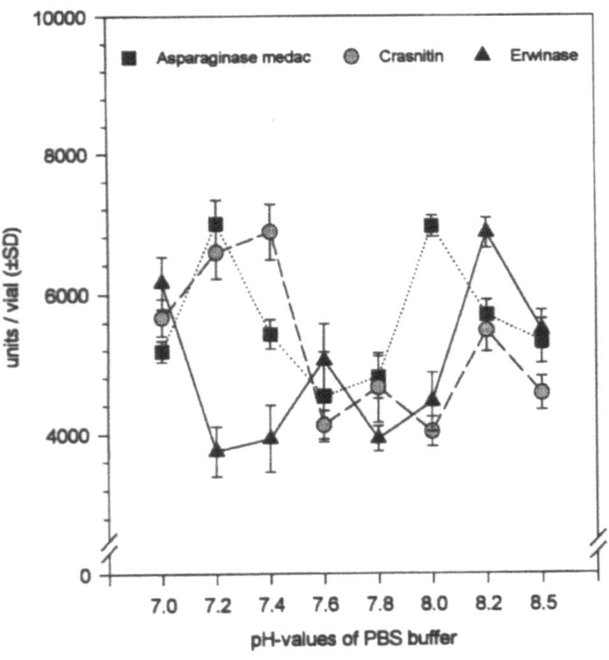

Fig. 3. Asparaginase activity of Asparaginase Medac (*Squares*) Crasnitin (*Circles*), and Erwinase (*Triangles*) measured in PBS buffer in the pH range of 7.0–8.5. Values are mean of all data ± SD, $n = 5$ of each Ase and each pH

chemical properties [5]. The activity depends on pH and buffer conditions. *Erwinia*-Ase is more sensitive to buffer conditions than *E.coli*-Ase. The addition of human and animal sera to *E.coli*-Ase has been shown to enhance the enzymatic activity in vitro [6] which is suggested to be due to a non-specific stabilization of the enzyme molecule. We detected the expected activity at pH 7.3 (Tris) and pH 8.5 (boric acid) and additional BSA. This resulted in a more reli-

Fig. 4. Enzyme activity of Asparaginase Medac (*Squares*) and Erwinase (*Triangles*) in various buffer conditions ($n = 5$). Values are mean ± SD. Buffer compositions are explained in Table 1

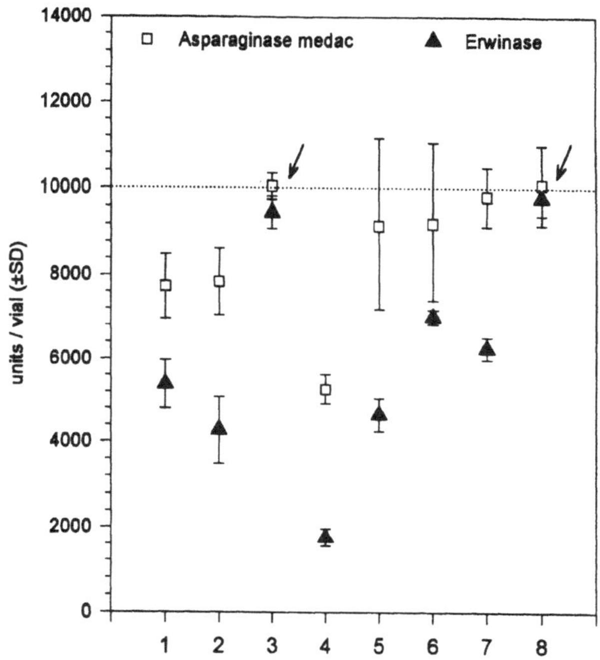

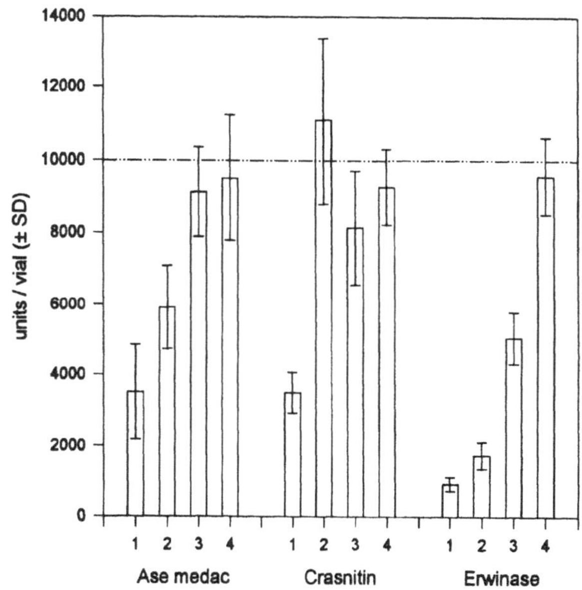

Fig. 5. Enzyme activity measured under the following buffer conditions: *1.* NaCl (0.9%), *2.* NaCl (0.9%) + BSA, *3.* human albumin, and *4* Tris (pH 7.3) + BSA. Asparaginase *Medac*-($n = 50$); Crasnitin-($n = 50$); Erwinase-($n = 50$). *Columns* are mean ± SD

able determination of enzyme activity, much closer to the specifications on the vials (100% ± 10%).

The enzyme activity of different Ases is to yield comparable results, if measured under the same conditions in vitro. For good comparability, we close the Tris + BSA buffer to test the activity in sera of patients treated with one of the different Ases.

Acknowledgments. The research project reported in this paper was supported by funds from the

Table 1. Buffer conditions used to compare the sensitivity of the different Ases to various conditions

Buffer	Molarity	pHvalue	Content per liter
Bayer	0.066 *M*	7.2	5.87Na_2HPO4, 4.49 g KH_2PO_4, 0.01%Brij 35
PBS	0.01 *M*	7.2	6.78 g NaCl, 1.42 g Na_2HPO_4, 0.41 g KH2PO4
MSD	0.015 *M*	7.3	1,82 g Tris, 150 mg BSA
Saline	0.15 *M*	7.4	NaCl 0.9%
Saline+BSA	0.15 *M*	7.4	NaCl 0.9%, 150 mg BSA
Kyowa	0.1 *M*	8.0	8.90 g Na2HPO4, 6.81 g KH2PO4
Porton I	0.2 *M*	8.5	12.8 g boric acid, 2.0 g NaOH
Porton II	0.2 *M*	8.5	12.8 g boric acid, 2.0 g NaOH, 150 mg BSA

Federal Department of Research and Technology (BMFT) and Medac GmbH, Hamburg. The responsibility for the contents of this publications rests with the authors.

References

1. Broome JD. Evidence that the L-asparaginase of guinea pig serum is responsible for its antilymphoma effects. I. Properties of the L-aspararaginase of guinea pig serum in relation to those of the antilymphoma substance. J Exp Med 1963; 108: 99–120.
2. Broomme JD. Evidence that the L-asparaginase of guinea pig serum is responsible for its antilymphoma effects. II. Lymphoma 6C3HED cells cultured in a medium devoid of L-asparagine lose their susceptibility to the effects of guinea pig serum in vivo. J Exp Med 1963; 108: 121–148.
3. Mashburn LT, Wriston JC, Jr. Tumor inhibition effect of L-asparaginase from Escherichia coli. Arch Biochem Biophys 1964; 105: 450–452.
4. Asselin BL, Whitin JC, Coppola DJ, Rupp IP, Sallan SE, Cohen HJ. Comparative pharmacokinetic studies of three asparaginase preparation. J Clin Oncol 1993; 11: 1780–1786.
5. Wriston JC, Jr., Yellin TO. L-Asparaginase: a review. Adv Enzymol Relat Areas Mol Biol 1973; 39: 185–248.
6. Lee MB, Bolger CD, Bridges JM. Factors influencing the "in vitro" enhancement of L-asparginase activity. Biochim Biophys Acta 1971; 242: 226–229.

Acute Leukemias VI
Prognostic Factors
and Treatment Strategies
Büchner et al. (eds)

Influence of L-Asparaginase *Escherichia Coli* and *Erwinia* on Antithrombin III and Coagulation Factors During Induction Therapy of Acute Lymphoblastic Leukemia in Children

A. Krauze[1], M. Jeleńska[2], M. Palester-Chlebowczyk[2], and M. Ochocka[1]

Abstract. Activity of antithrombin (AT) III and factors, I,II,V,VII,X were investigated in a prospective study in two groups of children. The first group of 30 children received L-asparaginase *Escherichia coli*, the second group of 14 children received *Erwinia*. Both groups were treated according to protocol acute lymphoblastic leukemia Berlin–Frankfurt–Münster 86 (ALL-BFM 86). Coagulation factors were measured before the therapy, during the 1st, the 2nd and the 3rd weeks of therapy and after finishing treatment with L-asparaginase. Results were analyzed statistically. Our studies showed a significant decrease in the activity of AT III and fibrinogen during L-asparaginase therapy in the first group of patients. However, in patients receiving *Erwinia* there was no such significant decrease in the activity of AT III and fibrinogen.

Introduction

L-Asparaginase (L-aspa) is a very effective agent incorporated in most intensive chemotherapy schedules, usually as part of induction therapy of acute lymphoblastic leukemia (ALL) in adults and children [1–4]. This drug is an effective antileukemic agent that inhibits neoplastic cell growth by hydrolizing L-asparagine to L-aspartic acid [5, 6]. L-asparagine, a nonessential amino acid, is synthesized by mammalian cells. Malignant cells have a diminished capacity to synthesize L-asparagine and must depend upon on external supply from the extracellular fluid. As asparaginase depletes extracellular L-asparagine, normal cells which are actively synthesizing protein may not be able to synthesize sufficient L-asparagine and the lack of protein can be observed [7–10]. hypoalbuminemia, hypoinsulinemia, a low level of thyroine-binding globulin, and a number of factors involved in coagulation and fibrinolysis during treatment with L-aspa can be explained by this mechanism [11–21].

Clinically active asparaginases have been derived from *Escherichia coli* and *Erwinia chrysanthemii* [22–24]. This Prospective study was undertaken to detect changes in antithrombin III (AT III) coagulation factors I, II, V, VII, X and platelets level during *E. coli* and *Erwinia asparaginase* treatment according to protocol I ALL-Berlin–Frankfurt–Münster Study Group 86 (ALL-BFM 86). We studied 44 consecutive pediatric patients with ALL and determined AT III and coagulation factor (I,II,V,VII,X) changes that developed during treatment with vincristine, prednisone, daunorubidomycine, and L-aspa.

Materials and Methods

Forty-four newly diagnosed pediatric patients with ALL were treated a standard regimen according to ALL-BFM 86 to induce a bone marrow remission. They received vincristine 1.5

[1]Warsaw University Medical School, Department of Pediatric Hematology-Oncology, Dzialdowska 1, Warsaw, Poland
[2]Warsaw University Medical School, Department of Vascular Surgery and Transplantology, Banacha St. 1, Warsaw, Poland

mg/m^2 and daunorubidomycine 40 mg/m^2 weekly for four doses, prednisone 60 mg/m^2 daily for 40 days, and L-aspa 10 000 U/m^2 intravenously on days 18, 22, 25, 28, 31, 34, 37, and 40. The first 30 patients (group 1) received L-aspa *E. coli* (Kidrolase). The last 14 patients (group 2) received L-aspa *Erwinia* (Erwinase, Porton, USA).

No significant difference in the distribution of sex, age, and in mean values of hematological parameters was present between the two groups of patients. Age-matched normal control values were obtained from children who were having minor elective surgery. An additional 5-ml blood sample was drawn by venipuncture from these children at the time that preoperative blood work was drawn. Thirty age-matched children served as concurrent controls.

Venous blood samples were collected in 3.8% sodium citrate (90:10, v:v) before administration of the first L-aspa dose in the 1st, 2nd, and 3rd weeks. All blood samples were centrifuged within 1 h of collection at 2000 g for 10 min at 4°C.

Platelet counts were determined by standard methods. Serum fibrinogen degradation products were assessed semi-quantitatively (thrombo-Wellcotest). Fibrinogen was measured by immunodiffusion (Fibrinogen Reagent, Boehringer Mannheim, Germany) Antithrombin III activity was measured by a kinetic method on chromogenic substrate (Boehringer Mannheim, Germany). Antithrombin III antigen in plasma was determined by immunodiffusion (BioMerieux). Factor II activity was measured by the Soulier method, factor V activity by the Wolf method, and factor VII and X activity by the Koller method.

Results

Group 1 (Patients Receiving L-aspa *E. coli*)

In patients from group 1 plasma AT III activity-was within the normal ranges (average value 105% SD 16) before therapy with L-aspa *E. coli*. During the 1st and the 2nd weeks of therapy, AT III activity dropped significantly ($p<0.001$) from an average value 105% (SD 19) to 65% (SD 19), reaching a nadir value of 60.3% (SD 20) in the 3rd week of therapy.

One third of the patients had AT III activity lower than 55%. Two weeks after the last L-aspa infusion, 90% of the children reached normal activity of AT III 101% (SD 24) (Fig. 1). Antithrombin III antigen levels were virtually identical to the corresponding AT III activity levels in both groups of patients.

Hypofibrinogenemia was observed in 30% of the patients before L-aspa therapy, mean average value was 209 mg% (SD 92). After the onset of therapy fibrinogen concentration dropped significantly ($p<0.001$) to a mean value 90 mg% (SD 43), and reached a nadir value of 83% (SD 37) ($p<0.001$) in the 3rd week of therapy (Fig. 2). The mean value of factor II activity for the

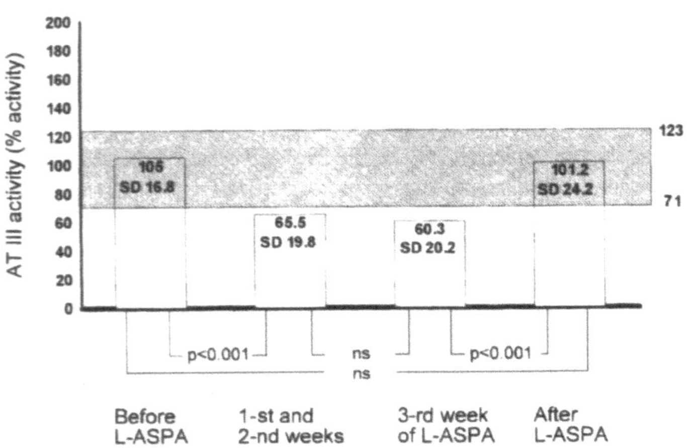

Fig. 1. Changes of plasma antithrombin III activity during L-aspa *E. coli* treatment. *Dashed area* represents the ranges observed in controls

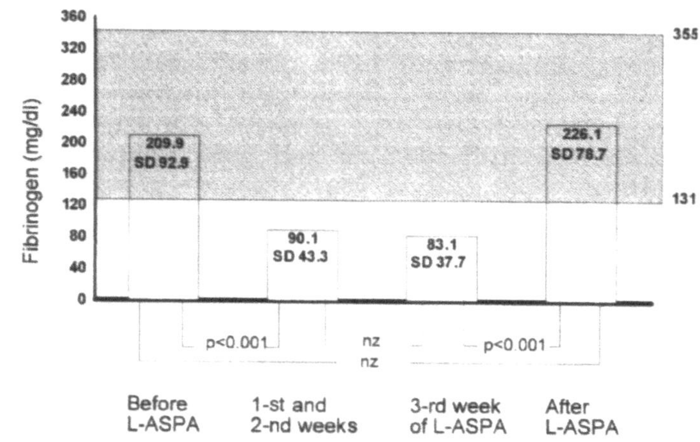

Fig. 2. Changes of fibrinogen concentration during L-aspa *E. coli* treatment. *Dashed area* represents the ranges observed in controls

group decreased to 92% (SD 27) in the first 2 weeks ($p<0.01$) and 87% (SD 31) in the 3rd week. This decrease was within normal ranges obtained from the control group (Fig. 3). The mean value of factor V activity decreased from 74% (SD 33) to 69% during L-aspa *E. coli* therapy and increased to higher than pretreatment mean values (97% SD 36) after the L-aspa was completed (Fig. 4). The mean value of factor VII and X activity was almost unchanged for the whole therapy (Fig. 5). The platelet count, which was low in both groups of patients at the beginning of L-aspa treatment as a consequence of disease and previous chemotherapy, gradually returned to normal levels by the end of L-aspa therapy (Figs. 6, 7).

Fibrinogen degradation products were normal (< 10 mg/l) and paracoagulation tests were negative in the both groups throughout the observation period (data not shown).

Group 2 (Patients Receiving L-aspa *Erwinia*)

In this group of patients, the decrease in the activity of AT III concentration was minimal from pretreatment mean value of 114% (SD 37)

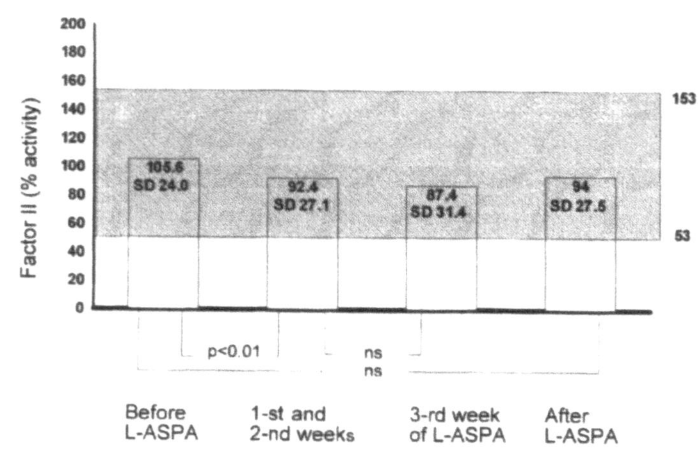

Fig. 3. Changes of factor II activity during L-aspa *E. coli* treatment. *Dashed area* represents the ranges observed in controls

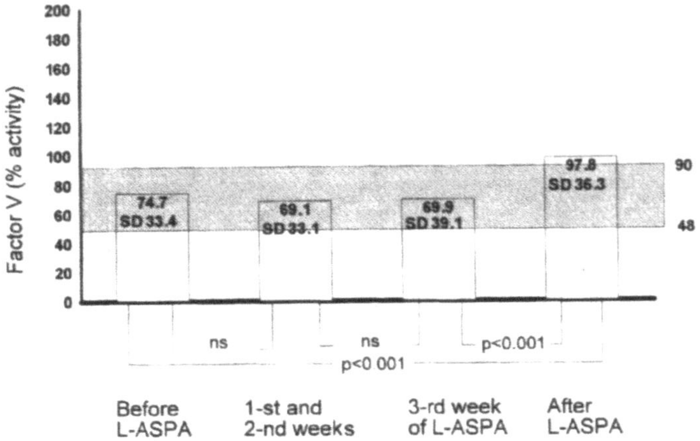

Fig. 4. Changes of factor V activity during L-aspa *E. coli* treatment. *Dashed area* represents the ranges observed in controls

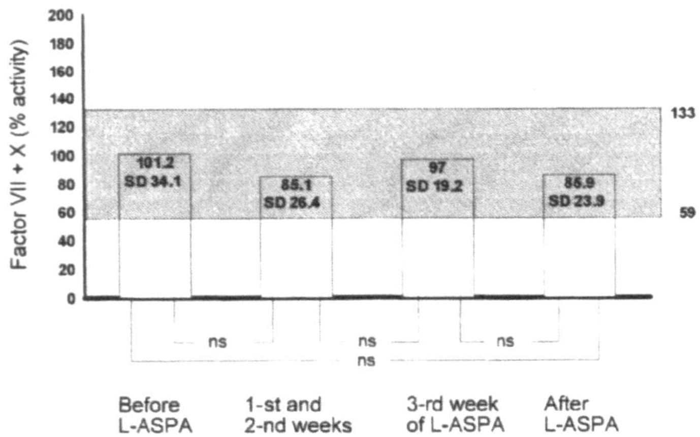

Fig. 5. Changes of factor VII + X activity during L-aspa *E. coli* treatment. *Dashed area* represents the ranges observed in controls

to 106% (SD 30) in the 3rd week of *Erwinia* therapy (Fig. 8). After the onset of *Erwinia* therapy, mean fibrinogen concentration dropped from 170 mg% to 164 mg% (SD 69) in the first 2 weeks and to 141 mg% (SD 92) in the 3rd week (Fig. 9). Minimal decrease of factor II activity from 113% (SD 36) to 96% (SD 20) was observed in the 1st and 2nd weeks (Fig. 10).

The mean value of factor V activity for the group increased steadily during the first 2 weeks of *Erwinia* therapy from 89% SD 32 to 110% SD 47 (Fig. 11). The mean value of factor VII+X activity decreased insignificantly from 101% SD 34 to 85% SD 26 in the first 2 weeks and increased to 97% SD 19 in the 3rd week (Fig. 12).

Discussion

Serious thrombosis or hemorrhage may occur in children during or shortly after L-aspa therapy for ALL [25–34]. We observed one patient who developed cerebral vein thrombosis while receiving L-aspa *E. coli* and was found to have a low level of AT III. Such observation prompted the broad evaluation of the hemostatic system

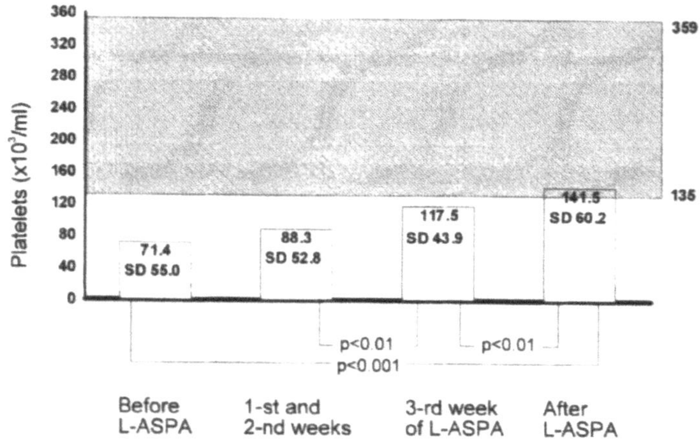

Fig. 6. Changes of platelets level during L-aspa *E. coli* treatment. *Dashed area* represents the ranges observed in controls

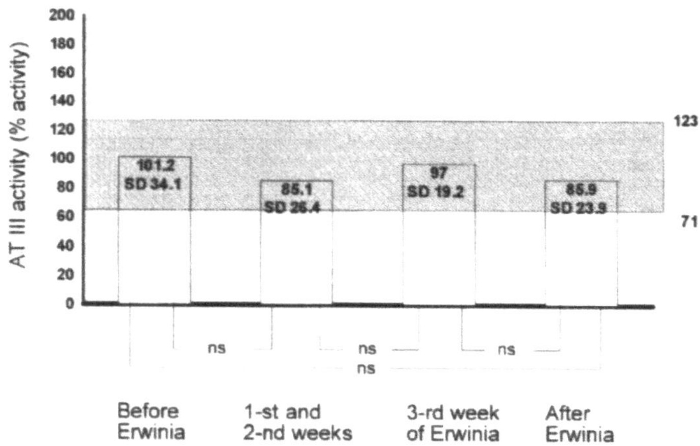

Fig. 7. Changes of platelets level during *Erwinia* treatment. *Dashed area* represents the ranges observed in controls

reported here. This study has demonstrated that treatment according to the ALL-BFM protocol I (induction phase) caused multiple coagulation changes in most of our 44 patients. Sutor et al. [35] reported that glucocorticoids alone (1–7 days of induction) had made fibrinogen drop and AT III rise. More severe alterations of AT III, fibrinogen, factors II, V, VII, and X were observed immediately following the start of therapy with L-aspa *E. coli*.

Influence of L-aspa E. coli on AT III and Factors I, II, V, VII, X. In the 1st and the 2nd weeks of L-aspa therapy, AT III activity dropped abruptly (mean average value 65%) in 70% of our patients, and this process was continued in the 3rd week (mean average value 60%). This decrease was statistically significant ($p < 0.001$). Ten children in this group had AT III activity below 50% (the lowest value was 26%). Our data confirm the observations of many authors [11, 14, 16, 18, 36–38] L-aspa depresses the concentration of various hemostatic proteins by inhibiting their synthesis. It is not known why the synthesis of certain proteins is impaired and synthesis of others is not. Correlation between the results of the func-

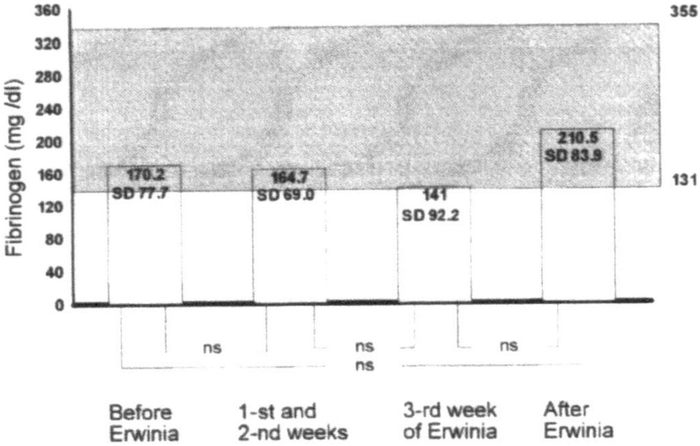

Fig. 8. Changes of plasma antithrombin III activity during *Erwinia* treatment. *Dashed area* represents the ranges observed in controls

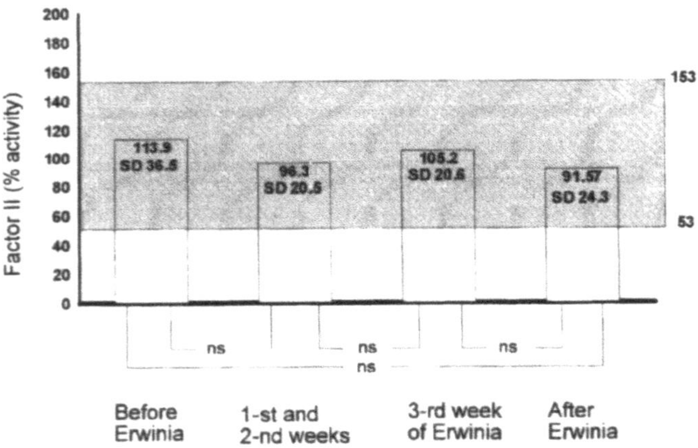

Fig. 9. Changes of fibrinogen concentration during *Erwinia* treatment. *Dashed area* represents the ranges observed in controls

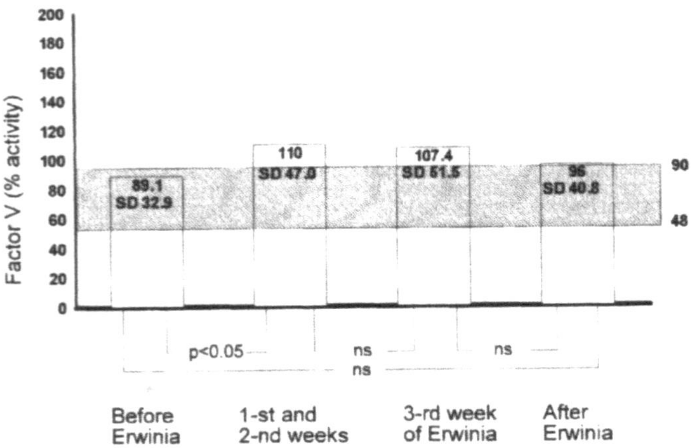

Fig. 10. Changes of factor II activity during *Erwinia* treatment. *Dashed area* represents the ranges observed in controls

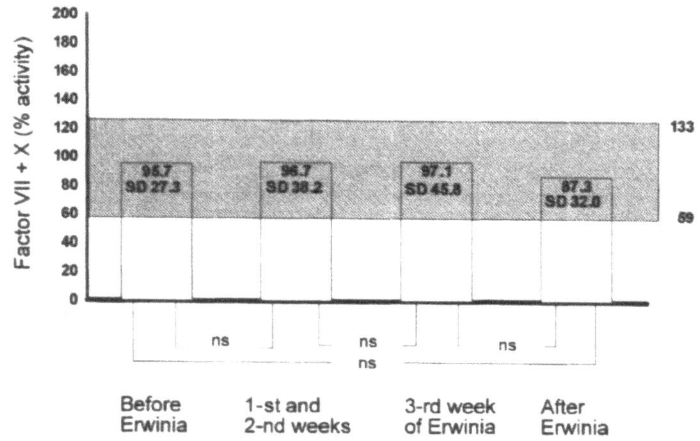

Fig. 11. Changes of factor V activity during *Erwinia* treatment. *Dashed area* represents the ranges observed in controls

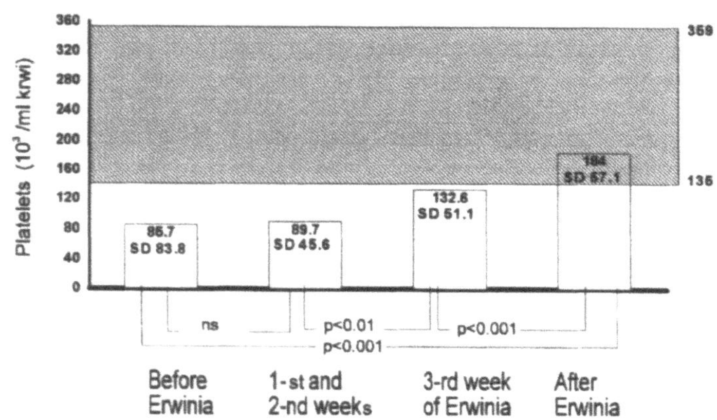

Fig. 12. Changes of factor VII + X activity during *Erwinia* treatment. *Dashed area* represents the ranges observed in controls

tional and immunologic assays for AT III also suggest deficient synthesis rather than synthesis of dysfunctional molecules [16]. Before L-aspa therapy 30% of our patients had hypofibrinogenemia, which could be caused by glucocorticoids [35]. During L-aspa therapy fibrinogen concentration dropped from an average mean value 209 mg% to 90 mg% in the first 2 weeks and 83 mg% in 3rd week. This is in agreement with the findings of others [12, 35, 36, 39]. Mean factor II activity for the group decreased significantly during therapy. The same observation was made by Priest [36]. Therapy with L-aspa *E. coli* was not associated with a marked reduction of the activity of factors V, VII, and X in our study and in the findings of the others [36, 37].

Influence of Erwinia on AT III and Factors I, II, V, VII, and X. In patients receiving *Erwinia*, there was no significant decrease in the concentration of fibrinogen and activity of AT III. This is in agreement with the findings of others [35]. Only O' Meara et al. [40] reported an increase of AT III concentration. In our study mean values of factors II, VII + X activities had only a borderline reduction while at the same time minimal increase of factor V activity was observed. Although both L-aspa *E. coli* and L-aspa *Erwinia* have a similar antitumor effect, the incidence of complications associated with the *E. coli* source of enzyme has been consistently higher [22, 24]. This may be attributable to:

1. Poorer penetration of tissue by *Erwinia* and greater confinement to the vascular system.
2. Asparagine synthetase induction may be enhanced by *Erwinia*, thereby protecting the liver from toxicity.
3. Significantly shorter $t_{1/2}$ of *Erwinia* [41].

Conclusion

1. Treatment according to protocol I ALL-BFM 86 including L-aspa *E. coli* caused multiple changes of hemostasis parameters especially AT III and fibrinogen.
2. Treatment including *Erwinia* induced only a borderline reduction of AT III and coagulation factors.
3. To avoid alteration of hemostasis the replacement of L-aspa *E-coli* by L-aspa *Erwinia* should be considered but in our opinion, because of a markedly shortened $t_{1/2}$ of *Erwinia*, the frequency of administration of this drug has to be changed.

References

1. Barr R.D., Deveber L.L., Pai K.M., Andrew M., Halton J., Cairney A.E., Witton A.C. Management of children with acute lymphoblastic leukaemia by Dana Farber Cancer Institute protocols. American Journal of Pediatric Hematology Oncology 1992;14:: 136-9
2. Clarkson B., Krakoff I., Burchenal J., Karnofsky D., Golbey R., Dowling M., Oettgen H., Lipton A. Clinical results of treatment with E. coli L-asparaginase in adults with leukaemia, lymphoma and solid tumors. Cancer 1970;25: 279–285
3. Jacobs P., Wood L. Treatment of acute lymphoblastic leukaemia. European Journal of Haematology 1992;49: 53–58
4. Ortega J.A., Nesbit M.E., Donaldson N.H.L-Asparaginase, vincristine and prednisone for induction of first remission in acute lymphocytic leukemia. Cancer Research 1977;37: 535–540
5. Broome J..D., Studies on the mechanism of tumor inhibition by L-asparaginase. Journal of Experimental Medicine 1968;127: 1055–1057
6. Prager M.D., Brachynsky N. Asparaginase synthetase in normal and malignant tissues, correlation with tumor sensitivity to asparaginase Arch. Biochem. Biophys. 1968;127: 645–647
7. Capizzi R.L., Holcenberg J.S. Asparaginase cancer medicine Vol 1. Third Edition edited by Lea and Febiger Philadelphia 1993 section XVI: 796–803
8. Chabner B.A., Myers Ch. E. Clinical pharmacology of cancer chemotherapy. L-Asparaginase. Principles and practice of oncology edited by De Vita V.T., Hellmann S., Rosenberg S.A. Lippincott Company 1986: 388–390
9. Kidd J.G. Regression of transplanted lymphoma induced in vivo by means of normal guinea pig serum. J. Exp. Med. 1953;98: 565–626.
10. Wade H.E., Elsworth R., Herbert D., Keppie J., Sargeant K.A. new L-asparaginase with antitumor activity. Lancet 1968;2: 776–780
11. Bauer K.A., Teitel J.M. Rosenberg R.D. L-Asparaginase induced antitrombin III deficiency. Evidence against the production of a hypercoagulable state. Thrombosis Research. 1983;29: 437–442
12. Bettigole R.E., Himelstein E.S., Oettgen H.F., Clifford G.O. Hypofibrynogenemia due to L-asparaginase; studies of fibrinogen survival using autologous 131J-fibrinogen blood. 1970;35: 195
13. Bezeaud A., Dronet L., Leverger G., Griffin J.H., Guillin M.C. Effect of L-asparaginase therapy for acute lymphoblastic leukemia on plasma vitamin K-dependent coagulation factors and inhibitors. Journal of Pediatrics 1986;108: 698–701
14. Conard J., Samame M., Bilsk-Pasquier G., Bousser J. Toxicite in vivo de la L-asparaginase sur les facteurs de coagulation et en particulier sur l'antitrombine III a propos de 25 observations. Coagulation 1971;4: 195–210
15. Dolowy W.D., Hensen D.V.M., Cornet J., Sellin H. Toxic and antineoplastic effects of L-asparaginase Cancer 1966;19: 1813–1819
16. Liebman H.A., Wada J.K., Patch M.J., McGehee W. Depression of functional and antigenic plasma antitrombin III due to therapy with L-asparaginase. Cancer 1982;50: 451–456
17. Lord V.J., Sutow W.W., Fernbach D.J. Toxicity of L-asparaginase in children with advanced leukemia. Cancer 1972;30: 339
18. Mielot F., Danel P., Bayer C., Coulombel L., Domergnes I., Tcherme G. Acquired deficiencies in AT III and C protein during treatment with L-asparaginase. Archives Francaises De Pediatrie 1987: 44: 161–165
19. Oettgen H.F., Stephenson P.A., Schwartz M.K., Leeper R.D., Tallal L., Toxicity of E. coli L-asparaginase in man. Cancer 1970;25: 253–258
20. Tallal L., Tan Ch., Oettgen H., Wolland N., McCarthy M., Helson L., Karnofsky D.A., Murphy M.L. Toxicity of E. coli L-asparaginase treatment of leukaemia and solid tumors in 131 children. Cancer 1970;25: 306–310
21. Saito M., Asakura H., Jokaji H., Uotani C., Kumabashiri K., Matsude T. Changes in hemostatic and fibrinolytic proteins in patients receiving L-asparaginase therapy. American Journal of Hematology 1989;32: 20–23
21. Vallenga E., Kluft C., Mulder N.H., Wijugaard S.G., Nieweg H.O. The influence of L-asparaginase ther-

apy on the fibrinolitic system. British Journal of Hematology 1984;57: 247–254
22. Billett A.L., Carls A., Gelber R.D., Sallan S.E. Allergic reactions to Erwinia asparaginase in children with ALL who had previous allergic reactions to Escherichia coli asparaginase. Cancer 1992;70: 201–206
23. North A.C.T., Wade H.E. Physicio-chemical studies of L-asparaginase from Erwinia carotovora. Nature 1969;224: 594–595
24. Ridgway D., Neerhout R.C., Bleyer A. Attenuation of asparaginase induced hyperglicemia after substitution of the Erwinia carotovora for the Escherichia Coli enzyme preparation. Cancer 1989;63: 561–563
25. Cairo M.S., Lazarus K., Gilmore R.L. Intracranial hemorrhage and focal seizures secondary to use of L-asparaginase during induction therapy of acute lymphoblastic leukemia. Journal of Pediatrics 1980;97: 829–833
26. Feinberg W., Swenson M. Cerebrovascular complications of L-asparaginase therapy. Neurology 1988; 38: 127–133
27. Foreman N.K., Mamomd H.H., Rivere G.K., Crist W.M. Recurrent cerebrovascular accident with L-asparaginase rechallenge. Medical Pediatric Oncology 1992;20: 534–532
28. Gugliotta L., Mazzucconi M.G., Leone G., Mattioli-Belmonte M., Defazio D., Annino Z., Tura S., Mandelli F. Incidence of thrombotic complications in adult patients with acute lymphoblastic leukaemia receiving L-asparaginase therapy during induction therapy, a retrospective study. The Gimema Group. European Journal of Haematology 1992;49: 63–66
29. Miniero R., Pastore G., Saracco P., Messina M, Fiandino G., Madon E. Hemostatic changes in children with acute lymphoblastic leukemia treated according to two different L-asparaginase schedules. American Journal of Pediatric Hematology-Oncology 1986;8: 116–120
30. Muttean W. Haemorrhagic complications of L-asparaginase therapy. Journal of Pediatrics 1983;102: 483–484
31. Shapiro A. Clarke S.L., Christian J.M., Odom L.F., Hathaway W.E. Thrombosis in children receiving l-asparaginase. The American Journal of Pediatric Hematology and Oncology 1993;15: 400–405
32. Steinherz P.G., Miller L.P., Ghavini F., Allen J., Miller D.R. Dural sinus thrombosis in children with acute lymphoblastic leukaemia. JAMA 1981;246: 2837–2839
33. Urban C., Sager W.D. Intracranial bleeding during therapy with L-asparaginase in childhood acute lymphoblastic leukaemia. European Journal of Pediatrics 1981;137: 323–327
34. Mondhiry Al. Hypofibrynogenemia associated with vincristine and prednisone therapy in lymphoblastic leukemia. Cancer 1975;35: 144–147
35. Sutor A.H., Niemeyer C., Santer S., Witt J., Rombach A., Brandis M., Riehm H. Gerinnungsveranderungen bei Behandlung mit den Protokollen ALL BFM 90 und NHL BFM 90 Klinische Padiatrie 1992;204: 264–273
36. Priest J.R., Ramsay N.K.C., Benett A.. Krint W., Edson J.R. The effect of L-asparaginase on antithrombin, plasminogen and plasma coagulation during therapy for acute lymphoblastic leukemia. The Journal of Pediatrics. 1982;100: 990–995
37. Ramsay N.K.C., Coccia P.F., Krivit W., Nesbit M.E., Edson J.R. The effect of L-asparaginase on plasma coagulation factors in acute lymphoblastic leukemia. Cancer 1977;40: 1398–1401
38. Schondorf H., Pralle H., Grauber M., Lasch H.G. Antitrombin III deficiency and thromboembolic complications under L-asparaginase treatment. Thrombosis and Haemostasis 1983; 50
39. Vicarioto M., Rosden A., Cappellato M.G., Zanesco L., Girolami A. Greater decrease of fibrinogen as compared to AT III in L-asparaginase treated leukaemia patients. Folia Haematologica-Leipz 1986;113: 663–669
40. O'Meara A., Daly M., Halinani F.H. Increased antitrombin III concentration in children with acute lymphoblastic leukaemia receiving L-asparaginase therapy. Medical and Pediatric Oncology 1988;16: 169–174
41. Asselin B.L., Whitin J.C., Coppola D.J., Ruppl P., Sallan S.E., Cohen H.J. Comparative Pharmacokinetic studies of three asparaginase preparations. 1993; J Clin Oncol: 11 1780–1786

Acute Leukemias VI
Prognostic Factors
and Treatment Strategies
Büchner et al. (eds)

Infusion Rate Does Not Influence Ifosfamide Side-Chain Metabolism

H. Silies[1,2], J. Boos[1], G. Blaschke[2], and H. Jürgens[1]

Abstract. Ifosfamide (IFO) undergoes metabolic activation by hydroxylation of the ring system to exert cytotoxic activity. A second metabolic pathway produces the cytostatically inactive metabolites 2-dechloroethylifosfamide (2-D-IFO) and 3-dechloroethylifosfamide (3-D-IFO) releasing chloroacetaldehyde. This pathway of side-chain metabolism has been discussed as a source of CNS and renal toxicity. As regards neurotoxicity, the incidence seems to be strongly schedule dependent.

We compared the urinary excretion of 2-D-IFO and 3-D-IFO on short-term and continuous ifosfamide infusion (3000 mg/m^2) and, in addition, schedules with dosages ranging from 400 mg to 3 g/m^2. Urine was sampled for up to 72 h and investigated by gas chromatography; 46.5% $\pm$ 13.2% of the applied dose could be recovered in the urine ($n = 26$ patients). The main metabolite was IFO (22.5% $\pm$ 8.5%) followed by 3-D-IFO (14.4% $\pm$ 4.2%), and 2-D-IFO (8.8% $\pm$ 3.4%). Neither the total amount formed nor the excretion kinetics of side-chain metabolites were found to be schedule dependent. Even with 1-h infusion, there was a lag of 3-6 h until excretion of side-chain metabolites set in. The excretion patterns of side-chain metabolites as well as unmetabolized IFO were nearly superimposable on short-term and on continuous infusion.

We conclude that differences in toxicity and efficacy cannot be explained by an influence of the application time on the metabolic profile of IFO.

Introduction

Ifosfamide (IFO) is a widely used anticancer drug from the group of oxazaphosphorines which also includes cyclophosphamide. Currently, IFO is used in first-line therapeutic regimens in approximately half of all children presenting with newly diagnosed cancer in Germany [1]. IFO is a prodrug and requires metabolic activation by hydroxylation of the ring system to exert a cytotoxic effect (see Fig. 1). 4-Hydroxy-ifosfamide (4-OH-IFO) is converted into tautomeric aldoifosfamide (ALDO-IFO) by opening of the oxazaphosphorine ring. Spontaneous elimination of acrolein (ACR) produces the alkylating compound isophosphoramide mustard [*N,N'*-bis(2-chloroethyl) -phosphoric acid diamide] (IFO-M). Further oxidation of 4-OH-IFO results in the inactive metabolites keto- and carboxyifosfamide [2,3] (see Fig. 1).

By an alternative metabolic pathway, IFO undergoes *N*-dealkylation to the cytostatically inactive metabolites 2-dechloroethylifosfamide (2-D-IFO) and 3-dechloroethylifosfamide (3-D -IFO) releasing chloroacetaldehyde [4]. These side-chain metabolites have been associated with CNS toxicity [5–8] and renal toxicity [9], effects not observed after cyclophosphamide. The incidence of neurotoxic side effects of IFO seems to be strongly schedule dependent, showing higher incidence on oral and short-term application [8]. On the other hand, the antitumor efficacy was also reported to be lower in patients on a continuous IFO application schedule [10].

[1]Department of Pediatric Hematology/Oncology, University of Münster, 48129 Münster, Germany
[2]Institute of Pharmaceutical Chemistry, University of Münster, 48129 Münster, Germany

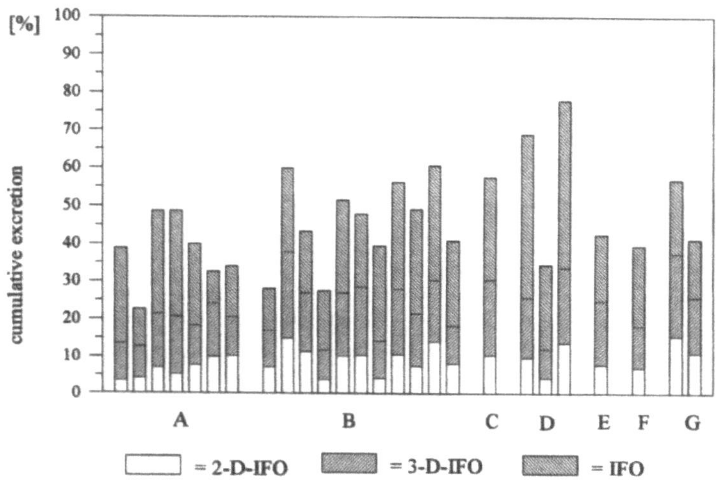

Fig. 1. Metabolism of ifosfamide

The present study was initiated to address the following questions:

- Is there a dose-dependent difference in the excretion of side-chain metabolites?
- Is there a schedule-dependent difference in the excretion of side-chain metabolites between short-term and continuous infusion of IFO?

Material and Methods

Patients and Study Design

The urinary output was completely collected during 26 cycles of IFO of 23 patients aged between 8 and 25 years and almost completely collected from another three patients during five cycles (Table 1). The patients were treated for osteosarcoma ($n=9$), rhabdomyosarcoma ($n=6$), Ewing's sarcoma ($n=4$), Askin tumor ($n=1$), clear cell sarcoma ($n=1$), neuroblastoma ($n=1$), B cell lymphoma ($n=1$) and acute lymphoblastic leukemia (ALL) relapse ($n=3$). The individual doses ranged from 400 mg/m^2 to 3000 mg/m^2. IFO was given by infusion at durations of 1 h to 3 days (continuous infusion). The treatment schedules and the cytostatically active comedication used are outlined in Table 1. Urinary fractions were collected at 3-, 6-, and 12-h intervals up to at least 23 h after the application when renal excretion was almost com-

Table 1. Dosage, scheduling, and cytostatic comedication used in the present study

Patients	Dose (mg/m^2 daily)	Days	Infusion	Other cytostatics
IS, DC, IF, RP, RS, SG, FS	3000	2	1h	Cisplatin
IK	3000	2	Continuous	Adriamycin, vincristine
MK	3000	3	Continuous	Adriamycin, vincristine
SJ, JB, JO, TL, RN, CK, CB, MT, AW	2000	3	1h	Etoposide, actinomycin, vincristine
LG	1500	5	Continuous	Vincristine, DTIC, adriamycin
DP	800	5	1h	Etoposide, ara-C, methotrexate
JN, EA, DH	400	5	1h	6-Thioguanine, VDS, methotrexate, daunorubicin, L-asparaginase

plete. The urinary fractions were immediately stored at −20°C. From each patient one spontaneous urine sample was collected before the IFO application as a reference sample.

Determination of IFO, 2-D-IFO and 3-D-IFO

Extraction Procedure. A sample of 500 μl urine was spiked with 25 μl of the internal standard solution containing the oxazaphosphorine trofosfamide (1 μg dissolved in 1 μl of methanol) (TROFO); the sample was shaken vigorously. After centrifugation the samples were transferred to extrelut-R-1 cartridges, and 3 ml dichloromethan/isopropanol (95:5 V/V) was added. After 5 min, the extraction procedure was repeated. After 10 min, the extraction solution was evaporated to dryness under a gentle stream of nitrogen. The residue was redissolved in 100 μl methanol, and the solution shaken vigorously.

Determination by Gas Chromatography. The simultaneous determination of IFO, 2-D-IFO, 3-D-IFO, and TROFO was done by separation on a fused silica capillary column (NB 1701, HNU, Nordion, 10 m × 0.32 mm ID × 0.25 μm film thickness). A gas chromatograph (Shimadzu GC 14A) equipped with a split-splitless injector and nitrogen-phosphorus-selective flame ionization detection (NPD) was used. The following temperature programme was applied: the starting temperature of the column was 140°C and raised to 175°C at 5°C/min, then maintained at 175°C for 3 min, the temperature was then raised to 200°C at 15°C/min and maintained for 8 min. The chromatograph was operated under the following conditions: temperature at the injection site, 200°C; temperature of the detector, 250°C; carrier gas, helium, flow rate 2.5 ml/min; flow detector gases, air at 0.6 bar, hydrogen at 0.6 bar, make-up gas (helium) at 35 ml/min; split injection at a ratio of 1:50; 1 μl of the extracted sample was injected in the gas chromatography system.

Validation. Standards were prepared by adding known amounts of 2-D-IFO, 3-D-IFO, IFO, and TROFO (which were kindly supplied by Asta Medica, Frankfurt, Germany) to urine samples obtained from volunteers. The concentration ranges used for calibration were 1–200 μg/ml urine for 2-D-IFO, 3-D-IFO, and IFO. Each calibration curve consisted of a total of seven values. All standards were run in triplicate. Quantitative estimation of drug and metabolite concentrations in the standard and the test samples were carried out according to the internal-standard ratio. The correlation coefficients for IFO and the dechloroethyl metabolites exceeded 0.999, so that there were linear peak area versus concentration curves.

The interassay coefficients of variation at the different concentrations averaged 5.57%, 6.49%, and 6.31%. The lower limits of detection at a peak-height to baseline-noise ratio of 3:1 was 200 ng/ml for 2-D-IFO, 3-D-IFO. The extraction recovery rates for 2-D-IFO, 3-D-IFO, IFO, and TROFO ranged between 97% and 99%.

Results

A total of 46.5 ± 13.2% of the applied dose could be recovered in the urine ($n = 26$ patients). The main metabolite was IFO (22.5% ± 8.5%) followed by 3-D-IFO (14.4% ± 4.2%), and 2-D-IFO (8.8% ± 3.4%) Figure 2 presents the cumulative excretion of IFO and the side-chain metabolites. The urinary excretion of each patient according to the application schedule is shown. No relationship could be found between the excreted amount of the side-chain metabolites and the application schedule.

The findings on evaluation of the total urinary excretion after different application patterns were to be confirmed by the comparison of the excretion kinetics. We compared the 2-D-IFO and 3-D-IFO excretion data of children treated with 3000 mg/m^2 per day IFO either by 1-h infusion or continuous infusion. This comparison included the patients IS, DC, IF,RP, and IK,as well as AH1, AH2, KK, IE, CT1, JP, PB2, and BB. The cumulative excretion data of the latter eight patients were given in a previous publication [11]. The excretion kinetics, shown in Figs. 3 and 4, are completely superimposable. The interindividual variability of each patient group for each determination time is indicated in the figures. Even with 1-h infusion there was a 3-6 h lag until dechloroethylation was apparent.

Discussion

Whereas some former published studies on the metabolism of IFO have shown wide interindividual variability [12,13], we found overall a

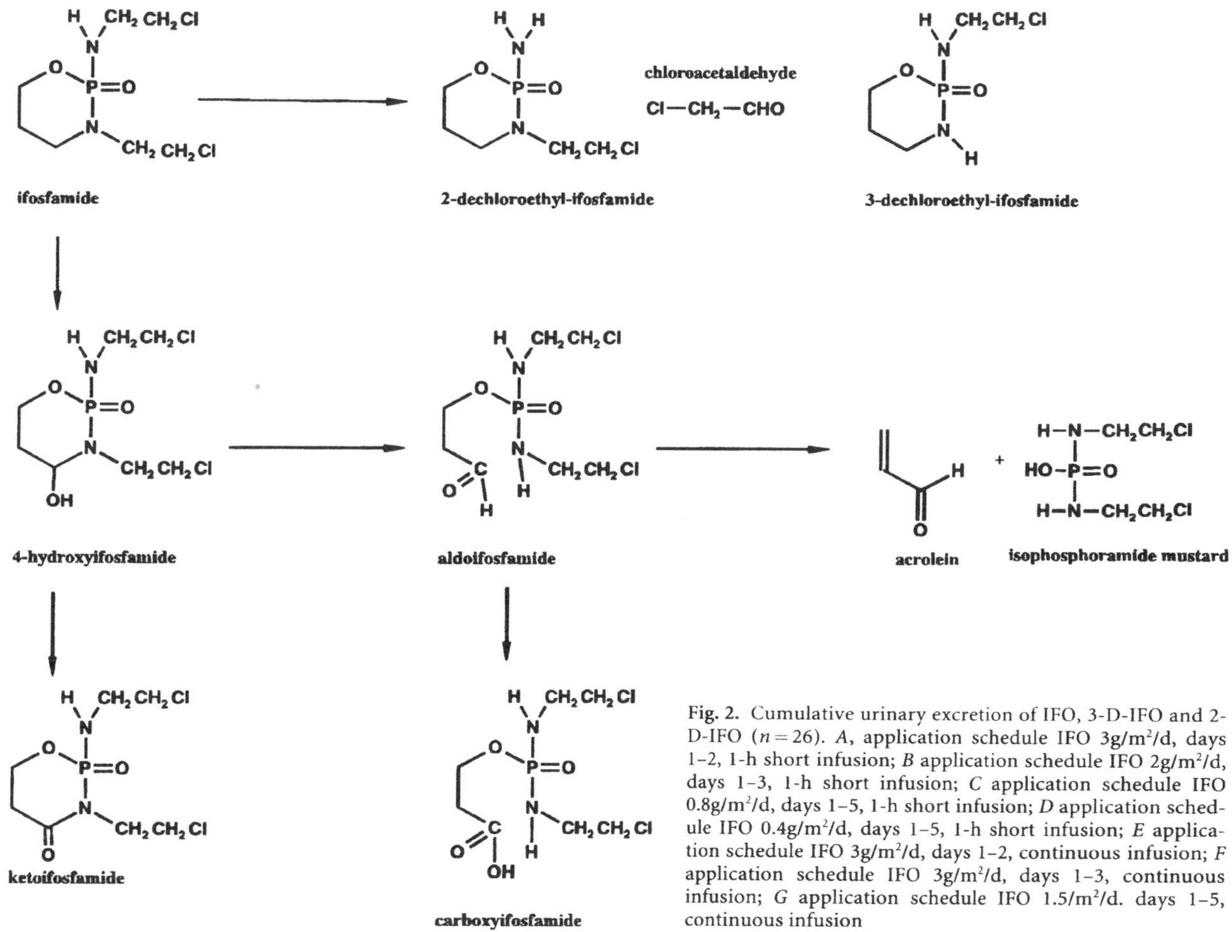

Fig. 2. Cumulative urinary excretion of IFO, 3-D-IFO and 2-D-IFO ($n = 26$). *A*, application schedule IFO 3g/m^2/d, days 1–2, 1-h short infusion; *B* application schedule IFO 2g/m^2/d, days 1–3, 1-h short infusion; *C* application schedule IFO 0.8g/m^2/d, days 1–5, 1-h short infusion; *D* application schedule IFO 0.4g/m^2/d, days 1–5, 1-h short infusion; *E* application schedule IFO 3g/m^2/d, days 1–2, continuous infusion; *F* application schedule IFO 3g/m^2/d, days 1–3, continuous infusion; *G* application schedule IFO 1.5/m^2/d. days 1–5, continuous infusion

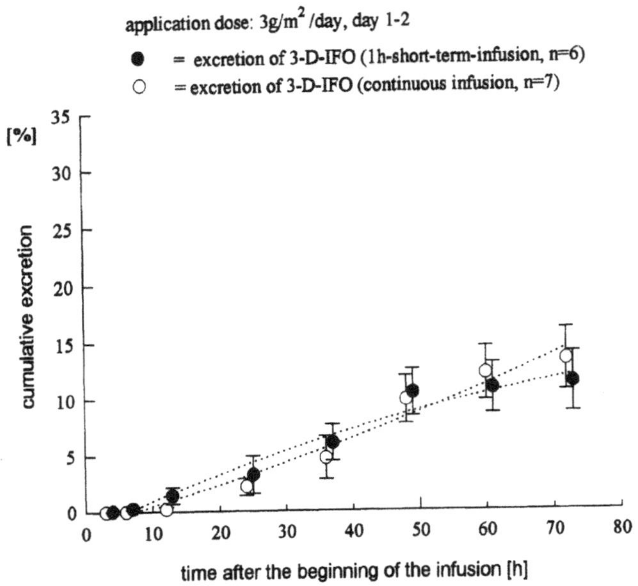

Fig. 3. Cumulative urinary excretion of 3-D-IFO during continuous (*open circles*, $n=7$) and short-term (*Solid circles*, 1-h infusion, $n=6$) IFO infusions according to the cumulative IFO dose per cycle. Application dose: 3g/m² per day per days

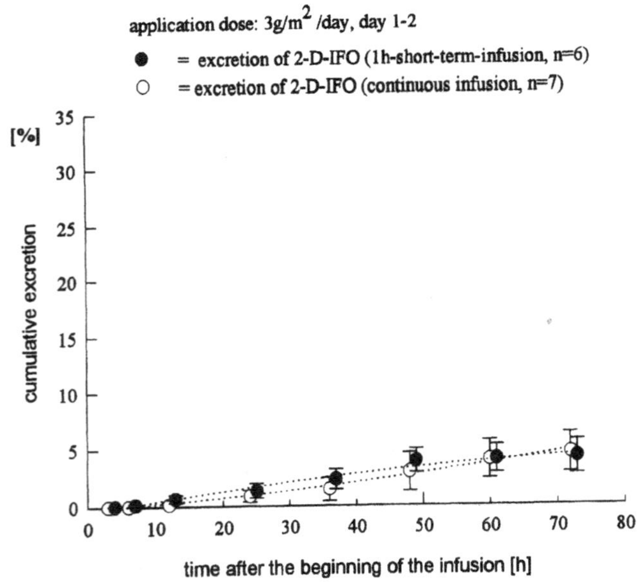

Fig. 4. Cumulative urinary excretion of 2-D-IFO during the continuous (*Open circles*, $n=7$) and short-term (*Solid circles*,1-h infusion, $n=6$) IFO infusions according to the total cumulative IFO dose per cycle. Application dose: 3g/m² per day on days 1–2

rather uniform pattern of excretion of unmetabolized IFO and *N*-desalkylated compounds. This was in accordance with our previous observation of the metabolism of IFO in 14 children [11]. The total amount excreted was similar to the results reported by other groups [14–16].

The phenomenon of autoinduction results in an increase of IFO metabolism to alkylating metabolites [17] as well as to the dechloroethylation products including chloroacetaldehyde [18]. The total IFO clearance on continuous infusion appeared to be higher in pediatric patients compared to adults [19] but was not different between short and long intravenous IFO infusion [20]. As the pathway of side-chain metabolism and the release of chloroacetaldehyde has been discussed as a source of CNS toxicity [5] and nephrotoxicity [9], the current investigation focussed on renal excretion of 2-D-IFO and 3-D-IFO. With regard to the indications of schedule-dependent toxicity [8] and efficacy [10] the excretion kinetics of these metabolites were compared on short-term versus continuous infusion.

No relationship, however, was found between the amount of the side-chain metabolites excreted and the application schedule (Fig. 2). Furthermore, the finding of an identical excretory pattern for IFO, 2-D-IFO, and the main side-chain metabolite 3-D-IFO does not suggest any significant differences in ring oxidation with formation of 4-OH-IFO either. Our data thus fail to support any association between differences in toxicity and clinical response and changes in metabolism with different infusion rates.

Moreover, the identical urinary excretory pattern of the substance proper and its metabolites suggests that a relationship between dosage schedule and renal toxicity is rather unlikely. Against this background, it is no surprise that children on regimens employing short-term, as compared to continuous, IFO infusion showed no differences in the pattern or incidence of renal impairment [21].

Acknowledgment. This research was financially supported by Asta Medica, Frankfurt.

References

1. Jürgens H, Treuner J, Winkler K, Göbel U (1989) Ifosfamide in pediatric malignancies. Semin Oncol 16 [Suppl 3]: 46–50
2. Connors TA, Cox PJ, Farmer PB, Foster AB, Jarman M (1973) Some studies of the active intermediates formed in the microsomal metabolism of cyclophosphamide and isophosphamide Biochem Pharmacol 23: 115–129
3. Hill DL, Russel Laster W, Kirk MC, El Dareer S, Struck RF (1973) Metabolism of iphosphamide [2-(2-chlorethylamino)-3-(2-chloroethyl)tetrahydro-2H-1,3-2-oxazaphorphorine-2-oxide] and production of a toxic iphosphamide metabolite. Cancer Res. 33: 1016-1022.
4. Norpoth K, Addicks Hw, Witting U, Müller G, Raidt H (1975) Quantitative Bestimmung von Cyclophosphamid, Ifosfamid, und Trofosfamid sowie ihrer stabilen Metabolite auf der DC-Platte mit 4-Pyridinaldehyd-2-benzothiazolyhydrazon (PHB). Arzneimittelforschung 25: 1331–1336.
5. Goren MP, Wright RK, Pratt CB, Pell FE: Dechloroethylation of ifosfamide and neurotoxicity Lancet 1986; ii: 1219–1220
6. Wainer IW, Ducharme J, Granvil CP, Truedeau M, Leyland-Jones B (1994) Ifosfamide stereoselective dechloroethylation and neurotoxicity. Lancet 343: 982–3
7. Lewis LD, Meanwell CA (1990) Ifosfamide pharmacokinetics and neurotoxicity. Lancet 335: 175-6
8. Cerny T, Castiglione M, Brunner K, Küpfer A, Matinelli G, Lind M (1990) Ifosfamide by continuous infusion to prevent encaphalopathy. Lancet 335: 175
9. Skinner R, Sharkey IM, Pearson ADJ, Craft AW: Ifosfamide, mesna, and nephrotoxicity in Children J. Clin. Oncol. 1993; 11: 173–190
10. Antman KH, Ryan L, Elias A, Sherman D, Grier HE (1989) Response to ifosfamide and mesna: 124 previously treated patients with metastatic or unresectable sarcoma. J. Clin Oncol 7: 126–131
11. Boos J, Welslau U, Ritter J. Blaschke G, Schellong G (1991) Urinary excretion of the enantiomers of ifosfamide and its inactive metabolites in children. Cancer Chemotherapy Pharmacol 28: 455–460
12. Lind J, Roberts HL, Thatcher N, Idle JR (1990) The effect of route of administration and fractionation of dose on the metabolism of ifosfamide. Cancer Pharmacol 26: 105–111.
13. Ninane J, Baurain R, Kraker J de, Frester A, Trouet A, Cornu G (1989) Alkylating activity in serum, urine and CSF following high-dose ifosfamide in children. Cancer Chemother Pharmacol 24 [Supp.]: 82–86.
14. Goren MP (1991) Determination of urinary 2- and 3- dechloroethylated metabolites of ifosfamide by high-performance liquid chromatography. J. Chromatogr, Biomed Appl 570: 351.
15. Misiura K, Okruszek A, Pankiewicz K, Stec WJ, Czownicki Z, Utracka B (1983) Stereospecific synthesis of chiral metabolites of ifosfamide and their determination in the urine. J Med Chem 26: 674.
16. Martino R, Crasnier F, Chouini-Lalanne N, Gilard V, Niemeyer U, de Forni M, Malet-Martino MC (1992) A new approach to the study of ifosfamide metabolism by the analysis of human body fluids with ^{31}P nuclear magnetic resonance spectroscopy. J Pharmacol Exp Ther 260: 1133.
17. Lewis LD, Fitzgerald DL, Harper PG, Rogers HJ (1990) Fractionated ifosfamide therapy produces a time-dependent increase in ifosfamide metabolism. Br J Pharmac 30: 725–32.
18. Kurowski V, Wagner T (1993) Comparative pharmacokinetics of ifosfamide, 4-hydroxyifosfamide, chloroacetaldehyde, and 2- and 3- dechloroethylifosfamide in patients on fractionated intravenous ifosfamide therapy. Cancer Chemother Pharmacol 33: 36–42.
19. Boddy AV, Yule SM, Wyllie R, Price L, Pearson AD, Idle JR (1993) Pharmacokinetics and metabolism of ifosfamide administered as a continuous infusion in children. Cancer Res 53: 3758–64.
20. Lewis LD, Fitzgerald DL, Mohan P, Thatcher N, Harper PG, Rogers HJ (1991) The pharmacokinet-

ics of ifosfamide given as short and long intravenous infusion in cancer patients. Br J Clin Pharmac 31: 71–82.
21. Rossi R, Gödde A, Kleinebrand A, Wygold T, Boos J, Riepenhausen M, Jürgens H (1994) The influence of push versus continuous ifosfamide infusion on the development of tubular damage. International Conference on Long-Term Complications of Treatment of Childhood and Adulescents for Cancer, Niagara Falls-New York (Abstr.#27)

Acute Leukemias VI
Prognostic Factors
and Treatment Strategies
Büchner et al. (eds)

Busulfan Pharmacology in Bone Marrow Transplantation Patients

V. Heinemann, K. Voges, J. Mittermüller H.-J. Kolb, K. Wachholz, W. Wilmanns, and U. Jehn

Abstract. Forty-three patients, 18 acute myeloid leukemia, 22 chronic myelogenous leukemia, two with refractory anemia with excess of blasts, and one patient with a diagnosis of thalassemia (median age 46 years, range 26–58 years) received high-dose busulfan as a conditioning regimen for bone marrow transplantation (32 allogeneic and 11 autologous). Busulfan was given at a dose of 1 mg/kg (2-mg tablets) every 6 h until a total dose of 16 mg/kg was achieved. Busulfan trough concentrations in plasma showed a considerable variability between different patients (14-fold), but also within the respective treatment courses (two-to seven fold). To allow a targeting of busulfan plasma concentrations by appropriate dose adjustment, it appeared necessary to reduce the intrapatient variability of busulfan plasma concentrations. We therefore evaluated the impact of food uptake on gastrointestinal absorption and pharmacokinetics of busulfan. Thirteen patients receiving enteral feeding were compared to 18 fasting patients who received parenteral feeding. In fact, interpatient and intrapatient variability was significantly decreased by parenteral feeding. However, trough values of busulfan were significantly lower in parenterally fed patients compared to enterally fed patients (350 vs. 500 ng/ml, $p < 0.001$). We further performed a longitudinal analysis of busulfan steady-state concentrations during the whole treatment period. The pharmacological evaluation of 30 patients demonstrated that mean busulfan steady-state concentrations significantly ($p = 0.01$) decreased from dose four to dose 15 (400 vs. 281 ng/ml). All patients received an anticonvulsant prophylaxis with phenytoin during busulfan treatment. Since steady-state busulfan concentrations did not decrease in ten additional patients who received diazepam as anticonvulsant prophylaxis, it was concluded that phenytoin, a known enzyme inducer, was responsible for enhanced hepatic metabolism of the drug and consequently induced an increased clearance of busulfan during the course of busulfan conditioning treatment.

Introduction

Busulfan is a bialkylating agent with known activity in chronic myelogenous leukemia (CML). This agent shows a predominant antihematopoietic activity, while immunosuppression is induced to a lesser extent [1]. High-dose busulfan is presently being evaluated as conditioning regimen for allogeneic and autologous bone marrow transplantation in hematologic malignancies. In this setting, busulfan substitutes total body irradiation prior to bone marrow transplantation [2]. Busulfan is applied orally at a dose of 16 mg/kg over 4 days. Owing to its oral application, bioavailability of busulfan may vary as a function of gastrointestinal absorption kinetics. Since busulfan is known to be lipophilic, drug absorption may further be determined by food composition. It has been reported that a relation exists between toxic side effects of busulfan, such as veno-occlusive disease of the liver, and the area under the concen-

Department of Hematology, III Med. Klinik, Klinikum Grosshadern, University of Munich, Germany

tration × time curve (AUC) of busulfan in plasma [3]. This study was therefore designed to monitor busulfan plasma concentrations following three lines of investigation. First, the effect of food uptake on busulfan plasma pharmacokinetics was studied. The primary goal of this analysis was to reduce the variability of gastrointestinal busulfan absorption. Second, we analyzed the relationship between busulfan trough levels in plasma and therapeutic outcome. Third, we evaluated the impact of concomitant anticonvulsant treatment on busulfan pharmacokinetics. Since phenytoin, in contrast to diazepam, is a known inducer of hepatic enzymes, and since busulfan is extensively metabolized by the liver, it was of interest to investigate if phenytoin would enhance busulfan metabolism as compared to diazepam.

Patients and Methods

Patients. Forty-three patients, 18 with the diagnosis of acute myelogenous leukemia (AML), 22 with the diagnosis of CML, two patients with the diagnosis of refractory anemia with excess of blasts (RAEBT), and one patient with the diagnosis of thalassemia were included into the study. Median age was 46 years (range 26–58 years). Thirty-two patients received allogeneic bone marrow transplantation, while 11 patients underwent autologous bone marrow transplantation.

Treatment Regimen. High-dose busulfan was administered orally at a daily dose of four times 1 mg/kg using 2-mg tablets until a total dose of 16 mg/kg was reached after 4 days of treatment. Intervals between busulfan doses were generally kept at 6 h. *Anticonvulsant prophylaxis* was performed in one group of patients ($n=33$) by administration of an oral dose of 300–400 mg/day, while the following group of patients ($n=11$) received oral diazepam prophylaxis at a daily dose of 25 mg.

Materials and Methods. Blood samples were taken before the start of the conditioning treatment and at 6-h intervals before each dose of busulfan. Blood was generally provided in Li-heparin-containing vials, and plasma was separated by centrifugation. Busulfan quantification in plasma was adapted from the method described by Blanz et al. [4]. In short, heparinized plasma samples were cleaned by solid-phase extraction using a Vac Elut system equipped with Bond Elut 1-ml C_8 cartridges (Analytichem International Handelsgesellschaft, Frankfurt, Germany).

High-performance liquid chromatography (HPLC) analysis was performed using a Waters Model 490E Detector, two Waters Model 510 pumps, (Fa. Waters, Eschborn, Germany), an automatic sample injector Waters 717, and the Maxima 3.10 software, an IBM computer-based program designed for pump control and chromatogram evaluation. Peak seperation was achieved by a 5-μm LiChrosorb CN analytical column and a guard column of 5-μm LiChrosorb CN (Grom, Herrenberg, Germany). Postcolumn derivatization was performed by use of a photochemical reaction chamber interposed between the analytical column and detector. The busulfan derivative 1,4-diiodobutane was separated under isocratic elution conditions with a water/acetonitrile solvent (70: 30, v: v) at a flow rate of 1 ml/min. For peak detection a wavelength of 226 nm was chosen. Quantification of busulfan was performed by external standard calculation using derivatized busulfan standards. The reproducibility of busulfan detection and quantification in plasma was reasonably good with a coefficient of variation of 4.4%. Data were submitted to a pharmacokinetic analysis using the IBM computer-based software TOPFIT.

Results

At the beginning of this study, all patients ($n=13$) received oral feeding during the busulfan conditioning treatment. Busulfan was generally administered at 6-h intervals at doses of 1 mg/kg, which were held constant throughout the treatment. Busulfan absorption kinetics showed a considerable intrapatient and interpatient variablity. With regard to the *intrapatient* analysis, steady-state concentrations of busulfan, measured on days 2-4, showed a two- to seven fold variability (data not shown). Between 13 different patients, steady-state concentrations varied by a factor of 14 (data not shown). From this it was concluded that the predictability of busulfan plasma concentrations within one patient and even more between different patients was so low that a reliable relation between dose and plasma concentration of busulfan could not be established. Under these conditions, a pharmacologically directed dose adjustment of busulfan appeared inappropriate.

Effect of Food Uptake on Busulfan Pharmacokinetics. Since busulfan is a lipophilic drug, it appeared likely that gastrointestinal drug absorption was greatly determined by concomitant food uptake. We therefore changed the feeding protocol during the conditioning treatment. To achieve a maximal uniformity of drug absorption, patients ($n = 18$) were kept in a fasting condition and were fed parenterally. Since the interval between oral busulfan uptake and peak concentrations of busulfan in plasma could not be reliably predicted, determinations of busulfan peak concentrations were omitted in the following patients. All subsequent measurements were therefore determinations of busulfan trough levels, each taken prior to the next oral dose. In fact, when busulfan steady-state levels were compared in orally fed and fasting patients, it became apparent that intrapatient ($p < 0.02$) and interpatient ($p < 0.04$) variability of trough concentrations was significantly reduced by the fasting condition. However, the lack of oral food uptake also induced a significant ($p = 0.0006$) decrease of mean plasma busulfan trough levels in the group of fasting patients as compared to the orally fed patients (350 ng/ml vs. 500 ng/ml) (Fig.1).

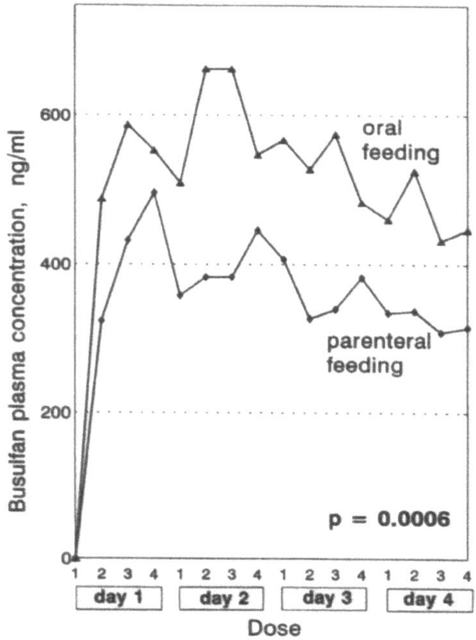

Fig. 1. Busuflan steady-state levels in relation to enteral ($n = 13$) vs. parenteral ($n = 18$) feeding

Effects of Busulfan Pharmacology on Treatment Effectivity. A further analysis evaluated the impact of busulfan pharmacology on treatment effectivity. To this end, we compared busulfan trough concentrations in 16 patients with ongoing disease-free survival to five patients who relapsed after bone marrow transplantation (median time to relapse = 14 months, range = 5–18 months). This evaluation demonstrated that busulfan trough concentrations were significantly ($p = 0.036$) greater in relapsed as compared to disease-free patients.

Effect of Phenytoin and Diazepam on Busulfan Pharmacokinetics. To evaluate the effect of anticonvulsant treatment with the enzyme-inducing agent phenytoin on busulfan plasma concentrations, an analysis of busulfan steady-state levels was performed in 30 patients (Fig. 2). It was demonstrated that in these patients mean busulfan plasma concentrations significantly ($p = 0.01$) decreased from dose four to dose 15 (400 ng/ml vs. 281 ng/ml). For comparison, busulfan

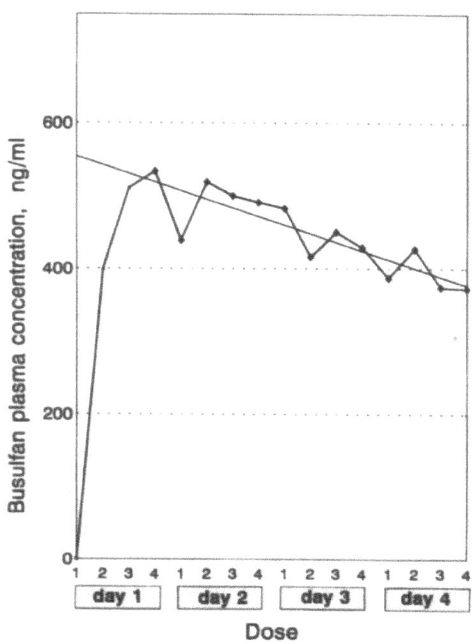

Fig. 2. Steady-state busulfan concentrations during phenytoin prophylaxis ($n = 30$)

steady-state levels were evaluated in ten patients who received anticonvulsant prophylaxis with diazepam. In this patient group, a decline of busulfan concentrations could not be observed (Fig. 3).

Discussion

The primary goal of this study was to introduce a pharmacologically directed adjustment of busulfan dosing during conditioning treatment for bone marrow transplantation. This approach had been prompted by reports indicating a correlation of busulfan-associated toxicity and the AUC of busulfan in plasma. An initial analysis of the plasma pharmacokinetics of busulfan in eight patients during days 1–4 of treatment came to the conclusion that absorption of the drug followed multicompartment kinetics and was highly variable in each patient. Considering two- to seven fold differences of steady-state concentrations in single patients, it was clear that a targeting of busulfan AUCs was not possible. Moreover, it was apparent that the great *interpatient* variability of busulfan bioavailability might also translate into a considerably variable effectivity of conditioning treatment.

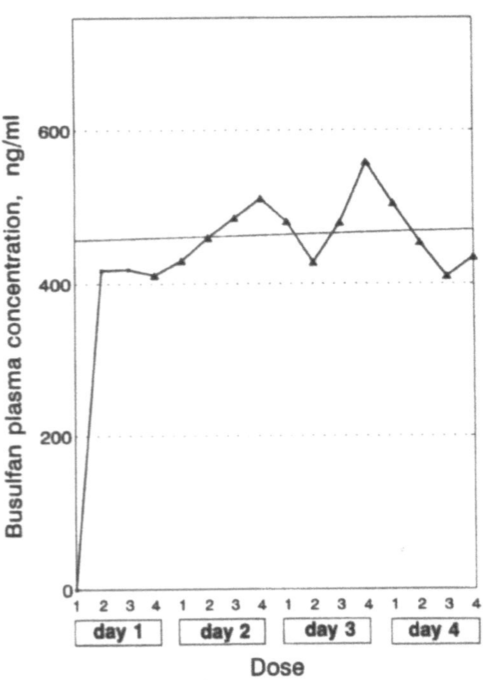

Fig. 3. Steady-state busulfan concentrations during diazepam prophylaxis ($n = 10$)

Consequently, the next step of investigation was to lower the *intrapatient* and *interpatient* variability of busulfan pharmacokinetics. Busulfan is a lipophilic drug. It was therefore assumed that differences in food composition might have an impact on gastrointestinal drug absorption. To evaluate the importance of food uptake we compared 13 orally fed patients with 18 fasting patients who received parenteral feeding. The fasting condition was chosen, on the one hand, to introduce an element of uniformity and, on the other hand, to investigate the true importance of food uptake.

In fact, it was shown that fasting induced a significant stabilization of busulfan trough concentrations during the course of treatment not only for single patients, but also in the interpatient comparison. Another effect of fasting was demonstrated to be a highly significant ($p = 0.0006$) decrease of busulfan bioavailability (Fig. 1). It may be hypothesized that gastrointestinal absorption of busulfan is improved in the presence of a lipophilic milieu which is provided by concurrent uptake of lipophilic food components.

Since fasting of patients improved the uniformity of busulfan pharmacology, but since it also decreased the trough concentrations, it was of interest to investigate the importance of busulfan trough levels for treatment outcome. Therefore, 16 patients with ongoing disease-free survival were compared to another five patients who relapsed after bone marrow transplantation. This analysis demonstrated that relapsed patients had greater busulfan trough levels than disease-free patients. It was concluded that at a busulfan dose of 4 × 1 mg/kg (days 1–4) through levels of busulfan were not determinants of treatment effectively. Further studies need to clarify if this also holds true for the relationship between busulfan peak concentrations and treatment outcome.

During the pharmacological analysis of 30 patients, it became apparent that busulfan steady-state levels continuously decreased in the course of treatment (Fig. 2). From dose four (day 1) to dose 15 (day 4) mean busulfan steady-state concentrations decreased by 27%. Elimination of busulfan from the plasma primarily occurs by metabolic conversion which in a rat model primarily takes place in the liver [5]. The decrease of busulfan steady-state concentrations may therefore be explained by an enhanced hepatic drug metabolism which initially had been assumed to be induced by an autoinduction of busulfan metabolism [6]. However, since all patients received anticonvulsant prophylaxis with phenytoin, a known enzyme-inducing agent, it was suggested that phenytoin might be responsible for an increased hepatic metabolism of busulfan [7-9]. To test this hypothesis, the following ten patients received diazepam for anticonvulsant prophylaxis (Fig. 3). In fact, a decline of busulfan plasma concentrations was not observed in this patient group. In conclusion, the enzyme-inducing activity of phenytoin most likely increases hepatic metabolism of busulfan and thereby decreases busulfan steady-state levels during the course of conditioning treatment. Since diazepam does not affect busulfan pharmacokinetics, this drug might be preferred for anticonvulsant prophylaxis during high-dose busulfan conditioning treatment.

References

1. Peters WP, Henner WD, Grochow LB, Olsen G, Edwards S, Stanbuck H, Stuart A, Gockerman J, Moore J, Bast RC, Seigler HF, Colvin OM. Clinical and pharmacological effects of high-dose single agent busulfan with autologous bone marrow support in the treatment of solid tumors. Cancer Res 47: 6402–6406, 1987
2. Santos GW, Tutschka PJ, Brookmeyer R, Saral R, Beschorner WE, Bias WB, Braine HG, Burns WH, Elfenbien GJ, Kaizer H, Mellits D, Sensenbrenner LL, Stuart RK, Yeager AM. Marrow transplantation for acute non-lymphoblastic leukemia after treatment with busulfan and cyclophosphamide. N Engl J Med 309: 1347–1352, 1983
3. Grochow LB, Jones RJ, Bundrett RB, Braine HG, Chen T-L, Saral R, Santos GW, Colvin OM. Pharmacokinetics of busulphan: correlation with veno-occlusive disease in patients undergoing bone marrow transplantation. Cancer Chemother Pharmacol 25: 55–61, 1989
4. Blanz J, Rosenfeld C, Proksch B, Ehninger G. Quantification of busulfan in plasma by high-performance liquid chromatography using postcolumn photolysis. J Chromatography 532: 429–437, 1990
5. Hassan M, Ehrsson H. Metabolism of ^{14}C-busulfan in isolated perfused rat liver. Eur J Drug Metab Pharmacokinet 12: 71–76, 1987
6. Hassan M, Öberg G, Ehrsson H, Ehrnebo M, Wallin I, Smedmyr B, Tötterman T, Eksborg S, Simonsson B. Pharmacokinetics and metabolic studies of high-dose busulfan in adults. Eur J Clin Pharmacol 36: 525–530, 1989
7. Fitzsimmons WE, Ghalie R, Kaizer H. Anticonvulsants and busulfan. Ann Intern Med 112: 552–553, 1990
8. Fitzsimmons WE, Ghalie R, Kaizer H. The effect of hepatic enzyme inducers on busulfan neurotoxicity and myelotoxicity. Cancer Chemother Pharmacol 27: 226–228, 1990
9. Hassan M, Ölberg G, Björkholm M, Wallin I, Lindgren M. Influence of prophylactic anticonvulsant therapy on high-dose busulphan kinetics. Cancer Chemother Pharmacol 33: 181–186, 1993

Acute Leukemias VI
Prognostic Factors
and Treatment Strategies
Büchner et al. (eds)

Topoisomerase II Activities in Human Leukemic Cells and Their Sensitivity to Anthracyclines and Podophyllotoxines

F. Gieseler[1], A. Glasmacher[2], D. Kämpfe[3], V. Nüßler[4], S. Valsamas[1], J. Kunze[1], and M. Clark[1]

Abstract. With the purpose of defining prognostic factors for cellular response to treatment with topoisomerase II (topo II) inhibitors, we determined topo II activities in human leukemic cells and the in vitro sensitivity of these cells to topo II inhibitors. The cells from 76 patients with chronic lymphocytic leukemia (CLL, $n=28$), chronic myelogonous leukemia (CML, $n=18$), and acute myeloid leukemia (AML, $n=30$) were examined. Fresh specimens from either peripheral blood or bone marrow were partially separated by Ficoll gradient and examined by light microscopy. Only samples with at least 80% of the cells of interest were taken into account. Either decatenation activity or relaxation activity after inhibition of topo I by camptothecin were determined in units by dilution. Under high-stringency conditions with 240 mm KGlu, two different topo II activities could be detected by their different pH optima. The activity, with its maximum at pH 8.9 (topo II α), could be inhibited by daunorubicin, doxorubicin, idarubicin, and etoposide. In contrast, the second activity with its maximum peak at pH 7.9 (topo II β) could not be inhibited. Although the topo II α activity seems to be the target substrate of these drugs, the topo II β activity is important for the sensitivity of the cells to daunorubicin and idarubicin. AML cells with a activity ratio of topo II α/β of > 1.51 were significantly more sensitive than cells with a ratio of ≤ 1.51 (daunorubicin $P=0.036$, idarubicin $P=0.164$). In CLL and CML, we found a positive correlation between the topo II β activity and the IC_{90} of anthracyclines and podophyllotoxines.

Obviously, the topo II α activity is inhibited by these drugs, but the survival of the cells notably depends on the topo II β activity, i.e., that cells with a high topo II β activity survive the treatment.

Introduction

Topoisomease II inhibitors belong to the most important cytostatic drugs. They are widely used in the therapy of leukemia. Nevertheless, we still do not know the exact molecular mechanisms of how they induce cell death. Cellular resistance to these drugs is one of the major problems in therapy and its prediction would be of high value. It is known that topo II is the target structure of acridines, epipodophyllotoxins, and anthracyclines [1, 2]. Two different isoforms named topo II α and topo II β and additional posttranscriptional modifications have been described [3, 6] Owing to these modification, there is no direct correlation between gene transcription and the activity of topos. This is one of the reasons why we determined the cellular activity of topo II. In this paper, we present the results of an ongoing study in which we looked for a correlation between the cellular sensitivity to topo II inhibitors and the activity of topo II in leukemic cells.

[1]Medizinische Poliklinik der Universität Würzburg, Germany
[2]Medizinische Klinik und Poliklinik der Universität Bonn, Germany
[3]Universitätsklinikum Kröllwitz, Halle, Germany
[4]Klinikum Großhadern, Medizinische Klinik III, Munich Germany

Material and Methods

We examined 76 samples from patients with acute and chronic leukemias. Fresh patient cells from peripheral blood or bone marrow were examined within 30 h. Cells were separated using a Ficoll gradient and standard methods. Aliquots were examined by light microscopy after preparing centrifuge slides and staining the cells. Only samples with >80% of the cells of interest were taken into account. The cells were washed twice with cold phosphate-buffered saline (PBS), resuspended in 3.5 ml lysine buffer (0.3 *M* sucrose; 0.5 m*M* EDTA pH 8.0; 60 m*M* KCl; 15 m*M* HEPES pH 7.5; μ*M* spermidine; 50 μ*M*. Lysis buffer—spermin 0.5ml containing 20 μl triton X-100 was added and then put on ice for 15 min. To prevent clumping, the cells were mixed gently several times. The optimal cell quantities, are 5×10^6–5×10^7 although as few as 1×10^6 cells may be used with good results (80%–90% nuclei recovery). After centrifugation the nuclei were resuspended in 100–500μl lysis buffer and then laid upon 1 ml lysis buffer with 30% sucrose in 1.5 ml reaction tubes, the nuclei were separated from cytoplasmic and membrane proteins by centrifugation. Nuclei were resuspended in extraction buffer (5m*M* $KHPO_4$, pH 7.4; 100 m*M* NaCl, 10 m*M* 2-mercaptoethanol, 5 μl/ml 200 m*M* phenylmethyl sulfonyl fluoride PMSF, in dimethyl sulphoxide DMSO) at a concentration of 3×10^7 nuclei/ml. one fifth volume 5 *M* NaCl was then slowly added and gently mixed. The extract was put on ice for 15 min before centrifuging. The supernatant was loaded on a mini-spin column containing 100 μl heparin sepharose in 5 m*M* $KHPO_4$, 50m*M* NaCl, pH 7.4 and washed with several volumes of the same buffer. The column was subsequently washed with 150 m*M* $KHPO_4$, 100 m*M* NaCl, pH 7.4. Topo II was eluted with 400 m*M* $KHPO_4$, 100 m*M* NaCl, pH 7.4. Relaxation and decatenation assays were done in 0.1 *M* bis-tris-propane, 1 m*M* $MgCl_2$, 15 μg bovine serum albumin (BSA), 1 m*M* adenosine 5^1 triphosphate (ATP), 5 m*M* dithiothrieitol (DTT), and L-glutamic acid monopotassium salt concentrations 120, 180, or 240 m*M* were used.

A sample of 200 ng kDNA was used for decatenation assays, 200 ng pBR322 with 1 μm camptothecin to inhibit topo I was used for relaxation assays. Incubation was done for 30 min at 37°C for all assays. Decatenation assays were incubated for an additional 30 min at room temperature with 4 μl 10 mg/ml proteinase K in 10% Sodium dodecyl sulphate (SDS). The samples were then heated to 65°C for 2–3 min before being run on a 1% tris-borate-EDTA-buffer agarose gel with 100 μl 5mg/ml ethidium bromide/liter TBE. Relaxation assays were run on 1% tris-acetate-EDTA-buffer agarose gels, the samples were not treated by proteinase/SDS to avoid a topo-I-induced open circular form. Gels were scanned using an Apple One Scanner and the amount of DNA quantified by gray scale analysis using the program NIH Image V1.42 on a Macintosh Powerbook 180.

Inhibition of topo isoactivities was performed with HL60 cells. The cells were incubated with idarubicin (200 ng/ml), daunorubicin (500 ng/ml), and etoposide (2500 ng/ml). Condition I is the control activity before incubation, condition II after 2.5 h incubation, condition III after 8 h incubation. After incubation, the cells were washed twice with buffer and then processed as described above.

In vitro determination of cellular sensitivity was done by incubation of the cells in various drug concentrations. Viability was examined by using the alamar blue assay which is a colorimetric determination of the ability of the cells to reduce a substrate analogue to the widely used methyl-thiazol-tetrazolium (MTT) assay [7].

Statistical analysis was done using the Mann-Whitney U test. Unit definition of topo II activity per 10^4 cells; 1 U topo relaxes 90% plasmid DNA; 200 ng pBr322 per lane; agarose 1% 20V (approximately 18 mAmp), 18 h; inhibition of topo I by 1 μm camptothecin.

Results

Two topo II activities could be found in all the cells we examined. We have previously described that, under the conditions we used,these activities can be discriminated without overlap by their pH optima [8, 9]. In order to find out which isoactivity is inhibited by anthracyclines and (epi) podophyllotoxines, we performed the experiments shown in Fig. 1. Tapoisomerase II alpha is the is the intracellular target for authracylines and epipodophyllotoxins in HL-60 leukemia cells.

The distribution of the cellular sensitivities was non-parametric for all cells. For this reason, we expressed the result in median and the 25% and 75% percentiles. Thirty samples from

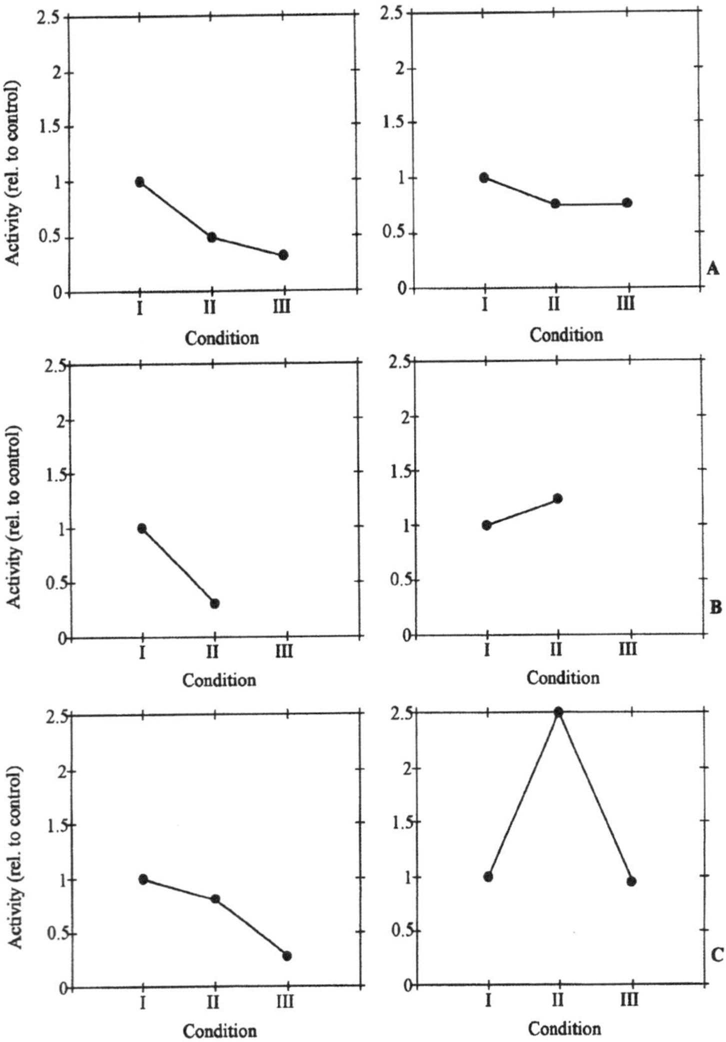

Fig. 1A–C. Topo II activities after incubation of HL 60 cells with topo II inhibitors. *Left*, topo IIα, pH 8.9; *Right*, topo II·, pH 7.9. **A** idarubicin; **B** daunorsicin **C** etoposide

patients with AML were examined. The sensitivities and topo II activities are shown in Table 1. Table 2 shows the statistically significant correlations. AML cells with a high topo II alphalbeta ratio (<1.51, median) were significantly they more sensitive to anthracyelines. Twently-eight samples from patients with CLL (Table 3) and 18 from patients with (Table 4) were examined. An in the samples from AML and CLL, we found no statistically significant relation between the LD_{90} drug sensitivities and the activity of topo II α The following drug sensitivities in CML. correlated significantly with the topo II β activity ($n=8$): daunorubicin (p value 0.08), idarubicin (p value 0.022), etoposide (p value 0.046), teniposide (p value 0.056).

Discussion

Seventy-six samples from patients with AML, CLL, and CML have been examined. In all examined leukemic cells, we found two topo II activities which could be separated by their different

Table 1. Sensitivities and topo II activities of AML cells[a] ($n = 30$)

	25th Percentile	Median	75th Percentile
Daunorubicin	58.59	375.15	3820.00
Doxorubicin	288.05	1685.50	13 470.00
Idarubicin	24.29	215.20	4920.50
Etoposide	22 035.00	42 845.00	72 967.50
Teniposide	5163.75	9246.00	11 772.50
Topo IIα	1.04	3.33	6.67
Topo IIβ	0.83	1.67	3.33
Ratio topo IIα/β	1.00	1.50	2.00

[a] Sensitivity (IC_{90} ng/ml), topo II activity (U).

Table 2. Statistically significant correlations (AML cells)[a]

	Ratio α/β ≤ 1.51	Ratio α/β > 1.51	p value
Daunorubicin	985.00	93.00	0.0364
Idarubicin	3626.00	41.00	0.0164

[a] Mann-Whitney U test, sensitivity (IC_{90} ng/ml), topo II activity (U).

Table 3. Sensitivities and topo II activities of CLL cells[a] ($n = 28$)

	25th Percentile	Median	75th Percentile
Daunorubicin	70.20	1946.00	8277.00
Doxorubicin	226.45	1994.00	28012.50
Idarubicin	84.69	1106.00	5657.00
Etoposide	18270.00	23980.00	54550.00
Teniposide	2630.00	5864.00	10970.00
Topo IIα	0.83	5.00	10.00
Topo IIβ	0.63	1.67	5.00
Ratio topo IIα/β	1.00	1.50	2.00

[a]Sensitivity (IC_{90} ng/ml), topo II activity (U).

Table 4. Sensitivities and topo II activities of CML cells [a] ($n = 18$)

	25th Percentile	Median	75th Percentile
Daunorubicin	623.25	7221.50	11137.50
Doxorubicin	3907.00	80460.00	163202.50
Idarubicin	1037.55	5022.00	10967.50
Etoposide	44320.00	83325.00	97745.00
Teniposide	6202.50	11375.00	20180.00
Topo IIα	0.47	1.25	3.12
Topo IIβ	0.42	1.25	3.12
Ratio topo IIα/β	0.83	1.14	2.00

[a] Sensitivity (IC 90 ng/ml), topo II activity (U).

pH optima in assay conditions with high ionic strength. One activity, topo II α, had it peak at pH 8.9; the second, topo II-β, peaked at pH 7.9. Incubation of HL 60 promyelocytic leukemic cells with drugs which are known to inhibit topo II resulted in the selective inhibition of the topo II α activity. Only idarubicin had a slight (less that 25%) inhibitory effect on the topo II β activity. At least 79% of the topo II α activity was inhibited by idarubicin, daunorubicin, and etoposide within 8 h after incubation of the cells. Although topo II α is the target activity for topo II inhibiting cytostatics, the topo II β activity seems to be important for the sensitivity of leukemic cells to treatment. The numbers of the examined leukemia samples are too small to form subgroups, which would probably increase the significance of statistical tests especially in heterogeneous cell populations such as CML samples. Nevertheless, neither in AML cells nor in CLL and CML cells did we find a relation ship between the topo II activity and the sensitivity of the cells. Howevers in the three leukemias we found a positive correlation either between the ratio of topo II α/β or directly with the topo II β· activity.

The inhibition of topos does not kill the cells directly, but the cellular response to the induced DNA damage plays an important role. This response depends on biological cellular factors such as differentiation, proliferation and the repair capacity [10–12]. Obviously, the inhibition of topo isoforms is not sufficient for cell death if the cell has enough topo activity left for the necessary DNA repair. In childhood ALL, the expression of topo II β could be correlated to cellular sensitivity to adriamycin and etoposide [13]. These findings support our results, although, due to posttranslational modifications, the gene expression and the activity of topos cannot be compared directly.

References

1. Zunio F, Capranico G. DNA toposiomerase II as the primary target of anti-tumor anthracyclines. Anticancer Drug Des 1990; 5(4): 307–17.
2. Zwelling LA, Estey E, Bakic M, Silbermann L, Chan D. Topoisomerase II as a target of Antileukemic Drugs. NCI Monogr. 1987; 4: 79–82.
3. Coderoni S, Paparelli M, Gianfranceschi GL. Specific regulatory role of phosphroylation of calf thymus DNA-topoisomerase I smaller forms on the relaxational activity expression. Phosphorylation role on Topo I smaller form activity. Mol Biol Rep 1992; 16(2): 75–80.
4. Davies SL, Jenkins JR, Hickson ID. Human cells express two differently spliced forms of topoisomerase beta mRNA. Nucl. Acid Res. 1993; 21: 3719–3723.
5. De Vore R, Corbett AH, Osheroff N. Phosphorylation of topoisomerase II by casein kinase II and protein kinase C: effects on enzyme-mediated DNA cleavage\religation and sensitivity to the antineoplastic drugs etoposide and 4'-(9-acridinylamino) methane-sulfon-m-anisidide. Cancer Res 1992; 52(8): 2156–61.
6. Tan KB, Dorman TE, Falls KM, et al. Topoisomerase IIa and Topoisomerase IIβ Genes: Characterization and Mapping to Human Chromosomes 17 and 3, Respectively. Cancer Research 1992; 52: 231–234.
7. Kaspers GJL, Veerman AJP, Pieters R, et al. In Vitro Cytotoxicity of Mitoxantrone, Daunorubicin and doxorubicin in Untreated Childhood Acute Leukemia. Leukemia 1994; 8(1(Jan.)): 24–29.
8. Gieseler F, Glasmacher A, Kämpfe D, et al. Topoisomerase II activities in AML-blasts and their correlation with cellular sensitivity to anthracyclines and epipodophyllotoxines. Leukemia 1996; 10: 46–53.
9. Clark M, Gieseler F. A method for the determination of topoisomerase II alpha and beta activity in patient cells. Proc AACR 1994; 34: 209.
10. Evan GI, Wyllie AH, Gibert CS, et al. Induction of apoptosis in fibroblasts by c-myc protein. Cell 1992; 69: 119–122.
11. Kamesaki S, Kamesaki H, Jorgensen TJ, Tanizawa A, Pommier Y, Cossman J. bcl-2 Protein inhibits etoposide-induced apoptosis through its effects on events subsequent to topoisomerase II-induced DNA strand breaks and their repair. Cancer Res. 1933; 53: 4251–4256.
12. Lotem J, Cragoe EJ, Sachs L. Rescue from programmed cell death in leukemic and normal myeloid cells. Blood 1991; 78: 953–956.
13. Brown GA, McPherson JP, Gu L, et al. Relationship of DNA topoisomerase II alpha and beta expression to cytotoxicity of antineoplastic agents in human acute lymphoblastic leukemia cell lines. Cancer Res 1995; 55(1): 78–82.

Acute Leukemias VI
Prognostic Factors
and Treatment Strategies
Büchner et al. (eds)

Quantitative Cytosine Arabinoside Metabolism in HL60 and Raji Cells Using a Novel High Performance Liquid Chromatography Assay for Detection and Quantitation of ^{3}H-Cytosine Arabinoside and Its Metabolites

J. Braess, J. Pförtner, C.C. Kaufmann, B. Ramsauer, M. Unterhalt, W. Hiddemann, and E. Schleyer

Abstract. An ion-pair high-performance liquid chromatography assay involving solid-phase scintillation detection was established for rapid identification and quantitation of all major metabolites of tritium-labeled cytosine arabinoside (ara-C) in an in vitro system. In a single run of 55 min ara-C, ara-CMP, ara-CDP-cholin, ara-CDP, ara-U, ara-UMP, ara-CTP, ara-UDP, and ara-UTP can be measured and quantitated. The presented method is fast, sensitive, with various limits of detection ranging from 40 to 200 pg (absolute), and highly reproducible. Metabolic profiles of HL60 and Raji cells following incubation with ara-C were established using this technique.

Introduction

Cytosine arabinoside (ara-C) is a widely used cytotoxic agent in the treatment of various hematological malignancies and comprises the background of therapy especially in acute myeloid leukemias (AML). Besides the kinetics of plasma concentrations, most investigators have focussed on the triphosphorylated metabolite of cytosine arabinoside (ara-CTP) which is considered to constitute the major determinant of cytotoxicity [8]. Several assays for the detection and quantitation of this substance have been published [9, 12, 13] and were used to analyze ara-CTP pharmacokinetics in relation to clinical response. A prospective comparative evaluation of 1.0 vs. 3.0 g/m^2 ara-C clearly indicated a superior response to high-dose therapy in selected patients with AML refractory to conventional therapies and, since at these plasma concentrations ara-CTP formation will be maximum, strongly suggests that additive mechanisms must be involved in ara-C-mediated cytotoxicity [2–4]. One potential way of action could be the impairment of cell membrane integrity through the interaction with phosphatidylcholin formation as suggested by recent investigations [1, 7]. Hence deeper insights into the intracellular metabolism of ara-C are needed to further elucidate its mechanisms of action.

In order to provide a means for a more exact and more specific evaluation of the intracellular metabolism of ara-C, a highly sensitive and specific high-performance liquid chromatography (HPLC) assay involving tritium labeled ara-C (^{3}H-ara-C) was developed for the quantitation of all major intracellular metabolites of ara-C. Using this assay the individual profiles of HL60 and Raji cells regarding their formation of intracellular metabolites of ara-C at a clinically relevant concentration of 1 µg/ml were evaluated. Kinetics of the intracellular formation of ara-C metabolites during dose escalation were established for Raji cells.

Method and Materials

Materials. Tritium-labeled cytosine arabinoside (^{3}H-ara-C) was purchased from Amersham (Great Britain). All nucleotides used as standards were provided by Sigma (Germany). Salts and reagents were of analytical quality and were

Department of Hematology and Oncology, University of Göttingen, Germany supplied by Merck (Darmstadt, Germany). All solvents (HPLC quality) were obtained from Baker (Gross-Gerau, Germany). PIC A low UV (tetrabutylammonium-phosphate) was purchased from Waters (Erkrath, Germany).

HPLC Apparatus. The chromatographic system involves an HPLC pump type 501 (Waters, Erkrath, Germany), a pulsation reducer type LP21 (Scientific Systems Inc., USA), a 500-µl injection loop (Macherey and Nagel, Düren, Germany), a low-pressure mobile phase selection valve (model 5011, Macherey and Nagel, Düren, Germany), an injection valve type 7125 (Rheodyne, Germany) and 1/16" HPLC capillaries. As solid phases a 30.5-min 5 µ C_{18} precolumn and a 250/1/4"/4,6-120-5µ C_{18} reversed phase column as the analytical column were used (both by Macherey and Nagel). Detection of the radioactive signal was performed by Ramona 92 scintillation counter (Raytest, Germany). While establishing the respective calibration curves for each metabolite a liquid scintillation counter type Mark III (Searle Analytic Inc; USA) was also used.

HPLC Conditions. Initially a weak eluent containing 0.0025 mol PIC A (also providing a 0.0001-mol phosphate buffer) and 0.2% acetonitrile at a pH of 3.0 is employed at a flow rate of 0.8 ml/min. After 18 min the flow rate is gradually increased to 1.5 ml/min in the course of one min. This flow is maintained for 27 min resulting in a total of 45 min for one analysis. After 13.5 ml of the first eluent have passed through the system, it is exchanged for the stronger one consisting of 0.1 mol KH_2PO_4, 0.005 mol PIC A, and 0.5% acetonitrile at a pH of 2.7. Nine minutes before the end of the analysis, the weak eluent is reconnected by switching the low pressure valve. After reequilibration and reduction of the flow to 0.7 ml/min, a new measurement can be started.

Solid Scintillation HPLC Detector. ^{3}H-ara-C and its metabolites are detected by a solid scintillation detector. This means a molecule like ara-CDP-cholin, even though more than twice the molecular weight of ara-C, will produce the same signal as the lighter molecule—because each molecule bears the same amount of radioactivity, i.e., one tritium atom. Therefore, ideally a calibration curve for ^{3}H-ara-C would be representative of the calibration curves of all its derivates and needs only be corrected for the different molecular weights.

Some of the negatively charged substances will interact with CaF_2 in the detector cell and will therefore produce some tailing of their respective chromatographic peaks. Whereas knowledge of the molecular weights of the respective substances will solve the first problem, the "tailing problem" is solved by the use of a liquid scintillation counter which is not influenced by this particular chemical interaction.

Liquid Scintillation Counter. In the case of the Mark III 6880 liquid scintillation counter, the signal of the counter is proportional to the number of emitting particles in the samples. Considering the relative molecular weights of the various compounds, the calibration curves for liquid scintillation detection can be interchanged. In the case of ara-C, which is available as a radioactive compound, a regular calibration curve could be derived from measurements of aqueous standards using the solid scintillation detector. In the case of the other compounds, an alternative method had to be used. During measurements of cell samples following incubation with tritium-labeled ara-C regular chromatograms via the solid scintillation detector were taken and at the same time on-line sampling of the eluent containing the respective front of the substance was performed. In this scenario all derivates of ^{3}H-ara-C will be formed intracellularly during the incubation process. Peaks are first identified via the chromatogram but then quantitated using liquid scintillation detection of the on-line samples. The amounts of substance found during liquid scintillation detection are then correlated with their respective Area under the peak during solid scintillation producing excellent correlations for all substances involved in more than 20 such experiments. The tailing problem was thus "circumvented" since liquid scintillation is not influenced by any possible interaction between the different metabolites and $CaFl_2$.

Peak Identification. In order to define the order of elution and to establish the exact retention times of ara-C and its metabolites an ultraviolet (UV) detector was set up immediately in front of the solid scientillation detector when developing this assay. With ara-C, ara-CTP, and ara-U being available as aqueous non-radioactive (and in the case of ara-C also as tritium labeled) standards, the retention times of ara-CMP, ara-CDP and ara-CDP-cholin were approximated by their cytidine analogues CMP, CDP, and CDP-cholin [13]. The relative positions of ara-UMP, ara-UDP, and ara-UTP in the order of elution were established by their respective uridine analogues UMP, UDP, and UTP which are commercially available. In order to present all these findings in a single graph, a complex measurement involving a mixture of an aqueous solution (containing ara-C, CMP, CDP-cholin, ara-U, CDP, UMP ara-CTP, UDP—plus uridine and dCTP as further landmarks) and a prepared sample of cells following incubation with ^{3}H-ara-C (therefore containing the tritium-labeled equivalents of these substances) was performed.

Cell Incubation. Raji, HL60, and K562 were used for validation of this assay; 0.5 × 10^6 cells of both cell lines/1ml RPMI medium were exposed to a concentration of 1 µg/ml ^{3}H-ara-C for 5 h. Dose escalation of 1, 2.5, 5, 12.5 and 25 µg/ml (a mixture of tritium-labeled and unlabeled ara-C) was performed for Raji cells in order to establish the kinetics of the formation of the various ara-C metabolites.

Sample Preparation. Cells were washed and then lyzed by adding 120 µl weak eluent. After final centrifugation of the sample, the eluent is separated from the cell debris, filtered, and then frozen at −20°C until analysis.

Results

Specificity

With detection depending on radioactivity, no coeluting substances but metabolites of ^{3}H-ara-C were detected. ^{3}H-ara-C was shown to have a retention time of 5:46 min with its deaminated metabolite ^{3}H-ara-U running at 13:22 min. The phosphorylated metabolites ^{3}H-ara-CMP, ^{3}H-ara-CDP, and ^{3}H-ara-CTP revealed retention times of 7:00, 15:32 and 23:76 min, respectively. ^{3}H-ara-CDP-cholin was detected at 7:46 min which is 0:52 min later than its cytidine equivalent CDP-cholin. A similar finding was observed for ^{3}H-ara-UMP which was preceded by UMP also by 0:52 min. A representative chromatogram illustrating these findings is shown in Fig. 1.

Intra- and Interday Variance, Recovery. Following incubation an aliquot of the cells was first washed and then measured via liquid scintillation counting without any prior sample preparation, thereby representing the total radioactivity contained in the cells. Cells were then prepared in the way described above and an aliquot was taken for measurement of the amount of tritium-labeled molecules. An average of 85% of the total radioactivity was thus shown to remain in the cell extract, another 10% was found in the cell pellet.

In order to demonstrate the intra- and interday variance of the assay ten cell incubations and measurements were performed on a single day for the former and another ten on 10 consecutive days for the latter. Following incubation the cells were pooled and then again separated into ten distinct samples in order to differentiate the variances resulting from sample separation and from the HPLC assay as such from variations due to incubation conditions. The variation coefficients representing both intraday and interday variances are given in Table 1 ranging from 9.8% as intraday variance for ara-CDP-cholin to 21.4% for ara-C (at a concentration of 100 pg).

Limit of Detection

A signal twice to six times the noise depending on the amount of tailing was defined as the limit of detection (LOD). The respective LODs for ara-C, ara-CMP, ara-CDP-cholin, ara-U, ara-CDP, ara-UMP, and ara-CTP were 40, 80, 70, 90, 100, 100, and 110 pg. Ara-UDP and ara-UTP were detected in few measurements and at very low concentrations. Since in these measurements they demonstrated a nearly identical chromatographic behavior (tailing) as their respective counterparts (ara-CDP and ara-CTP) but appeared later in the chromatogram, similar LODs of 150 pg for ara-UDP and 200 pg for ara-UTP were defined.

Quantitation

In the case of ^{3}H-ara-C a calibration curve using aqueous standards was combined with results of multiple cell incubations wherein ^{3}H-ara-C had not only been detected by HPLC solid scintillation detection but also had been quantitated via sampling and consecutive liquid scintillation counting. The excellent correlation (r=0.98) of

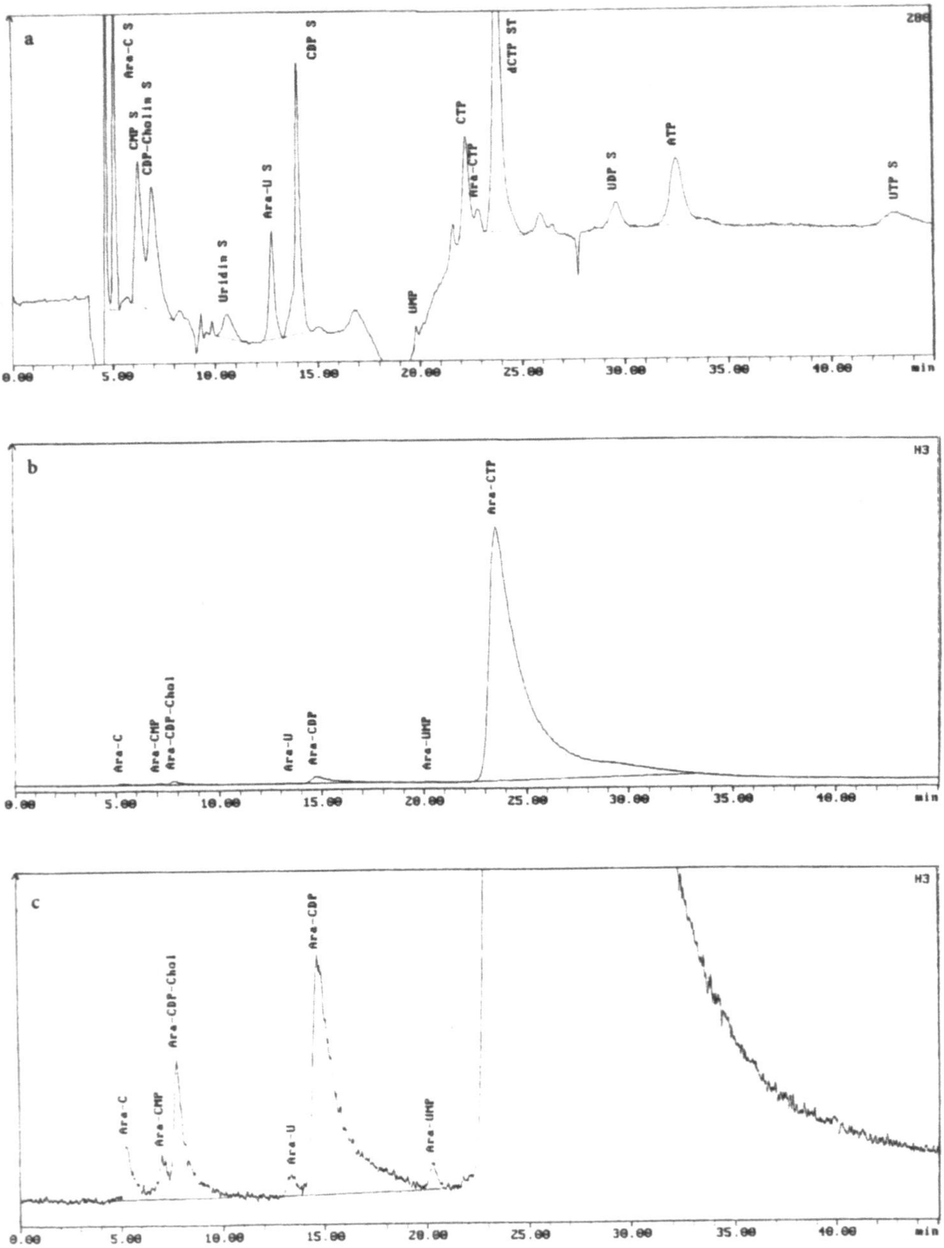

Fig. 1. **a** UV detection (280 nm) of a chromatogram of $0.5.10^6$ HL60 cells incubated with 1µg/ml^{3}H-ara-C for 5 h spiked with ara-C, CMP, CDP-cholin, uridine, ara-U, CDP, UMP, CTP, Ara-CTP, UDP, and UTP (marked with "S") **b** Simultaneous ^{3}H chromatogram with an ordinate ranging from 0 to 20000 counts per second. **c** Simultaneous ^{3}H chromatogram with an ordinate ranging from 0 to 600 counts per second

Table 1. Characteristics of the individual substances under the conditions of the presented HPLC assay

	^{3}H-ara-C	^{3}H-ara--CMP	^{3}H-ara--CDP-cholin	^{3}H-ara-U	^{3}H-ara--CDP	^{3}H-ara--UMP	^{3}H-ara--CTP
LOD (pg absolute)	40	80	70	90	100	100	110
AUP (pg)	5.02	2.93	3.18	3.50	16.09	1.96	50.48
Correlation coefficient (r)	0.98	0.99	0.98	0.92	0.96	0.73	0.98
Intraday variance (%)	21.4	16.4	9.8	17.7	13.2	11.4	12.0
Interday variance (%)	23.5	18.3	11.2	22.0	18.7	13.8	14.5
Retention time	5: 24	7: 04	7: 78	13: 34	14: 68	20: 28	23: 50

these results is shown in Fig. 2. A slope of 5.02 AUP/pg is found. Calibration curves for the other substances (Fig. 3) were obtained in an identical fashion (initial quantitation via liquid scintillation counting) resulting in slopes (AUP/pg) of 2.93 for ara-CMP, 3.18 for ara-CDP-cholin, 3.50 for ara-U, 16.09 for ara-CDP, 1.96 for ara-UMP, and 50.48 for ara-CTP. The correlation coefficients and variances for each substance are shown in Table 1. Quantitation of ara-UDP and ara-UTP is therefore restricted to determination of whether intracellular formation resulted in concentrations above or below 1.5 ng/ml.10^{7} cells and 2.0 ng/ml.10^{7} cells according to their respective LODs.

Linearity. Linearity of the HPLC analysis was demonstrated for each metabolite by defined

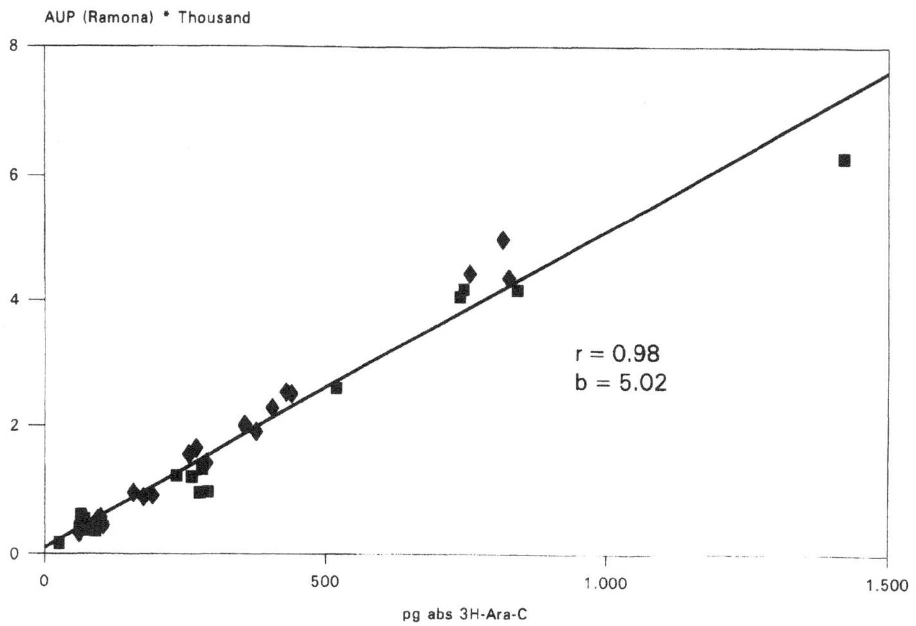

Fig. 2. Regression curve of aqueous ^{3}H-ara-C standards (*rhombi*) combined with the results of multiple intracellular ^{3}H-ara-C measurements of HL60, Raji and K562 samples *squares* following incubation with 1 μg/ml ^{3}H-ara-C for 5 quantitated by HPLC solid scintillation detection (*ordinate*) and liquid scintillation counting (*abscissa*)

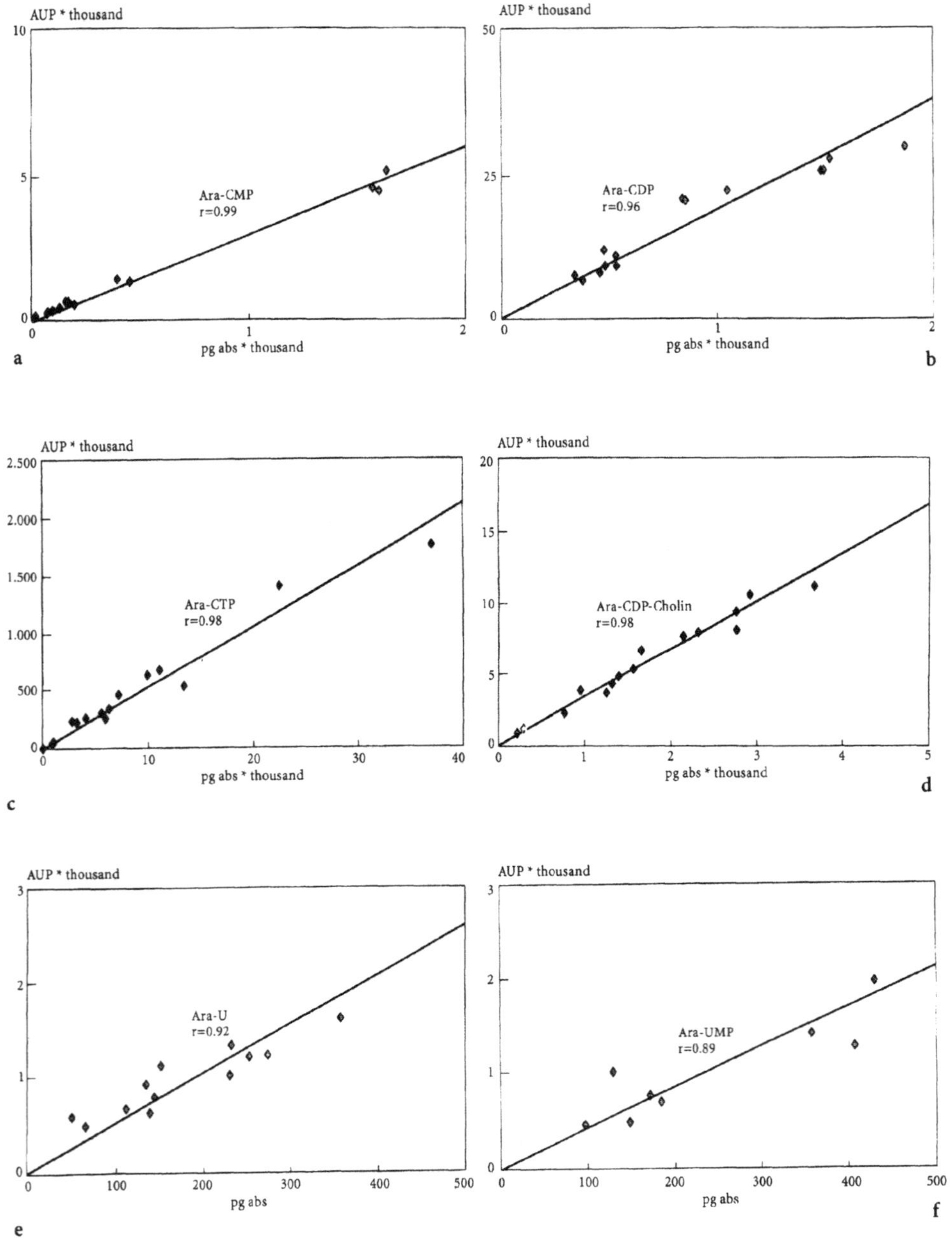

Fig. 3. Regression curves of ^{3}H-ara-C metabolites featuring the results of multiple measurements of HL60, Raji and K562 *samples* following incubation with 1 µg/ml ^{3}H-ara-C for 5 h quantitated by HPLC solid scintillation detection (*ordinate*) and liquid scintillation counting (*abscissa*)

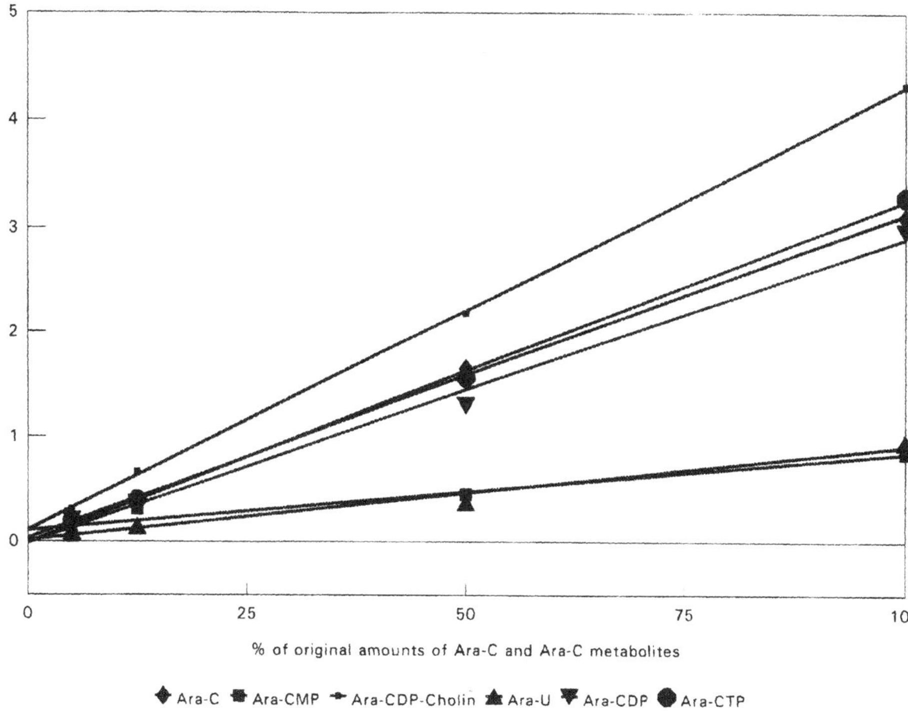

Fig. 4. Regression curves of ^{3}H-ara-C and its metabolites derived from a incubation of Raji cells with 1 µg/ml ^{3}H-ara-U for 5 h with subsequent dilution of sample aliquots (for increased clarity ara-CTP results were divided by five)

dilutions (100%, 50%, 12.5%, and 5% of the original sample) of two pooled samples (1 µg/ml ^{3}H-ara-C for 5 h). Figure 4 demonstrates the linear relation between the measured amounts of the metabolites and their respective dilutions with correlation coefficients ranging from 0.98 to 0.99.

Intracellular ara-C Metabolism in HL60 and RAJI Cells

The intracellular formation of ^{3}H-ara-C metabolites is demonstrated in Fig. 5. For both cell lines measurements were made in triplicate. In HL60 cells an average of 93 ng/ml × 10^7 cells (range 85–102) of ara-CTP was found with ara-C mono- and diphosphates, only reaching levels of 6 and 22 ng/ml × 10^7 cells (range 3–9 17–25), respectively. Ara-CDP-cholin levels are in a similar order at 17 ng/ml × 10^7 cells (range 15–19). In the case of Raji cells moderately higher levels of ara-CTP (139 ng/ml × 10^7 cells, range 125–147) are found. In relation to the triphosphate, the mono- and diphosphates are distinctly less at 7 (range 5–9) and 26 (range 22–29) ng/ml × 10^7 cells. Ara-CDP-cholin levels are higher at 68 (range 57–74) ng/ml × 10^7 cells reaching nearly 50% of the total amount of ara-CTP. In both cell-lines only minute amounts of ara-UMP were found with ara-UDP and ara-UTP remaining below the detection limit. During dose escalation in Raji cells, similar kinetics in the formation for all the various ara-C metabolities can be observed in Fig. 6.

Discussion

Quantitation of ara-CTP via HPLC measurements [12, 13] has led to valuable insights into the kinetics and mechanisms of ara-C cytotoxicity. Nevertheless major issues such as the reason for the efficacy of high-dose ara-C regimens and the membrane alterations during ara-C treatment probably mediated by ara-CDP-cholin

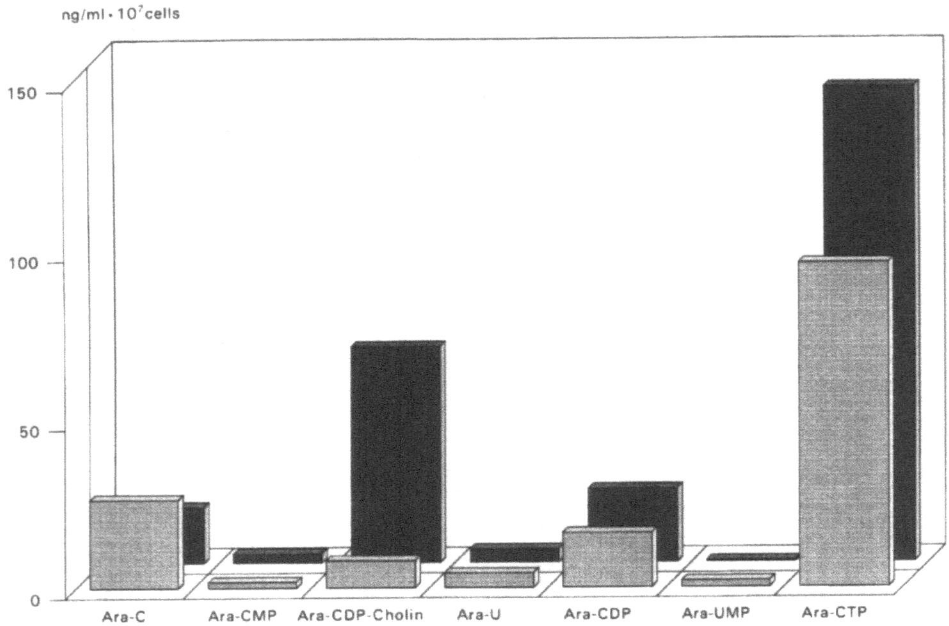

Fig. 5. Amounts of ^{3}H-ara-C and ^{3}H-ara-C metabolites in HL660 (light columns) and Raji (dark columns) cells after an incubation with 1 µg/ml ^{3}H-ara-C for 5 h

remain unclear. To address these topics, a more specific evaluation of the intracellular metabolism of ara-C is required. The present assay was developed in order to provide a means for a sensitive and exact quantitation of all major ara-C metabolites in an in vitro system using tritium-labeled molecules. Under these conditions, ara-C and eight metabolites (ara-CMP, ara-CDP, ara-CTP, ara-CDP-cholin, ara-U, ara-UMP, ara-UDP, and ara-UTP) can be separated and quantitated in a single run. The limits of detection range from 40 pg absolute for ara-C to 110 pg for ara-CTP. Solid scintillation detection provided a convenient and sensitive method of detection so that on-line sampling was only needed initially in order to provide the presented calibration curves for each substance. So far, no other successful attempts [12] for measurements of such a comprehensive panel of intracellular ara-C metabolites have been published.

For the validation of this assay, the metabolic profiles of two cell lines (HL60 and Raji) at one concentration and the kinetics of metabolite formation in Raji cells during dose escalation have been established. Both cell lines had an individual profile concerning the formation of ara-C metabolites and exhibited distinct differences between each other especially concerning ara-CDP-cholin formation. The metabolic profile—represented by the various relations of distinct metabolites to the major metabolite ara-CTP—was nearly constant during dose escalation in Raji cells.

The present assay therefore represents a tool that will provide a new scope in the investigation of the intracellular metabolism of ara-C. It will be used to investigate the differential ara-C metabolism in clinically relevant cell populations (leukemic blasts and normal bone marrow cells) and its possible impact on modified treatment protocols. Such a detailed and quantitative approach will be vital in addressing the issues of ara-C cytotoxicity in high-dose ara-C regimens when deoxycytidine kinase is saturated and in establishing the role of ara-CDP-cholin in the perturbation of cell membranes during ara-C treatment.

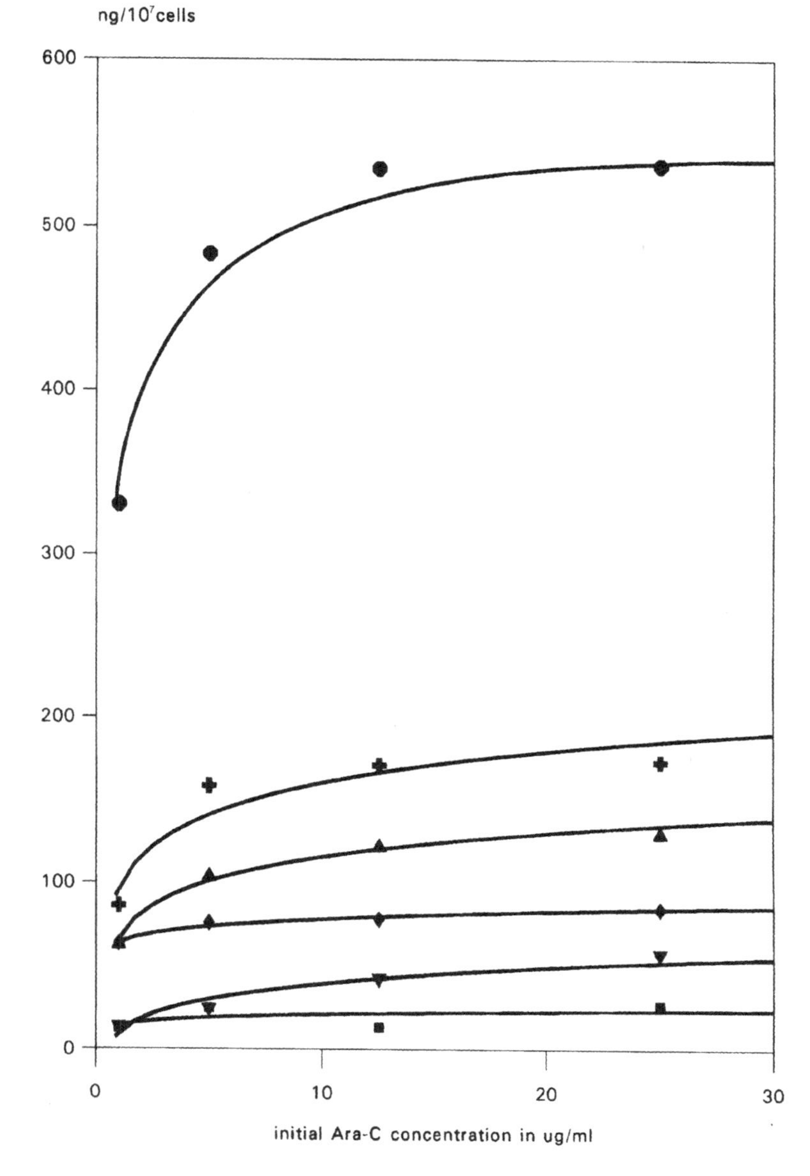

Fig. 6. Kinetics of the formation of ara-C metabolites during dose escalation in Raji cells dose (1, 2.5, 5, 12.5 and 25 μg/ml ara-C (labeled and unlabeled) for 5 h. *Triangles*, are-C; *inverted triangles*, are-CMP, *crosses*, arc-CDP-cholin; *squares*, are-U; *rhombi*, arc-CDP; *circles*, arc-CTP

References

1. Y. Azuma, Y. Onishi, Y. Mizuno, H. Kizaki, Immunopharmacology 26, 235–240 (1993)
2. R.L. Capizzi, M. Poole, M.R. Cooper et al, Blood 63, 694–700 (1984)
3. J.E. Curtis, H.A. Messner, M.D. Minde, S. Minking, E.A. McCulloch, Journal of Clinical Oncology 5, 532–543 (1987)
4. W. Hiddemann, C. Aul, G. Maschmeyer, R. Schönrock-Nabulsi, W.D. Ludwig, A. Bartholomäus, P. Bettelheim, K. Becker, L. Balleisen, B.

Lathan, H. Köppler, T. Grüneisen, R. Donhuisen-Ant, A. Reichle and Th. Büchner, Seminars in Hematology 28, 35–38 (1991)
5. W. Hiddemann, H. Kreutzmann, K. Straif, W.D. Ludwig, R. Mertelsmann, R. Donhuijsen-Ant, E. Lengfelder, Z. Arlin and T. Büchner, Blood 69, 744–749 (1987)
6. W. Hiddemann, E. Schleyer, M. Zühlsdorf, C. Rolf, U. Kewer, C. Uhrmeister, M. Kiehl, B. Wörmann and T. Büchner, Leukemia 12 (Vol. 6), 1273-1280 (1992)
7. G.L. Kucera and R.L. Capizzi, Cancer Research 52, 3886–3891 (1992)
8. D.W. Kufe and D.R. Spriggs, Seminars in Oncology 2, 33–48 (1985)
9. W. Plunkett, S. Chub and B. Barlogie, Journal of Chromatography 221, 425 (1980)
10. W. Plunkett, J.O. Liliemark, T.M. Adams, B. Nowak, E. Estey, H. Kantarjian and M. Keating, Cancer Research 47, 1–7 (1987)
11. W. Plunkett, J.O. Liliemark, E. Estey and M.J. Keating, Semin. Oncol., 14 (Suppl. 1) (1987) 157
12. R.L. Schilsky and F.S. Ordway, Journal of Chromatography 337, 63–71 (1985)
13. E. Schleyer, G. Ehninger, M. Zühlsdorf, B. Proksch and W. Hiddemann, Journal of Chromatography/Biomedical Applications 497, 109–120 (1989)

Acute Leukemias VI
Prognostic Factors
and Treatment Strategies
Büchner et al. (eds)

Role of Deoxycytidine Triphosphate for Feedback Regulation of Deoxycytidine Kinase and Phosphorylation of Cytosine Arabinoside in Whole Leukemic Cells

V. Heinemann[1], L. Schulz[2], A. Debus[1] W. Wilmanns[1,2], and R.D. Issels[1,2]

Abstract. Deoxycytidine (dCyd) kinase (dCK) is the rate-limiting enzyme in the activation of a variety of antimetabolites such as 1-β-D-arabino-furanosylcytosine (ara-C), 2′-chlorodeoxyadenosine or 2′, 2′-difluorodeoxycytidine. In vitro experiments with purified dCK led to the conclusion that dCK activity is tightly regulated by the concentration of deoxycytidine triphosphate (dCTP). This has, however, not been conclusively demonstrated in whole cells. In fact, hydroxyurea (HU), a potent inhibitor of ribonucleotide reductase (RR) depleted dCTP in CEM and Raji cells, but enhanced ara-CTP formation only in the latter cell line. In this study, we analysed dCK activity as a function of dCTP concentration in whole Raji cells and used ara-CTP formation as a measure of enzyme activity. Depletion of dCTP was achieved by three different drugs: HU, 3-deazauridine, and thymidine. 3-Deazauridine acts as an inhibitor of CTP synthetase, an enzyme converting CTP to UTP, while thymidine blocks CDP reduction. In Raji cells, HU (5 m*M*) depleted dCTP to 84% of control and increased dCK activity by 3.7-fold. On the other hand, thymidine (100 μ*M*) and 3-deazauridine (5 μ*M*) caused a reduction of the intracellular dCTP pool to 50% and 20%, respectively. However, dCTP depletion by the latter agents was not associated with an increase of dCK activity compared to control cells. We therefore concluded, that in Raji cells HU-mediated enhancement of dCK activity is not a result of lowered dCTP feedback on dCK. Enhanced ara-CTP formation may, however, be explained by the observation that HU decreased the intracellular dCyd pool, while this was not achieved by exposure to 3-deazauridine. We conclude that HU activates ara-C phosphorylation of dCK predominantly through a depletion of the competing dCyd pool. dCyd depletion is most likely caused by inhibition of the de novo pathway of dCTP synthesis and the associated compensatory activation of the dCTP salvage pathway. Intracellular depletion of dCyd may consequently be regarded as a necessary event which allows HU-mediated enhancement of dCyd analog phosphorylation. Agents which only deplete dCTP without affecting the dCyd pool may not modulate ara-C phosphorylation.

Introduction

Two pathways for cellular deoxycytidine triphosphate (dCTP) synthesis may be differentiated: the *de novo* pathway and the *salvage* pathway. The clinical importance of the dCTP salvage pathway is given by the fact that deoxycytidine (dCyd) analogs like cytosine arabinoside (ara-C) are activated via the salvage pathway. In fact, the non-toxic prodrug ara-C gains its cytotoxic activity only by phosphorylation to the 5'-triphosphate ara-CTP. Deoxycytdine kinase (dCK) is the rate-limiting enzyme for intracellular ara-CTP formation. In vitro experiments performed with purified dCK demonstrated that dCTP, the final product of phosphorylation, acts as a potent feedback inhibitor of this enzyme [1, 2]. The regulatory importance of dCTP was further supported by the observation that deple-

[1]Medizinische Klinik III, University Hospital Grosshadern, University of Munich, Germany
[2]GSF Institute for Clinical Hematology, Munich, Germany

tion of intracellular dCTP as induced by inhibition of the de novo pathway led to an increase of ara-C phosphorylation [3, 4]. Consequently, the working hypothesis was developed that the release of dCTP-mediated feedback inhibition was responsible for enhanced dCK activity. The present study investigates the role of dCTP for regulation of dCK activity in two cell lines, namely CCRF-CEM (T cell line) and Raji cells (B cell line). These cell lines are characterized by considerable differences of deoxynucleotide metabolism, specifically a faster turnover of dNTP in B cells, as opposed to T cells. The study is based on the assumption that common mechanisms of dCK regulation should be working in the cell lines tested. While dCTP depletion was observed in both cell lines when the de novo pathway was inhibited, enhancement of ara-C phosphorylation via the salvage pathway was observed only in Raji cells. It was therefore asked if mechanisms other than dCTP depletion alone may be responsible for the enhancement of ara-C phosphorylation when the de novo pathway is inhibited.

Materials and Methods

[^{3}H]dCyd (specific activity, 24.8 Ci/mmol) and [^{3}H]ara-C (specific activity, 29 Ci/mmol) were products from Amersham (Buckinghmshire, UK). Ara-C, deoxycytidine, hydroxyurea 3-deazauridine, and thymidine were purchased from Sigma Chemical Co., Inc. (St. Louis, MO, USA).

Cell Culture. CCRF-CEM cells and Raji cells were cultured in RPMI 1640 medium (Life Technology, Grand Island, NY, USA) at 37°C in a humidified atmosphere containing 5% CO_2. Cell cultures consistently tested negative for mycoplasma contamination. All experiments were performed with cell in the exponential growth phase. Cell number and mean cell volume were determined by a Coulter counter equipped with a model C-1000 particle analyzer (Counter Electronics Inc, Luton, UK).

Nucleotide Extraction and Analysis. Following incubation with drugs, monolayer cells were washed twice with ice-cold phosphate-buffered saline, and, after centrifugation, the pellet was extracted with 0.4 N $HClO_4$, as previously described [5]. The nucleoside triphosphates in the neutralized acid-soluble extract were analyzed by HPLC using a high-pressure liquid chromatograph (HPLC) equipped with two Waters model 510 pumps, a Waters model 490E detector, and the Maxima 3.10 software (Waters), and IBM computer-based program for pump control and chromatogram evaluation. Anion exchange chromatography was performed using a Partisil-10 SAX column (250 × 4 mm) (Whatman). Extracts of 0.1–10 × 10^6 cell equivalents were injected onto the column by means of the U6K-LC injection system. Cellular metabolites were separated by the procedures outlined below.

Determination of Nucleoside Triphosphates by Anion-Exchange HPLC. From an initial buffer composition of 65% buffer A (0.005 *M* $NH_4H_2PO_4$, pH 2.8) and 35% buffer B (0.75 *M* $NH_4H_2PO_4$, pH 3.49), a concave gradient (curve 9) was run at a rate of 3 ml/min for 30 min concluding with a composition of 100% buffer B. The amount of nucleoside triphosphate (NTP) was determined by external standard quantitation. The concentration of intracellular NTP was calculated by dividing the amount of NTP by the number of cell equivalents analyzed and the mean volume of the cellular H_2O.

Determination of Deoxynucleotides. Degradation of NTP in the $HClO_4$-soluble cell extracts was achieved by periodate oxidation as previously described [6]. The dNTP were separated on a Partisil-10 SAX column at a flow rate of 3 ml/min and a run time of 47 min. After an isocratic elution with 75% buffer A (0.005 *M* $NH_4H_2PO_4$, pH 2.8) and 25% buffer B (0.75 *M* $NH_4H_2PO_4$, pH 3.5) over 20 min, a linear gradient led to 21% buffer A and 79% buffer B (43 min).

Determination of Intracellular Deoxycytidine. A μ-Bondapak C_{18} column (Waters GmbH) was used for the separation of intracellular nucleosides. An initial buffer composition of 100% buffer A (0.5 *M* ammonium acetate, pH 6.8) was maintained over 10 min followed by a linear gradient reaching 40% buffer B (50% methanol) after 30 min. In all experiments analyzing intracellular nucleoside concentratios, incubations were terminated by use of ice-cold phosphate buffered saline (PBS) containing 10 μ*M* dipyridamole.

Results

Modulation of Intracellular ara-CTP Accumulation by Inhibition of Ribonucleotide Reductase. The goal of this experiment was to activate the dCTP salvage pathway by inhibition of the de novo pathway. Hydroxyurea, a known inhibitor of ribonucleotide reductase (RR) was used to inhibit the de novo dCTP synthesis. Cells were preincubated for 2 h with 5 m*M* HU, then ara-C (10 μ*M*) was added for a further 2 h, after which cellular dNTP and ara-CTP concentrations were analyzed. In control experiments, CEM cells accumulated greater ara-CTP concentrations (412 ± 43 μ*M*) than Raji cells (116 ± 6 μ*M*). After a 2-h preincubation with HU, intracellular ara-CTP formation remained essentially unchanged in CEM cells, while in Raji cells ara-CTP accumulation was enhanced by 3.7-fold. It was therefore concluded that inhibition of RR, by HU apparently does not have a uniform effect in all cell lines. The following experiments were designed to clarify the mechanisms responsible for the apparent differences of dCTP salvage regulation.

Intracellular Half-Life of dCTP. The intracellular half-life of dCTP was measured to develop an indicator for the cellular turnover of deoxynucleotides in the respective cell lines. To this end, cells were exposed for 2 h to [^{3}H]dCyd, and after washout the decay of intracellular [^{3}H]dCTP was determined. As expected, the intracellular half-lifes was greatest in the T-lymphoblastic CEM cells (75 min), while the respective half lifes of dCTP elimination were considerably shorter in Raji cells. Correspondingly, the pool size of dCTP under control conditions was greater in CEM cell (25 ± 5 μ*M*) than in Raji cells (2.5 ± 0.3 μ*M*). The faster turnover rate of dCTP correlated well with a shorter half-life of ara-CTP in Raji and HL-60 cells compared to CEM cells (data not shown).

Perturbation of the Cellular dCTP Pool by Inhibition of RR. Cells were exposed to 5 m*M* HU for 2 h after which intracellular concentrations of dCTP were analyzed as indicated in Materials and Methods. HU-mediated inhibition of RR reduced intracellular dCTP to 20% of control in CEM cells, while in Raji cells dCTP was decreased to 84% of control. This experiment demonstrated that, although dCTP depletion was greatest in CEM cells, it did not relate to a corresponding enhancement of dCK-mediated ara-C phopshorylation.

Effect of dCTP Depletion on Cellular ara-CTP Accumulation in Raji cells. The imporatance of dCTP for cellular ara-CTP formation was further analyzed in Raji cells in which inhibition of the de novo pathway and concomitant depletion of dCTP was achieved by preincubation of cells with three different agents. Thymidine acts as an inhibitor of CDP reduction. A 2-h pre-exposure of Raji cells to 100 μ*M* thymidine and a subsequent exposure to 10 μ*M* ara-C depleted the cellular dCTP concentration to 50% of control and decreased ara-CTP synthesis to 57% of control. In the following experiment, 3-deazauridine, a known inhibitor of CTP synthetase was used. This agent indirectly depletes dCTP via a CTP depletion. Preincubation with 5 μ*M* 3-deazauridine dCTP and subsequent exposure to 10 μM ara-C reduced dCTP to 20% of control, while ara-CTP formation remained at 90% of control. By contrast, HU only decreased dCTP to 84% of control, while ara-CTP formation was enhanced by a factor of 3.3. It may be concluded that also in a single cell line the degree of dCTP depletion cannot be simply related to the activity of ara-CTP formation by the salvage pathway.

Modulation of the Cellular dCyd Concentration by Inhibition of RR. Since dCTP, the final product of the salvage pathway, did not appear to be a good predictor in intracellular ara-CTP formation, the substrate level of the salvage pathway was analyzed with regard to the cellular dCyd concentration. In Raji cells, inhibition of ribonucleotide reductase decreased the cellular dCyd pool to 33 ± 12% of control. It was therefore hypothesized that a decreased cellular concentration of dCyd reduces the competition of intracellular dCyd and ara-C at the substrate level of dCK and may therefore allow more ara-C to be phosphorylated.

Discussion

The primary goal of this study was to elucidate the mechanism by which inhibition of the de novo pathway for dCTP synthesis activates intracellular ara-CTP formation via the salvage pathway in some, but not all, leukemia cell lines. Previous studies analyzing the regulation of purified (dCK) in vitro emphasized the regulatory importance of dCTP as a feedback inhibitor. The present analysis was performed in intact leukemia cells. HU, an effective inhibitor of RR, was used to inhibit the de novo pathway of dCTP synthesis. Intracellular ara-CTP accumulation served as an indicator for the activity of the dCTP salvage pathway.

When the de novo pathway was blocked by inhibition of RR, activation of the salvage pathway, i.e., a 3.7-fold enhancement of ara-CTP accumulation, was observed in Raji cells, but not in CEM cells. In the same experimental setting, HU lowered intracellular dCTP concentrations to 20% of control in CEM cells, but only to 84% of control in Raji cells.

It may be concluded that dCTP depletion is observed when the de novo pathway of dCTP synthesis is inhibited. However, the extent of dCTP depletion does not correlate with the activation of the salvage pathway and therefore does not predict the activity of ara-C phosphorylation by dCK. Enhanced ara-CTP accumulation during inhibition of RR can therefore not simply be explained by a release of dCTP-mediated feedback inhibition on dCK. The minor importance of dCTP for the regulation of dCK activity is further supported by the observation that in Raji cells only HU enhanced ara-CTP accumulation, while thymidine and 3-deazauridine did not increase dCK activity although cellular concentrations of dCTP were more extensively depleted by the latter drugs.

Since dCTP, the product of the salvage pathway, was an insufficient prognosticator for the activation of the salvage pathway and specifically for the activity of dCK, we analyzed the substrate level of dCK, namely, the effect of RR inhibition on the cellular dCyd concentration. This analysis demonstrated that HU depleted the cellular dCTP pool to 33% of control in Raji cells.

The cellular depletion of dCyd pool reduces the competition of dCyd and ara-C at the binding sites of dCK and may thereby allow an enhanced phosphorylation of ara-C. It is therefore concluded that inhibition of RR activates dCyd analog phosphorylation rather by a decrease of cellular dCyd than by a depletion of the dCTP pool. This hypothesis fits well with a report [7], obtained using purified dCK, starting that dCyd inhibits ara-C phosphorylation at a Ki value (0.17 μM) which was 40-fold lower than the Ki of dCTP (7.3 μM).

The question then arises why the dCyd pool was smaller in CEM cells compared to Raji cells. One explanation may be the short half-life, and consequently the fast turnover of dCTP in Raji cells. A fast turnover of dCTP may correspond to a great production of endogeneous dCyd [8] which then may compete with ara-C for phosphorylation. Owing to this element of competition, phosphorylation of ara-C via the salvage pathway is comparatively low in Raji cells. Additionally, it is conceivable that cells with a fast dCTP turnover need a correspondingly great activation of the salvage pathway when the de novo pathway is inhibited. By contrast, CEM cells are characterized by a rather slow turnover of dCTP, and a correspondingly low endogeneous dCyd production. Owing to a lower competition of ara-C with endogenous dCyd, a maximal activity of ara-C phosphorylation may be expected under control conditions. In fact, when RR is inhibited, these cells do not further activate the dCTP salvage pathway despite a considerable depletion of dCTP. Further studies are needed to evaluate if the differential mechanisms of dCK regulation observed in Raji and CEM cells will also apply for T cells and B cells in general.

Acknowledgment. This work was supported by the Deutsche Forschungsgemeinschaft, Grant He 2029/3-1.

References

1. Ives DH, Durham J P. Deoxycytidine kinase. III. Kinetics and allosteric regulation of the calf-thymus enzyme. J Biol Chem 245: 2285–2294, 1970
2. Cheng Y-C, Domain B, Lee L-S. Human deoxycytidine kinase. Purification and characterization of the cytoplasmic and mitochondrial isozymes from blast cells of acute myelocytic leukemia patients. Biochim Biphys Acta 481: 481–492, 1977
3. Grant S, Lehman C, Cadman E. Enhancement of 1-β-D-arabinofuranosylcytosine accumulation within L1210 cells and increased cytotoxicity following thymidine exposure. Cancer Res 40: 1525–1531, 1980
4. Plagemann PGW, Marz R, Wohlhueter R M. Transport and metabolism of deoxycytidine and 1-β-D-arabinofuranosylcytosine into cultured Novikoff rat hepatoma cells, relationship to phosphorylation, and regulation of triphosphate synthesis. Cancer Res 38: 978–989, 1978
5. Heinemann V, Hertel L W, Grindey G B, Plunkett W. Comparison of the cellular pharmacokinetics and toxicity of 2′,2′-difluorodeoxycytidine and 1-β-D-arabinosylcytosine. Cancer Res 48: 4024–4031, 1988
6. Heinemann V, Xu Y-Z, Chubb S, Sen A, Hertel L W, Grindey G B, Plunkett W. Inhibition of ribonu-

cleotide reduction in CCRF-CEM cells by 2'2'-difluorodeoxycytidine. Mol Pharmacol 38: 567–572, 1990
7. Coleman C N, Stoller R G, Drake J C, Chabner B A. Deoxycytidine Kinase: properties of the enzyme from human leukemic granulocytes. Blood: 791–803, 1975
8. Kubota M, Takimoto T, Tanizawa A, Akiyama Y, Mikawa H. Differential modulation of 1-β-D-arabinofuranosylcytosine metabolism by hydroxyurea in human leukemic cells. Biochem Pharmacol 37: 1745–1749, 1988

Acute Leukemias VI
Prognostic Factors
and Treatment Strategies
Büchner et al. (eds)

Drug Resistance Profile: Strongest Independent Prognostic Factor in Childhood Acute Lymphoblastic Leukemia in a BFM-Oriented Treatment Protocol

G.J.L. Kaspers[1], A.J.P. Veerman[1,2], R. Pieters[1], C.H. van Zantwijk[1], L.A. Smets[3], E.R. van Wering[2], A. van der Does-van den Berg[2]

Abstract. Cellular drug resistance is an important factor with respect to the response to chemotherapy. Its measurement may therefore provide prognostically significant information. We studied the relation between in vitro cellular drug resistance, measured with the methyl-thiazol-tetrazolium (MTT) assay, and clinical response to combination chemotherapy in 152 children with newly diagnosed acute lymphoblastic leukemia (ALL). Resistance to each of several drugs was significantly related to the probability of disease-free survival. Multiple regression analysis, however, showed that the combination of the data for Prednisolone, vincristine and L-asparaginase provided a drug resistance profile with an even better prognostic predictive value. This profile had prognostic independent significance superior to that of any other factor. The group with the most sensitive profile, 19% of all patients, had a 3-years probability of disease-free survival (pDFS) of 100%, the group with an intermediately sensitive profile, 41% of all patients, had a 3-years pDFS of 84%, and the group with the most resistant profile, 41% of all patients, had a 3-year pDFS of 39% ($p<0.001$). Treatment failure in childhood ALL can thus be predicted by in vitro determination of cellular drug resistance.

Introduction

In vitro cell culture drug resistance assays have a number of potentially valuable applications in leukemias, as well as in other malignancies. An important one is risk group stratification, based on the prognostic significance of these assay results. A large number of studies have reported significant correlations between results of in vitro drug resistance testing and the clinical outcome in childhood leukemia [1–5] and adult leukemia [6–13]. However, these studies were retrospective, often concerned small and heterogeneous patient groups, and tested few drugs. The purpose of the present study was to determine the relationship between in vitro cellular drug resistance and the clinical outcome after combination chemotherapy in large number of successively diagnosed children with acute lymphoblastic leukemia (ALL). We especially explored the possibility that combining the data for two or more single-tested drugs would provide additional prognostic information to that of the most predictive single drugs. In vitro drug resistance was assessed with the colorimetric methyl-thiazol-tetrazolium (MTT) assay [14–15].

Materials and Methods

Patients and Patient Samples. Eligible were children (age 0–18 years) with non-B ALL, newly diagnosed between 1989 and 1994. Bone marrow (BM) and peripheral blood (PB) samples and smears of patients were sent by local institutions

[1]Department of Pediatrics, Free University Hospital, De Boelelaan 1117, 1081 HV Amsterdam, The Netherlands
[2]Dutch Childhood Leukemia Study Group, The Hague, The Netherlands
[3]Netherlands Cancer Institute, Amsterdam, The Netherlands

to the Dutch Childhood Leukemia Study Group (DCLSG) laboratory for confirmation of the diagnosis ALL, French-American-British Group (FAB) classification and immunophenotyping as recently described [16]. Fresh samples of 152 children were sent by the DCLSG laboratory to the research laboratory for pediatric hemato-onco-immunology at the Free University Hospital in Amsterdam and successfully tested for in vitro drug resistance.

In Vitro Cellular Drug Resistance. This was measured with the 4-day colorimetric cell culture MTT assay, as previously described [14]. BM and PB ALL samples were evaluated together because they do not differ in drug resistance [17]. Twelve drugs were tested, each at six concentrations as previously described [18]. Methotrexate was not included in the panel because this drug is not cytotoxic to human leukemia samples in non-clonogenic assays [14,17]. The drug concentration lethal to 50% of the ALL cells—the LC_{50} —was used as a measure of resistance. Samples were considered evaluable if the drug-free control wells contained $\geqslant$80% leukemic cells before and $\geqslant$70% leukemic cells after 4 days of culture (as determined by morphology and immunology), and if the control optical density at day 4 exceeded 0.050. The MTT assay gives reliable results under these conditions [14, 19, 20]. The coefficient of variation of the optical density of the control wells in the successful assays is median 5.2% (range, 0.9–15.3%). The intra-assay variation (duplicates) and interassay variation (repeated testing of frozen sample) in LC_{50} values for all drugs are well within one dilution step [18].

Treatment and Treatment Outcome. Patients were treated according to DCLSG protocols (ALL-VII and ALL-VIII), which are based on treatment principles of the International Berlin-Frankfurt-Münster (BFM) Study Group, but without cranial irradiation. All patients first received a 1-week systemic monotherapy with prednisone. Patients were then stratified into one of three risk groups according to the clinical response to prednisone, BFM risk factor (based on peripheral leukemic cell count, and liver and spleen size), and response to induction chemotherapy, and received risk-adapted treatment. All drugs included in the in vitro panel were used in the treatment of at least some of the patients. Failure to achieve complete remission (CR) after induction chemotherapy (induction failure) was considered an event at day 0. Early death was defined as death before completion of induction therapy. Disease-free survival (DFS) was defined as the time from diagnosis to induction failure or relapse (leukemia-related events). For estimation of DFS, toxic deaths in remission were censored at the time of occurrence and early deaths at day 0. For analyses of DFS, patients who were disease free were censored at the time of latest follow up.

Statistics. Differences in distribution of variables were tested with the Mann-Whitney U (MWU) test or the χ^2 test. Estimates of event-free survival (EFS) and DFS (with standard errors, SE) were calculated according to the Kaplan-Meier product limit analysis [21]. Because toxic and early deaths are presumably unrelated to cellular drug resistance, in contrast to induction failures and relapses, results of DFS analysis are shown. Univariate and multivariate statistical comparisons of outcome were conducted by proportional hazard Cox regression analysis after stratification for risk group [22]. The model for multivariate analysis included the established conventional prognostic factors i.e., age, BFM risk factor, immunophenotype and DNA ploidy, and in vitro drug resistance. Information about karyotype was not available. Analyses were two-tailed at a significance level of 5%.

Results

In 152 patient samples at least one drug (depending on the amount of material available) was successfully tested. LC_{50} values varied markedly between the patient samples for all drugs. For each single drug, except prednisolone, patients were classified into three equally large groups (to avoid response-driven cut-off points) as sensitive (33% lowest LC_{50} values), intermediately sensitive (33% intermediate LC_{50} values), or resistant (33% highest LC50 values). For prednisolone these three groups were defined using the cut-off values obtained in our retrospective study to prospectively confirm those results and because the LC_{50} values for prednisolone in particular show a skewed distributioin [4].

Table 1 shows the pDFS at 3 years for sensitive, intermediately sensitive, and resistant

Table 1. The relationship between in vitro drug resistance and clinical outcome 3 years from diagnosis in 152 children with newly diagnosed ALL. Univariate analyses, stratified for protocol risk group

Drug	3-Year probability of disease-free survival			
	Sensitive (%)	Intermediate (%)	Resistant (%)	*p*-value[2]
prednisolone	100	78	33	<0.001
Dexamethasone	87	72	54	0.006
L-asparaginase	93	69	48	<0.001
Vincristine	92	61	62	0.002
Vindesine	85	64	68	0.056
Daunorubicin	83	72	56	0.04
Doxorubicin	82	72	61	0.017
Mitoxantrone	79	78	61	0.07
Mercaptopurine	80	78	63	0.15
Thioguanine	86	68	69	0.42
Cytarabine	74	82	55	0.30
Teniposide	82	68	65	0.20

patients for each drug, and *p* values. Of the other factors studied, only leukemic cell burden as expressed by the BFM risk factor had (borderline) prognostic significance (p=0.07), while sex, age, white blood cell count (WBC), FAB type, immunophenotype, and DNA ploidy had not. We next performed a multiple regression analysis including those drugs which all patients had received in the course of their treatment. The combination of in vitro results for prednisolone, L-asparaginase and vincristine provided prognostic information additional to that of the most predictive single drugs, prednisolone and L-asparaginase. For each of these three drugs patients were classsified according to the definitions mentioned above, and a sensitive result was counted as 1, an intermediate result as 2, and a resistant result as 3. For each patient a score was calculated by adding up these counts. Thus, the score ranged from 3 (sensitive to all 3 drugs) to 9 (resistant to all 3 drugs). Table 2 shows that an increase of this "drug resistance profile score" is associated with an increased event rate (χ^2=22.6, p=0.001). Three patient groups were defined arbitrarily. The group with the most sensitive profile (score 3 or 4), 19% of all patients, had a 3-year pDFS of 100%, the group with an intermediately sensitive profile (score 5 or 6), 41% of all patients, had a 3-year pDFS of 84% (SE 8%), and the group with the most resistant profile (score 7, 8 or 9), 41% of all patients, had a 3-year pDFS of 39% (SE 17%) ($p<0.001$). Figure 1 shows the Kaplan-Meier curves for these three groups. Multivariate analysis showed the prognostic independent significance of this drug resistance profile, being clearly superior to that of immunophenotype, the other factor with independent prognostic significance.

Table 2. Drug resistance profile (combined data for prednisolone, L-asparaginase, and vincristine) and the occurrence of leukemia-related events (no complete remission, relapse)

	Drug resistance profile score[a]						
	Most sensitive <-----> Most resistant						
	3	4	5	6	7	8	9
Patients(*n*)	5	17	20	28	23	13	12
Events(*n*)	0	0	3	5	12	5	6
Event rate (%)	0	0	15	18	52	38	50

[a] See text for details

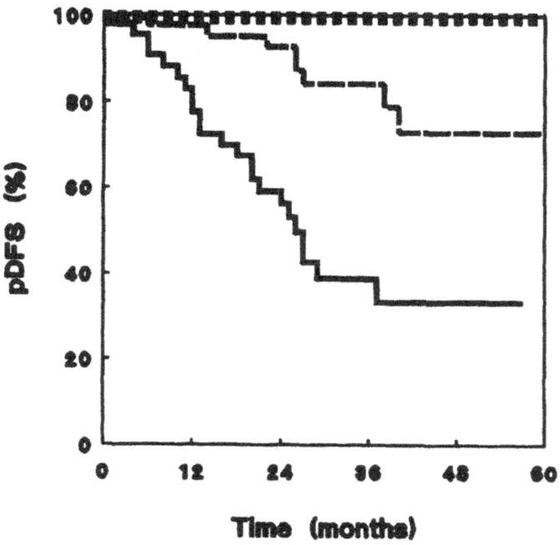

Fig. 1. Relationship between in vitro drug resistance profile, obtained by combining results for prednisolone, L-asparaginase, and vincristine (see text), and probability of disease-free survival in newly diagnosed childhood ALL. *Dotted line*, sensitive; *broken line*, intermediate; *solid line*, resistant. $p < 0.001$

Discussion

In the present study including 152 children with newly diagnosed ALL, increased in vitro resistance to each of the single drugs prednisolone, dexamethasone, L-asparaginase, vincristine, daunorubicin, and doxorubicin was significantly associated with a lower pDFS. After combining the results for prednisolone, L-asparaginase, and vincristine, a drug resistance profile emerged with prognostic independent significance superior to that of any other factor. The pDFS decreased markedly and significantly from the patients with a sensitive profile via patients with an intermediately sensitive profile to the group with a resistant profile (Fig. 1). Although the patient group was not entirely representative of the entire population of newly diagnosed patients (not shown), cellular drug resistance retained its prognostic significance at immunophenotype and risk-group stratified analyses.

The present study is the first to show in a large group of children with ALL treated with contemporary chemotherapy that in vitro cellular drug resistance testing provides significant information about the clinical outcome after combination chemotherapy. This confirms the results of a large number of retrospective studies which showed significant in vitro–in vivo correlations in smaller groups of childhood and adult leukemia [1–13]. Using similar cut-off points for sensitivity and resistance, we could confirm the significant relationship between in vitro resistance to prednisolone and clinical outcome in childhood ALL, as was found in our retrospective study on cryopreserved leukemic cells [4]. Our results, however, do differ for the other drugs which were tested in the retrospective study. This may be explained by differences in treatment and patient groups. Concerning the validation of the MTT assay, it is of importance that we also found a highly significant correlation between the antileukemic activity of prednisolone in vitro and the clinical response to monotherapy with that drug [23].

We conclude that the MTT assay provides drug resistance profiles which accurately predict the clinical outcome after chemotherapy in childhood ALL. The MTT assay may be a valuable tool for risk-group stratification. The success rate of the MTT assay is about 80% on fresh samples. In the remaining 20% of patients, stratification could be done using conventional criteria. The drug resistance profile can be obtained with fewer than 10 million leukemic cells. The presented data may stimulate studies regarding other potential applications of cellular drug resistance assays, such as rational improvements of current regimens, selection of patients for phase II trials or adjuvant chemotherapy, and assay-selected chemotherapy.

Acknowledgments. This work was financially supported by the Dutch Cancer Society (IKA 89-06) and by the project VONK (VU Onderzoek Naar Kinderkarker). Computer equipment was provided by Olivetti Nederland BV. The Dutch Childhood Leukemia Study Group (DCLSG) provided the patient samples. Board members of the DCLSG are H.van den Berg, M.V.A. Bruin, J.P.M. Bokkerink, P.J. van Dijken, K. Hahlen, W.A. Kamps, F.A.E. Nabben, A.Postma, J.A. Rammeloo, I.M. Risseeuw-Appel, A.Y.N. Schouten-van Meeteren, G.A.M. de Vaan, E.T. van't Veer-Korthof, A.J.P. Veerman, M. van Weel-Sipman, and R.S.Weening.

References

1. Hongo T, Fujii Y, Igarashi Y. An in vitro chemosensitivity test for the screening of anti-cancer drugs in childhood leukemia. Cancer 1990;65: 1263–72.

2. Asselin BL, Ryan D, Frantz CN, et al. In vitro and in vivo killing of acute lymphoblastic leukemia cells by L-asparaginase. Cancer Res 1989; 49: 4363–8.
3. Dow LW, Dahl GV, Kalwinsky DK, Mirro J, Nash MB, Roberson PK. Correlation of drug sensitivity in vitro with clinical responses in childhood acute myeloid leukemia. Blood 1986;68: 400–5.
4. Pieters R, Huismans DR, Loonen AH, et al. Relation of cellular drug resistance to long-term clinical outcome in childhood acute lymphoblastic leukaemia. Lancet 1991;338:399–403.
5. Smith PJ, Lihou MG. Prediction of remission induction in childhood acute myeloid leukemia. Aust N Z J Med 1986;16: 39–42.
6. Weisenthal LM, Dill PL, Finklestein JZ, Duarte TE, Baker JA, Moran EM. Laboratory detection of primary and acquired drug resistance in human lymphatic neoplasms. Cancer Treatm Rep 1986;70: 1283–95.
7. Bosanquet AG. Correlations between therapeutic responsé of leukaemias and in-vitro drug-sensitivity assay. Lancet 1991;337: 711–14.
8. Delmer A, Marie J-P, Thevenin D, Cadiou M, Viguie F, Zittoun R. Multivariate analysis of prognostic factors in acute myeloid leukemia: value of clonogenic leukemic cell properties. J Clin Oncol 1989;7: 738–46.
9. Gustavsson A, Olofsson T. Prediction of response to chemotherapy in acute leukemia by in vitro drug sensitivity testing on leukemic stem cells. Cancer Res 1984;44: 4648–52.
10. Lathan B, Von Tettau M, Verpoort K, Diehl V. pretherapeutic drug testing in acute leukemias for prediction of individual prognosis. Haematol Blood Transf 1990;33: 295–8.
11. Park CH, Amare M, Savin MA, Goodwin JW, Newcomb MM, Hoostraten B. Prediction of chemotherapy response in human leukemia using an in vitro chemotherapy sensitivity test on the leukemic colony-forming cells, Blood 1980; 55: 595–601.
12. Sargent JM, Taylor CG. Appraisal of the MTT assay as a rapid test of chemosensitivity in acute myeloid leukaemia. Br J Cancer 1989;60: 206–210.
13. Tidefelt U, Sundman-Engberg B, Rhedin AS, paul C. In vitro drug testing in patients mimicking in vivo intracellular drug concentrations. Eur J Haematol 1989;43: 374–84.
14. Pieters R, Loonen AH, Huismans DR, et al. In vitro sensitivity of cells from children with leukemia using the MTT assay with improved culture conditions. Blood 1990;76: 2327–36.
15. Veerman AJP, Pieters R. Drug sensitivity assays in leukaemia and lymphoma. Br J Haematol 1990;74: 381–4.
16. Van Wering ER, Brederoo P, Van Staalduinen GJ, Van Der Meulen J, Van Der Linden-Schrever BEM, Van Dongen JJM. Contribution of electron microscopy to the classification of minimally differentiated acute leukemias in children. Recent Results Cancer Res 1993;131: 77–87.
17. Kaspers GJL, Pieters R, Van Zantwijk CH, et al. In vitro drug sensitivity of normal peripheral blood lymphocytes and childhood leukaemic cells from bone marrow and peripheral blood. Br J Cancer 1991;64: 469–74.
18. Kaspers GJL, Kardos G, Pieters R, et al. Different cellular drug resistance profiles in childhood lymphoblastic and nonlymphoblastic leukemia: a preliminary analysis. Leukemia 1994;8: 1224–1229.
19. Kaspers GJL, Veerman AJP, Pieters R, et al. Mononuclear cells contaminating acute lymphoblastic leukaemic samples tested for cellular drug resistance using the methyl-thiazol-tetrazolium assay. Br J Cancer 1994;70: 1047–1052.
20. Pieters R, Huismans DR, Leyva A, Veerman AJP. Comparison of the rapid automated MTT-assay with a dye exclusion assay for chemosensitivity testing in childhood leukemia. Br J Cancer 1989; 59: 217–20.
21. Kaplan EL, Meier P. Nonparametric estimation from in-complete observations. J Am Stat Assoc 1958;53: 457–81.22.
22. Cox DR. Regression models and life tables. J R Stat Soc 1972;34: 187–220.
23. Kaspers GJL, Pieters R, Van Zantwijk CH, De Waal FC, Van Wering ER, Veerman AJP. Is resistance to prednisolone in vitro related to the response to prednisolone at initial diagnosis in childhood acute lymphoblastic leukemia? A preliminary analysis. In: Kaspers GJL, Pieters R, Twentyman PR, Weisenthal LM, Veerman AJP, eds. Drug resistance in leukemia and lymphoma. The clinical value of laboratory assays. Chur, Harwood Academic Publ., 1993: 321–8.

Acute Leukemias VI
Prognostic Factors
and Treatment Strategies
Büchner et al. (eds)

In Vitro Drug Sensitivity of Acute Myeloid Leukemic Cells Using the Methyl-Thazol-Tetrazolium Assay

A. Mestice, G. Specchia, M.R. Coppi, I. Attolico, A. Ricco, D. Pastore, A. Vaira, M.R. de Paolis, V. Caretto, and V. Liso

Abstract. Different assays (clonogenic, dye exclusion, etc.) have been developed to assess the chemosensitivity of malignant cells. The MTT assay, in particular, based on the reduction by living cells of MTT [3-4,5-dimethylthiazol-2-yl]-2,5-diphenyl tetrazolium bromide) to a formazan product, provides a simple, automated, and efficient method for chemosensitivity testing in leukemias.

In this study, in vitro drug sensitivity was assessed in the cells from 46 adult acute myeloid leukemias (AML). Dose-response curves were obtained for cytosine arabinoside (ara-C), daunorubicin (DNR), idarubicin (IDA), mitoxantrone (MIT), etoposide (VP-16). There were marked interindividual differences in leukemic cell survival (LCS) values (expressed as the percentage of cell survival with respect to the untreated controls). LCS was less than 50% in 30/46 samples (65%) tested with ara-C, in 38/41 (98%) with IDA, in 41/42 (98%) with DNR, in 40/46 (87%) with MIT, and in 30/45 (67%) with VP-16. The in vitro results were compared with the clinical response in 31 patients treated by combination chemotherapy according to GIMEMA protocols (AML 10 and P 491). The MTT test correlated with in vivo response in 18 (58%) out of 31 patients. Sensitive chemotherapeutic response in vitro but resistance in vivo was observed in 12 patients. Only one AML patient was found to be resistant in vitro and sensitive in vivo.

Our preliminary results suggest that the MTT assay may be useful in evaluating chemosensitivity in some AML patients, although further studies are needed to assess the clinical utility of in vitro chemosensitivity tests.

Hematology Service, University of Bari, 70124 Bari, Italy

Introduction

Different assays have been developed to assess the chemosensitivity of malignant cells. Although the clonogenic test is considered the gold standard because it tests the sensitivity of stem cells, it is limited by its "low plating efficiency" and long incubation time [1–3]. The differential staining cytotoxicity (DiSC) assay is a short-term test but it is time consuming and subject to observer error. [4,5]. The methyl-thiazol-tetrazolium MTT colorimetric assay tests the viability of cells by measuring the reduction of 3-[4,5-dimethylthiazol-2-yl]-2,5-diphenyl tetrazolium bromide to an insoluble colored formazan precipitate by means of dehydrogenase, enzymes which are active only in viable cells [6–8]. The concentration of formazan can be measured by spectrophotometry at 540 nm. This assay is particularly interesting as it is simple, automated, rapid, and reproducible.

In this study we assessed drug sensitivity in cells from 46 patients with acute myeloid leukemia (AML) treated according to GIMEMA protocols (AML 10, P 491) [9]. The in vitro results were compared with the clinical response in 31 patients selected for homogeneous drug use in vivo and in vitro.

Materials and Methods

Cells. Bone marrow (BM) or peripheral blood (PB) samples were taken from 46 patients with AML diagnosed according to French-American-British (FAB) criteria [10]. Mononuclear cells were isolated by Ficoll density gradient centrifugation and washed twice; then they were resuspended in Iscove's modified Dulbecco's medium supplemented with 20% heat-inactivated fetal calf serum (FCS) and gentamycin. Adherent cells were removed by incubating the cells in medium with 10% FCS for 24 h in a plastic culture flask, at 37°C, in a fully humidified atmosphere with 5% CO_2.

Reagents and Drugs. The following drugs were used: cytarabine (aRA-C), mitoxantrone hydrochloride (MIT), daunorubicin hydrochloride (DNR), etoposide (VP-16), idarubicin (IDA). MTT was obtained from Sigma (St. Louis, MO, USA).

Cellular Drug Resistance Testing. The test was performed within 24 h of collection of the sample. BM and PB samples were evaluated together, since their drug resistance does not differ. All samples tested with the MTT assay contained >90% leukemic cells after isolation, and cell viability (tripan blue exclusion) was always >90%. A sample of 90 µl cell suspension (2-4 $\times 10^6$ cells/ml) was added to 10 µl of drug solution in 96-well round-bottomed microculture plates. Each drug was tested in three concentrations in triplicate; the highest dose in vitro was ten times the one in vivo. Four drug-free wells were used to determine the control cell survival. The plates were incubated in humidified air containing 5% CO_2 for 2 days at 37°C. Then 10 µl MTT solution (5 mg/ml) was added and, after shaking the plates until the cell pellet was resuspended, they were incubated for an additional 4 h. The formazan crystals were dissolved with 100 µl dimethyl sulphoxide (DMSO). The optical density (OD) of the wells, which is linearly related to the cell number, was measured with a spectrophotometer at 540 nm. Leukemic cell survival (LCS) was calculated by the equation: LCS = (OD treated wells/mean OD control wells) × 100 [11, 12].

Clinical Evalution. The clinical correlation was evaluated only when cells were tested in vitro for at least all the drugs used in vivo.

Statistical Analysis. Statistical anaylsis of the in vitro-in vivo relationship was performed with χ^2 contingency table analysis [13].

Results

Forty-six patients with AML were included in our study: 22 males and 24 females with a median age of 61 years (range 22-85 years); the white blood cell count (WBC) ranged from 1.1 to 140.7×10^9/l (median 12.2×10^9/l); 37 patients were at onset and nine at first relapse; there were two M0, two M1, 24 M2, eight M4, seven M5, three M6 cases according to the FAB clssification (Table 1).

Only tests with OD control >0.150 were taken into account. A linear correlation between cell number/well and OD values was found within the range of cellular concentrations used: at lower concentrations the test is not reproducible, while at higher concentrations the curve reaches a plateau.

All drugs showed concentration-dependent cytotoxicity. There was no difference between control LCS (100%) and LCS values with drugs at the lowest concentration (0.001 µm) while in almost all cases LCS was <50% at 10 µm; there was a wide range of LCS (11%-242%) at 0.1µm drug concentration.

Cells were considered sensitive when (LCS) was <50% (Fig. 1). In vitro sensitivity was 50% in 30/46 (65%) samples tested with a RA-C, in 30/45 (67%) with VP-16, in 38/41 (93%) with IDA, in 41/42 (98%) with DNR, and in 40/46 (87%) with MIT. In sensitive cases, median LCS was 28 (range 10-48) for a RA-C, 31 (range 11-49) for VP-16, 26 (range 11-49)for IDA, (range 11-49) for DNR, and 26 (range 8-49) for MIT (Table 2). Individual correlations were evaluated

Table 1. Clinical features of 46 AML patients

Patients (*n*)	46
Male/female (*n*)	22/4
Age—Median (years)	61
Range (years)	22-85
Hemoglobin—Median (g/dl)	9.1
Range (g/dl)	4.4-14.1
WBC $\times 10^9$/I—Median	12.2
Range	1.1-140.7
Platelets $\times 10^9$/I	36.5
	3-307
Onset/relapse (*n*)	37/9
FAB M0 (*n*)	2
M1 (*n*)	2
M2 (*n*)	24
M4 (*n*)	8
M5 (*n*)	7
M6 (*n*)	3

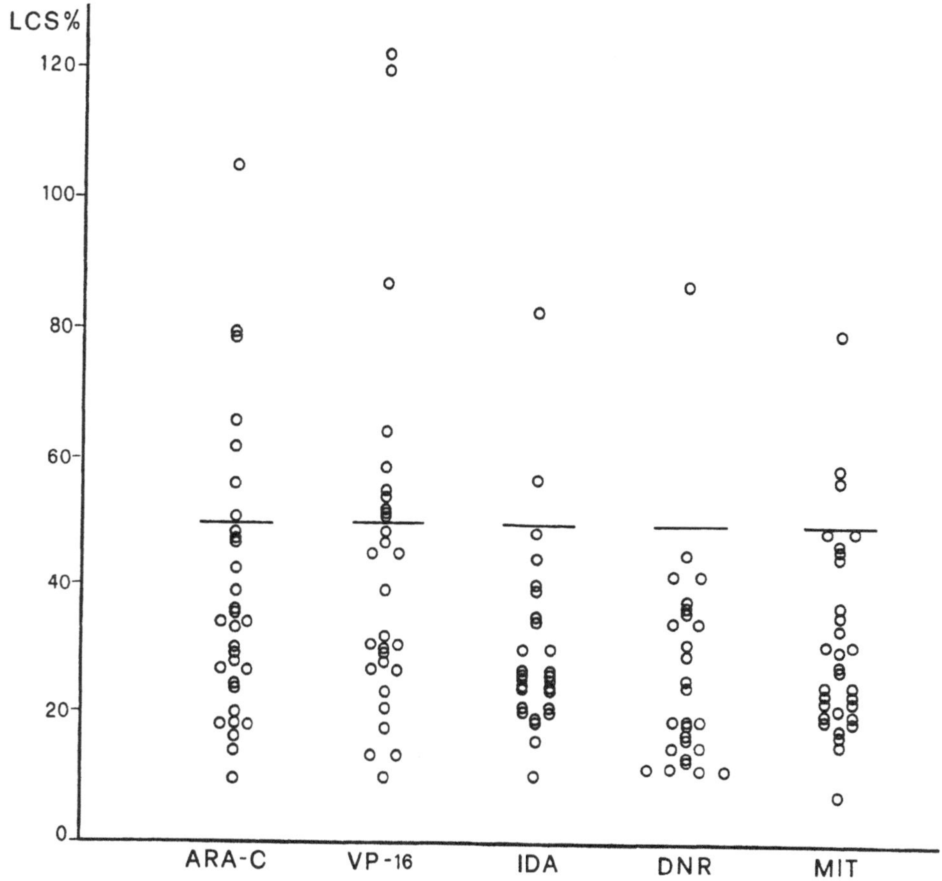

Fig. 1. LCS values of a RA-C, VP-16, IDA, DNR, and MIT at high concentration on cells from AML patients

Table 2. In vitro drug sensitivity according to MTT test

Drug	Sensitivity		LCS	
	(%)	(*n*)	range	median
Ara-C	65	30/46	28	10–48
VP-16	67	30/45	31	11–49
IDA	93	38/41	26	11–49
DNR	98	41/42	23	11–49
MIT	87	40/46	26	8–49

in 31 patients selected according to the criteria described above; among these patients, one was found to be resistant and 30 sensitive in vitro. In vivo, 12 patients had resistant disease (RD) and 19 achieved complete remission (CR). The MTT test correlated with the in vivo response in 18 out of 31 patients (58%); 12 patients showed sensitive chemotherapeutic response in vitro and resistance in vivo (39%) and only one patient was resistant in vitro and sensitive in vivo (3%) ($p < 0.005$).

Discussion

The standard way to validate the in vitro drug sensitivity assay is by demonstrating its predictive ability in a prospective study of patients in treatment with antiblastic drugs. The aim of the present study was to evaluate the MTT assay in AML. The MTT assay enables a very large number of cells to be processed using an objective endpoint [11, 14]. Since it is a short-term test, should its ability to predict clinical responses be found reliable, it would constitute an aid in identifying most active treatment schema. A number of reports have already been published comparing the MTT with other short-term assays and a few studies have also indicated good correlation between in vitro sensitivity and long-term clinical response [15–18]. In particular; MTT has been reported to be efficient in predicting long-term response to chemotherapy in acute lymphoblastic leukemia and in AML. Furthermore, in previous studies the correlation of MTT results and clinical outcome confirmed that there were no false negatives [15, 19, 20].

In our experience of 46 AML samples, we found good correlation in 18 of 31 selected patients; of the remaining, 12 patients sensitive in vitro were not responsive to chemotherapeutic treatment while only one of the patient who achieved CR was found to be resistant in vitro. These results supported our opinion that drug sensitivity tests cannot be expected to predict the clinical outcome of remission induction therapy, which depends on a large number of clinical factors, apart from drug cytotoxicity. However, the cellular damage detected by the MTT assay may be influenced by temporary and reversible energy depletion of the cells investigated [21, 22]. Nevertheless, they can be useful for predicting a drug's ability to reduce leukemic cells in vivo.

We conclude that the clinical implication of in vitro chemosensitivity assays may include the exclusion of drugs with very low probability of clinical activity and the selection of in vitro senstive drugs with a probability of clinical response. Further studies, including in vitro and in vivo investigations, are needed to assess the clinical utility to chemosensitivity tests.

References

1. Weisenthal LM, Lippman ME (1985) Clonogenic and non-clonogenic in vitro chemosensitivity assay. Canc Treat Rep 69: 616–32
2. Karney DN, Winkler CF (1985) In vitro assays of chemotherapeutic sensitivity. In: Important advances in oncology. De Vita et al (eds). p.78 JB Lippincott: Philadelphia
3. Marie JP (1987) Prognostic value of clonogenic assay for induction for duration of complete remission in acute myelogenous. Leukemia 1: 121
4. Weisenthal LM,Marsden JA, Dill PL, Macaluso CK (1983) A novel dye exclusion method for testing in vitro chemosensitivity of human tumors. Canc Res 43: 749–57
5. Bird MC, Bosanquet AG, Gilby ED (1985) In vitro determination of tumor sensitivity in haematological malignancies. Haematol Oncol 3: 1–9
6. Berridge MV, An S. Tan. (1993) Characterization of the cellular reduction of 3-(4,5-dimethylthiazol-2-yl)-2,5-diphenyltetrazolium bromide (MTT): Subcellular localization, substrate dependence, and involvement of mitochondrial electron transport in MTT reduction. Arch. Biochem. Biophys. 303: 474–82
7. Mossmann T (1983) Rapid colorimetric assay for cellular growth and survival: application to proliferation and cytotoxicity assays. Imm Meth 65: 55
8. `Pieters R, Huisman DR, Leyva A, Veerman AJP (1988) Adaptation of a rapid tetrazolium based (MTT-) assay for chemosensitivity testing in childhood leukaemia. Cancer Lett 41: 323
9. Zittoun R, Liso V, Mandelli F, Rotoli B, de Witte T et al. (1992) Intensive consolidation chemotheraphy versus standard consolidation maintenance in acute myelogenous leukemia (AML) in first remission: an EORTC/GIMEMA phase III trial (AML 8B). Leukemia 6: Suppl 2: 120–3
10. Bennett JM, Catovsky D, Daniel MT, Flandrin G, Galtan DAG, Gralnik HR, Sultan G (1976) Proposal for the classification of the acute leukemias. Br J Haematol 33: 451–58
11. Pieters R, Huismans DR, Leiva A, Veerman AJP (1989) Comparison of the rapid automated MTT assay with a dye exclusion assay for chemosensitivity testing in childhood leukemia. Br J Cancer 59: 217–20
12. Kaspers GJL, Kardos G, Pieters R, van Zantwijk CH, Klumper E, Hahlem K, de Waal FC, van Wering ER, Veerman AJP (1994) In vitro cytotoxicity of mitoxantrone, daunorubicin and doxorubicin in untreated childhood acute leukemia. Leukemia 8: 24–29
13. Colton T (1974) Statistics in medicine. Little, Brown, Boston
14. Bird MC, Forskit S, Gilby ED, Bosanquet AG (1986) The influence of sample source and cell concentration of in vitro chemosensitivity of haematological tumors. Br. J.Cancer 53: 539
15. Sargent JM, Taylor CG (1989) Appraisel of the MTT assay as a rapid test of chemosensitivity in acute myeloid leukemia. Br.J Cancer 60: 206–10
16. Hwang W, Chen L, Huang S, Wang C, Tseng MT (1993) Prediction of chemotherapy response in human leukemia using in vitro chemosensitivity. Luek Res 17: 685–88
17. Bird MC, Bosanquey AG, Forskit S, Gilby ED (1988) Long term comparison of results of an in vitro drug sensitivity assay with patient response in lymphatic neoplasm. Cancer 61: 1104–9
18. Weisenthal LM, Dill PL, Finkelstein JZ, Duarte TE, Baker JA, Moran EN (1976) Laboratory detection of primary and acquired drug resistance in human lymphatic neoplasm. Cancer Treat Rep 70: 1283–88
19. Boekhorst PAW, Lowenberg B, Sonneveld P (1993) Enhance chemosensitivity acute myeloid leukemia by hematopoietic growth factors: a comparison of the MTT assay with a clonogenic assay. Leukemia 7: 1637–44
20. Kirkpatrick DL, Duke M, Goh TS (1990) Chemosensitivity testing of fresh human leukemia

cells using both a dye-exclusion assay and a tetrazolium dye (MTT) assay. Leukemia Res 14: 459–66
21. Larsonn R, Nygren P (1989) A semi-automated fluorometric method for determination of cytotoxicity and cellular proliferation of human tumor cell lines in microculture. Anticancer Res 9: 1111–20
22. Larsonn R, Jorgen K, Sandberg C, Nygren P (1992) Laboratory determination of chemotherapeutic drug resistance in tumor cells from patients with leukemia using a fluorimetric microculture assay (FMCA). Int J Cancer 50: 177–85

Acute Leukemias VI
Prognostic Factors
and Treatment Strategies
Büchner et al. (eds)

Does P-Glycoprotein Predict Response to Chemotherapy? Expression of P-Glycoprotein in Children's and Adults' Leukemia—Correlation with Clinical Outcome

S. Kaczorowski[1], M. Ochocka[2], M. Kaczorowska[3], and M. Matysiak[2]

Abstract. The purpose of this study was to define the expression of P-glycoprotein (P-gp) in healthy donors as well as in children's and adults' leukemia cases. Expression of P-gp was evaluated with three monoclonal antibodies (MAbs); C219, JSB-1, MRK-16 and immunocytochemical (IC) APAAP staining technique. Seventy-eight patients: 45 children, 33 adults as well as 27 normal healthy donors entered the study. Twenty-seven healthy donors' peripheral blood mononuclear cells (PBMC) were investigated by means of IC and FACScan analysis. Positive staining for P-gp was detected in 31% of children's and 33% of adults' leukemia samples by IC. No reactivity of the three MAbs was observed with PBMC by means of IC. Flow cytometry analysis with C219 MAb revealed staining for P-gp present on a subpopulation of lymphocytes and monocytes. P-gp (+) as well as P-gp (−) cases were compared in respect to clinical outcome, French-American-British (FAB) classification and blood group. Complete remission (CR) was achieved in 12/14 (85%) of children's and 9/11 (81%) of adults' P-gp (+) leukemia cases. Within the P-gp (−) leukemia cases, CR was observed in 24/29 (82%) and 18/22 (81%), respectively. Partial remission, relapse, resistance, and death were registered in 14% of children's and 18% of adults' P-gp (+) samples. In P-gp (−) cases these parameters were observed in 17% and 18%, respectively.

Introduction

Chemotherapy is still an important treatment method in the cure of acute and chronic leukemias. P-glycoprotein (P-gp) is one of the factors responsible for the lack of tumor sensitivity to cytotoxic drugs, potentially limiting their effectiveness in cancer chemotherapy. Malignant cells can become resistant to chemotherapy via numerous mechanisms. Most of them are well characterized: delivery of the cytostatic drugs, inactivation, excretion, and induction of other enzymes. Cross-resistance to multiple drugs, observed in clinical practice, can be mediated by more than one mechanism. The mechanism(s) underlying this clinical phenomenon are currently being studied in in vitro models. Treatment with one drug can cause cross-resistance to a wide variety of structurally unrelated drugs with a different mode of action [1]. Classic drug resistance has been shown to be associated with the expression of P-gp, the product of the mdr-1 gene [2, 3]. In humans there are two closely related genes, the mdr-1 and the mdr-3 [4]. Only the mdr-1 gene product has been linked to clinical and experimental multidrug resistance [5, 6]. Transfection experiments with mdr-1 gene provided the most direct evidence that P-gp overexpression is responsible for the MDR phenotype [2, 7]. The function of the mdr-3 gene and its product remains

[1]Department of Immunology, Maria Sklodowska-Curie Memorial Cancer Center and Institute of Oncology, Findera 101, 02-781 Warsaw, Poland
[2]Warsaw University Medical School, Department of Pediatric Hematology - Oncology, Dzialdowska 1, 01-184 Warsaw, Poland
[3]Department of Internal Medicine, Family Medicine, Postgraduate Medical Center, Czerniakowska 231, 00-416 Warsaw, Poland

unknown and it has been suggested that elevated mdr-3 gene expression could be implicated in drug resistance (decrease drug sensitivity) in chronic lymphocytic leukemia (CLL) [8]. The P-gp functions as an energy-dependent pump for the efflux of diverse anti-cancer drugs from MDR cells, i.e., antracyclines, podophyllins, and vinca alkaloids, drugs that are important in the treatment of leukemia. The physiologic role of P-gp and substrates for P-gp in normal cells are not known but it is quite likely that P-gp plays an important role as one of the transport mechanisms within the tissues, or serves as one of the mechanisms protecting normal or tumor cells from environmental toxins. The expression of P-gp is sometimes associated with the presence of P-gp mRNA and/or mdr gene amplification [13, 14]. P-gp is widely accepted, in in vitro models, as a factor responsible for generating the classical MDR phenotype [2, 6, 7]. The over-expression of P-gp and expression of the mdr-1 gene has been reported in drug-resistant cell lines as well as in normal tissue, leukemias, lymphomas, and solid tumors [5, 9, 10–12, 14–21]; however, the role of the P-gp in human tumors in vivo is currently being extensively studied [5, 10, 14, 17, 22–24].

Materials and Methods

Patients

A total of 45 children and 33 adults were entered into the study. Children's specimens were collected within a period of 2 years at different stages of disease: at diagnosis ($n=36$), at remission ($n=3$), at second ($n=4$), and at third relapse ($n=2$). The following cases were included: acute myeloid leukaemia (AML $n=8$), myelo-dysplastic syndrome (MDS, $n=1$), acute lymophocytic leukemia (ALL, $n=29$), chronic myelogenous leukemia (CML, $n=1$) and non-Hodgkin's lymphoma (NHL, $n=6$) (median age 8 years 9 months, range 1 year 8 months, 14 years 5 months).

Adults' material was retrieved from the blood bank, where it was collected at the stage of presentation and the following cases were examined: AML ($n=22$), MDS ($n=4$), ALL ($n=6$), CML ($n=1$) (median age 45 years 6 months, range 18–77 years). Peripheral blood mononuclear cells (PBMC) obtained from 27 healthy donors (ten children and 17 adults) were also included in the study. The diagnosis was made on the basis of bone marrow aspiration biopsy and the French-American-British (FAB) classification was used. A complete remission (CR) was determined as fewer than 5% of blasts counted in bone marrow smears [25]. Children's AML and ALL cases were treated according to the Berlin-Frankfurt-Münster (BFM) program. NHL patients were treated with COAMP. Adults with AML received treatment with either rubidomycin, vincristine, and cytarabine; or mitoxantrone, etoposide, and cytarabine; or thioguanine, cytarabine, and daunorubicin. ALL patients received treatment with daunorubicin, cyclophosphamide, vincristine, prednisone, and asparaginase.

Antibodies

Three monoclonal antibodies (MAbs), directed against three separate epitopes of P-gp were used. MAbs C219 (Centocor Diagnostics, Malvern, USA) [16] and JSB-1 (Sanbio/Monosan, The Netherlands) [26] react with the intracytoplasmic and MAb MRK-16 (kindly provided by Dr. T. Tsuruo, Cancer Chemotherapy Centre, Japanese Foundation for Cancer Research, Tokyo, Japan) [27] with the extracellular domain of the P-gp.

Preparation of Blast Cells

Peripheral blood mononuclear cells, obtained from patients and healthy donors, were separated by Ficoll/Hypaque (Pharmacia, Sweden) gradient centrifugation. After separation they were washed in phosphate-buffered saline (PBS); 1×10^6 cells were suspended in PBS and cytospins were prepared (Shandon, UK). Cytospins were dried and fixed in acetone for 5 min, wrapped in Parafilm (American Can Company) and stored at $-70°C$ until used.

Controls

Human myelogenous leukemia K562 vincristine (VCR)-sensitive and K562VCR vincristine-resistant cell lines were used as negative and positive controls, respectively. The K562VCR cell line was cultured in medium supplemented with vincristine (30 n*M*–150 n*M*). The K562VCR cell line had been shown to have elevated levels of mdr-1 transcripts by solution hybridization (personal communication, Dr. A. Gruber, Division of

Medicine, Karolinska Hospital, Stockholm, Sweden). Twenty-seven PBMC separated from healthy donors, ten children's and 17 adults' specimens, were also studied. Children's control PBMC were obtained from children hospitalized with diseases other than hematologic malignancies and adults' control PBMC from healthy volunteers. Neither group had received previous chemotherapy.

Immunocytochemical Staining and FACScan Analysis

Before immunostaining, the cytospins were fixed again in acetone for 5 min. They were rehydrated and primary MAbs C219, JSB-1, and MRK16 were applied. Negative controls included omission of primary antibody as well as reconstitution of primary MAbs with irrelevant immunoglobulins of the same isotype. The alkaline phosphatase anti-alkaline phosphatase (APAAP) method was used [28]. The slides were evaluated by light microscopy. PBMC obtained from healthy donors were analyzed by means of immunocytochemistry (IC) and three MAbs as well as with FACScan (Becton Dickinson) and C219 MAb.

Evaluation

We considered cases positive for P-gp if they were positive with at least two MAbs. Intensity of staining was evaluated as strong, moderate, weak, and no staining on 200 cells counted at the light microscope in randomly selected high-power fields. Within the examined cases, the intensity and frequency of P-gp$^+$ cells were labeled as weak (range 9%–79%, median 38.2%) or moderate to strong (range 5% - 47%, median 13.6%). Occasionally, reactivity of one or two MAbs with single blast cells was detected. Commonly, weaker staining with C219 MAb in comparison with staining of JSB-1 and MRK-16 MAbs was observed. With C219 and JSB-1 cytoplasmic staining and with MRK-16 MAbs membrane staining was seen. A dot-like, Golgi-associated staining with JSB-1 and granular intracytoplasmic staining with C219 and JSB-1 MAbs were also observed.

Results

Reactivity of MAbs with Controls. The vincristine-resistant K562VCR and vincristine-sensitive K562 cell lines showed consistent reactivity with three antibodies. The intensity of staining, within the P-gp$^+$ control slides, varied from weak to strong. Regularly in the K562VCR cell line, included as a positive control for P-gp staining, we detected a subpopulation of cells that do not display any reactivity with the three antibodies. These data were verified by FACScan analysis. Immunoreactivity of K562VCR (30 n*M*) and K562VCR (150 n*M*) cell sublines with C219 antibody varied from 15% to 25% and from 73% to 95% of positive cells, respectively. No reactivity was detected with PBMC from 27 healthy donors using IC and three MAbs. Similarly to the pilot study performed with control K562 and K562VCR cell lines, we also analyzed PBMC from healthy donors by FACScan. We observed reactivity of C219 MAb with subpopulation of lymphocytes: it ranges from 0.21% to 6.6%, median 0.94%, and in monocytes it ranges from 1.53% up to 13.6%, median 2.86%.

Reactivity of MAbs with Leukemia Cases. Positive for P-gp staining was detected in 14/45 (31%) children's samples. P-gp staining was detected in 11/36 (30%) children's specimens at presentation and in three of nine cases (33%) during remission or relapse. One case was investigated twice within an interval of 13 months both at presentation and in relapse, in both staining for P-gp was positive. Positive for P-gp staining in adults' material was detected in 11/33 (33%) samples. This material is more homogenous than the children's since it was collected at presentation and retrieved from the blood bank.

Correlation of P-gp Staining with Outcome FAB Classification and Blood Group. A high rate of complete remission (CR) was achieved both in P-gp$^+$ and P-gp$^-$ cases. In P-gp$^+$ cases, CR was noticed in 12/14 (85%) children's and in 9/11 (81%) adults', in P-gp$^-$ specimens in 24/29 (82%) and in 18/22 (81%), respectively. Partial remission, relapse, resistance, and death were observed in 14% children's and 18% adults' P-gp$^+$cases and in 17% and 18% P-gp$^-$ cases, respectively. We did not find any particular prevalence of distribution of P-gp$^+$ cases within examined types of leukemia. P-gp$^+$ staining was observed in approximately 33% of all the FAB subtypes of leukemia recorded. Moreover, we did not find any correlation between clinical response, blood group, and P-gp immunostaining.

Discussion

Although the reactivity of C219, JSB-1, and MRK-16 MAbs with the P-gp-dependent MDR cell line was well determined [16, 26, 27], the specificity of these antibodies has not yet been thoroughly characterized [18, 29, 30]. The C219 MAb seems to detect the highly conserved carboxy terminal part of the protein, found in three isoforms of P-gp [9, 34]. Thiebaut et al. [18] and Garberoglio et al. [35] report cross-reactivity of C219 MAb with 200-kDa (heavy chain) protein present in myosin molecules in the skeletal and heart muscle. Sonneveld et al. [8], Nooter et al. [31], and Herweijer et al. [32, 33] reported coexpression of mdrl and mdr3 mRNA in leukemia patients and elevated levels of mdr3 mRNA in advanced stages of CLL, hairy cell leukemia, prolymphocytic leukemia, as well as in other B cell hematologic malignancies. JSB-1 MAb reacts with an epitope distinct from the epitope recognized by C219 [29]. Finsta et al. [30] and Weinstein et al. [36] report predominant, Golgi-associated staining with C219 and JSB-1 MAbs and found reactivity of these MAbs on epithelial cells carrying antigens to blood group A. The MRK-16 MAb reacts with an epitope localized to the external surface of the cell membrane which shows a weak sequence homology between mdr-1 and mdr-3 gene [27, 37]. MAb MRK-16 in vitro can partially inhibit drug efflux from drug-resistant cells by binding to the external domain of the P-gp [38]. So far, several studies of multidrug resistance, related to the expression of P-gp or mdrl mRNA, in human leukemias have been reported [21, 24, 39–48]. The expression of P-gp or amplification of mdr-1 gene has been studied in hematologic malignancies and solid tumors using different techniques and authors presented contrary results [5, 10, 19, 21–24, 29]. Expression of P-gp, product of mdrl gene, in the classic MDR phenotype was widely accepted. Whether mdrl gene amplification or expression of mdrl mRNA is sufficient to confirm MDR phenotype is disputable. Holmes et al. [40] have reported amplification of mdr-1 gene without the presence of P-gp. Contrary results are reported by Ito et al. [39]. They found expression of P-gp without amplification of mdr-1 gene. A recent report [49] has pointed out the role of oncogenes and suppressor genes in the regulation of expression of mdrl gene. From these studies it is obvious that more complicated mechanisms are involved in mdr-1 gene regulation.

The present study reports expression of P-gp in one third of children's and adults' leukemia cases as detected with three MAbs. Immunoreactivity for P-gp was generally recognized on neoplastic cells, although positive for P-gp staining was also observed on some non-neoplastic cells such as lymphocytes and monocytes in healthy donor PBMC. Positive P-gp staining was detected with FACScan analysis but not with IC. Similar staining may also occur in hematologic malignancies in non-neoplastic cells such as lymphocytes, monocytes, macrophages, or reactive T cells, obscuring true expression of P-gp + in the tumor cells. Of note is the high level of mdrl gene found in normal PBMC, NK, CD8, and CD4 cells [50]. Kemnitz et al. [51] reported expression of P-gp in healthy donors PBMC, while Neyfakh et al. [52] reported the presence of a population of T lymphocytes, mostly T killers/suppressors and part of the helpers, bearing the MDR phenotype. Michieli et al. [48] report the reactivity of C219 and MRK 16 MAbs with PBMC obtained from healthy donors. Detection of the P-gp molecule in normal PBMC should be taken into consideration when P-gp staining is evaluated and the consequent interpretation of reactivity of MAbs directed to the P-gp molecule may be very difficult. This study reports variable expression of P-gp$^+$ cells, ranging from 9% to 79%, labeled as weak, and 5% to 47% , labeled as a moderate to strong staining. Musto et al. [24, 41] also reported a heterogeneous expression of P-gp$^+$ cells ranging from < 1% to 100% in various hematologic malignancies. We have documented variability in the intensity of staining with three antibodies which can be segregated by their decreasing reactivity or intensity of staining as MRK-16, JSB-1, and C219. Similar observations were reported by Goasguen et al. [43] and Kemnitz et al. [51].

The clinical importance of immunostaining, showing only a few positive cells, is still unclear. Detection of a single P-gp$^+$ cell or cluster of P-gp$^+$ cells could be an important factor in the further promotion of the MDR phenotype from detected scattered P-gp$^+$ cells. Clonal growth of P-gp positive cells among tumor cells raises the question whether one or 100 cells should be considered as a threshold level above which results can be enumerated as positive. In their studies Goasguen et al. [43] put the gate level at 1% of P-gp$^+$ cells, while Musto et al. [41] observed in 30% of examined cases P-gp expression in fewer than 1% of neoplastic cells. In our IC study we regarded a case as positive for P-gp in which the immunoreactivity was observed with at least two antibodies. The first detection of MDR phenotype with C219 MAb was reported by Ma et al. [42]. They found, in two longitudinally studied patients, an increasing proportion of P-gp$^+$ cells during chemotherapy; moreover, they showed that intensity of staining and the proportion of P-gp$^+$ cells correlated well with drug resistance.

The present study reports detection of P-gp$^+$ cells in approximately one third children's and one third adults' leukemia cases, which is similar to the results by Zhou et al. [46] who found low expression of P-gp in 27% newly diagnosed AML cases. Results similar to ours were reported by Goasguen et al. [43]. They found reactivity of two MAbs, C219 and JSB-1, in 17 out of 55 (30%) children's and adults' newly diagnosed leukemias. Musto et al. [41] demonstrated P-gp$^+$ staining with C219 MAb in 44% newly diagnosed leukemia samples. Kuwazuru et al. [44] detected P-gp$^+$ staining in 56% newly and 50% relapsed AML as well as in 36% newly and 50% relapsed ALL cases using the immunoblotting technique and C219 MAb. In the latter study by Musto et al., variable reactivity of C219 MAb was detected in leukemic samples ranging from 19% at diagnosis, 25% at remission, and in 40% at relapse [24]. Higher immunoreactivity of this antibody than we observed in our study may reflect either "true" expression of P-gp or cross-reactivity of C219 MAb with the mdr3 gene product present in some hematologic malignancies [8, 31–34].

We compared P-gp$^+$ and P-gp$^-$ staining with clinical response to chemotherapy. In both P-gp$^+$ and P$^-$gp - specimens we observed considerable response to chemotherapy with high frequencies of complete remission: 85% children's, 81% adults' and 82% children's, 81% adults' respectively. Resistance to chemotherapy defined as partial remission, resistance, and death, was evident in approximately 18% of the cases. Musto et al. [41] also found response to chemotherapy at high frequencies in (80%) of P-gp$^+$ cases and resistance in 20% cases. These authors report a higher incidence of relapsed patients, while during disease presentation or CR, P-gp was detected in leukemic cells [24]. Goasguen et al. [43] also report high incidence of CR in P-gp$^+$ and P-gp$^-$ cases, and found that CR was achieved in 92% children's and 56% adults' P-gp$^-$ and in 92% children's and 93% adults' P-gp$^+$ samples. Kuwazuru et al. [44] report higher refractoriness to chemotherapy in patients with P-gp$^+$ cases. However, contrary to results presented by Musto et al. [41] and Kuwazuru et al. [44], 2 years of follow up of our patients revealed that relapse in P-gp$^+$ patients occurred with low frequencies. Clinical follow up in children's and adults' leukemias reveals a good initial response to chemotherapy used in newly diagnosed leukemias.

In the present study we did not find any correlation between refractoriness to chemotherapy and P-gp$^+$ stainings. CR was completed in 85% P-gp$^+$ cases in comparison with relapse, partial remission, resistance, and death (14%). Almost the same clinical outcome was observed in P-gp$^-$ staining cases 85% vs. 17%, respectively. It is, however, possible that the presence of P-gp$^+$ cells might identify a subset of patients with a potential risk of relapse, but we have been unable to prove it in our investigations. These results raise the question of whether the expression of P-gp can be used as a single prognostic marker to detect the multidrug resistance phenomenon in vivo.

References

1. Riordan, J.R., Ling, V. Genetic and biochemical characterization of multidrug resistance. Pharmac. Ther., 1985, 28, 51–75
2. Deuchars, K.L., Ling, V. P-glycoprotein and multidrug resistance in cancer chemotherapy. Seminars in Oncology, 1989, 16, 156–165
3. Roninson, I. B. The role of the MDRI (P-glycoprtein) gene in multidrug resistance in vitro and in vivo. Biochem. Pharmacol., 1992, 43, 95–102
4. Chen, Ch., Chin, J.E., Ueda, K., Clark, D.P., Pastan, I., Gottesman, M.M., Roninson, I. B. Internal duplication and homology with bacterial transport proteins in the mdr1 (P-glycoprotein) gene from multidrug-resistant human cells. Cell, 1986, 47, 381–389
5. Goldstein, L.J., Galski, H., Fojo, A., Willingham, M., Lai, S.L., Gazdar, A., Pirker, R., Green A., Crist, W., Brodeur, G.M., Lieber, M., Cossman, J., Gottesman, M.M., Pastan, I. Expression of a multidrug resistance gene in human cancers. J. Natl. Cancer Inst., 1989, 81, 116-124
6. Van der Bliek, A.M., Baas, F., Van der Velde-Koerts, T., Biedler, J.L., Meyers, M.B., Ozols, R.F., Hamilton, T.C., Joenje, H., Borst, P. Genes amplified and overexpressed in human multidrug-resistant cell lines. Cancer Res., 1988, 48, 5927–5932
7. Shen, D.W., Fojo, A., Roninson, I.B., Chin, J.E., Soffir, R., Pastan, I., Gottesman, M.M. Multidrug

resistance of DNA-mediated transformants is linked to transfer of the human mdr1 gene. Mol. Cell. Biol., 1986, 6, 4039-4044
8. Sonneveld, P., Nooter, K., Burghouts, J.T., Herweijer, H., Adriaansen, H.J., van Dongen, J.J. High expression of the mdr3 multidrug-resistance gene in advanced-stage chronic lymphocytic leukemia. Blood, 1992, 79, 1496-1500
9. Cordon-Cardo, C., O'Brien, J.P., Boccia, J., Casals, D., Bertino, J.R., Melamed, M.R. Expression of the multidrug resistance gene product (P-glycoprotein) in human normal and tumor tissues. J. Histochem. Cytochem., 1990, 38, 1277-1287
10. Pileri, S.A., Sabattini, E., Falini, B., Tazzari, P.L., Gherlinzoni, F., Michieli, M.G., Damiani, D., Zucchini, L., Gobbis, M., Tsuruo, T., Baccarani, M. Immunohistochemical detection of the multidrug transport protein P170 in human normal tissues and malignant lymphomas. Histopathology, 1991, 19, 131-140
11. Thiebaut, F., Tsuruo, T., Hamada, H., Gottesman, M.M., Pastan, I., Willingham, M.C. Cellular localization of the multidrug-resistance gene product P-glycoprotein in normal human tissues. Proc. Natl. Acad. Sci. USA, 1987, 84, 7735-7738
12. Van Kalken, C.K., Giaccone, G., van der Valk, P., Kuiper, C.M., Hadisaputro, M.M.N., Bosma, S.A.A., Scheper, R.J., Meijer, C.J.L.M., Pinedo, H.M., Multidrug resistance gene (P-glycoprotein) expression in the human fetus. Am. J. Pathol., 1992, 141, 1063-1072
13. Shen, D.W., Fojo, A., Chin, J.E., roninson, I.B., Richert, N., Pastan, I., Gottesman, I. Human multidrug-resistant cell lines: increased mdr1 expression can precede gene amplification. Science, 1987, 232, 643-6445
14. Fojo, A.T., Ueda, K., Slamon, D.J., Poplack, D.G., Gottesman, M.M., Pastan, I. Expression of multidrug-resistance in human tumors and tissues. Proc Natl Ac Sci USA, 1987, 84, 265-269
15. Cordon-Cardo, C., O'Brien, J.P., Casals, D., Rittman-Grauer, L., Biedler, J.L., Melamed, M.R., Bertino J.R. Multidrug-resistance gene (P-glycoprotein) is expressed by endothelial cells at blood—brain barrier sites. Proc. Natl. Acad. Sci. USA, 1989, 86, 695-698.
16. Kartner, N., Evernden-Porelle, D., Bradley, G., Ling, V. Detection of P-glycoprotein in multidrug resistant cell lines by monoclonal antibodies. Nature, 1985, 316, 820-823
17. Schlaifer, D., Laurent, G., Chittal, S., Tsuruo, T., Soues, S., Muller, C., Charcosset, J.Y., Alard, C., Brousset, P., Mazerrolles, C., Delsol, G. Immunohistochemical detection of multidrug resistance associated P-glycoprotein in tumour and stromal cells of human cancers. Br. J. Cancer, 1990, 62, 177-182
18. Thiebaut, F., Tsuruo, T., Hamada, H., Gottesman, M.M., Pastan, I., Willingham, M.C. Immunohistochemical localization in normal tissues of different epitopes in the multidrug transport protein P170: evidence for localization in brain capillaries and crossreactivity of one antibody with a muscle protein. J. Histochem. Cytochem., 1989, 37, 159-164
19. Kaczorowski, S., Porwit, A., Christensson, B. Expression of P-glycoprotein in non-Hodgkin's lymphomas. Leukemia and Lymphoma, 1991, 5, 379-386
20. Ucci, G., Petrini, M., Riccardi, A., Invernizzi, R., Carulli, G., Luoni, R., Giordano, M., Danova, M. Expression of p170 protein in multiple myeloma: a clinical study. Hematol Oncol., 1992, 10, 213-220
21. Gruber, A., Vitols, S., Norgren, S., Arestroem, I., Peterson,- C., Bjoerkholm, M., Reizenstein, P., Luthman, H. Quantitative determination of mdr1 gene expression in leukaemic cells from patients with acute leukaemia. Br. J. Cancer, 1992, 66, 266-272
22. Pirker, R., Wallner, J., Geissler, K., Linkesch, W., Haas, O.A., Bettelheim, P., Hopfner, M., Scherrer, R., Havelec, L., Ludwig, H., Lechner, K. MDRI gene expression and treatment outcome in acute myeloid leukemia. J. Natl. Cancer Inst., 1991, 83, 708-712
23. Sato, H., Preisler, H., Day, Raza, A., Larson, R., Browman, G., Goldberg, J., Vogler, R., Grunwald, H., Gottlieb, A., Bennet, J., Gottesman, M., Pastan, I. MDRI transcript levels as an indication of resistant disease in acute myelogenous leukemia. Br. J. Haemat., 1990, 75, 340-345
24. Musto, P., Melillo, L., Lombardi, G., Matera, R., di Giorgio, D., Carotenuto, M. High risk of early resistant relapse for leukaemic patients with presence of multidrug associated P-glycoprotein positive cells in complete remission. Br J Haematology, 1991, 77, 50-53
25. Bennett, J.M., Catovsky, D., Daniel, M.T., Flandrin, G., Galton, D.A.G., Gralnick, H.R., Sultan, C. Proposals for the classification of the acute leukaemias (FAB) cooperative group. Br. J. Haematol., 1976, 33, 451-458
26. Scheper, J.R., Bulte, J.W.M., Brakkee, J.G.P., Quak, J.J., van der Schoot, E., Balm, A.J.M., Meijer, C.J.L.M., Broxterman, H.J., Kuiper, C.M., Lankelma, J., Pinedo, H.M. Monoclonal antibody JSB-1 detects a highly conserved epitope on the P-glycoprotein associated with multi-drug-resistance. Int. J. Cancer, 1988, 42, 389-394
27. Hamada, H., Tsuruo, T. Functional role for the 170- to 180-kDa glycoprotein specific to drug-resistant tumor cells as revealed by monoclonal antibodies. Proc Natl Acad Sci USA, 1986, 83, 7785-7789
28. Cordell, J.L., Falini, B., Erber, W.N., Ghosh, A.K., Abdulaziz, Z., MacDonald, S., Pulford, K.A.F., Stein, H., Mason, D.Y. Immunoenzymatic labeling of monoclonal antibodies using immune complexes of alkaline phosphatase and monoclonal anti-alkaline phosphatase (APAAP complexes). J. Histochem. Cytochem., 1984, 32, 219-229
29. Van der Valk, P., van Kalken, C.K., Katelaars, H. Broxterman, H.J., Scheffer, G., Kuiper, C.M., Tsuruo, T., Lankelma, J., Meijer, C.J.L.M., Pinedo, H.M., Scheper, R.J. Distribution of multi-drug resistance-associated P-glycoprotein in normal

and neoplastic human tissues. Analysis with 3 monoclonal antibodies recognizing different epitopes of the P-glycoprotein molecule. Annals of Oncol., 1990, 1, 56–64
30. Weinstein, R.S., Kuszak, J.R., Jakate, S.M., Lebovitz, M.D., Kluskens, L.F., Coon, J.S. ABO blood type predicts the cytolocalization of anti-P-glycoprotein monoclonal antibody reactivity in human colon and ureter. Hum Pathol., 1990, 21, 949-958
31. Nooter, K., Sonneveld, P., Janssen, A., Oostrum, R., Boersma, T., Herweijer, H., Valerio, D., Hagemeijer, A., Baas, F. Expression of the mdr3 gene in prolymphocytic leukemia: association with cyclosporin-A-induced increase in drug accumulation. Int J Cancer, 1990, 45, 626–631
32. Herweijer, H., Sonneveld, P., Baas, F., Nooter, K. Expression of mdrl and mdr3 multidrug-resistance genes in human acute and chronic leukemias and association with stimulation of drug accumulation by cyclosporine. J Natl Cancer Inst, 1990, 82, 1133–1140
33. Herweijer, H., Nooter, K., Beishuizen, A., Sonneweld, P., Oosrum, R.G., Hesseling-Janssen, A.L.W., van Dongen, J.J.M. Expression of mdrl and mdr3 multidrug-resistance genes in hairy cell leukemia. Eur J Cancer, 1991, 27, 297–298
34. Georges, E., Bradley, G., Geriepy, J., Ling, V. Detection of P-glycoprotein isoforms by gene-specific monoclonal antibodies. Proc Natl Ac Sci USA, 1990, 87, 152–156
35. Garberoglio, C., Dudas, M., Casper, E.S., Bertino, J., Cordon-Cardo, C. Expression of P-glycoprotein in normal muscle cells and myogenic tumors. Arch Patol Lab Med., 1992, 116, 1055–1061
36. Finstad, C.L., Yin, B.W.T., Gordon, C.M., Federici, M.G., Welt, S., Lloyd K.O. Some monoclonal antibody reagents (C219 and JSB-1) to P-glycoprotein contains antibodies to blood group A carbohydrate determinants: a problem of quality control for immunohistochemical analysis. J. Histochem. Cytochem., 1991, 39, 1603–1610
37. Sugawara, I., Kataoka, I., Morishita, Y., Hamada, H., Tsuruo, T., Itoyama, S., Mori, S. Tissue distribution of P-glycoprotein encoded by a multidrug-resistant gene as revealed by monoclonal antibody MRK16. Cancer Res., 1988, 48, 1926–1929
38. Georges, E., Tsuruo, T., Ling, V. Topology of P-glycoprotein as determined by epitope mapping of MRK-16 monoclonal antibody. J. Biol. Chem., 1993, 268, 1792-1798
39. Ito Y., Tanimoto, M., Kumazawa, T., Okumura, M., Morishima, Y., Ohno, R., Saito H. Increased P-glycoprotein expression and multidrug resistant gene (mdrl) amplification are infrequently found in fresh acute leukemia cells. Cancer, 1989, 63, 1534–1538
40. Holmes, J., Jacobs, A., Carter, G., Janowska-Wieczorek, A., Padua, R.A. Multidrug resistance in haemopoietic cell lines, myelodysplastic syndromes and acute myeloblastic leukaemia. Br J Haematology, 1989, 72, 40–44
41. Musto, P., Cascavilla, Di Renzo, N., Ladogana, S., La Sala, A., Melillo, L., Nobile, M., Matera, R., lombardi, G., Carotenuto, M. Clinical relevance of immunocytochemical detection of multidrug resistance associated P-glycoprotein in hematologic malignancies. Tumori, 1990, 76, 353–359
42. Ma, D.D.F., Davey, R.A., Harman, D.H., Isbister, J.P., Scurr, R.D., Makertich, S.M., Dowden, G., Bell, D.R. Detection of a multidrug resistant phenotype in acute non-lymphoblastic leukaemia. Lancet, 1987, 135–137
43. Goasguen, J.E., Dossot, J-M., Fardel, O., Le Mee, F., le Gall, E., Leblay, R., LePrise, P.Y., Chaperon, J., Fauchet, R. Expression of the multidrug resistance associated P-glycoprotein (P-170) in 59 cases of de novo acute lymphoblastic leukemia: prognostic implication. Blood, 1993, 81, 2394–2398
44. Kuwazuru, Y., Yoshimura, A., Hanada, S., Utsunomiya, A., Makino, T., Ishibashi, K., Kodama, M., Iwashashi, M., Arima, T., Akiyama, S-I. Expression of the multidrug transporter P-glycoprotein in acute leukemia cells and correlation to clinical drug resistance. Cancer, 1990, 66, 868–873
45. Michieli, M., Damiani, D., Geromin, A., Michelutti, A., Fanin, R., Raspadori, D., Russo, D., Visani, G., Dinota, A., Pileri, S. et al. Overexpression of multidrug resistance-associated p170-glycoprotein in acute non-lymphocytic leukemia. Eur J Haematol., 1992, 48, 87–92
46. Zhou, D.C., Marie, J.P., Suberville, A.M., Zittoun, R. Relevance of mdrl gene expression in acute myeloid leukemia and comparison of different diagnostic methods. Leukemia, 1992, 6, 879–885
47. Mizuno, Y., Hara, T., Nagata, M., Tawa, A., Tsuruo, T., Ueda, K. Detection of multidrug-resistant protein, P-glycoprotein in childhood leukaemia and lymphoma. Eur J Pediatr., 1991, 150, 416–418
48. Michieli, M., Raspadori, D., Damiani, D., Geromin, A., Gallizia, C., Michelutti, A., Fanin, R., Fasola, G., Russo, D., Tazzari, P., pileri, S., Mallardi, F., Baccarani, M. The expression of the multidrug resistance-associated glycoprotein in B-cell chronic lymphocytic leukemia. Br J Haematology, 1991, 77, 460–465
49. Kellen, J.A. Molecular interrelationships in multidrug resistance (Review). Anticancer Res., 1994, 14, 433–436
50. Drach, D., Zhao, S., Drach, J., Mahadevia, R., gattringer, C., Huber, H., Andreeff, M. Subpopulations of normal peripheral blood and bone marrow cells express a functional multidrug resistance phenotype. Blood, 1992, 80,2729–2734
51. Kemnitz, J., Freund, M., Dominis, M., Cohnert, T.R., Uysal, A., Georgii, A. Detection of cells with multidrug-resistant phenotype in myeloproliferative disorders before therapy. Hematologic Pathol, 1989, 3, 73–78
52. Neyfakh, A.A., Serpinskaya, A.S., Chervonsky, A.V., Apasov, S.G., Kazarov, A.R. Multidrug-resistance phenotype of a subpopulation of T-lymphocytes without drug selection. Exp. Cell Res., 1989, 185, 496–505

Acute Leukemias VI
Prognostic Factors
and Treatment Strategies
Büchner et al. (eds)

Clinical Relevance of P-Glycoprotein-Related Resistance in Patients with Acute Leukemia

V. Nüssler[1], R. Pelka-Fleischer[1], H. Zwierzina[2], C. Nerl[3], B. Beckert[1], F. Gieseler[4], D. Hölzel[5], G. Ledderose[1], E. Gullis[6], H. Sauer[1], and W. Wilmanns[1,6]

Abstract. P-glycoprotein (P-gp) is a crucial factor in the development of chemotherapy resistance in malignant disorders. Between 1989 and 1994 P-gp expression was prospectively studied in mononuclear bone marrow cells of 304 (221 acute myelogenous leukemia, AML; 83 acute lymphoblastic leukemia, ALL) patients. In 282 patients P-gp was investigated before and after therapy and in 22 patients only before therapy: 148 AML patients with the AML-6 protocol (European Organization for Research on Treatment of Cancer), containing daunorubicin, vincristine and conventional-dose cytarabine (ara-C); and 63 AML patients were treated with intermediate-dose ara-C plus amsacrine. A further 71 ALL patients were treated according to a German standard polychemotherapy protocol (Bundesgesundheitsministerium für Forschung and Technologie, BMFT04/1989). P-gp was determined by using monoclonal antibodies C219 and 4E3, and the cut-off point for P-gp overexpression was set at $\geqslant 10\%$. A significant ($p < 0.05$) difference in P-gp overexpression was demonstrated between AML (21.7%) and ALL (10.2%) patients at primary diagnosis and between primary diagnosis and relapse/refractoriness in AML (21.7%; 51.2%) and ALL (10.2%; 27.2%) patients. According to French-American-British (FAB) classification, P-gp overexpression was detected in AML patients significantly ($P < 0.05$) more frequently in classes M4, M5a, and M5b and less frequently in M3, as compared to other types. Of AML patients 35%, after therapy according to the AML-6 protocol, and 11.5%, after intermediate-dose ara-C plus amsacrine, as well as 7% of ALL patients after treatment developed P-gp overexpression. For AML patients with P-gp overexpression at primary diagnosis or early relapse/refractoriness, the predictive values for nonresponse to AML-6 protocol were 90% and 94%, respectively, while late-relapsed AML patients with P-gp overexpression had a significantly ($p < 0.05$) lower predictive value of 73% for nonresponse. Additionally, in refractory and late-relapsed P-gp-overexpressing AML patients treated with intermediate-dose ara-C plus amsacrine, the predictive values for nonresponse were 44% and 39%, respectively, significantly ($p < 0.05$) lower as compared to AML-6 protocol-treated refractory or late-relapsed AML patients. In P-gp-overexpressing treated ALL patients the predictive values of 50% and 55% for nonresponse were calculated at primary diagnosis and late relapse, respectively. We conclude that P-gp overexpression is a common phenomenon in AML patients at primary diagnosis or relapse, has an inverse influence on AML-6 treatment outcome, and should be taken into consideration in the development of new therapy strategies.

[1]Medizinische Klinik III, Klinikum Großhadern, Marchioninistr. 15, 80377 Munich, Germany
[2]Innere Medizin, Universitätsklinik Innsbruck, Anichstr. 35, 6020 Innsbruck, Austria
[3]I. Medizinische Abteilung, Krankenhaus Schwabing, Kölner Platz 1, 80804 Munich, Germany
[4]Medizinische Polyklinik, Klinikstr. 8, 97070 Würzburg, Germany
[5]IBE, Klinikum Großhadern, Marchioninistr. 15, 80377 Munich, Germany
[6]gsf-Forschungszentrum, Haematologikum, Marchioninistr. 25, 80377 Munich, Germany

Introduction

Polychemotherapy in adult acute leukemia patients has a complete remission rate of 58% to 80% [1–6]. Some 20% of these patients, however, are primarily refractory to treatment and an even higher percentage will be refractory in relapse [7]. Since the identification of a transmembrane glycoprotein known as 170 kd P-glycoprotein [8](P-gp) and coded by the multidrug-resistance (mdr)1 gene [9], the field of resistance research has focused on an intense in vitro and ex vivo characterization of the mechanism of P-gp-related resistance[10]. It is assumed that P-gp actively pumps P-gp-related substances (such as anthracyclines, vinca alkaloids, podophyllotoxins, paclitaxel, and actinomycin D) out of the cell in an (adenosine-s'-triphosphate ATP) dependent manner[11]. However, a few reports show that P-gp overexpression may also be associated with a decrease in drug influx [12].

A similar glycoprotein coded by the mdr2 (mdr3) gene is presumed to occur mainly in B cell neoplasms [13]. This glycoprotein has no relation to the resistance phenomenon caused by the mdr1-coded glycoprotein.

Many reports [14–49] have recently been published on P-gp expression in acute myelogenous leukemia (AML) and acute lymphoblastic leukemia (ALL). Most of these have failed to investigate a large number of patients with close follow-up according to the same treatment protocol. Furthermore, results are often not comparable because of the different methods used, and the definition of P-gp overexpression fluctuates in most publications. We used immunocytology as a simple and quick test, because it is easy to standardize.

This study aims to prove the incidence and clinical relevance of P-gp-related resistance in a large number of acute leukemia patients. The following questions were additionally addressed in our study: How is the cut-off point for P-gp overexpression defined? What is the incidence of P-gp expression in AML/ALL patients at primary diagnosis and in relapse or refractoriness? Does a particular group according to French–American–British (FAB) classification demonstrate P-gp-related resistance more often? Can P-gp overexpression be acquired by patients during treatment? Does intrinsic or acquired P-gp overexpression influence treatment outcome?

Materials and Methods

Patients. This study covers 304 acute leukemia patients including 92 AML patients at primary diagnosis and 129 AML patients in relapse/refractoriness, as well as 83 ALL patients, of whom 39 were at primary diagnosis and 44 in relapse (Table 1). Therapy-related leukemia or leukemia evolving from a myelodysplastic syndrome was excluded from this analysis. The age of AML patients ranged from 21 to 58 years and that of ALL patients from 19 to 53 years. Additionally, 22 healthy bone marrow (BM) donors were analyzed. P-gp expression of mononucleated BM cells was determined in 282 patients before and after therapy, provided that the leukocyte count was >1.5 g/l. However, in 22 patients P-gp expression was only measured before therapy (Table 1). P-gp expression was measured in fresh BM specimens, which were stored at room temperature for no longer than 3 days. No significant changes in P-gp expression value were seen (data not shown).

Treatment Protocols. AML patients were treated according to the European Organization of Research on Treatment of Cancer (EORTC) AML-6 protocol (study coordinator: R. Zittoun) [3] daunorubicin 45 mg/m^2 days 1–3; vincristine 1 mg/m^2, day 2; ara-C at 12-h intervals 50mg/m^2 and daily continuous infusions 100 mg/m^2, days 1–7) or according to a regimen using intermediate-dose cytarabine (ara-C, 1 g/m^2, days 1–6) and amsacrine (120 mg/m^2, days 5–7).

Acute lymphoblastic leukemia patients were included in the German BMFT[5] (Bundesgesundheitsministerium für Forschung and Technologie) study 04/1989 (study coordinator: D. Hoelzer). Treatment results were evaluated for response in relation of P-gp expression after an induction therapy with vincristine (2mg absolute/day) on days 1, 8, 15, 22; daunorubicin (45 mg/m^2) on days 1, 8, 15, 22; prednisone (60 mg/m) on days 1–28; and asparaginase (5000U/m^2) on days 15–28. In patients who achieved a partial remission (PR) only the induction protocol was repeated.

Evaluation Criteria. Two groups were defined for evaluation of treatment results. Patients achieving complete remission (CR) were compared with nonresponders, including PR, no change (NC), or progressive disease (PD). Early relapse is defined as relapse with in 6 months, and in relation there to late relapse as a relapse after more than 6 months. Refractoriness is determined as the primary NC or PD to chemotherapy.

Monoclonal Antibodies. MAb C219 (Centokor, Malvern, USA) is a mouse MAb (IgG2a class) directed toward an intracellular epitope of the human mdr1-encoded P-gp[50,51]. MAb C219, however, also recognizes the mdr2-encoded glycoprotein[52], and reaction with myosin [53] or contamination of some charges of purified MAb C219 with an anti-A blood group[54] antibody has been reported. MAb 4E3 is a mouse MAb directed toward an extracellular epitope of the human mdr1-encoded P-gp[55]. This MAb is also an IgG2a class antibody, which was originally a gift of Dr. Arceci (Dana-Faber Institute, Boston, USA) and was later ordered from Signet Laboratories, Inc., Dedham, MA,USA. MAb 4E3 specifically recognizes the human mdr1 P-gp but not the mdr2 product.

Cell Lines. Standardization was performed with human T-lymphoblastic leukemia cell line (CCRF-CEM) with low P-gp expression and its variants (CCRF-CEMACT400, CCRF-CEMVCR-1000; a gift from Dr. V. Gekeler, Byk Gulden, Constance, Germany) with P-gp overexpression between 95% and 100%. "ACT 400" or "VCR 1000" means actinomycin D (MSD, Sharp Dohme) at a concentration of 400 ng/m^2 or lincristine (Lilly, Germany) at a concentration of 1000 ng/ml as needed to maintain maximal P-gp expression in these cell lines.

P-gp Determination. Using MAb C219, P-gp was determined with the direct immunocytological method. Mononuclear BM cells were obtained with the standard Ficoll-Hypaque technique, washed twice with phosphate-buffered saline (PBS)+0.05% NaN3 and centrifuged at 200 *g* for 5 min. For fixation the mononuclear cells were resuspended in 70% cold methanol and incubated for 10 min at −20°C to permeabilize the cell membrane. The cells were then washed again twice in PBS+0.05% NaN3, centrifuged at 200 *g* for 5 min and resuspended in PBS+0.05% NaN3+0.5% Tween 20 for 10 min on ice. Cell suspensions were centrifuged at 200 *g* for 5 min, and pellets resuspended in PBS+0.05% NaN3+20% fetal calf serum (FCS) at a final concentration of 5×10^6 cells/ml. After 15 min on ice 1×10^6 cells were incubated for 1 h with 0.5 μg of the fluorescein isothiocyanate (FITC)-labeled MAb C219. For negative control, a separate tube was filled with the same concentration of an FITC MAb of the same isotype (IgG2a). After incubation in darkness on ice for 1h, cells were washed twice, resuspended in the above-mentioned solution, and evaluated with a flow cytometer (FACScan, Becton Dickinson, San Jose, USA) combined with LYSIS II computer software. P-glycoprotein was determined with the indirect immunocytological method using M Ab 4E3. For 4E3 estimation, mononuclear cells were concentrated and washed using the method for MAb C219 (see above). The pellets were resuspended in PBS+0.05% NaN3+20% FCS at a final concentration of 5×10^6 cells/ml. After 15 min on ice, 200 μl cell suspension was incubated with 5 μl MAb 4E3. For negative control 200 μl suspension was put in a separate tube without antibody. Both tubes were incubated on ice for 30–60 min. Samples were centrifuged and washed (see MAb C219). Pellets were resuspended and 1 μl FITC-conjugated secondary antibody (goat anti-mouse IgG2a, Sigma Immuno Chemicals, Deisenhofen, Germany) added. Both tubes were subsequently incubated on ice in darkness for 30–45 min. After the cells were washed once, they were resuspended for flow cytometric analysis with LYSIS II computer software.

Statistics. The U (Wilcoxon) test was used for comparison of patients' P-gp values (CSS software). Wilcoxon tests the hypothesis that there are no differences between two paired populations of ordered-metric scores. The test takes into account the magnitude of the differences between two paired variables; p values <0.05 were considered statistically significant. Assuming that P-gp expression correlates with the response/nonresponse ratio, a predictive value estimation for response in relation to normal P-gp expression was calculated as the ratio of responding patients to the total number of treated patients with normal P-gp expression. The predictive value for nonresponse in relation to P-gp overexpression is the ratio of nonresponding patients to the total number of treated patients with P-gp overexpression. Sensitivity for MAb C219 and 4E3 is the ratio between responding patients with normal P-gp expression and the total number of all responders. Specificity for MAb C219 and 4E3 is the ratio between nonresponding patients with P-gp overexpression and the total of all nonresponders.

Results

Cut-off Point for P-gp Overexpression

When using the direct and/or indirect immunocytology method with MAbs C219 and 4E3 in the mononuclear cell fraction of the BM, the cut-off point for P-gp positivity was set at ≥10%. The reason for this decision was that in 22 healthy persons P-gp expression in mononuclear BM cells ranged between 0% and 8% when using both MAbs. To further rule out the above-mentioned cross-reactivities of C219, MAb 4E3 was also used. In 83 examined specimens from ALL patients, correspondence of 4E3 versus C219 results was seen to be 98%. The 2% difference was seen in two B-ALL patients, where MAb C219 was positive (35% and 57%) and MAb 4E3 negative (2% and 3%), which can be interpreted as identification of the mdr2 glycoprotein. In 153 examined AML patients a total correspondence was seen between the results of MAbs C219 and 4E3. Therefore, all results for ALL patients were routinely measured with MAbs C219 and 4E3. For AML patients, however, P-gp expression was determined with MAb C219 and partially controlled with MAb 4E3.

P-gp Expression in AML, ALL Patients at Primary Diagnosis or Relapse/Refractoriness Before Therapy

Twenty (21.7%) of 92 AML patients with primary diagnosis were P-gp positive as compared to 129 AML patients at early relapse (≤6 months), refractoriness, or late relapse (>6 months), where 66 (51.2%) were P-gp positive (Fig.1). Of the 39 ALL patients with primary diagnosis, two T-ALL and two C-ALL patients (10.2%) were P-gp positive in comparison to 44 ALL patients in relapse, where 12 (27.2%) were P-gp positive (Fig. 1).

The difference in P-gp overexpression between primary diagnosis and relapse/refractoriness is significant ($p<0.05$) in AML and ALL patients. Regarding primary diagnosis, the difference between P-pg overexpression is also significant ($p<0.05$) in AML and ALL patients. The incidence of P-gp overexpression in AML patients in relapsed/refractory state is, however, not significant as compared to ALL patients at relapse/refractoriness diagnosis.

P-gp Expression Relation to FAB Classification in AML Patients and Immunophenotype in ALL Patients

The AML patient demonstrated a significantly ($p<0.05$) higher incidence of P-gp overexpression in FAB classifications M4, M5a, and M5b as compared to the remaining classes (Table 2). In contrast, FAB M3 AML patients had the signifi-

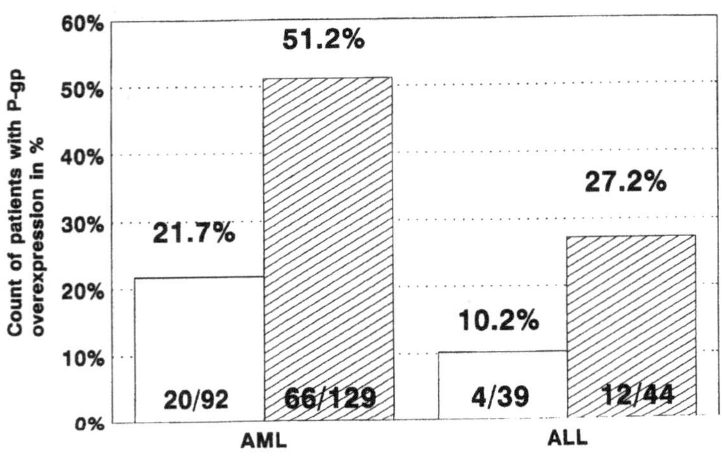

Fig. 1. P-gp expression in AML and ALL patients at primary diagnosis (*open columns*); or (*hatched columns*) relapse/refractoriness

Table 1. Overview of treated and untreated AML/ALL patients in relation to P-gp expression

Patients	Evaluated Patients (*n*)	Patients with P-gp overexpression:	
		(*n*)	(%)
AML at primary diagnosis treated with AML-6-protocol	92	20	22
AML at early relapse (< 6months) or refractoriness treated with AML-6-protocol	26	17	65
AML at late (> 6 months) relapse treated with AML-6-protocol	30	11	37
AML at refractoriness after AML-6-protocol treated with intermediate-dose ara-C plus amsacrine	19	16	84
AML at late relapse treated with intermediate-dose ara-C plus amsacrine	44	18	41
AML at late relapse treated according to protocols not included in this study[a]	10	4	40
ALL at primary diagnosis treated with BMFT protocol (induction part)	39	4	10
ALL at first late relapse treated with BMFT protocol (induction part)	32	9	28
ALL at late relapse treated according to protocols not included in this study[a]	12	3	25

[a]P-gp expression was determined before therapy.

Table 2. Distribution of AML patients at primary diagnosis and newly registered patients at relapse/refractoriness in relation to P-gp overexpression and FAB classification

FAB classification of AML patients	Examined patients (*n*)	Patients with P-gp overexpression	
		(*n*)	(%)
M1	34	12	35
M2	79	21	26
M3	12	2	17
M4	20	12	60
M4 E0	2	-	
M5a	7	5	71
M5b	7	5	71
M6	7	2	29
M7	3	1	33

cantly ($p < 0.05$) lowest incidence of P-gp overexpression (Table 2). For ALL patients, the different P-gp overexpression in relation to immunophenotype (Table 3) is not significant.

Follow-up of P-gp Expression Before and After AML-6 Protocol, Intermediate-Dose ara-C plus Amsacrine and BMFT Protocol Treatment

P-glycoprotein level was observed before and after each AML-6 therapy in 100 AML patients at primary diagnosis and relapse/refractoriness who had normal P-gp expression before treat-

Table 3. Distribution of examined ALL patients at primary diagnosis and newly registered patients at relapse/refractoriness in relation to P-gp overexpression and immunophenotype

Immunophenotype of ALL patients	Examined patients (n)	Patients with P-gp overexpression	
		(n)	(%)
C-ALL	43	4	9
T-ALL	22	8	36
NOALL	15	4	27
B-ALL	3	–	–

ment. P-gp overexpression was observed in 35 (35%) AML patients after one or two AML-6 protocol therapies. Twenty-nine (83%) of these 35 AML patients showed an increase in P-gp expression after the first AML-6 protocol therapy: 12 showed PR, 13 NC, and four PD. Six (17%) of these 35 AML patients exhibited an increase in P-gp in BM after the second AML-6 protocol therapy. All of these patients showed NC afterwards.

In three (11.5%) of 26 AML patients treated with intermediate-dose ara-C plus amsacrine, P-gp overexpression combined with PR was seen after the first therapy. Ten of these 26 patients were treated with a second regimen of intermediate-dose ara-C plus amsacrine, but no P-gp overexpression was observed.

Only four (7%) of the 58 ALL patients at primary diagnosis or relapse developed P-gp overexpression after induction therapy according to the BMFT protocol. None of them achieved CR.

The difference between acquisition of P-gp overexpression after therapy according to the AML-6 protocol as compared to the intermediate-dose ara-C plus amsacrine and BMFT protocol (induction part) is significant ($p < 0.05$).

P-gp Expression in Relation to Response of AML-6, Intermediate-Dose ara-C plus Amsacrine and BMFT Protocol Treatment

As shown in Table 1, 92 AML patients at primary diagnosis, 26 AML patients at early relapse/refractoriness, and 30 AML patients in late

Table 4. Overview of treated AML patients in relation to predictive values for response/nonresponse regarding P-gp expression

Patient groups	P-gp expression (%)	Responders (n)	Non-responders (n)	Total (n)	Predictive values (%)	(n)
AML at primary diagnosis and treated with AML-6 protocol	< 10	68	4	72	Response: 94.4	68/72
	⩾ 10	2	18	20	Nonresponse: 90.0	18/20
		70	22	92		
AML at early relapse or refractoriness and treated with AML-6 protocol	< 10	6	3	9	Response: 66.6	6/9
	⩾ 10	1	16	17	Nonresponse: 94.1	16/17
		7	19	26		
AML at late relapse treated with AML-6 protocol	< 10	10	9	19	Response: 52.6	10/19
	⩾ 10	3	8	11	Nonresponse: 72.7	8/11
		13	17	30		
AML at refractoriness after AML-6 protocol treated with intermediate-dose ara-C plus amsacrine	< 10	1	2	3	Response: 33.3	1/3
	⩾ 10	9	7	16	Nonresponse: 43.7	7/16
		10	9	19		
AML at late relapse treated with intermediate-dose ara-C plus amsacrine	< 10	11	15	26	Response: 42.3	11/26
	⩾ 10	11	7	18	Nonresponse: 38.8	7/18
		22	22	44		

relapse were treated with the AML-6 protocol. Nineteen refractory AML patients after AML-6 protocol therapy were treated with intermediate-dose ara-C plus amsacrine. Forty-four AML patients in late relapse were treated with intermediate-dose ara-C plus amsacrine. Thirty-nine ALL patients at primary diagnosis and 32 ALL patients in first late relapse were treated with the induction part of BMFT study 04/1989.

AML-6 Protocol Treatment. At primary diagnosis the predictive value for nonresponse in AML patients with P-gp overexpression was 90.0%, while for response in patients with normal P-gp expression it was 94.4% (Table 4). Test sensitivity (68/70 patients) and specificity (18/22 patients) reached a value of 97.1% and 81.8%, respectively. PR was seen in six of 18 nonresponding AML patients at primary diagnosis with P-gp overexpression. A reinduction AML-6 protocol therapy in these six patients resulted in four patients with NC and two with PD. Compared to the four nonresponding (PR) AML patients with normal P-gp expression, reinduction therapy demonstrated CR in two of these four patients. For AML patients at early relapse/refractoriness with P-gp overexpression, the predictive value for nonresponse was 94.1%, while for patients with normal P-gp expression the predictive value for response was 66.6%. Test sensitivity (6/7 patients) was 85.7%, test specificity (16/19 patients) 84.2%. Compared to the two latter patient groups, the predictive value for nonresponse in AML patients at late relapse with P-gp overexpression was 72.7%, thus significantly ($p = 0.048$) lower. The predictive value for response in relation to normal P-gp expression was 52.6%. Test sensitivity (10/13 patients) and test specificity (8/17 patients) were 76.9% and 47%, respectively.

Intermediate-Dose ara-C plus Amsacrine Treatment. Predictive values were calculated at 43.7% for nonresponse in refractory AML patients with P-gp overexpression and at 33.3% for response in relation to normal P-gp expression (Table 4.). Test sensitivity (1/10 patients) and test specificity (7/9 patients) were seen to be 10% and 77.7%, respectively. Predictive values of 38.8% for nonresponse and 42.3% for response were determined in relation to P-gp overexpression or normal P-gp expression for AML patients at late relapse. Test sensitivity (11/22 patients) and test specificity (7/22) were 50% and 31.8%, respectively. In AML patients at refractoriness and late relapse with P-gp overexpression a significant ($p < 0.05$) difference regarding predictive value for nonresponse was evaluated between AML-6 and intermediate-dose ara-C plus amsacrine treatment.

Induction Part of BMFT Study 04/1989. For ALL patients at primary diagnosis the predictive value for nonresponse in relation to P-gp overexpression was 50%, and for response with normal P-gp expression 71.4% (Table 5). Sensitivity (25/27 patients) and specificity (2/12 patients) were established at 92.6% and 16.6%, respectively. Predictive values for nonresponse with P-gp overexpression and response with normal P-gp expression were 55.5% and 65.2%, respectively, in ALL patients at late relapse. Test sensitivity (15/19 patients) and test specificity (5/13 patients) were 78.9% and 38.5%, respectively.

Table 5. Overview of treated ALL patients in relation to predictive values for response/nonresponse regarding P-gp expression

Patient groups	P-gp expression (%)	Responders (n)	Non-responders (n)	Total (n)	Predictive values		
						(%)	(n)
ALL at primary diagnosis and treated with BMFT protocol (induction part)	< 10	25	10	35	Response:	71.4	25/35
	≥ 10	2	2	4	Nonresponse:	50.0	2/4
		27	12	39			
ALL at first late relapse and treated with BMFT protocol (induction part)	< 10	15	8	23	Response:	65.2	15/23
	≥ 10	4	5	9	Nonresponse:	55.5	5/9
		19	13	32			

Discussion

The goal of this analysis of 304 acute leukemia patients was to substantiate the clinical relevance of P-gp. For this purpose, it was necessary to first define the cut-off point of P-gp overexpression according to our method. The described procedure using MAbs C219 and 4E3 defines P-gp overexpression at ≥ 10% positive cells in BM. The decision to use this method was made to ensure a simple and fast method, and to measure the target at the protein level. The use of MAb C219, however, presents a possible trap as it also recognizes the mdr2-coded glycoprotein. Therefore, MAb 4E3 was used to exclude cross-reactivities to the mdr2 gene product, especially in B-ALL patients in whom mdr2 gene product overexpression is more frequent [13].

Our data allows clinically relevant conclusions in the following direction. In AML patients FAB M4, M5a, and M5b, the frequency of P-gp overexpression is significantly higher, while it is significantly lower for FAB M3 as compared to the remaining FAB classes. This variable P-gp expression within the FAB classification of AML patients underscores the reports of other authors that P-gp expression may contribute to different responses to chemotherapy seen within FAB classes [48]. In ALL patients there is no significant difference within the immunophenotypic subtypes in relation to P-gp expression.

As P-gp overexpression in ALL patients at primary diagnosis is significantly less common as compared to AML patients, it is very probable that in ALL patients refractory to chemotherapy at primary diagnosis other resistance mechanisms are dominant, like DNA topoismerases, glutathione-S-transferase and multidrug-related protein (mrp) mechanisms [56–59]. Acquired P-gp-related resistance is significantly more common in relapsed/refractory AML than ALL patients. This fact and the significantly more frequent occurrence of P-gp overexpression in AML patients at primary diagnosis as compared to ALL patients supports the conjecture that AML patients are at greater risk of developing P-gp-related resistance.

Three different therapy protocols were applied in this analysis: strong P-gp transport-related drugs; AML-6 protocol containing two strong P-gp-related drugs like daunorubicin and vincristine; German standard ALL protocol, also containing daunorubicin and vincristine, but additionally asparaginase, a P-gp-nonrelated substance, and dexamethasone [60], which inhibit the P-gp-related drug transport mechanism. The third protocol used intermediate-dose ara-C plus amsacrine are two cytostatics not or only less well related to P-gp. In this respect, the three mentioned protocols can be ranked as P-gp-related, less well P-gp-related, and non-P-gp-related protocols for further discussion.

P-glycoprotein overexpression influences the outcome of AML patients at primary diagnosis and early relapse/refractoriness and treated with a P-gp-related protocol. A comparison of these results with the predictive value for nonresponse of AML patients with P-gp overexpression at late relapse demonstrated a significantly lower value. This indicates that, especially in late relapsed AML patients, the probable reason is multiple pretreatment; other resistance mechanisms are more dominant, like P-gp-related ones. In ALL patients no difference was observed between primary diagnosis and late relapse in relation to the predictive value for response in patients with P-gp overexpression. The probable reason is the additional use of different drugs not related to P-gp transport and the fact that in ALL patients a low incidence of P-gp overexpression was found. Additionally, the latter point is underscored by the low incidence of ocurrence of P-gp overexpression after German standard protocol therapy, as compared to the high incidence in AML patients treated with the AML-6 protocol.

Reasons for developing P-gp overexpression after therapy could be induction and/or selection of P-gp-positive cells. Induction of P-gp overexpression might be explained by mutations [61] or the action of cytotoxic drugs via a receptor [62] activating the mdr 1 gene. On the other hand, selection may be a result of selective reduction in the P-gp-negative blast population, therefore resulting in a relative increase in frequency of P-gp overexpression.A further aspect is the clinical relevance of P-gp overexpression in relation to P-gp-nonrelated therapy protocols. The significantly lower predictive values for nonresponse in AML patients at late relapse and refractoriness with P-gp overexpression treated with intermediate-dose ara-C plus amsacrine as compared to AML patients at late relapse and refractoriness treated with a P-gp-related protocol (AML-6) provide evidence for the subordinate role of P-gp in relation to a P-gp-nonrelated therapy. Surprisingly, however, a considerable number of these patients with P-gp overexpression do not respond to a P-gp-nonrelated therapy. This strengthens the hypothesis that P-gp can be a marker for several resistance mechanisms more than the P-gp-related resistance mechanism can be. This assumption is also supported by results of other authors [63–70] showing that P-gp overexpression might be combined with other resistance or regulation proteins like topoisomerase II, glutathione-S-transferase, metallothionein, c-fos or c-jun.

The consequence for clinical practice is that P-gp expression should be routinely established before and after treatment of acute leukemia patients, particularly in AML patients who are to be treated with a P-gp-related therapy. Our study shows that protocols containing daunorubicin/vincristine with a conventional dose of ara-C (like the AMl-6 protocol) should not be used in AML patients with P-gp overexpression. Like the results of other authors in vitro [71] and ourselves [72], with refractory multiply pretreated leukemia patients, P-gp-related drugs should be replaced with cytostatics that are not as well transported, or not at all, by *P*-gp. Because not enough experience with these drugs is available as yet, close screening is necessary in order to detect induction and/or selection of P-gp overexpression at an early time. Another therapeutic possibility is to combine protocols containing daunorubicin and/or vincristine with a P-gp modulator. These P-gp pump-blocking substances [73] might have the advantage that they do not induce and/or select P-gp overexpression and they also seem to have tolerable side effects. In this context, more clinical phase II and III studies are needed. Further intensive research should focus on examining methods that permit the full complexity of resistance mechanisms to cytostatic drugs to be analyzed.

References

1. Büchner T, Hiddemann W, Koch P, Pielken H, Urbanitz D, Kreutzmann H, Maschmeyer G, Wendt F, Kuse R, Thiel E, Ludwig W.D, Seibt H, Gassmann W, Löffler H, Aul C, Heyll A, Schneider W, Mertelsmann R, Anders C.H, Nowrousian M.R, Straif K, Vaupel H.A, Hossfeld D: The role of maintenance chemotherapy, immunotherapy, induction dose reduction in elderly patients and double induction in the treatment of adult acute myeloid leukemia. 4 randomized studies of the AML Cooperative Group. Neue therapeutische Strategien in der hämatologischen Onkologie. 36: 1,1989
2. Büchner T, Hiddemann W, Maschmeyer G, Ludwig W, Löffler H, Nowrousian M, Aul C, Heinecke A: How to improve therapy for adult acute myeloid leukemia. Studies of the AML-Cooperative-Group in the Federal Republic of Germany J. Cancer Res. clin. Oncol. 116: 97,1990.
3. Jehn U, Zittoun R, Suciu S, Fiere D, Haanen C, Peetermans M, Löwenberg B, Willemze R, Solbu G, Stryckmans P, EORTC Leukemia Cooperative Group: A randomized comparison of intensive maintenance treatment for adult acute myelogenous leukemia using either cyclic alternating drugs or repeated courses of the induction-type chemotherapy. AML-6 trial of the EORTC Leukemia Cooperative Group. Hemat. Blood Transfusion. 33: 277,1990
4. Thiel E, Kranz B.R. Raghavachar A, Bartram CR, Löffler H, Messerer D, Ganser A, Ludwig W.D. Büchner T, Hölzer D: Prethymic phenotype and genotype of pre-T (CD7 + /ER-) cell leukemia and its clinical significance within adult acute lymphoblastic leukemia. Blood. 37: 1247,1989
5. Hölzer D, Thiel E, Löffler H, Büchner T, Ganser A: Prognostic factors in a multicenter study for treatment of acute lymphoblastic leukemia in adults. Blood 71: 123,1988
6. Berman E, Hellar G, Santorsa J.A, McKenzie S, Gee T, Kempin S, Gulati S, Andreeff M, Kolitz J, Gabrilove J, Reich L, Mayer K, Keefe D., Trainor K, Schluger A, Penenberg D, Raymond V, O'Reilly R, Jhanwar S, Young Ch, Clarkson B: Results of a randomized trial comparing idarubicin and cytosine arabinoside with daunorubicin and cytosine arabinoside in adult patients with newly diagnosed acute myelogenous leukemia. Blood. 77: 1666,1991
7. Hiddemann W, Martin WR, Sauerland CM, Heinecke A, Büchner T: Definition of refractoriness against conventional chemotherapy in acute myeloid leukemia: a proposal based on the results of retreatment by thioguanine, cytosine arabinoside, and danorubicin (TAD 9) in 150 patients with relapse after standardized 1st line therapy. Leukemia 4: 184, 1990
8. Kartner N, Riordan JR, Ling V: Cell surface P-glycoprotein is associated with multidrug-resistance in mammalian cells. Science 221: 1285, 1983
9. Gros P, Croop J, Roninson I, Varshavsky A, Houseman D: Isolation and characterization of DNA sequences amplified in multidrug-resistant hamster cells. Proc Natl Acad Sci USA 83: 337, 1986
10. Gottesman MM: How cancer cells evade chemotherapy: Sixteenth Richard and Hinda Rosenthal Foundation Award Lecture[1]. Cancer Research 53: 747, 1993
11. Juranka PF, Zastawny RL, Ling V: P-glycoprotein: multidrug-resistance and a superfamily of membrane-associated transport proteins. FASEB J 3: 2583, 1989
12. Ramu A, Ramu N, Rosario LM: Circumvention of multidrug-resistance in P388 cells is associated

with a rise in the cellular content of phosphatidylcholine. Biochem: Pharmacol 41: 1455, 1991
13. Nooter K, Sonneveld P, Janssen A, Oostrum R, Boersma T, Herweijer H, Valerio D, Hagemeijer A, Baas F: Expression of the mdr3 gene in prolymphocytic leukemia; association with cyclosporin-A-induced increase in drug accumulation. Int J. Cancer 45: 626, 1990
14. Ma DDF, Scurr RD, Davey RA, Mackertich SM, Harman DH, Dowden G, Isbister JP, Bell DR: Detection of a multidrug resistant phenotype in acute non-lymphoblastic leukemia. Lancet i: 135, 1987
15. Fojo At, Ueda K, Salmon DJ, Poplack DG, Gottesman MM, Pastan I: Expression of a multidrug resistance gene in human tumors and tissues. Proc Natl Acad Sci USA 84: 265, 1987
16. Carulli G, Petrini M, Marini A, Ambrogi F: P-glycoprotein in acute lymphoblastic leukemia and in the blastic crisis of myeloid leukemia. N Engl J Med 319: 797, 1988
17. Yau L, Li D, Tsao J, Kuo T, Savaraj N, Lu K: Expression of P-glycoprotein (MDRl) gene in patients with leukemia. Blood 72(Suppl): 186, 1988
18. Funato T, Bando Y, Kato H, Tokuhiro H, Shimoda Y, Ohtani H: Analysis of P-glycoprotein in patients with acute leukemias by flow cytometry. Rinsho-Byori 37: 779, 1989
19. Goldstein LJ, Galski H, Fojo A, Willingham M, Lai SL, Gazdar A, Pirker R, Green A, Crist W, Brodeur GM, Lieber M, Cossman J, Gottesman MM, Pastan I: Expression of a multidrug resistance gene in human cancers. Cancer Inst 81: 116, 1989
20. Holmes J, Jacobs A, Carter G, Janowska-Wieczorek A, Padua RA: Multidrug resistancve in haemopoietic cell lines, myelodysplastic syndromes and acute myeloblastic leukemia. Br J Haematol 72: 40, 1989
21. Ito Y, Tanimoto M, Kumazawa T, Okumura M, Morishima Y, Ohno R, Saito H,: Increased P-glycoprotein expression and multidrug-resistant gene (mdrl) amplification are frequently found in fresh acute leukemia cells. Cancer 63: 1534, 1989
22. Mattern J, Efferth T, Bak M, Ho AD, Volm M: Detection of P-glycoprotein in human leukemias using monoclonal antibodies. Blut 58: 215, 1989
23. Rothenberg ML, Mickley LA, Cole DE, Balis FM, Tsuruo T, Poplack DG, Fojo AT: Expression of the mdr-1/p-170 gene in patients with acute lymphoblastic leukemia. Blood 74: 1388, 1989
24. Sugawara I, Kodo H, Ohkochi E, Hamada H, Tsuruo T, Mori S: High-level expression of MRK 16 and MRK 20 murine monoclonal antibody-defined proteins (170,000-180,000 P-glycoprotein and 85,000 protein) in leukemias and malignant lymphomas. Br J Cancer 60: 538, 1989
25. Ball ED, Lawrence D, Malnar M, Ciminelli N, Mayer R, Wurster-Hill D, Davey FR, Bloomfield CD: Correlation of CD34 and multi-drug resistance P170 with FAB and cytogenetics but not prognosis in acute myeloid leukemia (AML). Blood 76: 252a, 1990
26. Carulli G, Petrini M, Marini A, Vaglini F, Cracciolo F, Grassi B: P-glycoprotein and drug resistance in acute leukemias and in the blastic crisis of chronic myeloid leukemia. Haematologica 75: 516, 1990
27. Kato S, Nishimura J, Muta K, Yufu Y, Nawata H, Ideguchi H: Overexpression of P-glycoprotein in adult T-cell leukemia. Lancet 336: 573, 1990
28. Kuwazuru Y, Hanada S, Furukawa T, Yoshimura A, Sumizawa T, Utsonomiya A, Ishibashi K, Saito T, Uozumi K, Maruyama M, Ishizawa M, Arima T, Akiyama S: Expression of P-glycoprotein in adult T-cell leukemia cells. Blood 76: 2065, 1990
29. Kuwazuru Y, Yoshimura A, Hanada S, Utsonomiya A, Makino T, Ishibashi K, Kodama M, Iwahashi M, Arima T, AkiyamaS: Expression of the multidrug transporter, P-glycoprotein, in acute leukemia cells and correlation to clinical drug resistance. Cancer 66: 868, 1990
30. Musto P, Cascavilla N, Di Renzo N, Ladogana S, La-Sala A, Melillo L, Nibile M, Matera R, Lombardi G, Carotenuto M: Clinical relevance of immunocytochemical detection of multidrug-resistance-associated P-glycoprotein in haematological malignancies. Tumori 76: 353, 1990
31. Nooter K, Sonneveld P, Oostrum R, Herweijer H, Haganbeek T, Valerio D: Overexpression of the mdr 1 gene in blast cells from patients with acute myelocytic leukemia is associated with decreased anthracycline accumulation that can be restored by cyclosporin-A. Int J Cancer 45: 263, 1990
32. Redner A, Hegewisch S, Haimi J, Steinherz P, Jhanwar S, Andreff M: A study of multidrug resistance and cell kinetics in a child with near-haploid acute lymphoblastic leukemia. Leukemia Res 14: 771, 1990
33. Sato H, Gottesman MM, Goldstein LJ, Pastan I, Block AM, Sandberg AA, Preisler HD: Expression of the multidrug resistance gene in myeloid leukemias. Leukemia Res 14: 11, 1990
34. Chitnis M, Hedge U, Chavan S, Juvekar A, Advani S: Expression of the multidrug transporter P-glycoprotein and in vitro chemosensitivity: correlation with in vivo response to chemotherapy in acute myeloid leukemia. Sel Cancer Ther 7: 165, 1991
35. Marie JP, Zittoun R, Sikic BI: Multidrug resistance (mdrl) gene expression in adult acute leukemias: correlations with treatment outcome and in vitro drug sensivity. Blood 79: 586, 1991
36. Musto P, Melillo L, Lombardi G, Matera R, Di Giorgio G, Carotenuto M: High risk of early resistant relapse for leukaemic patients with presence of multidrug resistance associated P-glycoprotein positive cells in complete remission. Br J Heamatol 77: 50, 1991
37. Pirker R, Wallner J, Geissler K, Linkesch W, Haas OA, Bettelheim P, Hopfner M, Scherrer R, Valent P, Havelec L: MDRl gene expression and treatment outcome in acute myeloid leukaemia. J. Natl Cancer Inst. 83: 708, 1991
38. Campos L, Guyotat D, Archimbaud E, Calmard-Oriol P, Tsuruo T, Troncy J, Treille D, Fiere D: Clinical significance of multidrug resistance P-glycoprotein expression on acute nonlymphoblastic leukemia cells at diagnosis. Blood 79: 473, 1992

39. Campos L, Guyotat D, Jaffar C, Solary E, Archimbaud E, Treille D: Correlation of MDF/P-170 expression with daunorubicin uptake and sensitivity of leukemic progenitors in acute myeloid leukemia. Eur J Haematol 48: 254, 1992
40. Michieli M, Damiani D, Geromin A, Michelutti A, Fanin R, Raspadori D, Russo D, Visani G, Dinota A, Pileri S, Tsuruo T, Grandi M, Baccarani M, Tura S: Overexpression of multidrug resistance-associated p170-glycoprotein in acute non-lymphocytic leukemia. Eur J Haematol 48: 87, 1992
41. Tiirikainen MI, Syrjälä MT, Jansson SE, Krusius T: Flow cytometric analysis of P-glycoprotein in normal and leukemic cells. Ann Hematol 65: 124, 1992
42. Gruber A, Vitols S, Norgren S, Arestrom I, Peterson C, Bjorkholm M, Reizenstein P, Luthman H: Quantative determination of mdr 1 gene expression in leukaemic cells from patients with acute leukaemia. Br. J. Cancer 66: 266, 1992
43. Zhou DC, Marie JP, Suberville AM, Zittoun R: Relevance of mdr-1 gene expression in acute myeloid leukaemia and comparison of different diagnostic methods. Leukaemia 6: 879, 1992
44. Willman CL, Kopecky KJ, Weick J, Applebaum F, Grever MR, Head DR, Elias L, Balcerzak SP, Mills GM, Hynes HE: Biologic parameters that predict treatment response in de novo acute myeloid leukaemia (AML): CD34 but not multidrug resistance (mdr) gene expression is associated with a decreased complete remission (CR) rate and CD34+patients more frequently achieve CR with high dose cytosine arabinoside. Proc. ASCO 11: 262, 1992
45. Wittebol S, Te Boekhorst P, Hagemelier A, Van Dongen JJM, Schoester M, Sonneveld P: Expression of the multidrug resistance (MDR-1) phenotype in acute myelocytic leukaemia is associated with CD34 expression and monosomy 7 and predicts for poor survival. Blood 80: 202a, 1992
46. Wood P, Liu Yin JA, Burgess R: P-glycoprotein expression in adult acute leukaemias: correlation with treatment outcome. Proc. ISH p. 54, 1992
47. Goasguen J.E, Dossot J.M, Fardel O, Le Mee F, Le Gall E, Leblay R, Leprise, P.Y, Chaperson J, Fauchet R: Expression of the multidrug resistance-associated P-glycoprotein (P-170) in 59 cases of de novo acute lymphoblastic leukemia: prognostic implications. Blood 81: 2394, 1993
48. Miyachi H, Takemura Y, Yonekura S, Komatsuda M, Nagao T, Arimori S, Ando Y: MDR1 (multidrug resistance) gene expression in adult acute leukemia: correlations with blast phenotype. Int Journal of Hematology 57: 31, 1993
49. Hegewisch-Becker S, Fliegener M, Tsuruo T, Zeller W, Hossfeld D: K: Multidrug resistance (mdr1) in adult acute leukemia at diagnosis: correlation with response to induction chemotherapy. Onkologie 16: 264, 1993
50. Kartner N, Evernden-Porelle D, Bradley G, Ling V: Detection of P-glycoprotein in multidrug-resistance cell lines by monoclonal antibodies. Nature 316: 820, 1985
51. Georges E, Bradley G, Gariepy J, Ling V: Detection of P-glycoprotein isoforms by gene-specific monoclonal antibodies. Proc Natl Acad Sci USA 87: 152, 1990
52. Schinkel AH Roelofs MEM, Borst P: Characterization of the human MDR3 P-glycoprotein and its recognition by P-glycoprotein-specific monoclonal antibodies. Cancer Research 51: 2628, 1991
53. Dixon AR, Bell J, Ellis IO, Elston CW, Blamey RW: P-glycoprotein expression in locally advanced breast cancer treated by neoadjuvant chemotherapy. Br J Cancer 66: 537, 1992
54. Finstad CL, Yin BWT, Gordon CM, Federeci MG, Welt S, Lloyd KO: Some monoclonal antibody reagents (C219 and JSB-1) to P-glycoprotein contain antibodies to blood group A carbohydrate determinants: a problem of quality control for immunohistochemical analysis. The journal of Histochemistry and Cytochemistry 39: 1603, 1991
55. Arceci RJ, Stieglitz K, Bras J, Schinkel A, Baas F, Croop J: Monoclonal antibody to an external epitope of the human mdr1 P-glycoprotein. Cancer Research 53: 310, 1993
56. Gekeler V, Frese G, Noller A, Handgretinger R, Willisch A, Schmidt H, Muller CP, Dopfer R, Klingebiel T, Diddens H, Probst H. Niethammer D: Mdr1/P-glycoprotein, topoisomedrase an gultuatahions-s-glycoprotein, topoisomerase and glutathione-s-transferase: PI gene expression in primary and relapsed state adult and childhood leukemias. Br J Cancer 66; 507–517, 1992
57. Moscow JA, Fairchild CR, Maden MJ, Ransom DT, Wieand HS, O'Brien EE, Poplack DG, Cossman J, Myers CE, Cowan KH: Expression of anionic gluthatione-S-transferase and P-glycoprotein genes in human tissues and tumors. Cancer Res 49: 1422, 1989
58. Beck WT: Mechanisms of multidrug resistance in human tumor cells: the roles of P-glycoprotein, DNA topoisomerase II, and other factors. Cancer Treatment Reviews 17: 11, 1990
59. Krishnamachary N, Center MS: The MRP gene associated with a non-P-glycoprotein multidrug resistance encodes a 190-kDa membrane bound glycoprotein. Cancer Research 53: 3658, 1993
60. Nooter K, Sonneveld P: Clinical relevance of P-glycoprotein expression in haematological malignancies. Leukemia Research 18/4: 233, 1994
61. Zhao JY, Ikeguchi M, Eckersberg T, Tien Kuo M: Modulation of multidrug resistance gene expression by dexamethasone in cultered hepatoma cells. Endocrinology 133: 521, 1993
62. De Vita VT: The influence of information of drug resistance on protocol design. Ann Oncol 2: 93, 1991
63. Cornwell MM: The human multidrug resistance gene: sequences upstream and downstream of the initation site influence transcription. Cell Growth Diff 1: 607, 1990
64. Quantin B, Breathnach R: Epidermal growth factor stimulates transcription of the c-jun proto-oncogene in rat fibroblasts. Nature (Lond.) 334: 538, 1988

65. Tanaguchi H, Pyerin W: Glutathione-S-transferase is an in vitro substrate of Ca++-phospholipid-dependent protein kinase (protein kinase C). Biochem. Biophys. Res. Commun. 162: 903, 1989
66. Chambers TC, McAvoy EM, Jakobs JW, Eilon G: Protein kinase C phosphorylates P-glycoprotein in multidrug resistant human KB carcinoma cells. J. biol. Chem. 265: 7679, 1990
67. Teeter LD, Eckersberg T, Tsai Y, Kuo MT: Analysis of the Chinese hamster P-glycoprotein/multidrug resistance gene pgp1 reveals that the AP-1 site is essential for full promoter activity. Cell Growth Different. 2: 429, 1991
68. Nakagawa M, Schneider E, Dixon KH, Horten J, Kelley K, Marrow Ch, Cowan K. H: Reduced intracellular drug accumulation in the absence of P-glycoprotein (mdr1) overexpression in mitoxantrone-resistant human MCF-7 breast cancer cells. Cancer Research 52: 6175, 1992
69. Kamath N, Grabowski D, Ford J, Kerrigan D, Pommier Y, Ganapathi R: Overexpression of P-glycoprotein and alterations in topoisomerase II in P388 mouse leukemia cells selected in vivo for resistance to mitoxantrone. Biochem. Pharmacol 44: 937, 1992
70. Volm M: P-glycoprotein associated expression of c-fos and c-jun products in human lung carcinomas. Anticancer Res. 13: 375, 1993
71. Berman E, Mc Bride M: Comparative cellular pharmacology of daunorubicin and idarubicin in human multidrug-resistant leukemia cells. Blood 79: 3267, 1992
72. Nüssler V, Gieseler F, Pelka-Fleischer R. Gullis E, Zwiezina H, Bartl R, Abenhard W, Schmitt R Langenmayer I, Heinemann V, Kolb HJ, Wilmanns W: Pilot study with idarubicin monotherapy: response of multiply pretreated leukemia patients. (submitted).
73. Grunicke H, Überall F: Protein kinase C modulation. Sem Cancer Biol 3: 351, 1992

Acute Leukemias VI
Prognostic Factors
and Treatment Strategies
Büchner et al. (eds)

Lack of Correlation Between Multi-Drug Resistance Expression and Clinical Response to Chemotherapy in Patients with Acute Myeloid Leukemia

A. Schulz, P. Engling, Q. Cao, C. Scheid, V. Diehl, and P.D. Wickramanayake

Abstract. Expression of the multi-drug-resistance (MDR) protein gp170 encoded by the mdr1 gene has been implied to play a role in acute myeloid leukemia (AML) refractory to chemotherapy. We investigated MDR expression by flow cytometry and immunocytologically stained slides using the monoclonal antibodies MRK-16 and C-219, respectively, as well as RT-PCR in 15 patients (seven male, eight female) with AML. The median age was 49.5 years (range 22–75 years), the distribution according to the French–American –British (FAB) classification was M1: one case; M2: five cases; M3: one case; M4: three cases; M5: two cases; M6: one case; and one bispecific case. Induction chemotherapy consisted of thioguanine, cytosine arabinoside and daunorubicine (TAD-HAM) (nine cases) and idarubicin-fludarabine-cytidine arabinoside-filgrastim (granulocyte colony-stimulating factor) (Ida-FLAG) (six cases). The proportion of leukemic blasts in the bone marrow varied between 30% and 100% with a median of 95% . In seven patients who subsequently achieved complete remission (CR) 5%–47% (median 27%) of bone marrow cells were positive for MRK-16 compared to 9%–47% (median 29%) in eight patients without CR. The flow cytometry results were confirmed by immunocytochemistry and RT-PCR. A high percentage of $CD34^+$ cells was correlated with failure to achieve CR. Otherwise there was no correlation with age, FAB classification, or chemotherapy protocol. In conclusion, MDR expression does not seem to predict treatment failure in AML, independently of which method of detection is being used.

Introduction

Drug resistance remains a major problem in acute myeloid leukemia (AML). Knowledge of the exact nature of this resistance should help to devise ways for its reversal and thus improve the outcome of treatment.

The classical multidrug resistance (MDR) phenotype is an experimentally well-described entity including cross-resistance to several unrelated xenobiotics (like anthracyclines, vinca alkaloids, epipodophylline derivatives, actinomycin D, and colchicine) after prolonged in vitro exposure to these agents [2, 4, 8, 17]. It works with a decrease in intracellular drug accumulation due to the expression of the mdrl gene which codes for P-glycoprotein, a 170 kD transmembrane protein [8, 10, 17]. Recent reports have indicated that mdrl/gp170 overexpression is correlated with poor prognosis in AML, though the largest studies to date found no such correlation (1, 21).

In an attempt to determine the incidence and clinical relevance of mdr1 gene expression in AML and to find a reliable method to diagnose MDR phenotype, we investigated mdr1 gene expression in specimens obtained from 15 adult patients with de novo AML at diagnosis by using RT-PCR, immunocytology with the monoclonal

First Department of Internal Medicine, University Hospital Cologne, Joseph-Stelzmann-Str. 9, 50924 Cologne, Germany

antibody (MAb)C-219 and flow cytometry with MAb MRK-16 simultaneously.

Patients

Fifteen consecutive adult patients with AML were entered into the trial. No patient was pretreated with chemotherapy. After diagnosis, the patients were treated according to the protocol of the German Acute Myeloid Leukemia Cooperative Group (thioguanine–cytosine arabionoside–daunorubicin, TAD-9/HAM; nine patients) [5] or a new protocol for elderly or relapsed AML patients (Idarubian–fludarabine -cytidine arabinoside–filgrastim Ida-FLAG; six patients) [20]. Patient characteristics are shown in Table 1.

Material and Methods

All tests were performed in comparison with MDR^+ and MDR^- Chinese hamster ovarian cell line, and by its colchicin-selected MDR variant (CHO-RT), which was grown in the presence of doxorubicin (100 ng/ml) (obtained from R. Volm, Deutsches Krebsforschungs-Zentrum, Heidelberg, Germany).

Immunocytology. C-219, a MAb which reacts with a gp170 C terminal epitope of membrane internal surface [14] was used for immunocytology in all cases (Biomedical Diagnostics, Röderbach, Germany). For the alkaline phosphate anti-alkaline phosphatase (APAAP) technique, cytospin or bone marrow smear preparations were fixed in acetone for 20 min at room temperature and rinsed in tris buffered saline for 2 × 1 min. The MAb C-219 was applied at a final concentration of 100 µg/ml in a diluent solution containing 0.02% saponin for 60 min at 37°C in a humid chamber. The staining was performed by the APAAP method, as described by Cordell et al. [7], using the MAbs D605 and Z259 (Dako, Hamburg, Germany). Cytospin or bone marrow smear preparations unexposed to C-219, as well as exposed to irrelevant MAb, were processed simultaneously. Final preparations were counterstained with Gill's Haemalaun, mounted in kaiser glycerine, and examined in light microscopy by three independent observers. Cells were scored by comparison with CHO-RT cells, with normal leukocytes, and normal marrow cells as strongly positive (S), moderately positive (M), weakly positive (W), and negative (N). S cells were as positive as the majority of CHO-RT cells. W cells were slightly more positive than normal leukocytes. The proportion of S cells was counted on 500 blast cells or more.

Flow Cytometric Analysis of Blast Cells. MRK-16, a (MAb) which recognizes an external surface membrane component of gp170 [10] was used for flow cytometry in all cases (Dianova, Hamburg, Germany). Cells were washed in phosphate-buffered saline (PBS) without Ca^{2+} and Mg^{2+}. After washing the cells, a cell suspen-

Table 1. Patient characteristics

Patient no.	Sex	Age (years)	Morpholigical diagnosis (FAB)	Chemotherapy
1	M	75	M 2	Ida-FLAG
2	F	45	M 5	TAD/HAM
3	M	68	M 1	TAD/HAM
4	F	37	M 4	Ida-FLAG
5	M	48	M 2	TAD/HAM
6	M	64	M 6	TAD/HAM
7	F	48	M 4	Ida-FLAG
8	F	47	M 5	TAD/HAM
9	M	54	M 4	Ida-FLAG
10	M	51	M 3	TAD/HAM
11	F	61	M 2	Ida-FLAG
12	M	22	Biphenotypic	Ida-FLAG
13	F	42	M 2	TAD/HAM
14	F	60	M 1	TAD/HAM
15	F	39	M 2	TAD/HAM

sion of 1×10^5 cells/ml was prepared. A cell suspension of 50 µl was incubated with 20 µl (5 µg) MRK-16 for 30 min. at 4°C. After washing, the cell pellet was resuspended and incubated with 50 µl 1:100 (vol/vol) diluted fluorescein isothiocyanate (FITC)-conjugated rabbit antimouse IgG antiserum (Sigma Immunochemicals, Deisenhofen, Germany). Next, the cells were washed and incubated with phycoerythrin (PE)-conjugated HPCA-2 (anti-CD34 PE; Becton Dickinson, BD, Heidelberg, Germany) for 30 min at 4°C. An irrelevant, isotype-matched MAb was used as negative control. After washing, 20 000 events were counted using a FACScan flow cytometer (BD). Both FITC and PE fluorescence signals were logarithmically amplified. Other cell surface marker analysis was performed using directly conjugated MAbs (BD). The blast cell population was gated using scatter parameters. Data analysis was performed using FlowMate software (Dako, Hamburg, Germany).

C-DNA. Total cellular RNA was isolated from 2 ml 1×10^6 cells/ml using a modification of the acid guanidinium thiocyanate/phenol/chloroform extraction [6]. cDNA was synthesized with 5 µg total cellular RNA and 100 ng random hexadeoxynucleotide primer (Pharmacia) in 30 µl solution containing 50 m*M* Tris HCl (pH 8.3), 75 m*M* KC6, 3h mM $MgCl_2$, 10 m*M* dithiothreitol, 500 m*M* each dNTP, and 10 units Moloney murine leukemia virus reverse transcriptase (Bethesda Research Laboratories, USA; Pharmacia, Freiburg, Germany). After 1 h at 37°C, cDNA was stored at -20°C until use. Oligonucleotides were synthesized by MWG-Biotech (Munich, Germany).

Reverse Transcription Polymerase Chain Reaction. Polymerase chain reaction (PCR) was carried out with cDNA derived from 80 ng RNA, 1 unit AmpliTaq polymerase and reaction kits (Boehringer Mannheim, Germany) in a final volume of 25 µl. Each cycle of PCR included 45 s of denaturation at 94°C, 1 min of primer annealing at 60°C, and 2 min of extension/synthesis at 72°C. The number of cycles was 40. Mdrl-specific sequences were amplified by using the sensestand primer CCCATCATTGCAATAGCAGG (residues 2596–2615) and the antisense-strand primer GTTCAAACTTCTGCTCCTGA (residues 2733-2752) [16], which yield a 167-bp product. Each primer was added at 37.5 pmol per reaction. PCR products were separated on 1.5% agarose gels and stained with ethidium bromide. All the necessary precautions against contamination of PCRs [15] were rigorously applied.

Results

Incidence of mdr1 Gene Expression. Expression of mdrl was studied by staining of gp170 on blast cells by MAbs C-219 and MRK-16 as well as mdrl-mRNA measuring by RT-PCR in all patients. There was no correlation of gp170 expression with age, sex, or French–American–British or (FAB) classification. Patients with resistant or relapsed disease showed no higher incidence of mdrl gene expression: seven of eight specimens from patients with resistant or relapsed disease were mdrl-mRNA positive (analysed by RT-PCR), while this was the case for six of seven specimens from patients with complete remission (CR). No obvious correlation of mdrl gene expression to other surface markers (CD33, CD14, CD13, TdT, CD19, CD2) was found (data not shown). These data are summarized in Table 2.

Immunocytology(APAAP). The MDR-associated gp 170 was detectable by C-219 and APAAP in all cases, ranging from 1% to 51% reactive with the MAb C-219. More than 10% S blast cells were detectable in 12/15 cases (80%). No relationship from the presence and frequency of S cells to the phase of disease was detectable. S cells were found in all FAB subtypes, either at onset or in relapse. There was no detectable relationship between peripheral blood blast cell count and presence and proportion of S cells, especially in relapse.

Flow Cytometry. The results of flow cytometry using the MRK-16 MAb to detect gp 170 are summarized in Table 2. P-glycoprotein was detected in 13 of 15 bone marrow specimens tested using a cut-off value of 10%. The proportion of MRK-16-positive cells was lower than 10% in two cases, and ranged between 13% and 47% in the remaining cases. The proportion of CD34-positive cells was lower than 10% in four out of 15 cases, and ranged between 10% and 94% in the remaining 11 cases. No difference in incidence was observed between de novo AML and in relapse and there was no correlation with response. Table 2 shows a comparison of MRK-

Table 2. Results: C-219, MRK-16, and CD34 were counted as a percentage of stained blast cells

Patient no.	FAB	Response	Duration of CR (months)	PCR	C-219 (%)	MRK-16 (%)	CD34 (%)
1	M2	CR	12	pos	12	13.7	5.7
2	M5	NR		pos	27	24.8	60
3	M1	NR		pos	31	28.9	13.4
4	M4	CR	11	pos	51	47.2	73
5	M2	NR		pos	34	23.7	94
6	M6	NR		pos	33	34.4	34
7	M4	NR		pos	42	45.4	11
8	M5	NR		neg	1	5.2	82
9	M4	CR	>8	pos	20	22.7	11.1
10	M3	CR	>10	pos	22	24.8	3
11	M2	CR	>9	pos	41	46.8	25
12	biAL	CR	>10	neg	4	9.3	56.9
13	M2	CR	>8	pos	29	28.8	3.8
14	M1	CR	>7	pos	32	37.6	24.3
15	M2	CR	>7	pos	26	28.8	5

16 and CD34 as well as C-219 and PCR in all cases studied with both antibodies. Reactivity to MRK-16 and to CD34 was identical in patients who had never been treated and in those who had been treated with alkylating agents.

Polymerase Chain Reaction. Total cellular RNA was used to synthesize cDNA with a random hexadeoxynucleotide primer. cDNA was analysed using RT-PCR. Thirteen out of 15 blast cell samples expressed mdrl gene product as shown in Fig. 1.

Comparison of gp170 Expression Recognized by C-219 and MRK-16. There was agreement between the detection of mdrl gene expression by RT-PCR and C-219 as well as MRK-16 in 15 of 15 matched studies (13 positive, two negative).

CD34⁺ and mdrl Gene Expression and Clinical Outcome. The association of mdrl gene expression with CR rates after induction chemotherapy is shown in Table 2. The CR rate was not significantly different for patients with mdrl gene expression or patients with no detectable expression. Seven of eight patients with relapse or no response were positive for mdr1 gene expression whereas six of seven patients with CR were positive. Seven of eight nonresponders were positive for CD34 (median 60% stained blast cells), whereas four of seven responders were positive (median 24% stained blast cells).

Discussion

The precise mechanism of drug resistance in AML is still unknown. One possible mechanism may be the expression of the multidrug transporter gp170. In this study, we examined the presence of the P-glycoprotein in 15 consecutive patients with AML. Mdrl expression of bone marrow blast cells was determined by using RT-PCR, immunocytology with MAb C-219, and flow cytometry with MAb MRK-16 simultaneously. There was a good correlation between the different detection methods.

We found a high incidence of mdrl gene expression in AML patients, even for the newly diagnosed patients who had never recieved any chemotherapy. This finding differs from those of Goldstein et al. [9] and Ito et al. [13] who reported a very low incidence of mdrl gene expression. However, our result was consistent with other published studies, which detected mdr1 gene expression in 25%–70% of newly diagnosed AML patients [11, 18]. Furthermore, we found that there was no difference in the incidence of mdr1 gene expression between newly diagnosed patients and relapsed patients.

Our study did not confirm the direct relationship between mdrl gene expression and achievement of CR in patients with de novo AML. This was true for patients with newly diagnosed AML or in relapse. A meta-analysis of

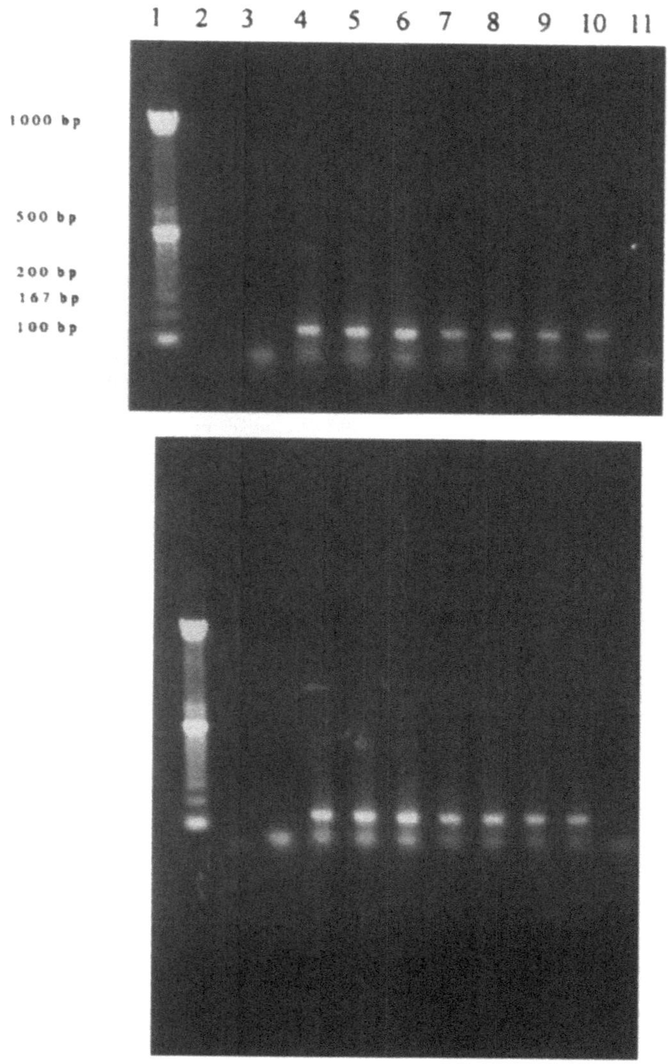

Fig. 1. RT-PCR of total cellular RNA from AML blast cell samples. *Line 1*, molecular weight markers; *line 2* h negative control; *lines 3–9* h patient blast cell samples; *line 10*, CHO-RT; *line 11* h CHO-WT

several studies showed an estimated risk of 0.68 for MDR-positive AML with respect to CR [12]. The two largest studies [1, 21] draw the conclusion that gp170 expression is not a prognostic factor in AML.

Our data suggest that MDR expression cannot be used to predict treatment outcome on an individual patient basis. This has to be seen in the context of a number of other molecular mechanisms of drug resistance which have been described so far, e.g., topoisomerase I and II, glutathione, multi-drug resistance-associated protein (MRP), and which all might be contributing to the phenomenon of clinical treatment failure [3, 19].

CD34 expression in leukemic blasts has been implicated as a negative prognostic factor independent of MDR1 [21], and we found higher levels of CD34 positivity in patients who failed to achieve CR (Table 2).

These results emphasize the need for further investigation to study the role of MDR in chemotherpy resistance.

References

1. Ball Ed, Miller R, Malnar M, Davey FR, Bloomfield CD (1990). Correlation of CD34 and multidrug resistance p170 with FAB and cytogenetics but not prognosis in acute myeloid leukemia (AML). Blood 76: 252a (abstract)
2. Bech-Hanson NT, Till JE, Ling V. (1976). Pleiotropic phenotype of colchicine-resistant CHO cells: cross resistance and collateral sensitivity J Cell Physiol 88: 23.
3. Beck WT (1989). Unknotting the complexities of multidrug resistance: the involvement of DNA topoisomerases in drug action and resistance. J. Natl Cancer Inst 81: 1683–1685.
4. Biedler JL, Riehm H (1970). Cellular resistance to actinomycin D in Chinese hamster cells in vitro: cross-resistance, radioautographic and cytogenetic studies Cancer Res 30: 1174.
5. Büchner T, Urbanitz D, Hiddemann W, Rühl H, Ludwig WD, Fischer J, Aul HC, Vaupel HA, Kuse R, Zeile G, Nowrousian MR, König HJ, Walter M., Wendt FC, Sodomann H, Hossfeld DK, von Paleske A, Löffler H, Gassmann W, Hellriegel KP, Fülle HH, Lunschken CH, Emmerich B, Pralle H, Pees HW, Pfreundschuh M, Bartels H, Koeppen KM, Schwerdtfeger R, Donhuijsen-Ant R, Mainzer K,Bonfert B, Köppler H, Zurborn KH, Ranft K, Thiel E, Heinecke A (1985). Intensified induction and consolidation with or without maintenance chemotherapy for acute myeloid leukemia (AML): two multicenter studies of the German AML Cooperative Group J Clin Oncol 3: 1583.
6. Chomczynski P, Sacchi N. (1987). Single-step method of RNA isolation by acid guanidinium thiocyanate-phenol-chloroform extraction. Anal Biochem 162: 156.
7. Cordell JL, Falini B, Erber WN, Ghosh AK, Abdulazis Z, Macdonald S, Pulford KAF, Stein H, Mason DY (1984). Immunoenzymatic labelling of monoclonal antibodies using immune complexes of alkaline phosphate and monoclonal anti-alkaline phosphatase (APAAP) complexes of J Histochem Cytochem 32: 219.
8. Deuchars KL, Ling V (1989). P-glycoprotein and multidrug resistance in cancer chemotherapy. Semin Oncol 16: 156.
9. Goldstein LJ, Galski H, Fojo A, Willingham M, Lai SL, Gazdar A, Pirker R, Green A, Crist W, Brodeur GM, Lieber M, Cossman J, Gottesman MM, Pastan I (1089). Expression of a multidrug resistance gene in human cancers. J. Natl Cancer Inst 81: 116.
10. Hamada H, Tsuruo T (1986). Functional role for the 170-180-kDa glycoprotein specific to drug-resistant tumour cells as revealed by monoclonal antibodies. Proc Natl Acad Sci USA 83: 7785.
11. Holmes J, Jacobs A, Carter G, Janowska-Wieczorek A, Padua RA (1989). Multidrug resistance in haemopoietic cell lines, myelodysplastic syndromes and acute myeloblastic leukaemia Br J Haematol 72: 40.
12. Holmes JA, West RR (1994). The effect of mdr 1 gene expression on outcome in acute myeloblastic leukaemia Br J Cancer 69(2): 382
13. Ito Y, Tanimoto M, Kumazawa T, Okumura M, Morishima Y, Ohno R, Saito H (1989). Increased P-glycoprotein expression and multidrug-resistance gene (mdrl) amplification are infrequently found in fresh acute leukaemia cells. Sequential analysis of 15 cases at initial diagnosis and relapsed stage. Cancer 63: 1534.
14. Kartner N, Everden-Porelle D, Bradley G, Ling V (1985). Detection of P-glycoprotein in multidrug-resistant cell lines by monoclonal antibodies. Nature 316: 820.
15. Kwok S, Higuchi R (1989). Avoiding false positives with PCR, Nature 339: 237–238.
16. Noonan KE, Beck C, Holzmayer TA, Chin JE, Wunder JS, Andrulis IL, Gazdar AF, Willman CL, Griffith B, Von Hoff DD, Robinson IB (1990). Quantitative analysis of mDR1 (multidrug resistance) gene expression in human tumours by polymerase chain reaction Proc. Natl Acad. Sci. USA 87: 7160.
17. Pastan I, Gottesman M (1987). Multiple drug resistance in human cancer. N Engl J Med 316: 1388.
18. Sato H, Preisler H, Day R, Raza A, Larson R, Browman G, Goldberg J, Vogler R, Grunwald H, Gottlieb A, Bennett J, Gottesman MM, Pastan I (1990). MDRI transcript levels as an indication of resistant disease in acute myelogenous leukaemia. Br J Haematol 75: 340.
19. Schneider E, Cowan KH, Bader H, Toomey S, Schwartz GN, Karp JE, Burke PJ, Kaufmann SH (1995). Increased expression of the multi-drug resistance associated protein gene in relapsed acute leukemia. Blood 85: 186.
20. Wickramanayake PD, Steinmetz HT, Katay I, Glasmacher A, Neufang A, Staib P, Schwonzen M, Diehl V (1994). Phase II trial of idarubicin, fludarabine cytidine arabinoside (aRA-C), and filgrastim (G-CSF) (Ida-FLAG) for treatment of poor prognosis acute myeloid leukemia. Blood 10: Suppl. 1: 618a (abstr).
21. Willman CL, Kopecky KJ, Weick J, Appelbaum F, Grever MR, Head DR, Elias L, Balcerak SP, Mills GM, Hynes HE (1992). Biologic parameters that predict treatment response in de novo acute myeloid leukaemia (AML): CD 34 but not multidrug resistance (mdr) gene expression is associated with a decreased complete remission (CR) rate and CD 34⁺ patients more frequently achieve CR with high dose cytosine arabinoside. Proc ASCO 11: 262.

Acute Leukemias VI
Prognostic Factors
and Treatment Strategies
Büchner et al. (eds)

Coexpression of mdr-1 and myc Genes in Relation to Prognosis in Acute Leukemia Patients

A. Zaritskey[1,3], I. Stuif[1], T. Bykova[1], A. Sominskaya[1], N. Anikina[3], and B. Afanasiev[2,3]

Abstract. Proliferative ability and resistance to chemotherapy (CHT) seem to be the major facilities of leukemic blast cells in relation to outcome of therapy. We have studied the expression of the myc gene in 27 de novo and 23 pretreated acute leukemia (AL) patients by hybridization in situ. It appeares that the predominant expression level of the mdr-1 gene (above the myc gene) correlates to resistance. The opposite situation (when the myc gene is predominant) correlates to tumor lytic syndrome and early death (ED) on CHT. Absence of overexpression of both mdr-1 and the myc gene is the most favorable type in relation to achieving complete remission (CR).

Introduction

The mdr-1 and myc genes are expressed in a number of both de novo and pretreated acute leukemia (AL) patients, these data have a prognostic significance [1–3]. It appeared that chemotherapeutic [CHT] regimens containing two drugs separately inducing mdr-1 gene expression (vinca alkaloid/epipodophylline derivate+antracycline) vs. one (an antracycline only) are more potent in inducing mdr-1 gene expression in both leukemic and normal cell clones [2]. Therefore mdr-1 gene overexpression is related to previous CHT and has an impact on the resistance of leukemic blasts to further CHT [1, 2, 4]. An expression of the myc gene reflects the proliferative capacity of a cell [5]. Therefore its overexpression in leukemic blasts may correspond to their expansion ability. In contrast to some other gene [6, 7], there are no data about mutual regulation of expression of mdr-1 and myc genes.

This study appears to be novel in coupling the genes which are not mutually regulated and which are responsible for the major facilities of leukemic cells—proliferation and drug resistance.

Methods and Patients

Twenty-one de nova and 13 pretreated acute myelogenous leukemia (AML) patients, and six de novo and ten pretreated acute lymphoblastic leukemia (ALL) patients were studied. Some of them were pretreated in other hospitals with standard and lower than standard regimens and did not achieve complete remission (CR). The number of resistant patients are artificially increased in this study because not all de novo patients with good response to cytostatic agents could be studied before the beginning of therapy, whereas leukemic cells in resistant patients were studied several times.

The hybridization in situ method for the detection of expression of studied genes was used [8] with slight modification.

The level of expression of genes was evaluated according to the following criteria: background value means 0–5 silver grains per cell; insignificant—6–15 grains per cell of a healthy

[1]Pavlov Medical University, St. Petersburg, Russia
[2]Petrov Scientific Oncology Institute, St, Petersburg, Russia
[3]The Centre for Advanced Medical Technology, St. Petersburg, Russia

donor. Expression exceeding 16 grains per cell was accepted as low and expression exceeding 30 grains per cell was accepted as high. The K 562 cell line was used as a positive control for myc gene expression.

Results and Discussion

We studied the level of myc gene expression in de novo and pretreated AL patients and found no differences in distribution of myc-positive patients in these groups, neither in AML nor in ALL (Table 1, $p > 0.05$).

The level of myc gene expression in de novo patients seemed to be higher than in pretreated ones (data not presented). We then studied myc gene expression in relation to prognosis (Table 2). Absence of myc gene expression correlated with obtaining CR in the total number of AML patients ($p < 0.01$). This correlation seemed to be valid for de novo patients ($p < 0.01$) and not statistically significant for the pretreated patients ($p > 0.05$). The main cause of worse clinical results in myc-positive (myc^+) patients was early death ED; (5/5 in myc^+ patients in comparison to 0/11 in myc-negative, (myc−) ones, $n = 21$, $p < 0.01$). This is not valid for the total population of leukemic patients, treated in our department ($7_{1/7}$, $n = 88$, $p < 0.01$).

We then tried to analyse the impact of myc gene overexpression on the results of different types of CHT (standard "7+3" based regimens vs. more intensive ones). These data are presented in Table 3. The expression of the myc gene had prognostic significance in patients treated by high-dose cytosine arabinoside (ara-C) regimens ($p < 0.01$) and not by standard ones ($p > 0.05$). At the same time, ED on standard dose ara-C regimens was observed in myc^+ patients only. It probably irelates to higher sensitivity of myc^+ blast cells to cytostatic agents. In contrast to AML patients, there was no prognostic significance of myc gene expression in ALL patients (data not presented, $p > 0.05$).

Table 1. The level of myc gene expression in de novo and pretreated AML and ALL patients

Cohorts of patients	Type of leukemia	Patients with different levels of myc gene expression	
		myc^+ (n)	myc^- (n)
De novo	AML	7	10
	ALL	1	5
Pretreated	AML	5	4
	ALL	3	7

Table 2. Myc gene expression and prognosis in de novo and pretreated patients

Results of therapy	Type of leukemia	Patients with different level of myc gene expression	
		myc^+ (n)	myc^- (n)
CR^+	De novo	3	8
	Pretreated	2	3
		5	11
CR^-	De novo	5	0
	Pretreated	3	1
		8	1

Table 3. Different CHT regimens and ED in AML patients

Types of therapy	Results of therapy	Patients with different levels of myc gene expression	
		myc$^+$ (*n*)	myc$^-$ (*n*)
Standard ($p > 0.05$)	CR$^+$	3	4
	ED	0	2
High dose ($p < 0.01$)	CR$^+$	6	1
	ED	0	3

We then compared mdr-1 and myc gene expression in different cohorts of AML and ALL patients (Tables 1,4). There were no differences in distribution of myc$^+$ patients between AML and ALL; the incidence of mdr-1$^+$ pretreated ALL patients was rather higher than in AML ones ($p < 0.05$). The reason for this phenomenon is unclear; it is probably related to more frequent use of two drugs known to turn on mdr-1 gene expression (vinca alkaloid/epipodophylline derivate+antracycline) in ALL treatment vs. predominantly an antracycline alone in AML CHT regimens.

Thereafter we evaluated coexpression of myc and mdr-1 genes (Tables 5, 6). There was a statistically significant correlation between mdr-1 and myc gene expression in AML ($p < 0.01$) but not in ALL ($p > 0.05$). Maybe the reason is the more frequent mdr-1 gene expression in ALL patients. As we have shown above, myc gene overexpression is a negative prognostic factor in relation to ED; myc$^+$ patients are considered to

Table 4. Comparison of mdr-1 gene in different cohorts of AML and ALL patients

Patients	Type of leukemia	Patients with different levels of mdr-1 gene expression	
		mdr-1$^+$ (*n*)	mdr-1$^-$ (*n*)
De nova	AML	3	16
	ALL	3	3
Pretreated	AML	4	8
	ALL	8	2

Table 5. of mdr-1 and myc genes in de novo and pretreated AML patients

Mdr-1 gene expression	Patients with different levels of myc gene expression**	
	myc$^+$	myc$^-$
mdr-1$^+$	4	1
mdr-1$^-$	3	13

**$p > 0.04$

Table 6. Coexpression of mdr-1 and myc genes in de novo and pretreated ALL patients

Mdr-1 gene expression	Patients with different levels of myc gene expression*	
	myc^{+}	myc^{-}
mdr-1^{+}	4	7
mdr-1^{-}	0	4

*$p > 0.05$

be hypersensitive to CHT, especially to intensive regimens. It is of no importance for resistance in AL patients.

Mdr-1 gene overexpression is one of the causes of drug resistance in AL patients (Table 7). Mdr-1^{+} patients appeared to be resistant more often than mdr-1^{-} ($p < 0.05$). Mdr-1 gene overexpression is of less importance for resistance on high-dose ara-C CHT regimens [9] and of no significance for ED (Table 7).

We have advanced a hypothesis of the significance of coexpression of mdr-1 and myc genes. First we compared the mdr-1^{+} myc^{+} group of patients with the mdr-1^{-}myc-one (Table 8). ED in the mdr-1^{+}/myc^{+} group seemed to be more frequent ($p < 0.05$), as was resistance, although the latter was not statistically confirmed. We then divided the population of myc^{+} patients into high expression (comparable to K 562 myc gene expression, myc-H) and low expression (myc-L) and studied the significance of coexpression of myc-L or myc-H with mdr-1 gene vs. myc/mdr-1-type of coexpression (Table 9).

The low level of myc gene expression was shown to be prognostic factor when expressed alone and was of no significance when coexpressed with the mdr-1 gene; the latter group of

Table 7. Results of CHT in relation to mdr-1 gene expression in AL patients

Results of CHT	Patients with different levels of mdr-1 gene expression	
	mdr^{+}	mdr^{-}
Resistance	7*	4*
Complete remission	3*	12*
Early death	1	3

*$p > 0.05$

Table 8. Impact of mdr-1 and myc gene coexpression on result of CHT

Results of CHT	Types of mdr-1 and myc-gene coexpression	
	mdr^{+}/myc^{+} (n)	mdr^{-}/myc^{-} (n)
Resistance	4	3
Complete remission	2*	11*
Early death	1*	0*

*$p < 0.05$

patients seemed to be more often resistant (not statistically significant).

In contrast to myc-L there was no statistical significance in comparing the myc-mdr-group with both the myc-H/mdr^{+} and myc-H/mdr-groups in relation to either resistance or ED.

We then tried to accumulate the data mentioned above (Table 10 Fig. 1). The main feature of the first group was rather high mdr-1 gene expression and low or an absence of myc gene expression. The clinical peculiarity of this group was a resistant type of response to CHT as compared to the second one ($p < 0.05$); the intensive CHT regimens would be of preference. The patients of the third group with a predominant myc gene expression above mdr-1 gene expression appeared to be hypersensitive to CHT with a high frequency of ED as compared to the former groups ($p < 0.01$). Such patients probably need prephase before intensive CHT. The mdr-1^{-} and myc patients had the most favorable prognosis.

Conclusions

1. There are no differences in myc gene expression in AML and ALL patients. Mdr-1 gene expression is significantly higher in pretreated ALL patients than in a corresponding cohort of AML patients.
2. Myc gene overexpression is a negative prognostic factor in AML patients. The high expression of myc gene correlates to ED and is of more prognostic importance on intensive CHT regimens.
3. The frequency of resistance to CHT is higher in patients with mdr-1^{+} cells.
4. Coexpression of mdr-1^{-} and the myc gene is more common for AML patients.

Table 9. Impact of coexpression of mdr-1 and low-expressed γ-myc gene (myc-L) on results of CHT

Results of CHT	Types of myc-L and mdr-1 gene coexpression		
	mdr-1 myc-L	mdr-1 myc	mdr-1 myc-L
Resistance	4	3	1
Complete remission	2	11*	0*
Early death	0	0*	1*

**$p < 0.01$

Table 10. Correlation of different types of myc-L, myc-H, and mdr-1 gene coexpression to results of CHT

Results of CHT	Different types of g-myc and mdr-1 gene coexpression		
	mdr /myc mdr /myc-L	mdr /myc	mdr /myc-H mdr /myc-L
Resistance	7*	3*	1
Complete remission	3*	11*	1*
Early death	0	0*	4*

$p < 0.05$

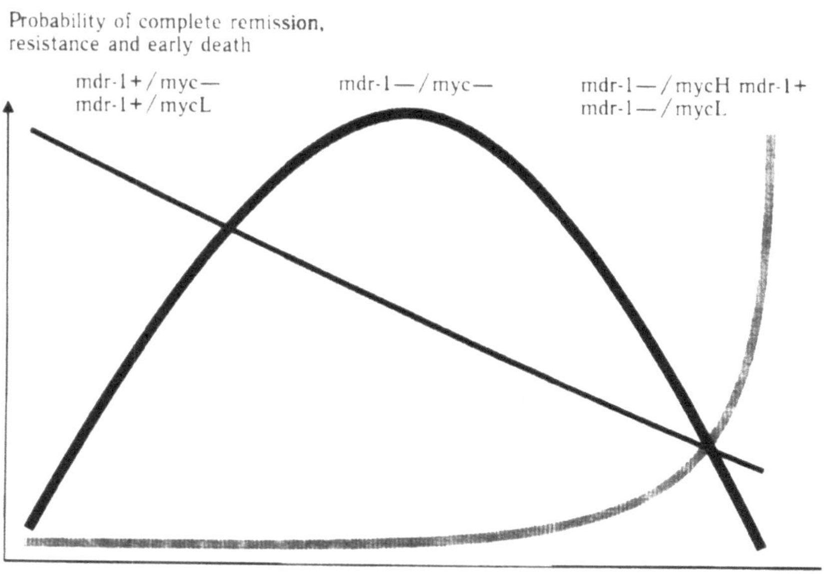

Fig. 1. Probability of different results of therapy in relation to types of mdr-1 and myc gene coexpression. *Thick dark line*, complete remission; *thin line*, resistance; *light line*, early death

5. Resistance in mdr-1$^+$ patients, depends on coexpression of the myc gene.

Acknowledgments. We are grateful to the staff of molecular biological laboratories of the BMT Center and the Petrov Scientific Oncology Institute for their help in performing the study. We also thank the city regional hematological outpatient department no2 for clinical studies of patients.

References

1. Zaritskey A., Afanasiev B. Clinical signisicance of p53 and mdr-1 gene expression in AML patients. Blut, N3, p.237, abstr. 668, 1994.
2. Zaritskey A., Bykova T., Stuif I., Sominskaya A., Medvedeva N., Anikina N., Afanasiev B. Prognoistic significance and relationship of myc and mdr-1 gene expression in adult acute leukemia. Modern Trends in Human Leukemia, 1995, in press.
3. Andreef M., Zhao S., Drach D., Hegewish S. et al. Expression of multidrug resistance and p53 genes in hematological cell systems: implications for biology and gene therapy. Cancer Bull, 1993, v.45, p131–138.
4. Drach D., Zhao Z., Drach Y., Mahadevia R., Gatringer C., Huber H., Andreef M. Subpopulations on normal peripheral blood and bone marrow cells express a functional multidrug resistant phenotype. Blood, 1992, v.80, p.2729.
5. Shidzinsky S., Brellwiz S., Feldman S.C., Watt R.A. Participation of c-myc-protein in DNA synthesis of human cells. Science, v.457, p.467, 1986.
6. Quesnel B., Preudhomme C., Oscier D., Lepelley P., Collyn-d'Hoghe M., Facon T., Zandecki M., Fenaux P. Overexpression of MDM-2 gene is found in some cases of haematological malignancies. Brit.J.Haem., v.88, p 415–419, 1994.
7. Ferrary S., Narni F., Mars W., Kaczmarek L., Wenturelly D., Anderson B. Calabretta B. Expression of growth factor regulated genes in human acute leukemias. Cancer Res., v. 46, p. 5162–5166, 1986.
8. Kanz L., Mielke R., Lonhr G. W., Fauser A. Detection of messenger RNAs within single hemopoietic cells by in situ hybridization on small slide areas. Exp. Hematol. v. 16, p.394–399 (1988)
9. Kiss C. Impaired capacity of multidrug resistance related cytotoxic drugs to inhibit colony formation of dexamethasone-resistant human leukemic cell lines. Cancer Invest. v. 11, p. 358–360 (1993)

ALL in Children

Acute Leukemias VI
Prognostic Factors
and Treatment Strategies
Büchner et al. (eds)

Risk Adapted Treatment in Childhood Acute Lymphoblastic Leukemia: Data from the Berlin–Frankfurt–Münster Group

M. Schrappe[1], A. Reiter[1], K. Welte[1], W.-D. Ludwig[2], J. Harbott[3], F. Lampert[3], G. Henze[4], and H. Riehm[1]

Abstract. Experience with approximately 3700 patients in the last four multicenter trials for childhood acute lymphoblastic leukemia (ALL) performed over the last 13 years by the Berlin–Frankfurt–Münster (BFM) study group established and reconfirmed basic knowledge on the risk of relapse. A series of randomized and prospective questions, however, allowed new insights into additional biological and therapy-related factors. In trials ALL-BFM 83, evidence was generated on the importance of delayed intensification, even for standard-risk ALL that was later confirmed in the following trial ALL-BFM 86. Patients with standard-risk ALL treated without reinduction therapy had an even higher risk of relapse than patients stratified into the medium-risk group. From 1981 to 1986. the impact of adequate maintenance therapy with 6-mercaptopurine (6-MP) and methotrexate (MTR) on event-free surival was evaluated by randomization of 18 vs. 24 months total therapy duration, proving the impact of prolonged exposure on disease-free survival. Also in trial ALL-BFM 83, the blast cell reduction after the 1 week of treatment with prednisone and MTX i.th. was prospectively evaluated to find a reliable prognostic parameter for early prediction of increased risk of relapse. Thus, a new independent risk factor called the "prednisone poor response"(PRED-PR) was generated that identified approximately 10% of all patients with ALL. The prognosis for this group, however, has not yet improved from the time of discovery in trial ALL-BFM 83, despite various attempts at treatment intensification. Patients in this group are predominantly boys, have an high initial leukemic cell burden, present with T cell ALL in 40% of the cases, and have an increased risk of remission failure. The probability of event-free survival (pEFS) in the group is less than 50%. Among these patients with PRED-PR, a subgroup can be identified that is at even higher risk of relapse: with the coexpression of myeloid markers on their blast population, T-ALL, or a very high White blood cell count (WBC). Translocation t(9; 22), the equivalent BCR-ABL recombination, or t(4;11) are, together with nonresponse to primary treatment, additional high-risk features that qualify any patient for maximum therapy, including allogeneic bone marrow transplantation (BMT). Despite the difficulties for high-risk patients a pEFS of 75% for the total study population is encouraging.

Introduction

Biological features at diagnosis of acute lymphoblastic leukemia (ALL) such as the age of the patient, white blood cell count (WBC), organ involvement, immunophenotype, and cytogenetics have been used by all major study groups to stratify treatment composition and intensity. However, recently treatment intensity has also

[1]Department of Pediatrics, Medizinische Hochschule Hannover, 30623 Hannover, Germany
[2]Department of Medical Oncology and Applied Molecular Biology, Röbert-Rossle-Clinic, Humboldt University, 13122 Berlin, Germany
[3]Department of Pediatrics, University Hospital, 35385 Gieβen, Germany
[4]Department of Pediatrics, Rudolf Virchow Medical Center, 13347 Berlin, Germany

turned out to be a major prognostic factor [1–4]. The Berlin–Frankfurt–Münster (BFM) group addressed the impact of treatment intensity in two randomized trials conducted from 1981 to 1986 [5, 6]. The prognostic influence of early treatment response was prospectively evaluated in trial ALL-BFM 83, and later utilized in trials ALL-BFM 86 and 90 to identify the group of ALL patients with the highest risk for relapse [3, 6]. For this patient group, which is characterized by an inadequate response to a brief induction prephase based on prednisone, very intensive chemotherapy can offer only limited efficacy resulting in event-free survival rates of 40%–50% but causing considerable toxicity. Therefore, in 1991 a randomized trial for high-risk patients was initiated to evaluate the effect of recombinant human ranulocyte colony-stimulating factor (r-metHuG-CSF, filgastrim) on myelosuppression and related complications, and on overall response rate to chemotherapy. This paper reviews the updated results of four trials of the BFM study group, reflecting the significant impact that treatment intensity and treatment response have on long-term outcome for children with ALL.

Patients and Methods

Between 1981 and 1994 more than 3500 patients with ALL were treated with four consecutive BFM protocols in up to 85 institutions in Germany, Switzerland, and Austria. Cytomorphology, immunology, cytogenetics, and DNA index were determined in central laboratories as previously described [3]. Life table estimates were based on the Kaplan-Meier method, and compared using the log-rank test. Therapy for patients with B precursor or T-ALL was risk adapted by stratifying according to the *BFM risk factor* (BFM RF) calculating the leukemic cell load at diagnosis:

$$RF = 0.2*\log(B+1)+0.06*L+0.04.S$$

Where B equals the number of leukemic blasts per microliter of peripheral blood; *L* and *S* are the enlargement of liver and spleen in centimeters below the costal margin [7]. Patients with B-ALL were treated with a different protocol [8]. Randomization and therapy were performed only after informed consent had been obtained. The major components of therapy have been published in details [3, 5, 9, 10].

To randomize for the duration of maintenance therapy, all patients of trials ALL-BFM 81 and 83 were recruited independently of their initial risk features: 764 patients were randomized shortly before the end of the 18th month of therapy to be continued on maintenance therapy with 6-mercaptopurine (6-MP) and oral methotrexate (MTX) up to a total therapy duration of 24 months, or to discontinue maintenance therapy after the 18th month of treatment.

In trial ALL-BFM 83,126 patients with standard-low risk (SR-L) ALL (BFM-RF <0.8, no initial CNS disease) were randomized (Fig. 1) during consolidation therapy to receive or not to receive reinduction therapy with protocol III (dexamethasone DEXA, 10 mg/m^2 per day on days 1–14; vincristine, VCR, 1.5 mg/m^2 on days 1+8; doxorubicin, DOXO, 30 mg/m^2 on days 1+8; L-asparaginase, L-ASP,10 000 U/m^2 on days 1,4,8,12; 6-thioguanine,6-TG, 60 mg/m^2 per day on days 15–29; cytarabine, ara-C, 75 mg/m^2 17–20, on days 24–27; ith. MTX on days 17+24). Reinduction therapy was scheduled to start 2 weeks after the end of consolidation therapy, that is, 23 weeks after diagnosis (arm SR-L/2). Patients randomized not to receive reinduction therapy (SR-L/1) were started directly on maintenance therapy with oral 6-MP and MTX 2 weeks after consolidation [5, 6]. Patients with SR-L ALL (RF < 0.8) were not treated with rein-

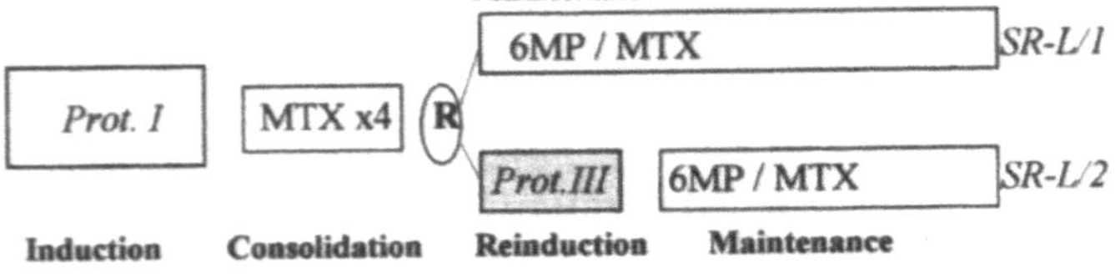

Fig. 1. Randomization of reinduction therapy in standard-low risk (*SR-L*) patients of trial ALL-BFM 83 (BFM-RF < 0.8). Reinduction therapy or beginning of maintenance therapy was scheduled for week 23

duction therapy in the subsequent trial ALL-BFM 86 until the follow up of trial ALL-BFM 83 revealed a significantly worse outcome for SR patients treated without reinduction [3]. Thereafter, all SR patients were treated in addition to induction and consolidation therapy with the reinduction element protocol II [5, 6, 9] that had been used in medium-risk (MR) and high-risk (HR) patients (drugs as in protocol III expect for: DEXA on days 1–21; DOXO and VCR on days 1, 8, 15, and 22; cyclophosphamide (CP) 1000 mg/m^2 on days 29).

The prospective evaluation of early prednisone (PRED) response in peripheral blood was initiated in trial ALL-BFM 83 [6]. All patients received one i. th. injection of MTX on day 1 and PRED at a dosage of 60 mg/m^2 per day for 7 days; in case of a large tumor load, initial dose reduction was permitted. On day 8 the number of leukemic blasts in the peripheral blood was determined. Risk-stratified treatment was continued with induction protocol I containing in addition to PRED L-ASP, daunorubicin (DNR), VCR, CP, ara-C, 6-MP, 1 and i. th. MTX. HR patients (BFM RF $> = 1.7$) were scheduled to receive a 5-day block containing intermediate-dose MTX, ara-C, teniposide, DEX and CP immediately following the PRED prephase. This block was to be repeated before starting protocol I[6].

Patients with $> = 1000$ leukemic blasts after the 7-day PRED prephase (PRED poor response, PR) were found to have a probability for event-free survival (pEFS) of less than 40% compared to nearly 70% for the complementary group. Therefore, the in vivo steriod response was utilized for treatment stratification in the subsequent trials ALL-BFM 86 and 90: Patients with PRED-PR qualified for intensified therapy in the HR group. In trial ALL-BFM 86, treatment for HR patients included in addition to induction by protocol I and reinduction by protocol II intensified consolidation with protocol E containing high-dose (HD)-PRED, HD-MTX, ifosfamide (IFO), HD-ara-C, and mitoxantrone [3]. In trial ALL-BFM 90 [10] another approach using short but highly intensive blocks applied after a 5-week induction therapy was chosen for HR patients [10].

In trial ALL-BFM 90, patients qualified for the HR group were randomized to receive or not to receive nine cycles of r-metHuG-CSF (filgastrim) between intensified consolidation elements. These 6-day chemotherapy block contained DEXA, HD-ara-C, HD-MTX, IFO, L-ASP, DNR, VCR, vindesine (VDS), 6-MP, 6-TG, and etoposide [10]. G-CSF (5 μg/kg/d) was started 1 day after the end of each block, and continued for 14 days, in the case of unsatisfactory neutrophil recovery for up to 21 days.

Results

Treatment Duration

A total of 764 patients were randomized in trials ALL-BFM 81 and ALL-BFM 83 for 18 vs. 24 months of total therapy duration. All other patients ($n = 345$) were chosen for one or other treatment arm (145 patients for 18 months, 200 patients for 24 months). All events prior to the 18th month of therapy are censored in this analysis. Thus, the probability for event-free interval (pEFI) is 79% after a medium observation time of 10 years (range 8–12 years) for patients randomized for 24 months, but only 71% for patients randomized for 18 months ($p = 0.0097$) as demonstrated in Fig. 2 and Table 1. The majority of late relapses occurred in patients with B precursor ALL, thus extended maintenance therapy could prevent a signficant portion of relapses in that subgroup: pEFI is 72% for 24 months vs. 62% for 18 months ($p = 0.01$). In contrast, patients with T-ALL rarely experienced a relapse more than 18 months after diagnosis. Comparing the randomized groups within the various risk groups defined by cell load at diagnosis (BFM-RF), the effect of prolonged maintenance ther`apy can be demonstrated for all risk groups, but only in the HR group is the extended therapy significantly ($p = 0.02$) superior to that of 18 months (pEFI 78% vs. 68%). The long-term observation reveals that patients defined as MR or HR ALL by a BFM-RF $> = 1.2$ who entered this randomization fared just as well as those with SR/intermediate-risk features (defined in this trial by a BFM-RF < 1.2): pEFI in MR/HR patients is 71%/80%, and in SR patients 71%/79% for 18/24 months of treatment, respectively. Nearly the same results were observed in patients who were not randomized for treatment duration and who were chosen for 18 or 24 months of treatment.

Reinduction Therapy

On the basis of results favorable to reinduction therapy that were generated in HR patients in

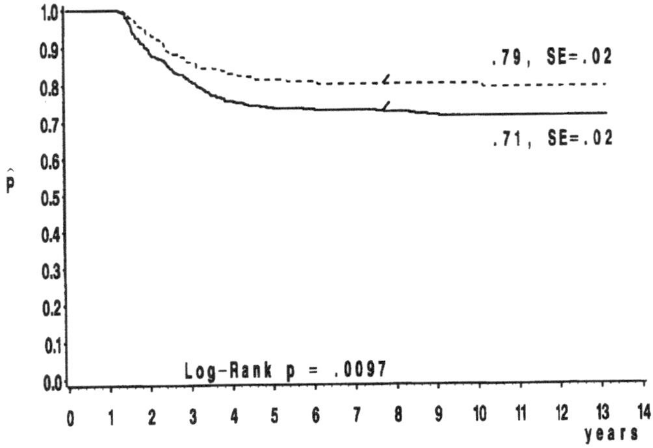

Fig. 2. Event-free interval from month 18 in patients randomized for duration of maintenance therapy in trials ALL-BFM 81 and 83. *Solid line*, 18 months (n = 390, 275 in CCR); *broken line*, 24 months (n = 374, 296 in CCR)

Table 1. Characteristics and outcome in patients randomized for treatment duration in trials ALL-BFM 81 and 83

	Treatment duration			
	18 Months		24 Months	
	(n)	(%)	(n)	(%)
Patients	390		374	
Male/female	220/170 (Ratio 1.29: 1)		207/167 (Ratio 1.24: 1)	
Distribution in risk groups:				
SR / MR / HR[a]		63.3/32.3/4.4		65.2/29.4/5.3
Death in CR	3	0.8	–	
Relapses	107	27.4	77	20.6
Isolated BM	66	16.9	43	11.5
Isolated CNS	7	1.8	8	2.1
Isolated testes	8	3.6[c]	5	2.4[c]
Combined BM/CNS	17	4.4	13	3.5
Other	9	2.3	8	2.1
Patients in CCR	275	70.5	296	79.1
LFU	5		1	
pEFI (SE)[b]	0.71	0.02	0.79	0.02

Patients were randomized in the 18th month after diagnosis, only events after the 18th month were evaluated.
[a]SR, standard and intermediate risk (BFM RF < 1.2); MR, medium risk (RF 1.2– < 1.7); HR, high risk (RF > = 1.7).
[b]pEFI at 12 years (median observation time 10 yrs); SE, standard error.
[c]Percentage of male patients only.

previous ALL-BFM trials [11] and owing to inconclusive results in SR patients with regard to the efficacy of reintensification in trials ALL-BFM 79 and 81 [5, 12], a randomized evaluation of the influence of reinduction therapy (delayed intensification) on remission duration in low-risk (LR) patients was initiated in trial ALL-BFM 83. LR patients defined by a BFM RF < 0.8 were characterized by a WBC < 10 000 in 95% of patients, an adequate PRED response in all patients, and by one quarter the patients being older than 10 years. However, in two thirds of the patients for whom data are available a DNA index of < 1.16 was found. After a median observation time of nearly 10 years (range 8.5–11.5 years), stable results can be presented: LR patients had a significantly worse outcome when treated without reinduction element protocol III (SR-L/1) than patients who received delayed reintensification (SR-L/2) as demonstrated in Table 2.

The negative result in SR-L/1 is mainly due to an excessive rate of systemic relapses that occurred up to 5 years from diagnosis. There were also more relapses with CNS involvement in group SR-L/1. With regard to testes, no relapses were observed in either arm. No patient died due to toxicity. Similar results were observed in those patients for whom one of the two treatment options was chosen. Thus, intensive reinduction therapy with protocol III could safely prevent more than half of the relapses that were seen in patients without reinduction therapy. The late incidence of relapses made it difficult to recognize this result early enough before trial ALL-BFM 86 was initiated.

In trial ALL-BFM 86, SR patients (BFM-RF <0.8, no T-ALL, good PRED response) were scheduled to receive HD-MTX (4×5 g, 24-h infusion , instead of 4×0.5 g as in trial 83) in consolidation therapy but not to receive delayed intensification. Figure 3 demonstrates the significantly ($p = 0.0001$) inferior outcome (pEFS) of 109 patients treated from October 1986 until March 1988 who did not receive delayed intensification with protocol II when compared to 175 patients who were treated with reinduction therapy after amendment to the protocol from April 1988 until March 1990. Both groups are comparable with regard to WBC, age, sex, and DNA index. In the cohort of patients who did not receive protocol II the rate of relapses was near-

Table 2. Replapses in *randomized* standard-low risk (SR-L) patients (RF <0.8) in trial ALL-BFM 83

Reinduction (protocol III)	SR-L/1 No		SR-L/2 Yes	
	n	(%)	*n*	(%)
Patients	66		60	
Relapses	27	40.9	10	16.7
Isolated BM	18	27.3	5	8.3
Isolated CNS	1	1.5	-	
Combined BM/CNS	6	9.1	2	3.3
Other	2	3.0	3	5.0
In CCR	39	59.1	50	83.3
pEFS (SE)	0.59	0.06[a]	0.83	0.05[a]

[a]The differences of pEFS at 10 years is significant: $p = 0.0023$ (log-rank test). SE, standard error.

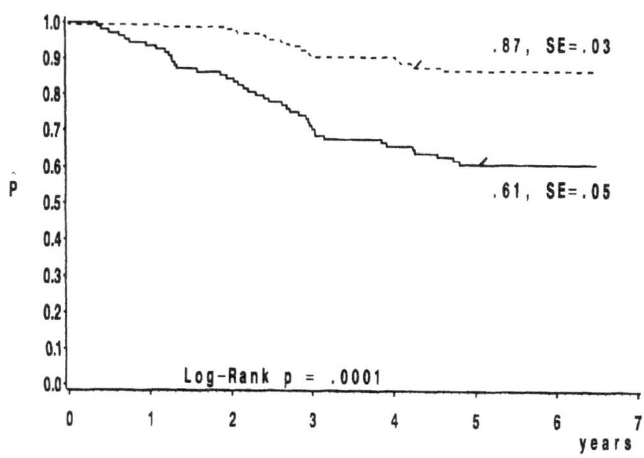

Fig. 3. Event-free survival in patients of trial ALL-BFM 86 treated without reinduction therapy (*solid line*; $n = 109$, 63 in CCR) or with reinduction therapy (*broken line*; $n = 175$, 146 in CCR)

ly four times higher than in the group of patients treated with protocol II. The majority of relapses in that group was observed in the bone marrow (BM) and in the testes, whereas the rate of CNS relapses did not increase significantly [3]. This might have been due to the newly introduced HD-MTX given in consolidation therapy.

Early Response to PRED

Analysis of early therapy response to 7 days of PRED and one i.th. injection of MTX that had prospectively been evaluated in trial ALL-BFM 83 [6] identified a novel poor prognosis marker that was more predictive of relapse than any other marker used thus far: 8% of the patients formed a small poor risk group that was characterized by the presence of ≥1000 leukemic blasts per microliter of peripheral blood after 1 week of PRED (PRED-PR). After a median observation time in trial ALL-BFM 83 of approximately 10 years, the pEFS for patients with PRED-PR is 39%, compared to 66% in patients with adequate response to PRED. No other mathematical model or any other single factor could describe a group of patients that was as large and had a prognosis of less than 50% pEFS. Reflecting the reliability of this method that has been applied in 2851 patients since 1983, 8%–10% of the patients have always been identified as PRED-PR in all subsequent trials. In addition, some characteristics have constantly been observed in these trials [3, 6, 10] that indicate that this parameter is associated with some well-known poor risk features (Table 3).

Any treatment variation or intensification that was applied in trials ALL-BFM 86 and 90 for patients with PRED-PR did not significantly alter the outcome of this group as shown in Fig. 4. The life table also demonstrates that relapses in this HR group consistently occur in the first 30 months after diagnosis. However, treatment stratification utilizing the PRED response selected a large favorable group of T-ALL patients: 73% of all T-ALL patients were characterized by

Table 3. Patient characteristics according to prednisone response in three ALL-BFM trials 83, 86 and 90

Patient characterstics	PRED-PR $n=268$ (%)	PRED-GR $n=2583$ (%)
Boys	67	55
WBC > 50000 per µl	62	16
T-ALL	45	10
No CR after 5-week induction	16	0.9
pEFS (SE)[a]	0.48 (0.05)	0.78 (0.02)

[a]Result from trial ALL-BFM 86 (6-year EFS). PRED-PR, prednisone poor response; PRED-GR, prednisone good response; (for definitions see text).

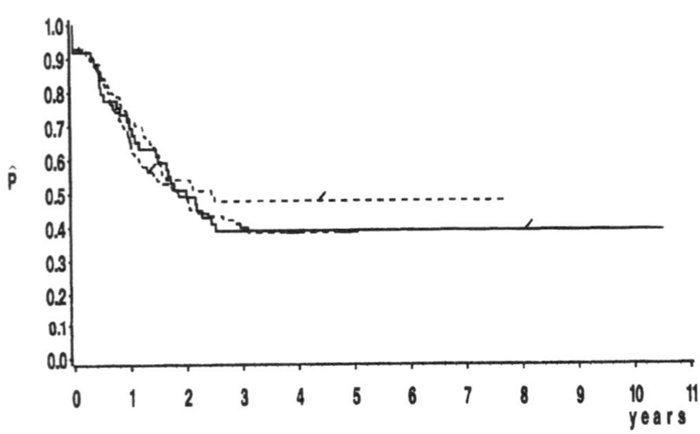

Fig. 4. Event-free survival in high-risk ALL patients characterized by poor prednisone response treated in three consecutive ALL-BFM trials between 1983 and 1993: no significant difference between the three groups (log-rank test)

an adequate PRED response and were successfully treated in trial ALL-BFM 86 resulting in a 6-year EFS of 84% [3].

The group of patients with PRED-PR can be divided into two subgroups with significantly different outcomes. The following *additional* features were found in trial ALL-BFM 86 to increase the risk of relapse for patients with PRED-PR [3]:

- large leukemic cell mass: BFM-RF> =1.7
- T-ALL
- Pre-pre-B-ALL
- Coexpression of myeloid marker(s)
- No remission on day 40 of induction

These characteristics qualified any patient with PRED-PR for an "unfavorable" HR group, and thus eligible for HLA-matched sibling bone marrow transplantation (BMT) in first complete remission (CR). In addition, independently of the PRED response, patients with no remission after 5 weeks of induction therapy and patients with cytogenetic or molecular-genetic evidence of translocations t(9; 22) or t(4; 11) qualified for allogeneic HLA-matched sibling donor BMT in first CR in trial ALL-BFM 90.

Some characteristics and the treatment results of the unfavorable and favorable PRED-PR groups in trial ALL-BFM 86 are shown in Table 4 illustrate the negative selection achieved by the above-listed criteria.

Morbidity of High Treatment Intensity

In trial ALL-BFM 90, the effect of r-metHuG-CSF on treatment morbidity and on response to chemotherapy was investigated in HR patients. These patients mainly qualified for high-intensity treatment due to a PRED-PR. The following significantly different results were observed in the G-CSF-treated group [13]:

- Lower incidence and shorter (threefold) duration of febrile neutropenia
- Fewer culture-confirmed infections
- Lower antibiotic use

It also appeared that a tighter adherence to the treatment schedule was facilitated even though this had not been an objective of the study. The incidence of relapses was not increased in the G-CSF-treated group. Thus, the application of G-CSF seems to be an efficient way to decrease morbidity of highly intensive chemotherapy in ALL. The use of G-CSF may allow an enhancement of treatment intensity that could help to overcome resistant disease in HR ALL.

Discussion

The prognostic significance of leukemia-specific biological factors is undoubted; therefore, initial diagnostic procedures have to aim at obtaining as much information as possible to use the combination of immunological, cytogenetic, and molecular-genetic findings for optimal risk adjustment of therapy. Especially in large multicenter trials, however, there are technical and logistic limitations to obtaining all this information. With the exception of rather rare, well-defined cytogenetic abnormalities, easily available factors such as WBC, age, and sex have also successfully been used for reasonable risk

Table 4. Characteristics and outcome of patients with unfavorable and favorable PRED-PR response in trial ALL-BFM 86

Patient characteristics	Unfavorable PRED-PR $n=59$ (%)	Favorable PRED-PR $n=36$ (%)
Boys	58	47
WBC > 50 000/μl	73	44
Age < 1 year	17	11
Relapses	46	31
pEFS (SE)[a]	0.37 (0.06)	0.62 (0.08)

[a]pEFS at 8 years; log-rank test $p=0.02$. Unfavorable PRED-PR, PRED-PR *plus* one of the following additional features: BFM-RF> =1.7, T-ALL, pre-pre-B-ALL, coexpression of myeloid markers, no remission on day 40 of induction. Favorable PRED-PR, only PRED-PR, no other risk features.

assessment [2, 14–16]. Analysis of early therapy response has provided an additional instrument to detect increased risk of failure in ALL therapy [6, 17].

Treatment intensity is well known to have a major impact on EFS in leukemia treatment [1–3, 14, 15, 18–20]. Two randomized trials of the ALL-BFM group demonstrated that rather late intensification of treatment is effective in preventing some subsequent relapses. First, extension of the maintenance therapy from 18 to 24 months can decrease the rate of relapses from 1: 4 to 1: 5 in an unselected population of children with ALL (Table 1). This first randomized evaluation of the role of maintenance therapy for remission duration demonstrated the advantage of 24-month maintenance therapy which reduced the rate of relapses for both sexes by approximately 7%. The advantage was independent of the initial BFM RF but limited to patients with B precursor ALL. This result was not imparied by any increase in toxic events.

The second randomized trial focused on the reduction of acute and late toxicity for SR patients by limiting the use of all cytostatic drugs except for oral 6-MP and MTX. The short repetition of the induction therapy given from week 23 to week 27 in SR-L patients could cut down the relapse rate from 40% to 16% (ALL-BFM 83). This was unintentionally confirmed in the subsequent trial ALL-BFM 86 in which delayed intensification had initially been omitted. A comparison of the end results in trials ALL-BFM 83 and 86 in SR-L patients treated without or with delayed intensification reveals very similar results: patients treated with delayed intensification had a final result of >80% pEFS, whereas those who were treated without reinduction had a final pEFS that was inferior by 25%. This result was even inferior to that of MR patients, and nearly as poor as that of the HR group. Even though trial ALL-BFM 86 was not a randomized study, there cannot be any doubt that reinduction therapy as provided by protocol II is able to decrease the incidence of relapses sharply in SR ALL patients. It seems possible that the more intensive therapy (HD-MTX, protocol II instead of protocol III) for SR patients as provided in trial ALL-BFM 86 will have prevented more relapses than the treatment in ALL-BFM 83 because at this point only 11.4% relapses have been registered in trial 86 compared to 22.1% in the total group SR-L/2 of trial 83. The outcome of the SR patients in trial ALL-BFM 86 treated with reinduction therapy appears quite favorable considering the fact that this group of patients contained a large number of patients characterized by a DNA index of<1.16 which is regarded in general to be an adverse prognostic factor [21].

The evaluation of the in vivo sensitivity to PRED allowed the identification of a well-defined HR group representing 9% of the total patient population. In a multivariate analysis performed on 848 patients of trial ALL-BFM 86, the PRED-PR was found to be a strong predictor of treatment failure together with WBC>20000, or WBC>200000. Another response parameter, i.e., the presence of>5% blasts in the BM on day 40 of induction therapy, was the strongest negative prognostic parameter [3]. The HR group as defined by the BFM group seems to be a group of patients which is primarily highly resistant to multichemotherapy as several attempts with HD chemotherapy that also included some alternative drugs such as mitoxantrone and IFO failed to improve the outcome of that group.

Since 1990 the early response to chemotherapy has been evaluated in the BM on day 15 of induction therapy in addition to the evaluation in the peripheral blood on day 8. Interim analysis indicates that a small subgroup of patients who have >25% blasts in the BM can be identified as appearing to have an inferior prognosis. However, the selection is not as accurate as the one provided by the PRED response in peripheral blood on day 8. Eventually, the evaluation of treatment response in the BM might help to describe subgroups at increased risk for relapse that are not identified by other factors.

Thus, it is quite easily possible to describe a LR group, and a HR group, but the characteristics of the intermediate or MR group that predict treatment failure are more difficult to define. The majority of relapses in an unselected group of patients will occur in individuals that were not previously identified as having special risk features as patients in the HR group. In trial ALL-BFM 86, 135 (58%) of 233 relapses (in 998 patients enrolled) occurred in MR patients, whereas 60 (25%) occurred in SR and 38 (16%) in HR patients. Identification of new biological markers as well as more subtle ways to detect resistance to chemotherapy are needed to prevent the large number of "unpredictable" relapses.

References

1. Sallan SE, Gelber RD, Kimball V, Donnelly M, Cohen HJ (1990) More is better! Update of Dana-Farber Cancer Institute/Children's Hospital childhood acute lymphoblastic leukemia trials. Haematol Blood Transfus 33: 459–466
2. Tubergen DG, Gilchrist GS, O'Brien RT, Coccia PF, Sather HN, Waskerwitz MJ, Hammond GD (1993) Improved outcome with delayed intensification for children with acute lymphoblastic leukemia and intermediate presenting features: a Children's Cancer Group phase III trial. J Clin Oncol 11: 527–537
3. Reiter A, Schrappe M, Ludwig W-D, Hiddermann W, Sauter S, Henze G, Zimmermann M, Lampert F, Havers W, Niethammer D, Odenwald E, Ritter J, Mann G, Welte K, Gadner H, Riehm H (1994) Chemotherapy in 998 unselected childhood acute lymphoblastic leukemia patients. Results and conclusions of the multicenter trial ALL-BFM 86. Blood 84: 3122–3133
4. Schmiegelow K, Pulczynska MK (1990) Maintenance chemotherapy for childhood acute lymphoblastic leukemia: should dosage be guided by white blood cell counts? Am J Pediatr Hematol Oncol 12: 462–467
5. Schrappe M, Beck J, Brandeis WE, Feickert HJ, Gadner H, Graf N, Havers W, Henze G, Jobke A, Kornhuber B, Kühl J, Lampert F, Müller-Weihrich St, Niethammer D, Reiter A, Rister M, Ritter J, Schellong G, Tausch W, Weinel P, Riehm H (1987) Die Behandlung der akuten lymphoblastischen Leukämie im Kindes- und Jugendalter: Ergebnisse der multizentrischen Therapiestudie ALL-BFM 81. Klin Pädiatr 199: 133–150
6. Riehm H, Reiter A, Schrappe M, Berthold F, Dopfer R, Gerein H, Ludwig R, Ritter J, Stollmann B, Henze G (1987) The in vivo response on corticosteroid therapy as an additional prognostic factor in childhood acute lymphoblastic leukemia (therapy study ALL-BFM 83). Klin Pädiatr 199: 151–160
7. Langermann H-J, Henze G, Wulf M, Riehm H (1982) Abschätzung der Tumorzellmasse bei der akuten lymphoblastischen Leukämie im Kindesalter: prognostische Bedeutung und praktische Anwendung. Klin Pädiatr 194: 209–213
8. Reiter A, Schrappe M, Ludwig WD, Lampert F, Harbott J, Henze G, Niemeyer CM, Gadner H, Muller Weihrich S, Ritter J, Odenwald E, Riehm H (1992) Favorable outcome of B-cell acute lymphoblastic leukemia in childhood: a report of three consecutive studies of the BFM group. Blood 80: 2471–2478
9. Riehm H, Gadner H, Henze G, Langermann H-J, Odenwald E (1980) The Berlin childhood acute lymphoblastic leukemia therapy study, 1970-1976. Am J Pediatr Hematol Oncol 2: 299–306
10. Schrappe M, Reiter A, Sauter S, Ludwig W-D, Wörmann B, Harbott J, Bender-Götze C, Dörffel W, Dopfer R, Frey E, Havers W, Henze G, Kühl J, Richter R, Ritter J, Treuner J, Zintl F, Odenwald E, Welte K, Riehm H (1994) Concept and interim analysis of trial ALL-BFM 90 for the treatment of children and adolescents with acute lymphoblastic leukemia: significance of therapy response in peripheral blood and bone marrow. Klin Pädiatr 206: 208–221
11. Lampert F, Henze G, Langermann H-J, Schellong G, Gadner H, Riehm H (1984) Acute lymphoblastic leukemia: current status of therapy in children. Recent Results in Cancer Research 93: 159–181
12. Henze G, Langermann H-J, Fengler R, Brandeis M, Evers KG, Gadner H, Hinderfeld L, Jobke A, Kornhuber B, Lampert F, Lasson U, Ludwig R, Müller-Weihrich S, Neidhardt M, Nessler G, Niethammer D, Rister M, Ritter J, Schaaf A, Schellong G, Stollmann B, Treuner J, Wahlen W, Weinel P, Wehinger H, Riehm H (1982) Therapiestudie BFM 79/81 zur Behandlung der akuten lymphoblastischen Leukämie bei Kindern und Jugendlichen: intensivierte Reinduktionstherapie für Patientengruppen mit unterschiedlichem Rezidivrisiko. Klin Pädiatr 194: 195–203
13. Welte K, Mempel K, Reiter A, Yakisan E, Odenwald E, Pfetsch M, Zwingers T, Schwab G, Riehm H (1993) A randomized phase III study of recombinant human granulocyte colony-stimulating factor (r-metHuG-CSF) in childhood high risk acute lymphoblastic leukemia. Blood 82 (Suppl.1): 194a(Abstract)
14. Schorin MA, Blattner S, Gelber RD, Tarbell NJ, Donnelly M, Dalton V, Cohen HJ, Sallan SE (1994) Treatment of childhood acute lymphoblastic leukemia: results of Dana-Farber Cancer Institute/Children's Hospital Acute Lymphoblastic Leukemia Consortium Protocol 85-01. J Clin Oncol 12: 740–747
15. Rivera GK, Raimondi SC, Hancock ML, Behm FG, Pui CH, Abromowitch M, Mirro JJ, Ochs JS, Look AT, Williams DL, et al (1991) Improved outcome in childhood acute lymphoblastic leukaemia with reinforced early treatment and rotational combination chemotherapy. Lancet 337: 61–66
16. Chessells JM, Richards SM, Bailey CC, Lilleyman JS, Eden OB (1995) Gender and treatment outcome in childhood lymphoblastic leukaemia: report from the MRC UKALL trials. Br J Haematol 89: 364–372
17. Gaynon PS, Bleyer WA, Steinherz PG, Finklestein JZ, Littman P, Miller DR, Reaman G, Sather H, Hammond GD (1990) Day 7 marrow response and outcome for children with acute lymphoblastic leukemia and unfavorable presenting features. Med Pediatr Oncol 18: 273–279
18. Gaynon PS, Steinherz PG, Bleyer WA, Ablin AR, Albo VC, Finklestein JZ, Grossman NJ, Novak LJ, Pyesmany AF, Reaman GH, et al (1993) Improved therapy for children with acute lymphoblastic leukemia presenting features: a follow-up report of the Children's Cancer Group Study CCG-106. J Clin Oncol 11: 2234–2242
19. Chessells JM, Bailey C, Richards SM (1995) Intensification of treatment and survival in all chil-

dren with lymphoblastic leukaemia: results of UK Medical Research Council trial UKALL X. Lancet 345: 143–148
20. Riehm H, Gadner H, Henze G, Kornhuber B, Lampert F, Niethammer D, Reiter A, Schellong G (1990) Results and significance of six randomized trials in four consecutive ALL-BFM trials. Haematol Blood Transfus 33: 439–450
21. Look AT (1988) The cytogenetics of childhood leukemia: clinical and biologic implications. Pediatr Clin NA 35: 723–741

Acute Leukemias VI
Prognostic Factors
and Treatment Strategies
Büchner et al. (eds)

Mechanisms of Treatment Failure in Childhood Acute Lymphoblastic Leukemia: Children's Cancer Group Initiatives

P.S. Gaynon[1], B.C. Bostrom[2], G.H. Reaman[3], H.N. Sather[4], M.E. Trigg[5], D.G. Tubergen[6], and F.M. Uckun[7]
for the Children's Cancer Study Group

Abstract. The Children's Cancer Group (CCG) has conducted clinical trials for children with newly diagnosed acute lymphoblastic leukemia (ALL) since 1968 and enrolled more than 12000 children. More than 1000 children were enrolled in 1994 alone. Prelimary analyses show a 4-years event-free survival of 74% for the current concluding CCG-1800 series and successive statistically significant 25% reductions in relative risk of failure over the last two series of studies. Several themes may be derived from this experience. (a) early response to therapy is a consistent determinant of outcome; (b) effective intensification of systemic therapy after induction reduces the likelihood of marrow and extramedullary relapse for patients with either favorable or unfavorable presenting features; (c) effective presymptomatic CNS therapy may be provided to all infants and most children without cranial irradiation. However, 18 Gy cranial irradiation may still be useful for a minority of children with higher-risk presenting features. Recent observations point to primary disease resistance to chemotherapy and unfavorable host thiopurine pharmacology as common mechanisms of treatment failure. Resistance to chemotherapy may be linked to resistance to apoptosis. Patients with primary disease resistance may be identified through in vitro assays or poor early marrow response and assigned to more prolonged, more rigorous intensification. We propose to employ laboratory assays of end-induction leukemic burden to measure the specific contribution of anti-CD19 pokeweed antiviral protein conjugate in the context of complex therapy in known resistant disease. Failure to achieve adequate intracellular levels of thiopurine metabolites may possibly be redressed by parentheral administration and/or substitution of 6-thioguanine (6-TG) for 6-mercaptopurine (6-MP). The reasons for treatment failure in cases of Philadelphia chromosome-positive ALL remain to be elucidated.

Introduction

Childhood acute lymphoblastic leukemia (ALL) is the single most common malignancy in children [1] and its incidence is increasing [2]. The Children's Cancer Group (CCG) has conducted clinical trials for children with newly diagnosed ALL enrolling more than 12000 children since 1968. Therapy has been allocated on the basis of estimated risk of relapse since 1976. Appendix 1 lists the more than 100 CCG treatment sites presently active in the United States, Canada, and Western Australia. More than 1000 children were enrolled in 1994 alone.

[1]University of Wisconsin, Madison, USA
[2]Children's Health Care, Minneapolis, USA
[3]Children's National Medical Center, Washington D.C., USA
[4]School of Medicine, University of Southern California, Los Angeles, USA
[5]University of Iowa, Iowa City, USA
[6]MD. Anderson Cancer Center, University of Texas, Houston, USA
[7]University of Minnesota, Minneapolis, USA

Despite important progress to date [3], the absolute *number* of children with ALL who relapse still exceeds the number of children with newly diagnosed acute myeloid leukemia, medulloblastoma, and osteosarcoma [1]. In CCG experience, approximately one half of relapses still derive from the two thirds of patients with favorable presenting features and one half of relapses from the one third of patients with unfavorable presenting features. The generally unsatisfactory outcome of children after relapse continues to contribute greatly to the overall morbidity and mortality of childhood cancer.

Figure 1 depicts the improvements in outcome achieved in successive studies over the past 17 years. Preliminary analysis shows an overall 4-year event-free survival (EFS) of 74% for the more than 3600 patients enrolled on the CCG-1800 series trial now completing accrual. Successive statistically significant and clinically important 25% reductions in the relative risk of adverse events have been achieved in each of the last two series of trials.

Several themes may be derived from this experience. Early response to therapy is a consistent determinant of outcome [4–9] which now may be linked to the chemosensitivity of leukemic blasts [10–12] and, perhaps, their threshold for apoptosis [13]. As first described by Riehm and his coworkers in the Berlin-Frankfurt-Münster (BFM) Group [14, 15], effective intensification of systemic therapy after induction therapy reduces the likelihood of marrow and extramedullary relapse for patients with either favorable or unfavorable presenting features [16–18]. Effective presymptomatic CNS therapy may be provided to all infants and most children without cranial irradiation [19–21]. However, 18-Gy cranial irradiation may still be useful for some children with higher-risk presenting features [20, 21]. With regimens containing cranial/spinal irradiation, patients with CNS leukemia at diagnosis achieve an EFS similar to that of patients with similar presenting features but without CNS leukemia at diagnosis [22].

Traditional clinical and laboratory presenting features such as age, gender, white blood cell count (WBC), platelet count, hemoglobin concentration, organomegaly, blast morphology, histochemistry, immunophenotype, ploidy, and karyotype have been studied intensively and used to group patients by estimated risk of relapse [23–26]. The best of these descriptors have significance in multivariate as well as univariate analyses and retain importance across a variety of studies over time. However, these empirical factors provide litle insight into the biologic mechanisms of treatment success or failure.

A simple model for treatment success or failure may be useful to explore the mechanisms of treatment failure and to generate testable hypotheses. The model includes disease, host, and environmental factors. The following is a review of the work of variety of individuals bear-

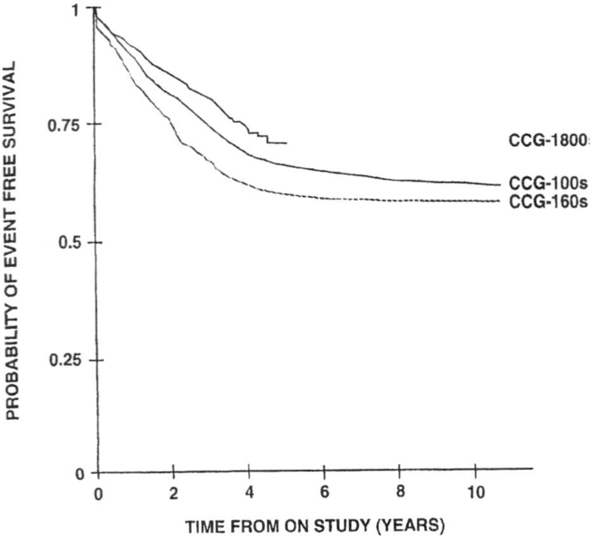

Fig. 1. EFS: CCG-1800 vs. 100 vs. 160 series. This figure represents the event-free survival of 10 305 patients treated on the CCG-160 series ($n = 2985$), CCG-100 series ($n = 3710$), and CCG-1800 series ($n = 3610$) studies. The standard error at 48 months is $\pm 0.92\%$, $\pm 0.77\%$ and $\pm 1.25\%$, respecively

ing on the mechanisms of treatment success and failure in childhood ALL and of current and planned CCG trials that seek to test these insights. We seek better, more precise means to identify those patients for whom current therapy is likely to be satisfactory or unsatisfactory and to evaluate interventions of possible benefit for patients for whom current therapy is inadequate.

Disease Factors

Blast Sensitivity to Chemotherapy

Resistance to chemotherapy, already present at diagnosis among the majority of the leukemic population, is a common cause of treatment failure. Resistance to chemotherapy may be manifest rarely as a failure to achieve remission or as a delay in achieving remission [27–33]. More often, it may be manifest as a poor initial response to therapy as determined by persistence of blasts in the peripheral blood [34–36] or bone marrow [4–9, 32] by light microscopy or by a relatively high leukemic burden in the bone marrow by laboratory means at the end of induction in patients in remission by conventional criteria [37, 38].

Almost all children with ALL achieve remission, but Jacquillat and colleagues [27] reported that children who achieved remission prior to day 14 of a vincristine, prednisone, and daunomycin induction had a better disease-free survival (DFS) than those who first achieved remission only at a later time during induction [27]. Similarly, Sallan and coworkers [28–30] found that children who required more than 30 days to achieve remission had an inferior DFS relative to those who achieved remission more rapidly. Persistence of $>$ 5% marrow blasts on day 28 of induction remains a strongly adverse finding on current CCG (H. Sather, personal communication), BFM [31, 32], and German COALL Study Group trials [33].

Resistance to chemotherapy may be assayed by means of the rapidity of the peripheral blood or bone marrow response. Over all risk groups on ALL-BFM 83, 8% of patients ($n = 630$) had a poor peripheral blood response, i.e., $\geqslant$1000 circulating blasts/µl on day 7 of therapy and contributed 21% of all relapses [34]. Among patients with favorable presenting features on a recent CCG trial for children with favorable presenting features, CCG-1881 ($n = 725$), 9% of patients had a poor marrow response i.e., $>$ 5% marrow blasts, on day 14 of therapy and contributed 27% of relapses [7]. Over all risk groups on ALL-BFM 90, 46% of evaluable patients ($n = 511$) had $>$5% marrow blasts on day 14 of therapy and contributed 75% of treatment failures; 16% had $>$20% marrow blasts on day 14 of therapy and contributed 46% of treatment failures. Conversely, 54% of patients had $<$ 5% blasts on day 14 and contributed only 25% of treatment failures [32].

Laboratory techniques have been employed to quantitate end-induction leukemic burden. Clinical correlations have been found in the settings of conventional chemotherapy and of bone marrow transplantation. Brisco and coworkers [37] were able to study 88 of 181 children with presenting WBC $<$100 000/µl and found a worse outcome for 38/88 children in whom leukemia could be detected at the end of induction by a polymerase chain reaction (PCR) based clonotypic assay on re-arranged immunoglobin heavy chain genes. Twenty-six of 38 relapsed compared to six of 50 with no detectable leukemia at the end of induction [37]. Uckun and coworkers [38] have reported the Minneapolis experience with the clonogenic FACS/LPC assay. Patients with higher leukemic burdens prior to autologous bone marrow transplantation (BMT) were more likely to relapse after BMT than were patients with lower leukemic burdens.

Resistance to chemotherapy may be assayed in vitro by means of the methyl-thiazol-tetrazolivn (MTT) assay [10–12] or assays of apoptosis [39]. Pieters and coworkers [10–12] assayed the 50% lethal concentration (LC_{50}) of prednisolone for blasts from 117 children with ALL at diagnosis utilizing the MTT assay. The median LC_{50} was-62 fold-higher for patients with a poor day 7 peripheral blood response. At 2 years, the DFS was 67% for patients with a prednisolone LC_{50} above the median and 98% for patients with an LC_{50} below the median ($p = 0.009$, relative risk 7!). The difference was preserved in multivariate analyses after adjustment for sex, WBC, BFM risk factor, French-American-British Group (FAB) blast morphology, immunophenotype, and DNA ploidy in multivariate analyses [10–12].

Resistance to therapy, whether measured by in vivo response or in vitro assay, is associated with conventional adverse prognostic factors.

These include extreme age (older or younger), higher WBC, FAB L2 morphology, T lineage, myeloid co-expression, and CD 10 negativity [11, 12, 40].

Prompt identification of patients with more resistant disease allows their assignment to more aggressive and hopefully more effective therapy. In planned CCG trials, in vitro assays of apoptosis, conventional early marrow evaluations, and laboratory determinations of end-induction and end-intensification leukemic burden will be explored in order to identify critical molecular markers and cellular characteristics and to establish useful proximal surrogate measures to sensitivity and ultimate outcome. Identification of critical features may provide molecular targets for future therapeutic interventions. We hope to establish end-induction leukemic burden as a useful surrogate for early evaluation of the specific contribution of novel interventions in the context of already complex therapy. Higher-risk patients with CD 19 positivity and a poor response on day 7 of therapy will be randomly assigned to receive or not to receive an anti-CD 19 pokeweed antiviral protein immunoconjugate [41–47] in addition to standard vincristine, prednisone, daunomycin, and L-asparaginase in induction. Event-free survival (EFS) will be followed as well as end-induction leukemic burden.

Treatment failure may be multifactorial. Inherent resistance to chemotherapy may exacerbate other potential causes of treatment failure. Rapid proliferation may accelerate recovery from chemotherapy-induced cytoreduction and compound the lesser cyto-reduction in resistant blast populations. If the typical cell in the leukemic population has increased resistance, then the presence of a yet more resistant subclone may be more likely. Patients with more resistant disease may be more vulnerable to poor patient compliance, unfavorable host pharmacokinetics or pharmacodynamics, choice of less effective therapy, and/or failure to deliver planned therapy.

Blast Growth Rate

Blasts with a greater net growth rate might better be able to recover from the effects of therapy. Net growth depends upon growth fraction, doubling time, and spontaneous cell death.

Masterson and coworkers [48] studied the cell cycle kinetics of blasts from patients with newly diagnosed and relapsed disease by means of double labeling with intravenous bromodeoxyuridine (labeling index) and tritiated thymidine (S-phase, T_s, and total cell cycle, T_c). Although labeling indices were similar, median T_s and T_c were significantly shorter among relapsed patients, 6.5 vs 12.0 h, and 26.5 vs 44.3 h respectively ($p < 0.04$) [49]. T_c was shorter for relapsed and "poor risk" patients than for "good risk" patients [50]. Paired diagnostic and relapse specimens from the same patients were not reported so that one cannot determine whether the more rapid T_s and T_c were characteristics that were already present at diagnosis or were new cellular properties that appeared only at relapse.

Trerè and coworkers [51] have evaluated the rapidity of proliferation of blast cells in childhood ALL by means of assessment of the area of silver-stained nucleolar organizer regions (AgNOR). This parameter has been shown to be directly related to cell doubling time. A random sample of 119 children was studied with 91 being designated "low proliferative" activity and 28 designated "high proliferative" activity. Relapses were about three times more common in the highly proliferative group which was more likely to include patients with FAB L2 morphology and T lineage phenotype. The prognostic significance of the AgNOR was preserved in multivariate analyses [51].

Several authors have linked net growth in in vitro and xenograft systems to outcome. Kumagai [52] reported that better recovery of B lineage blasts cultured on allogeneic bone marrow-derived stromal layers predicted an adverse prognosis. Compana and coworkers [53] found a correlation between higher expression of the anti-apoptotic protein *bcl-2* and better recovery in in vitro culture [53]. Similarly, Uckun and coworkers [54] found that the overt engraftment of blasts at diagnosis within 12 weeks in a SCID mouse model was an adverse prognostic factor for patients with conventional higher-risk presenting features and among patients with t(4: 11) [55].

The Children's Cancer Group is currently inoculating SCID mice with aliquots of blasts from cases of ALL at initial diagnosis. Plans call for similar inoculation at relapse so that initial presentation might be compared with early and late relapse. In addition to confirmation of the prognostic significance of overt engraftment, we seek to establish xenografts for cellular and molecular investigation and for future preclinical evaluation of candidate interventions.

Propensity for Progression

Disease-based prognostic factors rely on an assessment of the characteristics of blast cells sampled at diagnosis. Conceivably, however, relapse may arise from a subclone with critical properties that differ from those of the predominant leukemic population at diagnosis.

Blasts may acquire resistance through adaptive, epigenetic, and/or genetic mechanisms. For example, exposure to prednisone induces downregulation of glucocorticoid receptors and glucocorticoid resistance in surviving blasts [56, 57]. Resistance to therapy has been associated with emergence of subclones with loss of function of p53 or RB1, defective DNA repair, and/or loss of imprinting [58, 59]. Mutations of p53 were found in 12 of 53 cases at relapsed T cell ALL. Banked specimens from the time of initial diagnosis were available for nine of 12 cases. Abnormality of p53 was found in only one of nine cases. The presence of an abnormal p53 was associated with an inferior subsequent outcome [60].

Philadelphia chromosome-positive (PH^+) chronic myelogenous leukemia may provide an example of disease progression in its unpredictable, but inexorable stepwise evolution from chronic phase through an accelerated phase to blast crisis with accrual of additional cytogenetic abnormalities [61]. In the laboratory, leukemias induced with *v-abl* or BCR/ABL undergo a process of leukemic progression. Expression of ABL in and of itself is necessary but not sufficient for leukemic transformation. Subclones derived from murine bone marrow cells grown over a pre-established stromal feeder layer shortly after infection with Abelson virus-infected murine marrow cells are poorly tumorigenic but highly tumorigenic subclones emerge over time. Clonal proliferation, increased cloning efficiency, accelerated proliferation, feeder-dependent agar growth feeder-independent liquid growth, and feeder-independent agar growth proceed full transformation in an ordered, stepwise manner. Changes in proliferative properties have genetic or molecular correlates [62].

Children with PH^+ ALL usually achieve remission despite a generally poor ultimate outcome [63–65]. Hongo et al.[66] found that blasts from newly diagnosed children with PH^+ ALL were sensitive to prednisolone on the MTT assay. Perhaps the propensity of this disease to acquire successively more therapy-resistant and aggressively proliferative characteristics accounts for the poor ultimate outcomes reported in most series.

A major future CCG laboratory initiative will be the comparison of blast characteristics, such as SCID mouse engraftment [54, 55] and patterns of tyrosine kinase expression [67] at presentation, early relapse, and late relapse. One might inquire as to what novel characteristics appear with disease progression and what the mechanisms of such progression are. Treatment strategies that are effective in overt relapse when the clinically resistant cells predominate may also be effective at presentation when the clinically resistant cells are more elusive.

Host Factors

Thiopurine Pharmacology

Children with ALL receive more days of treatment with thiopurine than with any other agent by a factor of at least 4. The variability of absorption of oral thiopurines—both 6-mercaptopurine (6-MP) and 6-thioguanine (6-TG)—is well known [68, 69]. Data consistently link outcome with erythrocyte accumulation of thiopurine metabolites [70, 71]. Specifically, Lilleyman and Lennard [71] found that only 12/79 patiens with erythrocyte thioguanine nucleotide concentrations above the median relapsed compared to 30/79 with concentrations below the median. Thus, 18/42 relapses (40%) might be attributed to inadequate intracellular levels of thiopurine metabolites.

Parenteral administration of thiopurine seems useful as a way to circumvent variable absorption. Such a strategy gained attention from the excellent though preliminary outcomes reported by Camitta and coworkers [72] in the Pediatric Oncology Group (POG) for children with favorable presenting features. The trial administered 6-MP 1 g/m^2 as an 8-h infusion every other week alternating with oral 6-MP.

However, the most appropriate schedule and duration of infusion remain unknown. Adamson and coworkers [73] examined 6-mp 2.4 g/m^2 by 48-h infusion in patients in relapse and found only one complete response and one partial response of 7 and 5 weeks, duration, respectively, among 40 children with relapsed ALL. A specific advantage for parenteral 6-MP remains to be demonstrated in a randomized trial.

The Children's Cancer Group is now evaluating parenteral 6-MP for children with ALL and favorable presenting features on CCG-1922. After a vincristine-prednisone—L-asparaginase (VPL) induction, patients in remission are randomly assigned to daily oral 6-MP × 12 weeks or to weekly parenteral 6-MP 1 g/m^2 every week by 10-h infusion × 11 infusions. Preliminary pharmacology data are becoming available but outcome data will require another 7 years.

Substitution of 6-TG for 6-MP may provide higher intracellular levels of critical metabolites. 6-MP is a pro drug which requires a three-step conversion to become its active moiety, 6-thioguanine monophosphate, while the pro drug 6-TG requires only a single step [74]. 6-MP is more vulnerable to xanthine oxidase in food and intestinal mucosa. Adamson and coworkers [75] found that in vitro leukemic cell lines were ten fold more sensitive to 6-TG than to 6-MP and the cytoxicity was less dependent on the duration of exposure. Assaying levels in the same patients, Lennard and coworkers [74] found that levels of red blood cell 6-TG nucleotides are approximately four fold higher with oral 6-TG than with oral 6-MP. In a randomized trial, Janka-Schaub and coworkers [76] found similarly that levels of 6-TG nucleotides were six fold higher with 6-TG. The role of the methylated metabolites which are present at high concentrations with 6-MP remains controversial [77]. A comparison of oral 6-MP and oral 6-TG is planned for the next CCG trial for lower-risk patients. Parenteral 6-TG is also available but similar critical questions with regard to schedule and duration of infusion remain [78, 79].

L-Asparaginase Antibodies

Repeated or prolonged courses of L-asparaginase are a component of the successful BFM [14–18, 32, 33] and Dana Farber Cancer Institute [80, 81] regimens. However, a substantial subset of patients may develop anti-asparaginase immunoglobulin G(lgG) antibodies after exposure to native *Escherichia coli* asparaginase with or without clinical allergy. The presence of these antibodies may alter asparagine pharmacology and asparagine depletion [82], and perhaps treatment success. Cheung and coworkers [83] found antibodies in six of 13 patients in first remission. Four of six patients with antibodies relapsed versus none of seven with no antibodies.

Kurtzberg and coworkers [84] found such antibodies in two thirds of patients in second relapse. Patients with antibodies had a lower response rate to subsequent therapy.

In the next trial for higher-risk patients CCG plans to survey patients for development of antibody and seek to confirm any prognostic significance in a population that will receive multiple exposures to L-asparaginase. Should such antibodies be detected, one might next ask whether native *Erwinia* asparaginase [85] or polyethylen glycol conjugated (PEG) asparaginase [82] are similarly immunogenic and whether patients with or without antibodies might benefit from substitution of a non-cross-reactive agent. The pharmacology and toxicity of PEG and *Erwinia* asparaginase will be compared in patients after clinical allergy in a proposed CCG initiative.

Patient Compliance

Much of ALL continuation therapy is taken at home by the child under the supervision of his or her family. The success of this therapy depends on compliance. DFS was compromised when doses were systematically halved [86] or when the duration of therapy was decreased from 2 years to 18 months [14] or from 3 years to 2 years [87]. Several groups have correlated ultimate outcome to red blood cell concentrations of 6-TG nucleotides which are determined by host compliance as well as by pharmacodynamics. However, DFS was not improved when the level of acceptable myelosuppression was increased on the POG ALinC-12 study. The authors cite erosion of discipline in maintaining the specified difference between treatment plans [88].

Davies and coworkers [89] found that six of 22 patients on a constant prescribed dose of 6-MP had fluctuations in the concentrations of drug metabolites best explained by partial compliance. In this era of intensive therapy, the number of children who suffer relapse because of inadequate compliance remains a fascinating question.

Environmental Factors

Supportive Care

The level of intensity of therapy chosen must be balanced by the availability and the will to provide appropriate supportive care so that the cure rate is not eroded by toxic deaths. The optimal balance may change as we improve our ability to support patients through more intensive therapy. The optimal balance may change with changing national priorities and resources.

Treatment

Treatment is the most importance prognostic factor. Without treatment, ALL is an invariably lethal disease. Improvements in treatment over the past 17 years have halved the incidence of treatment failure on CCG trials.

Protocol II: Delayed Intensification

In 1970, Riehm and the BFM Group [90] introduced an intensive induction/consolidation regimen denoted protocol 1. In 1976, a second intensive phase, protocol II, was added [91]. Among patients at higher risk of relapse, the EFS of the first cohort vs. the second cohort was 38% vs. 64% in a historical comparison ($p=0.001$).

Following preliminary experience in CCG-193P, a feasibility trial of therapy based on ALL-BFM 76 [92], CCG compared BFM-type therapy to more conventional therapy in two higher-risk subsets between 1983 and 1988, CCG-106 and CCG-123. CCG-106 enrolled patients with WBC $\geqslant 50000/\mu l$ or FAB L2 blast morphology while excluding patients with lymphomatous features [93]. The 7-year EFS was 63% for patients who received BFM-type therapy and 42% for patients who received "standard" therapy on CCG-106 ($p=0.006$) [17]. On CCG-123 for children and adolescents with lymphomatous features, BFM-type therapy was superior to LSA2L2 with or without cranial irradiation. At 9 years the EFS was 65%, 48%, and 42%, respectively, for this largely T lineage subset [18]. The advantage for BFM-type therapy extended to survival in both trials. Similar benefit was shown for the intensive New York (NY) 1 regimen [17, 18, 94].

Among 1675 patients with intermediate presenting features, CCG-105 tested the components of the BFM 76 regimen, intensive induction/consolidation (modified protocol I) and delayed intensification (modified protocol II) [16]. Large numbers and persistent follow up has allowed the ultimate identification of moderate but clinically important differences. The 5-year EFS was 61%, 67%, 72%, and 73% for control, protocol I only, protocol II only, and protocol I+II, respectively ($p=0.006$). Somewhat surprinsingly, the benefit of protocol II alone was very similar to that of protocols I and II together (risk ratio 0.9).

An interaction of age and systemic treatment was observed [16]. Among children < 10 years of age on Ccg-105 ($n=1256$), the 5-year EFS was 61%, 68%, 77%, and 73% for control, protocol I only, protocol II only, and protocol I and II, respectively ($p=0.002$). Protocol II alone was as effective as protocols I and II together.

Among children $\geqslant 10$ Years of age ($n=348$), the power of the comparison was severely limited by sample size [16]. However, patients appeared to require both protocols 1 and II together to derive benefit. The 5-Year EFS was 57%, 64%, 57%, and 73% for control, protocol I only, protocol II only, and protocols I + II, respectively ($P=0.24$).

Given these results, patients with the most favorable conventional presenting features were randomly allocated to receive or not to receive protocol II on the suceeding CCG-1881 trial. This trial enrolled 779 patients and was closed to accrual in 1992. No statistically significant differences have yet emerged, but such differences may be slow to emerge in such lower-risk subsets [15].

On CCG-1891, the CCG-100 series intermediate-risk group was redefined to exclude patients older than 10 years. When the trial was begun, definitive data from CCG-105 was not yet available. However, ALL-BFM 83 results [15] and the emerging, though not yet statistically compelling trend on CCG-105 encouraged continued pursuit of a post-induction intensification strategy. Between 1990 and 1993, 1211 patients were enrolled on CCG-1891. All patients receive a three drug VPL induction, i.th. methotrexate alone as pre-symptomatic CNS therapy, and at least one administration of protocol ll. Double administration of protocol II was tested in one experimental arm and every 3 weeks vincristine/prednisone pulses during maintenance in the other. CCG-1891 is now in follow up. Statistically significant differences have yet to emerge.

CCG-1882 accrued patients at higher risk of relapse because of WBC or older age but excluded infants and patients with lymphomatous features [18]. Over 1100 patients were entered from 1989 to 1995.After the initiation of induction with VPL plus daunomycin (VPLD), a day 7 marrow sample was evaluated and patients we stratified as good or poor early responders when marrow blasts were, < 25% or ⩾25%. Approximately 70% of patients were good responders (see below). Slow responders completed induction and were then randomly assigned to continue a CCG-modified BFM program, i.e, protocol Ib and II, or to a CCG further modified BFM program which we call "augmented BFM" Augmented BFM diverges from standard BFM on day 49 of therapy, 6 weeks after the day 7 marrow determination.

Patients on the standard regimen interrupted therapy after completion of the 2-week each cyclophosphamide (day O), cytosine arabinoside (days 1–4 and 8–11), and thiopurine (days 1–14) pulse in consolidation (protocol lb) and in delayed intensification (protocol llb) to allow for recovery of peripheral counts. The delay was about 14 days. Patients on the augmented regimen received weekly vincristine × two doses and asparaginase three times a week × six doses during this interval (protocol Ib[1], IIb; (Fig. 2).

Patients on the standard regimen received daily oral 6-MP and weekly oral methotrexate for 8 weeks between consolidation (protocol IB) and delayed intensification (protocol II). Patients on the augmented regimen instead received five pulses of vincristine, escalating parenteral methotrexate with no rescue, and L-asparaginase on the Capizzi I schedule [46] (Fig. 3).

The duration of post-induction intensification was increased from 4 months on the standard regimen to 10 months on the augmented regimen (Fig. 4). Delayed intensification (protocol II) was administered twice at 4 and 8 months from diagnosis. Patients received two five-pulse courses of Capizi l.

The initial 100 slow early response patients on CCG-1882 were assigned to the augmented regimen as a feasibility cohort. Subsequently, slow early response patients were randomly allocated to the standard or augmented regimen. No statistically significant difference has yet emerged among the 200 randomized patients. Table 1 compares the number of administered doses of various agents in the initial 10 months of therapy on the standard and augmented regimens. In the next CCG trial for patients with higher-risk presenting features, those with a rapid early response will be randomly assigned to the standard CCG-modified

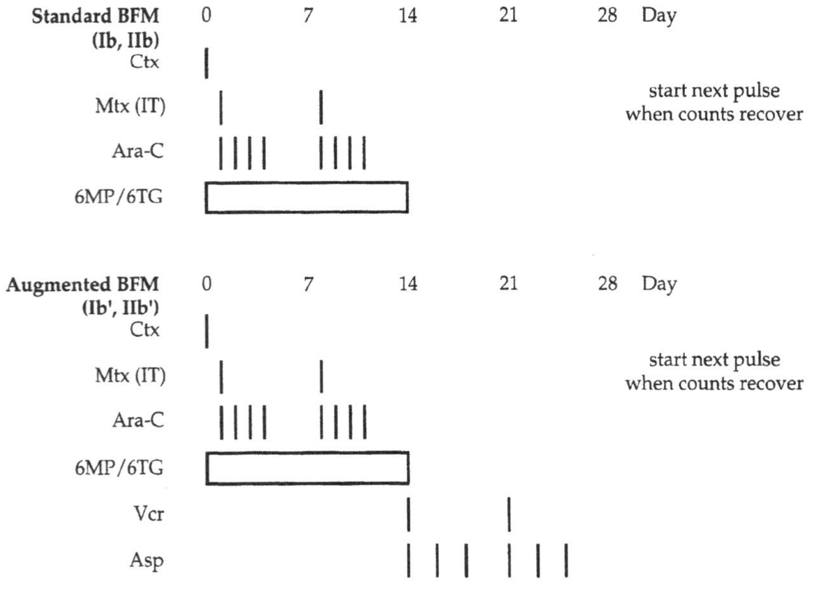

Fig. 2. Standard vs. augmented CCG-modified BFM therapy. Cyclophosphamide/cytosinearabinoside/ thiopurine pulses consolidation (protocol Ib) and re-consolidation (protocol IIb). Protocol Ib: 2nd month of protocol I; Protocol IIb: 2 month of delayed intensification. *Ctx*, cyclophosphamide; *Mtx*, methotrexate; *ARA-C*, cytosine arabinoside; VCR, vincristine; ASP, asparaginase

BFM therapy, prolonged intensive therapy (i.e., double administration of delayed intensification or protocol Ih), enhanced but brief intensive therapy (i.e., single administration of protocol II with additional vincristine/L-asparaginase and Capizzi I [95] in interim maintenance as above), or prolonged and enhanced intensive therapy (full augmented regimen). This study opened in the summer of 1995.

Vincristine/Prednisone Pulses

Currently, all children on CCG ALL protocols receive vincristine/prednisone pulses in maintenance. Between 1978 and 1981, CCG randomly enrolled 699 patients with favorable presenting features on CCG-161. Patients were randomly allocated to receive or not to receive vincristine/prednisone pulses every 4 weeks in maintenance. Early analyses showed no benefit but a statistically significant and clinically important difference in EFS ultimately emerged. Patients who received pulses had an EFS at 8 years of 79% vs. 61% for patients who received

Table 1. Number of doses—(standard vs. augmented BFM)(first 10 months of treatment)

	Standard BFM (*n*)	Augmented BFM (*n*)	Change (*Factor*)
Vincristine	11	28	2.5
Prednisone/ dexamethasone	69	70	1.0
Anthracycline	7	10	1.4
Asparaginase	15	55	3.7
Cyclophasphamide	3 4	1.3	
Ara-C	24	32	1.3
Methotrexate (p.o.)	16		
Methotrexate I.V.a		10	
6-MP/6-TG	161	56	.3

[a]No Rescue.

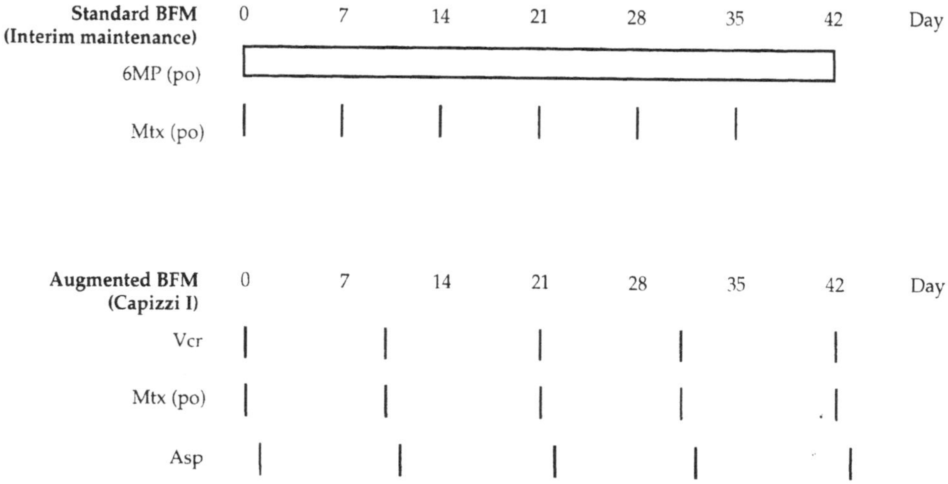

Fig. 3. Standard vs. augmented CCG-modified BFM therapy: interim maintenance and Capizzi I. *Mtx*: methotrexate; *Vcr*: vincristine; *Asp*: asparaginase

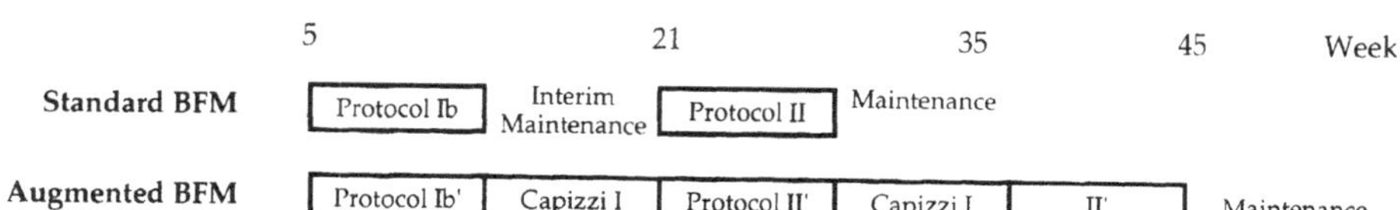

Fig. 4. Standard vs. augmented CCG-modified BFM therapy: overview of treatment plan, *Protocol Ib*, consolidation (CCG version of BFM protocol Ib); Protocol II, delayed intensification (CCG version of BFM protocol II); *Protocol Ib*, augmented consolidation (CCG version of augmented Protocol Ib; Protocol II, (see Fig. 2) augmented delayed intensification (CCG version of augmented Protocol II; see Fig. 2); *Capizzi*, see Fig. 3

no pulses. Curiously, the EFS advantage found on CCG-161 has not translated into a survival advantage even with a greater than 12-year follow up [19].

The Associazione Italiana di Ematologia ed Oncologia Pediatrica (AIEOP) 7601 study similarly found a better EFS for vincristine/prednisone pulses [96]. On the other hand, ALL-BFM 79 found no advantage for three vincristine/prednisone pulses in the 1st year of remission among 199 standard risk patients (BFM risk factor <2.0) (76% vs. 71% at 7 years, $p=0.44$) [15]. Vincristine every 3 weeks is a component of the Dana Farber Cancer Institute 81-01 and 85-01 regimens [80, 81]. CCG-1891, which enrolled more than 1200 intermediate-risk patients between 1990 and 1993, included a comparison of vincristine/prednisone pulses given every 3 or 4 weeks in maintenance and is currently in follow up.

Glucocorticosteroids

Recent data suggest that dexamethasone may be superior to prednisone in childhood ALL. Glucocorticosteroids, primarily prednisone, have been a component of ALL therapy for at least 40 years [97]. Balis and coworkers [98] showed that dexamethasone is less bound to protein and provides higher CNS levels. Pieters and coworkers [99] reported that dexamethasone was 35-fold more potent than prednisoloneh in vitro. The Dutch ALL VI trial introduced dexamethasone in place of prednisone and obtained an impressive benefit relative to historical controls [100]. The CCG-1922 study for patients with favorable presenting features includes a randomized comparison of dexamethasone and prednisone. Accrual is ongoing.

With more prolonged use of high-dose or more potent glucocorticosteroids, avascular necrosis of bone has become increasingly evident [101], especially among adolescents and young adults. This, together with knowledge of the rapid ligand-induced down-regulation of glucocorticosteriod receptors [56, 57] has raised questions as to the necessity of prolonged 3-4 week courses of continuous treatment. The BFM 87 relapse study [102] employed prednisone at 100 mg/m^2 per day on day 0-6 and 14-20 in induction rather than a more conventional day 0-27 schedule. This intermittent schedule might reduce the incidence of avascular necrosis of bone.

CNS Therapy

Over the past 20 years, CNS therapy has increased in efficacy and decreased in morbidity. In 1976, pre-symptomatic cranial irradiation was reduced from 24 to 18 Gy with no apparent detriment relative to historical controls [103]. In 1978, the conventional mg/m^2 dosage schedule of i.th. methotrexate was replaced by an age-based dosage schedule based on considerations of CSF volume. The cumulative rate of CNS relapse subsequently fell from 13% to 7%, but no corresponding improvement in EFS was seen [104]. Some benefit may have been seen with the addition of maintenance i.th. methotrexate to whole brain irradiation in older and higher-risk children (H. Sather, personal communication).

Cranial irradiation may be safely avoided for more than three quarters of children with ALL. CCG-161 showed that cranial irradiation could be replaced with maintenance i.th. methotrexate in children with the most favorable presenting features [19]. CCG-105 extended this observation to a large group, i.e., children aged ≥ 1 year and < 10 years with WBC < 50000/ml, but only when patients received improved systemic therapy. With standard therapy the life table estimates of EFS and CNS relapse-free survival for patients with cranial irradiation were 71% and 92% and for patients with maintenance i.th. methotrexate 63% and 82%. With intensive therapy the life table estimates of EFS and CNS relapse-free survival were 78% and 95% for patients with cranial irradiation and were 80% and 94% for patients with maintenance i.th. methotrexate [20]. Current plans for the next CCG lower-risk trial include a comparison of i.th. single-agent methotrexate and triple i.th. therapy [105],i.e., methotrexate, hydrocortisone, and cytosine arabinoside, in the context of current systemic therapy. The better schedule for maintenance i.th. therapy, e.g., every 8 weeks vs. every 12 weeks remains a question of current interest.

Some subsets of patients may still benefit from cranial irradiation. Substitution of maintenance i.th. methotrexate for cranial irradiation for adolescents and young adults between 10 and 21 years of age with WBC, $<50000/\mu l$ on CCG-105 resulted in a decrease in overall EFS from 60% to 53% ($P=0.04$) but very similar rates of CNS relapse-free survival; 90% and 91% [20]. CCG-123 enrolled patients with lymphomatous features, three quarters of whom had T cell immunophenotype. This subgroup has had a particularly high incidence of CNS relapse on past CCG trials. A number of patients were randomly assigned to receive LSA2L2 therapy with or without cranial irradiation. All patients received i.th. methotrexate every 8 weeks in maintenance. The cumulative rate of CNS relapse was 12% and 24% with and without cranial irradiation although the effect on EFS was smaller [18].

The CCG-1882 study enrolled children and adolescents with age ≥ 10 years or WBC $\geq 50\,000/\mu l$ while excluding those with lymphomatous features. Patients with a rapid day 7 marrow response all received CCG-modified BFM therapy and maintenance i.th. methotrexate but were randomly assigned to receive either cranial irradiation or additional i.th. methotrexate. This randomization was halted in accordance with prospective statistical stopping rules when the EFS was 82% for patients who received cranial irradiation vs. 70% for patients who received only i.th. methotrexate ($p = 0.004$). Differences were most marked for children with WBC $\geq 100000/\mu l$ and/or age $\geq$ 10 years [21].

The morbidity of 18 Gy cranial irradiation remains at issue. Mulhern and coworkers [105–107] found similar effects in patients who received cranial irradiation and those who received i.th. methotrexate. CCG-105NP, currently ongoing, seeks to measure the neurocognitive effects of CNS-directed therapy longitudinally comparing 18 Gy cranial irradiation and maintenance i.th. methotrexate.

In 1984 Poplack and coworkers [108] showed that very high-dose methotrexate, 33.6 g/m^2, was as effective a pre-symptomatic CNS therapy as 24 Gy cranial irradiation plus i.th. methotrexate and less neurotoxic. Subsequently this intervention has been employed successfully for infants and other children with either favorable or unfavorable presenting features as a component of complex therapies [109, 110]. However, it has not been successful for children with CNS disease at diagnosis. On other CCG trials which employ craniospisal irradiation, the outcome of children with CNS disease at diagnosis is similar to that of children with similar age and WBC and no CNS disease [22].

Bone Marrow Transplantation

The role of BMT in childhood ALL remains to be defined [111–120]. Increasing experience with alternative stem cell sources, e.g., purged autologous marrow [121, 122], autologous circulating stem cells [123], and matched unrelated marrow donors [124, 125], has broadened options. CCG is examining the role of conventional sibling donor BMT in first remission for children with very high-risk features on CCG-1921, specifically t(4: 11),t(9: 22), hypodiploidy (modal chromosome number < 44), age $\geq$ 10 years and WBC $\geq 200000/\mu l$, marrow blasts $> 5\%$ on day 28 of induction; and infants meeting one or more of the following criteria: CD 10 negativity, WBC $\geq 100\,000/\mu l$ and/or $>$ 5% marrow blasts on day 14 of therapy. In conjunction with POG, the planned new infant trial will provide matched sibling donor or matched unrelated donor BMT of infants with t(4: 11) in first remission. CCG-1941, the new study for children with marrow relapse within 12 months of the completion of therapy, will allocate all children with family marrow donors to BMT and randomize others to chemotherapy or to BMT employing an alternative marrow source. We will seek health status endpoints in addition to more conventional DFS end points [127, 128].

Physician Compliance/Modification for Toxicity

Therapy must be administered to have benefit. Physicians adapt protocol therapy to the specific clinical courses of their patients in an attempt to prevent, moderate, or treat morbidity. Hale and Lilleyman [129] attribute the better outcome seen in British trials after 1980 to a 22% increase in the amount of 6-MP actually administered. Of the 22% change, 9% could be attributed to changes in protocol dose and schedule and 13% could be attributed to new and more stringent guidelines for modification of dose.

Early or excessive leucovorin rescue may erode any benefit from intermediate-dose methotrexate. Jürgens and coworkers [130] reviewed treatment administered on the German COALL 82 and 85 trials. They found no correlation between steady-state methotrexate level and outcome. However, they found a statistically significant difference in outcome between patients who began rescue sooner than 43 h after initiation of the methotrexate infusion and patients who began leucovorin later, 76% vs. 42% at 8 years ($p < 0.05$). Patients who received more leucovorin tended to have a worse outcome although differences did not reach statistical significance.

The Future

Despite past triumphs and continued overall success, childhood ALL continues to contribute greatly to the overall mobility and mortality of childhood cancer because of its high incidence relative to other childhood malignancies. Calls to abandon further efforts in this disease would consign a large number of children to treatment failure and deny an opportunity to gain important insight into the mechanisms of treatment success and failure that may have implications beyond childhood ALL. Past success may provide direction for future efforts.

The chemosensitivity of the leukemic population at diagnosis is an important determinant of outcome. Novel agents are needed that differ not only in their molecular targets but in their dependence on the cellular mechanisms of apoptosis. Manipulation of the cellular threshold for apoptosis is an inviting strategy. The Dutch experience with the MTT assay raises hopes that clinical peripheral blood or marrow response can be replaced with more precise laboratory methods and more precise identification of patients likely to have better or worse outcome with current therapies. Quantitation of end-induction leukemic burden may allow for rapid evaluation of the contribution of novel agents in the context of complex therapy—a major challenge in childhood ALL. The day 7 marrow evalution will allow the planned CCG higher-risk study to limit randomization to immunotoxin to the higher-risk $CD19^+$ population with known resistant disease as demonstrated by a poor day 7 response.

Disease-based prognostic factors rely on an assessment of the characteristics of blast cells at diagnosis. However, relapse may sometimes arise from a subclone, not present or simply not identified at diagnosis, with critical properties that differ from those of the predominant leukemic population. Additionally, all disease-based prognostic factors are influenced by the interplay of host and environmental factors. Host differences include individual variability in pharmacokinetics and pharmacodynamics, e.g., thiopurines [70, 71], development of high-titer antibody against native *E.Coli* L-asparaginase [82, 83], and compliance with therapy. Environmental factors include choice of therapy, physician compliance, and supportive care. Further evolution of post-induction intensification may further improve EFS. One can only hope that better understanding of the mechanisms for treatment success and failure will lead to effective new strategies.

References

1. Young JL, Gloeckler Ries L, Silverberg E, et al.: Cancer incidence, survival, and mortality for children younger than age 15 years. Cancer 1986; 58: 598–602.
2. Bleyer WA: What can be learned about childhood cancer from "Cancer Statistics Review 1973–1988." Cancer 1993; 71: 3229–3236.
3. Rivera GK, Pinkel D, Simone JV, et al.: Treatment of acute lymphoblastic leukemia: 30 years' experience at St. Jude Children's Research Hospital. N Eng J Med 1993; 329; 1289–1295.
4. Miller DR, Leikin S, Albo V, et al.: Prognostic factors and therapy in acute lymphoblastic leukemia of childhood: CCG-141; a report from Childrens Cancer Study Group. Cancer 51: 1041–1049, 1983.
5. Miller DR, Coccia PF, Bleyer WA, et al.: Early response to induction therapy as a predictor of disease-free survival and late recurrence of childhood acute lymphoblastic leukemia: a report from Childrens Cancer Study Group. J Clin Oncol 1989; 7: 1807–1815.
6. Hammond GD, Sather H, Nesbit M, et al.: Analysis of prognostic factors in acute lymphoblastic leukemia. Med Pediatr Oncol 1986; 14: 124–134.
7. Hutchinson R, Bertolone S, Cooper H, et al.: Early marrow response predicts outcome for patients with low-risk ALL: results of CCG-1881. Proc Am Soc Clin Oncol 1994; 13: 319.
8. Gaynon PS, Bleyer WA, Steinherz PG, et al.: Day 7 marrow response and outcome for children with acute lymphoblastic leukemia and unfavorable presenting features. Med Pediatr Oncol 19909; 18: 273–279.
9. Steinherz P, Gaynon P, Breneman J, et al.: Early marrow response is a powerful predictor of outcome in acute lymphoblastic leukemia patients with unfavorable presenting features. Proc Am Assoc Cancer Res 1994; 35: 240
10. Pieters R, Kaspers GJL, Klumper E, et al.: Clinical relevance of in vitro drug resistance testing in childhood acute lymphoblastic leukemia: the state of the art. Med Pediatr Oncol 1994; 22: 299–308.
11. Pieters R, Kaspers GJL, van Wering ER, et al.: Prospective study of the in vitro prednisolone resistance in childhood acute lymphoblastic leukemia: a new risk factor in BFM-oriented treatment. Blood 1993; 82: 194a.
12. Kaspers GJL, Pieters R, van Zantwijk CH, et al.: Resistance to prednisolone (PRD) in vitro: a new prognostic factor in childhood acute lymphoblastic leukemia (ALL) at initial diagnosis. Proc Am Soc Clin Oncol 1993; 12: 320.

13. Schuler D, Szende B, Borsi J, et al.: Clinical studies of apoptosis in acute lymphoid leukemia. Med Pediatr Oncol 1993; 21: 558.
14. Riehm H, Feickert H-J, Schrappe M, et al.: Therapy results in five ALL-BFM studies since 1970: implications of risk factors for prognosis. Haematol Blood Trans 1987; 30: 139–146.
15. Henze G, Fengler R, Reiter A, et al.: Impact of early intensive reinduction therapy on event-free survival in children with low-risk acute lymphoblastic leukemia. Haematol Blood Trans 1990; 33: 483–488.
16. Tubergen DG, Glichrist GS, O'Brien RT, et al.: Improved outcome with delayed intensification for children with acute lymphoblastic leukemia and intermediate presenting features: a Childrens Cancer Group phase III trial. J Clin Oncol 1993; 11: 527–537.
17. Gaynon PS, Steinherz PG, Bleyer WA, et al.: Improved therapy for children with acute lymphoblastic leukemia and unfavorable presenting features: a follow-up report of the childrens Cancer study CCG-106. J Clin Oncol 1993; 11: 2234–2242.
18. Steinherz P, Gaynon P, Breneman J, et al.: Acute lymphoblastic leukemia (ALL) with lymphomatous features at diagnosis in children. Proc Am Soc Clin Oncol 1992; 11: 280.
19. Bleyer WA, Sather HN, Nicherson HJ, et al.: Monthy pulses of vincristine and prednisone prevent bone marrow and testicular relapse in low-risk childhood acute lymphoblastic leukemia: a report of the CCG-161 study by the Childrens Cancer Study Group. J Clin Oncol 1991; 9: 1012–1021.
20. Tubergen DG, Gilchrist GS, O'Brien RT, et al.: Prevention of CNS disease in intermediate-risk acute lymphoblastic leukemia: comparison of cranial radiation and intrathecal methotrexate and the importance of systemic therapy: a Childrens Cancer Group report. J Clin Oncol 1993; 11: 520–526.
21. Nachman J, Sather H, Lukens S (sic), et al.: Cranial radiation (CRT) improves event free survival (EFS) for high risk patients with acute lymphoblastic leukemia (ALL) showing a rapid response (RR) to BFM induction chemotherapy. Proc Am Soc Clin Oncol 1994; 13: 317.
22. Cherlow JM, Sather H, Steinherz P, et al.: Craniospinal irradiation for acute lymphoblastic leukemia at diagnosis—a report from the Childrens Cancer Group. submitted for publication.
23. Kalwinski DK, Roberson P, Dahl G, et al.: Clinical relevance of lymphoblast biological features in children with acute lymphoblastic leukemia. J Clin Oncol 1985; 3: 477–484.
24. Pui C-H, Crist WM, Look AT: Biology and clinical significance of cytogenetic abnormalities in childhood acute lymphoblastic leukemia. Blood 1990; 76: 1449–1463.
25. Bleyer WA: Acute lymphoblastic leukemia in children. Cancer 1990; 65: 689–695
26. Trueworthy R, Shuster J, Look T, et al.: Ploidy of lymphoblasts is the strongest predictor of treatment outcome in B-progenitor cell acute lymphoblastic leukemia of childhood: a pediatric Oncology Group study. J Clin Oncol 1992; 10: 606–613.
27. Jacquillat C, Weil M, Gemon M-F, et al.: Combination therapy in 130 patients with acute lymphoblastic leukemia (protocol 06 LA 66-Paris). Cancer Res 1973; 33: 3278–3284.
28. Sallan SE, Camitta BM, Cassady JR, et al.: Intermittent combination chemotherapy with adriamycin for childhood acute lymphoblastic leukemia: clinical results. Blood 1978; 51: 425–433.
29. Hitchcock-Bryan S, Gelber R, Cassady JR et al.: The impact of induction anthracycline on long-term failure-free survival in childhood acute lymphoblastic leukemia. Med Pediatr Oncol 1986; 14: 211–215.
30. Sallan SE, Hitchcock-Bryan S, Gelber R, et al.: Influence of intensive asparaginase in the treatment of childhood non-T-cell acute lymphoblastic leukemia. Cancer Res 1983; 43: 5601–5607.
31. Reiter A, Schrappe M, Ludwig W-D, et al.: Chemotherapy in 998 childhood acute lymphoblastic leukemia patients. Results and conclusions of the multicenter trial ALL-BFM 86. Blood 1994; 84; 3122–3133.
32. Schrappe M, Reiter A, Sauter S, et al.: Konzeption und Zwischenergebnis der Therapiestudie ALL-BFM 90 zur Behandlung der akuten lymphoblastischen Leukämie bei Kindern und Jungendlichen: die Bedeutung des initialen Therapieansprechens in Blut und Knochenmark. Klin Pädiatr. 1994; 206: 208–221, 1994.
33. Janka-Schaub GE, Stührk H, Kortüm B, et al.: Bone marrow blast count on day 28 as the single most important prognostic factor in childhood acute lymphoblastic leukemia. Haematol Blood Trans 1992; 34: 233–237.
34. Riehm H, Reiter A, Schrappe M, et al.: Die corticosteriod-abhängige Dezimierung der Leukämiezellzahl im Blut als Prognosefaktor beider akuten lymphoblastishchen Leukämie im Kindesalter (Therapiestudie ALL-BFM 83). Klin Pädiat 1986 199: 151–160.
35. Rautonen J, Hovi L, Siimes MA. Slow disappearance of peripheral blast cells: an independent risk factor indicating poor prognosis in children with acute lymphoblastic leukemia. Blood 71: 989–991. 1988.
36. Gaijar A, Ribeiro R, Hancock M, et al.: Persistence of circulating blasts after one week of intensive remission induction therapy confers a poor prognosis in childhood acute lymphoblastic leukemia (ALL). Blood 84: 515a (abstract 2044).
37. Brisco MJ, Don J, Hughes E, et al.: Outcome prediction in childhood acute lymphoblastic leukaemia by molecular quantification of residual disease at the end of induction. Lancet 1993; 343: 196–200.
38. Uckun FM, Kersey JH, Haake R, et al.: Pretransplantation burden of leukemic progenitor

cells as a predictor of relapse after bone marrow transplantation for acute lymphoblastic leukemia. N Eng J Med 1993; 329: 1296–1301.
39. Uckun FM, Tuel-Ahlgren L, Song CW, et al.: Ionizing radiation stimulates unidentified tyrosine-specific protein kinases in human B-lymphocyte precursors, triggering apoptosis and clonogenic cell death. Proc Natl Acad Sci (USA) 1992; 89: 9005–9009.
40. Nachman J, Lukens J, Gaynon P, et al.: Predictors of slow early response (SER) to BFM induction therapy in children and young adults with acute lymphoblastic leukemia (ALL). A report from Childrens Cancer Group (CCG). Blood 1992; 8O: 257a.
41. Uckun FM, Frankel A: The current status of immunotoxins: an overview of experimental and clinical studies as presented at the third international symposium on immunotoxins. Leukemia 1993; 7: 341–348.
42. Frankel AE: Immunotoxin therapy of cancer. Oncology 1993; 7: 6978, 1993.
43. Uckun FM, Chelstrom LM, Irvin JD, et al.: In vivo efficacy of B43 (anti-CD19) pokeweed antiviral protein immunotoxin against BCL-1 murine B-cell leukemia. Blood 1992; 79: 2649–2661.
44. Uckun FM, Manivel C, Arthur D, et al.: In vivo efficacy of B43(anti-CD19) pokeweed antiviral protein immunotoxin against human pre-B cell acute lymphoblastic leukemia in mice with severe combined immunodeficiency. Blood 1992; 79: 2201–2214.
45. Uckun FM, Chelstrom LM, Finnegan D et al.: Effective immunochemo-therapy of CALLA$^+$ Cm$^+$ human pre-B acute lymphoblastic leukemia in mice with severe combined immunodeficiency using B43 (anti-CD 19) pokeweed antiviral protein immunotoxin plus cyclophosphamide. Blood 1992; 79: 3116–3129.
46. Jansen B, Uckun FM, Jaszcz WB, et al.: Establishment of a human t(4;11) leukemia in severe combined immunodeficient mice and successful treatment using anti-CD19 (B43)-pokeweed antiviral protien immunotoxin. Cancer Res 1992; 52: 444406–412.
47. Uckun FM, Ramsay NKC, Mahmoud H, et al.: Immunotoxin therapy of relapsed B-lineage ALL: a clinical phase I dose escalation trial of B43 (anti-CD19) pokeweed antiviral protein (PAP) immunotoxin. Blood (in press).
48. Masterson M, Lampkin B, Yousuf N. et al.: In vivo cell cycle characteristics of pediatric leukemia patients. Exp Hematol 1992; 20: 1184–1187.
49. Masterson M, Raza A, Yousuf N et al.: Cell cycle Kinetics of relapsed pediatric acute lymphoblastic leukemia (ALL) patients. Blood 1991; 78: 40a (abstract).
50. Masterson M, Raza A, Yousuf N et al.: Cell cycle Kinetics in pediatric acute lymphoblastic leukemia (ALL): relationship to ploidy and immunophenotype. Blood 1991; 78: 40a (abstract)
51. Trere D, Pession A, Basso G, et al.: Prognostic relevance of pretreatment proliferative rapidity of marrow blast cells in childhood acute lymphoblastic leukaemia. Br J Cancer 1994; 70: 1198–1202.
52. Kumagai M, Manabe A, Behm FG, et al.: In vitro leukemic cell growth on stroma predicts outcome in childhood B-lineage acute lymphoblastic leukemia (ALL). Blood 1994; 84: 516a (abstract).
53. Compana D, Coustan-Smith E, Manabe A, et al.: Prolonged survival of B-lineage acute lymphoblastic leukemia cells is accompanied by overexpression of *bcl-2* protein. Blood 1993; 81: 1025–1031
54. Uckun FM, Sather H, Reaman G, et al.: Leukemic cell growth in SCID mice as a predictor of relapse in high-risk B-lineage acute lymphoblastic leukemia. Blood 1995; 85: 873–878.
55. Uckun FM, Downing JR, Chelstrom LM, Gunther R, Ryan M, Simon J, Carroll AJ, Tuel-Ahlgren L, and Crist WM: Human t(4;11)(q21;q23) acute lymphoblastic leukemia in mice with severe combined immunodeficiency. Blood 84: 859–865, 1994.
56. Bellingham DL, Sar M, Cidlowski JA: Ligand-dependent down regulation of stably transfected human glucocorticoid receptors is associated with the loss of functional glucocorticoid responsiveness. Mol Endocrinol 1992; 6: 2090–2102.
57. Burnstein KL Cidlowski JA: At the cutting edge. The down side of glucocorticoid receptor regulation. Mol Cell Endocrinol 1992; 83: C1–C8.
58. Cline MJ: The molecular basis of leukemia. N Eng J Med 1994; 330: 328–336.
59. Rainier S, Feinberg AP: Genomic imprinting, DNA methylation, and cancer. JNCI 1994; 86: 753–759.
60. Diccianni MB, Yu J, Hsiao M, et al.: Clinical significance of p53 mutations in relapsed T-cell acute lymphoblastic leukemia. Blood 1994; 84: 3105–3112.
61. Mills KI, Benn P, and Brinie GD: Does the breakpoint within the major breakpoint cluster region (M-bcr) influence the duration of the chronic phase in chronic myeloid leukemia? An analytical comparison of current literature. Blood 1991; 78: 1155–1161.
62. Clark SS and Liang Y: Increased detection of specific tyrosine phosphoproteins correlates with tumor progression of Abelson-virus-infected lymphocytes. Blood in press
63. Dow LW, Tachibana N, Raimondi SC, et al.: Comparative biochemical and cytogenetic studies of childhood acute lymphoblastic leukemia with the Philadelphia chromosome and other 11q22 variants. Blood 1989; 73: 1291–1297.
64. Crist W, Shuster J, Jackson D, et al.: Philadelphia chromosome positive childhood acute lymphoblastic leukemia: clinical and cytogenetic characteristics and treatment outcome. A Pediatic Oncology Group study. Blood 1990; 76; 489–494.
65. Russo C, Carroll A, Kohler S, et al.: Philadelphia choromosome and monosomy 7 in childhood acute lymphoblastic leukemia: a Pediatric Oncology Group study. Blood 1991; 77: 1050–1056.

66. Hongo T, Fujii Y, and Yajima S: In vitro chemosensitivity of childhood leukemic cells and relationship to the clinical courses. International Symposium on the Clinical Value of Drug Resistance Assays in Leukemia and Lymphoma. March 16, 1992, Amsterdam, The Netherlands, p.23.
67. Uckun FM, Burkhardt AL, Jarvis L, et al.: Signal transduction through the CD19 receptor during discrete developmental stages of human B-cell ontogeny. J Biol Chem 1993; 268; 21172-21184.
68. Koren G, Ferrazini G, Sulh H, et al.: Systemic exposure to mercaptopurine as a prognostic factor in acute lymphocytic leukemia in children. N Eng J Med 1990; 323: 17-23.
69. Lennard L, Lilleyman JS: Variable mercaptopurine metabolism and treatment outcome in childhood lymphoblastic leukemia. J Clin Oncol 1989; 7: 1816-1823.
70. Bostrom B, Erdmann GR: Association of relapse with mercaptopurine (6MP) cellular pharmacokinetics (CPK) in children with acute lymphoblastic leukemia (ALL). Proc Am Soc Clin Oncol 1992: 11: 278.
71. Lennard L and Lilleyman JS: . Mercaptopurine metabolism and risk for relapse in childhood lymphoblastic leukaemia. Lancet 1994; 343: 1188-1190.
72. Camitta B, Leventhal B, Lauer S, et al.: Intermediate-dose intravenous methotrexate and mercaptopurine therapy for non-T, non-B acute lymphocytic leukemia of childhood: a Pediatric Oncology Group study. J Clin Oncol 1989; 7: 1539-1544.
73. Adamson PC, Zimm S, Ragab AH, et al.: A phase II trial of continuous-infusion 6-mercaptopurine for childhood leukemia. Cancer Chemother Pharmacol 1992; 30: 155-157,1992.
74. Lennard L, Davies HA, Lilleyman JS: Is 6-thioguanine more appropriate than 6-mercaptopurine for children with acute lymphoblastic leukemia. Br. J Cancer 1993; 68: 186-190.
75. Adamson PC, Poplack DG, Balis FM: The cytotoxicity of thioguanine versus mercaptopurine in acute lymphoblastic leukemia. Leuk Res 1994; 18: 805-810.
76. Janka-Schaub GE, Erb N, Harms D: Randomized comparison of 6-mercaptopurine (6-MP) vs 6-thioguanine (6-TG) in maintenance treatment of childhood acute lymphoblastic leukemia (ALL): differing metabolism and hematologic toxicity. Med Pediatr Oncol 1994; 23: 197.
77. Bostrom B, Erdmann G: Cellular pharmacology of 6-mercaptopurine in acute lymphoblastic leukemia. Am J Pediatr Hematol Oncol 1993; 15: 80-86.
78. Kovach JS, Rubin J, Creagan ET, et al.: Phase I trial of parenteral 6—thioguanine given on 5 consecutive days. Cancer Res1986; 6: 5959-5962.
79. Powell BL, Lyerly ES, Motsinger CP, et al.: Phase I study of continuous infusion 6-thioguanine in acute leukemia. Proc Am Soc Clin Oncol 1993; 12: 165.
80. Clavell LA, Gelber RD, Cohen HJ, et al.: Four-agent induction and intensive asparaginase therapy for treatment of childhood acute lymphoblastic leukemia. N Eng J Med 1986; 315: 657-663.
81. Schorin MA, Blattner S, Gelber RD, et al.: Treatment of childhood acute lymphoblastic leukemia: results of Dana-Farber Cancer Institute/Children's Hospital acute lymphoblastic leukemia consortium protocol 85-01. J Clin Oncol 1994; 12: 740-747.
82. Asselin BL, Whitin JC, Coppola DJ, et al.: Comparative pharmacokinetic studies of three asparaginase preparations. J Clin Oncol 1993; 11: 1780-1786.
83. Cheung NK, Chau IY, Coccia PF: Antibody response to Escherichia coli L-asparaginase: prognostic significance and clinical utility of antibody measurement. Am J Pediatr Hematol Oncol 1986; 8: 99-104.
84. Kurtzberg J, Asselin B, Pollack B, et al.: PEG-L-asparaginase (PEGasp) vs native E. coli asparaginase (asp) for reinduction of relapsed acute lymphoblastic leukemia: POG #8866 phase II trial. Proc Am Soc Clin Oncol 1993; 12: 325.
85. Eden OB, Shaw MP, Lilleyman JS, et al.: Non-randomized study comparing toxicity of Escherichia coli and Erwinia asparaginase in children with leukaemia. Med Pediatr Oncol 1990; 18: 497-502.
86. Pinkel D, Hernandez K, Borella L, et al.: Drug dosage and remission duration in childhood acute lymphocytic leukemia. Cancer 1971; 27: 247-256.
87. Trigg ME, Sather H, Coccia P, et al.: Duration of maintenance therapy for childhood acute lymphoblastic leukemia. Proc Am Soc Clin Oncol 1993; 12:324 (abstract).
88. van Eys J, Berry D, Crist W, et al.: Treatment intensity and outcome for children with acute lymphoblastic leukemia of standard risk. Cancer 1989; 63: 1466-1471.
89. Davies HA, Lennard L, and Lilleyman JS: Variable mercaptopurine metabolism in children with leukaemia: a problem of non-compliance? BMJ 1993; 306: 1239-1240.
90. Riehm HJ, Langermann HJ, Gadner H, et al.: The Berlin childhood acute lymphoblastic leukemia therapy study, 1970-1976. Am J Pediatr Hematol Oncol 1980; 2: 299-306.
91. Henze G, Langermann HJ, Brämswig J, et al.: Ergebnisse der Studie BFM 76/79 zur Behandlung der akuten lymphoblastischen Leukämie bei Kindern und Jugendlichen. Klin Pädiat 1981; 193: 145-154.
92. Gaynon PS, Bleyer WA, Steinherz PG, et al.: Modified BFM therapy for children with previously untreated acute lymphoblastic leukemia and unfavorable prognostic features: report of the Childrens Cancer Study Group study CCG-193P. Am J Pediatr Hematol Oncol 1988; 10: 42-50.
93. Steinherz PG, Siegel SE, Bleyer WA, et al.: Lymphomatous presentation of childhood acute lym-

phoblastic leukemia: a subgroup at high risk for treatment failure. Cancer 1991; 68: 751-758.
94. Steinherz PG, Gaynon P, Miller DR, et al.: Improved disease free survival of children with acute lymphoblastic leukemia at high risk for early relapse with the New York regimen—a new intensive therapy protocol: a report from the Childrens Cancer Study Group. J Clin Oncol 1986; 4: 744-752.
95. Baum E, Nachman J, Ramsay N, et al.: Prolonged second remission in childhood acute lymphocy leukemia. a report from the Childrens Cancer Study Group. Med Pediatr Oncol 1983; 11: 1-7.
96. Paolucci G, Masera G, Vecchi V, et al.: Treating childhood acute lymphoblastic leukemia (ALL): summary of ten years' experience in Italy. Med Pediatr Oncol 1989; 17: 83-91.
97. Gaynon PS, Lustig RH: The use of glucocorticoids in acute lymphoblastic leukemia of childhood: molecular, cellular, and clinical considerations. Am J Pediatr Hematol Oncol (in press).
98. Balis F, Leste CM, Chrouses GP, et al.: Differences in cerebrospinal fluid penetration of corticosteroids: relationship to the prevention of meningeal leukemia. J clin Oncol 1987; 5: 202-207.
99. Pieters R, Kaspers GJL, van Wering ER, et al.: Dexamethasone is much more potent than prednisolone in the assumed equivalent doses in childhood leukemia. Proc Am Soc Clin Oncol 1992; 11: 282.
100. Veerman AJP, Hählen K, Kamps WA, et al.: Dutch Childhood Leukemia Study Group; early results of study VI (1984-1988). Haematol Blood Trans 1990; 33: 473-477
101. Murphy RG, Greenberg ML: Osteonecrosis in pediatric patients with acute lymphoblastic leukemia. Cancer 1990; 65: 1717-1721.
102. Bührer C, Hartmann R, Fengler R, et al.: Superior prognosis in combined compared to isolated bone marrow relapses in salvage therapy of childhood lymphoblastic leukemia. Med Pediatr Oncol 1993; 21: 470-476.
103. Nesbit ME, Sather HN, Robison LL, et al: Presymptomatic central nervous system therapy in previously untreated childhood acute lymphoblastic leukaemia: comparison of 1800 rad and 2400 rad: a report for Childrens Cancer Study Group. Lancet 1983; 1: 461-466.
104. Bleyer WA, Coccia PF, Sather HN, et al.: Reduction in central nervous system leukemia with a pharmacokinetically derived intrathecal methotrexate dosage regimen. J Clin Oncol 1983; 1: 317-325.
105. Camitta B, Mahoney D, Leventhal B, et al.: Intensive intravenous methotrexate and mercaptopurine treatment of higher-risk non-T, non-B acute lymphocytic leukemia: a Pediatric Oncology Group study. J Clin Oncol 1994; 12: 1383-1389.
106. Mulhern RK, Wasserman AL, Fairclough D, and Ochs J: Memory function in disease-free survivors of childhood acute lymphoblastic leukemia given CNS prophylaxis with or without 1,800 cGy cranial irradiation. J Clin Oncol 6: 315-320, 1988.
107. Ochs J, Mulhern R, Fairclough D, Parvey L, Whitaker J, Ch'ien L, Mauer A, and Simone J: Comparison of neuropsychologic functioning and clinical indicators of neurotoxicity in long-term survivors of childhood leukemia given cranial radiation or parenteral methotrexate: a prospective study. J Clin Oncol 1991; 9: 145-151.
108. Mulhern R, Fairclough D, and Ochs J: A prospective comparison of neuropsychologic performance of children surviving leukemia who received 18-Gy, 24-Gy or no cranial irradiation. J Clin Oncol 1991; 9: 1348-1356.
109. Poplack DG, Reaman GH, Bleyer WA, et al.: Central nervous system (CNS) preventive therapy with high dose methotrexate (HDMtx) in acute lymphoblastic leukemia (ALL): a preliminary report. Proc Amer Soc Clin Oncol 1984; 3: 204
110. Poplack DG, Reaman GH, Bleyer WA, Feusner J, Odom L, Steinberg S, Sather H, and Hammond D: Successful prevention of central nervous system (CNS) leukemia without cranial radiation in children with high risk acute lymphoblastic leukemia (ALL): a preliminary report. Proc Am Soc Clin Oncol 1989; 8: 213.
111. Reaman G, Lange B, Feusner J, et al.: Intensive systemic and intrathecal chemotherapy improves the outcome for infants with acute lymphoblastic leukemia (ALL). Proc Am Soc Clin Onco 1989; 8: 211.
112. Ramsay NKC, Kersey JH: Indications for marrow transplantation in acute lymphoblastic leukemia. Blood 1990; 75: 815-818.
113. Pinkel D: Allogeneic bone marrow transplantation in children with acute leukemia: a practice whose time has gone. Leukemia 1989; 3: 242-224.
114. Kersey JH: Reply to Dr. Donald Pinkel. Leukemia 1989; 3: 394-395.
115. Chessels JM: A reply to D Pinkel: allogeneic bone marrow transplantation in childhood leukemia: another form of intensive therapy. Leukemia 1989; 3: 543-544.
116. Pinkel D: Bone marrow transplantation in children. J Pediatr 1993; 122: 331-341.
117. Graham-Pole J: Treating acute lymphoblastic leukaimia after relapse: bone marrow transplantation or not.Lancet 1989; ii: 1517.
118. Butturini A, Rivera GK, Bortin, MM, and Gale RP: Which treatment for childhood acute lymphoblastic leukaemia in second remission. Lancet 1987; i: 429-432.
119. Butturini A and Gale RP: Chemotherapy versus transplantation in acute leukemia. Br.J Haematol 72: 1-8, 1989.
120. Barrett AJ, Horowitz MM, Pollock BH, et al.: Bone marrow transplants from HLA-identical sibling as compared with chemotherapy for children with acute lymphoblastic leukemia in second remission. N Eng J Med 1994; 331: 1253-1258.
121. Chessels JM, Bailey C, Wheeler K, et al.: Bone marrow transplantation for high-risk childhood lymphoblastic leukaemia first remission: experi-

ence in MRC UKALLX*. Lancet 1992; 340: 565-568.
122. Sallan SE, Niemeyer CM, Billett AL, et al.: Autologous bone marrow transplantation for acute lymphoblastic leukemia. J Clin Oncol 1989; 7: 1594-1601.
123. Billett AL, Kornmehl E, Tarbell NJ, et al.: Autologous bone marrow transplantation after a long first remission for children with recurrent acute lymphoblastic leukemia. Blood 19o93; 81: 1651-7.
124. Takaue Y, Watanabe A, Murakami T, et al.: High-dose chemotherapy and blood stem cell autografts for children with first relapsed acute lymphoblastic leukemia: a pilot study of the children's Cancer and Leukemia Study Group of Japan (CCLSG). Med Pediatr Oncol 1994; 23: 20-25.
125. Vowels MR, Lam Po, Tang R, Mameghan H, et al.: Bone marrow transplantation in children using closely matched related and unrelated donors. Bone Marrow Transplant 1991; 8: 87-92.
126. Kernan NA, Bartsch G, Ash RC, et al: Analysis of 462 transplantations from unrelated donors facilitated by the National Bone Marrow Donor Program. N Eng J Med 1993; 328: 593-602.
127. Barr RD, Furlong W, Dawson S, et al.: An assessment of global health status in survivors of acute lymphoblastic leukemia in childhood. Am J Pediatr Hematol Oncol 1993; 15: 284-290.
128. Feeny D, Barr RD, Furlong W, et al.: The comprehensive assessment of health status in survivors of childhood cancer: application to high-risk acute lymphoblastic leukaemia. Br J Cancer 1993; 67: 1047-1052.
129. Hale JP and Lilleyman JS: Importance of 6-mercaptopurine dose in lymphoblastic leukaemia. Arch Dis Child 1991; 66: 462-466.
130. Jürgens H, Janka G, Ibrahim M, et al.: Prognostic significance of exposure to intermediate-dose methotrexate in children with standard risk ALL: the COALL 82/85 experience. Haematol Blood Trans 1992; 34: 338-342.

Appendix I

CCG Treatment Sites as of October 1, 1994

A.B. Chandler Medical Center—University of Kentucky
Albany Medical Center
Albert Einstein Medical Center
Allan Blair Cancer Centre
Baystate Medical Centre
British Columbia Children's Hospital
Brookdale Hospital Medical Center
Brooklyn Hospital Center
C.S. Mott Children's Hospital
Cardinal Glennon Children's Hospital
Cedars-Sinai Medical Center
Children's Health Care, Minneapolis
Children's Medical Center Dayton
Children's Center for Cancer and Blood Disorders
Children's Hospital and Medical Center, Seattle
Children's Hospital Medical Center of Akron
Children's Hospital of Austin at Brackenridge
Children's Hospital of Columbus
Children's Hospital of Denver
Children's Hospital of Los Angeles
Children's Hospital of Oakland
Children's Hospital of Orange County
Children's Hospital of Philadelphia
Children's Hospital of Pittsburgh
Children's Hospital of Western Ontario
Children's Hospital-King's Daughters
Children's Medical Center of Dayton
Children's Memorial Hospital of Omaha
Children's Mercy Hospital of Kansas City
Children's National Medical Center of Washington DC
Columbia Presbyterian College of Physicians and Surgeons
Dakota Clinic
Dakota Midwest Cancer Institute
David Grant USAF Medical Center
Deaconess Medical Center
Doernbecher Childrens Hospital—Oregon HSU
Duluth Clinic
East Tennessee Children's Hospital
Fred Hutchinson Cancer Research Center
Medical Center of Delaware—Alfred I Dupont Institution
Geisinger Medical Center
Georgetown University Medical Center
Grands Rapids Clinical Oncology Program
Group Health Cooperative of Puget Sound
Gundersen Clinic Ltd.
Harbor/UCLA Medical Center
Henry Ford Hospital
Hershey Medical Center
Huntington Memorial Hosptial
Indiana University—Riley Children's Hospital
Izaak Walton Killam Hospital
Janeway Child Health Center
North Shore University Hospital—Cornell University Medical Center
Kalamazoo Comm Clinical Oncology Program
Kaiser Permanente Med Group Inc—Northern CA
Kosair Children's Hospital
Loma Linda University Medical Center
Loyola University Medical Center

Lutheran General Children's Medical Centers
M.D. Anderson Cancer Center
Manitoba Cancer Fd/Children's Hospital/U of Manitoba
Marshfield Clinic
Mary Bridge Hospital
Mayo Clinic and Foundation
Medical College of Georgia
Medial College of Ohio
Memorial Sloan Kettering Cancer Center
MeritCare Hospital CCOP
Methodist Hospital
MetroHealth Medical Center
Michigan State University
Montefiore Medical Center
New York Hospital—Cornell University Medical Center
New York Medical College
New York University Medical Center
Newark Beth Israel Medical Center
Overlook Hospital
Phoenix Children's Hospital
Presbyterian/St. Lukes Medical Center and CHOA
Primary Children's Medical Center
St. Mary's Hosptial Medical Center (Dean Medical Center
St. Paul Children's Hospital
Southern California Permanente Medical Group CA
Southern Illinois University School of Medicine
Southwest Cancer Center—Texas Tech/Lubbock
Southwest Texas Methodist Hospital
Sunrise Children's Hospital, Sunrise Hopital and Medical Center
The Children's Mercy Hospital
The Cleveland Clinic Foundation
Tulane University Medical School
UCLA School of Medicine
UCSF School Of Medicine
University of California—Irvine
University of Chicago Medical Center
University of Connecticut Health Center
University of Illinois
University of Illinois—Rockford
University of lowa Hospitals and Clinics
University of Medical and Dental-New Jersey
University of Minnesota Hospital and Clinic
University of Nebraska Medical Center
University of North Carolina at Chapel Hill
University of Wisconsin Children's Hospital and Clinics—Madison
Valley Children's Hospital
Vanderbilt Children's Hospital
William Beaumont Hospital
Western Reserve Care System—Tod Children's Hospital

Acute Leukemias VI
Prognostic Factors
and Treatment Strategies
Büchner et al. (eds)

Risk-Adapted Treatment for Acute Lymphoblastic Leukemia: Findings from St. Jude Children's Research Hospital

C.-H. Pui[1,4,5], G.K. Rivera[1,5], M.L. Hancock[2], J.T. Sandlund[1,5], R.C. Ribeiro[1,5], J.M. Boyett[2], M.V. Relling[3,5], W.E. Evans[3,5], and W.M. Crist[1,5]

Abstract. Data from St. Jude Total Therapy Study XI were analyzed to identify clinical and biologic features with prognostic significance. Results of this analysis, along with information available in the literature, led us to redefine lower-risk acute lymphoblastic leukemia (ALL) by the following features: DNA index between 1.16 and 1.60, or age 1–9 years plus white blood cell count (WBC) $< 50 \times 10^9$/l; absence of CNS leukemia, testicular leukemia, T-cell immunophenotype, and adverse genetic features {(i.e., BCR-ABL [t(9; 22)], ALL-1-AF4 [t(4; 11)], or E2APBX1 [t(1; 19) in pre-B ALL])}; and < 5% leukemic blasts in bone marrow aspirate on day 15 of remission induction. Based on these criteria, approximately 50% of newly diagnosed ALL cases would be classified to have lower-risk leukemia, and their projected long-term event-free survival approaches 90%. This new classification schema is being applied in our current risk-adapted clinical protocol for ALL (Study XIIIB).

Introduction

Contemporary chemotherapy will cure as many as 70% of children with acute lymphoblastic leukemia (ALL) [1, 2]. Recognition of the heterogeneity of this disease and the relationship of its clinical and biologic features to prognosis has made it clear that a uniform approach to therapy is no longer acceptable [3]. Current emphasis is placed on early and rigorous assessment of the relapse hazard in individual patients to ensure appropriately intensive therapy for subgroups at high risk of treatment failure and to permit attempts to reduce toxicity in those likely to fare well with standard therapy. In our current Total Therapy Study XIIIB, patients are assigned to higher-or lower-risk groups based on their presenting clinical features (age, leukocyte count, and presence or absence of central nervous system or testicular leukemia), biologic features of the leukemic cells (DNA index, immunophenotype, and genotype), and early response to treatment (Table 1). In this aritcle, we will discuss the rationale for this risk classfication schema and summarize supporting data from Study XI.

Materials and Methods

Patients and Treatment. From February 1984 to September 1988, 358 consecutive patients younger than 19 years old with newly diagnosed ALL were enrolled on St. Jude Total Therapy Study XI [4] after signed informed consent was obtained from them or from parents/guardians. The protocol was approved by the hospital's institutional review board and the National Cancer Institute. Induction treatment consisted of prednisone, vincristine, daunorubicin, asparaginase, teniposide, and cytarabine. On

[1]Department of Hematology-Oncology, St. Jude's Children's Research Hospital, Memphis, TN, USA
[2]Department of Biostatistics, St. Jude's Children's Research Hospital, Memphis, TN, USA
[3]Department of Pharmaceutical Science, St. Jude Children's Research Hospital, Memphis, TN, USA and
[4]Department of Pathology and Laboratory Medicine, St. Jude Children's Research Hospital, Memphis, TN, USA
[5]University of Tennessee, Memphis, College of Medicine, Memphis, TN, USA

Table 1. Critera for lower-risk ALL

1. DNA index ≥1.16 and ≤1.60, or age 1–9 years plus WBC <50 × 10^9/l and
2. Absence of:
(a) CNS 3 status (defined as ≥5 WBC/μl with detectable blasts in cerebrospinal fluid cytospin or presence of cranial nerve palsy)
(b) testicular leukemia
(c) T-cell immunophenotype
(d) adverse genetic features {i.e., *BCR-ABL* [t(9; 22)], *ALL1-AF4* [t(4; 11)], or *E2A-PBX1* [t(1; 19) in pre-B ALL])}
(d) ≥5% leukemic blasts in bone marrow aspirate on day 15 of remission induction

completion of consolidation therapy with high-dose methotrexate, 39 patients with lower-risk ALL received standard 120-week continuation therapy with 6-mercaptopurine daily plus methotrexate weekly for 3 weeks, alternating with 1 week of prednisone daily and vincristine once a week in the 4th week. The remaining 69 lower-risk patients and 233 higher-risk patients received continuation treatment with four pairs of drugs rotated weekly or every 6 weeks: etoposide plus cyclophosphamide, 6- mercaptopurine plus methotrexate, teniposide plus cytarabine, and prednisone plus vincristine.

Statistical Analysis. Life-table estimates of event-free survival (EFS) were derived by the method of Kaplan and Meier and compared with the log-rank test. Early death or failure to enter remission was considered an event at zero time. At the time of analysis, the median follow up of patients remaining in remission was 8.6 years.

Results and Discussion

Clinical Risk Features

Various cooperative groups and individual medical centers have used different prognostic factors in risk assignment. Until recently, there was not even consensus regarding the most basic clinical features — leukocyte count and age. To facilitate comparison of treatment results, participants in a workshop sponsored by the United States National Cancer Institute recommended uniform cutpoints for age and leukocyte count for cases of B-lineage ALL, after reviewing collective outcome data [5]. Participants agreed that "lower-risk" cases are defined by age 1–9 years and presenting leukocyte count $<50 \times 10^9$/l. Based on these criteria, two thirds of B-lineage cases in St. Jude Total Therapy Study XL would have been classified as lower-risk ALL.

These patients have a 5-year EFS estimate (±SE) of 86% ±3%. By contrast, higher risk cases (age <1 year or ≥10 years or leukocyte count $\geq 50 \times 10^9$/l) have a 5-year EFS of 62% ±5% (Fig. 1).

Traditionally, CNS leukemia is defined by the presence of at least five leukocytes per microliter of cerebrospinal fluid and identification of leukemic blast cells in a cytocentrifuged sample of cerebrospinal fluid, or by cranial-nerve palsies. Patients with CNS leukemia at diagnosis require intensified therapy to optimize the likelihood of cure. In a retrospective anlaysis of our Study XI, we found that patients with *any* number of leukemic blast cells in the cerebrospinal fluid were at increased risk for CNS relapse when cranial irradiation was given on a delayed schedule [6]. We therefore proposed a new classification for CNS disease status at diagnosis: CNS 1 (no blasts), CNS 2 (<5 leukocytes per microliter of cerebrospinal fluid with blasts), and CNS 3 (traditionally defined CNS leukemia).

Our reanalysis of Study XI showed that patients with CNS 2 or CNS 3 status had not only a significantly increased risk of CNS relapse ($p<0.0001$, Fig. 2) but a lower EFS ($P=0.0001$, Fig. 3). CNS 2 status was not predictive of CNS relapse in the Childrens Cancer Group (CCG) 105 study for intermediate-risk ALL [7], but was associated with a significantly higher early CNS relapse rate in our recently completed Study XII [8] and in the Pediatric Oncology Group (POG) study 8602 (AlinC-14) [9], when compared to patients with CNS 1 status. We attribute this apparent discrepancy to differences in patient populations, systemic chemotherapy, and methods and timing of CNS-directed treatment. Cranial irradiation was given early to half of the CCG patients (all with intermediate-risk ALL) but none of the POG study group. In the St. Jude

Fig. 1. Kaplan-Meier estimates (± SE) of EFS for B-lineage cases with lower- or higher-risk ALL, defined by age and leukocyte count. *Numbers on curves* reflect results at 5 and 10 years

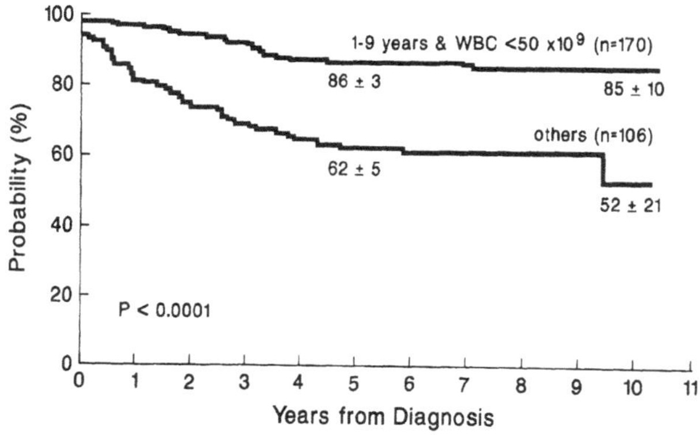

Fig. 2. Kaplan-Meier analysis of survival without isolated CNS relapse according to CNS status at diagnosis (see text for definitions). *Numbers on the curves* reflect results at 5 years

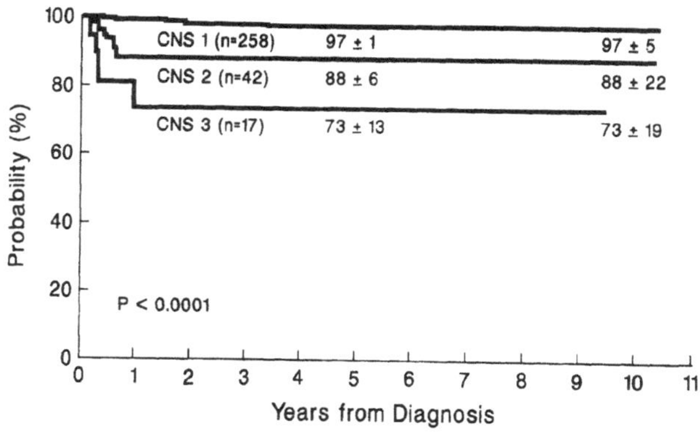

Fig. 3. Kaplan-Meier anlaysis of EFS according to CNS status at diagnosis. *Numbers on curves* reflect results at 5 and 10 years

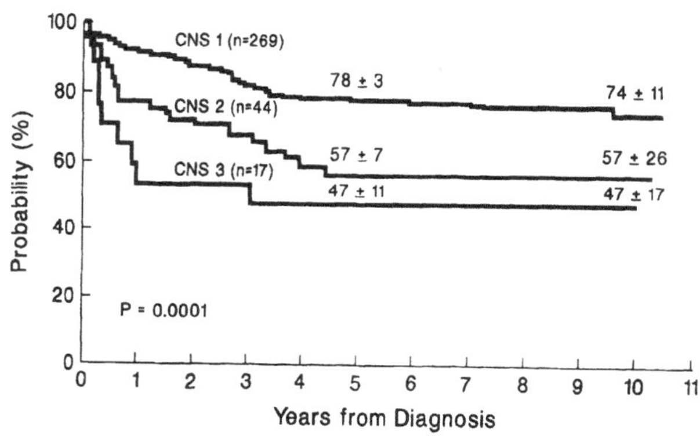

studies, cranial irradiation was given to higher-risk cases but was not scheduled until the end of 1 year of continuation therapy.

As a result of these findings, Total Therapy Study XIII was revised to provide early, more intensive CNS-directed therapy for *all* patients with any blast cells identified in the cerebrospinal fluid at diagnosis (CNS 2 and CNS 3 status). We subsequently found that increased vigilance in examinations of cerebrospinal fluid substantially increased the proportion of patients in the CNS 2 group. In the current study (XIIIB), CNS 2 patients receive more intensive triple intrathecal therapy, but cranial irradiation (18 Gy) is used only in cases with other adverse features (i.e., B-lineage ALL with leukocyte count $\geq 100 \times 10^9$/l, T-cell ALL with leukocyte count $\geq 50 \times 10^9$/l, and Philadelphia chromosome-positive cases). Patients with CNS 3 status are treated on the higher-risk protocol and receive both cranial irradiation (24 Gy) and more intensive systemic therapy.

Immunophenotype and Genotype

In Study XI, children with T-cell ALL had a significantly poorer EFS than those with B-lineage (early pre-B or pre-B) immunophenotypes, in part due to a higher CNS relapse rate ($p<0.0001$, Fig. 4). However, two recent studies have produced excellent treatment results for T-cell ALL: 7-year EFS of 70% ± 10% in the Dana Farber Cancer Institute/Children's Hospital ALL Consortium Protocol 85–01 [10] and 6-year EFS of 67% ± 5% in the Berlin-Frankfurt-Münster (BFM) 86 protocol [11]. The improved outcome was attributed to the intensive use of asparaginase and doxorubicin following induction therapy in the former study and to the introduction of high-dose methotrexate (5 g/m^2 as a 24 h infusion) in the latter. In our recent randomized study of high-dose versus lower-dose methotrexate "upfront window therapy" (i.e., prior to multiagent remission induction in newly diagnosed ALL), the accumulation of methotrexate and its active polyglutamate metabolites in blast cells was significantly higher in B-lineage than T-cell cases [12]. However, in T-cell blasts, high-dose methotrexate produced concentrations comparable to those in B-lineage blasts treated with lower-dose methotrexate, further supporting the use of high-dose methotrexate in treating patients with this immunophenotype. In our current study, T-cell cases are treated with more intensive therapy on the higher-risk protocol, which incorporates ten courses of high-dose methotrexate during the 1 year of continuation therapy and asparaginase during reinduction treatment.

We (and others) have shown that a leukemic cell DNA index between 1.16 and 1.60 is associated with a favorable prognosis [13]. In fact, among B-lineage cases with a favorable DNA index, age and leukocyte count at diagnosis had only a marginal impact on treatment outcome in our Study XI (Fig. 5) and in the POG Study 8602 [14]. More importantly, a favorable DNA index is associated with an excellent treatment outcome, even when patients receive antimetabolite-based therapy [14]. The biologic basis for this finding is not clear, but could be related to the tendency of hyperdiploid blasts to accumulate increased amounts of methotrexate and its polyglutamates [12,15], as well as their marked propensity for apoptosis [16]. Thus, we consider patients with a favorable DNA index to have lower-risk ALL, regardless of their age and leukocyte count, provided they do not have any of the other adverse features listed in Table 1. Among cytogenetic subgroups, cases with the Philadelphia chromosome or the t(4;11) have an extremely poor prognosis[17,18], although some patients with these translocations remain in long-term complete remission after treatment on our Study XI [19] (Fig. 6). The intensified treatment in that study also appeared to nullify the poor prognosis previously ascribed to the t(1;19). However, it is important to distinguish t(1;19) cases with the early pre-B phenotype from those with the pre-B phenotype. The former cases lack *E2A-PBX1* chimeric transcripts and their hybrid protein products, and appear to have a favorable prognosis with antimetabolite-based therapy [20]. Moreover, cases with these translocations may be missed by cytogenetic analysis, even in centers with a high suc-

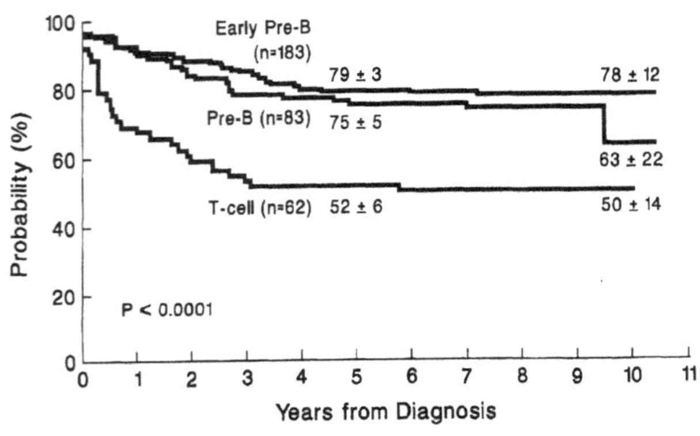

Fig. 4. Kaplan-Meier anlaysis of EFS according to leukemic cell immunophenotype. *Numbers on curves* reflect results at 5 and 10 years

cess rate in characterizing leukemic cells [21]. Hence, we now perform prospective molecular anlaysis to detect the *BCR-ABL*, *ALL1-AF4* and *E2A-PBX1* chimeric transcripts associated with the t(9; 22), t(4; 11), and t(1; 19), respectively.

Early Response to Therapy

Early treatment responses have previously been shown to be important predictors of treatment outcome in childhood ALL [22]. We found that, in Study XI, the presence of ⩾5% blast cells in bone marrow aspirates after 2 weeks of remission induction therapy has independent adverse prognostic significance [4] (Fig. 7). Hence, pati-

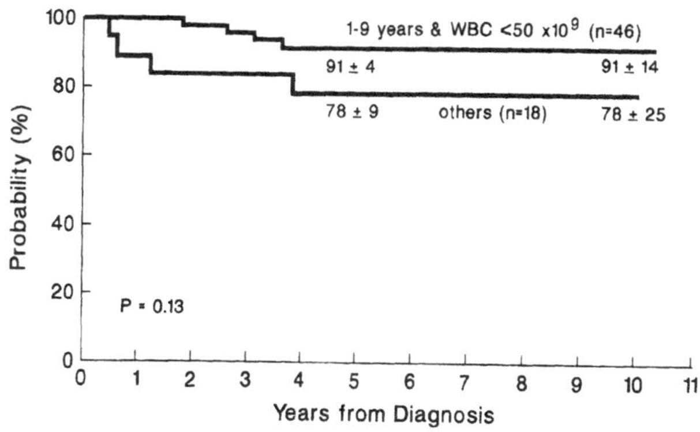

Fig. 5. Kaplan-Meier analysis of EFS among B-lineage cases with a favorable DNA index ⩾ 1.16 and ⩽ 1.60, according to age and leukocyte count. *Numbers on curves* reflect results at 5 and 10 years

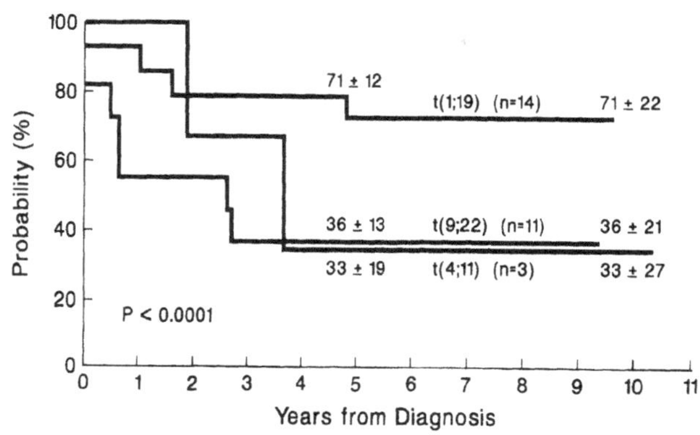

Fig. 6. Kaplan-Meier analysis of EFS according to karyotype. *Numbers on curves* reflect results at 5 years

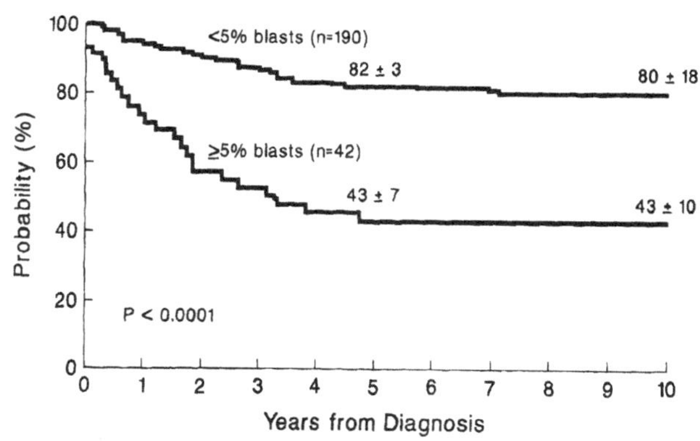

Fig. 7. Kaplan-Meier analysis of EFS according to the presence or absence of 5% or more blasts in bone marrow aspirates at day 15 of remission induction treatment. *Numbers on curves* reflect results at 5 and 10 years

ents with ⩾5% bone marrow blasts at day 15 are considered at higher risk, regardless of their initial status in our current study.

Projected Risk Distribution

With the use of the risk criteria discussed here and listed in Table 1, we anticipate that approximately equal members of newly diagnosed cases of ALL will fall into the lower— and higher-risk groups. When we retrospectively applied these criteria to patients treated on Study XI, we found that lower-risk cases had a long-term EFS approaching 90% (Fig. 8).

Total XIIIB Study Design and Rationale

In the Total XIIIB protocol, patients are stratified by risk criteria at diagnosis and randomized to receive upfront window therapy with (a) high-dose intravenous 6-mercaptopurine alone; (b) high-dose intravenous methotrexate followed by high-dose intravenous 6-mercaptopurine; or (c) lower-dose methotrexate followed by highdose intravenous 6-mercaptopurine. Pharmacokinetic and pharmacological studies are performed using bone marrow blasts obtained 20 h from the start of 6-mercaptopurine treatment to provide information on the optimal dosage and combination of these agents. Induction/consolidation treatment (Table 3), based on the therapy in Study XI, begins 72 h after the start of 6-mercaptopurine treatment and is identical for all patients. This regimen was chosen because of its potential contribution to the overall improved outcome in Study XI (Table 2).

Continuation therapy is based on risk status. The lower-risk group receives antimetabolite-based treatment, reinforced by pulses of dexamethasone plus vincristine every 4 weeks and high-dose methotrexate every 8 weeks (Table 4) —treatment components that have been shown to improve prognosis in lower-risk patients [23, 24]. We also included a reinduction/intensification treatment early during continuation ther-

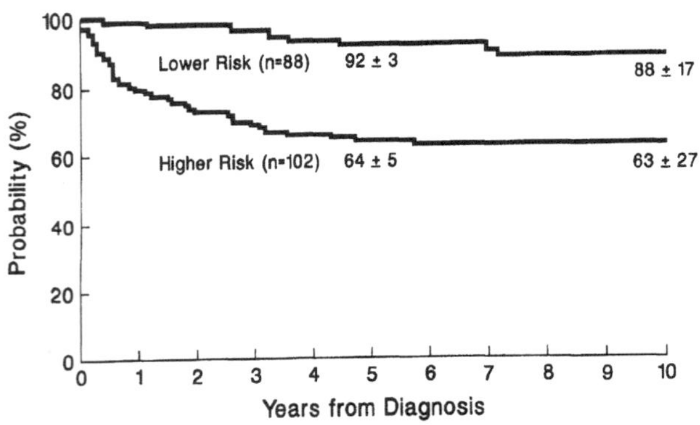

Fig. 8. Kaplan-Meier anlaysis of EFS in the Total XI study according to the new risk classification (see text). *Numbers on curves* reflect results at 5 and 10 years

Table 2. Five-year event-free survival (±SE) of 276 B-lineage cases in Study XI by age and leukocyte count at diagnosis

Leukocyte count	Age (years)				
	<1	1–2	3–5	6–9	⩾10
$<10\times10^9$/l					
EFS(%)	100	87±7	94±3	80±9	77±7
Percentage of patients(%)	1	9	18	7	13
$10–49\times10^9$/l					
EFS(%)	33±19	77±9	88±5	77±11	60±14
Percentage of patients(%)	1	8	15	5	4
$\geqslant 50\times10^9$/l					
EFS(%)	17±11	67±10	71±12	13±8	57±19
Percentage of patients(%)	2	8	5	3	3

Table 3. Study XIIIB: remission induction and consolidation therapy (8 weeks)

Therapy	Days
Prednisone	1–28
Vincristine	1,8,15,22
Daunorubicin	1,8
Asparaginase	2,4,6,8,10,12
Etoposide plus cytarabine	22,25,29
High-dose methotrexate plus mercaptopurine	43,50

Table 4. Study XIIIB: continuation therapy for lower-risk ALL (120 weeks)

Week	Therapy
1	6-Mercaptopurine + methotrexate
2	6-Mercaptopurine + methotrexate
3	6-Mercaptopurine + methotrexate
4	Dexamethasone + vincristine
5	6-Mercaptopurine + methotrexate
6	6-Mercaptopurine + methotrexate
7	6-Mercaptopurine + high-dose methotrexate+triple intrathecal[a]
8	Dexamethasone + vincristine
16–21	Repeat induction.

[a]Omitted after 1 year.

apy, as this component of therapy was credited with an improved outcome in the BFM 86 and Medical Research Council (MRC) UKALL X protocols that extended to lower-risk patients [11, 25]. For higher-risk cases, continuation is based on the weekly rotation arm of Study XI (see Table 5).This regimen included etoposide, given on a schedule associated with a low risk of secondary acute myeloid leukemia in the earlier study [26]. To improve survival, we have included high-dose methotrexate and repeated induction therapy to further intensify treatment during the 1 year of continuation therapy, and substituted dexamethasone for prednisone.

Table 5. Study XIIIB: continuation therapy for higher-risk ALL (120 weeks)

Week	Therapy
1	Etoposide + cyclophosphamide
2	6-Mercaptopurine + methotrexate
3	Methotrexate + cytarbine
4	Dexamethasone + vincristine
5	Etoposide + cyclophosphamide
6	6-Mercaptopurine + high-dose methotrexate[a] +triple intrathecal[a]
7	Etoposide + cytarabine
8	Dexamethasone + vincristine
16–21	Repeat Induction
55–57	CNS irradiation (very high risk only)

[a]Omitted after 1 year.

Study XIIIB should provide valuable information regarding the optimal use of antimetabolities and epipodophyllotoxins. The treatment plan should also substantially reduce the late sequelae of therapy for childhood ALL, especially for patients with lower-risk disease without compromising cure rates.

Future Considerations

A recent analysis of data from our Study XI identified the persistence of circulating blast cells at day 8 of multiagent remission induction therapy as a significant, independent adverse prognostic factor [27]. If confirmed in other studies, this measurement will be valuable because of its simplicity and the early information it may provide. In Study XII, the growth of leukemia cells on stromal-cell culture correlated with treatment outcome. That is, higher cell recovery after in vitro culture was significantly correlated with poorer EFS [28]. Further, the assay identified the few hyperdiploid cases that have had an adverse event. This method is attractive because, until recently, it has been difficult to assess the growth potential of leukemic lymphoblasts due to their rapid death in vitro by apoptosis. Finally, $P16^{INK4a}/MTS1$ was recently found to be one of the most commonly deleted tumor suppressor genes in childhood ALL [29,30]. Homozygous deletion of this gene correlated with T-cell phenotype, non-hyperdiploid karyotype, and poorer EFS. Ultimately, these newly identified prognostic factors may further refine risk assessment.

Acknowledgment. Supported by grants (PO1 CA 20180, R37 CA 36401, R29 CA 51001, P30 CA 21765) from the National Cancer Insitute and by the American Lebanese Syrian Associated Charities (ALSAC). We thank Christy Wright for editorial review.

References

1. Pui C-H, Crist WM (1994) Biology and treatment of acute lymphoblastic leukemia. J Pediatr 124: 491–503

2. Pui C-H, Crist WM. Treatment of childhood leukemias. Current Opinion on Oncology (in press).
3. Pui C-H. Childhood leukemias. N Engl J Med (in press).
4. Rivera GK, Raimondi SC, Hancock ML, Behm FG, Pui C-H, Abromowitch M, Mirro J Jr, Ochs JS, Look AT, Willimas DL, Murphy SB, Dahl GV, Kalwinsky DK, Evans WE, Kun Le, Simone JV, Crist WM (1991) Improved outcome in childhood acute lymphoblastic leukaemia with reinforced early treatment and rotational combination chemotherapy. Lancet 337: 61–66
5. Smith M (1994) Toward a more uniform approach to risk-classification and treatment assignment for children with acute lymphoblastic leukemia (ALL). ASCO Educational Book. pp 124–130.
6. Mahmoud HH, Rivera GK Hancock ML, Krance RA, Kun LE, Behm FG, Ribeiro RC, Sandlund JT, Crist WM, Pui C-H (1993) Low leukocyte counts with blast cells in cerebrospinal fluid of children with newly diagnosed acute lymphoblastic leukemia. N Engl J med 329: 314–319
7. Gilchrist GS, Tubergen DG, Sather HN, Coccia PF, O'Brien RT, Waskerwitz MJ, Hammond GD (1994) Low numbers of CSF blasts at diagnosis do not predict for the development of CNS leukemia in children with intermediate-risk acute lymphoblastic leukemia: a Childrens Cancer Group report. J Clin Oncol 12: 2594-2600
8. Mahmoud H, Relling M, Lie Q, Evans W, Kun L, Head D, Furman W, Ribeiro R, Kalwinsky D, Rivera G, Crist W, Pui C-H (1994) Presence of leukemic blasts in cerebrospinal fluid (CSF) is predicitive of central nervous system (CNS) relapse in childhood lymphoblastic leukemia. Proc ASCO 13: 319
9. Lauer S, Shuster J, Krichner O, Kiefer G, Pullen J, Camitta B, Land V, Pediatric Oncology Group (POG) (1994) Prognostic significance of cerebrospinal fluid (CSF) lymphoblasts (LB) at diagnosis (dx) in children with lymphoblastic leukemia (ALL). Proc ASCO 13: 317
10. Schorin MA, Blattner S, Gelber RD, Tarbell NJ, Donnelly M, Dalton V, Cohen HJ, Sallan SE (1994) Treatment of childhood acute lymphoblastic leukemia: results of Dana-Farber Cancer Insitute/ Children's Hospital Acute Lymphoblastic Leukemia Consortium Protocol 85-01. J Clin Oncol 12: 740–747
11. Reiter A, Schrappe M, Ludwig W-D, Hiddemann W, Sauter S, Henze G, Zimmermann M, Lampert F, Havers W, Niethammer D, Odenwald E, Ritter J, Mann G, Welte K, Gadner H, Riehm H (1994) Chemotherapy in 998 unselected childhood acute lymphoblastic leukemia patients. Results and conclusions of the multicenter trial ALL-BFM 86. Blood 84: 3122–3133
12. Synold TW, Relling MV, Boyett JM, Rivera GK, Sandlund JT, Mahmoud H, Crist WM, Pui C-H, Evans WE (1994) Blast cell methotrexate-polyglutamate accumulation in vivo differs by lineage, ploidy, and methotrexate dose in acute lymphoblastic leukemia. J Clin Invest 94: 1996–2001
13. Pui C-H, Crist WM, Look AT (1990) Biology and clinical significance of cytogenetic abnormalities in childhood acute lymphoblastic leukemia. Blood 76: 1449–1463
14. Trueworthy R, Shuster J, Look T, Crist W, Borowitz M, Carroll A, Frankel L, Harris M, Wagner H, Haggard M, Mosijczuk A,. Pullen J, Steuber P, Land V (1992) Ploidy of lymphoblasts is the strongest predictor of treatment outcome in B-progenitor cell acute lymphoblastic leukemia of childhood: a Pediatric Oncology Group study. J Clin Oncol 10: 606–613
15. Whitehead VM, Vuchich M-J, Carroll AJ, Lauer SJ, Mahoney D, Shuster JJ, Payment C, Koch PA, Akabutu JJ, Bowen T, Kamen BA, Ravindranath Y, Emami A, Beardsley GP, Pullen DJ, Camitta B (1994) Accumulation of methotrexate polyglutamates (MTXGPS) in lymphoblasts, ploidy and trisomy of both chromosomes 4 and 10 in childhood B-progenitor cell acute lymphoblastic leukemia (ALL): a Pediatric Oncology Group study. Blood 84(Suppl 1): 515a
16. Campana D, Kumagai M, Manabe A, Murti KG, Behm FG, Mahmoud H, Raimondi SC (1993) Hyperdiploid acute lymphoblastic leukemia (ALL): a distinct biological entity with marked propensity to programmed cell death. Blood 82(Suppl 1): 49a
17. Fletcher JA, Tu N, Tantravahi R, Sallan SE (1992) Extremely poor prognosis of pediatric acute lymphoblastic leukemia with translocation (9; 22): updated experience. Leukemia and Lymphoma 8: 75–79
18. Pui C-H, Frankel LS, Carroll AJ, Raimondi SC, Shuster JJ, Head DR, Crist WM, Land VJ, Pullen DJ, Steuber CP, Behm FG, Borrowitz MJ (1991) Clinical characterisitics and treatment outcome of childhood acute lymphoblastic leukemia with the t(4;11)(q21;q23):a collaborative study of 40 cases. Blood 77: 440–447
19. Roberts WM, Rivera GK, Raimondi SC, Santana VM, Sandlund JT, Crist WM, Pui C-H (1994) Intensive chemotherapy for Philadelphia-chromosome-positive acute lymphoblastic leukaemia. Lancet 343: 331–332
20. Pui C-H, Raimondi SC, Hancock ML, Rivera GK, Ribeiro RC, Mahmoud HH, Sandlund JT, Crist WM, Behm FG (1994) Immunologic, cytogenetic, and clinical characterization of childhood acute lymphoblastic leukemia with the t(1; 19) (q23; p13) or its derivative. J Clin Oncol 12: 2601–2602.
21. Pui C-H, Behm FG, Downing JR, Hancock ML, Shurtleff SA, Ribeiro RC, Head DR, Mahmoud HH, Sandlund JT, Furman WL, Roberts WM, Crist WM, Raimondi SC (1994) 11q23/*MLL* rearrangement confers a poor prognosis in infants with acute lymphoblastic leukemia. J Clin Oncol 12: 909–915
22. Miller DR, Coccia PF, Bleyer WA, Lukens JN, Siegel SE, Sather HN, Hammond GD (1989) Early response to induction therapy as a predictor of disease-free survival and late recurrence of childhood acute lymphoblastic leukemia: a report from the Childrens Cancer Study Group. J Clin Oncol 7: 1807–1815

23. Veerman AJ, Hählen K, Kamps WA, Vanleeuwen EF, deVaan GA, Vanwering ER, Vanderdoes-Vandenberg A, Solbu G, Suciu S (1990) Dutch Childhood Leukemia Study Group: early results of Study ALL VI (1984–1988). Haematol Bluttransfus 33: 473–477
24. Pui C-H, Simone JV, Hancock ML, Evans WE, Williams DL, Bowman WP, Dahl GV, Dodge RK, Ochs J, Abromowitch M, Rivera GK (1992) Impact of three methods of treatment intensification on acute lymphoblastic leukemia in children: long-term results of St. Jude Total Therapy Study X. Leukemia 6: 150–157
25. Chessells JM, Bailey C, Richards SM, for the Medical Research Council Working Party on Childhood Leukemia (1995): Intensification of treatment and survival in all children with lymphoblastic leukemia: results of UK Medical Research Council trial UKALL X. Lancet 345: 143–148
26. Pui C-H, Ribeiro RC, Hancock ML, Rivera GK, Evans WE, Raimondi SC, Head DR, Behm FG, Mahmoud HH, Sandlund JT, Crist WM (1991) Acute myeloid leukemia in children treated with epipodophyllotoxins for acute lymphoblastic leukemia. N Engl J Med 325: 1682–1687
27. Gajjar A, Ribeiro R, Hancock M, Rivera G, Mahmoud H, Sandlund J, Crist W, Pui C-H (1994) Persistence of circulating blasts after one week of intensive remission induction therapy confers a poor prognosis in childhood acute lymphoblastic leukemia (ALL). Blood 84 (Suppl 1): 515a
28. Kumagai M, Manabe A, Behm FG, Raimondi SC, Hancock M, Crist WM, Mahmoud H, Pui C-H, Campana D (1994) In vitro leukemic cell growth on stroma predicts outcome in childhood B-lineage acute lymphoblastic leukemia (ALL). Blood 84(Suppl 1): 516a
29. Okuda T, Valentine MB, Shurtleff SA, Hulshof MG, Komuro H, Raimondi SC, Pui C-H, Beach D, Sherr CJ, Look AT, Downing JR (1994) Frequent deletion of *INK4a/MTS1* in periatric acute lymphoblastic leukemia. Blood 84 (Suppl 1): 298a
30. Hebert J, Cayuela JM, Berkeley J, Sigaux F (1994) Candidate tumor-suppressor genes *MTS1* ($p16^{INK4A}$) and *MTS2* ($p15^{INK4B}$) display frequent homozygous deletion in primary cells from T- but not from B-cell lineage acute lymphoblastic leukemias. Blood 84: 4038–4044

Acute Leukemias VI
Prognostic Factors
and Treatment Strategies
Büchner et al. (eds)

Risk-Adapted Therapy for Acute Lymphocytic Leukemia: The Pediatric Oncology Group Experience

B. Camitta[1], A. Carroll[2], V. Land[3], S. Lauer[4] T. Look[5], D. Mahoney[6], J. Pullen[7], and J. Shuster[8]

Introduction

Long-term event-free survival (EFS) of children with acute lymphocytic leukemia (ALL) has improved from 5% in 1965 to 65%-70% today [1]. These results, achieved by an increased intensity of treatment, have been accompanied by an increased incidence of acute (myelosuppression, infection) and chronic (leukoencephalopathy, heart failure, second malignancy) complications [2-5]. This has led to the concept that treatment should be risk adapted. That is, the most intensive regimens should be reserved for patients with a poor prognosis while patients with a good prognosis may be treated effectively with less intensive therapy.

Prognosis in ALL depends upon a complex interaction of patient (age, gender, ethnicity, pharmacokinetics) and leukemia cell characteristics (white cell count, WBC; extramedullary disease; Lactate dehydrogenase, LDH; cell kinetics; ploidy; specific chromosome anomalies; surface markers) with therapy (intensive, multiagent, CNS prophylaxis; early blood or marrow response). These factors have been combined in multiple ways to define patient groups at lower and higher risk of treatment failure. This has made it difficult to compare results of protocols conducted at different centers.

The Cancer Therapy Evaluation Program (CTEP) of the National Cancer Institute (NCI) sponsored a workshop in September 1993 [6]. The goal of this meeting was to develop a more uniform approach to risk classification of children with ALL. Participants included the Children's Cancer Group (CCG), Dana Farber Cancer Institute (DFCI), the Pediatric Oncology Group (POG), and St. Jude Children's Research Hospital (SJCRH). Recommendations from this conference have been combined with studies of leukemia cell ploidy and cytogenetics to develop risk-adapted treatment strategies for POG.

Material and Methods

Statistical Methods

Actuarial (EF) curves were constructed by the method of Kaplan-Meier, with standard errors of Peto and coworkers. Multivariate analysis was conducted using the Cox proportional hazard model with forward variable selection.

[1]Midwest Children's Cancer Center, Medical College of Wisconsin, Milwaukee, WI, USA
[2]University of Alabama at Birmingham, Birmingham, AL, USA
[3]Children's Memorial Hospital, Northwestern University School of Medicine, Chicago, IL, USA
[4]Emory University School of Medicine, Atlanta, GA, USA
[5]St. Jude Children's Research Hospital, Memphis, TN, USA
[6]Baylor College of Medicine, Houston, TX, USA
[7]University of Mississippi Medical Center, Jackson, MS, USA
[8]Pediatric Oncology Group Statistical Office, Department of Biostatistics, University of Florida, Gainesville, FL, USA

Results and Discussion

Risk Classification Recommendations: CTEP/NCI Conference

Patient age and WBC at diagnosis are important prognostic factors in almost all studies of children with ALL. However, even these easily obtained parameters have been used in widely discrepant ways to define risk groups. For example, Table 1 shows criteria for lowest risk as employed by the NCI conferees.

In an attempt to develop uniform risk criteria using age and WBC at diagnosis, outcomes were tabulated for children with B-precursor ALL treated on recent protocols by CCG (100 and 1800 series) or POG (ALinC 14). Results are shown in Table 2. These data were then combined to produce simplified risk group as shown in Table 3. Conferees agreed to use these definitions in the design and reporting of clinical trials. It is interesting to note that the consensus risk group definitions are similar to those used

Table 1. Age and WBC criteria for lowest-risk Group. Adapted from [6]

Group	Age (years)	WBC (/μl)	Other factors
CCG	2–9	< 10000	No lymphoma syndrome Platelets > 10^5 if male
DFCI	2–8	< 20000	Remission by day 28 No CNS leukemia No mediastinal mass Not T-cell No t (9; 22)
POG	1–2, 6–10 3–5 Any age/WBC if DNA index is > 1.16	< 10000 < 100000	No CNS leukemia Not T-cell No t (9;22) or t (1;19)
SJCRH	1–10	< 25000	No CNS leukemia No t (9;22) or t (1;19) DNA index 1.16–1.60

Table 2. Four-year event-free survival of children with B-precursor ALL treated by CCG (100 and 1800 series) and POG (ALinC 14). Adapted from [6]

Age (years)	1–2		3–5		6–9		> 10	
	(*n*)	(%)	(*n*)	(%)	(*n*)	(%)	(*n*)	(%)
WBC (x103/μl)								
< 10	490	82.9	937	84.7	437	82.0	406	69.6
10-49.99	436	74.6	608	74.5	205	80.2	236	59.2
> 50	278	68.3	280	73.9	122	47.5	140	41.1

Table 3. Uniform age and WBC criteria for standard-and higher-risk B-precursor ALL adopted at the CTEP/NCI Workshop. Adapted from [6])

Risk group	Definition	4-Years% EFS	Percentage of patients
Standard	Age 1–9 years and WBC < 50000/μl	80.3	68
Higher	Age > 10 years or WBC > 50000/μl	63.9	32

at a workshop held at the Catholic University of Rome in October 1985 [7].

Several other factors may have prognostic significance in children with ALL. However, conferees felt that additional data were needed before incorporating them into risk group definitions. Agreement was reached to uniformly collect information on the items listed in Table 4. The prognostic import of each of these factors will be assessed in the setting of the age/WBC risk group definitions.

Ploidy (DNA Index)

A leukemic cell chromosome content greater than 50 is associated with a favourable prognosis in children with ALL (with the exception of rare tetraploid cases) [8]. Ploidy can be assessed within two to four chromosomes using flow cytometry. The ratio of the DNA content of leukemic G_0/G_1 cells to that of normal diploid cells is termed the DNA index. A DNA index > 1.16 corresponds to a modal chromosome number of 53. POG has previously shown that leukemic cell ploidy is a strong prognostic factor in ALL. Using age, WBC, and DNA index of marrow blasts at diagnosis, three subgroups of patients treated on the POG ALinC 14 study of B-precursor ALL (Table 5) were analyzed: (a) DNA index> 1.16, any age or WBC; (b) DNA index < 1.16, age> 11.0 years, WBC < 50000/μl; and (c) DNA index <1.16, age> 11.0 years and/or WBC> 50000/μl. These groups comprised 20%, 53% and 27% of the patients and had 4-year EFS rates (±SE) of 90.1% (6.3%), 80.5% (5.1%), and 50.4% (7.6%) [9]. It should be noted that a DNA index> 1.16 is seen in only 2% of children with T-cell ALL and in 3% of infants (age < 1.00) with ALL. Therefore ploidy is of limited value in these two groups.

Table 4. Prognostic factors to be uniformly collected in children with ALL. Adapted from [6]

1.	Age
2.	WBC
3.	DNA index (ploidy)
4.	Cytogenetics
5.	Immunophenotype (B-lineage vs. T-lineage)
6.	CNS status (no blasts vs. WBC < 5 with blasts vs. WBC > 5 with blasts)
7.	Early treatment response (day 7 or 14 marrow)

Trisomies of Chromosomes 4 and 10

In the POG ALinC 14 study of B-precursor ALL, trisomies of several individual chromosomes were associated with a favourable prognosis in univariate analyses. However, in that same study, trisomies of *both* chromosomes 4 and 10 was a very favourable prognostic factor that retained significance in multivariate analysis which also included: age, WBC, DNA index, gender, race, CD_{10}, CD_{24}, CD_{34}, pre-B phenotype and translocations [10].

Trisomies of both 4 and 10 are seen in 70% of patients with a DNA index > 1.16, but in only 4% with a DNA index ⩽1.16. Both the DNA index and trisomies of both 4 and 10 are signfi-

Table 5. ALinC 14 treatments

Type	Therapy
Induction	Prednisone, vincristine, asparaginase
CNS protection	Triple intrathecal (age adjusted)
Intensification (randomized)	A. IDMTX every 3 weeks × 6 B. A. + *E. coli* ASP every week × 24 C. IDMTX+ID-C every 3 weeks × 6 D. IDMTX+ID-C every 12 weeks × 6
Continuation	Weekly i.m. methotrexate+ daily oral mercaptopurine Vincristine+prednisone pulses at 8-16-week intervals × 8

IDMTX, intermediate-dose (1 gm/m^2) methotrexate i.v. in 24 h; ID-C, intermediate-dose cytosine arabinoside (1 gm/m^2) i.v. in 24 h (overlaps with last 12 h of IDMTX); *E. coli* ASP, *Escherichia coli* asparaginase (25000 units i.m.).

cant predictors of outcome. However, as shown in the ALinC 14 EFS curves in Fig.1, trisomies of both 4 and 10 is a more important predictor of outcome than the DNA index when informative cytogenetic results are available. Similar results are emerging from the ALinC 15 protocols, which use different intensification regimens.

As mentioned previously, a DNA index > 1.16 is unusual in children with T-ALL and in infants with ALL. Since trisomies of both 4 and 10 are rare when the DNA index is < 1.16, the presence of trisomies of both 4 and 10 is of limited value in these two groups.

Risk-Adapted Therapy for B-precursor ALL

The CTEP/NCI conference consensus definition of standard risk, trisomies of both chromosomes 4 and 10, and DNA index were used to retrospectively analyze outcomes of patients treated with the least intensive regimen of POG ALinC 14 (regimen A, Table 5). Selected patients satisfied the following criteria: (a) age 1.00 to 9.99 years; (b) WBC < 50000/μl; and (c) *either* trisomies of both chromosomes 4 and 10 *or* (if cytogenetics were normal or unknown) DNA index > 1.16. This subgroup has a 4-year EFS of 95% (SE ± 6%). We are currently prospectively treating this proposed very low-risk subgroup with a slight modification of ALinC 14 regimen A (POG ALinC 16, regimen 9201). The ability to cure a substantial proportion of children with relatively gentle chemotherapy would result in significant decreases in both toxicities (acute and long-term) and costs.

The consensus risk groups, trisomies of both chromosomes 4 and 10, and DNA index are being used to prospectively direct therapy on the POC ALinC 16 protocols for children with B-precursor ALL. The factors guiding these decisions are summarized in Table 6. Treatment regimens are summarized in Table 7. The percentage of patients assigned to the very low-risk (POG 9201), standard-risk (POG 9405), and higher-risk (POG 9406) studies is expected to be 20%, 50%, and 30%, respectively. From results of previous POG studies we estimate that long-term EFS will be 95%, 80%–85%, and 70%–75% in the very low-risk, standard-risk, and higher-risk cohorts. Overall EFS would then be 80%–84%. As can be seen, the intensity of therapy on these protocols is directly related to the risk of relapse. Thus, adapting the intensity of therapy to the risk of relapse. Thus, adapting the intensity of therapy to the risk of relapse holds promise to maximize cure while limiting exposure of patients to unnecessary toxicities.

Acknowledgment. This work was supported by grants CA-32053, CA-25408, CA-07431, CA-20549, CA-31566, CA-03161, CA-15989, and CA-29139 from the National Cancer Institute of the National Institutes of Health, Bethesda, MD and by the Midwest Athletes Against Childhood Cancer (MACC Fund).

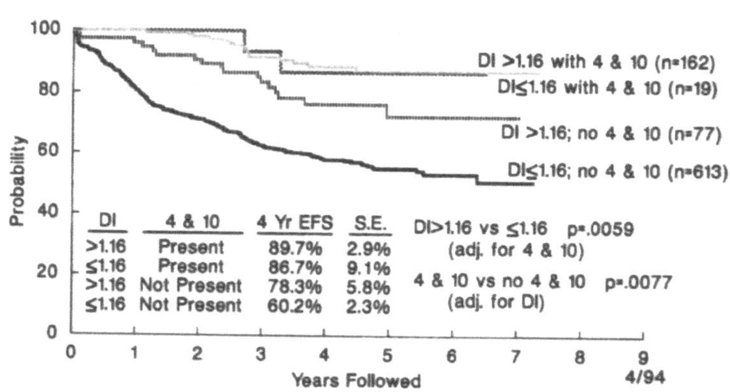

Fig. 1. EFS on the POG ALinC 14 protocol as a function of DNA index (DI) and trisomies of both chromosomes 4 and 10. Patients had B-precursor ALL and were > 1.00 year old. Patients with normal or unknown cytogenetics are not shown

Table 6. ALinC 16 treatment allocation algorithm

Consensus risk group	Cytogenetics	Trisomies 4/10	DNA index	Treatment[a]
Induction				
Post Induction				
Standard				3 Drugs
Higher or standard but+ CNS/testes				4 Drugs
Post Induction				
Standard	Abnormal	Present	Any	**9201 VLR**
		Absent	Any	9405 SR
	Normal/unknown	?	> 1.16	**9201 VLR**
		?	< 1.16	9405 SR
		?	Unknown	9405 SR
Higher	Abnormal	Present	Any	**9405 SR**
		Absent	Any	9406 HR
	Normal/unknown	?	> 1.16	**9405 SR**
		?	< 1.16	9406 HR
		?	Unknown	9406 HR
Any but CNS+ testes+ t(9;22) t(4;11) t(1;19)		Any	Any	9406 HR

[a] VLR, very low risk; SR, standard risk; HR, higher risk. **Bold type** indicates patients whose risk group (and therefore treatment intensity) is lowered by the presence of trisomies or an elevated DNA index.

Table 7. AlinC 16 treatments

Risk	Type	Therapy
very low		See regimen A, Table 5
standard	Induction	Prednisone, vincristine, asparaginase
	CNS protection:	triple intrathecal (age adjusted)[a]
	Intensification (randomized)	A. IDMTX (1 gm/m^2) + i.v. MP (1 gm/m^2) × 12 vs B. IDMTX (2.5/gm/m^2)+i.v. MP(1 gm/m^2) × 12
	Continuation	Weekly i. m. methotrexate (randomized) oral mercaptopurine 37.5 mg/m^2 bid vs 75 mg/m^2 qd.
Higher	Induction:	Prednisone, vincristine,asparaginase,daunorubicin
	CNS protection:	Triple intrathecal (age adjusted) [a b]
	Intensification doubly randomized)	Week 1–DMTX (1 vs. 2.5 gm/m^2) i.v. MP (1 gm/m^2) Week 2 – methotrexate p.o. mercaptopurine Week 3–arac-C (3 gm/m^2 i.v. q 12 h × 4) PEG asparaginase (1000 U/m^2 h 42) or ara-C (150 mg/m^2/24 h i.v. × 72 h) VM-26 (165 mg/m^2 i.v. days 1,2) Weeks 6,7–Same as weeks 1,2 Weeks 8–ara-C (150 mg/m^2/24 h i.v. × 72 h) Daunorubicin (3p mg/m^2 i.v. days 1,4) Prednisone (40 mg/m^2 p.o. days 1-8) Vincristine (1.5 mg/m^2 i.v. days 1,8) PEG asparaginase (2500 U/m^2 i.m. day 1) Repeat this 10-week cycle × 3 (total 30 weeks)
	Continuation	i.m. methotrexate weekly p.o. mercaptopurine daily

[a] Patients with CNS 2 status receive extra doses of i.th. medications.
[b] Patients with CNS 3 status receive craniospinal irradiation after completion of intensification; PE6, polyethylenglycol treated *E. coli* asparaginase; VM-26, teniposide.
IDMTX, intermediate-dose methotrexate, MP mercaptopurine; ara-C, cytosine arabinoside.

References

1. Pui C-H, Crist WM: Biology and treatment of acute lymphoblastic leukemia. J Pediatr 1994; 124: 491–503.
2. Neglia JP, Meadows AT, Robison LL, et al: Second neoplasms after acute lymphoblastic leukemia in childhood. N Engl J Med 1991; 325: 1330–6.
3. Ochs J, Mulhern R, Fairclough D, et al: Comparison of neuropsychologic functioning and clinical indicators of neurotoxicity in long-term survivors of childhood leukemia given cranial radiation or parenteral methotrexate: prospective study. J Clin Oncol 1991; 9: 145–51.
4. Kirk JA, Raghupathy P, Stevens MM, et al: Growth failure and growth hormone deficiency after treatment for acute lymphoblastic leukaemia. Lancet 1987; 1: 190–3.
5. Lipshultz SE, Colan SD, Gelber RD, Perez-Atayde AR, Sallan SE, Sanders SP: Late cardiac effects of doxorubicin therapy for acute lymphoblastic leukemia in childhood. N Engl J Med 1991; 324: 808–15.
6. Smith M: Towards a more uniform approach to risk-classification and treatment assignment for children with acute lymphoblastic leukemia (ALL). Am Soc Clin Oncol educational book. Dallas, TX, 1994; 124–30.
7. Mastrangelo R, Poplack D, Bleyer A, Ricardi R, Sather H, Dangio G: Report and recommendations of the Rome workshop concerning poor-prognosis acute lymphoblastic leukemia in children: biologic bases for staging, stratification treatment. Med Pediatr Oncol 1986; 14: 191–4.
8. Pui C-H, Crist WM, Look AT: Biology and clinical significance of cytogenetic abnormalities in childhood acute lymphoblastic leukemia. Blood 1990; 76: 1449–63.
9. Trueworthy R, Shuster J, Look T, et al: Ploidy of lymphoblasts is the strongest predictor of treatment outcome in B-progenitor cell acute lymphoblastic leukemia of childhood: Pediatric Oncology Group study. J Clin Oncol 1992; 10: 606–13.
10. Harris MD, Shuster JJ, Caroll A, et al: Trisomy of chromosomes 4 and 10 identifies children with B-progenitor cell acute lymphoblastic leukemia with a very low risk of treatment failure. A Pediatric Oncology Group study. Blood 1992; 79: 3316–24.

Acute Leukemias VI
Prognostic Factors
and Treatment Strategies
Büchner et al. (eds)

Treatment Results in Childhood B Non-Hodgkin Lymphoma with a Modified BFM Protocol in St. Petersburg

M. Belogurowa[1], B. Kolygin[2], G. Radulesku[1], M. Kirichenko[1], N. Klubovskaya[2], T. Victorovich[1], and A. Figursky[1]

Introduction

Intensive multiagent chemotherapy has resulted in remarkably improved event-free survival (EFS), approaching 80% in children with B non-Hodgkin lymphomas (B-NHL) [1, 2]. In contrast, conventional treatment of childhood B-NHL in St. Petersburg, especially in advanced stages, has continued to be associated with a poor prognosis, the overall long-term survival not exceeeding 40%. Reports of improved results obtained with Berlin-Frankfurt-Münster (BFM) regimens from Germany [2, 3] have motivated us to start treatment of children with B-NHL with a modified BFM 90 protocol [4].

Patients and Methods

Patients. From Feburary 1992 to November 1994, 23 newly diagnosed children with B-NHL (20 males, three females) aged 3-14 years were treated with a modified B-NHL BFM 90 protocol; 21 of the 23 patients had an abdominal tumor and two a primary tumor at the neck. Diagnosis of B-cell NHL was histologically confirmed in 20 patients and was based on French-American-British (FAB) L3 morphology [5] of lymphoblasts in malignant effusions in three patients. Immunohistochemical analyses were performed in ten cases. The tumors included were high-grade malignant B cell NHL according to the updated Kiel classification [6]. The extent of the disease was determined by physical examination, ultrasonography, X-ray, skeletal scintigraphy, scintigraphy with Ga-67, peripheral blood count, and examination of bone marrow and cerebrospinal fluid. Staging was performed according to the St. Jude staging system [7]. Three patients had stage II, ten stage III, and ten stage IV (two also with CNS involvement). All children were stratified into risk groups according to the criteria given by the original B-NHL BFM 90 protocol [4]: two patients had risk group 2, and 21 patients risk-group 3. Initial laparotomy was performed in 19 patients, in five of them as an emergency procedure.

Treatment. The following modifications of the original BFM 90 protocol were made: (a) the dosage of i.v. methotrexate (MTX) was reduced from 5 g/m^2 to 1 g/m^2 (24-h infusions) followed by 15 mg/m^2 citrovorum factor i.v. at 48 and 54 h; (b) in the two patients with initial CNS involvement an Ommaya or Rickham reservoir was not implanted; (c) only one double dose of cytosine arabinoside (ara-C)/MTX/Prednisone (PRED) was applied i. th. in all chemotherapy blocks, instead of two injections (blocks AA and BB) or instead of intraventricular chemotherapy (AA$_Z$ and BB$_Z$). Complete resection of abdominal primary tumors was performed in two patients. Seventeen patients underwent partial resection or biopsy. Both procedures entailed no postoperative complications, and chemotherapy was started without delay. Complete remission was defined as no evidence of localized disease

[1]Department of Pediatric Oncology and Hematology, Center of Advanced Medical Technologies, St. Petersburg, Russia
[2]Department of Pediatric Oncology, Petrov Research Institute of Oncology, St. Petersberg, Russia

(confirmed by computerized tomography in all patients) and absence of FAB L3 lymphoblasts in bone marrow, peripheral blood, and cerebrospinal fluid.

Results

Side Effects and Complications. Severe depletion of peripheral blood cells was frequently seen after chemotherapy. Transfusions of red blood cells and platelets were given to 60% of the patients after the first two blocks and to 30% after subsequent blocks. All patients developed neutropenia, 40% of them had different infectious complications (pneumonia, enterocolitis, sepsis, fever of unknown origin). One patient developed peritonitis (after the first AA block) due to perforation of the bowel. He received a colostomy and chemotherapy was continued. Stomatitis was observed in all patients after the first AA and BB blocks and only in one third of patients after subsequent blocks. The duration of cytopenia was longest after the first AA and BB blocks (median 8 days). After the second AA and BB blocks the average duration of bone marrow depression was 5 days, while after the third AA and BB blocks aplasia was observed only in two patients. After the CC block the bone marrow depression did not exceed 7 days. The average interval between the blocks was 25 days, so that delays longer than 10 days were not necessary. Two toxic deaths were observed: one 5-year-old boy with stage 3 abdominal B-NHL developed severe enterocolitis after the first AA block and died on the 18th day after the beginning of therapy. A 14 year-old girl with stage IV B-NHL died in complete remission (CR) due to candida sepsis after the fifth block of chemotherapy.

Treatment Results. Two patients were nonresponders and died due to progression of the disease (Table 1). One patient suffered early death due to enterocolitis. CR was attained in 20 patients (87%), after the first two blocks (AA and BB) in 15 patients and after the third and fourth blocks in five patients. One patient died in CR due to Candida sepsis. One patient developed a local abdominal relapse 6 months after diagnosis and died due to tumor progression. Eighteen patients are in continuous CR. As of 1 April, 1995, the probability of event-free survival [8] at 36 months (Kaplan-Meier analysis) is 78% (Fig. 1).

Table 1. Treatment results (as of 1.04.1995)

	(*n*)
Patients	23
Early death	1
Nonresponders (died)	2
Complete remission	20
Death in CR	1
Relapse (died)	1
In CCR	18

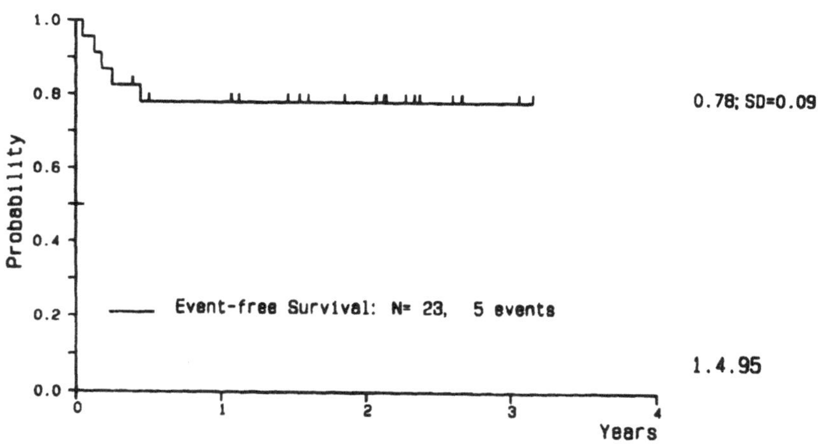

Fig. 1. Kaplan-Meier analysis [8] for event-free survival: the probability of survival in first remission after 6 months to 3 years is 78% (identical with probability of overall survival, not depicted here)

Discussion

The results obtained with the modified B-NHL-BFM protocol are clearly superior to the historical control of our group. As most relapses in B-NHL occur in the first 6 (-12) months [1-4], considerable changes in the results of our series are not expected.

The toxicity of the therapy is high, but can be kept within tolerable limits. Of course, final conclusions can be drawn only from a larger number of patients, which can be collected only in cooperative studies. Nevertheless, our preliminary results are encouraging. It will be of interest to evaluate the efficacy of 1 g/m^2 MTX instead of 5 g/m^2 in the modification of B-NHL-BFM 90 protocol. In conclusion, improved outcome in childhood B-NHL and the feasibility in a department whose members had no previous experience with such an intensive treatment regime was demonstrated.

Acknowledgment. The authors wasnt to express their gratitude to Priv.-Doz. Dr. Alfred Reiter, Hannover, Prof. Dr. Gritta Janka, Hamburg, Prof. Dr. Günther Schellong, Münster, and Dr. Martin Friedrichs, Moscow for their support by professional advice and material help.

References

1. Patte C., T. Philip, C. Rodary, J.M. Zucker, H. Behrendt, J.C. Gentet, J.P. Lamagnere, J. Otten, D. Dufillot, F. Pein, B. Caillou, J. Lemerle: High survival rate in advanced stage B-cell lymphomas und leukemias without CNS involvement with a short intensive polychemotherapy. Results from the French Pediatric Oncology Society of randomized trial of 216 children. J. Clin. Oncol. 9 (1991) 123-132
2. Reiter A., M. Schrappe, R. Parwaresch, G. Henze, St.Müller-Weihrich, S. Sauter, K.-W. Sykora, W.-D. Ludwig, H. Gadner, H. Riehlm: Non-Hodgkin's lymphomas of childhood and adolescence: results of a treatment stratified for biologic subtypes and stage — a report of the Berlin-Frankfurt-Münster group. J. Clin. Oncol. Vol. 13 (1995) 359-372
3. Reiter A., M. Schrappe, W.D. Ludwig, F. Lampert, J. Harbott, G. Henze, C. Niemeyer, H. Gadner, St. Müller-Weihrich, J. Ritter, E. Odenwald, H. Riehm: Favorable outcome of B-cell acute lymphoblastic leukemia in childhood: a report of three consecutive studies of the BFM group. Blood 80 (1992) 2471-2478
4. Reiter A., M. Schrappe, E. Yakisan, S. Sauter, W. Ebell, M. Zimmermann, W. Hartmann, B. Kremens, N. Kuhn, A. Claviez, A. Sauerbrey, P. Schmidt, St. Müller-Weihrich, T. Lieber, H. Riehm for BFM study group: Therapy of B-cell non-Hodgkin's-lymphoma (NHL) of childhood and adolescence: an interim analysis of study NHL-BFM 90. Part 3. Klin. Pädiatr. 206 (1994) 242-252
5. Bennet J.M., D. Catovsky, M.T. Daniel, G. Flandrin, D.A. Galton, H.K. Grabnick, C. Sultan: Proposals for the classification of the acute leukemias. French-American-British (FAB) co-operative group. Br. J. Hematol. 33 (1976) 451-458.
6. Standfeld A.G., J. Diebold, Y. Kapancy, G. Keleny, K. Lennert, O. Mioduszewska, H. Noel, F. Rilke, C. Sundstro, J.A.M. van Unnik, D.H. Wright: Updated Kiel classification. Lancet 1 (1998) 292-293
7. Murphy S.B.: Management of childhood non-Hodgkin's-lymphoma. Cancer Treat. Rep. 61 (1977) 1161-1173
8. Kaplan E.L., P. Meier: Nonparametric estimation from incomplete observation. J. Am. Stat. Assos. 53 (1958) 457-48

Acute Leukemias VI
Prognostic Factors
and Treatment Strategies
Büchner et al. (eds)

Similar Outcome in Boys with Isolated and Combined Testicular Acute Lymphoblastic Leukemia Relapse After Stratified BFM Salvage Therapy

C. Wolfrom[1], R. Hartmann[1], S. Brühmüller[1], R. Fengler[1], A. Reiter[2], J. Ritter[3], and G. Henze[1]
for the BFM Relapse Study Group

Introduction

Despite modern intensive treatment, relapses occur in about 25% children with acute lymphoblastic leukemia (ALL). After the central nervous system (CNS), the testes are the second most frequent site of an extramedullary relapse [1]. The incidence of testicular relapses has been decreased by intensification of front-line regimens, mainly by the introduction of intermediate-dose or high-dose methotrexate (MTX) [2-6]. When salvage therapy of an isolated relapse consisted of local treatment, alone or in combination with mild chemotherapy, a subsequent bone marrow relapse occurred in a high percentage of boys [3, 7-9]. Therefore, intensive systemic salvage therapy is necessary to achieve favorable results in boys with isolated as well as combined testicular relapse [10-13]. The aim of this study was to evaluate the efficacy of tumor load-adapated chemotherapy in boys with first overt testicular relapse, treated according to four consecutive Berlin-Frankfurt-Münster (BFM) relapse protocols.

Patients and Therapy

Eligible for this study were all boys up to 18 years of age with a first overt isolated or combined testicular relapse of non-B cell leukemia irrespective of the immune phenotype, first-line treatment, and site of initial manifestation of leukemia. Signed informed consent was obtained. In all trials, treatment was stratified according to time and location of the relapse. Early relapses at any time thereafter. Combined testicular relapse (CTR) were defined by bone marrow involvement exceeding 5% lymphoblasts. Accordingly, isolated testicular relapses (ITR) were diagnosed in cases of testicular leukemic infiltration without marrow involvement.

The study design is shown in Fig.1. Treatment started with multiagent chemotherapy courses. In trials ALL-REZ BFM 83, 85, and 87, two different courses R1 and R2, and in trial ALL REZ BFM 90 three different courses R1, R2, and R3 were given in alternating sequence with scheduled intervals of 3 weeks. Course R1 consisted of prednisone (or dexamethasone), mercaptopurine, vincristine, MTX, cytarabine, and asparaginase; course R2 of dexamethasone, thioguanine, vindesine, MTX, daunorubicin, ifosfamide, and asparaginase; and course R3 of dexamethasone, cytarabine, etoposide, and asparaginase. All courses except for R3 contained intermediate-dose or high-dose MTX. Intermediate-dose MTX was given at a dose of 500 mg/m^2 as a 24 h infusion in trial ALL-REZ BFM 83 and of 1 g/m^2 as a 36-h infusion in subsequent trials [14]. In trials ALL-REZ BFM 85 and 90, patients were randomized to receive intermediate-dose MTX (1 g/m^2 as a 36-h infusion) or high-dose MTX, which was dosed 12 g/m^2 as a 4-h infusion or 5 g/m^2 as a 24-h infusion, respectively [15].

[1]University Children's Hospital of Berlin Germany
[2]University Children's Hospital of Hannover, Germany
[3]University Children's Hospital of Münster, Germany

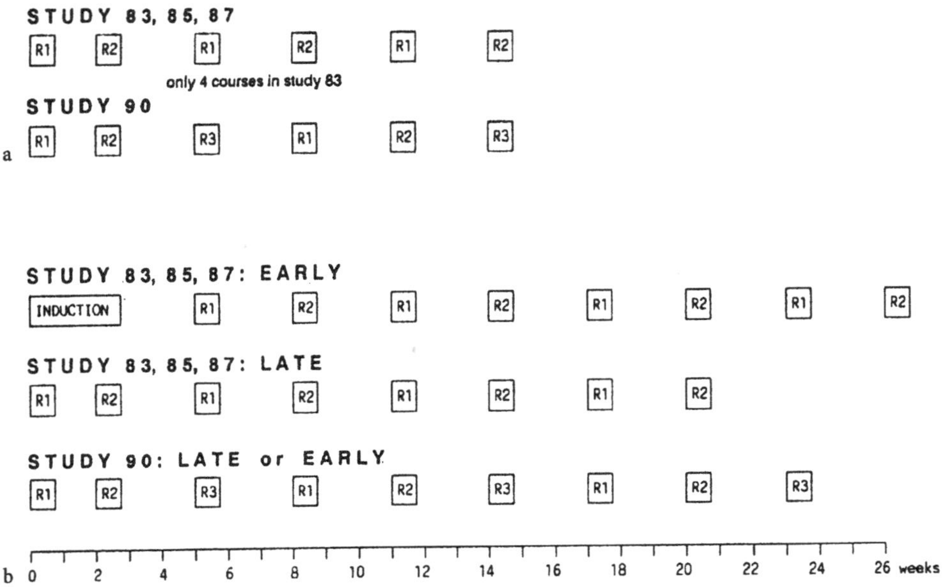

Fig. 1a,b. ALL-REZ BFM Study design; **a** ITR; **b** CTR

Boys with an ITR generally received six courses, seven patients received only four courses in the first trial. Depending on the time of relapse and study design, two or three additional courses (a total of eight or nine) were given to patients with concomitant bone marrow involvement. CNS prophylactic treatment consisted of intrathecal MTX in trials ALL-REZ BFM 83 and 85. In trials ALL-REZ BFM 87 and 90, triple intrathecal therapy (MTX, cytarabine, prednisone) was repeatedly administered during each course of chemotherapy, and patients with bone marrow involvement additionally received 12–18 Gy cranial irradiation. Conventional maintenance therapy with daily oral thioguanine and biweekly intravenous MTX was given for 1 year in ITR patients and for 2 years in CTR patients [14]. Bone marrow transplantation (BMT) was optional depending on the individual decision of patients,parents, and attending physicians. Allogeneic BMT was performed in 11 patients, for whom an HLA identical donor was available. In two boys autologous BMT was carried out.

Local treatment of an unilateral testicular relapse comprised orchiectomy of the involved testis and radiation (12–24 Gy) of the contralateral testis. In bilateral relapse, both testes were irradiated (24 Gy). Orchiectomy has been performed at diagnosis, and irradiation was applied after completion of the courses.

Results

Since 1983, a total of 114 boys with first overt testicular relapse, median age 7.6 years (range 1–16 years), have been treated according to the BFM relapse trials, 59 boys with ITR and 55 boys with CTR. All patients had received intensive front-line therapy, the majority (82%) according to BFM protocols. Patient characteristics are given in Table 1.

Of 114 boys 112 (98%) achieved complete remission (CR). Two patients with CTR did not respond to therapy. No induction death occurred. BMT was performed in 13 patients (11%). Excluding these patients from analysis did not change any of the results substantially. Three patients died in CR because of therapy-related complications, two after allogeneic BMT, and one after the third course of chemotherapy. In 46 patients, a second relapse occurred. Sixty-three patients are still in continuous CR after a median observation time of 5 years (range 1–10 years).

Event-free survival (EFS) rates at 8 years were 0.53 ± 0.07 in patients with ITR and 0.52 ± 0.07

Table 1. Patient characteristics

Testicular relapse	Isolated	Combined
Patients (*n*)	59	55
Age at relapse-Median	8.4	7.5
Range (years)	1–16	3–16
Duration of CR—Median,	30	33
Range, (months)	10–119	12–68
Time of relapse		
Early relapse (*n*)	32	15
Late relapse (*n*)	27	40
Immunological phenotype		
C-ALL (*n*)	35	36
Pre-B (*n*)	7	12
Pre-pre-B (*n*)	2	2
Hybrid (*n*)	1	–
T cell (*n*)	10	2
Not done	4	3
Treatment protocol		
ALL-REZ BFM 83 (*n*)	7	4
ALL-REZ BFM 85 (*n*)	0	5
ALL-REZ BFM 87 (*n*)	7	15
ALL-REZ BFM 90 (*n*)	35	31
BMT		
Allogeneic (*n*)	3	8
Autologous (*n*)	2	–

in patients with CTR (Fig. 2). Patients with late relapses occurring beyond 6 months after elective cessation of front-line therapy had a significantly better outcome than patients with early relapses (EFS 0.66 ± 0.06 vs.0.33 ± 0.07, $p < 0.001$, Fig.3). EFS rates of patients with early ITR (0.32 ± 0.09) and early CTR (0.37 ± 0.13) were virtually identical. Likewise, bone marrow involvement was not of statistical significance in patients with late relapses (EFS 0.78 ± 0.09 for ITR and 0.57 ± 0.08 for CTR, $p > .05$).

Discussion

In the experience of the BFM relapse trials, patients with bone marrow relapse and concomitant extramedullary involvement had a significantly better prognosis than patients with isolated bone marrow relapse [16]. The Pediatric Oncology Group reported significantly better results in boys with early ITR compared to boys with early isolated bone marrow relapse [12]. One explanation for the better outcome of patients with extramedullary relapses is that relapses originating from leukemic blast cells in the bone marrow are caused by selected drug resistant clones, whereas extramedullary relapses are caused by blasts, which are protected from the pressure of selection in a sanctuary and remain more susceptible to therapy. This implies that ITR or CTR are caused by leukemic blasts with other biological qualities than isolated bone marrow relapses.

This study was conducted to evaluate the efficacy of tumor load-adapted chemotherapy in boys with ITR and CTR and to prove whether concomitant bone marrow involvement has an impact on the prognosis. Regarding the etiology of testicular relapse, two theories are discussed. Testicular relapse could be caused by leukemic cells which hibernate in the testes and cause a systemic relapse by emigration and proliferation in the bone marrow. On the other hand, the testes could be a privileged site for an early

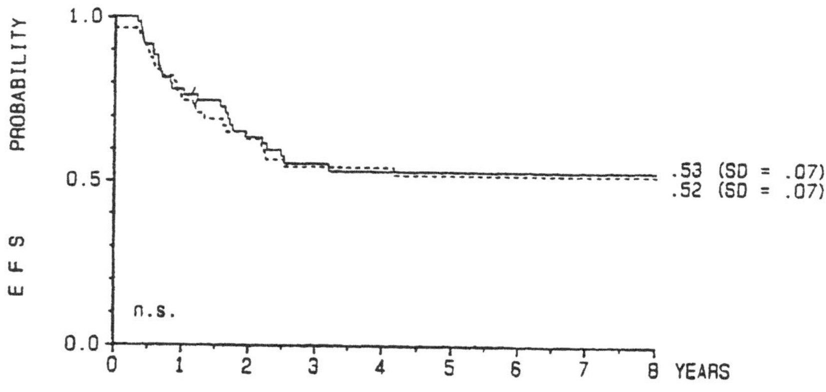

Fig. 2. Probability of EFS in boys with overt testicular relapse. The outcome of patients with ITR (*solid line*;$n = 59$; 33 in CCR) or CTR (*dotted line*; $n = 55$; 30 in CCR) identical . *Slash* indicates last follow up

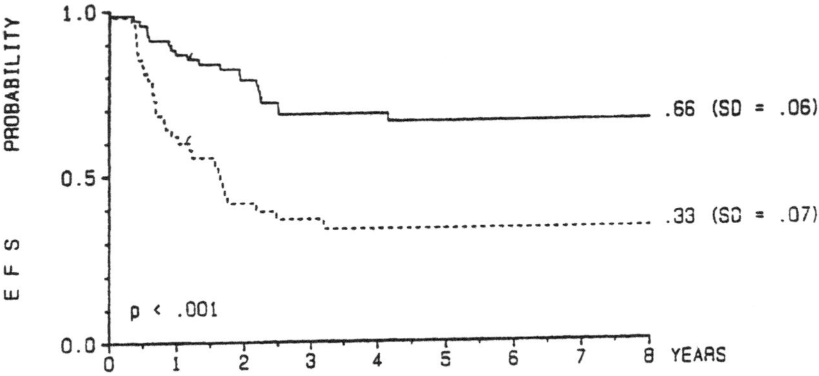

Fig. 3. Probability of EFS in boys with overt testicular relapse. Patients with late relapse (*upper curve*; $n = 67$; 46 in CCR) have a significanty better outcome than patients with early relapse (*lower curve*; $n = 47$; 17 in CCR). *Slash* indicates last follow up

manifestation of underlying systemic disease which could not evolve as a primary systemic relapse due to immunological or therapeutical systemic control of the disease. However, in ITR there is evidence that leukemic involvement is not restricted to the testes because involvement of abdominal lymph nodes, liver, and spleen were found at diagnosis and local treatment alone could not prevent subsequent bone marrow relapse in almost all cases [8, 17–20]. Therefore an ITR could be regarded as an early stage of a systemic relapse differing from a CTR by a lower leukemic cell burden.

In respect to the higher tumor cell load, ALL -REZ BFM protocols provide additional courses of chemotherapy for patients with CTR. The results of this study documented no singnificant difference in the outcome of patients with ITR and CTR. This was in agreement with the results of a previous analysis comparing the outcome of patients with ITR and CTR individually treated by intensive chemotherapy before 1982 [21].

Concerning the outcome of patients with CTR, there were no data available from comparable trials. The outcome of the patients with ITR is in accordance with the results of recent studies employing a similar therapeutic approach. In accordance with the results of these studies, duration of first remission was a main prognostic factor in the study presented here [10–13]. For boys with ITR occuring on therapy, EFS rates of 20% and 43% were reported [11, 13]. An EFS rate of 40% was observed for boys with an early ITR [12]. Boys with late testicular relapses had a substantial better outcome with an EFS rate of 84% at 4 years [11]. In a small group of ten patients relapsing later than 1 year after completion of therapy no subsequent relapse was observed [12].

The presented analyses show results obtained from a large cohort of boys with ITR or CTR. In summary, treatment according to the concept of the BFM relapse trials is effective in boys with testicular relapse. One third of patients with early relapse and two thirds of patients with late relapse can be rescued by salvage therapy. Irrespective of time of relapse, results are comparable in boys with and without concomitant bone marrow involvement. We conclude that patients with combined relapses may have a benefit from the additional courses of chemotherapy given in respect to the higher leukemic cell burden. On the other hand, testicular relapse, ITR as well as CTR, might be better accessible to treatment in general because they evolve from extracompartments and therefore leukemic cells may be less resistant.

Acknowledgment. Participating clinical centers and principal investigators: Aachen, R. Mertens; Aalen, B. Höhmann; Augsburg, E. Pongratz, Berlin, G. Henze; Berlin-Buch, W. Dörffel; Bonn, U. Bode; Bremen, H.-J. Spaar; Copenhagen, K. Schmiegelow; Dresden-Neustadt, V. Scharfe; Düsseldorf, U. Göbel; Erlangen, J.D. Beck; Essen, W. Havers; Frankfurt, B. Kornhuber; Freiburg, C. Niemeyer; Giessen, F. Lampert; Göttingen, M. Lakomek; Graz, C. Urban; Hamburg, G. Janka; Hannover, H. Riehm; Heidelberg, K.M. Debatin; Herdecke, C. Tautz; Kassel, H. Wehinger; Kiel,

R. Schneppenheim; Koblenz, M.Rister; Köln, F. Berthold; Linz, K. Schmitt; Ludwigshafen, H.C. Dominick; Lübeck, P. Bucsky; Mainz P. Gutjahr; Marburg, C. Eschenbach; München, C. Bender-Götze; München; S. Müller-Weihrich; München, R.J. Haas; Münster, H. Jürgens; Neunkirchen, E. Feldmann; Oldenburg; J. Drescher; Rostock, G. Eggers; Rotterdam, K. Hählen; Saarbrücken; R. Geib; Sankt Augustin, R. Dickerhoff; Stuttgart, J. Treuner; Trier, W. Rauh; Tübingen, D. Niethammer; Ulm, W. Hartmann; Wien, H. Gander; Wilhelmshaven, H.P. Krohn; Würzburg, J. Kühl; Wuppertal, B. Dohrn; Zürich, E. Frey This work was supported by grants from the Deutsche Krebshilfe.

References

1. Smith SD, Trueworthy RC, Klopovich PM, Vats TS, Snodgrass W: Management of children with isolated testicular leukemia. Cancer 54 (1984) 2854–2858
2. Brecher ML, Weinberg V, Boyett JM, Sinks LF, Jones B, Glicksman A, Holland JF, Freeman AI: Intermediate dose methotrexate in childhood acute lymphoblastic leukemia resulting in decreased incidence of testicular relapse. Cancer 58 (1986) 1024–1028
3. Russo A, Schiliro G: The enigma of testicular leukemia: a critical review. Med Pediatr Oncol 14 (1986) 300–305
4. Nesbit ME, Robison LL, Ortega JA, Sather HN, Donaldson M, Hammond D: Testicular relapse in childhood acute lymphoblastic leukemia: association with pretreatment patient characteristics and treatment. A report for Childrens Cancer Study Group. Cancer 45 (1980) 2009–2016
5. Bleyer WA, Poplack DG: Prophylaxis and treatment of leukemia in the central nervous system and other sanctuaries. Semin Oncol 1 (1985) 131–148
6. Moe PJ, Seip M, Finne PH: Intermediate dose methotrexate in childhood acute lymphocytic leukemia. Eur Paediatr Haematol Oncol 1 (1984) 113–118
7. Byrd RL: Testicular leukemia: incidence and management results. Med Pediatr Oncol 9 (1981) 493–500
8. Heaney JA, Klauber GT, Conley GR: Acute leukemia: diagnosis and management of testicular involvement. Urology 21 (1983) 573–577
9. Sullivan MP, Perez CA, Herson J, Silva-Sousa M, Land V, Dyment PG, Chan R, Ayala AG: Radiotherapy (2500 rad) for testicular leukemia: local control and subsequent clinical events: a Southwest Oncology Group study. Cancer 46 (1980) 508–515
10. Wofford MM, Smith SD, Shuster JJ, Johnson W, Buchanan GR, Wharam MD, Ritchey AK, Rosen D, Haggard ME, Golembe BL, Rivera GK: Treatment of occult or late overt testicular relapse in children with acute lymphoblastic leukemia: a Pediatric Oncology Group study. J Clin Oncol 10 (1992) 624–630
11. Uderzo C, Zurlo MG, Adamoli L, Zanesco L, Arico M, Calculli G, Comelli A, DiMontezemolo LC, DiTullio MT, Guazzelli C, Donfrancesco A, Werner B: Treatment of isolated testicular relapse in childhood acute lymphoblastic leukemia: an Italian multicenter study. J Clin Oncol 8 (1990) 672–677
12. Buchanan GR, Boyett JM, Pollock BH, Smith SD, Yanofsky RA, Ghim T, Wharam MD, Crist WM, Vietti TJ, Johnson W, Rivera GK: Improved treatment results in boys with overttesticular relapse during or shortly after initial therapy for acute lymphoblastic leukemia. A Pediatric Oncology Group study. Cancer 68 (1991) 48–55
13. Finklestein JZ, Miller DR, Feusner J, Stram DO, Baum E, Shina DC, Johnson DG, Gyepes MT, Hammond GD: Treatment of overt isolated testicular relapse in children on therapy for acute lymphoblastic leukemia. A report from the Childrens Cancer Group. Cancer 73 (1994) 219–223
14. Henze G, Fengler R, Hartmann R, Kornhuber B, Janka-Schaub G, Niethammer D, Riehm H: Six-year experience with a comprehensive approach to the treatment of recurrent childhood acute lymphoblastic leukemia (ALL-REZ BFM 85). A relapse study of the BFM Group. Blood 78 (1991) 1166–1172
15. Wolfrom C, Hartmann R, Fengler R, Brühmüller S, Ingwersen A, Henze G: Randomized comparison of 36-hour intermediate-dose versus 4-hour high-dose methotrexate infusions for remission induction in relapsed childhood acute lymphoblastic leukemia. J Clin Oncol 11 (1993) 827–833
16 .Bührer C, Hartmann R, Fengler R, Dopfer R, Gadner H, Gerein V, Göbel U, Reiter A, Ritter J, Henze G: Superior prognosis in combined compared to isolated bone marrow relapses in salvage therapy of childhood acute lymphoblastic leukemia. Med Pediatr Oncol 21 (1993) 470–476
17. Eden OB, Rankin A, Kay HE: Isolated testicular relapse in acute lymphoblastic leukaemia of childhood. Report on behalf of the Medical Research Council's Working Party on Leukaemia in Childhood. Arch Dis Child 58 (1983) 128–132
18. Kuo TT, Tschang TP, Chu JY: Testicular relapse in acute lymphocytic leukemia during bone marrow remission. Cancer 38 (1976) 2604–2612
19. Baum E, Heyn R, Nesbit M, Tilford D, Nachman J: Occult abdominal involvement with apparently isolated testicular relapse in children with acute lymphocytic leukemia. Am J Pediatr Hematol Oncol 6 (1984) 343–346
20. Mirro J, Wharam MD, Kaizer H, Zinkham W, Leventhal BG: Testicular leukemic relapse: rate of regression and persistent disease after radiation therapy. J Pediatr 99 (1981) 439–440
21. Fengler R, Henze G, Langermann HJ, Brämswig J, Jobke A, Kornhuber B, Ludwig R, Ritter J, Riehm H: Häufigkeit und Behandlungsergebnisse testikulärer Rezidive bei der akuten lymphoblastischen Leukämie im Kindesalter. Klin Padiatr 194 (1982) 204–208

Acute Leukemias VI
Prognostic Factors
and Treatment Strategies
Büchner et al. (eds)

Acute Cholecystitis Complicating Intensive Chemotherapy of Childhood Acute Lymphoblastic Leukemia

T. Urasiński[1], A. Brodkiewicz[1], A. Walecka[2], E. Kamieńska[1], J. Peregud-Pogorzelski[1], and J. Fydryk[1]

Abstract. Acute cholecystitis is a rare disorder in the pediatric age group over 10 years of age; female gender, obesity, and chronic hemolysis are considered to be predisposing factors. We report on three cases of acute cholecystitis complicating intensive chemotherapy of childhood acute lymphoblastic leukemia.

Introduction

The gastrointestinal tract is a common source of infection in neutropenic patients. Under normal conditions, the gastrointestinal mucosa acts as a mechnical barrier for external pathogens. In almost all leukemic patients it is disrupted or damaged from intensive chemotherapy, offering a potential site for bacterial, fungal, and viral colonization, invasion, and infection [1]. Acute cholecystitis is a rare disorder in the pediatric age group over 10 years of age; female gender, obesity, and chronic hemolysis are considered to be predisposing factors [2, 3]. We report on three cases of acute cholecystitis complicating intensive chemotherapy of childhood acute lymphoblastic leukemia (ALL).

Case Reports

Case 1. A 3-year-old girl, diagnosed as having low-risk ALL was treated with the ALL Berlin–Frankfurt–Münster (BFM) 86 protocol. On day 28 of protocol I she developed septic fever with chills and abdominal pain localized in the epigastric region, accompanied by nausea and vomiting and a positive Murphy sign. There were neither abdominal guarding nor jaundice. These symptoms occurred during granulocytopenia, after the seventh dose of L-asparaginase. Abdominal ultrasound revealed a distended gallbladder with a thickened wall. Blood culture was negative. The diagnosis of acalculous cholecystitis was made. Treatment with cephotaxime and metronidazole resulted in rapid resolution of all, including ultrasonographic, symptoms.

Case 2. A 4-year-old girl treated with the ALL-BFM 86 protocol for medium-risk ALL became neutropenic and febrile during protocol I, after the second dose of L-asparaginase. She complained of pain localized in the right abdominal quadrant, with a positive Murphy sign, nausea and vomiting. On physical examination, a tender mass was felt below the right costal margin. Abdominal ultrasound demonstrated an enlarged gallbladder with irregularity and thickening of its wall. Intravenous administration of carbenicillin and cephotoxim combined with metronidazole was followed by complete recovery and regression of abnormalities seen on ultrasound examination.

Case 3. A 10-year-old boy was treated with ALL-BFM 86 for standard-risk ALL. While neutropenic during protocol II, he developed septic fever and acute epigastric pain accompanied by nausea and vomiting. Physical examination

[1]Clinic of Pediatrics, Pomeranian Medical Academy, Szczecin, Poland
[2]Department of Radiology, Pomeranian Medical Academy, Szczecin, Poland

revealed abdominal tenderness and guarding, with a positive Murphy sign. A distended gallbladder with a thickened wall and no stones were seen on abdominal ultrasound. Treatment with cephotaxime plus metronidazole resulted in a brisk clinical recovery.

Comment

Acute cholecystitis is still a rare disorder, accounting for less than 1% of acute abdominal pain in children [1, 2, 4]. In most cases, it is rather a complication of underlying disease than an isolated disorder. Several authors have emphasized that many children with acute cholecystitis had acute systemic illness such as hemolytic disease, streptococcal septicemia or erysipelas. We previously reported on acute cholecystitis as a complication of Wilm's tumor or nephrotic syndrome [4].

It is suggested that the etiology is not entirely infectious, but rather results from associated dehydration and stagnation of bile. On the other hand, this dehydration and bile stagnation may predispose to infection [3, 5].

Acalculous cholecystitis can be a complication seen after bone marrow transplantation in adults with acute leukemia [6]. Leukemic infiltrates of the gallbladder presenting as acute cholecystitis are rarely seen in adult patients with relapsed acute leukemia [7, 8]. Reports on acute cholecystitis in children with leukemia are very limited [9].

Symptoms of acute cholecystitis in children are acute upper right quadrant or epigastric pain, and fever and vomiting similar to those seen in adults. This triad was observed in all our patients. It is worth noting that in all of them the Murphy sign was also positive. We share the opinion of Greenberg et al. [9] that ultrasonography should be the screening test for any child who presents with the above symptoms.

Three ultrasonographic signs are typical for gallbladder disease: a markedly thickened sonolucent gallbladder wall, a thickened hyperreflective irregular wall, and cholelithiasis. Most cases of cholecystitis in children are acalculous; thus particular attention should be directed towards evaluation of the gallbladder wall [9]. Changes were seen in all the patients, forming the basis for diagnosis. However, it must be kept in mind that other conditions such as ascites, hypoalbuminemia, cardiac failure, and renal disease can cause thickening of the gallbladder wall [10].

Conservative management rather than surgical intervention seems to be the treatment of choice in pediatric cancer patients with acute acalculous cholecystitis. Hydration, broad-spectrum antibiotics, and nasogastric decompression usually treat the acute process of cholecystitis [5]. This was seen in the patients reported; empiric antibiotics combined with other means of supportive therapy resulted in resolution of clinical symptoms and regression of ultrasonographic changes. This report aimed to draw attention to the fact that acute cholecystitis can be a septic complication in granulocytopenic children treated for ALL.

References

1. Freifeld AG, Hathorn JW, Pizzo PA. Infectious complications in the pediatric cancer patients. In: Pizzo, PA, Poplack DG.(eds.) Principles and practice of pediatric oncology. JB Lippincott Co, Philadelphia 1993, 987–1020.
2. Dutta T, George V, Sharma GD, Meenakshi PK. Gallbladder disease in infancy and childhood. Prog Pediatr Surg, 1975, 8, 109–118.
3. Andrassy RJ, Treadwell TA, Ratner IA, Buckley CJ. Gallbladder disease in children and adolescents. Am J Surg, 1976, 132, 19–21.
4. Walecka A, Brodkiewicz A. Zapalenie pęcherzyka żółciowego u dzieci. Pol Przeg Radiol, 1994, 1–2, 89–90.
5. Lange B, D'Angio G, Ross AJ III, O'Neill JA Jr, Packer RJ. Oncologic emergencies. In: Pizzo PA, Poplack DG.(eds.) Principles and practice of pediatric oncology. JB Lippincott Co, Philadelphia 1993, 951–972.
6. Pitkaranta P, Haapiainen R, Taavitsainen M, Elonen E. Acalculous cholecystitis after bone marrow transplantation in adults with acute leukemia. Eur J Surg, 1991, 157, 361–364.
7. Finlay DE, Mitchell SL, Letourneau JG, Longley DG. Leukemic infiltration of the gallbladder wall mimicking acute cholecysitis. Am J Roentgenol, 1993, 160, 63–64.
8. Hurley R, Weisdorf DJ, Jessurun J, Vercellotii GM, Miller WJ. Relapse of acute leukemia presenting as acute cholecystitis following bone marrow transplantation. Bone Marrow Transplant, 1992, 10, 387–389.
9. Greenberg M, Kangarloo H, Cochran ST, Sample WF. The ultrasonographic diagnosis of cholecystitis and cholelithiasis in children. Radiology, 1980, 137, 745–749.
10. Patriquin HB, DiPietro M, Barber FE, Teele RL. Sonography of thickened gallbladder wall: causes in children. Am J Roentgenol, 1983, 141, 57–60.

Acute Leukemias VI
Prognostic Factors
and Treatment Strategies
Büchner et al. (eds)

Prognostic Significance of Peanut Agglutinin Binding in Childhood T-Cell Acute Lymphoblastic Leukemia

G.J.L. Kaspers[1], A.J.P. Veerman[1,2], E.R. van Wering[2], B.E.M. van der Linden-Schrever[2], C.H. van Zantwijk[1], A. van der Does-van den Berg[2], and R. Pieters[1]

Abstract. We previously reported the favorable prognosis associated with positive peanut agglutinin (PNA) binding in childhood T-cell acute lymphoblastic leukemia (ALL), and hypothesized that this may be related to glucocorticoid sensitivity. The purposes of this prospective study involving 43 children with newly diagnosed T-cell ALL were to determine the relation between PNA binding and in vitro resistance to prednisolone (PRD) and dexamethasone (DXM), in vivo response to a systemic PRD monotherapy (plus one intrathecal injection with methotrexate) and to multidrug chemotherapy. PNA positivity was found in 28 (65%) out of the 43 cases. PNA-negative samples in vitro were not more resistant to PRD or DXM than PNA-positive samples. However, in 38 evaluable T-cell ALL patients, nine out of 13 PNA-negative cases were poor responders to PRD in vivo, while all 25 PNA-positive cases were good responders to PRD in vivo ($p<0.0001$). PNA-positive patients had a 3.4-fold (95% confidence interval, CI, 1.1–10.4, $p=0.03$) lower relative risk of any event than PNA-negative patients. The 3-year probability of event-free survival was 0.81 for PNA-positive patients and 0.40 for PNA-negative patients. In conclusion, PNA positivity is a marker for a subgroup of T-cell ALL patients who are very likely to respond well to systemic PRD monotherapy. In addition, PNA positivity is a favorable prognostic factor regarding event-free survival in childhood T-cell ALL.

Introduction

Peanut agglutinin (PNA) is a lectin derived from the plant *Arachus hypogea*, which binds to terminal nonreducing galactose residues on the cell membrane. It has especially been used to characterize thymocytes and lymphocytes [1, 2]. Subsequently, PNA binding was introduced to study leukemias, among other hematopoietic malignancies [3–10]. We showed in a previous retrospective study [9] that PNA positivity is mainly found in childhood acute lymphoblastic leukemia (ALL) of the T-cell immunophenotype and is associated with a good prognosis in this subgroup. Immature thymocytes, which are PNA-positive, are more sensitive to glucocorticoid-induced cell lysis than mature thymocytes, which are PNA negative [1, 11, 12]. We therefore hypothesized that the good prognosis associated with PNA positivity may be due to a relative sensitivity to glucocorticoids [9].

The purposes of this prospective study were to determine the relationship between PNA binding and clinical and cell biological features, in vitro resistance to predniso(lo)ne (PRD) and dexamethasone (DXM), in vivo response to systemic monotherapy with PRD accompanied by one intrathecal injection with methotrexate (MTX), and response to multidrug chemotherapy. PNA binding was assessed in 43 samples of children with newly diagnosed T-cell ALL.

[1] Department of Pediatrics, Free University Hospital, De Boelelaan 1117, 1081 HV Amsterdam, The Netherlands
[2] Dutch Childhood Leukemia Study Group, The Hague, The Netherlands

Materials and Methods

Patients and Patient Samples. Eligible were children (age 0–18 years) with T-cell ALL, newly diagnosed between 1989 and 1993. Bone marrow (BM) and peripheral blood (PB) samples as well as smears of children with ALL, obtained at diagnosis, were sent by local institutions to the central laboratory of the Dutch Childhood Leukemia Study Group (DCLSG) for confirmation of diagnosis, French-American-British (FAB) classification [13] and immunophenotyping [14]. A leukemia was considered to be a T-cell ALL if the malignant cells were positive for terminal deoxynucleotidyl transferase, cytoplasmic CD3, and CD7. A part of each sample with sufficient cells was sent to the research laboratory for pediatric hemato-onco-immunology at the Free University Hospital in Amsterdam for in vitro drug resistance testing.

PNA Binding. Cytocentrifuge preparations were fixed in buffered formaldehye acetone (pH 7.4, 4°C, 30s), rinsed in water, washed in PBS (pH 7.4), and incubated with 50 µl PNA (DAKO, ITK Diagnostics, De Kwakel, The Netherlands) at room temperature for 30 min. After this incubation, preparations were washed twice and incubated with 50 µl peroxidase-conjugated rabbit anti-PNA antiserum with 2% pooled AB human serum added, again washed with PBS (2 ×) and stained with diaminobenzidine 0.5 mg/ml with 0.05 *M* imidazole in 0.05 *M* Tris hydrochloride buffer (pH 7.6) and 0.02% H_2O_2 for 10 min at room temperature. Cells were counterstained with hematoxylin. If ≥20% of the malignant cells were positive for PNA, a sample was considered to be PNA positive, a similar definition as used in our retrospective study [9].

In Vitro Cellular Drug Resistance. This was measured with the methyl-thiazol-tetrazolium (MTT) assay, as described previously [15]. Briefly, leukemic cells were cultured in RPMI 1640 (Dutch modification, Gibco, Uxbridge, UK) with 20% fetal calf serum and other supplements [15] and incubated with PRD and DXM, each in six different concentrations in duplicate in wells of microculture plates at 37°C in humidified air with 5% CO_2. After 4 days, MTT (Sigma, St. Louis, MO, USA) was added to the wells for 6 h. MTT is reduced to colored formazan crystals by living cells only. The crystals were dissolved with acidified isopropanol. Formazan was quantitated using a spectrophotometer (Bio-tek Instruments Inc., Winooski, USA). The optical density is linearily related to the cell number [16]. Leukemic cell survival was calculated by the equation: (mean optical density treated wells/mean optical density control wells) × 100%. The drug concentration lethal to 50% of the cells—the LC_{50}—was used as measure of resistance. Samples were considered evaluable if they contained ≥80% leukemic cells before and ≥70% leukemic cells after 4 days of culture time, and if the control optical density exceeded 0.050 [15]. Since sample source does not influence the results of the MTT assay, BM and PB samples were evaluated together [17].

Treatment. Patients were treated according to current DCLSG protocols, which are based on Berlin-Frankfurt-Münster treatment principles but without cranial irradiation. All patients received a 7-day systemic monotherapy with PRD (60 mg/m^2 per day), and one injection with MTX intrathecally on day 1 of the PRD window. Patients were then stratified into one of three risk groups according to the in vivo response to PRD monotherapy, BFM risk factor (based on peripheral leukemic cell count, and liver and spleen size) [18], and response to induction chemotherapy and received risk-adapted treatment. In vivo PRD poor response was defined in the protocol as ≥1000 leukemic cells/mm^3 PB on day 8, and in vivo good PRD response as <1000 leukemic cells/mm^3 PB on day 8. Complete remission was defined as fewer than 5% leukemic blasts in representative BM with megakaryocytes and granulocyte precursors present with some degree of maturation and no manifestation of leukemia elsewhere. Failure to achieve complete remission after induction chemotherapy (induction failure) was considered an event on day 0. Early death was defined as death before completion of induction therapy. Event-free survival (EFS) was defined as time from diagnosis to induction failure, relapse, death from any cause, or to second malignancy, or time to latest contact for event-free patients.

Statistics. Statistical analysis was done with CSS and EGRET software. Differences in distribution of variables were tested with the Mann-Whitney U test or the χ^2 test. Estimates of EFS (with standard error, SE) were calculated according to the Kaplan-Meier product limit analysis [19]. Statistical comparisons of outcome were conducted by the proportional hazard Cox regression analysis [20]. Relative risks for PNA-positive patients relative to PNA-negative patients indicate the proportional increase or decrease in risk of failure at any time, and are given with a 95% confidence interval (CI). Analyses were two-tailed at a significance level of $p = 0.05$.

Results

PNA Binding and Clinical and Cell-Biological Features. Out of 43 cases, 28 (65%) showed positive binding to PNA. The characteristics of the PNA-positive and PNA-negative patients did not differ significantly with respect to age, sex, white blood cell count, BFM risk factor, or FAB type. However, the white blood cell count showed a trend ($p = 0.10$) of being higher in PNA-negative cases (median 91.2, range 5.3–729 × 10^9/l) than in PNA-positive cases (median 48.3, range 4.6–900 × 10^9/l).

PNA Binding and In Vitro Cellular Drug Resistance. This relationship could be studied in 28 cases. PNA-positive and PNA-negative cases did not differ in cellular resistance to PRD or DXM (Table 1).

PNA Binding and In Vivo Response to Systemic PRD Monotherapy. The in vivo response to systemic PRD monotherapy could be evaluated in 38 patients (Table 2). Nine (69%) out of 13 PNA-

Table 1. Relationship between PNA binding and in vitro cellular resistance to glucocorticoids in childhood T-cell ALL samples

Drug	PNA binding	LC_{50} values		*n*	*p* value
		Median (μg/ml)	Range (μg/ml)		
Prednisolone	Positive	121.9	.05–1500	13	0.85
	Negative	86.5	.26–1500	12	
Dexamethasone	Positive	6.0	.05–6	13	0.61
	Negative	2.0	.002–6	15	

Table 2. In vivo response to systemic predniso(lo)ne (PRD) monotherapy and multidrug chemotherapy in children with T-cell ALL, divided into PNA-positive and PNA-negative patients

	PNA positive	PNA negative	*p* value
n	28	15	
In vivo PRD response			<.0001
Evaluable (*n*)	25	13	
Poor (*n*)	0	9	
(%)	25	69	
Good (*n*)	100	4	
(%)		31	
Follow up			
Median months	31	30	.21
Range (months)	15–58	16–60	
Events			.024
Evaluable (*n*)	26	15	
No complete remission (*n*)	0	1	
(%)		7	
Relapse (*n*)	4	5	
(%)	15	33	
Early death (*n*)	0	1	
(%)		7	
Toxic death (*n*)	1	1	
(%)	4	7	

negative T-cell ALL patients showed a poor response, compared to none out of 25 PNA-positive cases ($p < 0.0001$, Fig. 1).

PNA Binding and In Vivo Response to Multidrug Chemotherapy. This could be evaluated in 41 patients, with a median follow-up from diagnosis of 30 months (range 14–60). The events that have occurred so far are listed in Table 2. The event rate was lower in PNA-positive (five out of 26, 19%) than in PNA-negative (eight out of 15, 53%) T-cell ALL patients ($p = 0.024$). PNA-positive T-cell ALL patients had a 3.4-fold (95% CI 1.1–10.4, $p = 0.03$) lower risk of any event than PNA-negative T-cell ALL patients. The 3-year probability of EFS was 0.81 for PNA-positive and 0.40 for PNA-negative patients (Fig. 2). In a multivariate analysis including BFM risk factor, clinical response to PRD and PNA binding only PNA binding was an independent prognostic factor for EFS.

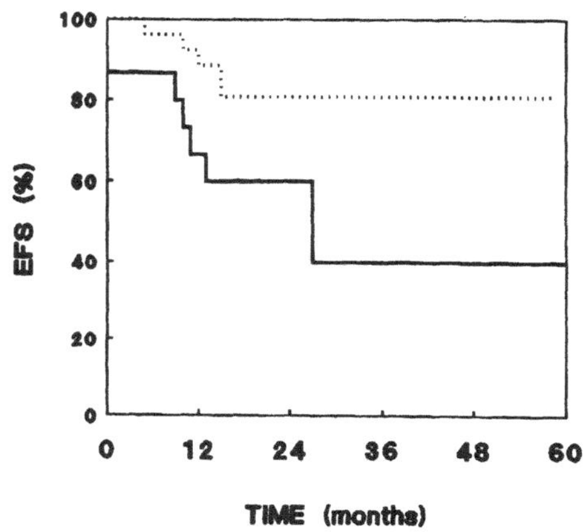

Fig. 2. Relationship between PNA binding and probability of EFS in newly diagnosed T-cell ALL; $p = 0.03$. *Dotted line*, PNA$^+$ T-ALL, $n = 26$; *solid line*, PNA$^-$ T-ALL, $n = 15$

Discussion

The results of this prospective study confirm those of our previous study, i.e., that T-cell ALL patients with positive PNA binding have a better prognosis than PNA-negative T-cell ALL patients. We hypothesized that this may be explained by a relative sensitivity of PNA-positive cells to glucocorticoids [9]. Glucocorticoid sensitivity, whether assessed in vitro or in vivo, is associated with a good prognosis in childhood ALL [21–23]. However, PNA-positive T-ALL cells were not more sensitive to glucocorticoids in vitro than PNA-negative T-ALL cells. In contrast to this, there was a highly significant relationship between PNA binding and in vivo response to a 1-week systemic PRD monotherapy, given together with one intrathecal injection with MTX. All of the PNA-positive patients showed a good in vivo response to PRD, while 69% of PNA-negative patients showed a poor response. This discrepancy between the in vitro and in vivo results is remarkable because we previously reported a significant correlation between in vitro resistance to PRD and the in vivo response to PRD in childhood ALL [24]. Moreover, the in vitro drug resistance MTT assay we used is a reliable and objective assay [25] and the results predict the clinical outcome in childhood ALL [22]. This discrepancy may be explained by the systemic antileukemic activity of MTX administered intrathecally [26–28] which does influence the in vivo response to PRD [29] but does not play a role in our results regarding in vitro resistance to PRD or DXM. According to this hypothesis, PNA-positive ALL cells should be more sensitive to MTX or at least to the combination of PRD and MTX than PNA-negative ALL cells. Another explanation for the discrepancy between the in vitro and in vivo results concerning the relationship to PNA binding may be an influence of glucocorticoids on the redistribution of ALL cells. Such an

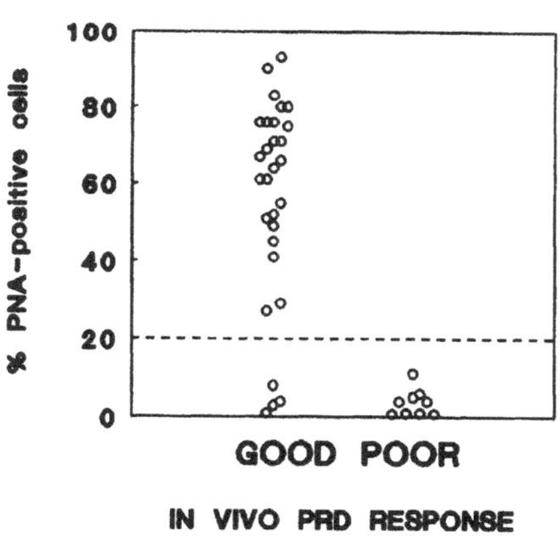

Fig. 1. Relationship between in vivo response to a systemic PRD monotherapy (plus MTX intrathecally) and PNA binding in newly diagnosed childhood T-cell ALL; $p < 0.001$. *circles*, childhood T-ALL, $n = 38$; *dotted line*, cut-off point for PNA positivity or negativity

effect, which does not play a role in our in vitro system, but which clinically may appear as a good response to PRD, has been reported for normal human lymphocytes [30]. According to this hypothesis, PNA-positive cells should be more susceptible to glucocorticoid-induced redistribution than PNA-negative cells.

The present study confirms our previous observation that PNA positivity predicts a good prognosis in T-cell ALL (Fig. 2), but now also prospectively in a larger number of patients and including multivariate analysis. Levin et al. [6] suggested that PNA-positive patients had a worse clinical outcome. However, they studied only 25 patients with a very short follow up and did not perform an analysis stratified for immunophenotype. Other authors who also studied PNA binding in large numbers of children with ALL did not report about its relationship with prognosis [4, 5].

The explanation for the relationship between PNA binding and prognosis may thus be related to resistance to MTX. However, PNA positivity may also be a marker for noncirculating cells [2, 31]. Weinberg et al. [10] reported that PNA-positive lymphomas had circulating blasts less often than PNA-negative lymphomas. In the present study, white blood cell count was higher in PNA-negative than in PNA-positive T-cell ALL patients, but the differences was not significant. We previously found no significant relationship between PNA binding and cell motility in the form of hand mirror cells [9].

We conclude that PNA positivity, especially frequent in T-cell ALL, is a marker for a subgroup of childhood T-cell ALL patients who are very likely to show a good in vivo response to a systemic PRD monotherapy given with MTX intrathecally. In addition, PNA positivity is a favorable independent prognostic factor with in T-cell ALL with regard to EFS.

Acknowledgments. This work was financially supported by Dutch Cancer Society (KWF/IKA 89-06) and VONK (VU Onderzoek Naar Kinderkanker). Board members of the Dutch Childhood Leukemia Study Group are H.van den Berg, M.V.A.Bruin, J.P.M.Bökkerink, P.J.van Dijken, K.Hählen, W.A.Kamps, F.A.E.Nabben, A.Postma, J.A.Rammeloo, I.M.Risseeuw-Appel, A.Y.N.Schouten-van Meeteren, G.A.M.de Vaan, E.T.van't Veer-Korthof, A.J.P.Veerman, M.van Weel-Sipman, and R.S.Weening.

References

1. London J, Berrih S, Bach J-F: Peanut agglutinin. I. A new tool for studying T lymphocyte subpopulations. J Immunol 121: 438–443, 1978
2. Reisner Y, Linker-Israeli M, Sharon N: Seperation of mouse thymocytes into two subpopulations by the use of peanut agglutinin. Cellular Immunol 25: 129-134, 1976
3. Barzilay M, Rosenthal E, Kende G, Reisner Y, Sharon N, Ramot B: Binding of peanut agglutinin to normal human lymphocytes and to leukemic cells. Leuk Res 6: 123–125, 1982
4. Dowell BL, Borowitz MJ, Boyett JM, Pullen DJ, Crist WM, Quddus FF, Russell EC, Falletta JM, Metzgar RS: Immunologic and clinicopathologic features of common acute lymphoblastic leukemia antigen-positive childhood T-cell leukemia. Cancer 59: 2020–2026, 1987
5. Haar JL, Raynor RH, Russell EC, Bhatnagar AS, Mohanakumar T: Ultrastructural analysis of acute lymphoblastic cells: peanut lectin binding correlates with degree of differentiation of the leukemic cells. Exp Hematol 13: 169–173, 1985
6. Levin S, Russell EC, Blanchard D, Mc Williams NB, Maurer HM, Mohanakumar T: Receptors for peanut agglutinin (Arachus hypogea) in childhood acute lymphoblastic leukemia: possible clinical significance. Blood 55: 37–39, 1980
7. Newman RA, Delia D: Analysis of the binding of peanut agglutinin (PNA) to leukaemic cells and its relationship to T-cell differentiation. Immunology 49: 147–152, 1983
8. Richard Y, Boumsell L, Lemerle J, Valensi F, Bernard A: Probing human malignant T cells with lectins: a comparison with their surface antigen patterns defined by monoclonal antibodies. Leuk Res 6: 307–312, 1982
9. Veerman AJP, Hogeman PHG, Huismans DR, Van Zantwijk CH, Bezemer PD: Peanut agglutinin, a marker for T-cell acute lymphoblastic leukemia with a good prognosis. Cancer Res 45: 1890–1893, 1985
10. Weinberg DS, Ault KA, Pinkus GS: Circulating malignant cells in non-Hodgkin's lymphoma: correlation with binding by peanut agglutinin. Blood 72: 698–704, 1988
11. Provvedini DM, Sakagami Y, Manolagas SC: Distinct target cells and effects of 1α,25-dihydroxyvitamin D3 and glucocorticoids in the rat thymus gland. Endocrinology 124: 1532–1538, 1989
12. Ranelletti FO, Pintelli M, Iacobelli S, Musiani P, Longo P, Lauriola L, Marchetti P: Glucocorticoid receptors and in vitro corticosensitivity of peanut-positive and peanut-negative human thymocyte subpopulations. J.Immunol 127: 849–855, 1981
13. Bennett JM, Catovsky D, Daniel MT, Flandrin G, Galton DAG, Gralnick HR, Sultan C: The morphological classification of acute lymphoblastic leukemia: concordance among observers and clinical correlations. Br J Haematol 47: 553–561, 1981

14. Van Wering ER, Brederoo P, Van Staalduinen GJ, Van Der Meulen J, Van Der Linden-Schrever BEM, Van Dongen JJM: Contribution of electron microscopy to the classification of minimally differentiated acute leukemias in children. Recent Results Cancer Res 131: 77-87, 1993
15. Pieters R, Loonen AH, Huismans DR, Broekema GJ, Driven MWJ, Heyenbrok MW, Hählen K, Veerman AJP: In vitro sensitivity of cells from children with leukemia using the MTT assay with improved culture conditions. Blood 76: 2327-2336, 1990
16. Pieters R, Huismans DR, Leyva A, Veerman AJP: Adaptation of the rapid automated tetrazolium dye based MTT assay for chemosensitivity testing in childhood leukemia. Cancer Lett 41: 323-332, 1988
17. Kaspers GJL, Pieters R, Van Zantwijk CH, De Laat PAJM, De Waal FC, Van Wering ER, Veerman AJP: In vitro drug sensitivity of normal peripheral blood lymphocytes and childhood leukaemic cells from bone marrow and peripheral blood. Br J Cancer 64: 469-474, 1991
18. Riehm H, Feickert H-J, Schrappe M, Henze G, Schellong G: Therapy results in five ALL-BFM studies since 1970: implications of risk factors for prognosis. Haematol Blood Transf 30: 139-146, 1987
19. Kaplan EL, Meier P: Nonparametric estimation from incomplete observations. J Am Stat Assoc 53: 457-481, 1958
20. Cox DR: Regression models and life tables. J R Stat Soc 34: 187-220, 1972
21. Riehm H, Reiter A, Schrappe, Berthold F, Dopfer R, Gerein V, Ludwig R, Ritter J, Stollmann B, Henze G: Die corticosteroid-abhängige Dezimierung der Leukämiezellzahl im Blut als Prognosefaktor bei der akuten lymphoblastischen Leukämie im Kindesalter (Therapiestudie ALL-BFM 83). Klin Pädiatr 199: 151-160, 1986
22. Pieters R, Huismans DR, Loonen AH, Hählen K, Van Der Does-Van Den Berg A, Van Wering ER, Veerman AJP: Relation of cellular drug resistance to longterm clinical outcome in childhood acute lymphoblastic leukaemia. Lancet 338: 399-403, 1991
23. Kaspers GJL, R Pieters, Van Zantwijk CH, ER Van Wering, A Van Der Does-Van Den Berg, AJP Veerman: Resistance to prednisolone (PRD) in vitro: a new prognostic factor in childhood acute lymphoblastic leukemia (ALL) at initial diagnosis. Proc Am Soc Clin Oncol 12: 320, 1993 (abstract)
24. Kaspers GJL, Pieters R, Van Zantwijk CH, De Waal FC, Van Wering ER, Veerman AJP: Is resistance to prednisolone in vitro related to the response to prednisolone at initial diagnosis in childhood acute lymphoblastic leukemia? A preliminary analysis in: Kaspers GJL, Pieters R, Twentyman PR, Weisenthal LM, Veerman AJP (eds): Drug resistance in leukemia and lymphoma. The clinical value of laboratory assays. Chur, Harwood Academic Publ., 1993, p 321-328
25. Veerman AJP, Pieters R: Drug sensitivity assays in leukaemia and lymphoma. Br J Haematol 74: 381-384, 1990
26. Bleyer WA, Dedrick RL: Clinical pharmacology of intra-thecal methotrexate. I. Pharmacokinetics in nontoxic patients after lumbar injection. Cancer Treatm Rep 61: 703-708, 1977
27. Jacobs SA, Bleyer WA, Chabner BA, Johns DG: Altered plasma pharmacokinetics of methotrexate administered intrathecally. Lancet 1: 465-466, 1975
28. Thyss A, Munzer C, Mechinaud-Lacroix F, Boutard P, Suciu S, Solbu G, Tokaji E, Philippe N, Otten J, for the EORTC C.L.C.G.: Intrathecal methotrexate (i.t. MTX) is an important factor of the response to the so-called "corticoid prephase" of the BFM protocol for ALL in the EORTC 58 881 trial. Med Pediatr Oncol, 21: 539, 1993 (abstract number 31)
29. Simmons ED, Somberg KA: Acute tumor lysis syndrome after intrathecal methotrexate administration. Cancer 67: 2062-2065,1995
30. Cohen JJ: Lymphocyte death induced by glucocorticoids. In Schleimer RP, Claman HN, Oronsky AL (eds): Anti-inflammatory steroid action. Basic and clinical aspects. San Diego, CA Academic Press Inc., 1989, pp 111-131
31. Rose ML: Binding of peanut lectin to lymphocytes: a marker of immaturity. Immunol Today 3: 6-8, 1982

Acute Leukemias VI
Prognostic Factors
and Treatment Strategies
Büchner et al. (eds)

Longitudinal Study of Cognitive, Motor, and Behavioral Functioning in Children Diagnosed with Acute Lymphoblastic Leukemia: A Report of Early Findings from the Childrens Cancer Group

T.A. Kaleita[1], D.G. Tubergen[2], J.A. Stehbens[3], W.E. MacLean[4], R.B. Noll[5], J.M. Cherlow[6], N.L. Cantor[7], P.N. Chang[8], R.T. O'Brien[7], F.B. Ruymann[9], H.N. Sather[10], E. Schwartz[11], J.K. Whitt[13], M.J. Waskerwitz[12], G.D. Hammond[10]

Abstract. Childhood acute lymphoblastic leukemia (ALL) was considered a fatal condition 40 years ago, but is curable in more than 70% of patients today. The survival rate is being improved by increasing the intensity of chemotherapy early in treatment. Risk factors for potential neurobehavioral sequelae from the most effective therapies continue to be defined. We present early findings from the first large-scale longitudinal study of neurobehavioral functioning (CCG-105NP) in childhood ALL patients from a randomized clinical trial (CCG-105). More than 200 patients (age range 1–18 years at diagnosis, $\bar{x} = 5.7$ years) with intermediate risk ALL were enrolled in the CCG-105NP study. These children had been randomized to: (a) one of four systemic chemotherapy approaches testing Childrens Cancer Group (CCG) versions of Berlin-Frankfurt-Münster (BFM) intensive and prolonged induction/consolidation (I/C) and delayed intensification (DI), separated and together; and (b) CNS-directed therapy using intrathecal methotrexate (IT MTX) alone throughout treatment versus 1800 cGy cranial irradiation (CXRT) and IT MTX during I/C and DI. They were examined at 9, 21, and 48 months after diagnosis. Comprehensive assessments included tests of early cognitive and motor development for pre-school patients, and intelligence, attention, visual-spatial perception, fine motor coordination, memory, language, school achievement, and social behaviour for school-age children and adolescents. At 9 months after diagnosis, preliminary data analyses possibly associated DI with fine motor difficulties in children 3–6.5 years of age. In addition, there were significant differences in cognitive and motor functioning between children who received CXRT and those in the same age range in the non-CXRT group. These test findings suggest that gross motor abilities and attentional processes were affected as early as 9 months after diagnosis. All treatment subgroup mean scores were in the average range. Longitudinal analyses of data from serial evaluations of patients will determine the persistence of these findings and the timing and occurrence of specific long-term neurobehavioral sequelae. Mediating factors such as age at diagnosis, gender, family socioeconomic status, and parental

[1]UCLA School of Medicine, Los Angeles, California, USA
[2]M.D. Anderson Cancer Center, Houston, Texas, USA
[3]University of lowa Hospital & Clinics, Iowa City, Iowa, USA
[4]Vanderbilt University, Nashville, Tennessee, USA
[5] Children's Hospital Medical Center, Cincinnati, Ohio, USA
[6]Long Beach Memorial Medical Center, Long Beach, California, USA
[7]Primary Children's Medical Center, Salt Lake City, Utah, USA
[8]University of Minnesota Medical Center, Minneapolis, Minnesota, USA
[9]Children's Hospital, Columbus, Ohio, USA
[10]University of Southern California School of Medicine, Los Angeles, California, USA
[11]University of Michigan, Ann Arbor, Michigan, USA
[12] Butterworth Hospital, Grand Rapids, Michigan, USA
[13]University of North Carolina, Chapel Hill, North Carolina, USA

education levels, as well as any interaction effects within the context of the clinical trial, will be analyzed more precisely than in previous studies. This could serve as a basis for future intervention efforts. These analyses of data are currently in progress.

Introduction

Acute lymphoblastic leukemia (ALL) in children has been changed from an almost universally fatal disease 40 years ago to a curable condition in over 70% of patients today. This improvement is the result of many factors, the major one being the introduction of more intensive therapy early in the course of treatment to prevent subsequent relapse in bone marrow, CNS, and other sites [1]. Intensity and success of ALL therapy have increased, concomitant with a concern for late effects such as cognitive, motor and behavioral sequelae. The most widely used treatment programs around the world for the management of ALL are Patterned after the Berlin-Frankfurt-Münster (BFM) regimens, which include intensified and prolonged induction and consolidation chemotherapy and early intensive reinduction [2]. Cranial irradiation (CXRT) is included in many, though not all, of the versions. A recent report from the Children's Cancer Group (CCG) indicated that children under 10 years of age with lower risk ALL can be effectively treated on BFM-derived therapy without CXRT [3]. This trial (CCG-105) also demonstrated that the effectiveness of CNS presymptomatic therapy, either CXRT with intrathecal (IT) methotrexate (MTX) or IT MTX alone, is enhanced by intensified systemic chemotherapy [4]. To date, there have been no reported randomized studies of the neurobehavioral effects of CNS-directed therapies including CXRT given in conjunction with BFM-derived systemic treatment.

Previous investigations into the impact of CNS-directed therapy on neurobehavioral functioning have relied primarily on retrospective reports [5]. Prospective, longitudinal studies are relatively few in number (see Table 1, which compares selected prospective studies to CCG-105NP). (See [5] for a complete review of most retrospective and prospective reports.) Methodological deficiencies in most of the published prospective reports limit interpretation and generalizability [6]. With few exceptions, these studies have included small sizes [7-11] and non-random assignment to CNS-directed treatments [8-13]. In some studies, controls or comparison groups have been lacking [11, 13], while in others, patients with malignancies other than ALL and, therefore, substantially different treatments have been used [8-10, 12]. In addition, many studies have been limited by the narrow range of neurobehavior assessed [14-16]. Others have not carefully considered the influence of inconsistent follow-up intervals on results [7, 11, 12, 16].

The CCG-105NP study was initiated as an extension of CCG efforts to refine CNS-directed therapy for ALL patients and to address methodological weaknesses in previous studies. It utilized a prospective longitudinal design with two evaluations during therapy and one performed after discontinuation of treatment. Each assessment included a comprehensive evaluation of cognitive, motor, and academic skills with a limited evaluation of behavior and social functioning at home and school. These repeated evalutions were planned to determine the timing and occurrence of deficits with respect to selected medical, patient and social factors. As mediating factors and interaction effects are defined within the context of the clinical trial, future intervention efforts can be developed.

The purpose of the present paper is: (1) to summarize the background and study plan of CCG-105NP; and (2) to present early findings from the prospective assessment of cognitive, motor, and behavioral functioning in children treated for childhood ALL.

Material and Methods

Patients

The CCG-105NP study formally opened in March 1986, and within a year was obtaining data from 16 of the more than 100 CCG institutions. Over 200 children ($\bar{x} = 5.7$ years old at diagnosis, range 1-18 years; 65% male, 35% female) diagnosed and treated for intermediate-risk ALL were enrolled. All patients were in first hematologic remission and without CNS involvement either at diagnosis or during the course of treatment. Children with pre-existing mental retardation or developmental language disorder, Down's syndrome, and those not sufficiently fluent in English were ineligible for this study.

Table 1. Prospective neurobehavioral studies of childhood acute leukemia patients

Study	Therapeutic trial (radiation dose)	Randomization to CNS Rx	Radiated patients (*N*)	Control groups[a]	Age at diagnosis (years)	Range of tests	Assessment intervals (years after) diagnosis)
Walther et al.[12]	Berlin ALL; Hamburg ALL St.Jude Total Therapy VIII (2400 cGy)	No	40	Lymphoma	Range: 3–19	1–7	Range: 1–8
Meadows et al.[7]	CCG-141 (2400 cGy)	Yes	23	IT MTX; Wilms	Median: 4.10	1,2,5,7,8	Range: 1–3
Berg et al.[13]	St. Jude Total Therapy IX (2400 cGy)	No	44	None	$\bar{x} = 7.0$	2,3,5,8	0.5,1.6,3.8
Stehbens et al.[8,9]	lowa ALL (2400 or 1800 cGy)	No	16	Solid tumors	$\bar{x} = 9.0$	2,8,9	0,1,3
Brouwers et al. [14,15]	CCG-191/NCI-77-02 [b] (2400 cGy)	Yes	–	HDMTX+ ITMTX	–	2,8	1,2,3.5
Copeland et al.[10]	Anderson ALL[c]	No	0	Sarcomo,lymphoma	$\bar{x} = 8.9$	2,4–8	0,1
Kaleita et al.[11]	UCLA BMT[d] (750cGy TBI)	No	2	None	$\bar{x} = <1$	1,2,5,7	Range: 0.2–5.3
Ochs et al.[16]	St. Jude Total Therapy X (1800 cGY)	Yes	23	IVMTX + ITMTX	Median: 4.6	2,8	Range: 1–7.8
CCG-105NP	CCG-105 (1800 cGy)	Yes	125	IT MTX	$\bar{x} = 5.7$	1–9	.75, 1.75,4

Range of tests:
1, early development; 2, intelligence; 3, attention; 4, visual-spatial perception; 5, fine motor coordination; 6, memory; 7, language; 8, school achievement; 9, behavior

[a] Note that control groups are designated either in terms of disease category or the CNS-directed chemotherapy (i.e., methotrexate) given to a comparison group treated for ALL

[b] Total number of patients reported on study = 33; mean age not reported

[c] Patients ($N = 19$) received CNS-directed treatment involving intrathecal methotrexate, cytosine arabinoside, and hydrocortisone

[d] Patients were treated with the University of California at Los Angeles pre-bone marrow transplant conditioning regimen, which included total body irradiation.

Comparability analyses of medical and demographic characteristics indicated that the patients studied on CCG-105NP were representative of all eligible patients entered on the therapeutic clinical trial, except for race (see Table 2). Study patients had a significantly higher percentage of Caucasian children and a lower percentage of Hispanic children. This difference was due to the requirement regarding fluency in English.

ALL Therapy: CCG-105

The CCG-105 study was a large randomized clinical trial of treatment for children with intermediate prognosis ALL [3, 4]. intermediate risk was defined by clinical and laboratory features (primarily age, gender, white blood cell count, and measurements of mass disease.) Over 1,600 patients were entered into this study between May, 1983 and April, 1989. The CCG-105 trial utilized a 4 × 2 factorial design, the first factor involving systemic chemotherapy and the second, CNS-directed treatment. Patients were randomly assigned to one of four chemotherapy regimens using CCG versions of BFM intensive and prolonged induction/consolidation plus delayed intensification (DI). Two of the regimens (A and B) included DI (Fig. 1) Patients were simultaneously randomly assigned to CNS-directed therapy consisting of either 1800 cGy CXRT plus IT MTX, given during induction, consolidation, and delayed intensification or IT MTX given throughout the course of treatment. The differences in CNS therapy between the most intensive systemic treatment arm and the least intensive systemic treatment arm are illustrated in Fig. 2. Males in the study received 3 years of maintenance treatment and females 2 years of therapy, measured from the beginning of interim maintenance (regimens A and B) or maintenance (regimens C and D).

Schedule of Assessment

Patients enrolled on CCG-105NP were given a baseline neurobehavioral assessment at 9 mon-

Table 2. Comparability analyses of medical and demographic characteristics

	CCG-105NP	*CCG-105*
Age at diagnosis		
<6 years	73%	65%
6–9 years	10%	13%
10+ years	17%	21%
Mean WBC at diagnosis	14,700	14,100
Day 14 marrow		
M1	93%	90%
M2	7%	7%
M3	0%	2%
*Race		
White	93%	75%
Black	2%	5%
Other	5%	20%
Treatment groups (CXRT)		
Randomized to CXRT	46%	50%
Randomized to no CXRT	54%	49%
Treatment groups (chemotherapy)		
Randomized to full BFM	23%	25%
Randomized to early BFM	27%	25%
Randomized to late BFM	25%	25%
Randomized to standard radiotherapy	25%	25%

CCG-105NP patients studied neurobehaviorally were compared to their non-participating counterparts in the same age range. This latter group consisted of all other patients enrolled on the CCG-105 therapeutic clinical trial. All patients were in continuous complete remission for the first 9 months of treatment, since patients had to reach that length of time in remission before they could be enrolled in CCG-105NP.
* $p < .0001$ (chi-square)

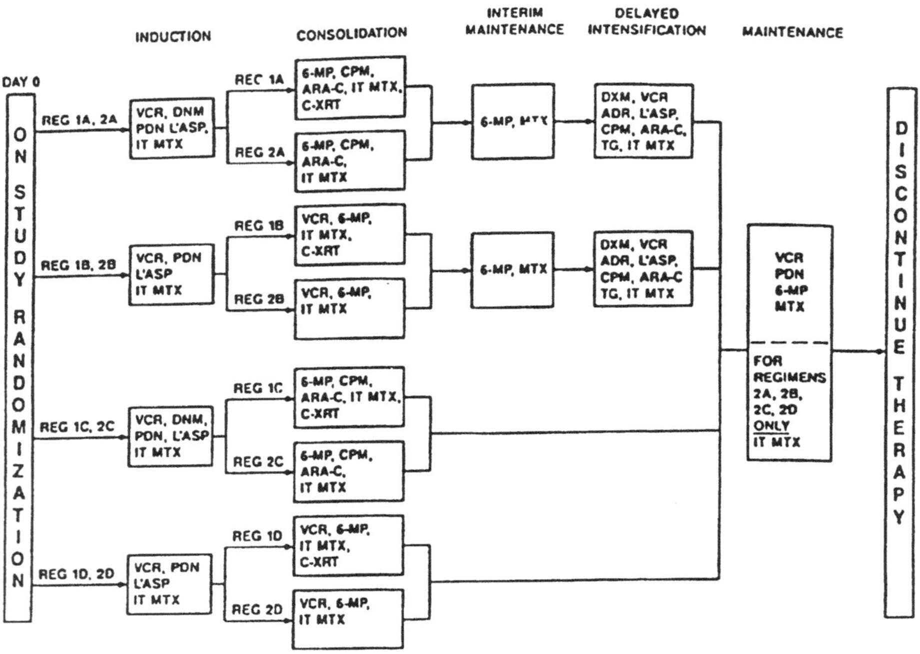

Fig. 1. Schematic diagram of the therapy in CCG-105. The 2 × 4 design tests two forms of CNS-directed therapy and four systemic chemotherapy regimens. VCR, vincristine; DNM, daunorubicin; PDN, prednisone; L'ASP, asparaginase; MTX, methotrexate; 6-MP, mercaptopurine; CPM, cyclophosphamide; ARA-C, cytarabine; DXM, dexamethasone; ADR, doxorubicin; TG, thioguanine (reprinted from [4], with permission)

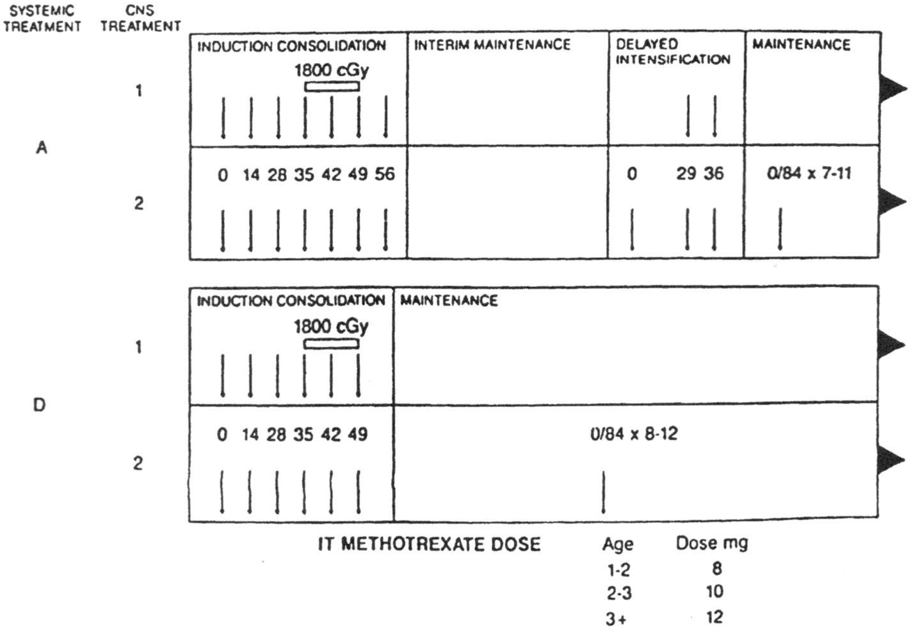

Fig. 2. Timing and dose of CNS-directed therapy for the most intensive systemic arm (regimen A) and the least intensive systemic arm (regimen D). CNS treatment 1 includes CXRT therapy; CNS treatment 2 provides IT MTX during all phases of treatment (reprinted from [4], with permission)

ths after diagnosis, because an earlier CCG/NCI study (CCG-191/NCI-77-02) had indicated that neurobehavioral status was stable over the first year after diagnosis [14, 15]. A second assessment on therapy at 21 months after diagnosis was planned for all children. A final assessment was planned for all children at 48 months after diagnosis, long after discontinuation of systemic treatment when any transient peripheral nervous system effects would likely be resolved and CNS effects would likely appear. A neurologic examination, scheduled on the same day as each neurobehavioral assessment in original study design, was discontinued entirely after review of findings from 100 patients revealed only decreased reflexes in the lower extremities. The sequence of treatment randomization and neurobehavioral assessment was as follows:

CCG-105		CCG-105:		CCG-105NP:		CCG-105NP
Patient entry	→	4 × 2 randomization systemic chemotherapy and CNS-directed therapy	→	On–therapy assessments at 9 and 21 months post diagnosis	→	Follow-up assessment at 48 months post diagnosis

and the expense. Four psychologists on the CCG-105NP study committee prepared a comprehensive manual of test administration and scoring methods for the neurobehavioral tests and parent-completed questionnaires.

The combination of tests was selected to provide a comprehensive assessment of neurobehavioral functioning and to address questions related to sequelae within the context of the clinical trial. Intelligence and academic achievement have been the most commonly assessed abilities in reports of neurobehavioral effects of childhood ALL and its therapy. These abilities, as well as cognitive and motor development in pre-school age children, were measured with some of the most widely accepted tests in their respective age ranges. Late neurobehavioral sequelae reported in ALL patients have most often included significant visual-spatial and visual-motor deficits, attentional and memory abnormalities, and learning difficulties [5]. These abilities were assessed by a more comprehensive and refined set of measures than previously used in other studies. Tests of receptive language at semantic and syntactic levels, measuring vocabulary and grammatic comprehension, respectively, were included, but not at the phonemic level, as speech discrimination abnormalities have rarely been reported in ALL patients. Expressive functions (e.g, naming and fluency) often sensitive to brain injuries of many etiologies [17] were also assessed. Social and behavioral functioning was assessed by two parent- and one teacher-completed checklists, all with proven reliability and validity in child development research. Tests in the CCG-105NP study have been utilized with numerous pediatric patient groups, including children with head trauma, developmental delays, and learning difficulties [18].

Tests selected for the neurobehavioral assessments are listed below. For the reader, they have been categorized according to the primary neurobehavioral system assessed by each test. In some past and future data analyses, various tests

Neurobehavioral Tests and Parent-Completed Questionnaires

Neurobehavioral measures that assess a broad range of higher cortical abilities were used in the CCG-105NP study. In addition to standardized intelligence tests, measures to assess cognitive and motor development in pre-school age children, as well as attention, visual-spatial perception, visuoconstructive and fine motor coordination, expressive and receptive language abilities, memory, school achievement, and behavior in older children were included. Neurocognitive, motor, and behavioral measures were selected from the many suitable ones using several criteria: (1) availability of normative standards on normal children; (2) availability of measures that are reasonably comparable across the developmental period of the children enrolled on study; and (3) availability of objective scoring criteria. Practical considerations, such as time required to administer the neurobehavioral test protocol, also influenced the choice of procedures. Other considerations included ease of test administration in a uniform manner, the amount of equipment needed,

and subtests (e.g., in the Wechsler scales) may be broadly categorized, as a single test may involve more than one neurobehavioral system. For example, the Trail Making Test is considered a measure of complex attention/concentration, but it also involves visual-spatial perception, fine motor coordination, and language[17]. The age range designated for use of each test is expressed in years. Note that the protocol of tests for an individual patient depended on chronological age at the time of testing. Additional information about each test, including normative data, is referenced accordingly.

Early cognitive and motor development

Minnesota Child Development Inventory (1.0–3.0)[19]

McCarthy Scales of Children's Abilities (3.0–6.5)[20]

Intelligence

Wechsler Intelligence Scale for Children - Revised (6.5–17.0)[21]

Wechsler Adult Intelligence Scale - Revised (17.0 & above)[22]

Attention/concentration

Freedom from Distractibility Triad (6.5 & above) [18]

Trail Making Test (7.0 above)[23]

Visual spatial perception

Visual Form Discrimination—F (6.0 & above) [24]

Visual memory

Visual Form Discrimination—G (6.0 & above) [24]

Revised Visual Retention Test (8.0 & above) [25]

Visuoconstructive/fine motor coordination

Developmental Test of Visual-Motor Integration (4.0 & above)[26]

Grooved Pegboard (5.0 & above)[27]

Language—receptive

Peabody Picture Vocabulary Test—Revised (4.0 & above) [28]

Token Test for Children (4.0 & above)[29]

Language—expressive

Rapid Automatized Naming (5.0 & above) [30]

Word Fluency (6.0 & above)[31]

Auditory memory

Sentence Repetition (4.0 & above)[32]

Rey Auditory Verbal Learning (6.0 & above)[33]

Academic achievement

Reading/Understanding (7.0 & above)[34]

Wide Range Achievement Test—Revised (6.0 & above)[35]

Behavior and social functioning

Child Behavior Checklist—Parent (4.0 & above)[36]

Child Behavior Checklist—Teacher (6.0 & above)[37]

Personality Inventory for Children—Short Form (4.0 & above)[38]

Following receipt of informed consent, each patient was assessed with an age-determined protocol from the tests above, and the parent/caretaker accompanying the child completed a sociodemographic questionnaire, requesting information about occupation, a brief description of job duties, and education. Each parent's employment status was rated according to the Revised Duncan Scale, TSE12, an occupation-based measure of social status [39]. This system was selected because of its current approach to social stratification and to the increasing complexities of parental socioeconomic status and its association to neurobehavioral development. The sociodemographic questionnaire was completed at each assessment. In addition, a two-way release of information was requested from each parent/caretaker of school-age patients to obtain grades, school achievement test results, completion of Child Behavior Checklist-Teacher, and to provide a report to the patient's school, if desired.

Results

Analyses have focused on data obtained at 9 months after diagnosis. The CCG-105 therapeutic trial has shown that DI in the BFM regimens is a critical treatment component for improved survival [3]. Thus, in addition to CXRT vs no CXRT analyses, developmental outcome indices in two age groups were compared using analysis of variance tests for the DI and no DI groups to determine whether the additional chemotherapy in that phase of treatment had any early effects on neurobehavioral functioning. Analysis of covariance tests (ANCOVA) were performed to determine any influence of age, gender and socioeconomic factors. Since the 9-month data were to represent "baseline" functioning for the longitudinal aspects of the study, few, if any, differences were anticipated between treatment sub-groups.

At 9 months after diagnosis, preliminary data analyses revealed only one significant difference in neurobehavioral functioning possibly associated with DI. Children 3–6.5 years old ($\bar{x} = 4.62$ years, $SD = 0.94$) who received DI performed significantly less well on the Beery Developmental Test of Visual Motor Integration than children who did not receive DI ($p < .02$). There were no significant differences between the groups on the McCarthy Scales of Children's Abilities. Peabody Picture Vocabulary Test—Revised, or Token Test. Means and standard deviations of the neurobehavioral tests for the 3–6.5 year old age group with regard to the DI vs. no DI comparison are presented in Table 3. There were no significant differences in cognitive and motor functioning associated with DI in patients 6.5 years old and above.

With respect to analyses concerning CXRT vs. no CXRT, there were statistically significant differences on the Motor Scale Index of the McCarthy Scales of Children's Abilities ($F(1,71) = 4.42$; $p < .05$) and the Token Test, a test of attention and syntax comprehension ($F(1,49) = 4.72$; $p < .05$) for children 3–6.5 years of age [40]. Children who received CXRT and IT MTX performed less adequately than children who received only IT MTX as CNS-directed therapy. These differences were independent of the child's age, gender, and family socioeconomic status. Means and standard deviations for the neurobehavioral tests with regard to the CXRT vs. no CXRT comparison for children 3–6.5 years of age are presented in Table 4. In contrast, the number of significant differences ($n = 3$) in neurobehavioral test performances in children 6.5 years old and above (chronological age $\bar{x} =$ 12.2 years) was approximately that expected by chance [41]. Data for the older group of subjects are presented in Tables 5 and 6.

In summary, findings from analyses at 9 months after diagnosis of ALL showed no significant effects of DI on cognitive functioning in two age groups. There was a possible effect of DI on fine motor coordination in the children 3–6.5 years of age. Similarly, there were significant differences on cognitive and motor tests between children 3–6.5 years old who received CXRT when those in the non-CXRT group, suggesting that gross motor abilities and attentional processes were affected at 9 months after diag-

Table 3. Neurobehavioral test performance of children 3-6.5 years old with ALL at 9 months after diagnosis comparison by delayed intensification (regimens A and B) vs no delayed intensification (regimens C and D)

Neurobehavioral test	Delayed intensification		No delayed intensification	
	Mean	SD	Mean	SD
MSCA GCI ($N = 74$)	98.83	(16.69)	101.82	(17.20)
Verbal	50.51	(9.45)	53.36	(11.78)
Perceptual-performance	47.46	(10.35)	50.05	(10.20)
Quantitative	48.60	(9.03)	48.72	(8.86)
Memory	47.34	(8.35)	49.15	(8.47)
Motor	43.83	(9.82)	46.97	(9.50)
Token Test ($N = 51$)	499.19	(6.43)	500.04	(5.71)
PPVT-R ($N = 52$)	102.67	(14.61)	101.16	(15.30)
VMI ($N = 50$)*	7.48	(2.50)	9.32	(2.51)

Not all patients have reported results from all tests
MSCA, McCarthy Scales of Children's Abilities; GCI, General Cognitive Index; PPVT-R, Peabody Picture Vocabulary Test'Revised; VMI, Beery Developmental Test of Visual-Motor Integration.
*$p < .02$

Table 4. Neurobehavioral test performance of children 3-6.5 years old with ALL at 9 months after diagnosis: comparisons by CNS-directed treatment regimen

Neurobehavioral test	CXRT plus IT MTX		IT MIX	
	Mean	SD	Mean	SD
MSCA GCI ($N=74$)	97.13	(19.27)	103.67	(13.67)
Verbal	50.51	(11.57)	53.51	(9.81)
Perceptual-performance	47.19	(11.51)	50.46	(8.74)
Quantitative	47.11	(10.08)	50.22	(8.00)
Memory	47.64	(9.47)	48.94	(7.25)
Motor*	43.16	(9.66)	47.83	(9.32)
Token Test ($N=51$)*	498.00	(6.41)	501.56	(5.04)
PPVT-R ($N=52$)	101.85	(16.58)	102.04	(13.02)
VMI ($N=50$)	8.23	(2.47)	8.58	(2.87)

Not all patients have reported results from all tests
*$p<.05$ Adapted from: MacLean et al. Arch Neuro 52: 156-160 Copyright 1995, the American Medical Association.

Table 5. Intelligence and academic achievement test performance of children 6.5 years old and above with ALL at 9 months after diagnosis: comparisons by CNS-directed treatment regimen

Neurobehavioral test	CXRT plus IT MTX ($N=23$)	IT MTX ($N=19$)	F^a
WISC-R/WAIS-R			
VIQ	107.4	103.7	0.40
PIQ	108.4	101.8	1.73
FSIQ	108.9	103.1	1.32
WRAT-R			
Reading	98.0	99.3	0.04
Spelling	95.6	95.9	0.01
Arithmetic	97.4	98.9	0.64
K-ABC			
Reading/ understanding	108.0	111.3	0.64

Scores are mean standard scores, independent of socioeconomic status and age
Adapted from [41]. Copyright 1994, Lawrence Erlbaum Associates, Inc.
[a]Based on analysis of covariance with family socioeconomic status and patient chronological age as covariates
*$p<.05$ WISC-R, Wechsler Intelligence Scale for Children—Revised;
WAIS-R, Wechsler Adult Intelligence Scale—Revised;
WRAT-R, Wide Range Achievement Test—Revised;
K-ABC, Kaufman Assessment Battery for Children

nosis. In patients 6 years old and above, ANCOVA tests associated family socioeconomic status (17 of 40 test comparisons, $p<.05$) and age (11 of 40 test comparisons, $p<.05$) with neurobehavioral outcome at 9 months after diagnosis, regardless of CNS treatment regimen. These findings are not surprising, as age at diagnosis of ALL has often been associated with neurobehavioral test performance [5], and numerous studies involving medical conditions have shown that family member characteristics may affect measures of child development [18]. How these factors mediate developmental outcome will require analyses with data from subsequent examinations.

Table 6. Neurobehavioral test performance of children 6.5 years old and above with ALL at 9 months after diagnosis: comparisons by CNS-directed treatment regimen

Neurobehavioural test	CXRT plus IT MTX ($N=23$)	IT MTX ($N=19$)	F
Attention/Concentration			
WISC-R/WAIS-R (scaled score)			
Arithmetic	10.9	10.7	0.01
DigitSpan	9.4	9.4	0.06
Coding/Digit Symbol	10.6	9.5	1.48
Trail Making A (time)	18.4	21.3	1.32
Trail Making B (time)	52.9	47.3	0.44
Visual spatial perception			
VFD-F (raw score)	13.0	14.3	1.21
WISC-R/WAIS-R (scaled score)			
Picture Completion	10.8	10.5	0.06
Visual memory			
VFD-G (raw score)	11.1	12.3	0.01
Visual Retention Test (raw score)	6.8	6.1	0.00
Visuoconstructive/fine motor coordination			
VMI (standard score)	9.2	7.8	1.72
Grooved Pegboard (time)			
Dominant hand	59.5	66.6	3.00
Non-dominant hand	66.9	72.1	2.28
WISC-R WAIS-R (scaled score)			
Block Design	11.1	10.5	0.33
Object Assembly	12.3	10.0	7.12*
Picture Arrangement	11.1	10.6	0.22
Language, receptive			
PPVT-R (standard score)	104.4	105.4	0.02
Token Test (age-scaled score)	501.0	502.6	0.80
Language, expressive			
Rapid Automatized Naming (time)			
Numbers	29.8	23.4	1.09
Letters	33.5	24.3	0.94
Colors	42.3	37.6	0.39
Objects	53.1	47.7	0.56
Word Fluency (total raw score)	30.6	30.0	0.80
WISC-R/WAIS-R (scaled score)			
Similarities	11.7	11.5	0.06
Vocabulary	11.4	10.9	0.15
Comprehension	11.2	10.2	0.90
Auditory memory			
Sentence Repetition (raw score)	12.8	14.2	4.02*
Rey AVLT (raw score)			
Trial 1	5.4	6.6	1.77
Trial 2	8.0	9.1	0.17
Trial 3	9.8	9.8	0.63
Trial 4	10.5	11.2	0.22
Trial 5	10.8	12.4	4.30
Delayed Recall	10.1	10.4	4.68*

Table 6 (*Contd.*)

Neurobehavioural test	CXRT plus IT MTX ($N=23$)	IT MTX ($N=19$)	F
Long term memory			
WISC-R/WAIS-R (Scaled score)			
Information	10.2	9.2	0.60

Scores are mean raw, standard, or scaled scores, as indicated, independent of socioeconomic status and age. Time is indicated in seconds, with higher scores representing poorer performance.
Adapted from [41] Copyright 1994, Lawrence Erlbaum Associates, Inc.
*$p=.05$ VFD, Visual For, Discrimination; Rey AVLT, Rey Auditory Verbal Learning Test
[a]Based on analysis of covariance with family socioeconomic status and patients chronological age as covariates

Discussion

The few significant findings associated with the use of DI and CXRT reported here should be considered with some caution, as no other prospective study has reported such early effects of these treatments on children's neurobehavioral functioning. Previously published research would strongly suggest that neurobehavioral sequelae will become apparent with subsequent assessments, especially in younger children and those patients who received CXRT as a part of CNS-directed treatment [5]. The long-term effects of DI are more uncertain, however, particularly when combined with CNS-directed therapy including CXRT. The early finding associated with DI reported here is most likely due to transient peripheral nervous system effects of the vincristine doses (1.5 mg/m^2, 2.0 mg maximum) during induction and DI for patients on regimens A and B. (An additional dose of vincristine was given during consolidation to patients on regimen B.) If this finding is, indeed, peripheral in nature, these effects would be expected to resolve after discontinuation of treatment. If, however, this finding is proven to include CNS abnormalities, we speculate that vincristine and dexamethasone, both given systemically in DI, play a major role in producing these effects, because of physiologic evidence documenting penetration of the blood-brain barrier [42, 43].

CCG-105NP is the largest neurobehavioral study of childhood leukemia patients ever conducted, with findings relevant to cognitive, motor, and behavioral functioning, both at home and school. We are unaware of any other prospective neurobehavioral study within the context of childhood ALL featuring randomized assignment to both intensified systemic chemotherapy and CNS-directed treatment regimens. The CCG-105NP study focuses primarily on comparisons of cognitive, motor, and behavioral functioning of patients receiving CNS-directed therapy consisting of IT MTX, with or without 1800 cGy CXRT. Almost all previously published studies of neurobehavioral outcome concern patients treated with 2400 cGy (see Table 1 for selected prospective studies). One recently published report from a randomized trial using 1800 cGy CXRT [44] found no significant differences associated with age at diagnosis and comparable decreases in cognitive functioning and arithmetic achievement, whether or not CXRT was part of the treatment [16]. That study, like many others of its kind before it, described neurobehavioral outcome in limited terms (IQ and academic achievement) and provided no information upon which to generate any educational or psychosocial interventions.

The CCG-105NP study cannot be compared to others of its kind for additional reasons. More specifically, the substantial differences in systemic ALL therapy given to patients in previous studies compound the methodologic problems summarized earlier to make generalization of findings even more difficult. Most systemic chemotherapy schedules now include prolonged and intensified chemotherapy early in treatment, while duration of maintenance has been reduced for some trials. The considerable variation among therapy regimens depends also on definitions of risk and the treatment strategies of a pediatric cancer centre or cooperative group. The most important aspect of current ALL therapy which may affect neurobehavioral outcome is the timing and the frequency of IT MTX doses, which are now derived from age and CNS volume rather than from body surface area [45]. This factor, and intensive BFM systemic chemotherapy, have yet to be studied in terms of neurobehavioral sequelae. Thus, our study of ALL patients following intensive and prolonged induc tion/consolidation and delayed intensification is contemporary and, at the same time, addresses methodological weaknesses in previous studies.

For a significant proportion of ALL patients considered at high risk of treatment failure, CXRT plays vital role in modern treatment regimens designed to produce long-term survival. In some high-risk groups, however, very high dose intravenous MTX combined with IT MTX [46], intermediate dose MTX[47], or triple IT therapy [48] has been used effectively for CNS-directed treatment. For other high-risk subgroups, recent therapeutic trials indicated that CXRT cannot be eliminated without possible compromise in patient outcome. For example, in CCG-123, patients with lymphomatous presentation, a sub-group with a high rate of CNS relapse, were shown to benefit from CXRT if they received less than optimal systemic chemotherapy [49]. Another randomized therapeutic trial, ALL-BFM 81, showed that in a group of standard-risk patients, a subset had significantly higher event-free survival ($p < .0003$) when CXRT was included in CNS directed treatment [2]. Subsequent ALL-BFM trials have retained CXRT in all but the best prognosis category, and have tested a lower dose of CXRT (1,200 cGy vs 1,800 cGy) [50]. An optimal therapeutic dose of CXRT (i.e., the lowest dose which permits satisfactory freedom from CNS relapse) has not been determined.

Results from the CCG-105NP study should prove helpful in judging the risk-benefit issue in the higher risk ALL populations, where some degree of disease-free survival advantage may come from using CXRT. This study also provides a longitudinal perspective of any neurobehavioral effects associated with intensified systemic chemotherapy and IT MTX, with or without CXRT. Clinical researchers can then evaluate such disease-free survival advantage relative to other potential issues in patient funztioning associated with the addition of irradiation treatment.

Acknowledgments. The authors are very grateful to Lucia Noll and Alan Nicoll, whose assistance and expertise are considered special contributions to the preparation of this manuscript.

References

1. Henze G., Langermann H.J., Bramswig J., Breu H., Gadner H., Schellong G., Welte K., Riehm H. (1981). Ergebnisse der Studie BFM 76/79 zur Behandlung der akuten lymphoblastischen Leukämie bei Kindern und Jugendlichen. Klin Pädiat 193: 145–154.
2. Riehm H., Gadner H., Henze G., Kornhuber B., Lampert F., Niethammer D., Reiter A., Schellong G. (1990). Results and significance of six randomized trials in four consecutive ALL-BFM trials. In Büchner T., Schellong G., Hiddemann W., Ritter J. (eds) Haematology and Blood Transfusion. Berlin, Springer-Verlag: 33: 439–450.
3. Tubergen D.G., Gilchrist G.S., O'Brien R.T., Coccia P.F., Sather H.N., Waskerwitz M.J., Hammond G.D.(1993). Improved outcome with delayed intensification for children with acute lymphoblastic leukemia and intermediate presenting features: A Children Cancer Group Phase III Trial. J Clin Oncol 11: 527–537.
4. Tubergen D.G., Gilchrist G.S., O'Brien R.T.,Coccia P.F., Sather H.N., Waskerwitz M.J., Hammond G.D. (1993). Prevention of CNS disease in intermediate-risk acute lymphoblastic leukemia: comparision of cranial radiation and intrathecal methotrexate and the importance of systemic therapy. A childrens Cancer Group report. J Clin Oncol 11: 520–526.
5. Stehbens J.A., Kaleita T.A., Noll R.B., MacLean W.E., O'Brien R.T., Waskerwitz M.J., Hammond G.D. (1991). CNS prophylaxis of childhood leukemia: What are the long-term neurological, neuropsychological and behavioral effects? Neuropsych Rev 2: 147–177.
6. Butler R.W., Copeland D.R.(1993). Neuropsychological effects of central nervous system prophylactic treatment in childhood leukemia: methodological considerations. J Ped Psych 18: 319–338.
7. Meadows A.T., Massari D.J., Fergusson J. (1981). Declines in IQ scores and cognitive dysfunction in children with acute lymphocytic leukemia treated with cranial irradiation. Lancet 2: 1015–1018.
8. Stehbens J.A., Kisker C.T., Wilson B.K. (1983). Achievement and intelligence test-retest performance in pediatric cancer patients at diagnosis and one year later. J Ped Psych 8: 47–56.
9. Stehbens J.A., Kisker C.T. (1984). Intelligence and achievement testing in childhood cancer: Three years post diagnosis. JDBP 5: 184–188.
10. Copeland D.R., Dowell R.E., Fletcher J.M., Sullivan M.P., Jaffe N., Cangir A., Frankel L.S., Judd B.W. (1988). Neuropsychological test performance of

pediatric cancer patients at diagnosis and one year later. J Ped Psych 13: 183–196.
11. Kaleita T.A., Shields W.D., Tesler A., Feig S.A. (1989). Normal neurodevelopment in four young children treated with bone marrow transplantation for acute leukemia or aplastic anemia. Pediatrics 83: 753–757.
12. Walther B., Gutjahr P., Beron G. (1981). Therapiebegleitende and überdauernde neurologische und neuropsychologische Diagnostik bei akuter lymphoblastischer Leukämie im Kindesalter. Klin Pädiat 193: 177–83.
13. Berg R.A., Ch'ien L.T., Bowman W.P., Ochs J., Lancaster W., Goff J.R. (1983). The neuropsychological effects of acute lymphoblastic leukemia and its treatment-a three year report. Intellectual functioning and academic achievement. Clin Neuropsych 5: 9–13.
14. Brouwers P., Moss H., Reaman G., McGuire T., Turpin E., Libow J., Tarnowski K., Bleyer A., Feusner J., Ruymann F.B., Miser J., Hammond D., Poplack D. (1987). Central nervous system preventive therapy with systemic high dose methotrexate vs cranial irradiation and intrathecal methotrexate: longitudinal comparison of effects of treatment on intellectual function of children with actue lymphoblastic leukemia. Proc Am Soc Clin Oncol 6: 158.
15. Brouwers P., Moss H., Reaman G., McGuire T., Turpin E., Libow J., Tarnowski K., Bleyer A., Feusner J., Ruymann F.B., Miser J., Hammond D., Poplack D. (1988). Central nervous system preventive therapy with systemic high dose methotrexate versus cranial radiation and intrathecal methotrexate: comparison of effects of treatment on academic achievement in children with acute lymphoblastic leukemia. Proc Am Soc Clin Oncol 7: 176.
16. Ochs J., Mulhern R., Fairclough D., Parvey L., Whitaker J., Ch'ien L., Mauer A., Simone J. (1991). Comparison of neuropsychologic functioning and clinical indicators of neurotoxicity in long-term survivors of childhood leukemia given cranial radiation or parenteral methotrexate: a prospective study. J Clin Oncol 9: 145–151.
17. Lezak M. (1983). Neuropsychological assessment (2nd ed.) New York: Oxford University Press.
18. Sattler J.M. (1988). Assessment of children (3rd edition). San Diego: Jerome M. Sattler, Publisher.
19. Ireton H. Thwing E. (1974). Minnesota Child Development Inventory. Minneapolis: Behavior Science Systems.
20. McCarthy D.(1972). McCarthy Scales of Children's Abilities. New York: The Psychological Corporation.
21. Wechsler D. (1974). Wechsler Intelligence Scale for Children—Revised. New York: Psychological Corporation.
22. Wechsler D. (1981). Wechsler Adult Intelligence Scale—Revised. New York: Psychological Corporation.
23. Klonoff H., Low M. (1974). Disordered brain function in young children and early adolescents: Neuropsychological and electroencephalographic correlates. In Reitan R., Davison L. (eds) Clinical neuropsychology: current status and applications. Washington, D.C.: V.H. Winston and Sons, pp. 167–178.
24. Benton A., deHamsher K., Varney N., Spreen O. (1983). Contributions to neuropsychological assessment. New York: Oxford University Press.
25. Benton A. (1974). Revised Visual Retention Test: clinical and experimental applications (4th ed.). New York: Psychological Corporation.
26. Beery K. (1982). Revised administation, scoring, and teaching manual for the Developmental Test of Visual-Motor Integration. Cleveland: Modern Curriculum Press.
27. Trites R.L. (1977). Neuropsychological test manual. Ottawa: Royal Ottawa Hospital.
28. Dunn L., Dunn L. (1981). Peabody Picture Vocabulary Test. Circle Pines, MN: American guidance service.
29. De Simoni F.G. (1978). The Token Test for children. Hingham, MA: Teaching Resources.
30. Denckla M., Rudel R. (1974). Rapid 'automatized' naming of pictured objects, colors, letters, and numbers by normal children. Cortex 10: 185–202.
31. Spreen O., Gaddes W. (1969). Developmental norms for 15 neuropsychological tests age 6 to 15. Cortex 5: 171–191.
32. Carmichael J.A., MacDonald J.W. (1984). Developmental norms for the Sentence Repetition Test. J Consult Clin Psych 52: 476–477.
33. Rey A. (1964). L'examen Clinique en Psychologie. Paris: Presses Universitaires de France.
34. Kaufman A., Kaufman N. (1983). Kaufman Assessment Battery for Children. Circle Pines, MN: American Guidance Service.
35. Jastak J.F., Jastak S. (1978). Wide Range Achievement Test—Revised Edition. Wilmington, DE: Jastak Associates, Inc.
36. Achenback T.M. (1991a). Manual for the Child Behavior Checklist/4-18 and 1991 Profile. Burlington, VT: University of Vermont Department of Psychiatry.
37. Achenbach T.M. (1991b). Manual for the Teacher's Report Form and 1991 Profile. Burlington, VT: University of Vermont Department of Psychiatry.
38. Wirt R.D., Seat P.D., Broen W.E., Lachar D. (1981). Personality Inventory for Children. Los Angeles: Western Psychological Services.
39. Stevens G., Featherman D. (1981). A revised socioeconomic index of occupational status. Soc Sci Res 10; 364–395.
40. MacLean W.E., Noll R.B., Stehbens J.A., Kaleita T.A., Schwartz E., Whitt J.K., Cantor N.L., Waskerwitz M.J., Ruymann F.B., Novak L.J., Woodard A., Hammond G.D. for the Children's Cancer Group (1995). Neuropsychological effects of cranial irradiation in young children with acute lymphoblastic leukemia 9 months after diagnosis. Arch Neuro 52: 156–160.
41. Stehbens J.A., MacLean W.E., Kaleita T.A., Noll R.B., Schwartz E., Cantor N.L., Woodard A., Whitt J.K., Waskerwitz M.J., Ruymann F.B., Hammond

G.D.(1994). Effects of CNS prophylaxis on theneuropsychological performance of children with acute lymphoblastic leukemia: nine months post diagnosis. Child Health Care 23: 231-250.
42. Kaleita T.A., Nuwer M., Falk P., Kiersch M.E., Shields W.D. (1988). Neuropsychologic and neurophysiologic CNS abnormalities associated with vincristine during therapy for acute lymphoblastic leukemia. Med Ped Onc 16: 450-451.
43. Balis F.M., Lester C.M., Chrousos, G.P. (1987). Differences in cerebrospinal fluid penetration of corticosteroids: possible relationship to the prevention of meningeal leukemia. J Clin Oncol 5: 202-207.
44. Abromowitch M., Ochs J., Pui C., Kalwinsky D., Rivera G., Fairclough D., Look T., Hustu O., Murphy S.B., Evans W.E., Dahl G., Bowman, W.P., (1988). High dose methotrexate improves clinical outcome in children with acute lymphoblastic leukemia: St. Jude Total Therapy Study X. Med Ped Onc 16: 297-303.
45. Bleyer W.A., Coccia P.F., Sather H.N., Level C., Lukens J., Niebrugge D.J., Siegel S., Littman P.S., Leikin S., Miller D.R., Chard R.L., Hammond G.D. (1983). Reduction in central nervous system leukemia with a pharmacokinetically derived intrathecal methotrexate dosage regimen. J Clin Oncol 1: 317-325.
46. Reaman G., Lange B., Feusner J., Heerema N., Steinherz P., Albo V., Zeltzer P., Kaleita T., Bleyer W.A., Sather H., Hammond D. (1989). Intensive systemic and intrathecal chemotherapy improves the outcome for infants with acute lymphoblastic leukemia. Proc Am Soc Clin Oncol 8: 211.
47. Moe P., Seip M., Finne P., Kolmannskoq S. (1984). Intermediate dose MTX in childhood acute lymphoblastic leukemia. Eur Pediatr Haematol Oncol 1: 113-118.
48. Pullen J., Boyett J., Shuster J., Crist W., Land V., Frankel L., Iyer R., Backstrom L., van Eys J., Harris M., Ravindranath Y., Sullivan M. (1993). Extended triple intrathecal chemotherapy trial for prevention of CNS relapse in good-risk and poor-risk patients with B-progenitor acute lymphoblastic leukemia. A Pediatric Oncology Group Study. J Clin Oncol 11: 838-849.
49. Cherlow J.M., Steinherz P.G., Sather H.N., Gaynon P.S., Grossman N.J., Kersey J.M., Johnstone H.S., Breneman J.C., Trigg M.E., Hammond G.D.(1993). The role of radiation therapy in the treatment of acute lymphoblastic leukemia with lymphomatous presentaion: a report from the Childrens Cancer Group. Int J Rad Oncol Biol Phys 27: 1001-1009.
50. Bührer C., Henze G., Hofmann J., Reiter A., Schellong G., Riehm H. (1990). Central nervous system relapse prevention in 1165 standard risk children with acute lymphoblastic leukemia in five BFM trials. In Büchner T., Schellong G., Hiddermann W., Ritter J.(eds) Haematology and Blood Transfusion. Berlin, Springer-Verlag: 33: 500-503.

ALL in Adults

Acute Leukemias VI
Prognostic Factors
and Treatment Strategies
Büchner et al. (eds)

Treatment of Biologically Determined Subsets of Acute Lymphoblastic Leukemia in Adults: Cancer and Leukemia Group B Studies

R.A. Larson[1], R.K. Dodge[2], C.D. Bloomfield[3], and C.A. Schiffer[4]

Abstract. The Cancer and Leukemia Group B (CALGB) has conducted a series of prospective clinical trials in adults with acute lymphoblastic leukemia (ALL). The impact of certain clinical and biological characteristics on the outcome of intensive chemotherapy has been investigated. In this report, the prognostic features of 379 patients entered onto two sequential trials (CALGB 8811 and 9111) are described. A total of 325 (86%) patients achieved a complete remission (CR). A higher CR rate was observed in younger patients (93% for those <30 years old, 86% for those 30–59 years old, and 64% for those ≥60 years old; $p<0.001$), and in those who had a mediastinal mass (98%) or blasts with a T-cell immunophenotype. A total of 83% of B-lineage and 94% of T-cell ALL patients achieved a CR ($p=0.04$). Co-expression of myeloid antigens did not affect the CR rate or remission duration. Of those with cytogenetic or molecular evidence of the Philadelphia (Ph) chromosome, 76% and 87% of those without such evidence achieved a CR ($p=0.08$). The median survival for all patients is 28 months, and 47% (95% confidence interval, CI, 40%–54%) of all patients are estimated to be alive at 3 years. The median remission duration for the 325 CR patients is also 28 months. Favourable pretreatment characteristics relative to remission duration or survival are younger age, the presence of a mediastinal mass, white blood cell (WBC) count <30000/µl, T or TMy immunophenotype, and the absence of the Ph chromosome. The estimates for the proportion surviving at 3 years are 66% for patients <30 years old, 36% for those 30–59 years old, 84% for those with a mediastinal mass, 54% with WBC <30000/µl, 65% with T or TMy antigen expression, and 52% for those who lack the Ph chromosome. Twenty-two patients (6%) had no unfavourable prognostic features and have an estimated probability of survival at 3 years of 91% (95% CI, 66%–98%). Patients with high-risk features are now being selected for additional therapy.

Introduction

The Cancer and Leukemia Group B (CALGB) has conducted a series of clinical trials in adults with acute lymphoblastic leukemia (ALL) with several specific aims. The primary objective has been to increase the initial complete response rate since the potential for cure exists only after a complete response. Secondly, several postremission regimens have been evaluated for their ability to prolong relapse-free survival by using multi-agent intensive consolidation chemotherapy. Thirdly, the impact of certain biological characteristics, such as immunophenotype, cytogenetics, and molecular genetic features, has been investigated in order to identify more homogeneous subsets of ALL of prognostic importance. Details of these studies have been published [1–8]. This report describes what we have learned.

[1]Section of Hematology/Oncology, Department of Medicine, The University of Chicago, Chicago, IL 60637, USA
[2]The Cancer and Leukemia Group B Statistical Center, Durham, NC 27705, USA
[3]Roswell Park Cancer Institute, Buffalo, NY 14263, USA
[4]University of Maryland Cancer Center, Baltimore, MD 21201, USA

Throughout each of these group-wide studies, there has been central review of pretreatment bone marrow samples for morphology and cytochemical features. In addition, two central laboratories have performed immunophenotyping by flow cytometry. A large series of prospectively studied patients with adult ALL whose lymphoblasts expressed one or more myeloid antigens was described by the CALGB in 1987 [4]. Our findings indicated that myeloid antigen expression occurred more frequently in adult ALL than previously realized, and identified possible high-risk subgroups that could not be defined by conventional cytologic and cytochemical evaluations. Using the treatment prescribed in study 8011, the presence of myeloid antigens was associated with a lower complete remission (CR) rate and shorter survival [4].

More recently, a subset of acute leukemia has been identified as minimally differentiated acute myeloid leukemia and later defined by the French-American-British (FAB) Cooperative Group as AML-MO [9]. These malignant cells lack lymphoid surface markers but usually have FAB-L2 morphology and are negative for myeloperoxidase or Sudan Black B reactivity. Thus, patients with AML-MO have often found their way into ALL clinical trials in the past where their outcome has been poor. FAB-MO cases by definition do not express lymphoid-specific markers. They may be positive for terminal deoxynucleotidal transferase (TdT) reactivity and CD7 expression, but these markers are not specific for lymphoblasts. In contrast, these AML-MO cells are positive for CD13 or CD33 or other myeloid markers, suggesting a minimal level of differentiation along the granulocytic pathway. When we carefully exclude such patients with minimally differentiated AML (FAB type MO) and use more intensive chemotherapy, we now find no important differences in the response rates, remission duration, or survival of ALL patients who have co-expression of CD13 or CD33 [4,6]. In general, the course of these patients appears to be determined by their lymphoid lineage, that is, B-lymphocyte or T-cell.

For several years, the CALGB has performed molecular analyses on pretreatment leukemia samples in central laboratories to determine in a prospective fashion the incidence and prognostic importance of immunoglobulin and T-cell receptor gene rearrangements and the BCR-ABL rearrangement associated with the Philadelphia (Ph) chromosome [5-7]. These results have been compared to cytogenetic data obtained through the central CALGB karyotype review process. In a prospective trial, molecular methods detected the BCR-ABL fusion gene in 30% of ALL cases, compared to cytogenetic detection of the Ph chromosome in 23% [5]. The Ph chromosome and/or the BCR-ABL rearrangement were found in almost half of the B-lineage ALL cases but in none of the T-cell cases. The majority of the BCR-ABL-positive cases (76%) were of the p190 subtype. Despite a nearly equivalent CR rate, the disease-free survival of Ph^+ ALL patients was clearly inferior to those without this genetic mutation [5,6]. Indeed, once this subgroup is reliably identified and considered separately, the estimated 3-year survival of the remaining B-lineage ALL patients improves and does not differ significantly from the survival of similarly evaluated patients with T-lineage ALL [6].

In this report, we describe the outcome of 379 adults with ALL treated in two sequential CALGB trials (8811 and 9111) using an intensive remission induction and consolidation chemotherapy program, followed by maintenance therapy lasting for 2 years from diagnosis. Detailed univariate and multivariate analyses have been performed to evaluate the impact of pretreatment clinical and biological characteristics of each patient as a determinant for their response, remission duration, and overall survival [6].

CALGB Studies 8811 and 9111

Patient Selection

Patients were eligible if they had untreated ALL of any of the three FAB subtypes or acute undifferentiated leukemia. Patients were registered by telephone with the CALGB Statistical Office prior to treatment. The diagnosis of ALL was confirmed by central review of blood smears and bone marrow specimens for cytologic and cytochemical features according to the FAB criteria [10]. Central immunophenotyping and pathology review were required. It was recommended that pretreatment blood and bone marrow specimens be submitted for cytogenetic analysis, including central review of the karyotypes (CALGB study 8461), and for molecular analysis for the presence of the BCR-ABL fusion gene (CALGB study 8762). Leukemia cells were analyzed in the central laboratory by Southern blot and pulsed field gel electrophoresis and polymerase chain reaction for rearrangements within the BCR gene according to previously reported methods, using conditions which will detect both the p190 and the p210 subtypes [5]. A lumbar puncture for cerebro spinal fluid (CSF) examination was not recommended at diagnosis for asymptomatic patients. However, patients with symptomatic central nervous system (CNS) leukemia were not excluded but received additional CNS therapy. All patients were older than 15 years, had adequate renal and hepatic function (< two fold elevated above the normal range unless felt to be due to leukemia infiltration), and had provided informed consent.

Immunophenotyping (CALGB study 8364) was performed in two central CALGB laboratories. In a small number of cases where the pretreatment specimen was not evaluable in the central laboratory, immunophenotyping data from the local institutions were used after central review. Flow cytometric analysis and a panel of monoclonal antibodies were used for indirect immunofluorescence. The criterion for surface marker positivity was expression by at least 20% of the leukemia blast cell population. B-lineage antigen expression was defined as CD19 or CD20 positivity; T-lineage antigen expression as CD5 or CD2 reactivity; and myeloid antigen (My) expression as CD13 or CD33 positivity. Expression of the common ALL antigen (CALLA) was assessed by CD10 reactivity. Cases expressing combinations of both B-lineage and T-lineage antigens were classified as BT, BTMy, or miscellaneous. Cases expressing surface membrane immunoglobulin (SmIg) were considered FAB-L3 (Burkitt-type ALL) and were not included among the other B-lineage cases in subsequent analyses. Patients with myeloperoxidase-negative blasts that expressed only myeloid antigens (and not B- or T-lymphoid antigens) were reclassified as AML-MO and deemed to be ineligible.

Treatment Protocol

The chemotherapy drugs and dosages used in the induction, consolidation, and maintenance phases of treatment on study 8811 are listed in Table 1 [6]. Study 9111 used exactly the same chemotherapy regimen but, in addition, patients were assigned in a double-blind fashion prior to treatment to receive filgrastim (granulocyte-colony stimulating factor, G-CSF) or a placebo during the induction and early intensification courses (i.e., during the first 3 months of treatment) [8].

The total duration of treatment was 24 months. Testicular biopsies were not required at the end of therapy, and testicular radiation was not given prophylactically. Radiation therapy was not used to treat mediastinal masses. Patients who had an isolated CNS relapse while continuing in marrow remission were counted as failures; however, they continued to receive systemic chemotherapy on protocol after suppression of CSF lymphoblasts with additional intrathecal chemotherapy. No hematopoietic growth factors were used in study 8811, and none were used in study 9111 after completion of the first 3 months of chemotherapy. Co-trimoxazole or aerosolized pentamidine were recommended for pneumocystis prophylaxis, starting in course 3. The use of oral non-absorbable antibiotics, the management of febrile episodes and transfusions, and the use of hospitalization were not prescribed by the protocols but rather left to institutional guidelines.

Data Audit

Personnel in CALGB Central Data Management were responsible for quality assurance for all clinical data submitted for this study. Eligibility criteria were verified for all patients, and an evaluation of treatment, response, and toxicity was made by the study chair (R.A. Larson). In addition, as part of the group data monitoring program, members of the CALGB Data Audit Committee made periodic site visits to all institutions to verify compliance with Federal regulations and protocol requirements, including eligibility, treatment, response data, and follow up. All radiotherapy portals and dosimetry records for the cranial irradiation were centrally reviewed for quality control by the Quality Assurance Review Center in Providence, Rhode Island.

Response Criteria

Patients were considered to be in CR when the neutrophil count was > 1500/μl, the platelet count was > 100000/μl, the results of bone marrow examination were normal (including <5% blasts and >25% cellularity), and all extramedullary disease had resolved. Patients with

Table 1. Chemotherapy regimen for acute lymphoblastic leukemia in adults

	Route	Dosage	Given on days
Course 1: induction (4 weeks)			
Cyclophosphamide*	i.v.	1200 mg/m^2	1
Daunorubicin*	i.v.	45 mg/m^2	1,2,3
Vincristine	i.v.	2 mg	1,8,15,22
Prednisone*	p.o./i.v.	60 mg/m^2/d	1–21
L-Asparaginase	s.c.	6000 IU/m^2	5,8,11,15,18,22
*For patients ⩾60 years old			
Cyclophosphamide		800 mg/m^2	1
Daunorubicin		30 mg/m^2	1,2,3
Prednisone		60 mg/m^2/d	1–7
Course 2: early intensification (4 weeks, repeat once)			
Intrathecal methotrexate		15 mg	1
Cyclophosphamide	i.v.	1000 mg/m^2	1
6-Mercaptopurine	p.o.	60 mg/m^2/d	1–14
Cytarabine	s.c.	75 mg/m^2/d	1–4, 8–11
Vincristine	i.v.	2 mg	15,22
L-Asparaginase	s.c.	6000 IU/m^2	15,18,22,25
Course 3: CNS prohylaxiz and interim maintenance (12 weeks)			
Cranial irradiation		2400 cGy	1–12
Intrathecal methotrexate		15 mg	1,8,15,22,29
6-Mercaptopurine	p.o.	60 mg/m^2/d	1–70
Methotrexate	p.o.	20 mg/m^2	36,43,50,57,64
Course 4: late intensification (8 weeks)			
Doxorubicin	i.v.	30 mg/m^2	1,8,15
Vincristine	i.v.	2 mg	1,8,15
Dexamethasone	p.o.	10 mg/m^2/d	1–14
Cyclophosphamide	i.v.	1000 mg/m^2	29
6-Thioguanine	p.o.	60 mg/m^2/d	29–42
Cytarabine	s.c.	75 mg/m^2/d	29–32, 36–39
Course 5: prolonged maintenance (until 24 months from diagnosis)			
Vincristine	i.v.	2 mg	1 of every 4 weeks
Prednisone	p.o.	60 mg/m^2/d	1–5 of every 4 weeks
Methotrexate	p.o.	20 mg/m^2	1,8,15,22
6-Mercaptopurine	p.o.	60 mg/m^2/d	1–28

>25% lymphoblasts remaining in the bone marrow after course 1 were removed from the protocol study. All patients were required to have achieved a CR by half-way through course 2 in order to remain on the study.

Statistical Methods

The proportion of patients achieving a CR to the induction regimen was the primary outcome measure for these studies. The duration of CR and length of survival were additional outcome measures. Differences in proportions of complete responders among patient subgroups were analyzed using Fisher's exact test. The duration of CR was defined to be the time from achieving a CR to relapse (bone marrow, blood, CNS, or testicular), death, or date of last follow up. Patients still at risk, lost to follow up, or withdrawn for bone marrow transplantation (BMT) were censored for the analysis of remission duration. Survival was defined as the time from study entry to death or date of last follow up. Probabilities of surviving and remaining in CR were estimated by the Kaplan-Meier method. Confidence intervals (CI) of 95% for these probabilities and the median survival times were obtained using the method of Simon and Lee. In instances where the median was not defined, the estimate was reported to be greater than the smallest possible time. Differences in survival or remission duration between patient subgroups were tested using the log-rank statistic, adjusted for multiple comparisons where appropriate.

In accordance with the study objectives, the prognostic significance of age, white blood cell

(WBC) count, platelet count, mediastinal mass, organomegaly, lymphadenopathy, FAB classification, immunophenotype, cytogenetics, and molecular analysis was assessed with respect to CR rate and remission duration and survival. For the joint analysis of these variables, regression analyses were used. The analysis of CR rate was carried out using the logistic regression model, while the analyses of CR duration and survival were carried out using the Cox proportional hazards regression model. All reported p values are nominal two-sided values. Analysis was based on all data available as of February 10, 1995.

Results

Patient Accrual

Between September, 1988 and June, 1991, 214 patients were entered on CALGB study 8811 from 25 main member institutions and their affiliated hospitals. Between June, 1991 and June, 1993, 198 patients were entered on CALGB study 9111. After central review of all data, 197 patients and 182 patients, respectively, were eligible and evaluable. These two patient cohorts from sequential trials have been combined for this report because there were no marked differences in eligibility and treatment, and no statistically significant differences have yet been observed in their estimated remission durations nor survivals.

Patient Characteristics

The 379 eligible patients ranged in age from 16 to 80 years, with a median age of 34 years; 53 patients (14%) were 60 years or older. There were 220 males (58%) and 159 females. The performance status was 0 or 1 in 308 patients (81%) and 2–4 in 71 patients. A total of 55% of patients had a fever or infection prior to chemotherapy. Initial WBC counts ranged from 200 to 475000/µl (median 17000/µl), platelet counts from 4000 to 557000/µl (median 50000/µl), and hemoglobin from 4.0 to 16.6 gm/dl (median, 9.7 gm/dl).

Effects of Age, Mediastinal Mass, and WBC Count on Outcome of Therapy

A total of 325 (86%) of the 379 eligible patients achieved a CR (Table 2); 237 (74%) of the responders were in CR within 30 days from the first treatment, 88 (26%) required more than 30 days, either because of slow recovery of marrow cellularity and blood counts or because additional chemotherapy (i.e., course 2) was required. There is a statistically significant difference in remission duration in favor of the rapid respon-

Table 2. Clinical characteristics in relation to complete remission rates, remission durations, and survivals

Parameter	(n)	CR			Remission duration		Survival	
		(n)	(%)	p	Median months	p	Median (months)	p
Total	379	325	86		28		28	
Age (years)								
<30	159	148	93	<.001	35	.003	56	<.001
30–59	167	143	86		25			22
⩾60	53	34	64		8		4	
Mediastinal mass								
Present	44	43	98	.02	>28	.002	>30	<.001
Absent	324	272	84		24		22	
Lymphadenopathy								
Present	140	125	89	.13	>32	.60	39	.04
Absent	223	186	83		26			23
WBC								
<30 000/µl	240	212	88	.002	34	.001	43	<.001
⩾30 000/µl	130	105	81		14		17	
Time to CR								
⩽30 days			237		34	.03	47	.10
>30 days			88		20		30	

ders, but as yet the difference in the proportion of patients alive at 3 years is not statistically significantly different (56% vs. 48%).

Treatment response was a function of age; 93% of patients less than 30 years old achieved a CR compared to 86% of those aged 30–59 years and only 64% of those 60 years and older ($p < 0.001$). Increasing age also had highly significant unfavourable effects on the remission duration and on survival (Table 2).

Forty-four patients (12%) had a mediastinal mass, and 98% of these patients achieved a CR. This was significantly better than the 84% CR rate for those without a mediastinal mass ($p = 0.02$). The presence of a mediastinal mass prior to treatment also had a significant effect on long-term outcome; 66% of these patients were estimated to remain in continuous CR at 3 years ($p = 0.002$), and 84% were estimated to be surviving at 3 years ($p < 0.001$).

A total of 240 patients (65%) had a WBC count $< 30000/\mu l$ at diagnosis, and 88% of these patients achieved a CR. This was significantly better than the 81% CR rate for those with WBC 30,000/μl ($p = 0.002$). In addition, a lower leukocyte count had significant effects on remission duration and survival; 49% of those with WBC $\geqslant 30{,}000/\mu l$ were estimated to be in continuous CR at 3 years ($p = 0.001$), and 54% were estimated to be alive at 3 years $p < 0.001$).

A multivariate analysis was performed for survival estimates, based on 359 patients with complete information for age, sex, presence of a mediastinal mass, lymphadenopathy, leukocytes, and platelets. A stepwise Cox regression analysis identified age, mediastinal mass, and leukocyte count as significant variables in this group of patients. The risk of dying was two fold greater for patients $\geqslant 60$ years old compared to those less than 60 ($p < 0.001$). After adjusting for age, the risk of dying was 4.6-fold greater for those patients without a mediastinal mass compared to those with a mediastinal mass ($p < 0.001$). After adjusting for age and a mediastinal mass, the leukocyte count remained significant, and the risk ratio was 1.9 for patients with WBC $\geqslant 30{,}000/\mu l$ ($p < 0.001$).

Effects of Morphology and Immunophenotype on Outcome

A total of 325 patients could be classified by the pathology review committee using the FAB criteria; 153 patients (41%) were L1, 160 (43%) were L2, and 12 (3%) were L3. Morphological subtyping could not be accomplished in 44 cases (12%), usually because of inadequate marrow aspirate samples, and these were considered unclassifiable acute leukemia. Ten cases were not evaluable for central review.

The CR rate (87%) was exactly the same for the patients with L1 or L2 morphology. There were no statistically significant differences in the remission durations nor in the survivals between these two groups, although trends were present in both outcome measures in favour of the FAB-L1 subset. Patients with FAB-L3 morphology were considered separately because of their small number and also because another CALGB study (9251), specifically designed for these patients, opened for accrual during the study period for these protocols. Ten (83%) of the 12 patients identified by morphology and immunophenotyping as L3 ALL achieved a CR, but the median remission duration was only 3 months, and the median survival was only 6 months.

Immunophenotyping data were available for 264 patients (Table 3). The CR rate was 94% for the 67 patients with a pure T-cell or TMy immunophenotype. This was significantly better than the 83% CR rate for 197 patients with a precursor B-cell or BMy immunophenotype ($p = 0.04$).The remission duration was significantly longer for patients with a T or TMy immunophenotype than for the B-lineage patients; 60% were estimated to remain in continuous CR at 3 years compared to 40% of the latter group ($p = .02$). Survival was also significantly better for the patients with a T or TMy immunophenotype; 65% were estimated to be alive at 3 years compared to 37% of those with a B or BMy immunophenotype ($p < 0.001$). Using this treatment regimen, co-expression of a myeloid antigen on the lymphoblast surface appeared not to alter the outcome. In a multivariate analysis, after adjusting for age, mediastinal mass, and leukocytes, the risk of dying was 1.8-fold greater for patients with a B or BMy immunophenotype compared to those with a T or TMy immunophenotype ($p = 0.03$).

Impact of Cytogenetics and Molecular Analyses on Outcome

Cytogenetic information is available for 165 patients (Table 4). In addition, molecular analyses have been completed on 80 patients. Taken

Table 3. Effects of morphology and immunophenotype on treatment outcome

Parameter	(*n*)	CR			Remission duration		Survival	
		(*n*)	(%)	*p*	Median (months)	*p*	Median (months)	*p*
FAB subtype								
L1	153	133	87	1.00	35	.06	39	.09
L2	160	139	87		21		23	
Immunophenotype								
B	150	126	84	.02	23	.09	19	<.001
T	51	50	98		>28		>40	
BMy	47	38	81		20		22	
TMy	16	13	81		>40		>40	
B or BMy	197	164	83	.04	24	.02	19	<.001
T or TMy	67	63	94		>30		>40	

Table 4. Detection of the Philadelphia chromosome or the BCR-ABL fusion gene and treatment outcome

Parameter	(*n*)	CR			Remissionduration		Survival	
		(*n*)	(%)	*p*	Median (months)	*p*	Median (months)	*p*
Cytogenetics								
Ph^+	48	36	75	.07	10	.01	13	.001
Ph^-	117	102	87		24		23	
Molecular								
$BCR\text{-}ABL^+$	22	15	68	.12	7	<.001	11	<.001
$BCR\text{-}ABL^-$	58	49	84		>30		>30	
Either method								
$Ph^+/BCR\text{-}ABL^+$	55	42	76	.08	9	<.001	13	<.001
Negative	141	123	87		31		38	

together, 55 patients have been identified to have the Ph chromosome or BCR-ABL rearrangement, and 141 patients have been evaluated by one or both of these tests and found not to have this genetic mutation. The CR rate was 76% for the $Ph^+/BCR\text{-}ABL^+$ patients compared to 87% for those without this mutation. This difference was not statistically significant ($p = 0.08$). However, both remission duration and survival were markedly different between these two groups ($p < 0.001$ for both). Only 17% of the patients with $Ph^+/BCR\text{-}ABL^+$ ALL were estimated to remain in continuous CR at 3 years (95% CI, 6%–40%) compared to 48% (95% CI, 37%–59%) of those who were negative by at least one genetic test. Only 16% (95% CI, 7%–32%) of those with either a Ph chromosome or a BCR-ABL rearrangement were estimated to be alive at 3 years compared to 52% (95% CI, 41%–62%) of those who were negative. However, after adjusting for age alone, the presence of Ph/BCR-ABL positivity loses most of its significance for the estimate of survival ($p = 0.06$).

Patients with a t(4;11) or a MLL gene rearrangement (in chromosome band 11q23) are another cytogenetic subset with a poor outcome [6, 11]. Eleven such patients were reported to be enrolled on these protocols (Table 5). Nine were female; five had WBC >200000/μl. All had a B-lineage immunophenotype. Five patients died during the induction chemotherapy or had refractory disease. Of the six complete responders, three have relapsed and two died after BMT.

Cumulative Adverse Risk Factors

It is interesting to consider the number of adverse features that an individual patient had at

Table 5. ALL patients with a t(4;11) or a MLL rearrangement (CALGB 8811/9111)

Age	Sex	WBC (per µl)	Immunophenotype	FAB	Treatment outcome	Survival (months)
64	F	392 200	B	L1	Died in induction	<1
18	F	297 200	B	L1	CR	50+
19	F	253 000	B	L1	CR; relapse (5 months)	9
43	M	19 600	B	L1	Died in induction	<1
61	M	209 800	BMy	L2	Refractory	2
24	F	72 300	B	L1	CR; relapse (3 months)	6
35	F	26 400	B	L1	CR; BMT	14
71	F	251 000	B	L2	Died in induction	<1
29	F	45 300	B	L1	Refractory	4
35	F	800	B	L2	CR; BMT	8
31	F	62 600	BMy	Mixed	CR;PBSCT; Relapse	15

Cases were identified by cytogenetics or molecular analysis at diagnosis or at relapse. Not all data listed were centrally reviewed [6,10]. FAB, morphology subclassification; CR, complete remission; BMT, bone marrow transplant; PBSCT, autologous peripheral blood stem cell transplant.

diagnosis. For this analysis, four adverse features were considered: age ⩾60 years, absence of a mediastinal mass, WBC ⩾30000/µl, and adverse laboratory features (either L3 morphology, B or BMy immunophenotype, or the Ph chromosome). Thus, the only patients removed from this analysis are the few who lack clinical information regarding a mediastinal mass or the pretreatment WBC count, and those who are missing all three values for FAB morphology, immunophenotype, and cytogenetics/molecular results. Table 6 and Fig. 1 show the survival estimates for 353 patients by the number of adverse features at diagnosis. Patients who have adverse biological features tend to have multiple adverse clinical features. Twenty-two patients (6%) had no unfavorable prognostic factors and had an estimated probability of survival at 3 years of 91% (95% CI, 66%–98%). Alternatively, none of the 13 patients with all four adverse risk factors survived longer than 17 months.

Discussion

The aim of CALGB study 8811 was to develop an aggressive multi-agent treatment that would improve the remission induction rate and the survival of adults with ALL. The aim of CALGB study 9111 was to evaluate the ability of G-CSF to increase the remission induction rate further by reducing the duration of neutropenia, and thereby the morbidity and mortality of treatment. Preliminary data from our study and two other randomized clinical trials, suggest that the concurrent use of G-CSF may improve the ability to deliver intensive chemotherapy more safely [8, 12, 13]. The follow-up periods for these trials

Table 6. Impact of four adverse features on the outcome of treatment on CALGB 8811/9111

Adverse features (n)	Patients (n)	Adverse Features				Estimated survival at 3 years (95%-CI)	
		Age >60	WBC >30 000/µl	No mediastinal mass	Laboratory features	(%)	(%)
0	22	0	0	0	0	91,	66–98
1	83	1	16	63	3	64,	51–75
2	146	12	25	145	110	49,	36–61
3	89	25	68	89	85	21,	12–35
4	13	13	13	13	13		0

[a]Adverse laboratory features include L3 morphology, or B/BMy immunophenotype, or Ph^+/$BCR\text{-}ABL^+$genetics.

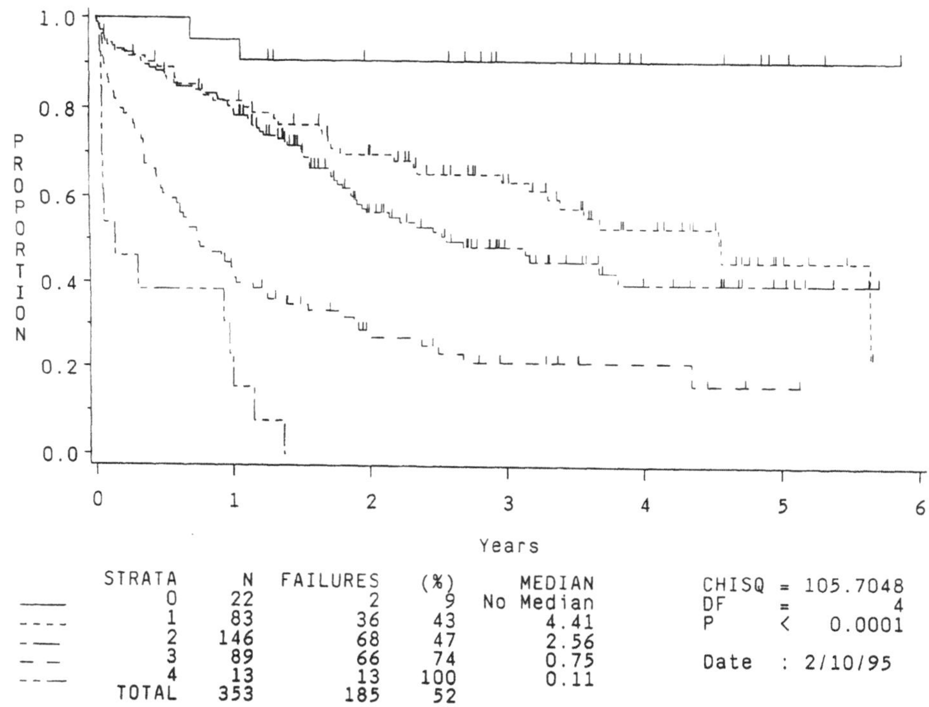

Fig. 1. The survival of 353 patients with ALL treated on CALGB studies 8811 and 9111 differed according to the number of adverse features that an individual patient had at diagnosis: age ⩾60 years, absence of a mediastinal mass, WBC ⩾30 000/μl, or adverse laboratory features (either L3 morphology, or B/BMy immunophenotype, or the Ph chromosome)

are still short, however, and the full impact of the use of G-CSF during the treatment of adults with ALL remains to be determined.

Twelve percent of our patients had prominent mediastinal adenopathy. Surprisingly, we found that this is predictive of a favorable outcome, with an influence on remission rate, duration of remission, and survival in multivariate analyses [6]. Most previous studies of adult ALL have failed to identify mediastinal enlargement as an important factor. A trend similar to ours seemed apparent in an older German study, but it did not reach statistical significance [14]. Furthermore, in our study, lymphadenopathy, another manifestation of leukemia mass, had a favorable effect on survival in a univariate, but not multivariate, analysis. The favorable outcome associated with a mediastinal mass using this treatment regimen may be due in part to the favorable effect of the T-lineage immunophenotype, since the large majority of the patients with a mediastinal mass had T-cell antigen expression. The median age of the patients with a mediastinal mass did not differ from the group overall nor was their median WBC count lower. None, however, had the Ph chromosome.

Biological characteristics of the disease continue to be powerful determinants of response. As yet, no chemotherapy regimen has effectively cured patients with the Ph chromosome. In our study, fewer than 20% of these patients are estimated to survive more than 3 years. The proportion of patients with the Ph chromosome increases with age, and more than 40% of ALL patients > 50 years old have this mutation. Thus, this abnormality may be in part responsible for the poor prognosis of older adults with ALL. Recent data suggest that approximately one third of Ph^+ ALL patients can be cured using allogeneic BMT. At this time, CALGB study 9113 is investigating allogeneic transplantation, early in first CR, using total body irradiation and high-dose etoposide for Ph^+ patients who have an HLA-identical sibling. Patients with a t(4;11) or other high-risk features are also eligible for this BMT trial.

Burkitt-type (L3) B-ALL also had a poor outcome using this treatment program. Approximately 5% of adults with ALL have this subtype, which is characterized by the t(8;14) or one of its variants [t(2;8), t(8;22)]. Ten of 12 L3 patients achieved a CR using this induction regimen, but remissions were very short (median, 3 months). Currently, the CALGB is investigating the use of a short, intensive chemotherapy program, using high doses of ifosfamide/cyclophosphamide with high-dose methotrexate and cytarabine, etoposide, and doxorubicin for patients identified at diagnosis with either ALL-L3 morphology or Burkitt lymphoma. Preliminary data (study 9251) suggest a high CR rate and durable remissions in many of these patients.

In order to improve the outcome of all adults with ALL, it will be increasingly important to stratify treatment groups by prognostic characteristics, particularly age, mediastinal mass, WBC, immunophenotype, and genetic abnormalities. Risk factor assessments must makeuse of clinical measurements or technological resources widely available to community hematologists, and then they must be validated prospectively. For patients with a favorable prognosis, the intensive chemotherapy developed in studies 8811 and 9111 can be recommended, and it is possible that additional refinements in therapy and supportive care may improve results further. The CALGB has recently completed a pilot study (9311) using the immunotoxin anti-B4 blocked ricin (immunogen) for patients with B-lineage ALL in first remission. As yet, no outcome data are available from this trial.

Patients in the high-risk subgroups clearly require different treatment. Unfortunately, the majority will not have an allogeneic bone marrow donor available. Thus, the challenge of developing new treatment strategies for these patients remains.

Acknowledgments. We gratefully knowledge the essential contributions of Dr. Frederick R. Davey and the CALGB Pathology Committee, the CALGB Correlative Sciences Committee, and the chairmen of the ancillary laboratory studies for this work: Dr. Robert E. Sobol, Dr. Stanley R. Frankel, and Dr. Carleton C. Stewart (CALGB 8364), Dr. Diane C. Arthur (CALGB 8461), and Dr. Carol A. Westbrook and Dr. Wendy Stock (CALGB 8762). We appreciate the assistance of Gwennelle Clark and Audrey Byrd (CALGB Data Management Center) for expert data coordination, and Susan Jarman for the preparation of the manuscript. We thank our co-investigators in the CALGB and the many treating physicians, cytogeneticists, research nurses, data managers, and patients without whom these trials could not have been completed. This work was supported in part by grants CA 31946, CA 31983, CA 33601, CA 37027, CA 37055, and CA 41287 from the National Cancer Institute.

References

1. Gottlieb AJ, Weinberg V, Ellison RR et al. (1984) Efficacy of daunorubicin in the therapy of adult acute lymphocytic leukemia: a prospective randomized trial by Cancer and Leukemia Group B. Blood 64: 267–274.
2. Cuttner J, Mick R, Budman DR et al. (1991) Phase III trial of brief intensive treatment of adult acute lymphocytic leukemia comparing daunorubicin and mitoxantrone: a CALGB study. Leukemia 5: 425–431.
3. Ellison RR, Mick R, Cuttner J et al. (1991) The effects of postinduction intensification treatment with cytarabine and daunorubicin in adult acute lymphocytic leukemia: a prospective randomized clinical trial by Cancer and Leukemia Group B. J Clin Oncol 9: 2002–2015.
4. Sobol RE, Mick R, Royston I et al. (1987). Clinical importance of myeloid antigen expression in adult acute lymphoblastic leukemia. N Engl J Med 316: 1111–1117.
5. Westbrook CA, Hooberman AL, Spino C et al. (1992) Clinical significance of the BCR-ABL fusion gene in adult acute lymphoblastic leukemia: a Cancer and Leukemia Group B study (8762). Blood 80: 2983–2990.
6. Larson RA, Dodge RK, Burns CP et al. (1995) A five-drug remission induction regimen with intensive consolidation for adults with acute lymphoblastic leukemia: Cancer and Leukemia Group B. Blood 85: in press.
7. Bloomfield CD, Wurster-Hill D, Peng G et al. (1990) Prognostic significance of the Philadelphia chromosome in adult acute lymphocytic leukemia. In Gale RP, Hoelzer D (eds): Acute lymphoblastic leukemia. UCLA Symposium on Molecular and Cellular Biology, New Series, Volume 108. New York, NY, Liss, pp 101–109.
8. Larson RA, Linker CA, Dodge RK, et al. (1994) Granulocyte-colony stimulating factor (filgrastin; G-CSF) reduces the time to neutrophil recovery in adults with acute lymphoblastic leukemia receiving intensive remission induction chemotherapy: Cancer and Leukemia Group B study 9111. Proc Am Soc Clin Onc 13: 305 (#995).

9. Lee EJ, Pollak A, Leavitt RD et al. (1987) Minimally differentiated acute nonlymphocytic leukemia: a distinct entity. Blood 70: 1400–1405.
10. Bennett JM, Catovsky D, Daniel MT et al. (1981) The morphologic classification of acute lymphoblastic leukemia. Concordance among observers and clinical correlations. Br J Haematol 47: 553–561.
11. Stock W, Thirman MJ, Dodge RK et al. (1994) Detection of MLL gene rearrangements in adult acute lymphoblastic leukemia. A Cancer and Leukemia Group B study. Leukemia 8: 1918–1922.
12. Ottmann OG, Hoelzer D, Gracien E et al. (1993) Concomitant R-metHuG-CSF (filgrastim) and intensive chemoradiotherapy as induction treatment in adult ALL: a randomized multicenter phase II trial. Blood 82 (Suppl 1):193a, (#757).
13. Ohno R, Tomonaga M, Kobayashi T, et al. (1990) Effect of granulocyte colony-stimulating factor after intensive induction therapy in relapsed or refractory acute leukemia. N Engl J Med 323: 871–877.
14. Hoelzer D, Thiel E, Löffler M et al. (1988) Prognostic factors in a multicenter study for treatment of acute lymphoblastic leukemia in adults. Blood 71: 123–131.

Acute Leukemias VI
Prognostic Factors
and Treatment Strategies
Büchner et al. (eds)

Treatment of Acute Lymphoblastic Leukemia in the Elderly: Results of the GIMEMA 0288 > 60 Years Trial

F. Mandelli, L. Annino, M.L. Vegna, A. Ferrari, F. Di Raimondo, R. Invernizzi, S. Ladogana, E. Miraglia, M. Montillo, F. Nobile, A. Peta, A. Recchia, G. Specchia, and A. Tabilio
for the GIMEMA Cooperative Group, Italy

Introduction

In the past decade acute lymphoblastic leukemia (ALL) in the elderly was considered a rare condition so that these patients were usually neglected in multiinstitutional studies [1-3] or were generally enrolled in the trials for all adult ALL [4-6].

When patients >60 years were treated like other adult ALL patients (> 15 years) the results were disappointing since the complete remission (CR) rate ranged from 35% to 58% [4-6]; induction death rate was high, strictly limiting the possibility of achieving CR and median survival remained short, less than 6 months.

This may discourage hematologists from enrolling these patients in the present intensive trials, preferring to treat them with palliative intent, i.e., conventional two-drug therapy consisting of vincristine (VCR) + prednisone (PDN) or personalized therapy.

In this way two goals were not attained: first, the treatment results did not improve [7]; secondly, the real incidence of older ALL patients remained underestimated. To date the incidence of ALL patients > 60 years is estimated to range from 16% to 31% of ALL adult cases [8].

In 1988 the GIMEMA Group initiated, in the context of the ALL 0288 trial, a specific treatment regimen for patients > 60 years. As of September 1994 these patients represented 10% of all adult ALL cases enrolled in the abovementioned trial. The specific goal of the protocol for elderly patients was to test its efficacy in inducing and maintaining CR, but especially its feasability in a population which would be unable to tolerate a 3-year chemotherapy regimen.

Material and Methods

In January 1988 the second national trial—ALL 0288—was initiated. In this trial, which was previously detailed [9], a treatment regimen for patients older than 60 years of age was established. This regimen consists of a 7-day PDN pretreatment followed by conventional four-drug induction, involving VCR, PDN, daunorubicin (DNR), and L-asparaginase (ASP). Patients who do not achieve CR follow salvage chemotherapy which consists of mitoxantrone and intermediate-dose of cytosine arabinoside (ID-AC). As post-remission chemotherapy, patients are treated as for all other adult ALL cases enrolled in the GIMEMA ALL 0288 trial, except that they are continued on conventional maintenance according to protocol (Fig. 1). From January 1988 to September 1994, 80 consecutive ALL patients over 60 years of age were enrolled in this protocol, which is still open.

Statistical Methods. Statistical analysis was done using the SAS package (SAS Institute, Inc., Cary, North Carolina, USA). Single factors were studied for their influence on remission rate by means of the chi-square test. Event-free, disease-free and overall survival were calculated using the product limit technique. To compare curves between two or more groups, the long-rank pro-

Department of Hematology, Universita Roma-La Sapienzia, Via Benevento 6, 00161 Rome, Italy

Fig. 1. Schema of protocol *P*, prednison; *V*, vincristine; *D*, daunorubicin; *A*, asparaginase; *AC*, cytosine arabinoside; *IDAC*, Intermediate-dose cytosine arabinoside; *MT*, mitoxantrone; *MTX*, methotrexate; *6-MP*, mercaptopurine; *L-VAMP*, vincristine, *ID*-methotrexate, cytosine, carabinoside, and desametazone; leucoverin

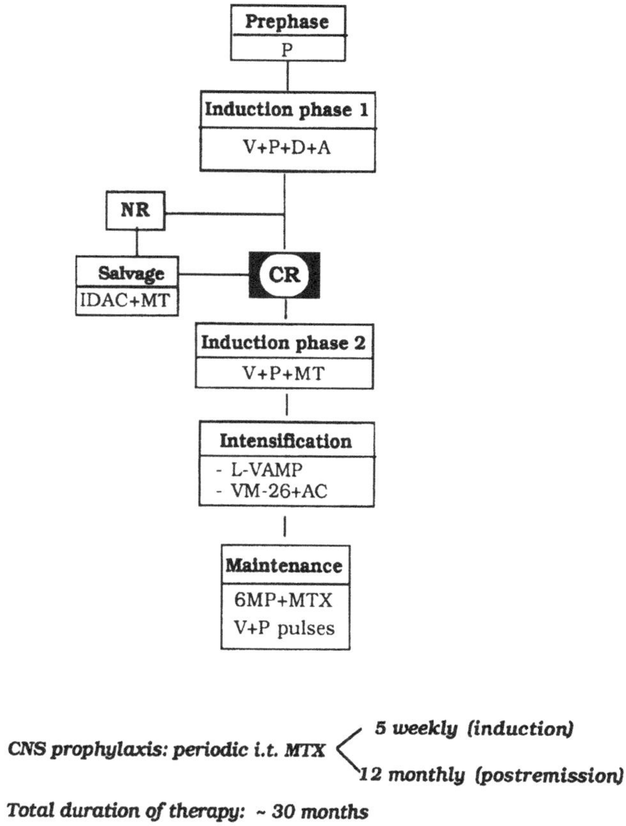

cedure was applied. Multivariate analysis to correlate various factors simultaneously with response to induction or event-free survival was performed using the linear logistic or the proportional hazard model, respectively. No patient was excluded from the analysis of the study.

Results

Patient Characteristics. As of September 1994, among 800 consecutive adult ALL patients, 80 (10%) patients over 60 years old had been included in the protocol. Out of these, 32 were males; median age was 64.9 years (range 60.1–78.2). At diagnosis, median white blood cell count WBC count was 11.5 × 10^9/l (range 0.4–290 × 10^9/l); three patients exhibited a mediastinal mass, only one a CNS involvement. A predominant L2 French-American-British (FAB) morphology (65%) was encountered compared with L1 FAB ALL (32%); two patients were classified as L3, while only two were not classifiable. B-lineage ALL and T-lineage ALL constituted 70% and 19%, respectively, of all cases, only one case was classified as hybrid leukemia and another one was acute undifferentiated leukemia (AUL). Finally, 9% of cases were not classifiable. Regarding performance status (PS), 12 (15%) patients showed a PS 3 and 4. Cytogenetic analysis was not carried out routinely so that only 28 cases were studied. No metaphases were found in ten; of the other 18 in whom karyotypic analysis was available six were normal, five showed aspecific abnormalities, and seven were Philadelphia chromosome (Ph1) positive (Table 1).

Response to Treatment. Among the 80 patients enrolled, 77 were considered evaluable for induction response; of the remaining, one was withdrawn because of early death and two refused treatment. After induction phase 1, 36 (47%) patients achieved CR, nine (12%) were

Table 1. Patient characteristics

Patients	(n)	80
Males	(n)	32
	(%)	40
Age—Median (Years)		64.9
Range (years)		60.1–78.2
WBC—Median ($\times$ 10^9/1)		11.5
Range ($\times$ 10^9/L)		0.4–290
FAB		
L1	(n)	25
	(%)	31
L2	(n)	51
	(%)	64
L3	(n)	2
	(%)	2.5
Not known	(n)	2
	(%)	2.5
Phenotype		
B-lineage	(n)	56
	(%)	70
T-lineage	(n)	15
	(%)	19
My+	(n)	1
	(%)	1
AUL	(n)	1
	(%)	1
Not known	(n)	7
	(%)	9
Mediastinal mass	(n)	3
	(%)	4
CNS involvement		
No	(n)	73
Yes	(n)	1
Performance status (WHO)		
3	(n)	10
4	(n)	2
Cytogenetics		28
Ph1 $^+$	(n)	7(4 p190$^+$)

refractory, and 32 (41%) died during induction (Table 2). Among the seven Ph1-positive ALL, four patients achieved CR, two were refractory, and one died during induction. Among the nine resistant patients, five followed salvage chemotherapy; only one of these achieved CR.

Table 2. Response to induction

	(n)	(%)
Evaluable patients	77	
Complete remission	36	47
Resistant	9	12
Induction deaths	32	41

The main induction death (ID) cause was infection (14 patients); six died because of hemorrhage, five of hepatic toxicity, and one of stroke, paralytic ileus, and leukemia, respectively. Among the 36 CRs, ten (28%) went off the study early because of chemotherapy-related toxicity (eight) or protocol violation two; three patients died in CR from infection. Nine patients—four in early post-CR phase and five during maintenance therapy- relapsed; two of these relapses were isolated CNS relapse. During maintenance therapy one patient was withdrawn because of toxicity. At the time of the present analysis, 13 patients (36%) of all complete remitters are alive without evidence of disease; three of them went off therapy. Survival was short-lived in these older patients with 27% and 19% of them remaining alive at 1 and 2 years, respectively (Fig. 2). At the same times, 24% and 13% of patients were event-free survivors (Fig. 3).

Factors Associated with Outcome. In our cohort of patients, age, as revealed in univariate analysis, was the main prognostic factor influencing the achievement of CR. Age of 70 years or older was associated with no CR achievement due to ID ($p=0.02$). With respect to phenotype, T cell immunophenotype was shown to be associated with a lower CR rate due to both ID and resistant disease ($p=0.05$); whereas, poor PS higher initial WBC count (WBC count $> 50 \times 10^9/1$), and prednisone pretreatment response were shown not to influence CR achievement significantly (Table 3). In multivariate analysis, age, initial WBC count, PDN pretreatment response and immunophenotype were tested to demonstrate their influence on event-free survival (EFS). Age was confirmed to be the only independent prognostic factor on EFS ($p=0.008$) (Table 4).

Discussion

The best therapeutic approach in elderly ALL patients still remains an open issue. Physicians still debate whether to treat them in a curative or palliative way. Among the curative approaches, the vincristine-adriamycin-dexamethasone (VAD) regimen was recently shown effective in inducing 58% CR rate [8]. Milder treatment consisting of VCR+PDN is considered a palliative therapy [7, 10]; though in one study this approach was nearly as high as the curative one, inducing a 53% CR rate [11].

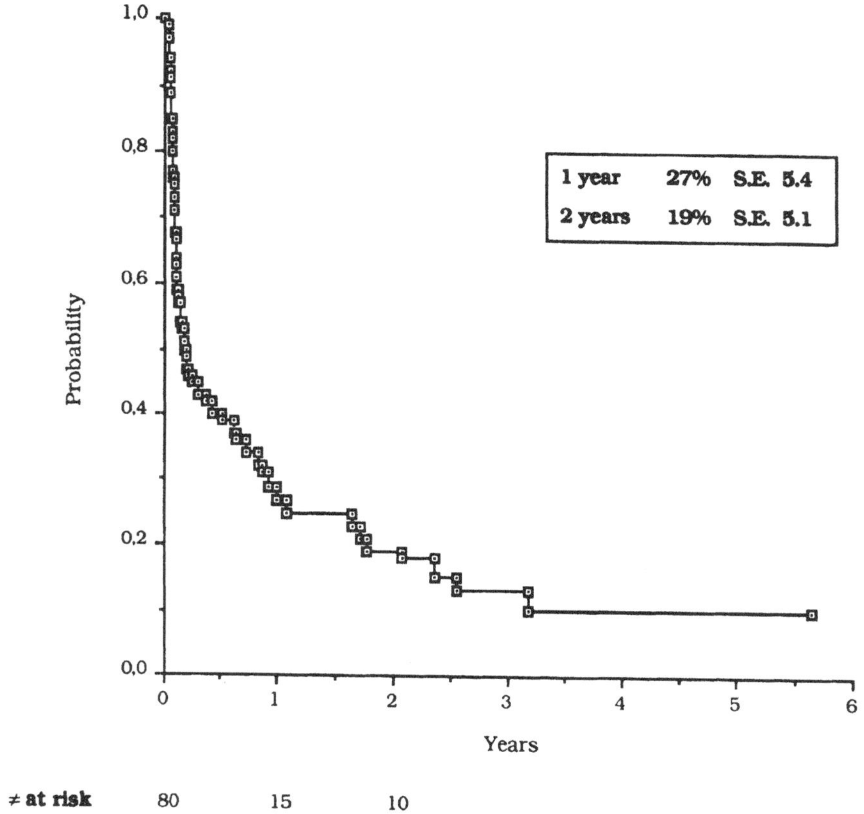

Fig. 2. Overall survival

It has been recently proposed that a possible therapeutic strategy for elderly patients may consist of conventional induction and consolidation, with the addition of growth factors, followed by a prolonged non-toxic conventional maintenance [8]. However, this type of post-induction therapy is considered inappropriate for most older patients; thus alternative novel agents or therapeutic approaches, strictly correlated to the biological characteristics of the disease, are suggested [12].

The GIMEMA ALL 0288 > 60 years has been, to our knowledge, the first multicenter trial specifically designed for the treatment of elderly patients. The goals of this present trial were to evaluate the bilogical characteristics of the disease, the response rate, and the feasibility and tolerance of a protocol lasting 3 years.

Regarding biological characteristics at the time of diagnosis, we were not able to find any significant difference with respect to our adult series of patients [9]. The distribution of immunophenotype in evaluable patients and WBC at diagnosis did not seem to show any peculiarity. However, T-lineage ALL incidence appeared higher (19%) in our series compared to other elderly ALL series [7, 10, 13, 14].

Unfortunately, cytogenetic studies were attempted on only 28 patients, seven of whom were Ph1 chromosome positive, which is fewer than that expected [15]. Thus, there were insufficient numbers to give any information on prognostic significance of cytogenetic and molecular abnormalities on disease outcome.

Overall CR rate was 47%, which compares favorably with CR rates recorded in other similar series [6, 7, 10, 12]. The ID) rate was 41% and the main ID cause was infection. This poor result, which was comparable to that observed in other single or multiinstitutional trials also involving younger patients [4, 5, 6, 12], could be attributed both to the fact that all the oldest

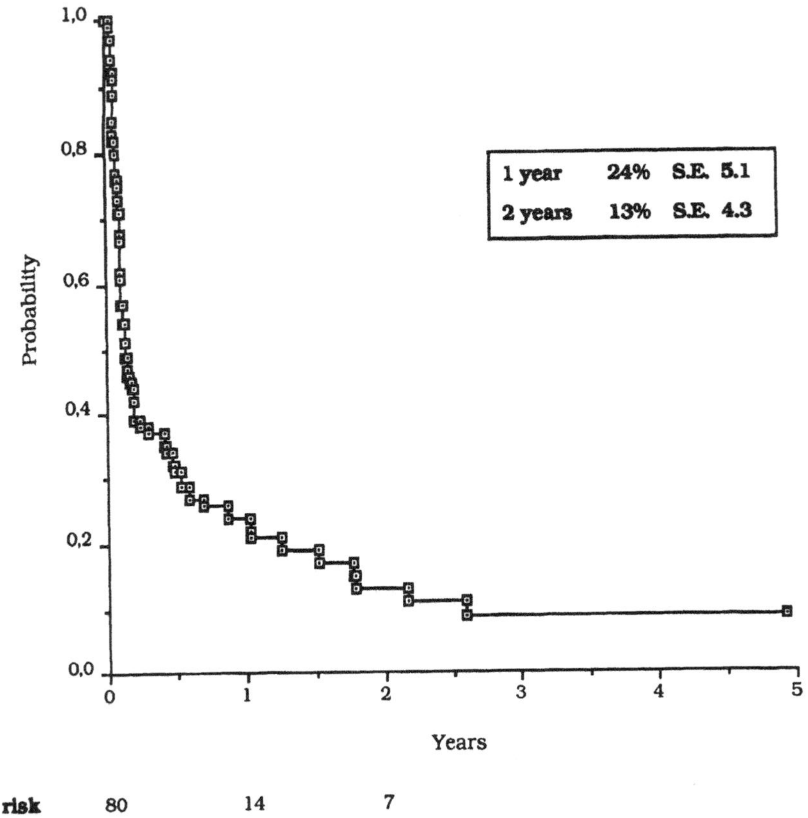

Fig. 3. Event-free survival

Table 3. Prognostic factors influencing complete remission

	Induction death		Resistant		CR		Total	p value
	(n)	(%)	(n)	(%)	(n)	(%)		
Peripheral blasts								
< 1000	24	49	2	4	23	47	49	n.s.
> 1000	4	25	6	37	6	37	16	
	28	43	8	12	29	45	65	
WBC								
< 50000	24	40	6	10	30	50	60	n.s.
> 50000	8	47	3	18	6	35	17	
	32	42	9	12	36	47	77	
Phenotype								
B-lineage	18	34	6	11	29	55	53	0.05
T-lineage	9	60	2	13	4	27	15	
	27	40	8	12	33	48	68	
Age								
< 70 years	26	37	9	13	36	51	71	0.02
> 70 years	6	100	–	–	–	–	6	
	32	41	9	12	36	47	77	
Performance status (WHO)								
0-1-2	26	42	6	10	30	48	62	n.s.
3-4	4	40	2	20	4	40	10	
	30	42	8	11	34	47	72	

Table 4. Proportional hazard model in EFS

	Relative risk	Confidence limits	*P*
Age (years)	1.13	1.03–1.25	0.008
WBC (x 10^9/l)	1.00	0.99–1.00	0.737
Peripheral blasts (× 10^9/l)			
< 1.0	1		
> 1.0	0.76	0.35–1.65	0.493
Immunophenotype			
B-lineage	1		
T-lineage	1.80	0.86–3.73	0.115

(> 70 years) patients died during induction and that the growth factors were employed in only few cases. It has recently been shown that, in elderly patients, growth factors have a significant impact on CR rate by reducing the ID rate [16]. But chemotherapy-related toxicity remains a problem not only limited to the induction phase. In our cohort of patients, out of 36 CRs, three died early in CR (during consolidation) because of cytopenia-related infections. Thus it may be argued that growth factors must be employed for supportive care not only during the induction but also during consolidation phase.

Two-year prolonged maintenance was shown to be a well-tolerated therapy since out of 12 patients who continued maintenance, only one was withdrawn due to toxicity; furthermore, three patients completed treatment and they are presently off therapy in first CR from 39+, 60+, and 67+ months.

It has been postulated that ALL in the elderly may be intrinsically different from that in younger patients [12] and that it is a stem cell disorder. This may explain the increased occurrence of Ph1 chromosome, as well as the different response to treatment observed in elderly patients.

In our series, CR achievement appeared significantly influenced by age and immuophenotype, while PDN pretreatment response did now show, unlike in our younger patients [9], any impact on this. Multivariate analysis confirmed age as the only independent prognostic factor influencing EFS.

What conclusions can be drawn from the experience of this protocol? With the present induction, admistered with curative intent, 47% of patients entered into remission; this constitutes an acceptable result. Furthermore, the relapse rate (25%) is lower than that observed in other series [6,12]. The main issue is chemotherapy-related death: probably this may be bypassed by means of a standardized use of growth factors.

Neverthless, the problem persists for the oldest patients (> 70 years) who can continue to be enrolled in this trial but more cautiously. Probably for this subset an alternative, less intensive approach may be desirable. Prolonged conventional maintenance was confirmed to be useful and well tolerated as a therapeutic approach in these patients.

The main criticism, emerging from this study is related to the incidence (10%) of ALL in the elderly; this may be understimated due to the fact that when the program was initiated in 1988, physycians were reluctant to refer elderly patients for intensive treatment. In fact, in a Italy a National Registry of Acute Leukemias was begun in July 1992. As of September 1994, among 488 adult ALL registered, 121 (25%) were older than 60 years, so the incidence of this disease seems to have increased since a peer diagnostic evaluation was conducted. The suggestions of this present trial could prove useful in future therapeutic trends for this particular group of patients.

References

1. Linker CA, Levitt LJ, O'Donnel M et al.: (1987) Improved results of treatment of adult acute lymphoblastic leukemia Blood, 69: 1242.
2. Hoelzer D, Thiel E, Loffler H et al.: (1988) Prognostic factors in a multicenter study for treatment of acute lymphoblastic leukemia in adults Blood, 71: 121–131.
3. Cassileth PA, Anderson JW, Bennet JM et al.: (1992) Adult acute lymphocytic leukemia: the Eastern Cooperative Oncology Group experience Leukemia, 6, (Suppl2): 178–181.
4. Gaynor J, Chapman D, Little C et al.: (1988) A cause-specific hazard rate analysis of prognostic factors among 199 adults with acute lymphoblastic leukemia: the Memorial Hospital experience since 1969" Journal of Clinical Oncology, 6, 6: 1014-1030.
5. Hussein KK, Dahlberg S, Head D et al.: (1989) "Treatment of acute lymphoblastic leukemia in adults with intensive induction, consolidation and maintenance chemotherapy. Blood, 73, 1: 57–63.
6. Ellison RR, Mick R, Cuttner J et al.: (1991) "The effect of post induction intensification treatment with cytarabine and daunorubicin in adult acute lymphoblastic leukemia: a prospective randomized

clinical trial by Cancer and Leukemia Group B" Journal of Clinical Oncology, 9:2002–2015.
7. Taylor PRA, Reid MM, Bown N et al.: (1992)" Acute lymphoblastic leukemia in patients aged 60 years and over: a population-based study of incidence and outcome" Blood, 7: 1813–1817.
8. Kantarjian HM, O'Brien S, Smith T et al.: (1994) "Acute lymphocytic leukemia in the elderly characteristics and outcome with the vincristineadriamycin-dexamethasone (VAD) regimen. British Journal of Haematology, 88: 94–100.
9. Mandelli F, Annino L, Vegna ML et al.: (1992) "GIMEMA ALL 0288: a multicentric study on adult acute lymphoblastic leukemia. Preliminary results." Leukemia, 6, Supll 2: 182–185.
10. Spath-Schawalbe E, Heil G, Heimpel H et al.: (1994) "Acute lymphoblastic leukemia in patients over 59 years of age. Experience in a single center over a 10-year period." Annals of Hematology, 69: 291–296.
11. Ferrari A, Annino L, Crescenzi S et al.: (1995) "Adult lymphoblastic leukemia in the elderly: results of two different approaches in 49 patients during a twenty-five period." Submitted
12. Taylor PRA, Reid MM and Proctor SJ (1994) "Acute lymphoblastic leukemia in the elderly" Leukemia and Lymphoma, 13: 373–380.
13. Dellanoy A. Ferrant A, Bosly A et al.: (1990)" Acute lymphoblastic leukemia in the elderly" European Journal of Haematology, 45: 90–93.
14. Virgilio JF, Moscinski C, Ballaster OF et al.: (1993)" Acute lymphocytic leukemia (ALL) in elderly patients" Hematological Oncology, 11: 121–126.
15. Secker-Walker LM, Craig JM, Hawkins JM et al.: (1991) "Philadelphia-positive acute lymphoblastic leukemia in adults: age distibution, BCR breakpoint and prognostic significance" Leukemia, 5, 3: 196–199.
16. Larson RA, Linker LA, Dodge RR et al.: (1994)" Granulocyte colony stimulating factor (filgrastim) reduces the time of neutrophil recovery in adults with acute lymphoblastic leukemia receiving intensive remission induction chemotherapy: Cancer and Leukemia Group B study 91-11" PROC AM SOC CLIN ONCOL 13:305 (Abstr 995)

Acute Leukemias VI
Prognostic Factors
and Treatment Strategies
Büchner et al. (eds)

Allogeneic and Autologous Bone Marrow Transplantation and Chemotherapy in First Remission of Adult Acute Lymphoblastic Leukemia: Results of the LALA 87 Trial of the French Group

D. Fière, J.P. Vernant, J. Reiffers, J.M. Miclea, F. Witz, F. Rigal Huguet, C. Danaila, and E. Lepage
for the French Group for Treatment of Adult ALL

Abstract. In a prospective study of 317 acute lymphoblastic leukemia (ALL) patients aged 15–40 years and in complete remission, 257 had a potential donor and one HLA typing analysis; A total of 116 patients were allocated to the allogeneic bone marrow transplantation (BMT) arm and 141 to a control group. In parallel, all patients without an identical donor were randomized to autologous BMT or classical chemotherapy. There is no difference in the two trials between the arms in overall survival. However, for high-risk ALL there is a better survival favoring the allogeneic BMT group. Autologous BMT has outcomes at least similar to classical chemotherapy. Classicial chemotherapy is effective in T-ALL.

Introduction

Improvement of the percentage of long-term survivors in adult acute lymphoblastic leukemia (ALL) remains a major goal in a disease in which 5-year survival stands at 20%–40% [1, 2]. In post-induction, early chemotherapy intensification, allogeneic or autologous bone marrow transplantation (BMT) have induced a better outcome but their respective indications remain controversial [3–8]. In a prospective study, the French group for the treatment of adult ALL has evaluated these three treatment regimens. Results may contribute to defining an adapted strategy able to improve the outcome of furture patients. The design and results of the multicentric LALA 87 protocol have recently been reported [9–110 and are shown in Fig. 1.

The present paper focuses on the outcome of patients 15–40 years old, who were allocated after HLA typing to allogeneic BMT in the case of an identical sibling or to a control group if no donor was found; all patients without a donor were randomized to autologous BMT or classical chemotherapy. The median follow up was 60 months.

Materials and Methods

Patients

From November 1986 to July 1991, 634 patients with ALL L1 or L2 aged 15–60 years were entered in the prospective study (LALA 87). A total of 572 patients were evaluable and 436 achieved a complete remission (CR); 317 patients were 15–40 years old and scheduled for HLA typing. However, 33 patients had no sibling and HLA typing was not performed in 27: all these patients were excluded. Among 257 patients with HLA typing, 116 had an identical donor and were entered in to the allogeneic BMT arm, 141 patients without a donor were entered into the control group. These two groups constituted the allogenic BMT trial.

A total of 201 patients without an identical sibling were scheduled for randomization between autologous BMT and chemotherapy in the autologous BMT trial. As the randomization took place during the second chemotherapy consolidation course, given as a result of early relapses or other causes, only 143 patients were

Hôpital Edouard Herriot, Lyon, France

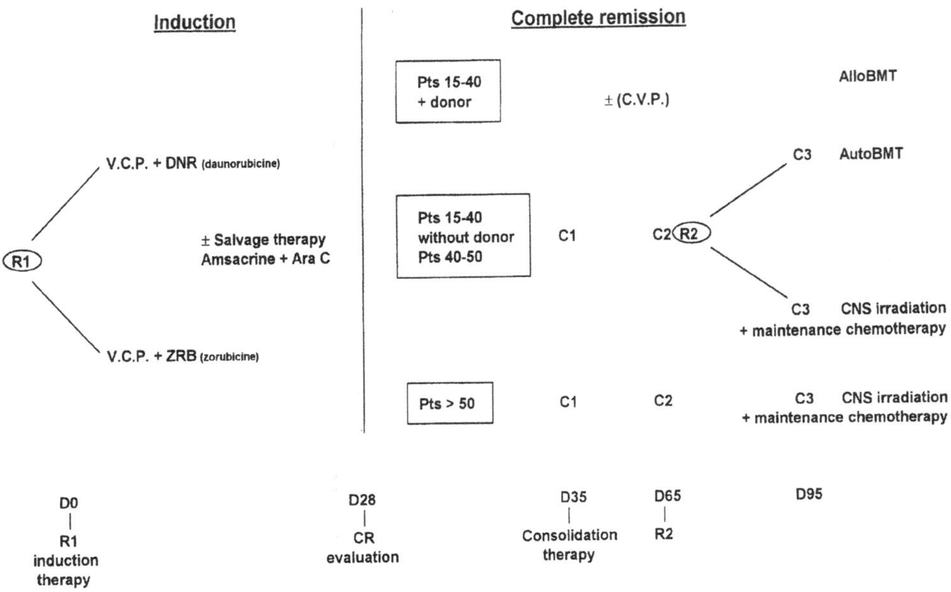

Fig. 1. Design of the multicentric LALA 87 protocol. *R1*, first randomization; *R2*, second randomization; *V.C.P.*, vincristine 1.5 mg/m², cyclopsphamide 600 mg/m², prednisone 60 mg/m², *C.V.P.*, cyclophosphamide 600 mg/m², vincristine 1.5 mg/m², prednisone 60 mg/m²; *C.*, consolidation; *Pts*, patients+age; *DNR*, daunorubicin; *ZRB*, zorubicin;

randomized, 73 in the autologous BMT arm and 70 in the chemotherapy arm.

Treatment

In the allogeneic BMT arm, patients received an allogeneic transplantation after one course, on day 35 from the beginning of induction therapy, with Prednisone 60 mg/m² on days 1–8, Vincristine 1.5 mg/m² on days 1 and 8 and Cyclophosphamide 600 mg/m² on days 1 and 8. The Seattle conditioning regimen of Cyclophosphamide 60 mg/kg for 2 days together with total irradiation was used [12]. Prevention of graft-versus-host disease was left to the choice of the physician with a recommended therapy consisting of Methotrexate plus Cyclosporin.

In the autologous BMT arm, patients received three monthly consolidation courses with Daunorubicine 60 mg/m² or Zorubicin 120 mg/m² on day 1, depending on the anthracyclin given during induction, Cytarabine 60 mg/m² on days 3–7 and Asparaginase 1000 U/kg on days 8–12.

After randomization at the beginning of the second course of consolidation, bone marrow was harvested 20–30 days later, and followed by the third course of consolidation. Bone marrow purging was performed according to the initial leukemia phenotype. The conditioning regimen was the same as in the allogeneic BMT arm. No further therapy was given after infusion of the marrow. In the chemotherapy arm, patients received the same three consolidation courses followed by maintenance therapy which consisted of eight courses of the modified L10 protocol [13]. Treatment regimens are summarized in Table 1.

Classification According Risk Factors

Patients are stratified, according to criteria reported in the literature in to high-risk and standard—risk ALL. High-risk ALL is defined as any patient with at least one of the following factors: (a) presence of Philadelphia chromosome (Ph1), (b) no luekemia (defined by a CD10-CD20- phenotype) or undifferentiated leukemia; (c) common leukemia with at least one adverse prognostic factor: age > 35 years, white blood cell (WBC) count > 30 × 10.9/I, or time to CR achievement greater than 4 weeks [14].

Statistical Analysis

The end point was overall survival. Survival duration was calculated from the date of CR achievement until death or the date when last known

Table 1. Post-Remission treatment Regimens-LALA 87

Allogeneic BMT arm
- Before day 90
- After a short consolidation course (CVP)
- Conditioning: cyclophosphamide 60 mg/kg on days 1,2, total body irradiation
Autologous BMT arm
- 3-Monthly consolidation courses—c1, c2, c3
- marrow harvesting between c2 and c3
- purging with (CD10, CD19) for B-ALL or (CD2, CD5, CD7) for T-All or mafosfamide for other cases
- Conditioning: cyclophosphamide 60 mg/kg on days 1,2 total body irradiation
Chemotherapy arm
- 3-monthly consolidation courses—c1, c2, c3
- maintenance chemotherapy with c10-modified regimen for 8 courses

CVP, Cyclophoshphamide 600 mg/m^2, vincristine: 1.5 mg/m^2, prednisone 60 mg/m^2.

alive. Survival curves were estimated using the product-limit method of Kaplan and Meier [15]. Differences between survival curves were tested for significance using the log-rank test [16]. All analyses were performed on an intention-to-treat basis. Statistical analysis was conducted using BMDP statistical software (BMDP statistical sofware, Los Angeles, CA, USA).

Results

Pretreatment Characteristics

In the allogeneic BMT trial, 96 out of 257 patients were stratified into the high-risk ALL group with 41 patients in the BMT arm and 55 in the control group. In the autologous BMT trial 48 out of 143 patients had high-risk ALL. In each trial there was a highly significant difference for outcome between the high and standard-risk groups. In each treatment arm, the percentage of patients with B or T leukemia cell lineage was not statistically different, and neither was the distribution of high-risk patients.

Overall Survival

Allogeneic BMT Trial. Using an intension-to-treat analysis there was no statistical difference between the two groups for disease free survival (DFS) with a median of 24 months for the BMT group versus 22 months for the control group ($p = .01$). There was also no difference in the overall survival (Fig. 2)($p = .08$).

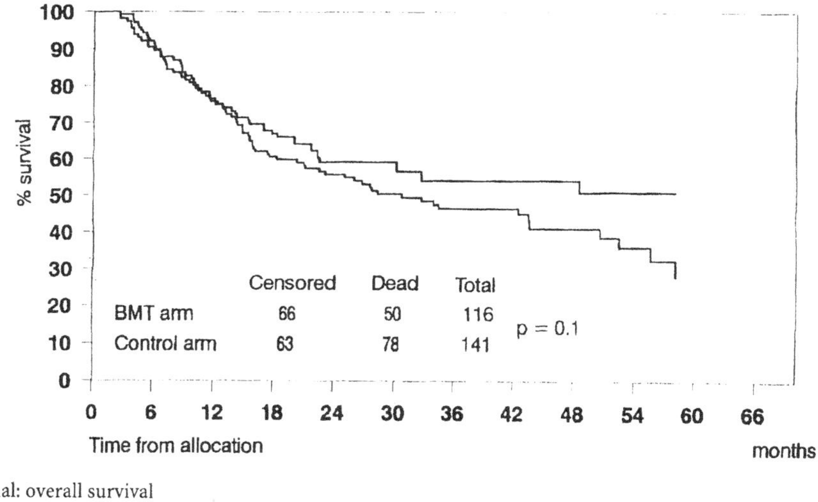

Fig. 2. BMT trial: overall survival

Autologous BMT Trial. Similarly, there was also no difference between the autologous BMT and chemotherapy arms with a median survival of 30 months for the chemotherapy arm versus 55 months in the autologous BMT arm ($p = 0.45$).

Survival According to Initial Risk Criteria. When outcome is compared in the allogeneic BMT trial, there is a best overall survival (Fig. 3)($p = 0.03$) and also a best DFS ($p = 0/01$) favoring BMT in high-risk patients. For standard risk, there is no difference in DFS and survival. In the autologous BMT trial no statistical difference appears in high-as well as in standard-risk patients between the autologous and chemotherapy randomized arms.

Survival According to treatment Arm and Initial Leukemic Lineage. Figs. 4–6 show the survival curve of patients included in the two trials stratified in each arms according to B or T cell lineage ALL. A major difference appears in the chemotherapy arm where the median survival for T-ALL is 84 months versus 25 months in B-ALL. For allogeneic and autologous BMT the median survival is superior in T versus B but the difference is not significant.

Discussion

The group of studied patients were a selected group of young ALL patients achieving a CR

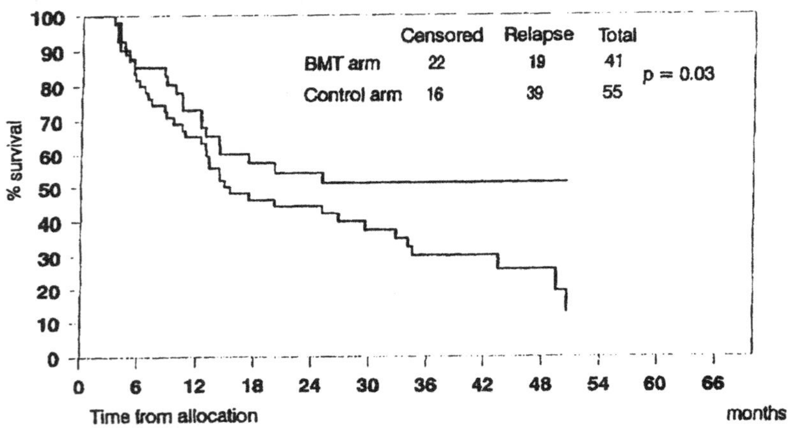

Fig. 3. BMT trial overall survival. High risk ALL

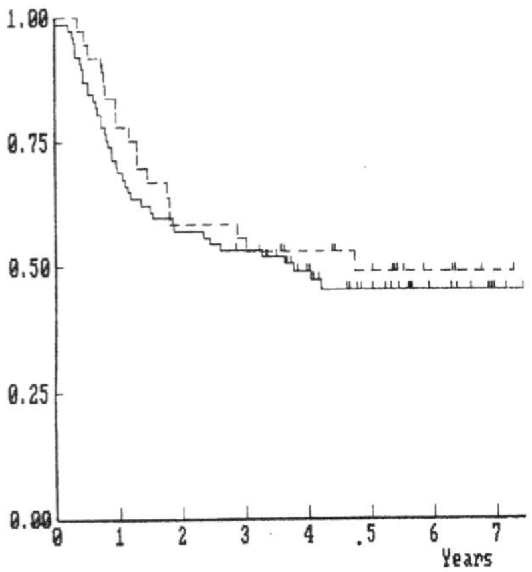

Fig. 4. LALA 87—B/T ALL: allogeneic BMT arm. *Solid line*, B-ALL; *broken line*, T-ALL. $p = 0.5583$

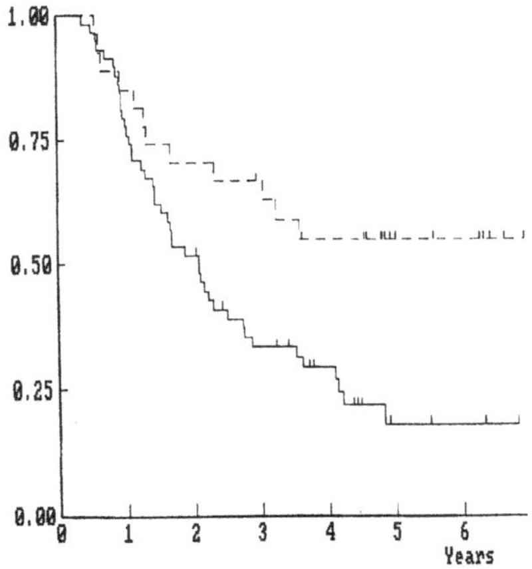

Fig. 5. LALA 87—B/T ALL: chemotherapy arm. *Solid line*, B-ALL; *broken line*, T-ALL. $p = 0.0073$

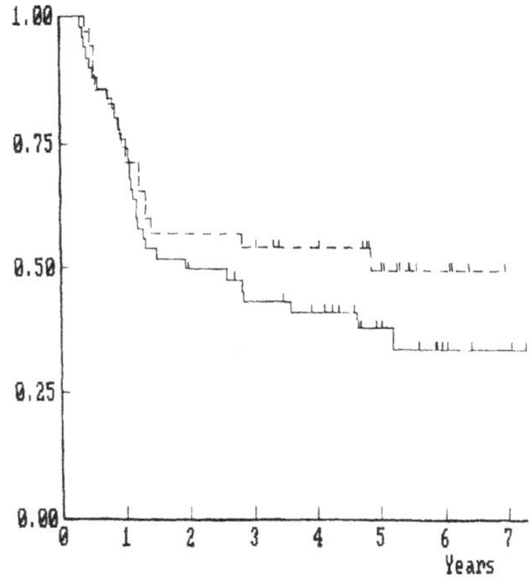

Fig. 6. LALA 87—B/T ALL: autologous BMT arm. *Solid line*, B-ALL; *broken line*, T-ALL. $p = 0.2578$

and, for patients without an identical sibling donor, who must be randomized during the second chemotherapy consolidation course; reasons for exclusion of patients were early relapse or patients in poor clinical status. Overall, the comparison of the development of patients receiving allogeneic BMT versus controls, or of patients randomized autologous BMT and classical chemotherapy does not show a statistically significant difference in outcome. However, two important points can be drawn from the two studies: (a) in the high-risk group of patients, allogeneic BMT appears as the best therapeutical strategy; (b) classical chemotherapy for T-ALL is a better regimen in first CR than BMT.

Another conclusion is that autologous BMT has at least similar outcomes to classical chemotherapy in ALL in first remission and needs to be further evaluated.

References

1. Champlin R, Gale RP: Acute lymphoblastic leukemia. Recent advances in biology and therapy. Blood 73; 2051-2066 1989.
2. Hoelzer D, Gale RP: Acute lymphoblatic leukemia in adults. Recent progress, future directions. Semin Hematol 24: 37-39, 1987
3. Gaynor J, Chapman D, Little et al.: A cause specific hazard rate analysis of prognostic factors among 199 adults with acute lympboblastic leukemia: the Memorial Hospital experience since 1969. J Clin Oncol 6: 1014-1030, 1988.
4. Linker CA, Levitt LY, O'Donnell M et al.: Treatment of adult acute lymphoblastic leukemia with intensive cyclical chemotherapy. A follow up report. Blood 78: 2814-2822, 1991
5. Gorin NC, Aegerter P, Auvert P et al: Autologous bone marrow transplantation (ABMT) for acute leukemia in remission: 5th European survey. Evidence in favor of marrow purging. Influence of retransplant intervals. Bone Marrow Transplant 3: 39-41, 1988 (sup. 1)
6. Kersey JH, Weisdorf D, Nesbit ME et al.: Comparison of autologous and allogeneic bone marrow transplantation for treatment of high risk refractory acute lymphoblastic leukemia. N Engl J Med 317: 461-467, 1987
7. Santos GW, Yearger AM, Jones RJ: Autologous bone marrow transplantation. Ann Rev Med 40: 99-112, 1989
8. Blume KG, Forman SJ, Snyders DS et al.: Allogeneic bone marrow transplantation for acute lymphoblastic leukemia during first complete remission. Transplantation 3:389-392, 1987
9. Fière D, Lepage E, Sebban C et al.: Adult acute lymphoblastic leukemia a multicentric randomized trial testing bone marrow transplantation as post remission therapy. J Clin Oncol 11: 1990-2001, 1993
10. Boucheix C, David B, Sebban C et al.: Immunophenotype of adult acute lymphoblastic leukemia, clinical parameters, and outcome: an analysis of a prospective trial including 562 tested patients (LALA 87). Blood 84: 1603-1612, 1994
11. Sebban C, Lepage E, Vernant JP et al.: Allogeneic bone marrow transplantation in adult acute lymphoblastic leukemia in first complete remission: a comparative study. J Clin Oncol 12: 2580-2587, 1994
12. Thomas ED, Sanders JE, Flournoy N et al.: Marrow transplantation for patients with acute lympboblastic leukemia in remission. Blood 54:468-476, 1979
13. Schauer P, Arlin ZA, Mertlesmann et al.: Treatment of acute lymphoblastic leukemia in adults. Results of the L10 and L10M protocol. J Clin Oncol 1: 462-470, 1983
14. Hoelzer D, Thiel E, Löffler H et al.: Prognostic factors in a multicenter study for treatment of acute lymphoblastic leukemia in adults. Blood 71: 123-131, 1988
15. Kaplan EL, Meier P: Non parametric estimation from incomplete observations. J Am Stat Assoc 53: 457-481, 1958
16. Peto R, Pike ML, Armitage P et al.: Design and analysis of randomized clinical trials requiring prolonged observation of each patient. Br J Cancer 35: 1-39, 1977

Acute Leukemias VI
Prognostic Factors
and Treatment Strategies
Büchner et al. (eds)

Bone Marrow Transplantation Versus Chemotherapy in Acute Lymphoblastic Leukemia. Joint Trial of the Medical Research Council (UKALL-12) with the United States Eastern Cooperative Oncology Group E2993

A.H. Goldstone, H.M. Lazarus, I.M. Franklin, S. Richards, J.W. Anderson, and J.M. Rowe

Background

Although the remission rate of adult patients with acute lymphoblastic leukemia (ALL) is high at >75%, most patients eventually relapse. The prevention of relapse by consolidation therapy is difficult and controversial, and with chemotherapy alone 5-year (DFS) disease free survivals have been in the range of 10%–42%. The use of allogeneic bone marrow transplantation (BMT) may result in a 40%–60% DFS with an actuarial relapse rate of between 10% and 40% with more than 90% of the recurrences occuring within the first 2 years. However, more than 50% of adults with ALL are more than 40 years old and in this age group allogeneic BMT still has substantial hazards. Autologous BMT is another alternative approach to consolidation therapy and the European BMT (EBMT) Registry of more than 200 patients in first complete remission (CR) showed a 41% DFS rate at 56 months for standard-risk patients transplanted in first CR. There was no statistical difference in those receiving purged or non-purged marrow and the 4 year probability of relapse was only 26% ±12% in this group. We have considered a randomised trial along the same basic pattern as the Medical Research Council Acute Myeloid Leukemia-10 (MRC AML-10) trial to establish the value of autologous and allogeneic BMT in first CR versus consolidation chemotherapy for adult patients between 15 and 56 years.

Objectives

The objectives of this study have been to investigate in a randomised controlled trial the outcome of treatment with allogeneic BMT in comparison with either myeloablative chemotherapy (etoposide, VP-16, + total body irradiation, TBI) with autologous BMT or intensive consolidation and maintenance chemotherapy. Patients in whom the Philadelphia chromosome is detected either cytogenetically or by molecular biological methods are in addition eligible to receive an allogeneic bone marrow transplant from a matched unrelated donor and to receive alpha-interferon during maintenance.

The trial design is that all eligible patients will receive uniform induction based on the Berlin-Frankfurt-Münster (BFM) protocol (Fig. 1). All patients receive a course of high-dose methotrexate to decrease the risk of CNS relapse from potential bone marrow contamination with residual disease at the time of bone marrow harvesting. Patients without a compatible donor and under 50 years of age will have marrow harvested and cryopreserved, and they can then be randomised to either myeloablative chemo/-radiotherapy with autologous BMT or four courses of intensive consolidation and maintenance therapy. Patients with a donor will be allocated to allogeneic BMT and patients who are Philadelphia positive without a matched donor are eligible for a transplant from a matched unrelated donor. If Philadelphia-positive patients do not have a potential donor, they

Department of Clinical Haematology, University College Hospital, Grafton Way, London WCIE 6AU, UK

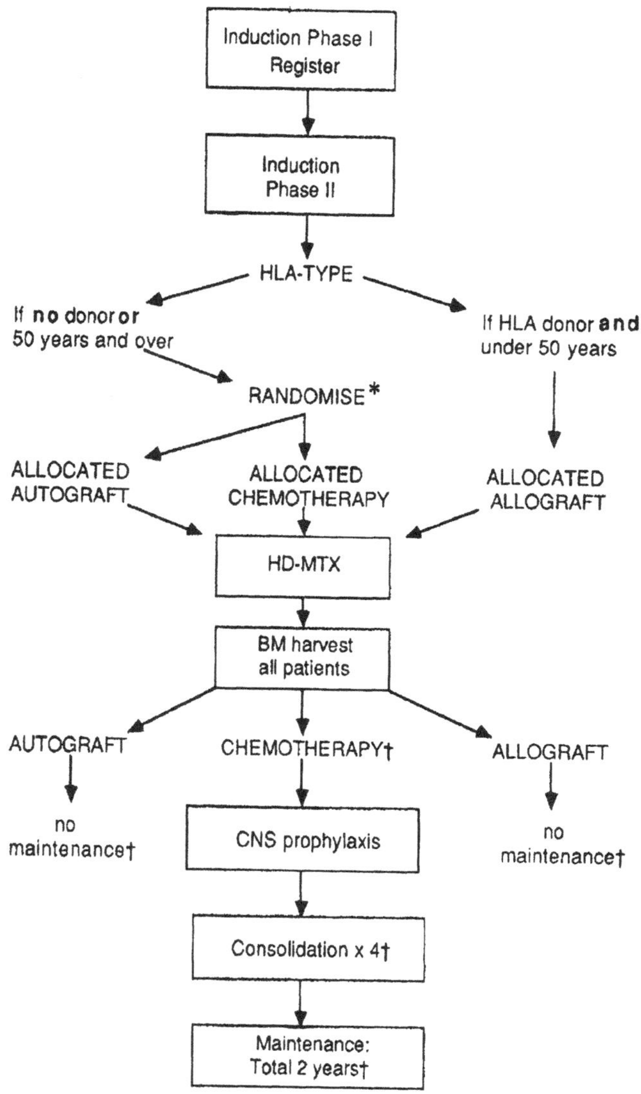

Fig. 1. Summary of UKALL-12/ECOG. Dagger, Philadelphia-positive patients receive a-interferon for 15 montsh after transplant or consolidation. *Asterisk*, Philadelphia-positive patients with no matched donor, a MUD transplant may be considered

are also randomised to myeloablative chemotherapy and autologous BMT.

Induction Chemotherapy

The induction chemotherapy is divided into two phases. Phase 1 consists of standard daunorubicin, vincristine, prednisolone and L-asparaginase. Phase II, beginning 1 month later, consists of cyclophosphamide, cytosine arabinoside, 6-mercaptopurine and intrathecal methotrexate. The intensification module with high-dose methotrexate begins 2 weeks after completion of phase II of induction, i.e. at the beginning of week 11 and ends at week 14. The dose of methotrexate is 3 g/m^2 i.v. given three times in the intensification course and accompanied by L-asparaginase 10000 units i.m. on each of the 3 days following the methotrexate. Leucovorin rescue, 50 mg/m^3 i.v. is given 36 h after finishing the methotrexate.

First Intensification Therapy

Following successful completion of phase I and phase II of induction and high-dose methotrexate, every patient has a bone marrow harvest, other than those with an HLA—identical sibling under 50 years who receive high-dose VP-16 and TBI, and allogeneic BMT. Patients less than 50 years without an HLA-matched donor and randomised to receive autologous BMT following VP-16/TBI or to receive consolidation and maintenance chemotherapy. The consolidation chemotherapy consists of four cycles; cycle 1, vincristine, cytosine, VP-16 and dexamethasone; cycle 2, cytosine and VP-16; cycle 3 daunorubicin, cyclophosphamide, cytosine, 6-thioguanine (6-TG); cycle 4, cytosine, VP-16(identical with cycle 2).

Management of Philadelphia-Positive Disease

Patients initially follow the trial protocol up to and including the high-dose methotrexate, the following options should be explored in Post-induction mangement:

1. The availability of a matched sibling donor if the patient is under the age of 50 years.
2. The availability in first CR of a matched unrelated donor. Such transplants should be considered.
3. All remaining patients are eligible for randomisation between chemotherapy and autologous BMT.
4. All patients will receive an additional 15 months of interferon therapy.

Statistical Considerations

To demonstrate a 60% improvement in 5-year survival from 25% on one treatment to 40% on the other requires 500 patients to have a 95% chance of detecting this difference. For 40% improvement in survival from 25% to 35%, this would require approximately 1000 patients to have a 95% chance of detecting this difference. Per year there are 170 cases of ALL in the United Kingdom between the ages of 15 and 59 and we hope for 130 registrations per year from the UK and bout 70 from the Eastern Cooperative Oncology Group (ECOG). The actual accrual over the first 2 years is shown in Fig. 2.

Results

Data are available on the first 148 patients. Of these 135 remitted (91%); Of these 135, 81 were in remission by day 21, and 21 not in remission by day 21. Data on the other 33 in terms of remission day are not yet known. Of the 21 who were not in remission at day 21, 12 remitted by day 28 and eight are unknown in relation to the time of remission.

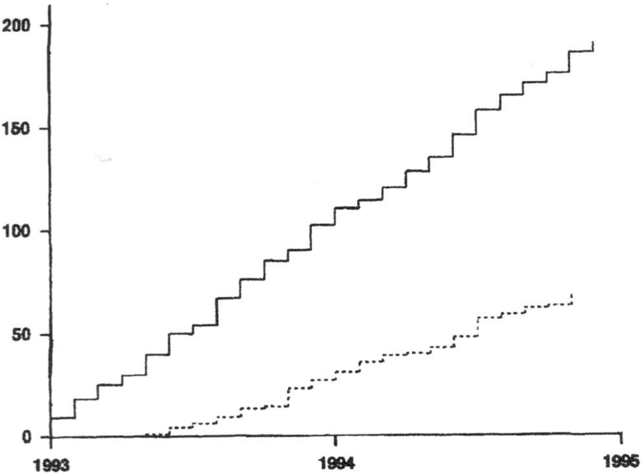

Fig. 2. ALLXII and ECOG—accumulative accession rate. *Solidline*, ALLXII; *Dottedline*, ECOG

Early Problems with the Study

A small number of cases of L-asparaginase—induced thrombophilia have been seen—in particular sagittal sinus thrombosis. It has been agreed that it is important to monitor antithrombin III, fibrinogen and partial thromboplastin time. Significant infection with pneumocystis and with aspergillus has been seen during induction and specific efforts are being taken with prophylaxis. There have been significant delays in haematological recovery from high-dose methotrexate. Whilst the United Kingdom group has been giving VP-16 before the TBI, it was discovered that the ECOG group were giving VP-16 after TBI.

Discussion

It has been found feasible to mount a collaborative trial between a major American cooperative group and the United Kingdom MRC. Remission rates at over 90% are high and this is satisfactory. The hospitalisation times for phase I and phase II are more than 28 days in each phase for the majority of patients. Investigators consider the protocol at least as intensive as the induction for adult AML. This is the first major collaborative randomised study which chooses a marrow transplant from an unrelated donor as a potential early option for a subgroup of patients, i.e. those with the Philadelphia chromosome. The trial as currently accruing will recruit a total of 500–600 patients within 4 years from starting.

Bcr-abl translocations will be detected by Polymerase chain reaction in a central laboratory. Assays will be sequentially performed in Philadelphia-positive patients throughout their treatment. The monitoring of minimal residual disease in known Philadelphia-positive patients is also being carried out.

Acute Leukemias VI
Prognostic Factors
and Treatment Strategies
Büchner et al. (eds)

Bone Marrow Transplantation for Philadelphia Chromosome Positive Acute Lymphoblastic Leukemia

M. Stockshläder[1], S. Hegewisch-Becker[2], W. Krüger[1], A. Dieck[1], M. Hoffknecht[2], C. Berger[1], B. Kohlschütter[1], H. Martin[4], S. Peters[1], H. Kabisch[3], R. Kuse[5], H.J. Weh[2], D.K. Hossfeld[2], and A. Zander[1]

Abstract. The outcome of 14 bone marrow transplantations (BMT; four autologous, ten allogeneic) for Philadelphia chromosome-positive acute lymphoblastic leukemia (ALL) was anlyzed. Preparative regimens consisted of etoposide (VP-16; 30–45 mg/kg; $n = 14$), cyclophosphamide (120 mg/kg; $n = 14$), and total body irradiation (TBI, 12 Gy; $n = 13$) or busulfan (16 mg/kg; $n = 1$). All patients receiving autologous marrow were in complete remission CR; three in first CR, one in second CR) at the time of BMT. For allogeneic BMT (nine related, one unrelated donor), seven patients were in first CR, two patients in first refractory relapse, and one patient in second relapse. With a median follow up of 503 days (range 93–1522 days), eight out of 14 patients are alive in CR (six out of ten patients receiving allogeneic and two out of four patients receiving autologous BMT). Disease-free survival at 38 weeks is 46%. Major causes of death were relapse ($n = 3$) and transplant-related toxicity (graft-versus-host disease), venous occlusive disease, sepsis; $n = 3$). All patients tested for the bcr/abl rearrangement by RT-PCR were negative 4 weeks post-BMT. Two of the three patients who subsequently relapsed were repeatedly PCR positive prior to relapse (test not done in the third). Considering the negligibly low curability of Philadelphia-positive ALL with conventional chemotherapy regimens, our data support the concept of early ($\geqslant$ first CR) BMT [allogeneic > autologous (purged)] following triple therapy with TBI, VP-16, and cyclophosphamide.

Introduction

The Philadelphia chromosome (Ph[1])[1], the product of a reciprocal translocation of distal segments of the long arms of chromosomes 9 and 22 [t(9; 22)(q34; q11)] [2] occurs in more than 95% of patients suffering from chronic myelogenous leukemia (CML), and in 2%–6% of children and 13%–32% of adults suffering from acute lymphoblastic leukemia (ALL) [3–4]. The translocation involves the movement of most of the *abl* protooncogene on chromosome 9 to the breakpoint cluster region (*bcr*) gene on chromosome 22 (the first exon, minor BCR region) or the second or third exon (major BCR region) [5,6]. Expression of the fused genes results in a chimeric 8.5-kb mRNA [7] which encodes a hybrid protein of 210 kd (p210)[8] with increased tyrosine kinase activity [9]. Most childhood Ph[1]-positive ALL and approximately half of adult Ph[1]-positive ALL patients have a translocation site different from that of CML and a more 5' bcr exon is used in the formation of the fused bcr-abl gene [4, 10]. This results in a

[1]BMT-Center, University Hospital Eppendorf, Martinistr. 52, 20246 Hamburg, Germany
[2]Department of Hematology and Oncology, University Hospital Ependorf, Martinistr. 52, 20246 Hamburg, Germany
[3]Department of Pediatric Oncology, University Hospital Eppendorf, Martinistr. 52, 20246 Hamburg, Germany
[4]Department of Hematology, Internal Medicine, J.W. Goethe University, Theodor-Stern-Kai 7, Frankfurt, Germany
[5]Department of Hematology, AK St. Georg, Lohmühlenstr. 1, 20251 Hamburg, Germany

smaller bcr-abl mRNA of 7 kb encoding a 190-kd protein (p190) [11,12].

Philadelphia-positive ALL has a poor prognosis in children and adults, this is independent of age and white blood cell (WBC) could [13, 14]. Although approximately 70% of patients achieve remission with chemotherapy, the median remission duration is less than 1 year and almost all relapse [15]. Bone marrow transplantation (BMT) has been reported to be an effective treatment for Ph[1]-positive ALL [16–24]. We analyzed the outcome of 14 patients with Ph[1]-positive ALL undergoing autologous or allogeneic BMT. The results suggest that high-dose radiochemotherapy such as total body irradiation (TBI), cyclophosphamide, and etoposide (VP-16) followed by BMT might be the preferred treatment modality for Ph[1]-positive ALL.

Material and Methods

The records of 14 patients who underwent autologous or allogeneic BMT for Ph[1]-positive ALL at the BMT Center of the University Hospital Eppendorf between August 1990 and October 1994 were reviewed. Patient characteristics and conditioning regimens are depicted in Table 1. Ten patients underwent allogeneic BMT from HLA-identical donors (nine related, one unrelated) and four patients received autologous bone marrow. Graft-versus-host disease

Table 1. Patient and treatment characteristics of patients transplanted for Ph1-positive ALL ($n = 14$)

	Allogeneic BMT ($n = 10$)	Autologous BMT ($n = 4$)
Age		
Recipient		
Median (years)	31	34
Range (years)	2–46	6–48
Donor		
Median (years)	33	n.a.
Range (years)	7-65	n.a.
Sex		
Recipient		
Female	5	3
Male	5	1
Donor		
Female	7	n.a.
Male	3	n.a.
Disease status at the time of transplantation:		
First CR	7	3
First refractory relapse	2	–
Second CR	–	1
Second relapse	1	–
Duration of CR until transplantation		
Median (days)	55	221
Range (days)	47–171	172–377
Immunophenotype		
CALLA	8	4
pre-B	1	–
Biphenotypic	1	–
Conditioning regimen		
fTBI (3 × 2 × 2 G)	9	4
Busulfan (16 mg/kg)	1	–
Cytoran (100 mg/kg)	10	4
VP-16	10	4
30 mg/kg	3	1
45 mg/kg	7	3
ATG	3	–

(CVGD) prophylaxis consisted of cyclosporine A (CSA) plus short methotrexate (MTX) in all patients. Acute GVHD was diagnosed and graded according to the Glucksberg criteria [25] and was treated in both groups with methylprednisolone and/or anti-thymocyte globulin (ATG). The maximum grade of acute GVHD achieved by day 100 post transplant was recorded. Post-transplant supportive care has been described before [26]. Two patients undergoing autologous BMT received purged BM (one mafosfamide, one immunological). Because of delayed engraftment the patient who received mafosfamide-purged marrow was treated with a marrow boost of unpurged back-up marrow (case record submitted). One patient who received an allogeneic BMT relapsed on day 165 post BMT and was treated with busulfan (14 mg/kg), VP-16 (30 mg/kg), and subsequent infusion of granulocyte colony-stimulating factor (G-CSF)-mobilized peripheral stem cells (sum of four harvests: 26.6*10^8 mononuclear cells/kg body weight, BW and 2.13*10^6 colony-forming unit —granulocyte—macrophage(CFU-GM)/kg BW, respectively) from the marrow donor.

RT-PCR Analysis. RT-PCR was performed as previously described using primers that will detect all rearrangements within the bcr. Briefly, total cellular RNA was isolated according to the guanidine isothiocyanate phenol/chloroform method. cDNA was synthesized with a cDNA synthesis kit (Boehringer Mannheim Corp., Indianapolis, IN, USA) according to the manufacturer's protocol using 1 µg total cellular RNA. PCR was performed in a final volume of 100 µl with 100 ng cDNA using a Gene Amp PCR kit (Perkin-Elmer Cetus, Norwalk CT, USA). A total of 40 cycles was performed. The conditions for amplification and the primer sequences for p210 and p190 have been described [27, 33]. As a positive control for the procedure, a second RT-PCR was performed on the same reverse transcriptase reaction products using abl-specific primers [33]. PCR products were visualized by electrophoresis in ethidium bromide-stained 2% agarose gels. Southern blotting and bybridzation for detection of bcr rearrangements were done as described [11] using junctional probes that had been end-labeled with ^{32}P-adenosine-5'-triphosphate(^{32}P-ATP).

Statistical Analysis. The disease-free survival (DFS) estimate was calculated by the product-limit estimates of Kaplan and Meier [28].

Results

Patient Characteristics and Engraftment. The characteristics of the 14 patients are depicted in Table I. Time to engraftment was defined as the number of days from marrow transplantation until the absolute neutrophil count was sustained above 0.2 and 0.5×10^9/l. The results are summarized in Table 2. One patient who died on day 21 due to *Candida krusei* sepsis was not evaluable. All patients receiving an allogeneic BMT and one patient undergoing autologous BMT were treated with the hematopoietic growth factor G-CSF.

Hepatic Toxicity. Hyperbilirubinemia developed in nine patients receiving allogeneic and one patient receiving autologous BM during the first 28 days post BMT. Severe hyperbilirubinemia defined as maximum serum bilirubin > 5 mg/dl and 10 mg/dl occurred in three and two patients receiving allogeneic BMT, respectively. For allogeneic BMT, median maximum serum bilirubin was higher for patients receiving 45 mg/kg VP-16 than for patients receiving 30 mg/kg VP-16: 3.5 mg/dl (range 1.8–21.6 mg/dl) vs. 1.5 mg/dl (range 1.1–4.0 mg/dl). For patients receiving 45 mg/kg VP-16, median maximum serum bilirubin was higher for patients receiving an allogeneic graft than for patients undergoing autologous BMT: 3.5 mg/dl (range 1.8–21.6 mg/dl) vs 1.0 mg/dl (range 0.9–1.5 mg/dl).

Table 2. Engraftment

	Allogeneic BMT	Autologous BMT
ANC > 0.2* 10^9—Median (days)	16	16
Range (days)	12–24	12–17
ANC > 0.5* 10^9—Median (days)	18	20
Range (days)	13–25	14–20

Graft-versus-Host Disease. Eight patients developed acute GVHD. GVHD grade ≥ II occured in seven patients (six grade II, one grade III). The median day of onset of acute GVHD was day 10 (range 7–19). Four of eight evaluable patients (50%) developed chronic GVHD.

Detection of the bcr-abl RNA by RT-PCR. The PCR amplification of cDNA prepared directly from clinical samples reliably distinguishes the three known species of BCR-ABL mRNA that are transcribed from the Ph[1] chromosome. As depicted in Table 3, the chimeric bcr-abl mRNA was detected by PCR in all tested patients ($n=11$) prior to transplantation. In five patients the translocation involved the major BCR region, in five patients the minor BCR region, and in one patient the major and minor BCR region. Examination of the karyotype of this patient revealed that cells contained two Ph[1] chromosomes. Four weeks after transplantation, none of the tested patients was positive. In patients, GG and SX who relapsed (day 144 and day 165, respectively) RT-PCR had become positive (day 86 and day 67, respectively) prior to relapse (58 and 98 days earlier). Patient CC who relapsed on day 110 tested negative by PCR 1 week before relapse, however, Patient MK who has been repeatedly positive by PCR analysis (3 and 6 months) after transplantation remains in unsustained complete remission (275 days). Patient BL who received autologous mafosfamide-purged BM and a boost of unpurged autologous BM has been repeatedly positive (day 84, day 795) and negative (day 11, day 24, day 230, day 489, day 887, day 1126, day 1489) by RT-PCR, but remains in complete remission (1522 days). Her case will be reported separately.

Survival. Within the first 100 days post transplant, only one patient who received allogeneic bone marrow died giving a day-100 survival of 90% for the allogeneic and for all autologous bone marrow recipients. Four patients relapsed 108, 110, 144, and 165 days after BMT, respectively. Three of these patients died of relapse (days, 205,

Table 3. bcr-abl RT-PCR of 11 Ph[1]-positive ALL patients undergoing DMT

Patient initials	Sub-type Age Years	Before BMT	4 Weeks post BMT	3 Months post BMT	4–6 Months post BMT	7–12 Months post BMT	Later
Autologous BMT							
BL	p190 25	+	Neg	+	Neg	ND	n/+n/n/n
MK	p210 6	+	Neg	+	+		
GG	p210 43	+	Neg	+	R+	+ Died	
Allogeneic BMT							
CC	p210	+	Neg	Neg R	+	ND	Died
IE	p190+ 2 p210	+	Neg	Neg	Neg	Neg	
MF	p190 36	+	Neg	Neg	Neg	Died	
HH	p190 33	+	Neg	Neg	Neg	Neg	
SK	p190 22	+	ND	Neg	ND	ND	Neg
BS	p210 29	+	ND	Neg	ND	Died	
SX	p210 47	+	Neg	+	R +	2nd Tx	
KN	p190 28	+	ND	Neg	ND	ND	Neg

+, RT-PCR positive; neg, RT-PCR negative; ND, not determined; n, negative; R, relapse; Tx, transplantation.

259, and 420) and one patient received a second transplant. Main causes of death in both groups included GVHD, sepsis, venous occlusive disease (VOD), and relapse. Of the 14 patients, eight (57%) are alive and in continuous remission with a minimum follow-up of 93 days (median 503 days). The estimated overall survival of the entire group at 60 weeks is 52% (Fig. 1).

Discussion

In this retrospective analysis of 14 patients with Ph[1]-positive ALL, we found that improved relapse-free survival was associated with BMT in first completed remission. Eight patients survive with a median follow up of 443 days. Three patients died of transplant-related complications and three of relapse. Eight of ten patients were transplanted within 6 months after achieving first complete remission. Early transplantation seems to be important considering the only short median remission duration of 22 weeks [15]. BMT leads to substantially prolonged DFS and cure. Earlier studies have shown similar results [18, 19, 24, 29].

The effectiveness of fractrionated TBI and high-dose VP-16 as a conditioning regimen for advanced leukemias and high-risk ALL has been reported presiously [24, 30, 31]. We also included also high-dose VP-16 into the standard preparative regimen of TBI and cyclophosphamide. The impact of the two different concentrations (30 vs. 45 mg/kg) of VP-16 on leukemia-free survival can not be determined because of the small patient number. It appears, however, that the higher dose of VP-16 leads to more severe hepatotixicity judged by the incidence of severe hyperbilirubinemia and VOD. The potentially higher incidence of transplant-related complications caused by further dose escalation has to be weighed against a potentially lower relapse rate.

As shown in earlier studies [29], PCR can be used as a tool for monitoring minimal residual disease in Ph[1]-positive ALL. In our study, 11 tested patients were PCR positive prior to BMT and converted to PCR negative 4 weeks after transplantation indicating the effectiveness of the preparative regimen. One patient was positive for both p190 and p210 as has been reported previously [12, 15, 32]. Two patients who became PCR positive upon further follow up subsequently relapsed (58 and 98 days later) indicating that molecular relapse after BMT correlates with clinical relapse in Ph[1]-positive ALL, as has been suggested before [29]. One patient who has repeatedly tested positive by PCR remains in hematological remision 7 months after the first PCR positivity, however.

Another patient who has remained disease-free for more than 50 months has also been PCR

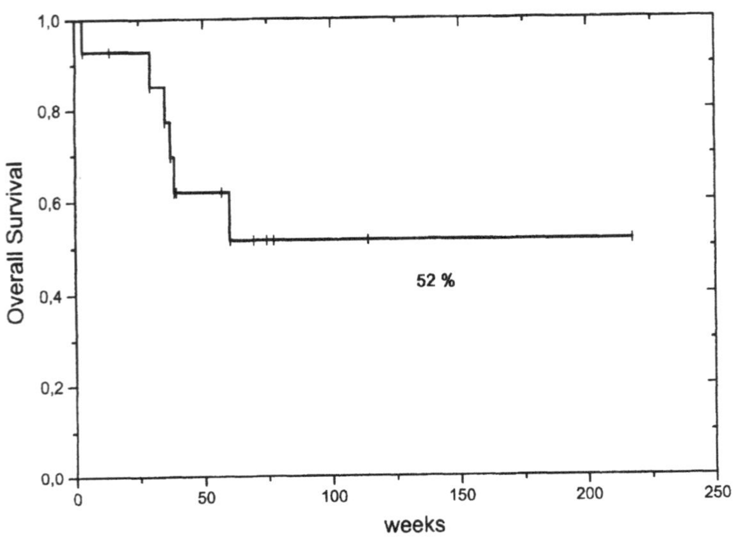

Fig. 1. BMT for Philadelphia chromosome-positive ALL

positive on several occasions post BMT. Why in these two cases molecular relapse has not preceded hematological relapse remains to be determined. Since these two patients received an autologous BMT, a potential alloreactive immune response controlling a leukemic clone can hardly be invoked. Whether it reflects the prolonged survival of "maglignant" cells or suggests that the engrafting immune system may be important in eliminating residual Ph[1]-positive cells for "cure" requires further investigation [33].

There are several caveats regarding out study. The patient group under study is relatively small and the observation time is still limited. Nevertheless, a combination of TBI, cytoxan (CTX), and VP-16 appears to be an effective preparatory regimen for Ph[1]-positive ALL. From our data we cannot recommend the best dose of VP-16.

Considering the poor prognosis for patients with this variant of ALL, BMT performed early during the course of the disease may currently be the treatment of choice. The poor prognosis of patients with Ph[1]-positive ALL also suggests that in the absence of a matched sibling donor, an unrelaterd donor should be sought or an autologous BMT performed (purged > unpurged).

Acknowledgments. We thank our BMT team members and nurses in the BMT unit for providing excellent care of our patients and the medical technicians for excellent work in the BMT laboratory.

References

1. Nowell PC and Hungerford DA. Chromosome studies on normal and luekemic human leukocytes. JNCI 1960, 25: 85.
2. Rowley JD. A new consistent chromosomal abnormality in chronic myelogenous leukemia identified by quinacrine fluorescence and Giemsa staining. *Nature* 1973, 243: 290–291.
3. Champlin RE and Golde DW. Chronic myelogenous leukemia: recent advances. *Blood* 1985, 65: 1039–1047.
4. Lestingi T, Hooberman A. Philadelphia chromosome-positive acute lymphoblastic leukemia. *Hem Onc Clin of North America* 1993, 7: 161–175.
5. de Klein A, van Kessel AG, GROSVELD et al. A cellular oncogene is translocated to the Philadelphia chromosome in chronic myelocytic leukemia. *Nature* 1982, 300: 765–767.
6. Groffen J, Stephenson JR, Heisterkamp N et al. Philadelphia chromosomal breakpoints are clustered within a limited region bor on chromosome 22. *Cell* 1984, 36: 93–99
7. Shtivelman E, Lifshitz B, Gale RP and Canaani E. Fused transcript of abl and bcr genes in chronic myelogenous leukemia. *Nature* 1985, 315: 550–554.
8. Ben-Neriah Y, Daley G, Mes-Masson AM: The chronic myelogenous leukemia-specific p210 protein is the product of the bcr/abl hybrid gene. *Science* 1986, 233: 212–233.
9. Konopka JB, Watanabe SM and Witte ON. An alteration of the human c-abl protein in K562 leukemia cells unmasks associated tyrosine kinase activity. *Cell* 1984, 37: 1035–1042.
10. Fainstein E; Marcelle C; Rosner A et al. A new fused transcript in Philadelphia chromosome positive acute lymphocytic leukemia. *Nature* 1987, 330: 386–388.
11. Kawasaki, Clark S, Coyne M et al. Diagnosis of chronic myeloid and acute lymphocytic leukemias by detection of leukemia-specific mRNA sequences amplified in vitro. *Proc Natl Acad Sci* 1988, 85: 5698–5702.
12. Hooberman A, Carrino J, Leibowitz D et al. Unexpected heterogeneity of BCR-ABL fusion mRNA detected by polymerasxe chain reaction in Philadelphia chromosome-positive acute lymphoblastic leukemia. *Proc Natl Acad Sci USA* 1989, 86: 4259–4263.
13. Jain K, Arlin Z, Mertelsmann R et al. Philadelphia chromosome and terminal transferase-positive acute leukemia: Similarity of terminal phase of chronic myelogenous leukemia and de novo acute presentation. *J Clin Oncol* 1983, 1: 669.
14. Mayer RJ. Acute lymphoblastic leukemia in adults. *Ann Intern Med* 1984, 101: 552.
15. Kantarjian H, Talpaz M, Dhingra K et al. Significance of the p210 versus p190 molecular abnormalities in adults with Philadelphia chromosome-positive acute leukemia. *Blood* 1991, 78: 2411.
16. Reece DE, Buskard NA, Hill RS et al. Allogeneic bone marrow transplantation for Philadelphia chromosome positive acute lymphoblastic leukemia. *Leuk Res* 1976, 10: 457.
17. Poynton CH and Barrett AJ. Relapsed acute lymphoblastic leukemia: evaluation of BMT in prolongation of unmaintained remission. *Bone Marrow Transplant* 1986, 1: 207.
18. Forman SJ, O'Donnell MR, Nademanee et al. Bone Marrow transplantation for patients with Philadelphia chromosome positive acute lymphoblastic leukemia. *Blood* 1987, 70: 587–588.
19. Barrett A. Horowitz M, ASH R et al. Bone marrow transplantation for Philadelphia chromosome positive acute lymphoblasitc leukemia. *Blood* 1992, 79: 3067–3070.
20. Forman S, O'Donnell M, Nademanee A et al. Bone marrow transplantation for patients with Philadelphia chromosome-positive acute lymphoblastic leukemia versus intensification chemotherapy for acute myelogenous leukemia in first remission: a prospective controlled trial. *Br J Hematol* 1988, 68: 219–226.

21. Hoelzer D. Change in treatment strategies for adult lymphoblastic leukemia according to prognostic factors and residual disease. *Bone Marrow Transplant* 1990, 6: 4.
22. Horowitz M, Messerer D, Hoelzer D et al. Chemotheray compared with bone marrow transplantation for adults with acute lymphoblastic leukemia in first remission. *Ann. Intern Med* 1991, 115: 13.
23. Wingard J, Piantadosi S, Santos G et al. Allogeneic bone marrow transplantation for patients with high-risk acute lymphoblastic leukemia. *J Clin Oncol* 1990, 8: 820.
24. Chao N, Forman S, Schmidt G et al. Allogeneic bone marrow transplantation for high-risk acute lymphoblastic leukemia during first complete remission. *Blood* 1991, 78: 1923–1927.
25. Glucksberg H, Storb R, Fefer A et al. Clinical manifestations of graft vs host disease in human recipients of marrow from HLA-matched sibling donors. *Transplantation* 1974, 18: 295.
26. Stockschläder M, Kalhs P, Peters S et al. Intravenous pentoxifylline failed to prevent transplantrelated toxicities in allogeneic bone marrow transplant recipients. *Bone Marrow Transplantation* 1993, 12: 357–362.
27. Hermans A, Gow J, Sellerie L et al. bcr-abl oncogene in Philadelphia chromosome-positive acute lymphoblastic leukemia. *Leukemia* 1988, 2: 628–633.
28. Kaplan E and Meier P. Nonparametric estimation from incomplete observations. *J AM Stat Assoc* 1958, 53: 457–481.
29. Miyamura K, Tanimoto M, Morishma Y et al. Detection of Philadelphia chromosome-positive acute lymphoblastic leukemia by polymerase chain reaction: possible eradication of minimal residual disease by marrow transplantation. *Blood* 1992, 79: 1366–1370.
30. Blume K, Forman S, O'Donnell M et al. Total body irradiation and high-dose etoposide: a new preparatory regimen for bone marrow transplantation in patients with advanced hematological malignancies. *Blood* 1987, 69: 1015–1020.
31. Schmitz N, Gassmann W, Rister M et al. Fractionated total body irradiation and high dose VP 16-213 followed by allogeneic bone marrow transplantation in advanced leukemias. *Blood* 1988, 72: 1567.
32. Hooberman A, Westbrook C, Davey F et al. Detection of Philadelphia chromosome in acute lymphoblastic leukemia by pulsed-field gel electrophoresis. *Blood* 1989, 74: 1101.
33. Roth M, Antin E, Bingham E, and Ginsburg D. Detection of Philadelphia chromosome-positive cells by the polymerase chain reaction following bone marrow transplantation for chronic myelogenous leukemia. *Blood* 1989, 74: 882–885

AML in Children

Acute Leukemias VI
Prognostic Factors
and Treatment Strategies
Büchner et al. (eds)

Childrens Cancer Group Studies in Acute Myeloid Leukemia, 1979–1995: Three Strategies That Have Worked

B. Lange[1], J. Buckley[2], B. Lampkin[3], M. Nesbit[4], and W.G. Woods[4] for the Childrens Cancer Group[5]

Abstract. Review of Childrens Cancer Group (CCG) randomized trials conducted since 1979 identifies three strategies that have led to incremental improvements in outcome: (a) allogeneic bone marrow transplantation (BMT) in first remission; (b) sequentially timed high-dose chemotherapy and the advent of more effective pre-and post-remission treatment; and (c) attenuation of maintenance therapy. Among patients treated from 1979 to 1983, the 5-year disease-free survival (DFS) following matched-related allogeneic transplantation was 45% and between 1983 and 1988, 46%. From 1983 to 1988 intensification therapy with sequentially timed high-dose cytosine arabinoside (ara-C) given on days 0,1 and 7 and 8 achieved a five-year DFS of 38% (p =.06 compared to BMT). Five-year post-remission survival with sequentially timed high-dose ara-C was 58% compared to 41% with conventionally timed day 0,1 and 28,29 ara-C (p=.05). Five-year survival following high-dose ara-C intensification was significantly lower after 16 months of maintenance therapy compared to no maintenance (44% vs. 68%, $p<.01$). Since 1979, the remission induction rate has ranged between 74% and 79%, even with kinetically based sequentially timed five-drug chemotherapy. However, post-remission DFS was significantly highr with sequentially timed induction therapy than with conventionally timed therapy: 60% vs. 37% at 3 years (p= .0002). With the combined use of sequentially timed induction therapy, matched-related BMT, and development of the best post-remission regimen from the current study. CCG acute myeloid leukemia (AML) therapy will potentially cure over half the children with (AML) by the year 1999.

Introduction

The Childrens Cancer Group (CCG) trial CCG-251, which opened in 1979, demonstrated the superiority of allogeneic bone marrow transplantation (BMT) over maintenance chemotherapy [1]. Allogeneic bone marrow transplantation has remained the standard to which other strategies have been compared in all subsequent CCG trials [2–5]. So far, no regimen has achieved a higher survival and disease-free survival (DFS) than matched-related allogeneic marrow transplantation.

In an attempt to develop myelosuppressive chemotherapy as effective as the myeloablation of marrow transplantation regimens, CCG investigated kinetically sequenced timing of high-dose phase-specific chemotherapy. In vitro studies have demonstrated recruitment and synchronization of acute myeloid leukemia (AML) blasts by scheduling successive pulses of cytosine arabinoside (ara-C) to coincide with entry of the blasts into S phase [6–9]. The optimal time between pulses of chemotherapy is about 6 days

[1]Children's Hospital of Philadelphia, Philadelphia, PA, USA
[2]University of California, Los Angeles, CA, USA
[3]Children's Hospital Medical Center, Cincinnati, OH, USA
[4]University of Minnesota Medical Center, Minneapolis, MN, USA
[5]Children's Cancer Group Operations, Arcadia, CA, USA

[6]. Kinetically sequenced therapy is a toxic, effective way to eradicate leukemic myeloblasts [7–10]. CCG-213P compared conventionally timed high-dose ara-C to sequentially timed high-dose ara-C during intensification. Sequentially timed high-dose ara-C was better [2,11]. CCG is now evaluating high-dose, sequentially timed chemotherapy in induction [5]. Again, sequential timing appears to be better.

The early protocols for AML therapy were adaptations of protocols for acute lymphoblastic leukemia (ALL). Hence, they included maintenance therapy, an intrinsic part of ALL therapy. CCG has examined maintenance strategies in AML since 1974 [1, 3, 12]. Those CCG trials where maintenance therapy was a randomized or controlled variable have not demonstrated a dose-response effect or any other measurable benefit from maintenance therapy [1, 3]. Therefore, CCG trials have successively and systematically attenuated maintenance therapy.

The goal of current CCG studies is to cure at least half the children with AML before the year 1999. To achieve this goal, CCG is building on three strategies that have worked consistently in CCG clinical trials of the past 15 years. These strategies are (a) allogeneic BMT in first remission, (b) high-dose, sequentially timed chemotherapy, and (c) attenuation of maintenance therapy. These three strategies have shortened the duration of AML therapy at the same time as they have increased its intensity. The review that follows tracks these strategies over 2 decades and 2009 eligible patients, identifies their contributions to cure, and argues for their continuation and further exploration in pediatric AML.

Methods

CCG Trials Evaluating Allogeneic BMT in First Remission: CCG-251, CCG-213, CCG-2861, and CCG-2891

Four successive CCG studies have included allogeneic BMT in first remission (Fig. 1) [1, 3–5, 13–15]. The major study question of the first, CCG-251, was whether allogeneic BMT in first remission brought about a better outcome than the best available maintanence chemotherapy. The second study, CCG-213, compared transplantation to intensification with the Capizzi II high-dose ara-C regimen [16, 17]. This regimen consists of high-dose ara-C 3 g/m^2 as a 3 h infusion every 12 h on days 0 and 1 and 7 and 8, and L-asparaginase 6000 U/m^2 at hour 42 on day 2 and day 8 [16, 17]. After completing two cycles of Capizzi II high-dose ara-C, patients receive 2 months of maintenance-like therapy consisting of pulses of four drugs every 28 days and daily 6-thioguanine (6-TG) and 3rd month of five-drug reinduction therapy [2]. The third study, CCG-2861, compared allogeneic BMT to autologous marrow (ABMT) purged with 4-hydroperoxycyclophosphamide (4-HC). Finally, the most recent study, CCG-2891, added a third alternative, the high-dose ara-C intensification complex.

Among the successive studies, induction regimens varied, as described in the next section and in the results. Cytoreduction and graft-versus-host prophylaxis varied also. In CCG-251 transplantation cytoreduction consisted of cyclophosphamide 60 mg/kg per day × 2 and 750–1000 cGy unfractionated total body irradiation [1, 15]. Initial graft-versus-host prophylaxis was methotrexate only [1, 3, 5, 13–15]. In CCG-213 cytoreduction included cyclophosphamide 60 mg/kg per day × 2 and 1200 CGY total body irradiation in six fractions [3,15]. Graft-versus-host prophylaxis was with cyclosporin and methotrexate [3,15]. In CCG-2861, transplantation cytoreduction included cyclophosphamide 50 mg/kg per day × 4 and busulfan 1 mg/kg every 6 h × 16 doses [5, 15]. Graft-versus-host prophylaxis consisted of methotrexate. In CCG-2891, transplantation cytoreduction and graft-versus-host prophylaxis were the same as in CCC-2861 [4, 5].

CCG AML Studies Evaluating Timed-Sequential Therapy: CCG-213P, CCG-213, CCG-2861

CCG AML Studies Evaluating Timed-Sequential Intensification Therapy with Capizzi II High-Dose ara-C/l-Asparaginase: CCG-213P, CCG-213 and CCG-2891. CCG-213P, a pilot study, compared administration of the drugs on days 0, 1, and 7 and 8 to days 0, 1 and 28 and 29, i.e., after marrow recovery [2,11]. The first cohort of patients received the days 0, 1, and 28 and 29 schedule; the second cohort, the timed-sequential schedule. After completing two cycles of high-dose ara-C, patients received the remainder of the high-dose ara-C complex. The days 0, 1, and 7 and 8 sequential schedule for ara-C was retained in CCG-213 and CCG-2891 [3–5].

CCG-2861 and CCG-2891: Five-Drug Timed-Sequential Induction Therapy. CCG-2861 was a pilot study assessing feasibility and toxicity of a timed-sequential dose-intensified five-drug regimen in induction followed by either matched-related allogeneic BMT or 4-HC-purged ABMT [4, 18]. The five-drug combination included dexamethasone, ara-C, 6-TG, etoposide, and rubidomycin (DCTER) [4]. The timed-sequential schedule mandated DCTER on days 0–3 and 10–13, irrespective of blood counts or clinical condition. CCG–2891 asked whether timed-sequential induction therapy improved remission induction rate and post-remission outcome [4, 5]. At diagnosis, patients were randomly assigned to receive DCTER according to either the timed-sequential schedule described above or a conventional schedule which prescribed the second cycle of DCTER on day or later depending on bone marrow status. Upon marrow recovery, patients received a second course of sequentially or conventionally timed DCTER. Patients in remission with a matched-related donor were allocated to allogeneic BMT; those without a donor were randomly assigned to 4-HC-purged ABMT or intensive chemotherapy.

CCG Trials Evaluating Maintenance Therapy: CCG-251, CCG-213P, and CCG-213

In CCG-251, patients in remission without a matched sibling donor were randomly assigned to one of two maintenance treatment plans. The eight-drug plan rotated pulses of ara-C and 5-azacytidine, prednisolone, 6-mercaptopurine, vincristine, and methotrexate; and carmustine (BCNU) and 6-TG. This combination was derived from VAPA therapy [1, 19]. The five-drug plan included vincristine on day 0, cyclophosphamide, ara-C, and 5-azacytidine on days 0–3 every 28 days, 6-TG daily. This regimen was derived from CCG-241 which showed the benefits of daily 6-TG [12]. In CCG-251, maintenance therapy lasted 2 years.

In CCG-213P, maintenance was not specified: patients or physicians elected to discontinue therapy after the high-dose ara-C intensification complex or to continue for 16 months using the four-drug pulse daily 6-TG regimen. CCG-213 randomly allocated patients to no maintenance or continuing for 16 months of maintenance after intensification.

Statistical Analysis

The definition of disease-free survival (DFS) is the time to relapse or death from any cause following remission induction. Survival time begins at the time the patient registers on the study. The major analyses are based on intent to treat. Where outcomes based on intent to treat differ substantially from outcomes according to treatment received, the latter results are also presented. Differences in proportions are tested using the χ^2 statistic or Fisher's exact test. The log rank statistic is used to compare survival and DFS [20–22]. The cure model measures outcome differences between transplantation and chemotherapy regimens and is used in analysis of CCG-251 and CCG-213 outcomes [23, 24].

Results

CCG AML Trials Evaluating Allogeneic BMT in First Remission

Figure 1 follows allogeneic BMT from 1979 to the present in studies CCG-251, CCG-213, CCG-2861, and CCG-2891. In CCG-251, of 490 eligible patients, 381 entered remission [1,25]. Eighty-nine patients had a matched sibling donor; 79 actually underwent transplantation. Of 266 patients 233 received chemotherapy. DFS and survival were significantly higher among transplanted patients at 5 and 8 years [1].

In CCG-213, of 591 eligible patients, 439 entered remission [3]. Of 113 patients with a matched sibling donor, 83 underwent transplantation. Of 298 patients without a donor, 225 participated in the randomized comparison of the high-dose ara-C intensification complex to allogeneic BMT (cf. next section) [3]. In CCG-213, the high-dose ara-C intensification complex achieved results closer to results of transplantation. When outcomes were analyzed according to intent to treat, 5 year DFS was 46% for transplantation and 38% for chemotherapy ($p = .06$; log-rank $= .27$) [3] (Fig. 5). When analyzed according to treatment received. 5 year DFS is 54% for transplantation and 36% for chemotherapy ($p = .001$ and log-rank $= .007$) [3] (not shown).

When only patients who received their randomized regimen were considered, 5-year DFS was 54% for transplantation and 37% for chemotherapy ($p = .002$ and log-rank $= .01$) [3]. Thus, allogeneic transplantation remained marginally superior,although the timed-sequential high-dose ara-C intensification complex narrowed the gap. In subsequent CCG studies, acute transplantation-related mortality has

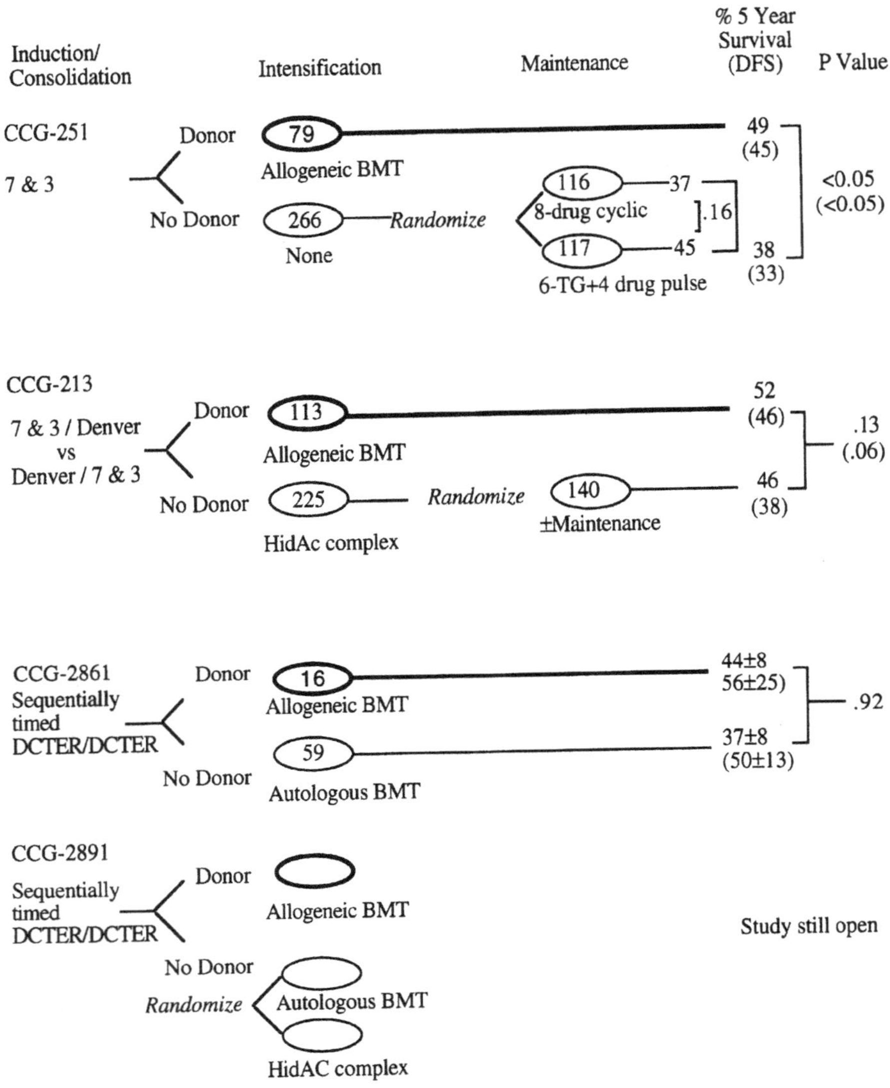

Fig. 1. Allogeneic bone marrow transplantation in CCG AML studies: acturial post-remission outcomes. Patient numbers are in *ovals. Bold lines* allogeneic bone marrow transplantation (*BMT*) involving sequentially timed induction therapy; *7&3* 7 days of cytosine arabinoside and 3 days of daunorubicin *DCTER* five drugs (dexamethasone, cytosine arabinoside, 6-thioguanine, etoposide, rubidomycin) [5]. *HidAc* high-dose cytosine arabinoside and L-asparaginase followed by three cycles of maintenance-like pulse chemotherapy [3,7,14,15]. Maintenance regimens are explained in Fig. 2

declined in each successive trial, so that in the present trial it is about 10%. This improvement in BMT may widen the gap again.

CCG AML Studies Evaluating Timed-Sequential Therapy: CCG-2861, CCG-2891, CCG-213-P, and CCG-213

CCG AML Studies Evaluating Capizzi II High-Dose ara-C/L-Asparaginase Timed-Sequential Consolidation Therapy: CCG-213P, CCG-213, and CCG-2891. The goal of the timed-sequential high-dose ara-C intensification complex was to bring about survival and DFS

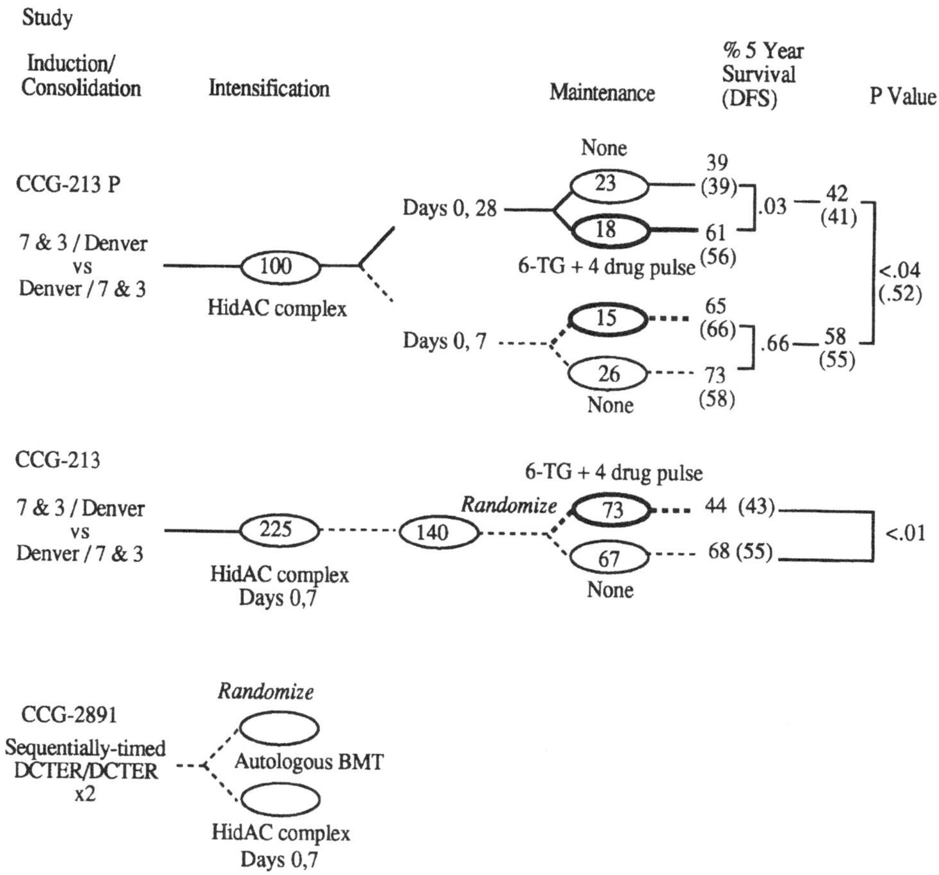

Fig. 2. Timed sequential intensification chemotherapy and attenuation of maintenance therapy in CCG AML trials: Acturial post-remission outcome following high-dose ara-C intensification therapy with or without maintenance therapy. *Broken lines* indicate timed sequential therapy. *Bold lines* indicate maintenance therapy, Patient numbers are in *ovals*. Four drug pulse+ 6-TG includes vincristine on day 0, cyclophosphamide, ara-C, and 5-*azacytidine* on days 0–3 every 28 days, and daily 6 TG. Ten-drug therapy consists of rotating pulses of ara-C and 5-azacytidine, predinsolone, 6-mercaptopurine, vincristine, and methotrexate, and lomustine and 6-TG. Maintenance continues for 2 years in CCG-251 and 16 months in CCG-213 and CCG-213P. *HidAC complex* high-dose ara-C/L-asparaginase followed by three cycles of maintenance chemotherapy (days 3, 7, 14, 15). Induction regimens are explained in Fig. 1

that approached those of marrow transplantation. The comparison of BMT and high-dose ara-C is in Fig. 1. Figure 2 tracks Capizzi II high-dose ara-C/L-asparaginase timed-sequential intensification therapy from CCG-213P through CCG-2891. Although not a randomized trial, CCG-213P prospectively compared a 6-day interval between pulses of high-dose ara-C/l-asparaginase to a 28-day interval. The 6-day interval effected a 5-year DFS of 61% compared to 45% for the 28-day interval ($p=.109$). Survival at 5 years was significantly higher with the 6-day interval: 58% vs. 41% ($p=<0.05$) [2]. The price of better long-term outcome with timed-sequential intensification was acute treatment-related mortality (three vs. none among 104 patients) [11].

CCG AML Studies Evaluating Five-Drug Timed-Sequential Induction Therapy: CCG-2861 and CCG-2891. To examine the role of the sequentially timed induction schedule on remission rate and long-term outcome, remission induction therapies in successive CCG trials were compared [1, 3, 25–27]. These trials manipulted the formulation and dose of anthracycline and added drugs to the standard 7 days of ara-C and 3 days of daunomycin. CCG-251 used the "7 and 3" paradigm, but with a relatively low dose of anthracycline, 30 mg/m^2 [1, 25]. CCG-213 compared 7 and 3, using daunorubicin 45 mg/m^2, to a combination of ara-C, daunorubicin, 6-TG, etoposide, and dexamethasone, called Denver, the precursor of the DCTER regimen [3, 18]. After two to three cycles of 7 and 3 as induction, patients received five-drug Denver as consolidation and vice versa [3]. Table 1 lists dose intensity during the first 14 days of therapy and the cumulative drug doses given before intensification in CCG studies CCG-251, CCG-213, and CCG-2891. Although the number of drugs, their cumulative doses, and their dose intensity in the first 14 days increased progressively among sequential studies, the remission induction rate remained fixed between 74% and 79%. Table 1 also shows that the induction mortality was higher with timed-sequential therapy than with the other induction regimens. However, greater durability of remission in the patients given sequentially timed induction offset the early mortality to provide an actuarial 3-year survival of 61%. Table 2 shows the blinded 3-year DFS rates in the three post-remission regimens in CCG-2891. The results of Table 1 and Table 2 demonstrate that induction therapy can influence the outcome of post-remission therapy with either transplantation or chemotherapy [2–5].

CCG AML Trials Evaluating Maintenance Chemotherapy

In CCG-251 no differences were found in survival or DFS at 3,5, and 8 years among patients who received monthly pulses of four drugs with daily 6-Ta compared to eight-drug cyclic therapy (Fig.1) [1]. CCG-213 and CCG-213P retained the simpler, less toxic four drugs with daily 6-TA regimen and shortened the duration of maintenance from 24 months to 16 months. Figure 1 shows that, with timed-sequential high-dose ara-C, maintenance and no maintenance achieved similar outcomes. However, with conventionally timed high-dose ara-C, maintenance

Table 1. CCG AML trials: (cumulative doses of drugs pre-consolidation and induction drug dose intensity during first 14 days of therapy (data from [1–5])

Study	251 7+3	213 7+3[a] Denver	213 7+3[a] Denver	2891 Conventional	2891 Timed-sequential
Cumulative					
mg/m^2					
Ara-C	1200–1400	2200–3100	2200–3100	3200	3200
DNM	70–180	294–490	294–490	320	320
VP-16		600–800	600–800	1600	1600
6-TG		800–1200	800–1200	2000	2000
Dex		48–72	48–72	96	96
Days 0–14[a]					
Ara-C	1 ×	1 × [a]	0.7 ×	2.3 ×	4.6 ×
DNM	1 ×	1.5 × [b]	0.7 ×	1.8 ×	3.6 ×
VP-16			1.0 ×	1.3 ×	2.6 ×
6-TG			1.0 ×	1.8 ×	3.6 ×
Dex			1.0 ×	0.8 ×	1.6 ×
Death (%)	10	12	6	5	14
Fail(%)	11	9	8	21	10
Remit (%)	79	79	76	74	78
3-Year survival from diagnosis	36±4	43±4	43±4	49±7	61±8

Poses and schedules of drugs in these protocols are as follows:
[a]1 × ara-C, 100mg/m^2 per day on days 0-7; 1 × DNM, 30mg/m^2 per day × 3; 1 × Dex, 10mg/m^2 per day × 3; 1 × 6-TG 100 mg/m^2 per day × 5; 1 × VP-16, 150 mg/m^2 × 2.
[b]On CCG-213, after two or three cycles, patients receiving Denver crossed over to "7+3" and vice versa. Hence the cumulative drug dose is the same for both regimens.

Table 2. Timed-sequential therapy in CCG-2891. Post-remission DFS following sequentially timed induction compared to conventionally timed induction therapy

Timing	Conventional (months)	Sequential (months)	p Value
Regimen X	49 ± 16	79 ± 14	0.013
Regimen Y	30 ± 17	39 ± 16	0.04
Regimen Z	52 ± 17	59 ± 18	0.12
Combined	37 ± 9	60 ± 9	0.0002

X,Y and Z refer to the blinded intensification regimens which are allogeneic BMT on ABMT or chemotherapy. Data are updated from [5].

was necessary. Figure 2 also shows that, with the high-dose ara-C complex as intensification, survival among patients receiving maintenance chemotherapy is significantly lower than among patients who receive none.

Comprehensive Improvement in Survival and DFS in CCG Studies, 1979-1995

Figures 3–6 show Kaplan-Meier estimates of actuarial survival DFS from the time of diagnosis and from the end of induction in CCG studies CCG-251, CCG-213P, CCG-213, CCG-2861, and CCG-2891. The figures document a steady significant improvement in survival and DFS.

Discussion

Randomized trials showing significant superiority of one treatment compared to another most powerfully argue for a cause and effect relationship between the strategy and the outcome. The results of CCG trials show that employment of three strategies, timed-sequential therapy, allogeneic BMT, and attenuation of maintenance therapy, occur concurrently with a progressive improvement in survival and DFS in children with AML treated in the CCG. In CCG-2891 the induction randomization between sequentially timed and conventionally timed chemotherapy has demonstrated that sequentially timed induction therapy increases the induction mortality rate, reduces the induction failure rate, has little effect on the remission induction rate, and substantially improves the post-remission outcome.

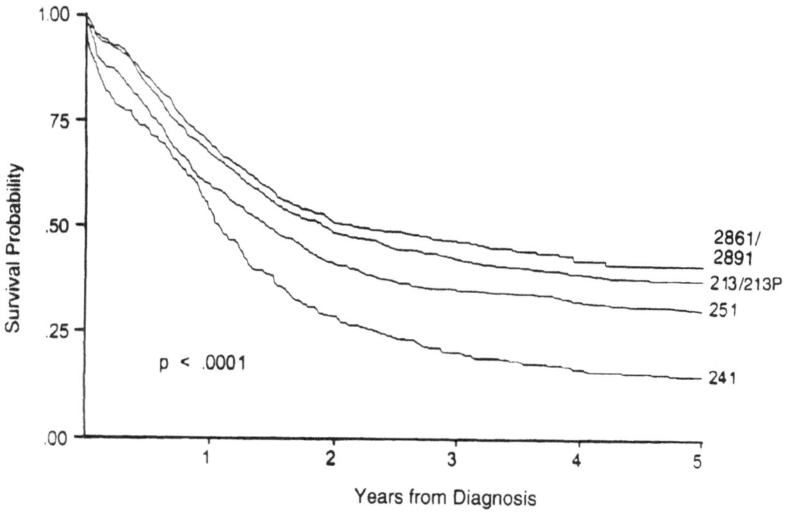

Fig. 3. Actuarial survival from diagnosis in six successive groups of AML trials

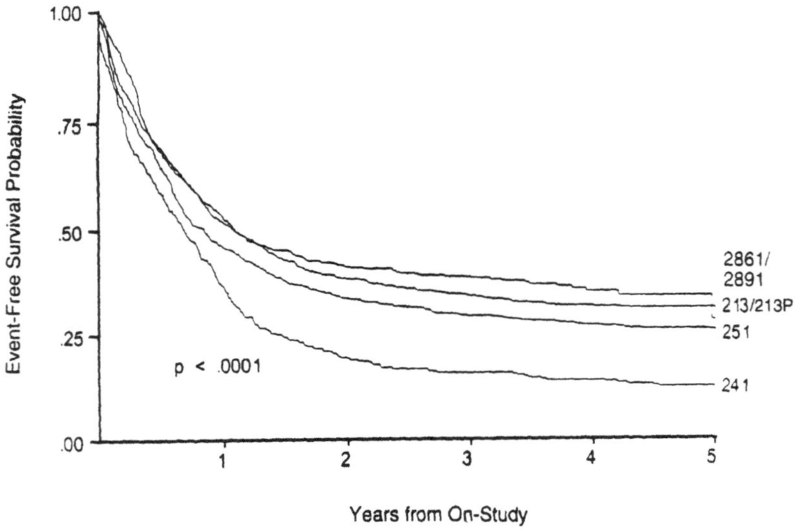

Fig. 4. Event-free actuarial survival from diagnosis in six successive CCG AML trials

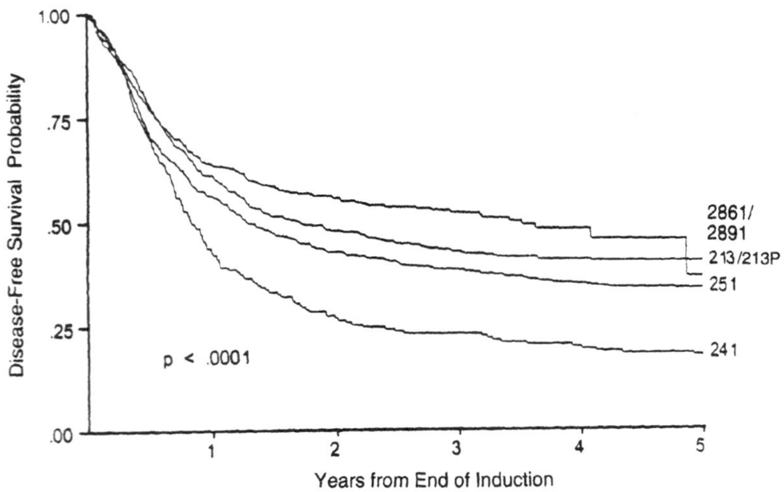

Fig. 5. Comparison of acturial disease-free survival from end of induction in six successive CCG AML studies

Post-remission outcome is improved regardless of post-remission therapy. Nonetheless, the differences in DFS among the randomized regimens in CCG-2891 indicate that a robust induction alone does not suffice. If induction alone determined outcome, in CCG-2891 all sequentially timed post-remission regimens would have similar outcomes as would all conventionally timed post remission regimens. Studies of timed-sequential therapy in adults with relapsed or recurrent AML support the conclusion that timed-sequential therapy contributes to better long-term outcome [28]. These findings have major implications for the comparison of BMT programs that are treating patients who have received a variety of induction therapies.

Several studies in adults with AML report the benefits of high-dose ara-C in intensification [29,30]. Remarkably, the Pediatric Oncology Group did not detect a benefit for high-dose ara-

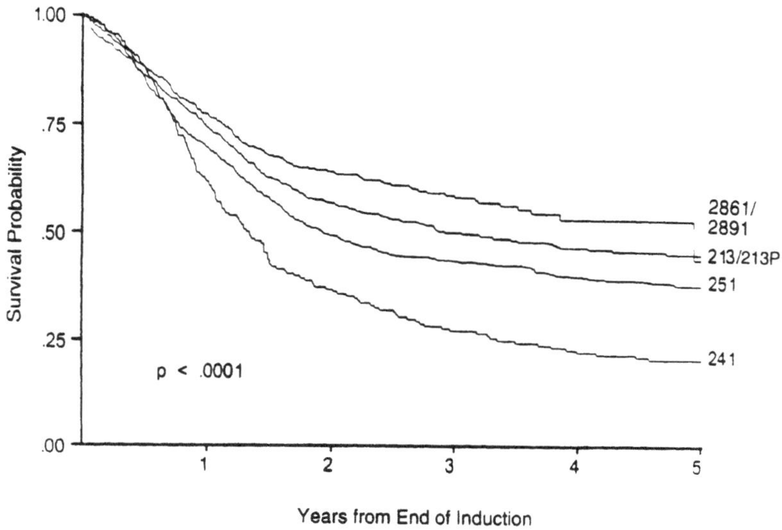

Fig. 6. Overall actuarial survival from end of induction in six successive groups of CCG AML trials

C in children [31]. Both dose and schedule may be important factors in determining outcome with high-dose ara-C. CCG-213P showed that dose alone, in the range of $12 g/m^2$ in 36 h does not guarantee a better outcome. Only when the sequence was repeated 6 days later were the benefits apparent.

Studies in AML of adults have not established a statistically significant benefit or a clinically important benefit to maintenance therapy in AML [32]. CCG-251 showed that there is no difference in outcome between a moderately intensive rotating eight-drug maintenance regimen and an ALL-like monthly pulse/daily 6-TG regimen. CCG-213 showed that, not only was maintenance therapy of no benefit, it actually reduced the survival in children with AML. The lack of obvious benefit of maintenance therapy in CCG trials has led to a progressive attenuation of maintenance from 2 years to 16 months and to a rudiment of maintenance-like therapy for 3 months after high-dose ara-C. Maintenance per se is eliminated in CCG-2891, but the high-dose ara-C complex still includes 3 months of maintenance-like therapy. The next CCG trial will eliminate this last vestige of maintenance.

To date, the Berlin-Frankfurt-Münster (BFM) AML trials have published the most successful results in AML [33, 34]. The approach to AML in children in the CCG contrasts sharply with that of the BFM group. First, CCG emphasizes timing and dose in induction. The BFM uses a more conventional induction. CCG relies on sequentially timed high-dose ara-C or BMT for intensification. The BFM trials have not found high-dose ara-C beneficial, especially when used to provide CNS prophylaxis [34]. Since CCG-251, CCG AML studies have protected the CNS with intrathecal and systemic therapy. Meanwhile, the BFM trials have shown that prophylactic cranial irradiation provides marrow prophylaxis. The BFM trials use a maintenance therapy similar to that which CCG has abandoned. These two contrasting approaches are both improving survival in AML. Only randomized trials focused on each of these differences will be able to sort out what to keep and what to discard.

In the United States, 5 year survival among children with AML has increased from 3% in 1963 to 31% in 1987, that is, a rate of progress of about 1% per year [35, 36]. In 1989, 5 year survival in CCG was 39%. In CCG-2891, the majority of events occur in the first 2 years from diagnosis; thus, early results of CCG-2891 predict a 5-year survival of nearly 50% among patients given intensively timed induction, that is, a steady but modest increase in the rate of progress. By incorporating sequentially timed induction and the two most effective regimens from the current CCG AML trial into the next trial, even with some regression to the mean, it may come to pass that over half the children with AML will be cured by the year 1999.

References

1. Nesbit M, Buckley J, Feig S, et al. Chemotherapy for induction of remission of childhood acute myeloid leukemia followed by marrow transplantation or multi-agent chemotherapy. J Clin Oncol 1994; 12(1): 127–135.
2. Wells R, Woods W, Lampkin B, et al. Impact of high-dose cytarabine and asparaginase intensification on childhood acute myeloid leukemia: a report from the Childrens Cancer Group. J Clin Oncol 1993; 11(3): 538–545.
3. Wells R, Woods W, Buckley J, et al. Treatment of newly diagnosed children and Adolescents with acute myeloid leukemia: a childrens Cancer Group Study. J Clin Oncol 1994; 12(11)L: 2367–2377.
4. Woods W, Kobrinsky N, Buckley J, et al. Intensively timed induction therapy followed by autologous or allogeneic bone marrow transplantation for children with acute myeloid leukemia or myelodysplastic syndrome: a Childrens Cancer Group pilot study. J Clin Oncol 1993; 11(8): 1448–1457.
5. Woods W, Kobrinsky N, Buckley J, et al. Timing intensive induction therapy improves post-remission outcome in acute myeloid leukemia irrespective of the use of bone marrow transplantation (BMT). Blood 1994; 84(10, Supplement 1): 232a.
6. Karp J, Donehower R, Burke P. An in vitro model to predict clinical response in adult acute myelogenous leukemia. Semin Oncol 1987; 14(2): 172–181.
7. Lampkin B, Nagao T, Mauer A. Synchronization and recruitment in acute leukemia. J Clin Invest 1971; 50: 2204–2214.
8. Lampkin B, Nagao T, Mauer A. Drug effect in acute leukemia. J Clin Invest 1969; 48: 1124–1130.
9. Lampkin B, McWilliams N, Mauer A, Flessa H, Hake D, Fisher V. Manipulation of the mitotic cycle in the treatment of acute myelogenous leukemia. Br,J Haematol 1976; 32: 29–40
10. Vaughan W, Karp J, Burke P. Two-cycle timed sequential chemotherapy for adult acute non-lymphocytic leukemia. Blood 1984; 64: 975–980.
11. Woods W, Ruymann F, Lampkin B, et al. The role of timing of high-dose cytosine arabinoside intensification and of maintenance therapy in the treatment of children with acute nonlymphocytic leukemia. Cancer 1990; 66(6): 1106–1113.
12. Baehner R, Bernstein I, Sather H, et al. Contrasting benefits of two maintenance programs following identical induction in children with acute nonlymphocytic leukemia. A report from the Childrens Cancer Study Group. Cancer Treat Rep 1984; 68: 1269–1272.
13. Feig SA, Lampkin BC, Woods WG, et al. Outcome of allogeneic bone marrow transplantation (BMT) in 156 children with acute non-lymphocytic leukemia. (ANLL) in first remission. Exp Hematol 1991; 19: 574,
14. Feig SA, Lampkin B, Nesbit ME, et al. Outcome of bone marrow transplantation during first complete remission of AML: a comparison of two sequential studies by the Childrens Cancer Group. Bone Marrow Transplantation 1993; 12: 65–71.
15. Feig S, Nesbit M, Lampkin B, et al. What is the optimal strategy to prevent relapse in children with acute myeloid leukemia? Tokyo: Excerpta Medica, Ltd., 1993. Cancer Chemotherapy: Challenges for the Future; vol.8.
16. Capizzi R, Poole M, Cooper M, et al. Treatment of poor risk acute leukemia with sequential high dose ara-C and asparaginase. Blood 1984; 63: 694–700.
17. Capizzi R, Davis R, Powell B, et al. Synergy between high-dose cytarabine and asparaginase in the treatment of adults with refractory and relapsed acute myelogenous leukemia–a Cancer and Leukemia Group B study. J Clin Oncol 1988; 6(3): 499–508.
18. Odom L, Morse H, Tubergen D, Blake M. Long-term survival in acute non-lymphoblastic leukemia. Med Pediatr Oncol 1988; 16: 248–254.
19. Weinstein H, Mayer R, Rosenthal D, et al. Treatement of acute myelogenous leukemia in children and adults. N. Engl J Med 1980; 303(9): 473–478.
20. Kaplan E, Meier P. Nonparametric estimation from incomplete observations. J Am Stat Assoc 1958; 53: 457–481.
21. Peto R, Pike M, Armitage P, et al. Design and analysis of randomized clinical trials requiring prolonged observation of each patient. II. Analysis and examples. Br J Cancer 1977; 35: 1–39.
22. Greenwood M. The errors of sampling of the survivorship tables. Reports on Public Health and Medical Subjects, His Majesty's Stationery Office, London, England, No. 33, Appendix 1, 1926.
23. Farewell V. The use of mixture models for the analysis of survival data with long-term survivors. Biometrics 1982; 38: 1041–1046.
24. Sposto R, Sather H, Baker S. A comparison of tests of the difference in the proportion of patients who are cured. Biometrics 1992; 48: 87–99.
25. Buckley JD, Chard RL, Baehner RL, et al. Improvement in outcome for children with acute non-lymphocytic leukemia: a report from the Children's Cancer Study Group. Cancer 1989; 63: 1457–1465.
26. Lange B, Lampkin B, Woods W, et al. Children's Cancer Study Group trials for acute non-lymphoblastic leukemia (ANLL) in children. New York: Wiley-Liss, Inc., 1990. Gale R, ed. Acute Myelogenous Leukemia: Progress and Controversies, pp.205–217.
27. Lange B, Woods W, Lampkin B et al. Childrens Cancer Study Group transplant trials for acute myeloid leukemia in children: a cross-study analysis of CCG-251, CCG-213, CCG-2861, and CCG-2891. In: Buchner T, Hiddlemann W, Wormann B, eds. Acute Leukemias IV: Prognostic factors and treatment strategies. Berlin: Springer Verlag, 1993: 724–733.
28. Archimbaud E, Thomas X, Leblond V, et al. Timed sequential chemotherapy for previously treated patients with acute myeloid leukemia: Long-term follow-up of the etoposide, mitoxantrone, and

cytarabine—86 trial. J Clin Oncol 1995; 13(1): 11-18.
29. Tallman M, Applebaum F, Amos D, et al. Evaluation of intensive postremission chemotherapy for adults with acute nonlymphocytic leukemia using high-dose cytosine arabinoside with L-asparaginase and amsacrine with etoposide. J Clin Oncol 1987; 5(6): 918-926.
30. Mayer R, Davis R, Schiffer C, et al. Intensive postremission chemotherapy in adults with acute myeloid leukemia. N Engl J Med 1994; 331(14): 896-903.
31. Ravindranath Y, Steuber CP, Krischer J, et al. High dose cytosine arabinoside for intensification of early therapy in childhood acute myeloid leukemia: a Pediatric Oncology Group study. J Clin Oncol 1991; 9: 572-581.
32. Champlin R, Gale R, Elashoff R, et al. Prolonged survival in acute myelogenous leukaemia without maintenance chemotherapy. Lancet 1984; April 21: 894-895.
33. Creutzig U, Ritter J, Schellong G, for the AML-BFM Study Group. Identification of two risk groups in childhood acute myelogenous leukemia after therapy intensification in study AML-BFM-83 as compared with AML-BFM-78. Blood 1990; 75: 1932-41.
34. Creutzig U, Ritter J, Zimmerman M, Schellong G. Does cranial irradiation reduce the risk for bone marrow relapse in acute myelogenous leukemia? Unexpected results of the childhood acute myelogenous leukemia study BFM-87. J Clin Oncol 1993; 11: 279-286.
35. Boring C, Squires T, Tong T. Cancer statistics. CA Cancer J Clin 1992; 42: 37
36. Miller B, Reis L, Hankey B, et al. SEER Cancer Statistics Review, 1973-1990. NCI-NIH Publication #93-2789 1993.

Acute Leukemias VI
Prognostic Factors
and Treatment Strategies
Büchner et al. (eds)

Intensified Early Therapy for Childhood Acute Myeloid Leukemia: Pilot Studies of the AIEOP Cooperative Group

S. Amadori, A.M. Testi, M.L. Moleti, A. Pession, R. Rondelli, and F. Mandelli
for the AIEOP Cooperative Group

Abstract. The efficacy and feasibility of two intensive three-drug (idarubicin, cytarabine, etoposide) induction courses were tested in two consecutive AIEOP pilot studies (LAM 92P, LAM 93P) for the treatment of acute myeloid leukemia (AML) in children. From April 1992 to March 1993, 20 patients aged <17 years from seven AIEOP centers entered study LAM 92P. Of the 19 evaluable patients, one died during induction (5%), three were resistant (16%), and 15 achieved complete remission (CR; 79%). Thirteen of the 15 responders completed the therapeutic program, including allogeneic bone marrow transplantation (BMT) in four and high-dose cytarabine (HiDAC) intensive postremission therapy in nine. One patient died in CR, five had recurrent disease, and seven remain in continuous CR (CCR) with a median follow up of 21 months.

In April 1993 a new pilot study (LAM 93P) was activated with the following main changes: exclusion of French-American-British classification (FAB) M3 and M3v; autologous BMT (ABMT) as postremission therapy. As of December 1994, 49 children were enrolled from 19 AIEOP centers. CR was achieved in 40 patients (82%). Seven children (14%) died during induction; two (4%) were resistant. Of the 34 responding patients evaluable for the follow up (six too early), four died in CR and four had early relapse (<2 months). Twenty-six children were submitted to transplant (15 ABMT, 11 BMT). One of them died in CR and six relapsed. Nineteen children are alive in CCR, with a median follow up of 6.5 months. Results suggest that aggressive induction treatment was highly effective in children with AML, but associated with severe toxicity and mortality. HiDAC and ABMT postremission therapies were feasible after such intensive induction.

Introduction

Despite recent advances in the treatment of children with acute myelogenous leukemia (AML), only one of three such patients can be expected to be a long-term survivor. Improvement in AML outcome over current treatment may depend on more effective induction therapy to attain higher complete remission (CR) rates and on more effective postremission approaches to reduce the risk of relapse. In recent years more potent induction regimens have been employed; the addition of etoposide (VP-16) and/or other drugs to the standard induction combination of cytarabine (ara-C) and anthracycline, and the intensification of chemotherapeutic induction schedules resulted in a more than 80% CR rate [1–5].

In an effort to improve the CR rate in children with AML, since April 1992 the Italian Hematology and Oncology Pediatric cooperative group (AIEOP) has conducted two consecutive pilot studies (LAM 92P, LAM 93P) exploring the feasibility of administering two intensive induction courses combining idarubicin (IDA), VP-16, and ara-C. The intensity of the second course was modulated on the basis of the response to the first one. In the first pilot study (LAM 92P), induction was followed (for patients lacking an HLA-matched sibling) by a single course of high-

Hematology Department of Human Biopathology, University "La Sapienza", Via Benevento 6, 00161 Rome, Italy

dose ara-C (HiDAC) and IDA as the sole post-remission therapy. In the second study (LAM 93P), the feasibility of autologous BMT (ABMT) was tested in children without an HLA-compatible sibling after the intensive induction therapy.

Materials and Methods

Patients younger than 16 years of age with newly diagnosed and previously untreated AML were eligible for the studies. The diagnosis of AML was made using accepted French-American-British (FAB) classification criteria. Smears of bone marrow and peripheral blood were submitted for central review by members of the Italian Leukemia Morphology Committee. All FAB subtypes were included in the first LAM 92P trial. FAB M3 and M3v were excluded from the second LAM 93P study. Myelodysplastic syndromes in a progressive phase (bone marrow blasts >25%) were included in both trials. Patients with blastic transformation of chronic myeloid leukemia, with concurrent malignancy and patients with Down's syndrome were excluded.

Therapy

The outlines of the two studies are illustrated in Fig. 1.

AIEOP LAM 92P. This protocol was opened in April 1992 and closed in March 1993. Seven selected AIEOP institutions participated to the study. Induction therapy consisted of two courses of IDA, ara-C, and VP-16 combination (ICE 3+5+10; ICE 2+3+7). Details regarding dosage and sequence of drugs and prophylactic CNS treatement are shown in Fig. 2. Children with CNS disease at diagnosis received weekly intrathecal therapy until CSF blast cells were eradicated plus further 2-weekly injections.

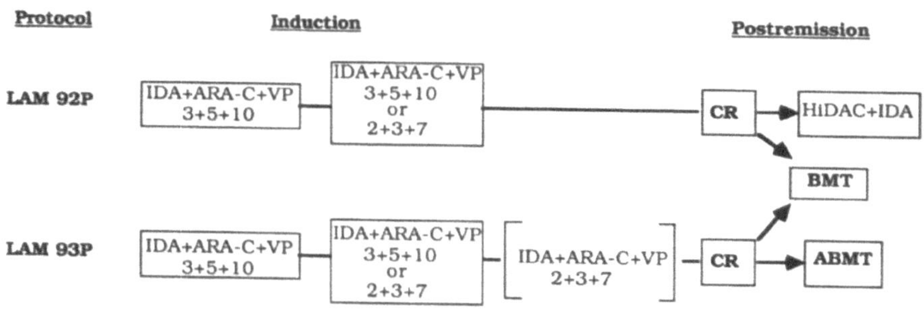

Fig. 1. AIEOP LAM 92P/93P'—Study designs

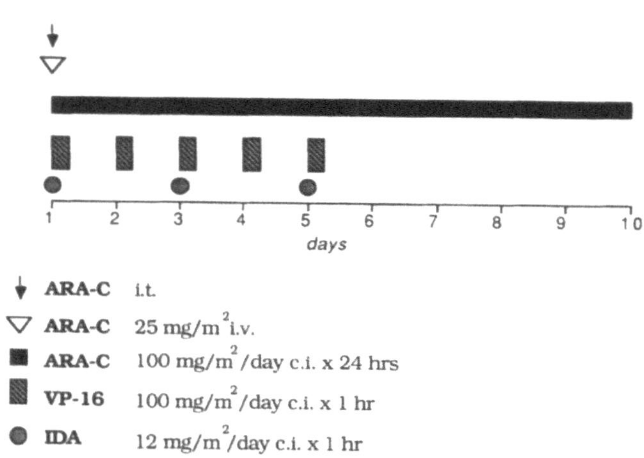

Fig. 2. AIEOP LAM 92P/93P'—induction schema

Bone marrow was evaluated on day 21 and repeated weekly if hypocellular and not evaluable. Children in CR after the first course proceeded to the second 2+3+7 ICE after hematological recovery and as soon as clinical conditions permitted. Patients with persistent leukemia or leukemic regrowth received, without any delay, the more intensive 3+5+10 ICE. If CR was not achieved after the second course, patients were regarded as "off protocol". Patients in CR with an HLA-compatible sibling were offered BMT; the other responding patients received a single course of very intensive postremission therapy with HiDAC (3 g/m^2 by 1h infusion every 12h × 12 doses) followed by IDA (8 mg/m^2 per day) for the next consecutive 3 days.

AIEOP LAM 93P. This new pilot study was activated in April 1993 with the following changes (a) FAB M3 and M3v patients were excluded; (b) the dose of IDA during induction was decreased (10 vs.12 mg/m^2 per day); (c) a third course of 2+3+7 ICE was added for patients requiring two courses to enter CR; (d) ABMT was considered as postremission therapy for all complete responders lacking an HLA-compatible sibling. Pretransplant conditioning was performed according to institutional preference. The study was extended to 19 AIEOP institutions and is still ongoing.

Supportive Care

Supportive care, including patient isolation procedures, methods of enteric decontamination, use of systemic antimicrobial therapy, use of central venous catheters, indications for blood products, was performed according to institutional preference, and was not prescribed in the protocol.

Statistical Analysis

Data were analyzed as of January 1, 1995. Disease-free survival (DFS) and overall survival were calculated by the product limit estimates of Kaplan-Meier. Terminal events, which were considered in the DFS determination, include relapse at any site or death from any cause.

Results

AIEOP LAM 92P

From April 1992 to March 1993, 20 consecutive patients aged less than 17 years were entered into the pilot study from seven selected AIEOP centers. The presenting characteristics of the 20 patients are listed in Table 1. There were 12 males and eight females; median age was 9 years, ranging from 1 month to 17 years. Five children had acute promyelocytic leukemia (M3 four patients, M3v one patient and seven presented with a recognizable monocytic component (M4 two patients, M5 five patients.) One registered patient with AML secondary to Ewing sarcoma and age > 16 years was ineligible for the study.

Of the 19 evaluable children, 15 (79%) achieved CR, including ten after the first course and two after the second one. In three children bone marrow after the first course was hypocellular, without leukemic cells, but not completely evaluable for response. One patient (5%) died during the first course induction from disseminated fungal infection. Three children had primary resistance (Table 2).

Table 1. Patient characteristics

	LAM 92P	LAM93P
Patients (*n*)	20	49
Male/Female (*n*)	12/8	23/26
Age		
Median (*n*)	9.0	9.1
Range (*n*)	0.1–17	0.1–16
Morphology (FAB)		
M1(*n*)	5	10
M2(*n*)	2	11
M3(*n*)	5	0
M4(*n*)	2	13
M5(*n*)	5	10
M6(*n*)	–	2
M7(*n*)	–	2
M0(*n*)	1	1
WBC × $10^9/l$		
Median	26.2	17.0
Range	1.2–227.0	1.9–700.0
CNS disease (*n*)	1	1
De novo AML (*n*)	19	47
Myelodysplastic disease secondary AML (*n*)	–	2
Ewing secondary AML (*n*)	1	–

Table 2. Induction results

	LAM 92P		LAM 93P		Total	
	(*n*)	(%)	(*n*)	(%)	(*n*)	(%)
Patients	20		49		69	
Evaluable	19		49		68	
Complete remission	15	79	40	82	55	81
First cycle	10		36		46	
Second cycle	2		4		6	
Not evaluable	3		-		3	
Early deaths	1	5	7	14	8	12
Nonresponders	3	16	2	4	5	7

Fever and suspected or proven infections were major complications during the induction period. In the 19 assessable patients there were eight cases of sepsis recorded: seven after the first course and one with the second course. Fungal infection was documented in four patients and caused patient's removal from the study in one case. Severe gastrointestinal toxicity (World Health Organization, WHO grade >3) was observed in the majority of patients (11 cases), life-threatening in five cases. Hepatic, renal, cardiac, and pulmonary toxicity were not considerable (Tables 3, 4).

Of the 15 children who entered CR, one suffered from an early relapse (2 months) and another was withdrawn from the study because of severe pulmonary fungal infection. The remaining 13 children completed the therapeutic program: nine received the intensive postremission treatment and four underwent BMT. One patient died in CR of disseminated fungal infection occuring during neutropenia induced by postremission chemotherapy. Five patients had recurrent disease in bone marrow at 3–12 months (one BMT, four chemotherapy). Seven patients are alive and in CCR with a median follow up of 21 months (range 2–27 months). The projected DFS is 46% at 2 years.

Table 3. Induction toxicity

	LAM 92P (*n*)	LAM 93P (*n*)
Patients	19	49
Sepsis		
Course 1	7	17
Course 2	1	7
Fungal infections		
Course 1	4	9
Course 2	2	6
Fever of unknown origin		
Course 1	7	24
Course 2	6	11
Hemorrhage (WHO > 3)		
Course 1	2	11
Course 2	0	2

Table 4. Type of toxicity (WHO)

	Grade 3 (n)	Grade 4 (*n*)	Grade 3 (*n*)	Grade 4 (*n*)
Gastrointestinal	6	5	15	6
Hepatic	1	-	3	–
Pulmonary	2	–	2	–
Cerebral seizure	–	–	1	-
Skin	1	–	4	–

AIEOP LAM 93P

From April 1993 to December 1994, 49 children were enrolled in this pilot study from 19 AIEOP centers. Patient's characteristics at diagnosis are shown in Table 1. Age ranged from 1 month to 16 years, with ten children aged less than 2 years; 23 children presented with M4-M5 FAB subtypes; two patients had AML secondary to myelodysplastic syndrome.

Forty children (82%) achieved CR, 36 after the first course and four after the second one. There have been seven (14%) induction deaths: five from infection, one from hemorrhage, and one from leukostasis. Most of deaths (six out of seven) occurred during the first induction cycle. There have also been two cases (4%) of primary resistant disease (Table 2).

Severe infectious complications were frequently observed. There were cases of 24 cases of sepsis (three fatal), 17 after the first cycle and seven after the second course. Fungal infections were also documented in 15 patients, causing death in two of them. Eleven patients experienced hemorrhage (WHO grade > 3), fatal in one of them.

As in the first trial, gastrointestinal toxicity was the only severe therapy-related extramedullary complication documented in 21 patients (WHO grade 4, six patients) (Tables 3, 4).

Of the 40 complete responders, 34 are evaluable for the follow up (six too early). Three children entered CR with the first course, died in CR (two infections, one hemorrhage) during the neutropenic phase induced by the ICE second course. Another patient who required two courses to achieve CR, died from infection during the third cycle. Four early bone marrow relapses (< 2 months) were observed. The remaining 26 children have already been submitted to transplantation, 15 autologous and 11 allogeneic. One patient died in CR from transplant-related toxicity. Relapses occurred in six children (five ABMT, one BMT) at 4–12 months (median 9 months). Bone marrow was the initial site of relapse in all patients, associated to testicular involvement in one of them. As of January 1, 1995, 19 children were alive in CCR, with a median follow up of 6.5 months (range 1–19 months). The projected DFS is 48% at 18 months.

Discussion

In the 10 year AIEOP experience (1982-1992), the conventional induction anthracycline plus ara-C association resulted in CR rates ranging from 65% to 80% in children with previously untreated de novo AML. The DFS rate ranged from 30% to 43% (at 2–7 years) but appears to be relatively stable despite the progressive intensification of postremission therapy [6–8]. In recent years, more potent induction regimens have been employed in pediatric AML in an attempt to increase the initial leukemic cell killing and consequently improve CR rate and duration of initial CR. Encouraging results, with a CR rate of more than 80%, have been reported by other cooperative groups utilizing a combination of three or more drugs administered in more intensive induction schedules [1–5]. In particular, in the Medical Research Council's randomized AML10 trial, the intensive 10 day, three-drug association (daunorubicin+ara-C+VP-16 or 6-thioguanine) resulted in a very high remission rate (91%) after one to three courses [1].

Based on these data, since April 1992 the AIEOP cooperative group has tested the feasibility and efficacy of intensive three-drug induction (IDA+VP-16+ara-C) administered according to the MRC AML10 schedule. IDA replaced daunorubicin in an attempt to increase the antileukemic efficacy and reduce cardiomiotoxicity. Two consecutive pilot studies, AIEOP LAM 92P and LAM 93P, were carried out. A total of 69 children from 21 AIEOP centers were enrolled in both studies. Fifty-five of the 68 evaluable patients achieved CR, with a CR rate of 81%. Induction failures were essentially represented by treatment-related deaths that occured in eight children (12%), mostly due to infections. The severe gastrointestinal toxicity, observed in 32 children, could explain the increased susceptibility to infections, often arising in the gastrointestinal tract. The induction-related toxicity also caused the death in CR of four patients and the removal from the study of another one.

Allogeneic marrow transplant was offered to responding children with an HLA-matched sibling. In the other responders, we tested two different postremission approaches: the intensive HiDAC plus IDA regimen in the first study and ABMT in the second one. Our aim was to explore the feasibility of both postremission modalities after the intensive induction regimen. A total of 24 children received post remission chemotherapy (nine cases) or ABMT (15 cases). Only one patient died from chemotherapy-related complications. As of January 1, 1995 seven of 15 patients treated in the first study and 19/34 evaluable patients from the second trial were alive and in CCR with a median follow up of 21 and 6.5 months, respectively. Owing to the short observation time and the small number of patients, the efficacy of both postremission approaches is not evaluable at the moment.

In summary, the intensive three-drug induction regimen demonstrated high antileukemic activity, resulting in an 81% CR rate in children with AML. However, severe treatment-related toxicity was observed, with 17% induction and remission deaths. Postremission therapy with either HiDAC or ABMT was feasible after such intensive induction.

Acknowledgments. This work was supported by a grant from the Consiglio Nazionale delle

Ricerche, Progetto Finalizzato "Applicazioni Cliniche della Ricerca Oncologica", sottoprogetto 11.n

References

1. Stevens RF, Hann IH, Wheatley K, Gray R (1992) Intensive chemotherapy with or without additional bone marrow transplantation in pediatric AML: progress report on the MRC AML 10 trial. Leukemia 6 (Suppl 2): 55–58
2. Woods WG, Kabrinsky N, Buckley J, Neudorf S, Sanders J, Miller L, Barnard D, Benjamin D, De Swarte J, Kalousek D, Shina D, Hammond GD, and Lange BJ (1993) Intensively timed induction therapy followed by autologous or allogeneic bone marrow transplantation for children with acute myeloid leukemia or myelodysplastic syndrome: a Childrens Cancer Group pilot study. J.Clin Oncol 11: 1448–1457
3. Nesbit ME, Buckley JD, Feig SA, Anderson JR, Lampkin B, Bernstein ID, Kim TH, Piomelli S, Kersey JH, Coccia PF, O'Reilly RC, August C, Thomas ED, Hammond GD (1994) Chemotherapy for induction of remission of childhood acute myeloid leukemia followed by marrow transplantation of multiagent chemotherapy: a report from the Childrens Cancer Group. J.Clin Oncol 12: 127–135
4. Ritter J, Creutzig U, Schellong G (1992) Treatment results of three consecutive German childhood AML trials: BFM-78, -83, and -87 Leukemia 6 (Suppl 2): 59–62
5. Weinstein H, Ravindranath Y, Krischer J, Steuber P. Civin C, Gresik M, and Vietti T (1992) The impact of early intensive therapy on event-free survival (EFS) in children with acute myeloid leukemia (AML). Leukemia 6 (Suppl 2): 52–54
6. Amadori S, Ceci A, Comelli A, Madon E, Masera G, Nespoli L, Paolucci G, Zanesco L, Vegna ML, Moleti ML, Testi AM, and Mandelli F (1990) Therapy of childhood acute myelogenous leukemia: an update of the AIEOP/LAM 8204 study. In: Buchner, Schellong, Hiddeman, Ritter (eds) Acute leukemias II. Springer-Verlag Berlin Heidelberg, pp 222–225 (Hematology and Blood transfusion, vol 33).
7. Amadori S, Testi AM, Arico'M, Comelli A, Giuliano M, Madon E, Masera G, Rondelli R, Zanesco L, and Mandelli F (1993) Prospective comparitive study of bone marrow transplantation and postremission chemotherapy for childhood acute myelogenous leukemia. J Clin Oncol 11: 1046–1054.
8. Amadori S, Giona F, Giuliano M, Moleti ML, Pession A, Rolla M, Rondelli R, Testi AM, Mandelli F (1992) Therapeutic strategies for postremission treatment in childhood acute myeloid leukemia (AML). The AIEOP experience 1987–1991. Leukemia 6 (Suppl 2): 44–47

Appendix

Portocols AIEOP LAM 92P/93P: Participating Institutions

Institutions
Clinica Pediatrica I, Bari
Clinica Pediatrica II, Bari
Clinica Pediatrica, Bologna
Clinica Pediatrica,Cagliari
Ospedale Civile, Catanzaro
Clinica Pediatrica,Firenze
Ospedale Gaslini, Genova
Ospedale Galliera,Genova
Clinica Pediatrica I, Napoli
Ospedale Pausilipon, Napoli
Clinica Pediatrica, Padova
Clinica Pediatrica, Palermo
Ospedali Riuniti, Parma
Clinica Pediatrica, Perugia
Ospedale Civile, Pescara
Cattedra Ematologia, Roma
Ospedale Bambino Gesù, Roma
Ospedale Civile, S.Giovanni Rotondo
Clinica Pediatrica, Sassari
Clinica Pediatrica, Torino
Clinica Pediatrica, Trieste
Investigators
F. Schettini, N. Santoro
A. Ceci, R. Colella
G. Paolucci, P. Rosito, A. Pession
P. F. Biddau, G. Murgia
S. Magro, C. Consarrino
G. Bernini, A. Lippi
P. Mori, E. Micalizzi
C. Cominetti
M.T. Di Tullio, F. Casale, P. Indolfi
V. Poggi, M.F. Pinta
L. Zanesco, C. Messina, G. Basso
M. Lo Curto, G. Milici
G. Izzi
R. Vaccaro, P. Zucchetti
G. Torlontano
F. Mandelli, S. Amadori
G. De Rossi, C. Miano
M. Carotenuto, S. Ladogana
T. Meloni, D. Gallisai
E. Madon, R. Miniero, E.Barisone
P. Tamaro, G. Zanasso

Acute Leukemias VI
Prognostic Factors
and Treatment Strategies
Büchner et al. (eds)

A Randomized Comparative Study of Purged Autologous Bone Marrow Transplantation Versus Intensive Multiagent Consolidation Chemotherapy in First Remission of Acute Myeloid Leukemia in Children (Pediatric Oncology Group Study—POG 8821)

Y. Ravindranath[1], A. Yeager,[2] C.P. Steuber,[3] J. Krischer,[4] M. Chang,[5] C.I. Civin,[6] J. Graham-Pole,[7] B. Camitta,[8] M. Gresik,[9] A. Carroll,[10] S. Raimondi,[11] S. Inoue[12], and H. Weinstein[13] for the Pediatric Oncology Group

Abstract. The role of autologous bone marrow transplantation (ABMT) for the treatment of children with acute myeloid leukemia (AML) is unknown. The POG 8821 AML study compared the efficacy of ABMT vs. intensive multiagent consolidation chemotherapy (ICT) as treatment for children with AML in first remission.

Methods. Remission induction therapy consisted of one course of daunorubicin, cytarabine and 6-thioguanine (DAT) followed by high-dose cytarabine (HdA; 3gm/m^2 every 12 h × 6 doses) and one course of etoposide plus azacytidine (VP/AZ). Randomization was performed after HdA. Allogeneic BMT was offered to patients with a matched sibling donor. Those not eligible for allogeneic BMT were randomized to receive either ICT (sequential courses of D/HdA, DAT, VP/AZ, HdA, DAT, VP/AZ), or ABMT after a preparative regimen of busulfan plus cyclophosphamide and 4-hydroperoxyocyclophosphamide-purged marrow.

Results. Between June 1988 and March 1993, 552 of 648 (85%) achieved remission (M1 marrow = 507 or M2a marrow = 45; 5–15% blasts). Patients undergoing non-protocol ABMT (19), and secondary AML (five) were not eligible for ABMT; 89 opted for allogeneic BMT; 19 others were removed from study prior to randomization. A total of 232/421 (55%) were randomized to ICT (117) or ABMT (115). The remaining patients non-randomly received ICT 189 (45%) because of Down's syndrome (28), refusal to be randomized (83), no funds to support ABMT (64), or no ABMT beds (14). The event-free survival (EFS) and survival for the entire group at 3 years were 34% and 42%, respectively. For the randomized patients, disease-free survival (DFS) was not statistically different when analyzed by intent to treat (3-year DFS: ICT 36% vs. ABMT 37%, log-rank test $p = 0.20$). Overall survival followed a similar pattern (3-year survival: ICT 44% vs. ABMT 40, log-rank test $p = 0.10$). There was a lower leukemia relapse rate but a higher treatment-related mortality in ABMT vs. ICT (15% vs. 2.7%, $p = 0.005$).

[1]Children's Hospital of Michigan, Detroit, MI, USA
[2]Johns Hopkins Oncology Center, Baltimore, MD, USA
[3]Baylor College of Medicine, Texas Children's Hospital, Houston, TX, USA
[4]POG Statistical Office, Gainesville, FL, USA
[5]POG Statistical Office, Gainesville, FL, USA
[6]Johns Hopkins Oncology Center, Baltimore, MD, USA
[7]University of Florida, Shands Teaching Hospital, Gainesville, FL, USA
[8]Midwest Children's Cancer Center, Milwaukee, WI, USA
[9]Baylor College of Medicine, Texas Children's Hospital, Houston, TX, USA
[10]University of Alabama, Sparks Center, Birmingham, AL, USA
[11]St. Jude Children's Research Hospital, Memphis, TN, USA
[12]Hurley Medical Center, Flint, MI, USA
[13]Dana-Farber Cancer Institute, Boston, MA, USA

Conclusions. Autologous BMT did not improve EFS when compared to intensive chemotherapy for children with AML in first remission.

Introduction

Despite intensification of post-remission chemotherapy, the event-free survival (EFS) in acute myeloid leukemia (AML) has plateaued at 35%–45% [1–7]. Pediatric Oncology Group (POG) surveys show that only 10%–15% of the children may have HLA-compatible siblings, thus limiting the option of allogeneic BMT (allo-BMT). Early results of 4-hydroxyperoxycyclophosphamide (4HC)-purged autologous bone marrow transplantation (ABMT) in first or subsequent remission were comparable to those achieved with allo-BMT [8, 9]. Thus, POG initiated a randomized study to compare 4-HC-purged ABMT and intensive consolidation chemotherapy (ICT) early in remission for children with AML.

Methods

The eligibility criteria for entering on the POG 8821 study were as follows: 18 years of age with previously untreated AML or secondary AML. The exclusions from randomization were: (a) no remission after induction course two; (b) no insurance or financial support; (c) intent to perform allo-BMT; (d) secondary AML; (e) Down syndrome and isolated chloroma. Both Down Syndrome [10] and isolated chloroma were added as exclusions after the protocol had been opened for a few months.

Treatment Regimen. The treatment schema is outlined in Fig. 1. The induction consisted of one standard 3+7 course of daunomycin,cytarabine (ara-C), and 6-thioguanine. Daunomycin was given at 45 mg/m^2 daily 3 and ara-C was given 100 mg/m^2 daily for 7 days by continuous infusion, and 6-thioguanine was given p.o. 100 mg/m^2 per day 7 days. This was followed by a course of high-dose ara-C 3 gm/m^2 every 12 h 6 doses. Patients who were in remission at the end of the second induction course (defined as M1 marrow or M2a marrow with < 15% blasts) were eligible for post-remission therapy. Children who had an HLA-compatible sibling donor were offered allo-BMT. All of those eligible for randomization, except for the exclusions as mentioned previously, were randomized to either the chemotherapy or ABMT arms. Both groups received one course of etoposide at 250 mg/m^2 daily 3 followed by azacytidine at 300 mg/m^2 on days 4 and 5. Patients randomized to intensive consolidation chemotherapy then received six additional courses of chemotherapy: daunomycin plus high-dose ara-C as described previously, 2 + 5 regimen of DAT, VP/AZ as previously noted, followed by high-dose ara-C for six doses, DAT (2 + 5), a VP/AZ.

CNS Prophylaxis. This consisted of i.t. ara-C (40 mg/m^2) on days 1 and 8 of the DAT induction course; two additional doses of i.t. ara-C were given on days 12 and 19 for patients with CNS disease at diagnosis. All patients also received i.t. ara-C on days 1 and 8 of the first VP/AZ course.

Autologous BMT. Patients randomized to autologous BMT received one consolidation course of

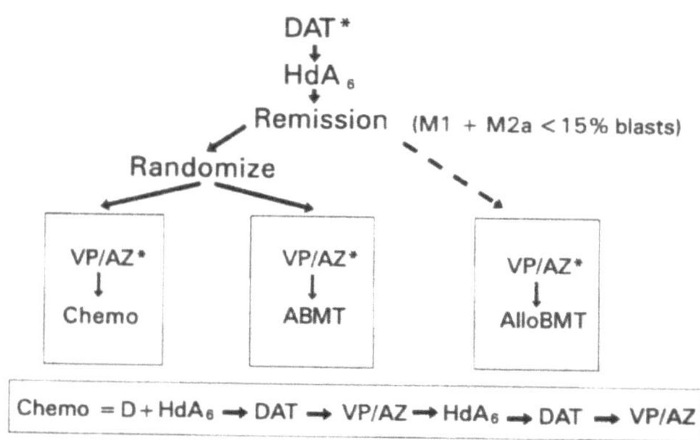

Fig. 1. Chemotherapy vs. ABMT for childhood AML: POG 8821—treatment schema. *Asterisk*, intrathecal ara-C x 2

VP/AZ. Upon count recovery, the marrow was harvested and purged with 4HC at a concentration of 100 µg/ml and an incubation hematocrit (Hct) of 5%–10% and stored. The preparative regimen consisted of the standard busulfan/cyclophosphamide. Patients opting for allo-BMT were recommended to go through one course of consolidation with VP/AZ as in the other treatment arms.

Results

Between June 1988 and March 1993, 666 patients were registered. This report describes preliminary analysis based on data as of October 1993. A total of 648 were evaluable (Fig. 2). There were 26 early deaths and 67 patients did not respond; 552 patients (86%) achieved remission (507 M1, and 45 M2a). Overall, 131 patients were excluded from randomization for the following reasons: 89 opted for allo-BMT, 18 additional patients had institutional non-protocol BMT, five for secondary AML, and 19 others for miscellaneous reasons; 421 patients, or 76% of those achieving remission, were eligible for randomization. Of these 421 patients, 232 (55%) were randomized: 117 to intensive consolidation therapy, and 115 to ABMT. A total of 189 cases (45%) were non-randomly assigned to chemotherapy because of refusal for randomization (89), Down syndrome (21), and others due to lack of funds (64) or lack of transplant beds (14).

Life Table Estimates of Survival. The survival data summarized here are based on data as of April 1994. The event-free survival (EFS) for the entire group was 37% at 3 years. The EFS by intent-to-treat for the randomized patients is shown in Fig. 3. As can be seen, the 3- year disease-free survival (DFS) from randomization for the chemotherapy patients was 37%, while that for the ABMT arm was 38%, the difference not being statistically significant. For patients undergoing allo-BMT ($n = 84$) the 3-year DFS was 51.3%.

Patterns of Failure. The pattern of failures in the two randomized study groups were different. Of particular interest is the fact more than a third of the patients randomized to the ABMT arm were removed from study prior to ABMT, primarily because of parental change of preference (17), relapse prior to bone marrow harvest (21), three patients were removed from the chemotherapy arm for allo-BMT, and three others had disseminated fungal sepsis. Thus, while 97% of patients on the chemotherapy arm received their assigned treatment (113/117), only 62% of the patients randomized to ABMT actually received their assigned treatment. The regimen-related mortality was also significantly higher in theABMT arm, nearly 14% compared

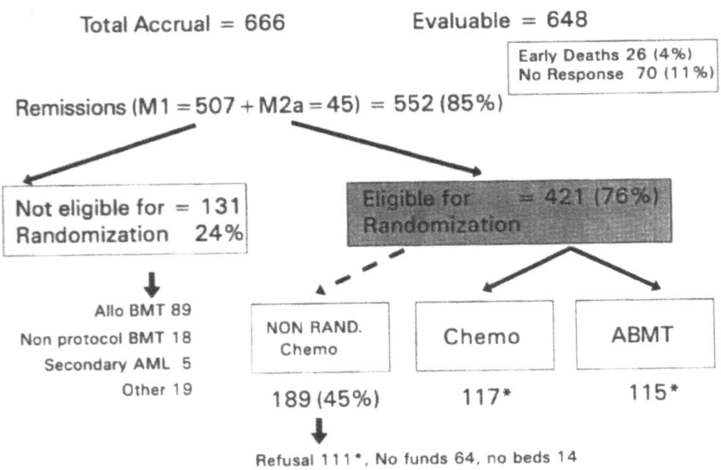

Fig. 2. Patient flow chart showing total registrations, evaluable patients, number of patients achieving remission, and subsequent disposition of patients. *Asterisk*, Down syndrome—21 non-randomized, four randomized to chemotherapy, two randomized to ABMT

Fig. 3. Disease-free survival by intent to treat. Disease-free survival estimates are calculated from the data of randomization and include toxic deaths and treatment failures

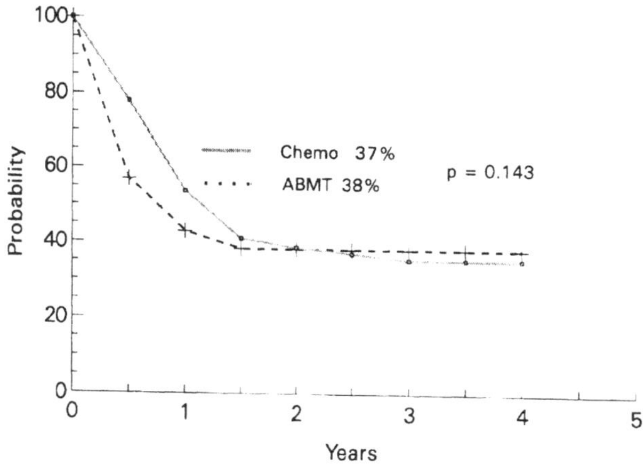

to 2% in the chemotherapy arm. The 14% mortality in the ABMT arm of this POG study is similar to the treatment-related mortality described in a recent report of ABMT experience from North American Bone Marrow Transplant Registry (NABMTR)[11]. The regimen-related mortality was 9% in a recent European study of adult AML patients having ABMT with unpurged marrow[12]. Although the study was designed for evaluation by intent-to-treat (Fig. 3), we also looked at the EFS in patients on the two randomized arms treated as assigned. The 3-year EFS as treated in the ABMT arm was 48% compared to 37% in the chemotherapy arm and 58% for allo-BMT patients; the difference was not statistically significant. In summary, for the entire group, the 3-year EFS from diagnosis and remission are 37% and 43%, respectively. For the randomized patients, EFS at 3 years for the chemotherapy and ABMT groups was not statistically different when analyzed by intent to treat or as treated. In the ABMT group, the regimen-related mortality was higher, nearly a third of all failures occurred before bone marrow harvest. Relapses post-auto BMT were rare after 18 months from randomization while the chemotherapy group continues to experience relapse up to 42 months. Allo-BMT patients had a superior EFS at 3 years compared to either ABMT or the chemotherapy patients.

Conclusions

The study underscores the logistics involved in designing a randomized trial comparing chemotherapy vs. bone marrow transplantation in childhood AML. Only 36% of the evaluable patients (232/648) were randomized. Further, only 62% of patients randomized to ABMT received their intended treatment. This, coupled with a high regimen-related mortality in the ABMT arm, affected the outcome of this study. Despite the use of three different intensive modes of therapy, the overall 3-year EFS remains unchanged at $< 40\%$, suggesting that new and novel approaches to therapy must be explored. New strategies during induction or in the post-remission phase of therapy are clearly needed to further improve these outcomes.

Acknowledgment. This work was supported in part by grants from the National Cancer Institute, Bethesda mD (CA-29691, CA-20549, CA-03161, CA-29139, CA-28476, CA-29281, CA-32053, CA 03161, CA-25408, CA-31566, CA-29691, CA-41573).

References

1. Weinstein HJ, Mayer RH, Rosenthal DS, et al.: Chemotherapy for acute myelogenous leukemia in children and adults. VAPA update. Blood 62: 315–319, 1983.
2. Grier H, Camitta B, Link M, Coral F, et al.: A seven-year experience with intensive post-remission chemotherapy for childhood acute myelogenous leukemia (AML). Blood 62 (suppl. 1): 203a, 1983.
3. Creutzig U, Ritter J, Riehm H, et al.: Improved treatment results in childhood acute myeloblastic leukemia: a report of the German Cooperative Study AML-BFM-78. Blood 65: 298–304, 1985.
4. Steuber CP, Civin C, Krischer J, Culbert S, Ragab A, Ruymann F, Ravindranath Y, Leventhal B, Wilkinson R, Vietti TJ: A comparison of induction

and maintenance therapy for acute non-lymphocytic leukemia of childhood: results of a Pediatric Oncology Group study. J Clin Onc 9: 247–258, 1991.
5. Nesbit ME Jr, Buckley JD, Feig SA, et al.: Chemotherapy for induction of remission of childhood acute myeloid leukemia followed by marrow transplantation or multiagent chemotherapy: a report from the Children's Cancer Group. J Clin Oncol 12: 127–135, 1994.
6. Woods WG,Ruymann FB, Lampkin BC, et al.: The role of timing high-dose cytosine arabinoside intensification and of maintenance therapy in the treatment of children with acute nonlymphocytic leukemia. Cancer 66: 1106–1113, 1990.
7. Ravindranath Y, Steuber CP, Krischer J, et al.: High-dose cytarabine for intensification of early therapy of childhood acute myeloid leukemia: a Pediatric Oncology Group study. *J Clin Oncol* 9: 572–580, 1991.
8. Yeager AM, Kaizer H, Santos GW, et al.: Autologous bone marrow transplantation in patients with acute lymphocytic leukemia using ex vivo marrow treatment with 4-hydroperoxycyclophosphamide. N Engl J Med 315: 142–147, 1986.
9. Applebaum FR, Cliff RA, Buckner DC, et al.: Allogeneic marrow transplantation for acute nonlymphoblastic leukemia after first relapse. Blood 61: 949–953, 1983.
10. Ravindranath Y, Abella E, Krischer J, Wiley J, Inoue S, Harris M, Chauvenet A, Alvarado CS, Dubowy R, Ritchey AK, Land V, Steuber CP, and Weinstein H: Acute myeloid leukemia (AML) in Down's syndrome is highly responsive to chemotherapy: experience on Pediatric Oncology Group AML Study 8498. Blood 80: 2210–2214, 1992.
11. Rowlings PA, Keating A, Horowitz MM, Zhang MJ, Armitage JO for the North American Bone Marrow Transplant Registry (NAABMTR): Autotransplants for acute myelogenous leukemia (AML) in North America. Proceedings of American Society of Clinical Oncology 13: 305 (Abs # 997), 1994.
12. Zittoun RA, Mandelli F, Willemze R et al.: for EORTC/GIMEMA groups: Autologous or allogeneic bone marrow transplantation compared with intensive chemotherapy in acute myelogenous leukemia. N Eng J Med 332: 217–223, 1995.

Appendix 1

Institution	PI	Grant No.
Albera Pediatric Oncology Consortium, Edmonton, Canada	Max Coppes	CA-53490
All Children's Hospital, St. Petersburgh, FL	Jerry Barbosa	
Baylor College of Medicine, Houston, TX	Philip Steuber	CA-03161
Boston Floating Hospital, Boston, MA	Cynthia Kretschmar	CA-53549
Bowman Gray School of Medicine, Winston, Salem, NC	Allen Chauvenet	CA-53128
Brooke Army Medical Center, Ft. Sam Houston, TX	Terry Pick	CA-28752
Cancer Center of Hawaii, Honolulu, HI	Robert Wilkinson	CA-28439
Carolinas Medical Center, Charlotte, NC	Barry Golembe	CA-15525
Children's Hospital and Health Center, San Diego, CA	Richard Kadota	CA-28439
Children's Hospital Greenville Health System, Greenville, SC	Cary Stroud	CA-53128
Children's Hospital of Michigan, Detroit, MI	Y. Ravindranath	CA-29691
Children's Hospital of New Orleans, LA	R.P. Warrier	
Children's Memorial Hospital, Chicago, IL	Morris Kletzel	CA-07431
Christ Hospital and Medical Center, Oak Lawn, IL	Sharad Salvi	CA-07431
City of Hope National Medical Center, Duarte, CA	Robert Chilcote	CA-32278
Cook-Ft. Worth Children's Medical Center, Ft. Worth, TX	Paul Bowman	CA-33625
Dana Farber Cancer Institute, Boston, MA	Holcombe Grier	CA-41573
Dartmouth - Hitchcock Medical Center, Lebanon, NH	Eric Larsen	CA-29293
Duke University, Durham, NC	Joanne Kurtzberg	CA-15525
East Carolina University School of Medicine, Greenville, NC	Tate Holbrook	CA-15515
Emory University School of Medicine, Atlanta, GA	Andrew Yeager	CA-20549
Fairfax Hospital, Falls Church, VA	Jay Greenberg	CA-28476
Hackensack Medical Center, Hackensack, NI	Michael Harris	
Hurley Medical Center, Flint, MI	Susumu Inoue	CA-29691
Joe Dimaggio Children's Hospital at Memorial, Hollywood, FL	Phillipa Sprinz	
Johns Hopkins University, Baltimore, MD	Cindy Schwartz	CA-28476
Kaiser Permanente Medical Center, Santa Clara, CA	Lily Young	CA-33603
Keesler Air Force Medical Center, Bilexi, MS	Thomas Abshire	CA-15989
MDA Cancer Center Orlando, Orlando, FL	Vincent Giusti	
Maine Children's Cancer Program, Portland, ME	Craig Hurwitz	CA-41573
Massachusetts General Hospital, Boston, MA	William Ferguson	CA-29293
McGill University, Montreal, Canada	Michael Whitehead	CA-33587
Medical College of Virginia, Richmond, VA	E. Clifton Russell	CA-28530

Medical University of South Carolina, Charleston, SC	Joseph Laver	CA-16388
Miami Children's Hospital, Miami, FL	Enrique Escalon	CA-29281
Midwest Children's Cancer Center, Milwaukee, WI	Bruce Camitta	CA-32053
Mount Sinai School of Medicine, New York, NY	Jeffrey Lipton	CA-38859
Naval Regional Medical Center, San Diego, CA	David Reardon	CA-28439
Nemours Children's Clinic, Jacksonville, FL	Paul Pitel	CA-29281
Oklahoma University Health Sciences Center, Oklahoma City, OK	Ruprecht Nitschke	CA-11233
Rhode Island Hospital, Providence, RI	Edwin Forman	CA-29293
Roswell Park Memorial Institute, Buffalo, NY	Martin Brecher	CA-28383
Rush-Presbyterian-St. Luke's Medical Center, Chicago, IL	Alexander Green	CA-07431
Sacred Heart Children's Hospital, Pensocola, FI	Thomas Jenkins	
St. Christopher Hospital, Philadelphia, PA	Edwin Douglass	CA-45261
St. Francis Regional Medical Center, Wichita, KS	David Rosen	CA-35431
St. John Hospital, Detroit, MI	Hadi Sawaf	CA-29691
St. Joseph's Cancer Institute, Tampa, FL	Cameron Tobbi	
St. Vincent Hospital, Green Bay, WI	Dorothy Ganick	CA-32053
Stanford University, Palo Alto, CA	Michael Link	CA-33603
State University of New York at Syracuse, Syracuse, NY	Ronald Dubowy	CA-28383
Swiss Pediatric Oncology Group, Bern, Switzerland	Hans Wagner	CA-53301
Tripler Army Medical Center, Tripler, HI	Shirley Reddoch	CA-28752
University of Alabama, Birmingham, AL	Robert Castleberry	CA-25408
University of Arizona Health Sciences Center, Tucson, AZ	John Hutter	CA-41188
University of Arkansas, Little Rock, AR	David Becton	CA-41188
University of California, Davis, Sacramento, CA	Jonathan Ducore	CA-58967
University of California, San Diego, CA	Faith Kung	CA-28439
University of Florida, Gainesville, FL	Paulette Mehta	CA-29281
University of Kansas, Kansas City, MO	Tribhawan Vats	CA-28841
University of Massachusetts Medical School, Worcester, MA	Molly Schwenn	CA-41573
University of Miami School of Medicine, Miami, FL	Stuart Toledano	CA-41082
University of Mississippi Medical Center, Jackson, MS	Jeanette Pullen	CA-15989
University of Missouri, Columbia, MO	Narollah Hakami	CA-05587
University of Fuerto Rico, San Juan, Puerto Rico	Nilka Barrios	
University of Rochester Medical Center, Rochester, NY	Reggie Duerst	CA-41573
University of South Alabama, Mobile, AL	Yih-Ming Yang	
University of South Florida, Tampa, FL	Eva Hvizdala	
University of Texas, San Antonio, TX	Paul Jon Thomas	CA-52771
University of Texas-Galveston, Galveston, TX	Mary Haggard	CA=03161
University of Texas-Southwestern Medical School, Dallas, TX	George Buchanan	CA-33625
University of Vermont College of Medicine, Burlington, VT	Joseph Dickerman	CA-29293
University of Virginia, Charlottosville, VA	Pedro de Alarcon	
Water Reed Army Medical Center, Washington, DC	David Maybee	CA-28752
Warren Clinics, Inc., Tulsa, OK	Gregory Kirkpatrick	CA-11233
Washington University School of Medicine, St. Louis, MO	Teresa Vietti	CA-05587
West Virginia University Health Science Center, Charleston, WV	Kenneth Starling	CA-15525
West Virginia University Health Services Center, Morgantown, WV	A. Kim Ritchey	CA-15525
Wilford Hall USAF Medical Center, Lackland AFB, TX	Tanya Trippet	
Yale University School of Medicine, New Havern, CT	Jack Van Hoff	CA-52317

Acute Leukemias VI
Prognostic Factors
and Treatment Strategies
Büchner et al. (eds)

Prognostic Factors and Treatment in Pediatric Acute Myeloblastic Leukemia: French Trials

G. Schaison, G. Leverger, G. Michel, T. Leblanc, D. Sommelet, I. Thuret, J. Landman-Parker, E. Le Gall, Y. Perel, E. Gluckman, J.P. Vannier, B. Nelken, A. Baruchel for the French Society of Pediatric Hematology and Immunology

Introduction

Acute myeloblastic leukemia (AML) accounts for less 25% of all cases of childhood leukemias. The homogeneous distribution contrasts with the well-known peak of incidence observed in acute lymphoblastic leukemia between the ages of 2 and 7 years.

Three major events have marked the evolution of leukemic treatments. First, the discovery that cytarabine (ara-C) used as a single agent enables 30% complete remission (CR) induction rate. Secondly, the fact that daunorubicin alone yields a 50% remission induction rate. These two findings have led to polychemotherapy, raising remission rate to 80% nowadays. The addition of 6-thioguanine or other agents in induction has not proved beneficial. However, the introduction of an intensive consolidation regimen with high-dose ara-C has improved the outcome [7, 9]. During induction and consolidation, supportive care has been found to facilitate the improvement of results. The third main advance in treatment is bone marrow transplantation (BMT) with an HLA-identical sibling [1–5]. In all studies BMT resulted in a significantly lower incidence of relapse.

We report here the outcome of 171 children with AML who were enrolled on the prospective French Protocol LAME 89/91. This protocol was designed to assess the comparative value of BMT when an HLA-compatible related donor was available versus an aggressive post-remission intensification including high-dose ara-C, asparaginase, and amsacrine.

Patients and Methods

Previously untreated AML with French-American-British (FAB) subtypes ranging from M1 to M7 and age less than 20 years were eligible. Patients with M0 or biphenotypic leukemia, myelodysplasia, secondary AML and patients with Down's syndrome were excluded. A total of 171 newly diagnosed children from 17 institutions were included between December 1988 and November 1993.

Induction Therapy. Induction chemotherapy was a combination of ara-C (200 mg/m^2 per day by continuous i.v. infusion from day 1 to day 7) and mitoxantrone (12 mg/m^2 on days 1–5). These drug doses were reduced to two thirds for children younger than 1 year of age. Bone marrow aspiration was performed on day 20 and patients who had more than 20% blasts received additional chemotherapy consisting of ara-C 200 mg/m^2 per day by continuous i.v. infusion for 3 days and mitoxantrone 12 mg/m^2 per day for 2 days.

Post-remission Therapy Design. Among 149 patients who achieved a CR, 32 had an HLA-identical sibling donor and were eligible to receive an allogeneic BMT early in first CR. None of these patients relapsed or died before the planned BMT and all were actually treated with BMT in first CR. One additional patient in first CR received a BMT from his one antigen HLA-mismatched father. This patient was analyzed in the BMT group, which consequently consisted of 33

Department of Pediatric Hematology, Saint Louis Hospital, 1, avenue Claude Vellefaux, 75010 Paris, France

children. The 116 remaining children (chemotherapy group) were treated according to the post-remission chemotherapy protocol. *Post-remission Chemotherapy Protocol: Consolidation Chemotherapy.* Two consolidation courses were given to patients without an HLA-matched donor. Consolidation 1 was a combination of etoposide (VP-16; 100 mg/m^2 per day i.v. from day 1 to day 4), ara-C (100 mg/m^2 per day as a continuous i.v. infusion from day 1 to day 4), and daunorubicin (40 mg/m^2 per day from day 1 to day 4). Consolidation 2, which was given after complete hematological recovery, consisted of two cycles of ara-C infusions (1 g/m^2 every 12 h × 4) administered at 7-day intervals (first cycle on days 1 and 2, second cycle on days 8 and 9), each cycle being followed by one dose of asparaginase at 6000 U/m^2. Between the two cytarabine cycles, children older than 1 year of age were treated with amsacrine at 150 mg/m^2 per day i.v. on days 4, 5, and 6, whereas younger children did not receive this medication.

Maintenance Chemotherapy. After consolidation chemotherapy, patients were treated with a 18-month maintenance program consisting of continuous oral 6-mercaptopurine 50 mg/m^2 per day and monthly pulses of subcutaneous ara-C 25 mg/m^2 twice a day for 4 days. In March 1991, a decision was made by the participating centers to randomize children to receive the maintenance chemotherapy versus not receiving any further treatment after consolidation 2. An interim analysis revealed no difference in relapse rate or disease-free survival (DFS) between these two groups. Consequently, all patients treated on the chemotherapy arm were analysed as a single group for the purpose of comparison with BMT, whether or not they received the maintenance program.

CNS Therapy. CNS prophylaxis was administered to patients with the M4 or the M5 FAB subtype and to patients with an initial white blood cell (WBC) count higher than 50×10^9/l. These patients received intrathecal chemotherapy (IT) with five doses of ara-C, methotrexate, and steroid. Patients with initial CNS involvement received three additional IT doses and 24-Gy cranial radiation after hematological recovery from consolidation 2.

Transplantation Methods. Among 33 transplanted children, 23 were conditioned with busulfan 16 mg/kg or 480 mg/m^2 and cyclophosphamide (Cy). Cy was given i.v. either at a dose of 60 mg/kg per day for 2 days or at 50 mg/kg per day for 4 days. Ten patients received a total body irradiation (TBI) containing regimen with Cy or with high-dose ara-C and melphalan. All patients received graft-versus-host disease (GVHD) prophylaxis consisting of cyclosporine A and a short course of methotrexate. The mean value of the interval from CR to transplantation was 80 ± 13 days. Most of patients received consolidation 1 before BMT.

Results

Patients Characteristics. Among 171 patients who were entered on the protocol, there were 83 boys and 88 girls with a mean age of 7.3 ± 0.7 years. Twenty-four children (14%) were less than 1 year old. Mean WBC count at diagnosis was 68.1 ± 13.8 × 10^9/l and the distribution of FAB subtypes was as follows: M1 ($n=23$), M2 ($n=37$), M3 ($n=12$), M4 ($n=41$, 12 of 41 patients with the M4eo subtype), M5 ($n=48$), M6 ($n=5$), and M7 ($n=5$). Bulky hepatosplenomegaly, defined as either spleen or liver enlargement below the umbilicus, was observed in 22 cases (13%). Twenty-two children (13 %) had initial CNS involvement. The characteristics of the patients in the two post-remission groups are listed in Table 1. The mean age was significantly lower in the chemotherapy group than in the BMT group ($p=0.04$). The percentage of patients less than 1 year old and the mean WBC count observed in the chemotherapy group were higher than in the BMT group, but these differences did not reach statistical significance. There were no differences between the two groups for the following characteristics: sex ratio, distribution of FAB subtypes, incidence of bulky hepatosplenomegaly and CNS involvement, and interval from the begining of induction to CR.

Remission Induction. A total of 149 of 171 children (87%) achieved a CR; 133 of them only received the standard 7-day induction course, whereas ten required the additional induction chemotherapy course. There were 22 failures (13%). They were secondary to resistant leukemia ($n=11$) or due to deaths during induction therapy ($n=11$).

Outcome for All Patients. The probability of DFS was 57% ± 9% at 3 years and 51% ± 13% at 4 years for the 149 patients who achieved CR after induc-

Table 1. Patient characteristics in the two post-remission groups

	BMT group ($n=33$)	Chemotherapy group ($n=116$)	Statistical significance
Age			
Mean[a] (years)	8.9 ± 1.5	6.8 ± 0.9	$P=0.04$[b]
Group			
< 1 year (*n*)	1	18	NS + ($p=0.08$)
(%)	3	16	
> 1 year (*n*)	32	98	
(%)	97	84	
WBC count at diagnosis			
Mean[a] ($\times 10^9$/l)	47.2 ± 24.5	62.6 ± 15.3	NS[b]
FAB subtype			
M5 (n)	10	31	NS[c]
(%)	30	27	
Meningeal involvement (*n*)	3	19	NS[d]
(%)	9	16	
Bulky disease (*n*)	1	16	NS[d]
(%)	3	16	
Interval induction–CR [days]	34.4 ± 2.6	37.1 ± 2.3	NS[b]

[a]Mean values ± their 95% confidence interval.
[b]Student's t test.
[c]χ^2 test
[d]Fischer exact test.
NS, not significant.

tion therapy. Overall event-free survival was 49% ± 9% at 3 years and 45% ± 11% at 4 years for the 171 patients entered into the protocol.

Relapse Rate. Five of 33 children in the BMT group relapsed, whereas 40 of 116 patients in the chemotherapy group had recurrence of their disease. The median value of the time interval from CR to relapse was 13 months (range 6–25 months) in the BMT group and 9 months (range 2–45 months) in the chemotherapy group. Most recurrences occurred in the bone marrow except for three patients who had isolated extramedullary relapses. Only one of 40 relapses observed in the chemotherapy group occurred before 80 days which was the mean value of the interval from CR to transplantation in the BMT group. The actuarial risk of relapse at 3 years was 22% ± 17% for the BMT group as compared to 43% ± 11% for the chemotherapy group (Fig. 1). The difference observed between the two groups was statistically significant ($p=0.025$).

Graft-Versus-Host Disease and Therapy-Related Mortality. Thirteen among 33 transplanted children (39%) developed acute GVHD (most of them grades 1 and 2). Chronic GVHD occurred in three of 32 patients (9%) who were assessable after day 100 post transplant. Only one patient in the BMT group died from a transplant-related complication. Seven patients in the chemotherapy group died in CR from infectious complications. Probability of therapy-related mortality TRM was 3% for the BMT group and 6.4% for the chemotherapy group (no statistical significance).

Disease-Free Survival. Twenty-seven children in the BMT group and 69 in the chemotherapy group were alive in continuous CR. The median follow-up duration from CR was 25 months in both groups. The Kaplan-Meier estimate of DFS at 3 years was 75% ±17% for the **BMT** group as compared to 51% ±10% for the chemotherapy group (Fig. 2) ($p=0.018$).

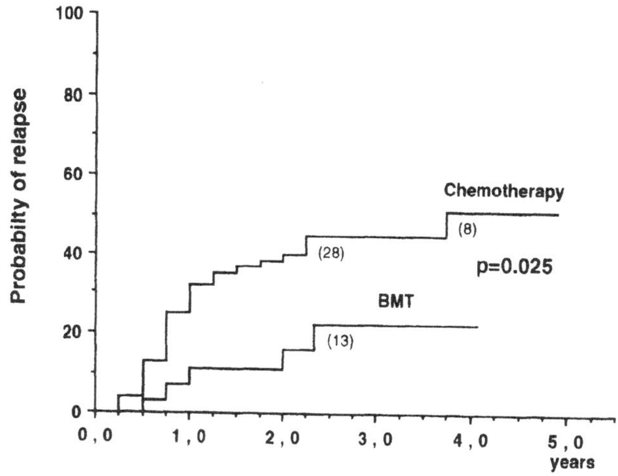

Fig. 1. Kaplan-Meier probability of relapse in the BMT group ($n=33$) and in the chemotherapy group ($n=116$). The comparison is made using the log-rank test. *Numbers in parenthesis* indicate the number of patients at risk at various time intervals

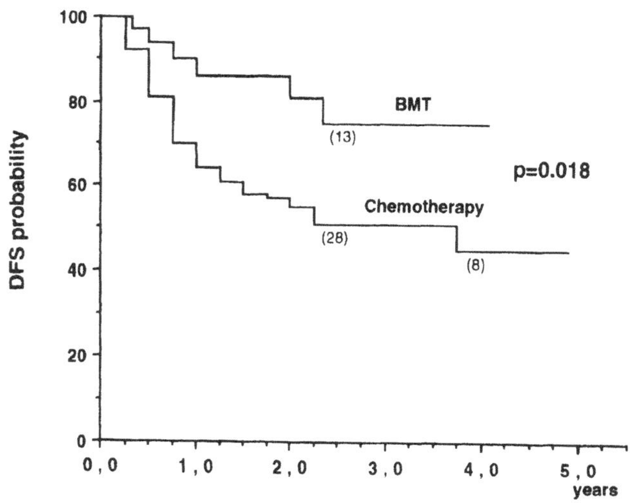

Fig. 2. Kaplan-Meier probability of DFS in the BMT group ($n=33$) and in the chemotherapy group ($n=116$). The comparison is made using the log-rank test. *Numbers in parenthesis* indicate the number of patients at risk at various time intervals

Prognostic Factors

Chemotherapy Group. In the univariate analysis, children less than 1 year old had a higher risk of relapse (71% versus 40% at 3 years, $p=0.001$) and a lower DFS (26% versus 55% at 3 years, $p=0.003$) than older children. The M5 subtype significantly affected the relapse rate (60% versus 40%, $p=0.006$) and DFS (36% versus 56%, $p=0.008$) when compared to other FAB subtypes. A WBC count higher than 50×10^9/l was associated with a high risk of relapse (61% versus 35%, $p=0.03$) but the impact on DFS did not reach the level of statistical significance. Meningeal involvement and bulky disease did not affect relapse risk or DFS. As shown in Table 2, only two factors were statistically significant in the multivariate analysis: age less than 1 year old and M5 subtype. Because children under 1 year of age had a poor prognosis when treated with chemotherapy alone and because the transplant group had a fewer proportion of such children than the chemotherapy group, we compared BMT to chemotherapy after excluding these children from both groups. When only children older than 1 year were analysed, DFS was 74% in the BMT group and 55% in the chemotherapy group ($p=0.07$). The relapse rate was 24% and 40% respectively ($p=0.09$).

BMT Group. FAB subtype (M5 versus others) and WBC count ($<$ versus $\geqslant 50 \times 10^9$/l) did not

Table 2. Multivariate analysis of prognostic factors for the probabilities of relapse and DFS in the chemotherapy group (Cox regression analysis)

Criteria	Relapse	DFS
Age at diagnosis (< vs. ≥ 1year)	$p=0.001$ RR = 3	$p=0.003$ RR = 2.52
FAB subtypes (M5 vs. others)	$p=0.03$ RR = 2.1	$p=0.03$ RR = 1.94
WBC count (< vs. ≥ 50×10^9/l	NS ($p=0.12$)	NS ($p=0.25$)
Hepatosplenomegaly	NS	NS
Meningeal involvement	NS	NS

Only patients who achieved CR and were treated in the chemotherapy arm were included in this analysis ($n=116$).
The p values < 0.05 were considered as statistically significant.
NS, not significant; RR, relative risk.

influence relapse risk or DFS. Children who received a TBI-containing regimen had a 64% probability of DFS and a 36% relapse rate; children who received busulfan and cyclophosphamide had a 81% probability of DFS and a 15% relapse rate (no statistical significance).

Comparison with Berlin-Frankfurt-Münster (BFM) Regimen. In the French and German [6] protocols, age is one of the most important prognostic factors and infants have a poor outcome compared to older children. According to the results of BFM-AML 3, two different risk groups, low and high, were identified. The low-risk group included FAB M1 with Auer rods, M2 with WBC less than 20 000, and M3 and M4 with eosinophilia. When using these parameters in the LAME protocol, we cannot differentiate two risk groups indicating that risk factors can only be regarded in the context of overall treatment strategy.

Discussion

This study was designed to evaluate the impact of allogeneic BMT on the outcome of children with AML in first CR. The relapse rate observed in the BMT group was lower than in the chemotherapy group (22.5% ± 17% versus 43% ± 11%). The difference was statistically significant in the univariate analysis as well as in the multivariate analysis. Three other studies comparing allogeneic BMT with consolidation have been reported [1, 2, 4]. All three revealed a significantly lower relapse rate in the BMT arm. However, high-dose ara-C was not used as consolidation in the treatment program. The effectiveness of this intensification in childhood AML has been clearly demonstrated by investigators from the Childrens Cancer Group (CCG) [5, 7, 8].

In our study, the given therapy corresponded with the intent to treat as none of the patients relapsed or died before their planned graft and all of them received BMT during first CR.

Many published studies have reported that the antileukemic effect of BMT was partially counterbalanced by a 25% risk of transplant-related mortality [2, 3, 4]. The transplant mortality in our trials was only 3% and this probability was not statistically different from the 6.4% risk of therapy-related mortality observed in the chemotherapy group. Transplant-related mortality has decreased dramatically for children who were transplanted during the years 1987–1990 as compared to patients grafted before 1987 (3% versus 36%, respectively [9]); other investigators have reported similar results [5]. It seems to us that shortening the interval from CR to transplant could have a favorable impact, probably by avoiding cumulative toxicity of several intensification regimens given before transplantation.

Our promising results suggest that allogeneic BMT in first CR remains the treatment of choice for improving DFS in children who have an HLA-identical sibling donor. The role of intensification, including high-dose ara-C, improves the results for patients lacking an HLA-matched sibling. CNS irradiation does not seem useful for patients without initial CNS involvement as there was no increased relapse rate in the CNS in nonirradiated patients. Finally, a 18-month maintenance program does not increase CR duration in patients receiving a chemotherapy program including two aggressive intensification regimens.

Acknowledgment. This work was supported by a grant from ARC.

References

1. Amadori S, Testi AM, Arico M et al.: Prospective comparitive study of bone marrow transplantation and post remission chemotherapy for childhood

acute myelogeneous leukemia. J Clin Oncol, 11: 1046–1054, 1993.
2. Dahl GV, Kalwinski DK, Mirpo J et al.: Allogeneic bone marrow transplantation in a program of intensive sequential chemotherapy for children and young adults with acute non-lymphocytic leukemia in first remission. J Clin Oncol, 8: 295–303, 1990.
3. Dinsmore R, Kirkpatrick D, Flomenberg N et al.: Allogeneic bone marrow transplantation for patients with acute non-lymphocytic leukemia. Blood, 63: 649–656, 1984.
4. Nesbit ME, Buckley JD, Feig SA et al.: Chemotherapy for induction remission of childhood acute myeloid leukemia followed by marrow transplantation or multiagent chemotherapy: a report from the Childrens Cancer Group. J Clin Oncol, 12: 127–135, 1994.
5. Woods WG, Kobrinky N, Buckley J et al.: Intensively timed induction therapy followed by autologous or allogeneic bone marrow transplantation for children with acute myeloid leukemia or myelodysplastic syndrome: a Children Cancer Group pilot study. J Clin Oncol, 11 : 1448–1457, 1993.
6. Creitzig U, Ritter J, Schellong G for the AML BFM Study Group. Identification of two risk groups in childhood acute myelogenous leukemia after therapy intensification in study AML BFM 83 as compared with study AML BFM 78. Blood, 75: 1932–1940, 1990.
7. Wells RJ, Woods WG, Lampkin BC et al.: Impact of high-dose cytarabine and asparaginase intensification on childhood acute myeloid leukemia: a report from the Childrens Cancer Group. J Clin Oncol, 11: 538–545, 1993.
8. Woods WG, Ruymann FB, Lampkin BC et al.: The role of timing of high dose cytosine arabinosie intensification and of maintenance therapy in the treatment of children with acute non-lymphoblastic leukemia. Cancer, 66: 1106–1113, 1990.
9. Michel G, Gluckman E, Blaise D et al.: Improvement in outcome for children receiving allogeneic bone marrow transplantation in first complete remission of acute myeloid leukemia. A report from the GEGMO. J Clin Oncol, 10: 1865–1869, 1992

Acute Leukemias VI
Prognostic Factors
and Treatment Strategies
Büchner et al. (eds)

Childhood Acute Nonlymphoblastic Leukemia — Results of the Austrian-Hungarian Acute Myeloid Leukemia Studies IGCI-84 and 90

F.M. Fink[1], G. Mann[2], P. Masát[3], E.R. Panzer-Grümayer[2], P. Kajtar, G. Kardos, C. Urban[5], D. Schuler[4], and H. Gadner[2], for the IGCI[a] Pediatric Study Group

Abstract. Between 1984 and 1992, 154 children and adolescents were registered to the two consecutive Austrian-Hungarian cooperative multicenter childhood acute nonlymphoblastic leukemia (ANLL), studies AML-IGCI-84 and 90. A total of 148 patients were evaluable for treatment response. Both protocols represented modifications of the German Berlin–Frankfurt–Minster (BFM) study protocols AML-BFM-83 and-87, respectively. Aclarubicin (ACR) was substituted for daunorubicin in the first-line induction protocol. In addition, two courses of high-dose cytosine arabinoside plus idarubicin or mitoxantrone, respectively, were given as early intensification in the IGCI-90 series instead of the late intensification courses of BFM-87. From IGCI-84 ($n=95$) to IGCI-90 ($n=53$) the remission rate improved from 67% to 77%, and probability of event-free survival (pEFS) from .30 to .37 (not significant, median follow up in complete remission (CR) 8.1 and 3.9 years, respectively). Remission duration was not improved (probability of event-free interval, pEFI, .44 vs. .48). A relatively high death rate in CR and the omission of cranial irrradiation in the second study may have been the main reasons for the lack of improvement of results.

Introduction

In the treatment of childhood acute nonlymphoblastic leukemia (ANLL), remission rates of 70% to more than 80% can be achieved by a variety of intensive induction chemotherapy regimens. A considerable percentage of children achieve long-term remissions and may be cured [1–10].

Aclarubicin (ACR)—a newer generation anthracycline antibiotic isolated from *Streptomyces galilaeus* [11]—was introduced into clinical use more than 10 years ago. Phase I and II studies had shown a significant antileukemic activity of the drug, particularly against ANLL [12–18]. Preclinical toxicity studies suggested that ACR was less cardiotoxic than the classical anthracycline antibiotics doxorubicin and daunorubicin [19–21].

From 1984 through 1992 154 children with ANLL were treated in two consecutive prospective multicentric studies. Both protocols—AML-IGCI-84 and AML-IGCI-90—included an ACR-based first-line induction therapy. The protocols aimed at remission rates and long-term survival comparable to the sister studies AML-BFM-83 and AML-BFM-87, respectively, together with the expectation of reduced cardiotoxicity by the substitution of ACR for DNR in the first therapy element.

[1]Department of Pediatrics, University of Innsbruck, Austria
[2]St. Anna Children's Hospital, CCRI, Vienna, Austria
[3]Teaching Hospital Szombathely, Hungary
[4]Semmelweis University Medical School, Budapest, Hungary
[5]Department of Pediatric Hematology/Oncology, University of Graz, Austria
[a]IGCI, Internationale Gesellschaft für Chemo- und Immunotherapie

Material and Methods

Patients and Diagnosis

A total of 154 children and adolescents with newly diagnosed untreated ANLL were registered (see Table 1 for a description of patient characteristics); 148 patients were evaluable for response to treatment. They were treated at 18 different pediatric institutions in Austria and Hungary. Leukemias were classified according to the cytological and cytochemical criteria of the French–American–British (FAB) group [22–24]. Children with Down's syndrome or severe underlying disease were excluded from the study. Standardized criteria for response evaluation were applied. Complete remission (CR) was defined as less than 5% blasts in the bone marrow aspirate together with recovery of normal hematopoiesis and clearance of all signs of extramedullary leukemic manifestations. Survival analysis was performed by the Kaplan–Meier life-table procedure [25]. Differences of survival between groups were analyzed by the log-rank test [26].

Table 1. Patient characteristics

	IGCI-84	IGCI-90
Patients registered (*n*)	97	57
Deaths before treatment (*n*)	2	4
Evaluable patients (*n*)	95	53
Males : females (*n*)	46 : 49	29 : 24
Age-median (years)	7.5	6.7
range (years)	0–17.9	0.3–16.6
Initial WBC (1/μl)	18 600	9800
WBC range (1/μl)	1400–1 35 0000	240–28 0000
CNS involvement (*n*)	3	3
FAB subtypes		
M1 (*n*)	29	18
M2 (*n*)	13	7
M3 (*n*)	1	1
M4 (*n*)	26	13
M5 (*n*)	20	9
M6 (*n*)	2	-
M7 (*n*)	4	5

Treatment—Study Design

The backbone of the protocols were the German Berlin–Frankfurt–Münster (BFM) therapy studies AML-BFM-83 and AML-BFM-87, respectively (Fig. 1) [2, 3]. In contrast to the original BFM protocols, however, all patients received a first induction (I1) consisting of cytosine arabinoside (ara-C), ACR, and etoposide (VP-16) (Fig. 2).

IGCI-84. All patients received I1 (Fig. 2). Children in CR after I1 proceeded to intensive consolidation. Children not in CR after I1 received an induction I2 (ADE protocol of AML-BFM-83 [2]): ara-C 100 mg/m^2 per day continuously i.v. on days 1 and 2, then 2 × 100 mg/m^2 per day i.v. on days 3–8, daunorubicin (DNR) 60 mg/m^2 perday i.v. on days 3–5, VP-16 150 mg/m^2 perday i.v. on days 4–6. After recovery from I1, or I1 plus I2, respectively, all children proceeded to the intensive BFM-83 consolidation: within 8 weeks this protocol incorporated prednisone 40 mg/m^2 daily p.o. on days 1–28, 6-thioguanine

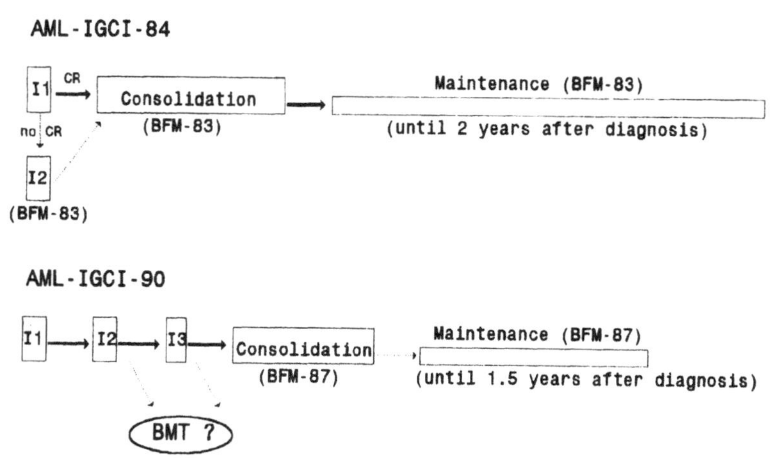

Fig. 1. Study designs

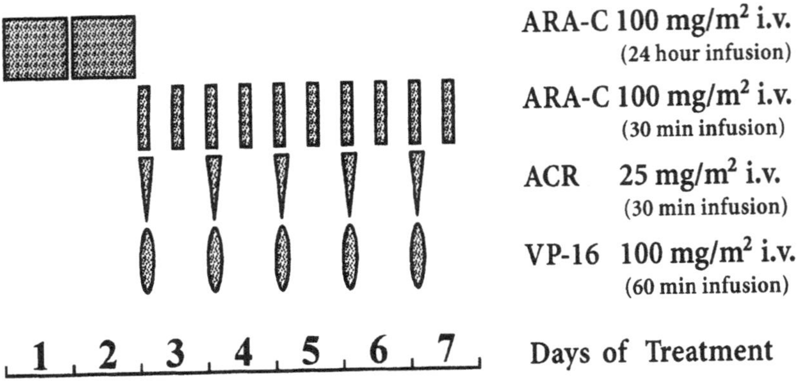

Fig. 2. Induction I1

(6-TG) 60 mg/m^2 daily p.o. on days 1–56, vincristine 1.5mg/m^2 i.v. and doxorubicin (ADR) 25 mg/m^2 i.v. on days 1,8,15,22, ara-C 75 mg/m^2 i.v. on 4 consecutive days starting on days 3, 10, 17, 24, 31, 38, 45, 52, respectively, cyclophosphamide 500 mg/m^2 i.v. on days 29 and 57, and age-dependent intrathecal ara-C on days 31, 38, 45, and 52. The consolidation protocol included cranial irradiation at an age-dependent dose (12–18 Gy)[2]. Low-dose maintenance with 6-TG and ara-C was given until 2 years from diagnosis and included intermittent ADR during the 1st year. I2, consolidation, and maintenance were original protocols of the study AML-BFM-83 [2].

IGCI-90. All patients received I1 with an increased ACR dose (30 mg/m^2 per day instead of 25 mg/m^2 per day). All children proceeded to I2 and I3 before the intensive consolidation (BFM-87, shortened by 2 weeks compared to IGCI-84/BFM-83 [3]) was started (Fig. 1). I2 consisted of ara-C 2 × 2g/m^2 per day i.v. on days 1–3, and idarubicin 10 mg/m^2 per day i.v. on days 2–4. I3 included ara-C 2 × 3g/m^2 per day i.v. on days 1 and 2, and mitoxantrone 12 mg/m^2 per day continuously i.v. on days 1 and 2 [27]. No prophylactic CNS irradiation was given. Low-dose maintenance (6-TG, ara-C) was adminstered until 1.5 years from diagnosis. Consolidation and maintenance were original protocol of the study AML-BFM-87 [3].

In both studies patients with high initial white blood cell counts (WBC) (>50 000/µl) and/or extensive organomegaly received a cytoreductive pretreatment with 6-TG and ara-C.

Results

The results of two consecutive studies are presented in Table 2. The remission rate of 67% in AML-IGCI-84 improved to 77% in AML-IGCI-90. The death rate in CR was high in both studies (8% and 12%, respectively). In the IGCI-84 series, 29 patients remain in continuous CR (CCR), in the IGCI-90 series 21 patients are currently in CCR. These figures include four and five patients undergoing transplantation in CR1, respectively. The median follow up in remission is 8.1 and 3.9 years, respectively.

Survival analyses failed to demonstrate a significant improvement of event-free survival (EFS, Fig. 3) or event-free interval (EFI, Fig. 4) (log-rank $p = .36$ and $p = .89$, respectively). For survival analyses patients undergoing transplantation in first remission (CR1) were censored at the date of grafting.

Table 2. Treatment results

		IGCI-84	IGCI-90
Complete remissions	(*n*)	64/95	41/53
	(%)	67	77
Relapses	(*n*)	27	13
Deaths in remission	(*n*)	5	5
BMT in CRI	(*n*)	7	7
Alive in CCR	(*n*)	29	21
Event-free survival [a]		.30(SE .05)	.37 (SE .07)
Event-free interval [a]		.44(SE .07)	.48 (SE .09)

[a]BMT patients censored at the date of grafting in CRI.

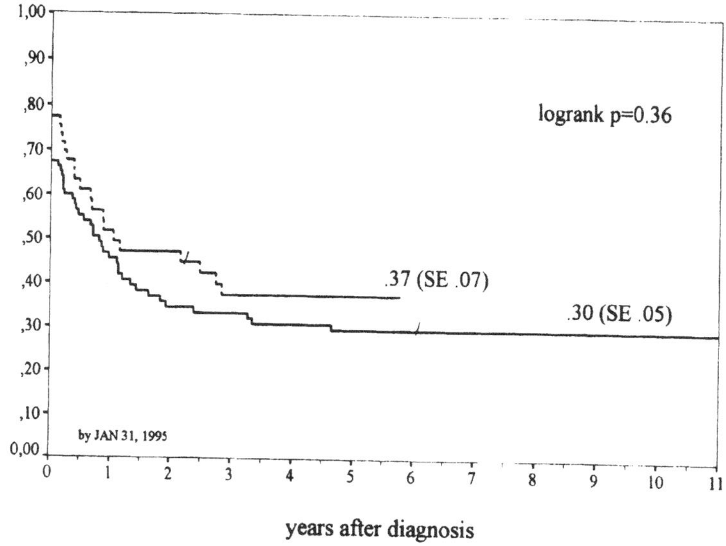

Fig. 3. Event-free survival: *broken line*, IGCI-90 ($n = 53$); *solid line*, IGCI-84 ($n = 95$)

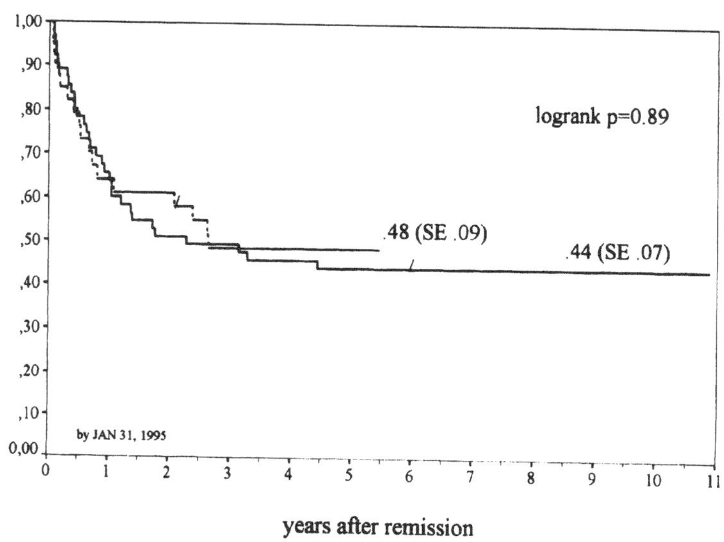

Fig. 4. Event-free interval: *broken line*, IGCI-90 ($n = 41$); *solid line*, IGCI-84 ($n = 64$)

Discussion

In both studies the ACR-based induction chemotherapy was effective. However, AML-IGCI-84 showed a high rate of early deaths, obviously impairing the remission rate. Improved control of induction toxicity led to an increased remission rate in the successor study AML-IGCI-90, the remission rate of 77% compares well with results achieved by other successful protocols for childhood ANLL [1–10].

The long-term results are also comparable with those of most pediatric studies for ANLL which published probalilities of EFS (pEFS) in the range of .20 to .40 and probabilities of EFI (pEFI) in the range of .40 to .50 [1, 4–10]. However, the German study AML-BFM-83—the most successful childhood ANLL study ever published—showed clearly better results with a pEFS of .49 (SE. 04) and a pEFI of .61 (SE .04) after 6 years [2, 3].

In adults, the value of ACR for the treatment of acute myelogenous leukemia (AML) has already been demonstrated in refractory disease as well as in front-line therapy. Phase I and II studies have demonstrated remission rates in the range of 20%–40% in patients with relapsed or refractory disease [12–18, 28]. In a recently published randomized trial, the ACR-containing induction course yielded a significantly higher remission rate than the one with daunorubicin [29].

The intensification of early postremission chemotherapy by the combined use of high-dose ara-C and newer-generation anthracyclines and related compounds (idarubicin and mitoxantrone, respectively) in the second series (IGCI-90) did not improve remission duration. A relatively high rate of deaths in CR may have been partially responsible. On the other hand, the elimination of cranial irradiation in our study AML-IGCI-90 may have impaired the systemic efficacy of the protocol. The importance of cranial irradiation in the systemic treatment of childhood ANLL has recently been demonstrated by the BFM group [30].

In conclusion, the two pediatric ANLL series IGCI-84 and -90 revealed results comparable to other successful protocols. In the light of the superior results of the original BFM trials. AML-BFM-83 and -87 [2–4], ACR-containing induction regimens remain approaches of second choice for childhood ANLL. Early intensification of postremission therapy did not improve remission duration, toxicity probably representing the main obstacle.

Acknowledgment. The authors wish to thank all the members of the IGCI pediatric study group in Austria and Hungary who cared for our patients for their cooperation.

References

1. Creutzig U, Ritter J, Riehm H, et al. (1985) Improved treatment results in childhood acute myelogenous leukemia. Blood 65: 298–304
2. Creutzig U, Ritter J, Schellong G (1990) Identification of two risk groups in childhood acute myelogenous leukemia after therapy intensification in study AML-BFM-83 as compared with study AML-BFM-78. Blood 75: 1932–1940
3. Ritter J, Creutzig U, Schellong G (1992) Treatment results of three consecutive German childhood AML trials: BFM-78, -83, and -87. AML-BFM-Group. Leukemia 6 (Suppl 2): 59–62
4. Buckley JD, Chard RL, Baehner RL, et al. (1989) Improvement in outcome for children with acute nonlymphocytic leukemia. A report from the Children's Cancer Study Group. Cancer 63: 1457–1465
5. Buckley JD, Lampkin B, Nesbit M, et al. (1989) Remission induction in children with acute nonlymphocytic leukemia using cytosine arabinoside and doxorubicin or daunorubicin: a report from the Childrens Cancer Study Group. Med Pediatr Oncol 17: 382–390
6. Nesbit ME, Buckley JD, Feig SA, et al. (1994) Chemotherapy for induction of remission of childhood acute myeloid leukemia followed by bone marrow transplantation or multiagent chemotherapy: a report from the Children's Cancer Group. J Clin Oncol 12: 127-135
7. Steuber CP, Civin C, Krischer J, et al.(1991) A comparison of induction and maintenance therapy for acute nonlymphocytic leukemia in childhood: results of a Pediatric Oncology Group study. J Clin Oncol 9: 247–258
8. Weinstein HJ, Mayer RJ, Rosenthal DS, et al. (1983) Chemotherapy for acute myelogenous leukemia in children and adults: VAPA update. Blood 62: 315–319
9. Grier HE, Gelber RD, Link MP, et al. (1992) Intensive sequential chemotherapy for children with acute myelogenous leukemia: VAPA, 80-035, and HI-C-Daze. Leukemia 6 (Suppl 2): 48–51
10. Chessells JM, O'Callaghan U, Hardisty RM (1986) Acute myeloid leukaemia in childhood: clinical features and prognosis. Br J Haematol 63: 555–564
11. Oki T, Matsuzawa Y, Yoshimoto A, et al. (1975) New antitumor antibiotics, aclacinomycin A and B. J Antibiot (Tokyo) 28: 830–834
12. Yamada K, Nakamura T, Tsurno T, et al. (1980) A phase II study of aclacinomycin A in acute leukemia in adults. Cancer Treat Rev 7: 177–182
13. Warrell RP, Arlin ZA, Zempin SJ, Young CW (1982) Phase I-II evaluation of a new anthracycline antibiotic, aclacinomycin A, in adults with refractory leukemia. Cancer Treat Rep 66: 1619–1623
14. Pedersen-Bjergaard J, Brincker H, Ellegard J, et al. (1984) Aclarubicin in the treatment of acute nonlymphocytic leukemia refractory to treatment with daunorubicin and cytarabine: a phase II trial. Cancer Treat Rep 68: 1233–1238
15. Machover D, Gastiaburu J, Delgado M, et al. (1984) Phase I-II study of aclarubicin for treatment of acute myeloid leukemia. Cancer Treat Rep 68: 881–886
16. Mitrou PS, Kuse R, Angers H, et al. (1985) Aclarubicin (aclacinomycin A) in the treatment of relapsing acute leukemias. Eur J Cancer Clin Oncol 21: 919–923
17. Dabich L, Bull FA, Beltran G, et al. (1986) Phase II evaluation of aclarubicin in refractory adult acute

leukemia: a Southwest Oncology Group study. Cancer Treat Rep 70: 967–969
18. Case DC, Ervin TJ, Boyd MA, et al. (1987) Phase II study of aclarubicin in acute myeloblastic leukemia. Am J Clin Oncol 10: 523–526
19. Dantchev D, Slioussarchouk V, Paintrand M, et al. (1979) Electron microsopic studies of the heart and light microscopic studies of the skin after treatment of golden hamsters with adriamycin, detrubicin, AD-32, and aclacinomycin. Cancer Treat Rep 63: 875–888
20. Wakabayashi T, Oki T, Tone H, et al. (1980) A comparative electron microscopic study of aclacinomycin and adriamycin cardiotoxicities in rabbits and hamster. J Electron Microsc 29: 106–118
21. Warrell RP Jr. (1986) Aclacinomycin A: clinical development of a novel anthracycline antibiotic in the hematologic cancers. Drugs Exptl Clin Res 12: 275–282
22. Bennett JM, Catovsky D, Daniel MT, et al. (1976) Proposals for the classification of the acute leukemias. French-American-British (FAB) cooperative groups. Br J Haematol 33: 451–458
23. Bennett JM, Catovski D, Daniel MT, et al. (1985) Proposed revised criteria for the classification of acute myeloid leukemia: a report from the French-American-British cooperative group. Ann Intern Med 103: 620–627
24. Bennett JM, Catovsky D, Daniel MT, et al. (1985) Criteria for the diagnosis of acute leukemia of megakaryocytic lineage (M7). A report of the French-American-British cooperative group. Ann Intern Med 103: 460–462
25. Kaplan E, Meier P (1958) Non-parametric estimation from incomplete observations. J Am Stat Assoc 53: 457-481
26. Peto R, Pike M C (1973) Conservatism of the approximation $\Sigma(O-E)^2/E$ in the logrank test for survival data or tumor incidence data. Biometrics 29: 579–584
27. Linkesch W, Thaler J, Gattringer C, Konwalinka G. Continuous infusion of mitoxantrone combined with high-dose cytarabine in refractory/relapsed acute myeloblastic leukemia. In: Büchner T, Schellong G, Hiddemann W, Ritter J (eds.): Haematology and blood transfusion 33, Acute leukemias II, pp 330–332, Springer, Berlin, Heidelberg, 1990
28. Rowe JM, ChangAY, Bennett JM (1988) Aclacinomycin A and etoposide (VP-16-213): an effective regimen in previously treated patients with refractory acute myelogenous leukemia. Blood 71: 992–996
29. Hansen OP, Pedersen-Bjergaard J, Ellegaard J, et al. (1991) Aclarubicin plus cytosine arabinoside versus daunorubicin plus cytosine arabinoside in previously untreated patients with acute myeloid leukemia: a Danish national phase III trial. The Danish Society of Hematology Study Group on AML, Denmark. Leukemia 5: 510–516
30. Creutzig U, Ritter J, Zimmermann M, Schellong G (1993) Does cranial irradiation reduce the risk for bone marrow relapse in acute myelogenous leukemia? Unexpected results of the Childhood Acute Myelogenous Leukemia Study BFM-87. J Clin Oncol 11: 279–86

Acute Leukemias VI
Prognostic Factors
and Treatment Strategies
Büchner et al. (eds)

Results of Intensive Chemotherapy of Acute Myeloblastic Leukemia in Children According to the Berlin–Frankfurt–Münster Strategy: A Single-Institution Trial

A.A. Maschan, L.V. Baydun, A.I. Karachunsky, M.J. Kharit, O.I. Kryzhanovsky, E.V. Samochatova, M.V. Timakova, T.V. Zhiganova, N.M. Zhestkova, and A.G. Rumjantsev

Abstract. In order to improve the poor results of treatment of childhood acute myeloblastic leukemia (AML), we applied the Berlin-Frankfurt-Münster (BFM) strategy for patients with AML admitted to the clinic of our institute. The reference group included 29 patients treated with courses "7+3" and "5+2" (conventional doses of cytosine arabinoside, ara-C, and daunorubicin). The results of this treatment were as follows: remission was achieved in 58.6% of patients relapse-free survival at 42 months was 21.4%. Between February 1990 and May 1994, a total of 46 consecutive patients with AML were treated according to the BFM strategy (compilcation from AML-BFM-83 and AML-BFM-87 studies); there were 17 males and 29 females. Mean age was 8 years (range 1–15 years). The French–American–British (FAB) subtype distribution was as follows: MO–4.25%, M1–6.45%, M2–19.1% M3–10.65%, M4–23.4%, M5–27.75%, M6–6.4%. All patients received an 8-day induction course: conventional doses of ara-C, daunorubicin 30 mg/m^2 daily-six doses, and etoposide 150 mg/m^2 a day—three doses. A six-drug (prednisolone; 6-mercapto-purine, 6-MP; vincristine; ara-C, cyclophosphamide; doxorubicin) consolidation course lasted 6 weeks. Twenty three patients received intensification therapy: 20 patients with high doses of ara-C plus etoposide and three patients with high-dose ara-C plus mitoxantrone. Twelve patients did not receive an intensification course. CNS prophylaxis included ara-C intrathecally and cranial gamma-irradiation (18 Gy). As a result of the treatment 35 patients (76%) achieved complete remission (CR). There were 11 induction failures: the toxic deaths (13%) and five primary refractory disease (10%). One patient died in CR after the intensification course. Of 34 patients completing the intensive phase of therapy, five patients relapsed (15%). The actuaial event-free survival is 63% at 51 months.

In conclusion our cohort of AML patients is characterized by a peculiar distribution of FAB subtypes with a prevalence of M4 and M5 subtypes needing intensive regimens of therapy. The BFM strategy of intensive treatment showed high efficacy in the presented group of patients with AML.

Introduction

In the past several years results of treatment of many children's cancers have improved. In acute myeloblastic leukemias (AML) treatment with cytosine arabinoside (ara-C) and optimal doses of anthracycline results in 75%–85% of complete remission (CR). About half of the remitters are presumed to achieve long-term survival and eventual cure with the use of modern forms of post-remission therapy. In our institute before 1990, 26 patients with AML received induction of remission consisting of conventional doses of ara-C and suboptimal doses (90–135 mg/m^2 bsa) of daunorubicin (DNR), according to the 7+3 scheme. Remission was maintained by several courses of the same drug association but on a reduced schedule (5+2). Such a treatment yielded 56.8% of CR

Institute of Children's Hematology, Moscow, Russia

and 21.9% of survival at 4 years in 26 patients treated between 1987 and 1990. Since 1990 we have begun to treate our AML patients according to the strategy of Berlin-Frankfurt-Münster (BFM) study group in order to improve such dismal results.

Patients and Methods

Forty-six consecutive pediatric patients with AML hospitalized at the clinic of our institute between February 1990 and May 1994 were included in the trial. Diagnostic procedures included morphological and cytochemical (myeloperoxidase, nonsepecific esterase with and without inhibition by NaF, Sudan black B in the cases of myeloper-oxidase negativity) identification of bone marrow aspirate in all patients. In 21 patients immunophenotyping of blast cells on was done on a FACS scan. Cytogenetics was done in 20 patients. Diagnostic lumbar puncture with cytospin of CSF was done in all patients. The diagnosis of acute nonlymphoblastic leukemia (ANLL) was established according to the revised criteria of the French-American-British (FAB) group [1, 2]. Initial CNS involvement was diagnosed by CSF containing any number of leukemia cells, unexplainable by contamination by peripheral blood, if CSF pleocytosis exceeded 5/μl and/or if signs of cranial nerve or spinal cord infiltration were present. Systemic relapse was stated if more than 25% of blasts were revealed in bone marrow (BM), CNS relapse was confirmed according to the above-mentioned criteria. Risk groups for treatment failure were defined according to the AML-BFM-83 study stratification [3]. Patients with FAB M1 with Auer rods, M2 with leukocytosis below 20000/μl, all patients with M3 and M4 eo were considered as a low-risk group, all other patients as high-risk group.

Treatment. All eligible patients received a three-drug containing induction (conventional doses of ara-C, DNR, and etoposide, VP-16), and a 6-week-six drug consolidation. After entering into CR 20 patients received intensification of treatment with high doses of ara-C (HD Ara-C) and VP-16 (Fig. 1), three patients received HD ara-C and novantrone; 12 patients did not receive intensification. Prophylactic treatment of CNS consisted of systematic intrathecal ara-C and cranial irradiation at an age-adapted dose. Maintenance therapy with daily 6-MP and a monthly 4-day cycle of ara-C lasted untill the 18 month after the beginning of induction [3].

Patients. Forty-six consecutive patients aged 1-15 years were included into the trial between February 1990 and May 1994. Patients characteristics are shown in Table 1 and Fig. 2. All patients were Caucasians, with a male:female ratio of 1:1.7 FAB subtypes of AML and stratification by risk group are shown in Figs. 2 and 3. Nineteen patients fulfilled the criteria of low risk, 27 patients were included in the high-risk group for treatment failure. Ten other patients with AML admitted to our clinic during the same period were treated according to the same protocol but are not included in this report because they were heavily pretreated before admission. Survival data are based on all 46 patients; the last update of the trial was December 31, 1994. The median follow-up duration is 21 months (range 1-55 months).

Statistics. Evaluation was made from the start of induction. Survival curves were constructed by the Kaplan-Meier method.

Results

Thirty-five of 46 patients entered into the trial achieved CR (76%). There were 11 induction failures—five toxic deaths (13%) and six refractory leukemias (11%). Overwhelming sepsis in three cases and severe hemorrage in two cases resulted in death. One of the remitters died of septic shock after the intensification course. Of 34 patients completing the intensive phase of treatment relapse occurred in six at 2.5-25 months after achievement of CR (Table 2). There were four systemic and two combined (BM+CNS; BM+peripheral chloroma) relapses. Three of the relapsed patients finally died of disease progression, but two are alive in second continuous remission(> 12 months) and one in third CR after salvage therapy. The curves of projected event-free survival (EFS) are shown in Figs. 4 and 5. Actuarial EFS (aEFS) for the whole group is 0.60 at 55 months, for the low-risk group the aEFS is 0.82 and for the high-risk group 0.47 at 55 months.

Fig. 1. Intensive phase of treatment according to AML BFM-87. *Drb*, daunorusicin; *VP-16*, etoposide; *cph*, cyclophosphamide; *Vc*, vincristine; *ADR*, doxorubicin; *Pr*, prednisolone

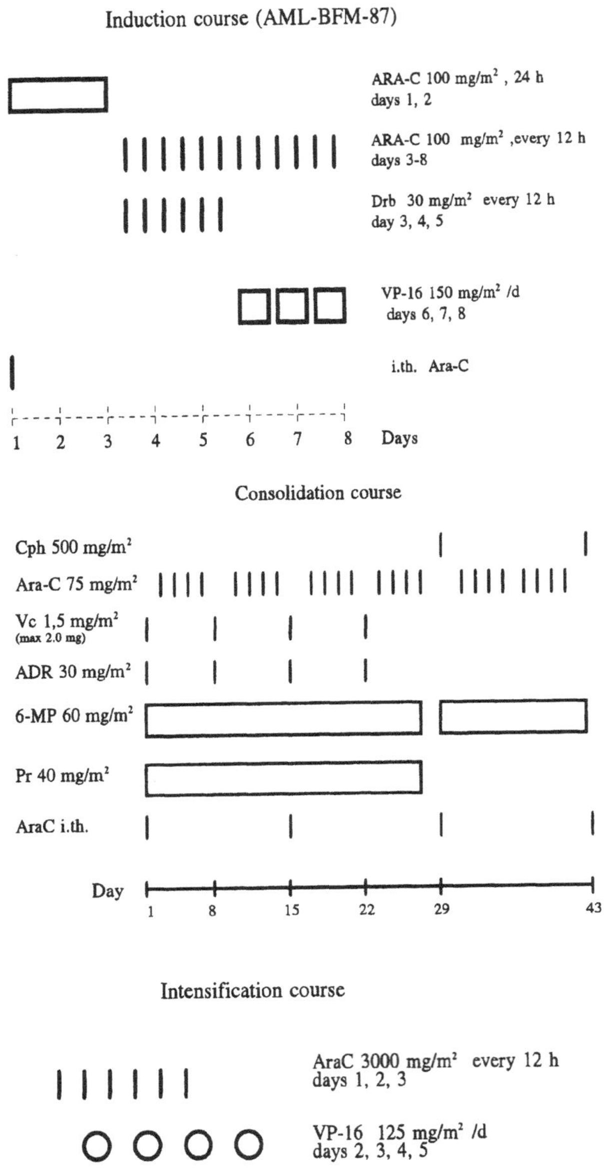

Table 1. Demographic characteristics of patients

Patients (*n*)	46
Male (*n*)	17
Female (*n*)	29
M:F ratio	1:1.7
Age	
Median(years)	8
Range(years)	1–14

Discussion

Before 1990 the results of treating children with AML in our institute were vey poor with a CR rate of 56% and relapse-free survival of 21%. On the one hand, it was due to inappropriate supportive care, resulting in high toxic mortality, and, on the other hand, to ineffective post-remission therapy. Considerable improvement of results has been achieved in the past 4 years

Fig. 2. Age distribution

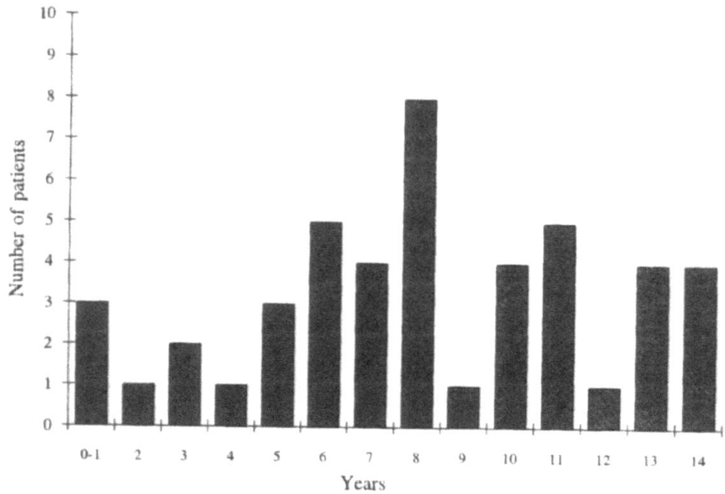

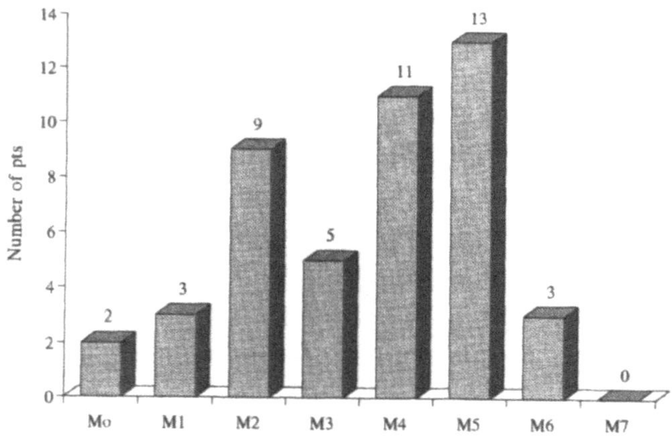

Fig. 3. Distribution according to FAB classification. Standard risk-17 patients; High—risk—29 patients

Table 2. Treatment results

	Patients(%) (*n*)
Total	46
Early deaths	6
Non-response	5
CR achieved	35 77.0
Death in remission	1
Relapse	6
CCR > 9 months(9–51)	24 57.6
LFU	3
Second CR	3

after the introduction of the BFM-AML-based program of chemotherapy. This treatment strategy of AML in children yields the best results worldwide, with an EFS rate approaching the magic 50% margin [4]. At the very beginning of trial our major fear was the high potential toxicity of this regimen and in fact during first 2 years of study the toxic mortality rate reached 25%. However, with the increase of standard of supportive measures, toxic mortality could be decreased to the very low level we achieved in 1993–1994 when no patients died from treatment-related causes. Although a considerable step forward in comparison with past experience, our results are still liable to criticism. First

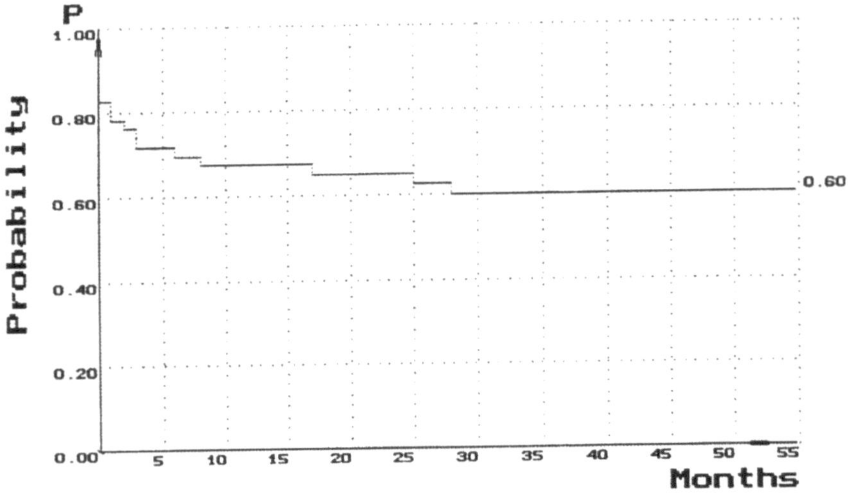

Fig. 4. EFS for all 46 patients during 55 months

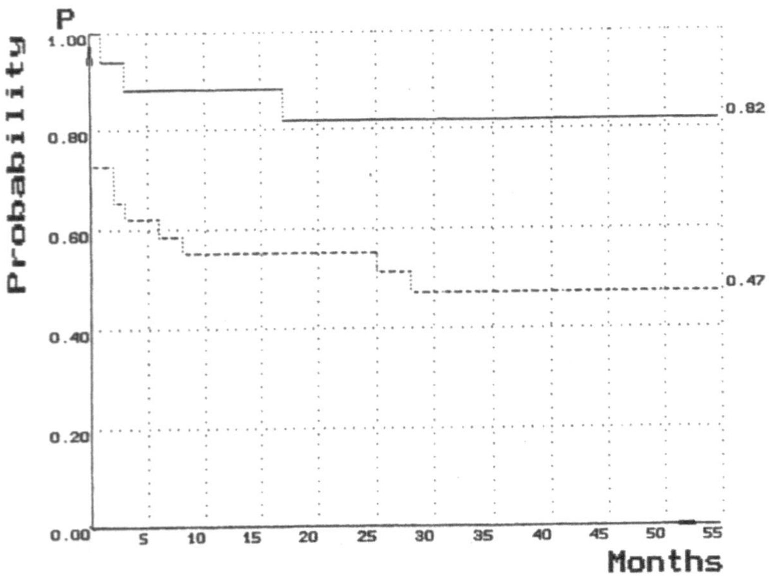

Fig. 5. AML standard risk (*solid line*); AML high risk (*broken line*)

of all, our analysis represents only interim results of treatment of a small group of patients with relatively short follow up and naturally the survival curves will be affected by inevitable adverse events. Secondly, being a large tertiary medical center, we probably do not deal with children at a very high risk of early treatment failure due to the impossibility of transferring them from local hospitals in our vast country. On the other hand, with such intensive therapeutic regimen as BFM-AML protocols, most relapses (up to 75%–90%) occur during first 2 years after the start of treatment. Thus we do not expect an excess of disease recurrences in our group of patients. Besides, children with adverse prognostic features cleary predominated in our group and therefore this cohort was probably balanced from the point of view of risk of treatment failure. The BFM-AML protocol represents one of the most successful attempts at "total therapy" of leukemia. However, it is still unclear what the main factors are in achieving such good results. Moreover, several therapy components are not widely used in the majority of modern protocols. First, the universal use of cranial gamma-irradiation [4]—given the high cure rate, it is expected that many survivors will suffer from some side effects of irradiation, including secondary tumors. Furthermore, it is unknown whether patients receiving such intensive chemotherapy really need any maintenance, which is simple and well tolerated but does not make treatment cheaper [5, 6]. Finally, there are some doubts about the rationality of incorporating such agents as vincristine and cyclophosphamide in the treatment of AML. Future trials would certainly answer such questions. Neverthelss, the BFM strategy of treating AML showed high efficacy and, in our opinion, deserves to be widely used until a more successful therapy is created.

Acknowledgments. The technical assistance of T. Churkina is gratefully acknowledged.

References

1. J. Bennett, D. Catovsky, M.T. Daniel et al. Proposed revised criteria for the classification of acute myeloid leukemia. Ann Int Med, 1985;103: 626–629
2. Bennett JM, Catovsky D, Daniel MT et al. Criteria for diagnosis of acute leukemia of megakaryocyte lineage (M7): a report of French-American British Cooperative Group Ann Intern Med 1985;103: 460
3. U. Creutzig, J. Ritter and G. Shellong. Identification of two risk groups in childhood acute myelogeneous leukemia after therapy intensification in study AML-BFM-83 as compared with study AML-BFM-78. Blood, vol.75 N10(May 15), 1990, 1932–1940
4. Cretzig U, Ritter J, Zimmermann and Shellong G. Does cranial irradiation reduce the risk of bone marrow relapse in acute myelogeneous leukemia? Unexpected results of the childhood acute myeloid leukemia study BFM-87. J Clin Oncol 1993, vol 11, N 2, 279–286
5. Preisler H, Davis RB, Krishner J et al. Comparison of three remission induction regimens and two postinduction strategies for the treatment of acute nonlymphocytic leukemia: a cancer and Leukemia Group B study. Blood, 1987, 69, 1441.
6. R.J. Wells, W.G. Woods, I.D. Buckley et al. Treatment of newly diagnosed children and adolescents with acute myeloid leukemia: Childrens Cancer Group study. J. Clin Oncol Vol 12, N 11(November), 1994; 2367-2377.

Acute Leukemias VI
Prognostic Factors
and Treatment Strategies
Büchner et al. (eds)

Down's Syndrome and Megakaryoblastic Leukemia

U. Creutzig[1], J. Ritter[1], C. Niemeyer[2], B. Stollmann-Gibbels[3], M. Zimmermann[1], I. Reinisch[4], and J. Harbott[4]

Abstract. Recent reports estimate an approximately 20-fold higher incidence of leukemia in children with Down's syndrome compared to non-Down's syndrome children and a marked increase of the megakaryoblastic subtype (FAB M7)[1]. Twenty-six of 42 children with Down's syndrome were enrolled in our studies since 1987 were classified as FAB M7 or presented with a preleukemic phase (myelodysplastic syndrome, MDS) with increased megakaryoblasts. All patients were under 3 years (0.4–2.6 median 1.8 years) and generally had a low leukocyte count (1.6–177 median $7.75 \times 10^3/mm^3$) and a low platelet count (4.0–210 median $26.0 \times 10^3/mm^3$). Karyotype abnormalities other than +21c or [t(21;21)c] were found in 11/15 patients, predominantly trisomies (8/15) involving the chromosomes #8 ($n=5$), #21 ($n=2$), #11 ($n=2$), #10, #14, #18, #19, and #22 ($n=1$). Only nine children initially presented with > 30% blasts in the bone marrow (BM). In ten patients diagnosis of M7 leukemia was based on morphology alone, and in 16 patients confirmed by immunophenotyping. A preleukemic phase with thrombocytopenia for at least 2 months was recorded in nine of the 17 patients presenting with a low blast count (≤30%) and myelodysplasia in the BM. Four children had a history of transient neonatal leukemia. Sixteen children were left untreated or received only minimal treatment and subsequently died due to progressing leukemia. In two of the untreated patients, a spontaneous improvement or a stable disease (with retinoids) lasting for several months was observed. Ten patients were treated. Three out of ten had an end-stage disease and received inadequate dosages of therapy and died early. Six of seven children treated according to the AML-BFM protocols including high-dose cytosine arabinoside were in continuous complete remission for 0.2–4.6 years. We conclude that M7 leukemia in Down's syndrome is often preceded by a preleukemic phase with thrombocytopenia. Patients treated according to the AML protocol showed good results. Further studies are warranted to clarify whether Down's syndrome patients with a preleukemic phase of M7 would also benefit from an early and intensive treatment.

Introduction

Recent reports estimate not only an approximately 20-fold higher incidence of leukemia in children with Down's syndrome compared to non-Down children but especially a marked increase (600x) of the megakaryoblastic subtype (French-American-British classification, FAB, M7)[1]. In addition, there are more unusual features of leukemia in children with Down's syndrome. These include (a) the phenomenon of transient myeloproliferation (TMD) in newborns, which normally disappears spontaneously [2], (b) the peak of incidence under 3 years of age [3]; and (c) the occurrence of a preleukemic

[1]University Children's Hospital, Münster, Germany
[2]University Children's Hospital, Freiburg, Germany
[3]University Children's Hospital, Essen, Germany
[4]University Children's Hospital, Gießen, Germany

(myelodysplastic, MDS) phase and difficulties in classifying the leukemia. According to the published literature [1, 4] as well as to our results, these features can be attributed to a high incidence of acute megakaryoblastic leukemia (FAB M7) in children with Down's syndrome.

While outcome in children with Down's syndrome and acute myeloid leukemia (AML) was thought to be poor, in the recent report of the Pediatric Oncology Group high rates of event-free survival with intensive AML treatment were reported [5]

In the present study, clinical, hematological, immunological, and cytogenetic features and outcome of 26 children with Down's syndrome and FAB M7 or a preleukemic phase with megakaryoblasts are described.

Patients and Methods

Between December 1986 and December 1994, 42 children with Down's syndrome were observed as non-protocol patients in the cooperative AML studies Berlin–Frankfurt–Münster (BFM)-87 and -93. Twenty-six of these patients were classified as FAB M7 or MDS/M7 (defined by <30% of megakaryoblasts in the bone marrow, BM). Acute leukemia and MDS were diagnosed according to the FAB criteria [6, 7].

Immunophenotyping was carried out at the central reference laboratory of the AML-BFM studies by W.-D. Ludwig, University Hospital Steglitz, Berlin. BM samples were centrally karyotyped in Gießen by J. Harbott, I. Reinisch, and F. Lampert. Chemotherapy was applied according to the protocols of studies AML-BFM-87[8] or the standard-risk arm of AML-BFM-93, which resembles the therapy of the preceding study but includes only one itensification block with high-dose cytosine arabinoside (ara-C) and etoposide (VP-16) (some patients received only essential parts of the protocol).

Results

Distribution of morphological subtypes in Down's syndrome patients showed a predominance of FAB M7 (including MDS/M7) subtypes, followed by atypical AML with immature and/or erythroid features, whereas typical FAB types (e.g., M1–M4 with positive peroxidase reaction) were only rarely found. Figure 1 compares 42 children with Down's syndrome with the non-Down patients of studies AML-BFM-87 and -93.

Initially, 17 of 26 patients with FAB M7 presented with a blast count ⩽30% and myelodysplasia in the BM. Only nine children showed an acute onset of leukemia with more than > 30% of blasts in the BM and usually a short history of a preceding thrombocytopenia (Tables 1 and 2). Interval from birth to thrombopenia varied between 0 and 30 months. In three children thrombopenia was already present at birth. Time of the MDS phase as confirmed by BM puncture until progressive disease with >30%

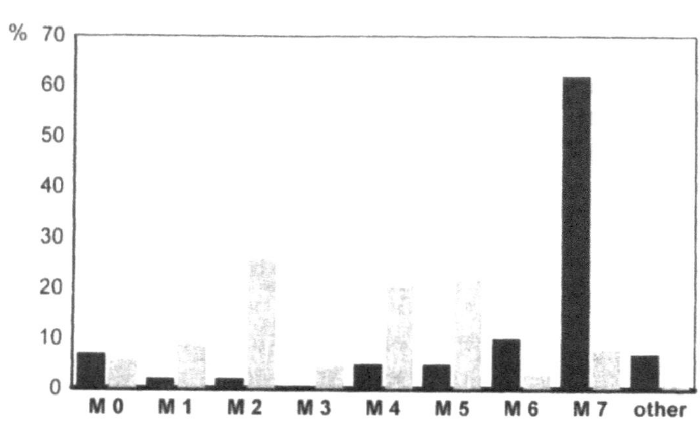

Fig. 1. Distribution of FAB types in children with Down's syndrome compared to non-Down patients of studies AML-BFM-87 and -93. *Dark columns*, Down's syndrome patients, $n=43$. *Light columns*, protocol patients, $n=478$

Table 1. Down's syndrome — FAB M7 — initial patient data

Patient no.	Age Gender (years)	WBC (mm³)	Blasts peripheral (%)	Platelets (mm³)	Hb (g/dl)	Blasts BM (%)	Biopsy data	Lineage-specific antigens	Karyotype	Diagnosis
Study AML-BFM-87										
1	1.5 f	9300	20	27000	11.3	20		n.d.	n.d.	MDS / M7
2	1.9 m	9700	2	87000	3.9	8 (− > 31)	Fibrosis/MPP	CD41/CD61	49,XY,+11,t(11;14)(p13;q117), +14,+21c	MDS / M7
3	1.7 f	5600	11	28000	6.0	10		CD41	n.d.	MDS / M7
4	0.4 f	7100	2	75000	9.9	8	Dysmegakaryopoesis	n.d.	47,XX,+21c	MDS / M7
5	1.0 f	6400	3	30000	7.9	45		n.d.	n.d.	M7
6	1.3 m	14300	10	4000	9.4	6		CD41 (16%)	47,XY, der(5)t(1;5)(q31;p14),+21c/, 47,XY,der(5)t(1;5)(q31;p14),	MDS / M7
7	2.7 m	9800	8	32000	11.8	24		n.d.	i(7)(q10),+21c,47,XY,+8,+21c	MDS / M7
8	0.9 m	57500	67	112000	11.2	56		CD41 (19%)	n.d.	M7
9	2.2 f	1600	6	15000	7.5	30		n.d.	48,XX,+8,+21c	(MDS) / M7
10	2.0 f	6800		44000	7.5	n.d.	MMP	CD61	n.d.	MDS /M7
11	2.4 m	4200	10	7000	5.4	90		CD41	48,XY,der(2)t(1;2)(q25;q37), +11,+21c	M7
12	1.4 f	3600	10	10000	7.5	25	Fibrosis/MMP	CD41 (15%);CDw42(28%) CD61 (24%)	47,XX,del(10)(q22),+21c	MDS / M7
13	1.7 m	177000	90	51000	3.0	91		CD41 (75%)	48,XY,+21,+21c	M7
14	2.0 m	9880	14	29000	14.6	54	No fibrosis	CD41 (25%)	48,XY,del(5)(p13),+8,+21c	M7
15	1.3 m	2800	0	18000	6.6	n.d.	Fibrosis/MMP		47,XY,+21c	MDS / M7
16	2.7 f	4700	22	2200	6.3	25		n.d.	49,X,t(X;13)(q11;p11),dup(1) (q25q43),+8,+10,+21c/49, idem,del(9)(p22)	MDS / M6 / M7
Study AML-BFM-93										
17	2.6 f	6000	1	25000	8.0	26	Fibrosis	CD61	n.d.	MDS / M7
18	2.3 f	3100	48	12000	5.6	60	Fibrosis	CD41/42, CD61	n.d.	M7
19	1.9 m	12800	10	45000	12	19		CD61	47,XY,+21c	MDS / M7
20	1.5 f	31500	22	210000	6	14		n.d.	n.d.	MDS / M7?
21	2.3 f	15500	11	12000	7	61		CD41/61	52,XX,+18,+19,+21,+22,+mar1 -3(cp11),+21c	M7
22	2.4 m	5400	5	8000	5	17		CD41	n.d.	MDS / M7
23	1.7 f	3500	6	20000	9	5		n.d.	48,XX,dup(1)(p32p36),+8, der(19)t(1;19)-(q23;p13),+21c	MDS / M7
24	2.1 m	4300	2	36000	11.1	13		(MPO-7)	n.d.	MDS / M7?
25	1.6 m	21000		8000	5	70		n.d.	n.d.	M0/M7?
26	1.9 f	8400	53	7000	9	35		CD61	46,XX,der(21)t(21;21)q10;q10)c	M7

MMP, megakaryocytic myeloproliferation; n.d., no data.

Table 2. Down's syndrome — FAB M7 — course of the disease

Patient No.	Age Gender (years)	Duration of thrombopenia before diagnosis	Therapy	Outcome	
				Survival (years)	Cause of death
Study AML-BFM-87					
1	1.5 f	Since birth	No chemotherapy	0.2	Progress, pneumonia
2	1.9 m	—	No chemotherapy, spontaneous remission (2x) (9 months + 13 months), chemotherapy after second relapse	2.8	Progress, bleeding
3	1.7 f	—	(6-TG, 40 mg)	0.6	Progress (94% blasts)
4	0.4 f	Since birth	No chemotherapy	1.2	Progress, bleeding (60% blasts)
5	1.0 f	3 months	(Retinoids)	1.2	Cardiac failure (vitium cordis); no progress of leukemia
6	1.3 m	2 months	6-TG	0.1	Progress
7	2.7 m	3 months	No chemotherapy	12 days	Progress
8	0.9 m	n.d.	No chemotherapy	0.1	Progress, sepsis, ileus
9	2.2 f	Prolonged progress	No chemotherapy	0.6	Progress
10	2.0 f	—	No chemotherapy	0.2	Progress, cardiac failure
11	2.4 m	—	AML-BFM-87	4.6+	—
12	1.4 f	10 months	ADE induction (therapy delayed)	10 days	Early death, cerebral bleeding
13	1.7 m		AML-BFM-87	1.9+	—
14	2.0 m	12 months	(Therapy delayed), consolidation, 1/3 dosage	1.3	Death in partial remission, sepsis, cardiac failure (vitium cordis)
15	1.3 m	15 months	No chemotherapy	1.3	Progress
16	2.7 f	1 month	Delayed minimal chemotherapy	0.4	Progress
Study AML-BFM-93					
17	2.6 f	Since 10 months	AML-BFM-93	1.2	Relapse after 7 months
18	2.3 f	TMD after birth, 3 months MDS	Consolidation (3 weeks)	0.1	Cerebral bleeding after i.t.ara-C
19	1.9 m	Since 5 weeks	No chemotherapy	0.1	Cardiac failure (vitium cordis)
20	1.5 f	(6 weeks)	AML-BFM-93	0.9+	—
21	2.3 f	(1 week)	AML-BFM-93	0.8+	—
22	2.4 m	(1 week)	AML-BFM-93	0.8+	—
23	1.7 f	Since birth	No chemotherapy	0.2	Progress
24	2.1 m	n.d.	No chemotherapy	0.3	Bleeding
25	1.6 m	Since birth	(TG/ara-C)	0.3	Progress
26	1.9 f	2 months	AML-BFM-93	0.2+	

TG/ara-C, thioguanine/cytosine arabinoside; TMD, transient myeloproliferative disease; n.d. = no data.

blasts in the BM varied from a few days to 15 months (patient, No. 15).

Owing to the low blast count in the BM, immunophenotyping of these blasts was not always predicative. In 16 patients, diagnosis of M7 was confirmed by expression of megakaryocytic associated antigens (CD41, CD42, CD61). In 12 of 14 patients at least one or two of three panmyeloid antigens (CD13, CD33, or CDw65) were expressed, and in nine of ten patients a coexpression of the T cell-associated antigen CD7 was observed.

Cytogenetic results could be obtained in 15 of 26 children. Fourteen of them showed a trisomy of chromosome 21 (+21c), whereas in one girl a Robertsonian translocation was found [t(21;21)c]. In addition to these constitutional aberrations, other acquired chromosomal abnormalities could be detected in 11 children. In the majority of patients (eight of 15), trisomies were found involving chromosomes #8 ($n=5$), #21 ($n=2$), #11 ($n=2$), #10, #14, #18, #19, and #22 ($n=1$).

Structural aberrations occurred in eight patients, leading to an ubalanced karyotype in seven, including three translocations, one duplication [dup(1q)], one isochromosome [i(7q)], and three deletions [del(5p), del(9p), del(10q)]. Except for the deletions, all abnormalities caused a partial trisomy either of long parts of chromosome #lq (Fig. 2) or the long arm of #7.

Outcome. Sixteen children did not receive any or only minimal treatment (Table 2). Twelve of them died subsequently within 12 days to 6 months. In three patients, duration until progressive disease was > 12 months, including one child with spontaneous improvement. Another patient who died from cardiac failure had a stable disease for several months under retinoid treatment. Ten children were treated according to the AML-BFM protocols. Three children with delayed onset and reduced dosages of chemotherapy died early. Six of the seven children receiving the protocol treatment, including high-dose ara-C were in continuous complete remission for 0.2 to 4.6 years. One child relapsed after 7 months.

Discussion

According to our results and those of Zipursky et al. [1], acute megakaryoblastic leukemia (FAB M7 or MDS/M7) is the predominant leukemic subtype in children with Down's syndrome. Compared to non-Down's syndrome patients with FAB M7 the following distinctive features could be found:

1. The occurrence of a preleukemic phase with abnormal megakaryopoesis (MDS/M7)
2. Differences in the morphology with dyserythropoetic features or atypical erythroblasts
3. Coexpression of the immunologic marker CD7
4. Numeric aberrations, trisomies in additional to +21c, but not the specific aberrations found in non-Down patients with M7

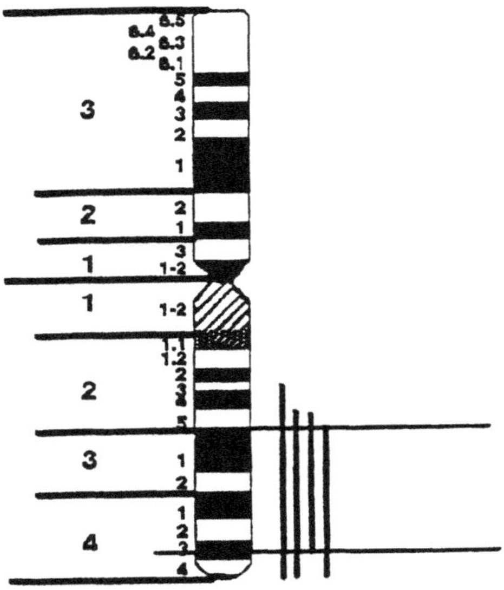

Fig. 2. Consensus region of chromosome 1 in four patients with Down's syndrome and partial trisomy 1

The description of a preleukemic phase of children with Down's syndrome and FAB M7 varied in the literature, probably due to the fact that this phase was usually asymptomatic or characterized only by thrombocytopenia. Furthermore, the duration of MDS before progression to FAB M7 with more than 30% blasts was unknown [1]. To our knowledge, this is the first report indicating that the preleukemic phase varies between 0 and 30 months, and that at least in three children thrombopenia had already been present at birth. In our series, the time of the MDS phase (confirmed by BM puncture) varied from several days to 15 months (median 3 months). According to case reports in the literature, progression to leukemia occurred within 6 or 11 months in two patients [1] or within 8-22 months in four [9] and two patients [10], respectively.

Differences in morphology and immunophenotyping in children with Down's syndrome compared to non-Down patients have been reported by Slordahl et al. [11], suggesting that acute megakaryoblastic leukemia in Down's syndrome is a mixed lineage leukemia with blasts presenting with cell surface antigens of the myeloid, lymphoid, and erythroid cells and therefore indicating the origin from an early progenitor cell with the capability of megakaryocytic differentiation. In our series, the most striking difference compared to non-Down patients with FAB M7 was the coexpression of the lymphoid marker CD7.

Similarly to these findings, karyotyping revealed that mainly trisomies in addition to +21c were seen but not the specific aberration t(1;22) which was found in non-Down infants with FAB M7 [12, 13]. The major difference, however, between FAB M7 and children with Down's syndrome compared to that in non-Down's syndrome children is a higher cure rate which was reported at least in some of these patients [1, 5], in contract to the poor response rate and low survival rate in non-Down children with FAB M7. Only four of 17 children treated according to study AML-BFM-87 were alive after 2 years (own results).

As so far mainly patients at the onset of acute leukemia have been treated with intensive chemotherapy and most of the children with Down's syndrome and MDS/M7 remained untreated or received only minimal chemotherapy, prognosis in these patients remains unclear. Depending on the time of the diagnositc BM puncture, the interval from diagnosis until progression varied from several days to more than year, and quite often, therapy was suspended due to the uncertain diagnosis. Another reason for retaining an AML-specific therapy was a well-known clinical and laboratory finding indicating deficiencies in humoral and cellular immunity in Down's syndrome, thus leading to a lower tolerance of intensive chemotherapy and a higher mortality rate from infections. Therefore, further studies are warranted to clarify whether children with Down's syndrome and a preleukemic phase of M7 could benefit from an early and adequate treatment.

In conclusion, acute megakaryoblastic leukemia is the predominant disorder in children with Down's syndrome. It is an unique disease occurring during the first 3 years of life with a preluekemic phase with abnormal megakaryopoesis and often with dyserythropoesis. Immunological features and chromosomal aberrations were different from those found in non-Down patients with M7. It is suggested therefore that chromosome 21 is involved in the development of the leukemic process in these patients.

Acknowledgments. We thank Elisabeth Kurzknabe und Petra Stappert for their excellent technical assistance and Christa Lausch for her valuable help in the management of the AML studies and the preparation of the manuscript.

References

1. Zipursky A, Thorner P, De Harven D, Christensen H, Doyle J (1994) Myelodysplasia and acute megakaryoblastic leukemia in Down's syndrome. Leuk Res 18: 163
2. Creutzig U, Ritter J, Vormoor J, Eschenbach C, Dickerhoff R, Burdach S, Scheel-Walter H-G, Kühl J, Schellong: G (1990) Transiente Myeloproliferation und akute myeloische Leukämie bei Säuglingen mit Morbus Down. Klin Pädiatr 202: 253
3. Robison LL, Nesbit MEJ, Sather HN, Level C, Shahidi N, Kennedy A, Hammond D (1984) Down syndrome and acute leukemia in children: a 10-year retrospective survey from Childrens Cancer Study Group. J Pediatr 105: 235
4. Zipursky A, Peeters M, Poon A (1987) Megakaryoblastic leukemia and Down's syndrome: a review. Pediatr Hematol Oncol 4: 21
5. Ravindranath Y, Abella E, Krischer JP, Wiley J, Inoue S, Harris M, Chauvenet A, Alvarado CS, Dubowy R, Ritchey AK, et al (1992) Acute myeloid leukemia (AML) in Down's syndrome is highly responsive to chemotherapy: experience on Pediatric Oncology Group AML Study 8498. Blood 80: 2210
6. Bennett JM, Catovsky D, Daniel MT, Flandrin G, Galton DAG, Gralnick HR, Sultan C (1985) proposed revised criteria for the classsification of acute meyloid leukemia. Ann Intern Med 103: 626
7. Bennett JM, Catovsky D, Daniel MT, Flandrin G, Galton DAG, Gralnick HR, Sultan C (1985) Criteria for the diagnosis of acute leukemia of megakaryocyte lineage (M7). A report of the French-American-British Cooperative Group. Ann Intern Med 103: 460
8. Creutzig U, Ritter J, Zimmermann M, Schellong G, for the AML-BFM Study Group (1993) Does cranial irradiation reduce the risk for bone marrow relapse in acute myelogenous leukemia (AML): unexpected results of the childhood AML study BFM-87. J Clin Oncol 11: 279

9. Broomhead A, Kwanyl F, Zell NA, Lamm-Po-Tan PR, O'Gorman HD (1985) Acute leukemia characterized by trisomy 8 in Down's syndrome. Psychology 17: 111 (Abstract)
10. Kaneko Y, Rowley JD, Variakojis D, Chilcote RR, Moohr JW, Patel D (1981) Chromosome abnormalities in Down's syndrome patients with acute leukemia. Blood 58: 459
11. Slordahl SH, Smeland EB, Holte H, Gronn M, Lie SO, Seip M (1993) Leukemic blasts with markers of four cell lineages in Down's syndrome ("megakaryoblastic leukemia"). Med Pediatr Oncol 21: 254
12. Carroll A, Civin C, Schneider N, Dahl G, Pappo A, Bowman P, Emami A, Gross S, Alvarado C, Phillips C, Krischer J, Crist WM, Head D, Gresik M, Ravindranath Y, Weinstein H (1991) The t(1;22)(p13; q13) is nonrandom and restricted to infants with acute megakaryoblastic leukemia: a Pediatric Oncology Group study. Blood 78: 748
13. Lion T, Haas OA, Harbott J, Bannier E, Ritterbach J, Jankovic M, Fink FM, Stojimirovic A, Herrmann J, Riehm HJ, Lampert F, Ritter J, Koch H, Gadner H (1992) The translocation t(1;22)(p13; q13) is a nonrandom marker specifically associated with acute megakaryocytic leukemia in young children. Blood 79: 3325

AML in Adults

Acute Leukemias VI
Prognostic Factors
and Treatment Strategies
Büchner et al. (eds)

Therapeutic and Prognostic Factors in the Management of Acute Myeloid Leukemia

T. Büchner, W. Hiddemann, B. Wörmann, H. Löffler, W. Gassmann, T. Haferlach, J. Goasguen, C. Fonatsch, R. Becher, D. Hossfeld, E. Lengfelder, W.-D. Ludwig, G. Maschmeyer, G. Innig, H.-C. Aul, A. Heyll, B. Lathan, R. Staib, K.-P. Hellriegel, H.-H. Fülle, A. Heinecke and M.C. Sauerland for the AML Cooperative Group

Abstract. The AML Cooperative Group in Germany studied the role of different intensities of induction therapy, all followed by similar postremission treatment. Of the 1034 patients of age 16–83 years. 33% were over age 60, 63% attained a complete remission, and the overall relapse-free surivival rate was 30% after 5 years. A significantly higher disease-free survival was predicted by: M3 morphology, a favorable karyotype including t(8;21), t(15;17), and inv(16); and the absence of dysmyelopoiesis. In contrast, dysmyelopoiesis; high serum lactic dehydrogenase; age over 64; and unfavorable karyotype, including abnormalities of chromosomes 5 or 7 and complex abnormalities all predicted a low relapse-free survival rate. No comparable impact on relapse-free survival was found from the two randomized different intensities of induction treatment in each age-group. Age, LDH, M3, and karyotype contributed to a prognostic index that identified good, intermediate, and poor prognostic groups. Patients older than age 60 showed significantly less frequently favorable and more frequently unfavorable karyotypes and received generally less-intensive induction treatment than younger patients did. We conclude from these results that, unlike some biologic disease characteristics, treatment variables are weak prognostic factors and high age per se may not be an independent factor of relapse-free survival.

Large controlled trials can act as important instruments to identify prognostic factors that determine the outcome of patients. On the basis of standardized diagnostic criteria and unbiased randomized treatment assignment, those prognostic factors can reflect the biology of the individual disease, which may have more impact on the effect of treatment than the actual treatment variables have.

In their 1986 trial, the AML Cooperative Group in Germany addressed questions about the role of different intensities of induction therapy, all of which were followed by similar postremission treatment. Since randomization was done before any treatment, there were no treatment-related exclusions, thus providing true intent-to-treat conditions. A total of 1034 patients from 60 centers throughout Germany entered the trial. Patients were randomized in two age groups: Those over age 60 were assigned to either standard-dose TAD (6-thioguanine, ara-C, and daunorubicin) chemotherapy or a reduced-dose regimen using daunorubicin at 30 mg/m^2 instead of 60 mg/m^2. Those aged 60 and younger were randomized between either standard-dose TAD followed by a second induction course of TAD or high-dose ara-C and mitoxantrone (HAM). All the younger patients received a second course of induction therapy; the older patients received a second induction course if required.

Sixty-three percent of the patients achieved a complete response. There were some differences in response in favor of the TAD-HAM sequence and full-dose TAD in the older patients. Once the patients were in remission, they all received TAD consolidation and monthly myelosuppressive maintenance treatment of reduced TAD courses for a total of 3 years. The 5-year, continuous relapse-free survival rate was 30% for the entire population of patients. There were no sig-

University of Münster, Germany

nificant differences between the randomized arms.

On the surface, the data in this study appear to show that age was the strongest prognostic factor. However, the study had an age-adjusted design, where the older patients received less treatment. Even in studies with a non-age-adjusted design, the elderly patients received less chemotherapy [1]. However, AML itself has biologic differences in younger and older patients. This can be seen in the chromosome abnormalities in these two age groups. Older patients almost never have the so-called favorable abnormalities, but the so-called unfavorable abnormalities occur three times as often in older as in younger patients. Karyotypes were very strong prognostic factors in this trial, making it possible to distinguish three clear prognostic groups: favorable, unfavorable, and an intermediate group that included both patients with normal or other abnorml karyotypes and patients in whom there was no karyotype available. Also noteworthy is that the favorable and unfavorable karyotypes were found in only 17% and 12%, respectively, on the entire population with karyotype available, meaning that the vast majority of patients cannot be classified by karyotype yet.

Table 1. Therapeutic and prognostic factors according to 5-year disease free survival

Factor	Probability of disease-free survival	*p*-value
M3 morphology	52%	0.0028
Favorable karyotype	43%	0.0004
Absence of dysmyelopoiesis (patients age < 60 years)	43%	0.0015
High dose induction (patients under age 60 years)	34%	n.s
Average patients	30%	
Standard dose induction (patients under age 60 years)	27%	n.s.
Dysmyelopoiesis	23%	0.015
Full dose induction (patients over age 60 years)	22%	n.s.
High LDH	20%	0.0002
Age over 64 years	18%	0.0001
Unfavorable karyotype	18%	0.0004
Reduced dose induction (patients over age 60 years)	17%	n.s.

LDH, lactic dehydrogenase.

The favorable karyotype, as shown previously by other studies and confirmed here, includes the translocation 15;17 and 8;21 and inversion 16 [2–6]. The unfavorable karyotype includes the abnormalities of chromosomes 5 or 7, the so-called complex abnormalities, and translocations involving 11q23 [2, 6, 7], although the data about their prognostic significance are conflicting.

In addition to the genotype identified by chromosome and molecular analyses, morphology also reflects some genotypes. For example, the M3 subtype [8–11], according to the French–American–British (FAB) classification, was predictive of a 5-year relapse-free survival rate significantly above the mean for the entire population. As shown by several groups [5, 8, 11], another morphologic entity that appears to reflect a favorable genotype in the M4Eo subtype in our study. However, there was no examination of eosinophils when the trial started so this is still under evaluation.

Another morphologic feature that may also reflect genotypes in AML is myelodysplasia. In particular trilineage dysplasia was found to predict a poor prognosis [12, 13]. There were almost no long-term remissions in this group.

In addition to parameters reflecting a genotype of the leukemic cells, there are also more functional parameters reflective of leukemic cell growth and cell burden. For example, lactic dehydrogenase (LDH) activity in serum prior to treatment [14, 15] was found to be the second strongest prognostic factor after age. Other adverse prognostic factors that have been identified are autonomous growth of colonies of leukemic cells without the addition of growth factors [16] and persistence of minimal residual disease [17–19]. Interestingly, the type of therapy was not found to be a prognostic factor.

All prognostic factors identified and their significance by univariate analysis are listed in Table 1.

According to a multivariate CART analysis [20] the hierarchy of prognostic factors, from highest to lowest, is as follows: (1) age, younger or older than 64 years; (2) LDH in both age groups; (3) in patients with a low LDH, presence of M3 morphology; and (4) favorable karyotypes. In younger patients with a high LDH, however, a higher platelet count was found to be indicative of a worse prognosis. The factors predictive of longer and shorter relapse-free survival are shown in Table 1.

In conclusion, unlike some biologic disease characteristics, treatment variables appear to be weak prognostic factors, and high age per se may not be an independent factor. Future trials will be challenged to complete this prognostic model in order to identify additional good-risk and poor-risk patients who remain hidden in the intermediate-risk group. Such information on karyotypes, morphology, dysplasia, and residual disease will help in the design of therapeutic strategies that treat patients according to their individual risk.

References

1. Mayer RJ, Davis RB, Schiffer CA et al.: Intensive postremission chemotherapy in adults with acute myeloid leukemia. N Engl J Med 6 (1994) 896–942
2. Fourth International Workshop on Chromosomes in Leukemia. Cancer Genet Cytogenet 11 (1984) 332–350
3. Arthur DC, Bloomfield CD: Partial deletion of the long arm of chromosome 16 and bone marrow eosinophilia in acute nonlymphocytic leukemia: a new association. Blood 61 (1983): 944–998
4. Le Beau MM, Larson RA, Bitter MA et al.: Association of an inversion of chromosome 16 with abnormal marrow eosinophils in acute myelomonocytic leukemia. N Engl J Med 309 (1983) 630–636
5. Larson RA, Williams SF, LeBeau MM, Bitter MA et al.: Acute myelomonocytic leukemia with abnormal eosinophils and inv(16) or t(16;16) has a favorable prognosis. Blood 68 (1986) 1242–1249
6. Berger R, Bernheim A, Ochoa-Noguera ME et al.: Prognostic significance of chromosomal abnormalities in acute nonlymphocytic leukemia: a study of 343 patients. Cancer Genet Cytogenet 28 (1987) 293–299
7. Yunis JJ, Brunning RD, Howe RB et al.: High-resolution chromosomes as an independent prognostic indicator in adult acute nonlymphocytic leukemia. N Engl J Med 311 (1984) 812–818
8. Schiffer CA, Lee EJ, Tomiyasu T et al.: Prognostic impact of cytogenetic abnormalities in patients with de novo acute nonlymphocytic leukemia. Blood 73 (1989) 263–270
9. Cunnigham I, Gee TS, Reich LM et al.: Acute promyelocytic leukaemia: treatment results during a decade at Memorial Hospital. Blood 73 (1989) 1116–1122
10. Bennett JM, Begg CB: Eastern Cooperative Oncology Group Study of the cytochemistry of adult acute myeloid leukaemia by correlation of subtypes with response and survival. Cancer Research 41 (1981) 4833–4837
11. Löffler H, Gassmann W, Jürgensen CH et al.: Clinical aspects of acute myelogenous leukaemias of the FAB-types M3 and M4Eo. Ann Hematol 36 (1994) 639–644
12. Estienne MH, Fenaux P, Preudhomme C et al.: Prognostic value of dysmyelopoietic features in de novo acute myeloid leukaemia: a report on 132 patients. Clin lab Haemat 12 (1990) 57–65
13. Kuriyama K, Tomonaga M, Matsuo T et al.: Poor response to intensive chemotherapy in de novo acute myeloid leukaemia with trilineage myelodysplasia. Br J Haematol 86 (1994) 767–773
14. Keating MJ, Smith TL, Kantarjian H et al.: Cytogenetic pattern in acute myelogenous leukemia: a major reproducible determinant of outcome. Leukaemia 2 (1988) 403–412
15. Büchner T, Hiddemann W, Wörmann B et al.: Factors determining therapeutic outcome in patients with AML. Blood 82 (suppl 1) (1993) 192a
16 .Löwenberg B, Putten WLJ, Touw IP et al.: Autonomous proliferation of leukemic cells in vitro as a determinant of prognosis in adult acute myeloid leukemia. N Engl J Med 328 (1993) 614–619
17. Reading CL, Estey EH, Huh YO et al.: Expression of unusual immunophenotype combinations in acute myelogenous leukaemia. Blood 11 (1993) 3083–3090
18. Wörmann B: Implications of detection of minimal residual disease. Curr Opin Oncol 5 (1993) 3–12
19. Wörmann B, Safford M, Koenemann S et al.: Prospective study on the clinical relevance of residual disease in patients with acute myeloid leukemia in complete remission. Hematology and Blood Transfusion 36 (1994) 675–680
20. Heinecke A, Sauerland M-C, Büchner Th for the AML Cooperative Group: Methods to detect prognostic factors in AML

Acute Leukemias VI
Prognostic Factors
and Treatment Strategies
Büchner et al. (eds)

Prognostic Factor Analyses in Acute Myeloid Leukemia: M.D. Anderson Experience

E. Estey, P. Thall, S. Kornblau, M. Andreeff, and M. Keating

Prognostic factor analyses in acute myeloid leukemia (AML) or other diseases serve at least two general purposes. First, they allow comparisons between a recently treated group and a previously treated group to be more accurate. Even in randomized trials that enroll fewer than 100–150 patients, comparison of prognostic characteristics in the various groups (covariate adjusting) is important. Second, prognostic factor analysis can identify patients who are highly unlikely to benefit from standard therapies and hence are candidates for experimental therapies.

At the M.D. Anderson Cancer Center prognostic factor anlayses have been undertaken for the last 15 years for the purposes described above. These analyses have been multivariate, i.e., the effects of different characteristics have been examined in relation to each other. For example, cytogenetics, antecedent hematologic disorder (AHD), bilirubin, age, fibrinogen, hemaglobin, and blood urea nitrogen (BUN) were each found to be independent predictors of complete remission (CR) [1], while performance status. bilirubin, age, neutrophil count, fibrinogen, albumin, hemaglobin, and creatinine were each found to be independent predictors of survival 28 days after start of chemotherapy [2]. These predictive "models" were based on patients who received more or less conventional regimens (ADOAP, AMSAOAP). Application of the models to a group of patients receiving an experimental therapy were used to derive, for example, an *expected* CR rate of 28-day survival rate had the patients given the experimental regimen received the standard regimen instead. This expected rate could be compared to the rate *observed* with the experimental therapy to produce an "O/E ratio," presumably a measure of the relative efficacy of the experimental and standard regimens. One problem with the O/E ratio is that it is difficult to provide a confidence limit about the ratio as the statistical variation in the expected rate is not accounted for. For this reason, use of prognostic factors to compare treatments is increasingly being done considering the treatments themselves as potential prognostic factors. In this approach patients receiving each of more than two treatments are lumped together, and treatment is considered along with non-treatment-related variables as a candidate to enter a prognostic factor model [3, 4].

Experience has also suggested that prognostic factor analysis can be improved in several ways. For example, consider an attempt to identify patients who remain alive and in initial CR 2 years after first treatment for newly diagnosed AML. After this time the probability of long-term disease-free survival exceeds 50% and so that endpoint can be taken as a measure of potential cure. A total of 879 patients with newly diagnosed AML were treated between 1980 and 1992 and 17% were alive in first CR more than 2 years later. Characteristics associated with this outcome (at $p < 10^{-3}$) are shown in Table 1. By combining several of these characteristics, groups with cure rates of about 40% can be identified (Table 2). However, these groups each

Departments of Hematology and Biomathematics, University of Texas M.D. Anderson Cancer Center, Houston, Texas, USA

Table 1. Characteristics associated with potential cure ($p<.001$)

	Percentage of all patients %	Cured %
Inv 16, t(8; 21), t(15; 17)	17	35
Normal, Insufficient	45	17
Other not -5/-7	24	11
-5/-7	13	4
Age <60 years	61	22
Polymorphonuclear leukocytes <1000	53	21
No AHD	66	20
Performance status <3	87	19

metaphases; or with other karyotypes, the four groups thus defined clearly have very distinct prognoses on day 1 of treatment, in CR, and for the first 9 months of CR. However, after 9 months in CR, the distinctions between them blur. In the meantime new variables measurable only after treatment begin to become important. An example is provided by a recent attempt to identify characteristics associated with achievement of CR on a second course of chemotherapy identical to the first course if the first course was unsuccessful [5]. Table 3 is a 2 × 2 table illustrating course 2 response by whether there were major complications on the first course and whether the patient received standard-dose cytosine arabinoside (ara-C) or high-dose ara-C. Clearly the occurrence of complications on course 1 augers poorly for response to course 2. However, this is statistically notable only in patients receiving high-dose ara-C. In other words, there is an *interaction* between course 1 and high-dose ara-C. Failure to test for such interactions can result in loss of prognostic information.

Table 2. Use of multiple characteristics to predict potential cure

Cytogenetics	Age (years)	Polymorphonuclear leukocytes	AHD	Performance status	Percentage of all patients (%)	Cured (%)
Good	<60	<1000	No	<3	9	41
Good	<60	<1000	No	>2	<1	0
Good	<60	<1000	Yes	<3	1	40
Good	<60	>1000	No	<3	3	39
Good	>59	<1000	No	<3	<1	20
Normal, intermediate	<60	<1000	No	<3	8	27

Table 3. Course 2 response by ara-C dose and course 1 complications

Ara-C dose	Course 1 complications		
	No (*n*)	Yes (*n*)	Total (*n*)
Standard	46/112(.41)	21/69(.3)	67/181(.37)
High	53/98(.54)	22/91(.24)	75/189(.4)
	99/210(.47)	43/160(.27)	142/370(.38)

Numbers in parentheses represent proportions (indices).

include only 1%–3% of all patients, whereas, as noted above, 17% of all patients fit into this potentially cured group.

How more such potentially cured patients can be identified forms the principal topic of this paper. One way is to use information gathered after treatment begins rather than focusing primarily on pre-treatment variables as the latter soon lose their predictive ability. For example, when patients are grouped for analysis by cytogenetics as either inv(16), t(8; 21), or t(15; 17); -5, 5q-, -7, 7q-; with normal or insufficient

Another issue is prognostic factor analysis is the choice of "cutpoints." This is illustrated by a recent analysis of the prognostic signification of CD 7 in newly diagnosed AML. Rather than use the traditional cutpoint of >20% vs. <20%, a systematic search was conducted to see which CD 7 percentage would give the best separation into two groups with different survivals after treatment, i.e., which cutpoint was associated with the lowest p value. This turned out to be >11% or <11%, at which cutpoint the p value was .08. However, because multiple analyses were performed, the p-value has to be adjusted upward as described by Altman et al. [6], in this case to .642. Another approach is to first construct a smoothed martingale residual plot which indicates how far each patient with an individual CD 7 value falls from the average survival. In the case of CD 7, this plot showed a crossing (change) from better to worse survival between a CD 7% percentage of 5%–15%. Searching for the optimal p-value can then be done within the small area where the crossing occurred necessitating less of a p-value adjustment.

A final issue in prognostic factor analyses is that some terms do not enter a model in linear fashion. An example is provided by the relationship between albumin and survival. Here examination of residual plots indicates that the effect of albumin on survival is negative at both low and high albumin levels. Under these circumstances, albumin is said to enter the model as a quadratic rather than a linear term.

In sum, prognostic factor analysis has proceeded a good deal in the last 15 years. We are using treatment itself as a covariate, are more aware of the time-dependent nature of covariates, the need to gather information after treatment begins, the need to account for interactions between covariates, the need to better dichotomize cutpoints and the need to determine if covariates are related in a linear, quadratic, or some other fashion to treatment outcome.

References

1. Keating M, Smith T, Kantarjian H, Cork A, Walters R, Trujillo J, McCredie K, Gehan E, Freireich E (1988) Cytogenetic pattern in AML: a major reproducible determinant of outcome. Leukemia 2: 403–412
2. Estey E, Smith T, Keating M, McCredie K, Gehan E, Freireich E (1989) Prediction of survival during induction therapy in patients with newly diagnosed AML. Leukemia 3: 257–263
3. Estey E, Thall P, Kantarjian H, O'Brien S, Koller C, Beran M, Gutterman J, Deisseroth A, Keating M (1992) Treatment of newly-diagnosed AML with GM-CSF prior to and during continuous-infusion high dose ara-C + daunorubicin: comparison to patients treated without GM-CSF. Blood 79: 2246–2255
4. Estey E, Thall P, Andreeff M, Beran M, Kantarijan H, O'Brien S, Escudier S, Robertson L, Koller C, Kornblau S, Pierce S, Freireich E, Deisseroth A, Keating M (1994) Use of G-CSF before, during, and after fludarabine + ara-C induction therapy of newly-diagnosed AML or MDS: comparison with fludarabine + ara-C without G-CSF. Journal of Clinical Oncology 12: 671–678
5. Ghaddar H, Pierce S, Kantarjian H, Keating M, Freireich E, Estey E (1994) Factors predicting response and disease-free survival after second course of induction chemotherapy in AML patients resistant to the first course Blood 84: 147a(ASH abstract # 574)
6. Altmann D, Lausen B, Sauerbrei W, Schumancher M (1994) Dangers of using optimal cutpoints in the evaluation of prognostic factors. Journal of the National Cancer Institute 86: 829-835

Acute Leukemias VI
Prognostic Factors
and Treatment Strategies
Büchner et al. (eds)

Intensified Therapy of Acute Myeloid Leukemia: Results of the German AML Cooperative Group

W. Hiddemann[1], A. Heinecke[2], and T. Büchner[2] for the German AML Cooperative Group

Introduction

After the major break throughs in the treatment of acute leukemias that occurred in the late 1970s and early 1980s, followed by several years of stagnation, new therapeutic perspectives have recently opened out and a further step forward now seems to be at hand.This progress has been achieved by further intenstification of AML therapy during both induction and postremission treatment, which has become feasible owing to several recent developments. These include the introduction of hematopoietic growth factors into AML therapy [1–3], improved management of infectious complications, and a better understanding of the pharmacokinetics and mechanisms of action of major antileukemic agents, cytosine arabinoside (AraC) in particular.

First studies with high-dose AraC in high-risk patients and patients with recurrent on refractory disease yielded promising results and prompted several groups to also introduce intensified regimens with high-dose AraC into first-line therapy [4–6]. Recently, significant prolongation of remission duration was reported by the CALGB for patients receiveing high-dose AraC during postremission therapy [7]. This approach also appeared beneficial when applied during induction and especially improved the outcome of patients with unfavorable cytogenetics [8, 9].

The concept of intensified treatment was also followed by the German AML Cooperative Group in a sequence of studies that were based on double induction as a new element of AML therapy in patients less than 60 years of age and the assessment of full-dose versus attenuated-dose anthracyclines in the older age goup [10–13].

Patients and Protocols

Double Induction for Patients Less Than 60 Years of Age. Patients under the age of 60 years with newly diagnosed AML were initially randomized to receive double induction therapy with the sequence of either TAT-TAD or TAD-HAM. Patients achieving complete remission all received one further course of TAD for consolidation and 3 years maintenance on alternating cycles of AraC plus daunorubicin, cyclophosphamide, or 6 thioguanine, as previously described in detail [10, 11, 13].

Induction with Full-Dose Versus Half-Dose Daunorubicin for Patients 60 Years of Age and Older. Patients aged 60 years or older with newly diagnosed AML were initially randomized to receive TAD induction therapy with either full-or half dose daunorubicin, i.e., 60 mg/m^2 perday versus 30 mg/m^2 perday, both given on days 3–5. During consolidation the same dose of daunorubicin as initially selected was given. Further postremission therapy was carried out as in younger patients.

Postremission Therapy with Monthly Maintenance Versus Intensified S-HAM Consolidation in Patients Less Than 60 Years of Age. After establishment of TAD-HAM as the standard induction regimen for patients less than 60 years of age, a subsequent study of the AMLCG addressed the question of monthly main-

[1]Department of Hematology, University of Göttingen, Germany
[2]Department of Oncology, University of Münster, Germany

tenance versus intensified S-HAM consolidation. For this purpose patients less than 60 years of age who achieved a complete remission after TAD-HAM induction were randomized to receive TAD consolidation and 3 years monthly maintenance or TAD consolidation followed by one course of S-HAM as second consolidation, only.

Results

Double Induction in Patients Less Than 60 Years of Age. Seven hundred and four patients aged from 16 to 59 years were randomized and evaluable as to response and toxicity. As shown in Table 1, a higher rate of complete remission was obtained with TAD-HAM, although the difference from the TAD-TAD arm was not significant. Most importantly, no increased mortality was encountered during TAD-HAM treatment, and failure from resistant leukemia also appeared to occur less frequently.

While the median remission duration was comparable, a favorable effect of TAD-HAM on long-term remission duration emerged (Fig. 1). At 7 years, continuing remissions were observed in 36 % of patients after induction with TAD-HAM, as compared to 24% after TAD-TAD induction.

A comparison of these results with the preceding AMLCG study in which patients received

Table 1. Results of intensification of AML therapy: double induction in patients less than 60 years of age

	TAD-TAD ($N=347$)		TAD-HAM ($N=357$)		p
	(n)	%	(n)	%	
Hypoplastic death	57	16	46	13	
Persistent leukemia	62	18	54	15	
Complete remission	228	66	257	72	n.s.
Complete remission if day 16 blasts > 40%	12	25	27	46	0.02

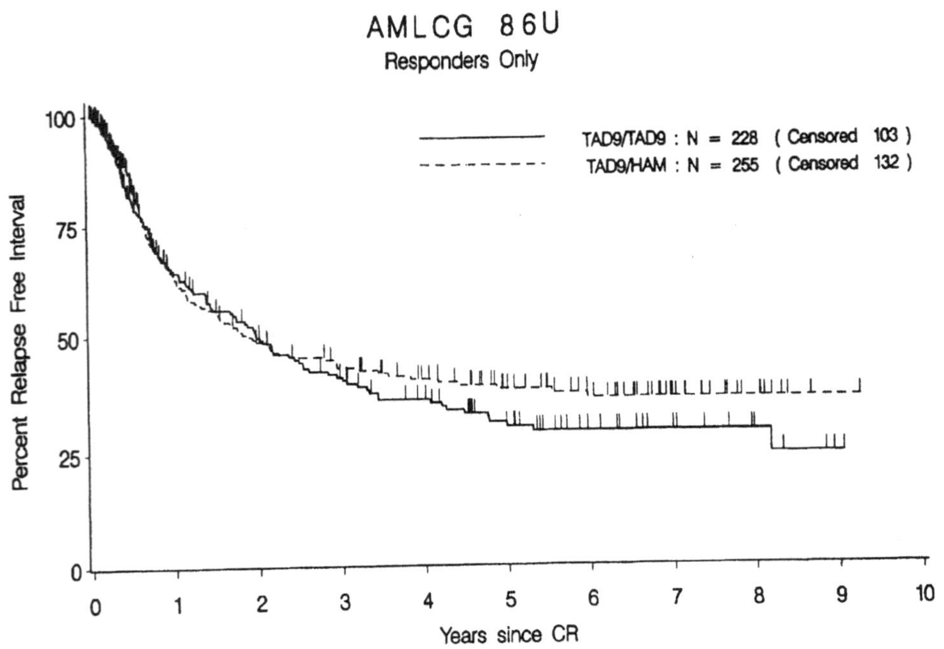

Fig. 1. Duration of remission after double induction therapy with TAD-TAD or TAD-HAM in patients less than 60 years of age

the identical postremission therapy but less intensive induction therapy revealed a significant improvement in of long-lasting remissions (Fig. 2) These data prompted the AMLCG to establish TAD-HAM double as the standard induction therapy during subsequent trials.

Induction with Full-Dose Versus Half-Dose Daunorubicin for Patients 60 Years of Age and Older. Two hundred and three patients aged 60–85 years were randomized and evaluable as to response and toxicity. For the higher dose group, assessment continued after the end of randomization and a further 137 cases were entered on this regimen. Table 2 indicates that a significantly higher rate of complete remission was achieved by full-dose daunorubicin, which was also associated with a lower rate of early deaths and failure from resistant disease. Patients achieving a complete remission experienced a comparable disease-free interval (Fig. 3).

Postremission Therapy with Monthly Maintenance Versus Intensified S-HAM Consolidation in Patients Less Than 60 Years of Age. One hundred and ninety-three patients underwent the TAD-HAM induction and were randomized between the two postremission therapies. One hundred and thirty-two (68 %) obtained complete remission. A preliminary evaluation on an intention-to-treat basis indicates no major differences in remission duration at the current time, suggesting that one course of intensified S-HAM therapy may be as effective as 3 years' monthly maintenance for postremission treatment (Fig. 4).

Table 2. Results of intensification of AML therapy: induction in patients 60 years of age and older

	TAD 60 ($N=237$)		TAD 30 ($N=103$)		P
	n	%	n	%	
Hypoplastic death	48	20	32	31	0.03
Persistent leukemia	59	25	28	27	0.60
Complete remission	130	55	43	42	0.03
Complete remission after one course	91	38	21	20	0.001

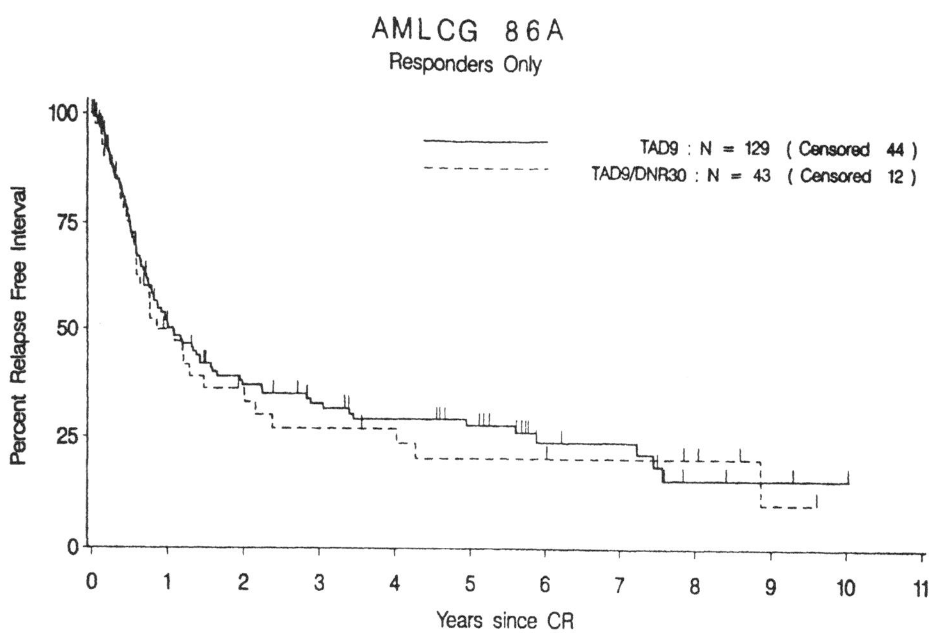

Fig. 2. Duration of remission after full-dose versus half-dose daunorubicin during TAD induction in patients 60 years of age or older

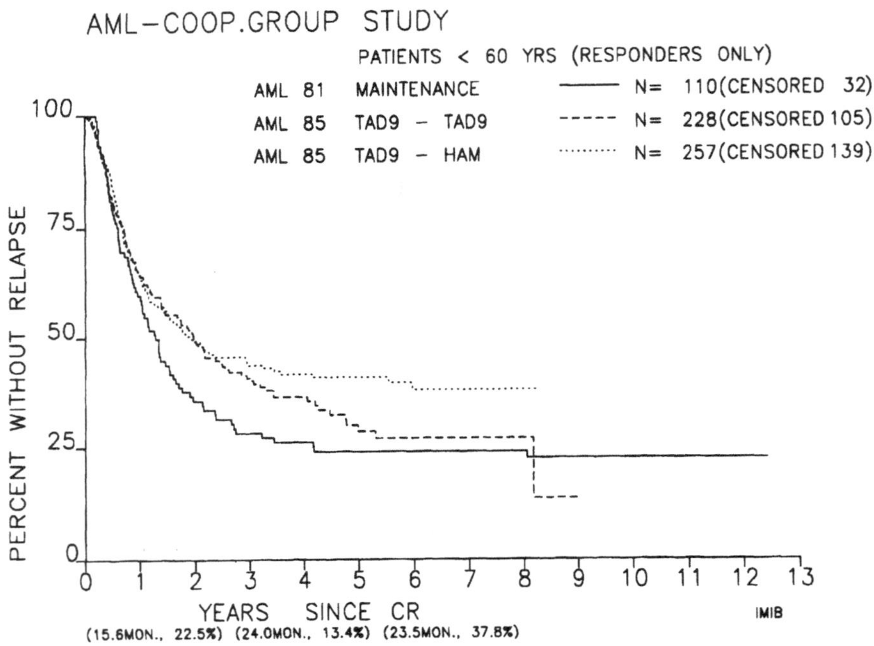

Fig. 3. Duration of remission after double induction and single induction in patients less than 60 years of age

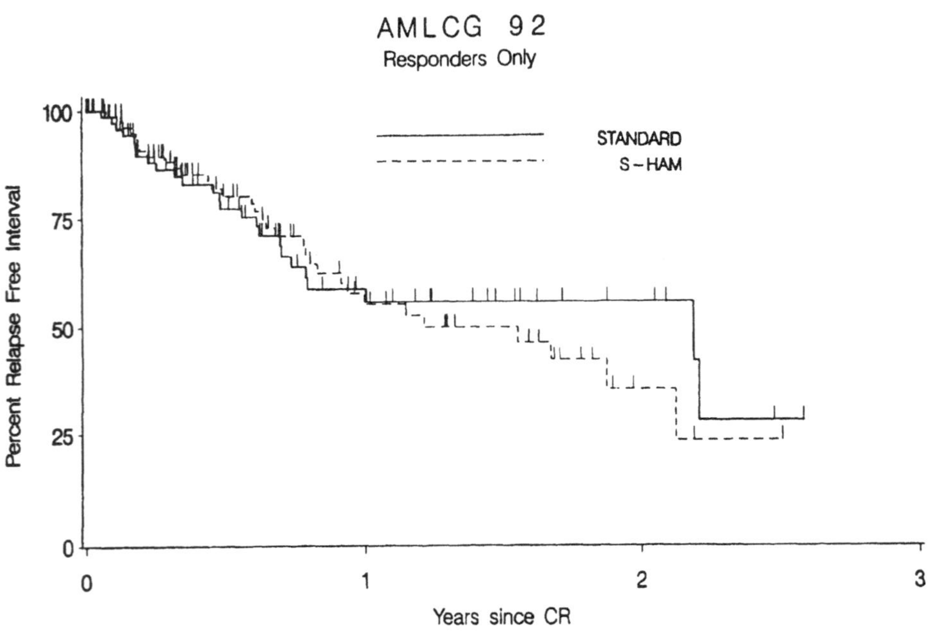

Fig. 4. Duration of remission after TAD-HAM induction and TAD consolidation followed by either monthly maintenance or S-HAM as second consolidation

Discussion

This overview of consecutive prospective studies of the German AML Cooperative Group indicates that a steady improvement of long-term outcome in adults with newly diagnosed AML is achieved by a gradual increase in treatment intensity. The reported data clearly indicate that this conclusion applies both to young and old patients. In both age groups higher remission rates and/or an improved duration of remission are achieved by intensified treatment. Remarkably, this advantage is not burdened with a higher rate of early deaths or toxicity, but on the contrary is associated with a lower frequency of total complications. This beneficial effect most probably results from the fact that a lower proportion of patients, especially in the older age group, require a second induction course for the achievement of complete remission, and thus experience a shorter duration of disease and treatment-associated critical cytopenia.

Independent of this effect, the results of double induction in younger patients exphasize the importance of initial intensification for the long-term outcome. This approach may be of varying relevance in different cytogenetic subgroups. Patients with unfavorable karyotypes appear to benefit more from high-dose AraC. They not only achieved a higher rate of complete remissions, but also experienced a prolongation of remission duration [8, 9]. This finding was also observed when high-dose AraC was administered during postremission treatment, while different effects were noted when the outcome of patients with favorable karyotypes was assessted [9, 14]. These findings emphasize our need to further understand the biology of different cytogenetic subgroups of AML and stimulate research into potential differences in the metabolism and mechanisms of action of AraC in AML.

References

1. Büchner T, Hiddemann W, Koenigsmann M et al. (1991) Recombinant human granulocyte-macrophage colony-stimulating factor following chemotherapy in patients with acute myeloid leukemia at higher age or after relapse. Blood 78: 1190–1197
2. Hiddemann W, Wörmann B, Reuter C et al. (1994) New perspectives in the treatment of acute myeloid leukemia by hematopoietic growth factors. Semin Oncol 21(6): 33–38, 1994.
3. Rowe J, Anderson J, Mazda JJ, et al. (1993) Phase III randomized placebo-controlled study of granulocyte-macrophage colony stimulating factor (GM-CSF) in adult patients (55–70 years) with acute myeloid leukemia (AML). A study of the Eastern Cooperative Oncology Group (ECOG). Blood 10: 1299.
4. Herzig RH, Wolff SN, Lazarus HM et al. (1983) High-dose cytosine arabinoside therapy for refractory leukemia. Blood 62: 361–369.
5. Hiddemann W, Kreutzmann H, Straif K et al. (1987) High-dose cytosine arabinoside and mitoxzantrone: a highly effective regimen in refractory acute myeloid leukemia. Blood 69: 744–749
6. Bishop JF, Young GA, Szer J et al. (1992) Randomized trial of high dose cytosine arabinoside (Ara-C) combination in induction in acute myeloid leukemia (AML). Proc ASCO 11: 849, 1992.
7. Mayer RJ, Davis RB, Schiffer CA et al. (1994) Intensive postremission chemotherapy in adults with acute myeloid leukemia. N Engl J Med 331: 896–903.
8. Garson QM, Matthews JP, Bishop JF et al. (1995) Prognostic significance of cytogenetic abnormalities in adult acute myeloid leukemia patients treated with high dose cytarabine. Blood 86 (10): 600a
9. Hiddemann W, Fonatsch C, Wörmann B et al. (1995) Cytogenetic subgroups of AML and outcome from high dose versus conventional dose Ara-C therapy as part of double induction therapy. Blood 86 (10), 267a
10. Büchner T, Hiddemann W, Schaefer UW et al. (1992) Combined effect of very early intensification and prolonged postremission chemotherapy in patients with AML. Leukemia 5: 68–70.
11. Büchner T, Hiddemann W, Löffler H et al. (1994) Double induction strategy in AML comparing high with standard dose Ara-C. Hematoxicity and antileukemic efficacy. Blood 84: 232a,
12. Büchner T, Hiddemann W, Wörmann B et al. (1994) Chemotherapy intensity and long-term outcome in AML. In Büchner T et al (eds). Acute leukemias IV; prognostic factors Springer Berlin Heidelberg pp513–518
13. Büchner T, Hiddemann W, Wörmann B et al. (1996) Hematologic and therapeutic effects of highdose AraC/mitoxantrone (HAM) in the induction treatment of patients with newly diagnosed AML. A trial by AML Cooperative Group. In Hiddemann W et al. (eds). Acute leukemias V; experimental approaches and management of refractory diseases Springer, Berlin Heidelberg, PP 595–598
14. Bloomfield CD, Lawrence D, Arthur DC et al. (1994) Curative impact of intensification with high-dose cytarabine (HiDAC) in acute myeloid leukemia (AML) varies by cytogenetic group. Blood 84 (10): 111a.

Acute Leukemias VI
Prognostic Factors
and Treatment Strategies
Büchner et al. (eds)

Intensified Induction Therapy in Acute Myeloid Leukemia

J.F. Bishop

Abstract. Optimal initial treatment has made a major impact on a number of curable cancers. To study methods to improve outcome in acute myeloid leukemia (AML), the Australian leukemia study group (ALSG) has intensified induction therapy in two consecutive randomized trials. In the first trial, patients were randomized to receive standard daunorubicin 50 mg/m^2 daily × 3 and cytarabine 100 mg/m^2 as a continuous infusion for 7 days (7–3) or 7–3 as above with additional etoposide 75 mg/m^2 daily × 7(7–3 vs. 7–3–7). Of 264 eligible patients the remission duration was significantly longer with 7–3–7. In a subset analysis patients aged <55 years had significantly superior survival on the etoposide arm. In a dose intensity multivariate anlaysis, we have shown that the initial dose of cytarabine and daunorubicin significantly influenced the duration of remission in AML. To test if cyratabine dose escalation in induction could influence outcome, the ALSG randomized 301 eligible de novo patients to either standard-dose cytarabine in the 7–3–7 regimen or to high-dose cytarabine at 3 g/m^2 twice daily on days 1, 3, 5, and 7 with daunorubicin and etoposide as above (7–3–7 vs. HIDAC-3-7). HIDAC-3-7 significantly prolonged remission duration with a median for HIDAC-3-7 of 45 months vs. 12 months for 7–3–7 ($p = 0.0004$). The percentage of patients who were relapse free at 5 years was 31% on HIDAC-3-7 and 25% on 7–3–7. The rate of relapse for HIDAC-3-7 patients was 0.53 relative to 7–3–7 patients and the rate of death was 0.86 relative to 7–3–7 patients. HIDAC-3-7 was associated with significantly more toxicity in induction with more leucopoenia, thrombocytopenia, nausea and vomiting and eye toxicity (all $p < 0.001$). Although both arms received the same post-induction therapy (5–2–5), patients who received HIDAC-3-7 in induction had significantly more myelosuppression. We conclude that intensifying induction therapy wtih etoposide and with high-dose cytarabine can significantly prolong relapse-free survival with increased but acceptable toxicity.

Introduction

Induction chemotherapy for acute myeloid leukemia (AML) has long been the prototype for the intensive chemotherapy, now widely used in the treatment of many cancers[1, 2]. Standard induction chemotherapy results in severe myelosuppression for 14–28 days[3]. This requires prolonged blood product support with red cells and platelets and prolonged use of multiple potent antibiotics. Major advances have been made in platelet transfusion therapy and control of sepsis [4, 5]. However, the successful support of severely myelosuppressed patients frequently produces difficult clinical problems.

It has been over 25 years since cytarabine was first shown to produce long-term survivors in AML [6]. The two drug combination of 7 days of cytarabin and 3 days of daunorubcin (7–3) has been used as standard induction therapy for many years and produced responses in 56%–66% of patients [1–3, 7]. Efforts to improve therapy with the addition of 6-thiogua-

Director, Sydney Cancer Centre, Royal Prince Alfred Hospital, Missenden Road, Camperdown, Sydney NSW 2050, Australia

nine [2, 8], lengthening the duration of cytarabine [2] or substituting daunorubicin [1] or amscrine [9] have not been successful strategies in randomized trials.

Idarubicin is an analogue of daunorubicin selected for its increased activity against leukemia cell lines in vitro. In four randomized studies idarubicin has been compared directly to daunorubicin in induction [10–13]. These studies show a variety of results, either improvement in response rates, response duration or survival were reported at least for younger patients [10–13]. The place of idarubicin compared to daunorubicin in induction is now the subject of an on-going meta-analysis.

Etoposide in Induction Therapy

Etoposide (VP16–213) is a semisynthetic derivative of podophyllotoxin that has been undergoing clinical evaluation since 1971. The in vitro synergism between etoposide and cytarabine in L1210 cells provides a rationale for the use of etoposide in leukemia. Moreover, the mechanism of action of etoposide differs from that of cytarabine and daunorubicin and its dose-limiting toxicity is myelosuppression [14–16]. Etoposide has been studied most extensively in AML

Etoposide has been used as a single agent in a variety of doses and schedules [17–32]. Most of the earlier studies involved heavily pretreated patients, and the dose and schedules used in these highly selected subjects were often suboptimal. Despite this disadvantage, etoposide has clearly demonstrated activity in AML, with 39 complete responses (CR) (17%) reported among the 233 patients treated [33]. Many more achieved demonstrable anti-leukemic effects that fell short of a CR. Two studies of etoposide alone as initial therapy in older patients have demonstrated clinically useful CR [29, 31].

Etoposide has been studied in relapsed and refractory patients in combination with cytarabine, daunorubicin, doxorubicin, aclacinomycin A, mitozantrone, and 5-azacytidine, among others. Amsacrine combinations have used etoposide in total doses of 500 to 630 mg/m^2, usually given as divided doses during 3–5 days. Following etoposide–amsacrine combinations, 28% of the patients achieved remissions of short duration (12–21 weeks) [34–37]. The combination was myelosuppressive, with marrow recovery occurring primarily in patients with CR. Gastrointestinal (GI) toxicity, particularly stomatitis and diarrhoea, was often dose-limiting.

Etoposide plus 5-azacytidine combinations have been studied in 162 patients and an overall CR rate of 49% has been reported [38–42]. The largest experience with this combination involves children, in whom it appears to be an active and tolerable regimen [40–42]. Those who achieved CR were cytopenic for a median of 32 days. Severe nausea and vomiting occurred in 39%, mucositis developed in 39% and was severe in 15% [42].

Etoposide in combination with conventional doses of an anthracycline and mitoxantrone has produced similar results in 146 relapsed or refractory patients, with 51% overall achieving CR[43–48]. Ho et al. [46] developed an active regimen of etoposide (100 mg/m^2 daily for 3 or 5 days) given with mitoxantrone (10 mg/m^2 daily for 5 days). The median duration of CR in that study was 4.7 months. The major toxicity, stomatitis, occurred in 67% but was severe (World Health Organisation, WHO,grade 3) in only 18% Etoposide (100 mg/m^2 once or twice daily for 5 days) has also been given with high-dose cytrabine (2 mg/m^2 during 3 h twice daily for 5 days) [49]. Of 41 patients treated, 63% achieved a CR, with a median response duration of 34 weeks for refractory and 19 weeks for relapsed patients.

Many combination regimens for AML have included etoposide plus cytarabine and either doxorubicin or daunorubicin [44, 45, 50–52]. The dose of etoposide has varied from 60 to 100 mg/m^2 for 5–7 days. Of 218 patients treated with these combinations, 70% achieved CR. These programs were well tolerated in general, but severe stomatitis (WHO Grade 3–4) was seen in 33% of patients who received etoposide at 10 mg/m^2 daily for 7 days [44].

Finally, etoposide has been added to intensify other induction regimens in AML [53, 54]. Although these regimens have yielded high response rates, the remission durations have been average. Kalwinsky et al. (53) reported only 33% of patients relapse free at 2 years.

These regimens have shown a high degree of activity in the phase II studies discussed. However, the specific contribution of etoposide to these multidrug regimens remains unclear.

Baldini et al. [55] compared a standard daunorubicin, cytarabine, and 6-thioguanine (DAT) regimen for four courses with the same chemotherapy alternated with vindesine, cytarabine and etoposide (DAT/VAE) for four courses in 156 patients with untreated AML. The regimens appeared to be equivalent without significant differences in CR rate, relapse-free survival or overall survival. However, the doses of daunorubicin and cytarabine in the alternating arm were only 66% and 80%, respectively, of the doses in the standard DAT arm. Thus, reduced-dose DAT plus VAE was equivalent to full-dose DAT.

The Australian Leukemia Study Group (ALSG) compared standard-dose daunorubicin and cytarabine given for 7 and 3 days (7–3), respectively, with the same drugs at full dose with etoposide added during a 7-day period (7–3–7) in a randomized trial in 264 patients [3, 33]. Etoposide was given at a dose of 75 mg/m^2 for the 7 days (525 mg/m^2 per course and was added to both induction and consolidation treatment. The CR rates were not significantly different, with CR occurring in 56% of 7–3 patients and 59% of 7–3–7 patients. There was, however, a significant prolongation of remission duration in the etoposide arm (median 12 months with the 7–3 regimen compared with 18 months on 7–3–7; log-rank test, $p = 0.01$) although not of overall survival. A hypothesis-testing subset analysis, performed to identify patients who may have received the most benefit from etoposide, indicated that younger patients appeared to benefit most. Patients younger than 55 years of age treated with 7–3–7 has prolonged remission duration (median 12 months with 7–3 vs. 27 months with 7–3–7: $p = 0.04$).

Multiple linear regression analyses of prognostic factors influencing remission duration confirmed the importance of etoposide in significantly influencing remission duration, independently of other factors.

The addition of etoposide was well tolerated overall, with equivalent hematologic toxicity on induction but significantly increased myelosuppression during consolidation therapy. Stomatitis did not increase overall, but in the subset of older patients (55 years of age or older) the incidence of WHO Grade 3 or 4 stomatitis was significantly higher.

It has been suggested that etoposide is most effective in myelomonocytic leukemia [16, 17]. In this trial [3], however, there were 85 patients classified as French–American–British (FAB) M4 or M5 and the benefits of etoposide were not confined to these patients. Neither was there evidence of additional benefits in this FAB subset compared with other subsets.

The 50% increase in median remission duration produced in this trial was a major clinical benefit of these patients. Although subset analysis indicated a significant survival benefit in younger patients, this advantage was short-term at 5 years there were no significant differences insurvival.

Dose and Dose Intensity in AML

It has been suggested that the dose of chemotherapy delivered over a period of time, or the dose intensity (DI), has an important influence on outcome in a number of tumours. Hryniuk et al. [56, 57] have suggested the DI delivered influences response rates and survival in breast and ovarian cancer. Similar correlations may exist between the DI of mustine, vincristine, procarbazine, prednisolone (MOPP) chemotherapy and survival in retrospective analyses of patients with advanced Hodgkin's disease [58, 59]. However, a meta-analysis of the DI of chemotherapy regimens in small cell lung cancer has failed to demonstrate any correlation with outcome[60]. In some of these DI analyses, the protocol dose planned has been used rather than the actual dose delivered although in a smaller number of studies similar correlations have been made with actual dose delivered.

From these data it is unclear whether dose, duration of dosing or the rate of dose delivery (DI) are the most important dose delivery parameters. It is possible that different dose delivery parameters have different effects in different tumours or chemotherapy regimens.

Influence of Dose and DI of Induction and Consolidation Chemotherapy on Relapse Rates in 264 De Novo Patients with AML on the ALSG Etoposide Study [3,61]. Cox proportional hazards regression models were used throughout to identify prognostic factors, including dose delivery paramters, influencing the rate of relapse. Of 152 patients who achieved a CR, 104 relapsed with a median duration of CR of 15.8 months. Actual dose delivered was prospectively documented. Cox regression analysis identified the most significant prognostic factors jointly influencing duration of CR as performance status ($p < 0.0001$), percentage peripheral blood blast count ($P = 0.0015$), 7–3–7 treatment arm ($p = 0.0075$), age < 40 years ($p = 0.022$) and induction-dose cytarabine plus daunorubicin ($p = 0.029$). In this analysis patients randomized to the 7–3–7 arm had an estimated 43% reduction in the relapse rate and each 10% reduction of doses of cytarabine and daunorubicin was associated with an estimated 45% increase in the relapse rate. The number of induction courses, delays in treatment and induction DI did not significantly influence the duration of CR nor did any of the consolidation treatment parameters. In conclusion, the authors suggested that the addition of etoposide and delivery of full induction doses of cytarabine and daunorubicin were the most important treatment parameters influencing the duration of CR. The importance of the dose of cytarabine in remission duration has provided an additional rationale for the use of high-dose cytarabine in induction therapy.

High-Dose Cytarabine Intensification of Induction Therapy

A rationale for using a higher dose of cytarabine is that there appears to be a steep dose response curve for cytarabine in experimental tumour systems [62, 63]. Patients whose myeloblasts formed and retained higher levels of cytarabine 5'-triphosphate had higher CR rates. Thus, high-dose cytarabine could overcome clinical resistance by this and other mechanisms. Early clinical studies in AML suggested that high-dose cytarabine with amsacrine produced high response rates in refractory and heavily pretreated patients [64]. High-dose cytarabine has subsequently been successfully used in a number of combinations in relapsed patients and as post-induction therapy in phase I and II studies [65–67].

In a large ALSG study [68], patients aged 15–60 years, presenting with newly diagnosed AML, were randomised to receive either high-dose cytarabine, 3 g/m^2 every 12 h on days 1, 3, 5 and 7 for eight doses, daunorubicin 50 mg/m^2 on days 1–3, etoposide 75 mg/m^2 on days 1–7 (HIDAC-3-7) or standard-dose cytarabine 100 mg/m^2 continuous intravenous infusion for 7 days with daunorubicin and etoposide at the same dose and schedule as above (7–3–7). Patients could receive a second or third induction course if CR was not achieved. All patients received the same post-induction consolidation therapy (5–2–5) for two courses. Eligible patients had no prior chemotherapy or myelodysplastic disease. Patients have been followed for a median of 54 months. Of 301 patients treated, CR was achieved in 71% with HIDAC-3-7 and 74% with 7–3–7. For patients in CR, the estimated median remission duration was 45 months with HIDAC-3–7 and 12 months with 737 ($p=0.0005$ univariate analysis, $p=0.0004$ multivariate analysis). The estimated percentange of patients relapse free 5 years after achieving a CR was 49% on HIDAC-3-7 and 24% on 7–3–7. Patients in CR tended to survive longer with HIDAC-3-7 but there were no overall survival differences between the two arms. HIDAC-3-7 was associated with significantly more toxicity in induction with more leukopenia, thrombocytopenia, nausea and vomiting, and eye toxicity (all $p < 0.001$) but a similar incidence of severe CNS and cerebellar toxicity compared to 7–3–7. The consolidation treatment was the same in both arms but caused significantly more leukopenia and thrombocytopenia in patients previously treated with HIDAC-3-7 induction ($p < 0.0001$). The authors concluded that a dose–effect relation exists for cytarabine in AML and that HIDAC-3-7 prolongs remission duration and disease-free survival and is tolerable when used as initial induction therapy in patients with de novo AML.

In the ALSG study, the schedule of eight doses of high-dose cytarabine two doses per day on alternate days was modified from the six doses successfully given by Mayer et al. [66] without major CNS toxicity. This strategy obviously carried the risk that high-dose cytarabine was reduced to a less effective dosage. This study has shown that this dose and schedule of high-dose cytarabine can be successfully given in a large cooperative group setting. However, the South-West Oncology Group (SWOG) study [69] of high-dose cytarabine in induction appeared to be associated with unacceptable toxicity using a 12-h daily schedule. Based on intracellular pharmacology, lower doses of high-dose cytarabine could be equally effective [70].

The results of the ALSG high-dose cytarabine trial are complementary and remarkably similar to those recently reported by Mayer et al. [71] using high-dose cytarabine as post-induction therapy. In that study, patients in remission received six doses per course of high-dose cytarabine, 3 gm/m^2, compared with an intermediate dose of cytarabine of 400 mg/m^2, and standard-dose cytarabine of 100 mg/m^2. Patients on high-dose cytarabine received four courses or 24 treatments. While only 56% of patinets were able to complete the four courses of high-dose cytarabine, more cytarabine was given than in the study conducted by the ALSG. The high-dose cytarabine significantly improved disease-free survival and overall survival when compared to conventional-dose cytarabine. The disease-free survival of patients on high-dose cytarabine was 44% at 4 years for patinets aged $\leqslant 60$ years, censoring patients who received a bone marrow transplant. In the ALSG study, the disease-free survival at 4 years was 43% overall for patients on HIDAC-3-7. Censoring for marrow transplant patients, the disease-free survival was 44% at 4 years. Comparing HIDAC-3-7 and 7-3-7, the hazard ration for disease-free survival was 0.63. In the study by Mayer et al. [71], high-dose cytarabine post induction resulted in a similar hazard ratio for disease-free survival of 0.67.

The results of these two studies compare favourably with those of autologous bone marrow transplantation with relapse-free survival rates of 25%–50% at 3 years [72]. They may compare favourably with 50% relapse-free survival seen with allogeneic transplantation if selection factors such as age, performance status, length of time after CR and tolerance to previous therapy are taken into account [73]. Mayer et al. reported few relapses after 20 months. However, relapses were seen at 36 months in the ALSG study, so that further follow up will be required to determine if the remissions noted are as durable as those seen with transplantation.

A three-arm post-induction by the Eastern Cooperative Oncology Group (ECOG) compared a single course of high-dose cytarabine, 3 g/m^2 for 12 doses plus amsacrine, weekly standard-dose cytarabine plus 6-thioguanine and allogeneic bone marrow transplantation [74]. The event-free survival for patients aged less than 60 years in CR who received high-dose cytarabine and amsacrine was 28% (Standard error 11%). There was no difference in outcome in the ECOG subset of patients aged less than 41 years treated with either high-dose cytarabine, amsacrine or allogeneic bone marrow transplantation although only 83 patients were compared. These results may be similar to those reported by Mayer et al. [71]

It is clear from a number of studies that the benefits of intensified therapy in AML are confined to younger patients [3, 66, 71]. In patients receiving the three-drug combination with etoposide (7–3–7), the prolongation of relapse-free survival was more marked and the survival advantage seen over a standard two-drug therapy was confined to younger patients aged less than 55 years [3]. Mayer et al. [71] stratified their patients according to age, reported no benefit in patients over 60 years of age and could not deliver high-dose cytarabine in that older age group. This study was age limited but younger patients fared better with higher response rates. Thus, intensive therapy cannot be generally recommended for older patients.

A more fundamental issue raised by this study and those of post-induction intensification is when in the chemotherapy cascade should therapy in AML be intensified [71, 74, 75]. Treatment could be theoretically intensified during the induction phase, immediately after remission, or after 2–3 months of preparative regimens, as in some transplantation programs. The advantages of giving intensive therapy to patients in remission are that the marrow contains a normal proportion of hematopoietic cell progenitors and the patients' general condition is better. Thus, intensive treatment is better tolerated and less dangerous during remission than during induction. However, 30%–40% of patients on standard regimens never have a remission and will never have the chance of benefiting from new improved intensified therapies that may develop in the future. Other curable tumours, such as testicular cancer and some lymphomas, appear to benefit from optimal initial treatment. Less high-dose cytarabine may be required when used in one or two courses in induction, as in the ALSG study, compared to the planned 24 doses used in the study by Mayer et al. The disadvantage remains the initial toxicity of intensified induction. There may be subsets of patient in whom it is safe or desirable to intensify induction and others where such intensification is contra-indicated.

Regardless of its optimal position in the chemotherapy program, it is now clear that a dose–response relation exists for cytarabine in AML. This has important implications for intensifying induction and post-induction therapies and in designing optimal preparative regimens for transplantation.

References

1. Yates J, Glidewell O, Wiernik PH, Cooper MR, Steinber D, Dosik H, Levy R, Hoagland C, Henry P, Gottlieb H, Cornell C, Berenberg J, Hutchinson JH, Raich P, Nissen N, Ellison RR, Frelick R, James GN, Falkson G, Silver RT, Haurani F, Green M, Henderson E, Leone L, Holland JF: Cytosine arabinoside with daunorubicin or adriamycin for therapy of acute myelocytic leukemia: CALGB study. Blood 60: 2, 454-462, 1982.
2. Priesler H, Davis RB, Kirschner J, Dupre E, Richards F, Hoagland HC, Kopel S, Levy RN, Carey R, Shulman P, Gottlieb AJ, McIntyre OR: Comparison of three remission induction regimens and two post induction strategies for the treatment of acute non-lymphocyte leukemia: CALGB study. Blood 69: 5, 1441-1449, 1987.
3. Bishop JF, Lowenthal RM, Joshua D, Matthews JP, Todd D, Cobcroft R, Whiteside MG, Kronenberg H, Ma D, Dodds A, Herrman R, Szer J, Wolf MM, Young G. Etoposide in acute non-lymphocytic leukemia. Blood 75, 27-32, 1990.
4. Bishop JF, McGrath K, Wolf MM, Matthews JP, De Luise T, Holdsworth R, Yuen K, Veal M, Whiteside MG/M^2, Cooper IA, Szer J. Clinical factors influencing the efficacy of pooled platelet transfusions. Blood 71: 383-387, 1988.
5. Bishop JF, Matthews JP, McGrath K, Wolf MM, Yuen K. Factors influencing 20 hour increment following platelet transfusions. Transfusion 31: 392-396, 1991.
6. Ellison RR, Holland JF, Weil M et al. Arabinisyl cytosine: a useful agent in the treatment of acute leukemia in adults. Blood 32: 507-23, 1968.
7. Mayer RJ, Davis RB, Schiffer CA, Berg DT, Powell BL, Schulmane P, Omura GA, Moore JO, McIntyre OR, Frei E. Intensive postremission chemotherapy in adults with acute myeloid leukemia. New Engl J. Med 331: 896-903, 1994.
8. The Finnish Leukemia Group: The effect of thioguanine on a combination of daunorubicin, cytarabine and prednisolone in the treatment of acute leukemia in adults. Scand J Haematol 23: 124-128, 1979.
9. Clarkson BD, Gee T, Mertelsmann R et al. Current status of treatment of acute leukemia in adults: an overview of the Memorial experience and review of the literature. Crit Rev Oncol Hematol 4: 221-48, 1986.
10. Berman E, Heller G, Santorsa J. McKenzie S, Gee T, Kempia S, Guiati S, Andreef M, Kolitz J, Gabrilore J, Reich L, Mayer K, Keefe D, Trainor K, Schluger A, Penenber D, Raymond V, O'Reilly R, Jhanwar S, Young c, Clarkson B. Results of a randomized trial comparing idarubicin and cytosine arabinoside with daunorubicin and cytosine arabinoside in adult patients with newly diagnosed acute myelogenous leukemia. Blood 77: 1666-1674, 1991.
11. Mandelli F, Petti M, Ardia A, Di Pietro N, Di Raimondo F, Ganzina F, Falconi, Geraci E, Ladogana S, Latagliata R, Malleo C, Nobile F, Petti N, Rotoli B, Specchia G, Tabilio A, Resegotti L. A randomised clinical trial comparing idarubicin and cytarabine to daunorubicin and cytarabine in the treatment of acute non-lymphoid leukaemia. Eur J Cancer 27: 750-755, 1991.
12. Wiernick P, Banks P, Case D, Arlin Z, Periman P, Todd M, Ritch P, Enck R, Weitberg A. Cytarabine plus idarubicin or daunorubicin as induction and consolidation therapy for previously untreated adult patients with acute myeloid leukemia. Blood 79: 313-319, 1992.
13. Vogler W, Velez-Garcia E, Weiner R, Flaum M, Bartolucci A, Omura G, Gerber M, Banks P. A phase III trial comparing idarubicin and daunorubicin in combination with cytarabine in acute myelogenous leukemia: a South eastern Cancer Study Group study. Clin Oncol 10: 1103-1111, 1992.
14. Rivera G, Avery T, Roberts D. Response of L1210 to combination of cytosine arabinoside and VM-26 or VP16-213. Eur J Cancer 11: 639-647; 1975.
15. Loike J. VP 16-213 and podophyllotoxin. A study on the relationship between chemical structure and biological activity. Cancer Chemother Pharmacol 7: 103-111; 1982.
16. Cavalli F. VP16-231 (etoposide): a critical review of its activity. Cancer Chemother Pharmacol 7: 81-85; 1982.
17. European Organisation for Research on the Treatment of Cancer, clinical screening group (1973). Epipodophyllotoxin VP16-213 in the treatment of acute leukemias, haematosarcomas and solid tumours. Br Med J 3: 199-202; 1973.
18. Mathe G, Schwarzenberg L, Pouillart P et al. Two epipodophyllotoxin derivations. VM26 and VP16-213 in the treatment leukemias, hematosarcomas and lymphomas. Cancer 34: 1985-988; 1974.
19. Jungi WF, Senn HJ, Erste Resultate mit dem Epipodophyllotoxin VP16-213 bei der Behandlung akuter Leukämie. Schweiz Med Sochesnschr 105: 1365-1369: 1975.
20. Cavalli F, Sonntag RW, Brunner KW. Epipodophyllotoxin-Derivat VP16-213 in acute nonlymphoblastic leukaemia (letter) Br Med 3: 227; 1975.
21. Falkson G, Van Dyk JJ, Van Eden ED et al. A Clinical trial of oral form of 4-demethyl-epipodophyllotoxin-d-ethylidene glycoside VP 16-213, Cancer 35: 1141-1144; 1975.
22. McKenna RW, Bloomfield CD, Dick F et al. Acute monoblastic leukemia: diagnosis and treatment of 10 cases. Blood 46: 841-494; 1975.
23. Bernasconi C, Lazzarino M, Morra E. The use of epipodophyllotoxin derivative (VP16-213) in the treatment of acute monocytic leukemias. In: Stacker A, Hocker P, eds. Erkrankungen der Myelopoese. Munich: Urban and Schwatzenberg. 224-227; 1976.
24. Smith IR, Gerben ME, Clinic HM et al. VP16-213 in acute myelogenous leukemia. Postgrad Med J 52: 66-69; 1976.
25. Chard RL, Drivit W, Bleyer WA et al. Phase II study of VP16-213 in childhood malignant disease:

a Childrens Cancer Study Group report. Cancer Treat Rep 63: 17555–1759; 1979.
26. Van Echo DA, Wiernik Ph, Aisner J. High dose VP16–213 (NSC141540) for the treatment of patients with previously treated acute leukemia. Cancer Clin Trials 3: 325–328; 1980.
27. Karp G, Antman K, Canellos G. VP16–213: a phase II trial using a weekly schedule. Cancer Clin Trials 4: 465–467; 1981.
28. Rivera G, Bowman WP, Lok AT et al. Single-agent and combination chemotherapy with etoposide in acute leukemias of childhood. Cancer Treat Rev (Suppl) 9: 53–57; 1982.
29. Evans JPM, Prentice HG. Remission induction in acute myeloid leukaemia with oral etoposide. Lancet ; : 1345–1346; 1982.
30. Bennett JM, Lymmann GH, Cassileth PA. A phase II trial of VP16–213 in adults with refractory acute myeloid leukemia. Am J Clin Oncol 7: 471–473; 1984.
31. Mailliard JA, Letendre L, Dalton RJ et al. Phase II trial of VP-16 in the treatment of acute nonlymphocytic leukemia in blast crisis of chronic granulocytic leukemia. Med Pediatr Oncol 14: 306–309; 1986.
32. Nishikawa A, Nakmura Y, Nobori U et al. Acute monocytic leukemia in children. Cancer 60: 2146–2149; 1987.
33. Bishop JF, Lowenthal R, Joshua E, Matthews JP, Wolf MM <Cooper IA> Etoposide in leukemia. Cancer 67: 285–291, 1991.
34. Letendre L, Hinemann V, Hoagland C et al. Phase I study of VP-16 (etoposide) and amsacrine (AMSA) in the treatment of refractory acute leukemia. Med Pediatr Oncol 13: 232–234; 1985.
35. Tschopp L, von Fliedner VE, Sauter C et al. Efficacy and clinical cross-resistance of a new combination therapy (AMSA/VP16) in previously treated patients with acute nonlymphocytic leukemia. J Clin Oncol 4: 318–324; 1986.
36. Abrams RA, Hanson G, Anderson T. Phase II study of combination chemotherapy with etoposide and amsacrine in relapsed adult leukemia. Cancer Treat Rep 70 (4): 535; 1986.
37. Hiddemann W, Urbanitz O, Preusser P et al. Treatment of refractory acute myeloid leukemia with AMSA and VP16-213 in combination. Results of a clinical phase I/II study. Haematol Oncol 7: 267–273; 1989.
38. Van Echo DA, Lichtenfeld KM, Wiernik PH. Vinblastine 5-azacytindine and VP16-213 therapy for previously treated patients with acute nonlymphocytic leukemia. Cancer Treat Rep 61(8): 1599–1601; 1977.
39. Suater C, Fehr J, Frick P et al. Acute myelogenous leukemia. Successful treatment of relapse with cytosine arabinoside. VP16-213, vincristine and vinblastine (A-triple V). Eur J Cancer Clin Oncol 18(8) 733–737; 1982.
40. Look AT, Dahl GV, Kalwinsky D et al. Effective remission induction of refractory childhood acute non-lymphocytic leukemia by VP16-213 plus azacytidine. Cancer Treat Rep 65: 995–999; 1981.
41. Kalwinsky DK, Dahl GC. Mirro J et al. Induction failures in childhood acute nonlymphocytic leukemia: etoposide 5-azacytidine for cases refractory to daunorubicin cytarabine. Med Pediatr Oncol 14: 245–250; 1986.
42. Hakami N, Look AT, Steuber PC et al. Combined etoposide and 5-azacytidine in children and adolescents with refractory or relapsed acute non-lymphocytic leukemia. A Pediatric Oncology Group study; J Clin Oncol 5: 1022–1025; 1987.
43. Carella AM, Santini G, Gikordano D et al. Idarubicin alone or in combination with cytarabine and etoposide (3 + 3 + 5 protocol) in acute non-lymphocytic leukemia (letter). Leukemia Res 9(5); 631; 1985.
44. Bishop JF, Joshua DE, Lowenthal RM et al. A phase I-II study of cytosine arabinoside, daunorubicin and VP16-213 in adult patients with acute non-lymphocytic leukemia. Aust NZ J Med 16: 48–51; 1986.
45. Bern MM, Wallach SR, Arkin CF et al. Etoposide in combination with cytarabine, doxorubicin and 6-thioguanine for treatment of acute non-lymphoblastic leukemia in a protocol adjusted for age. Cancer Treat Rep 71; 201–203; 1987.
46. Ho AD, Lipp T, Ehninger G et al. Combination of mitoxantrone and etoposide in refractory acute myelogenous leukemia. An active well tolerated regimen. J Clin Oncol 6: 213–217; 1988.
47. Rower JM, Chang AYC, Bennett JM, Aclacinomycin A and etoposide (VP-16-213): an effective regimen in previously treated patients with refractory acute myelogenous leukemia. Blood 71(4): 992–996; 1988.
48. Lazzarino M, Morra E, Alessandrino EP et al. Treatment of relapsed or refractory acute myeloid leukemia in adults. Bone Marrow Transpl (Suppl) 4: 121–123; 1989.
49. Gore M, Powles R, Lakhami A, et al. Treatment of relapsed and refractory acute leukemia with high-dose cytosine arabinoside and etoposide. Cancer Chemother Pharmacol 23: 373–376; 1989.
50. Dubovsky D, Kernoff L, Jacobs P. Rapid remission induction in adult acute non-lymphocytic leukaemia. Eur J Cancer 14: 1179–1183; 1978.
51. Kurrle E, Ehninger G, Freund M et al. A multicentre study of intensive induction and consolidation therapy in acute myelogenous leukaemia. Blut 56: 233–236; 1988.
52. Carella AM, Pungolino E, Pratti G et al. Idarubicin in combination with etoposide and cytarabine in adult non-lymphocytic leukaemia (ANLL). Bonw Marrow Transpl (Supple) 4: 50–51; 1989.
53. Kalwinsky D, Mirro J, Schell M et al. Early intensification of chemotherapy for childhood acute non-lymphoblastic leukemia: improved remission induction with a five drug regimen including etoposide. J Clin Oncol 6(7): 1134–1143; 1987.
54. Amadori S, Ceci A, Comelli A et al. Treatment of acute myelogenous leukemia in children: results of the Italian co-operative study AIEOP/LAM 8204. J Clin Oncol 5: 1356–1363; 1987.
55. Baldini G, Bacgarani M, Cavazzini G et al. Treatment of acute non-lymphocytic leukemia:

results of a prospective trial of daunorubicin, arabinosyl cytosine and 6-thioguanine (DAT) versus DAT plus vindesine and etoposide. Haematologica 72: 431–471; 1987.
56. Hryniuk W and Bush H. The importance of dose intensity in chemotherapy of metastatic breast cancer. J Clin Oncol 2: 1281–1287; 1984.
57. Levin L, and Hryniuk W. Dose intensity analysis of chemotherapy regimens in ovarian carcinoma. J Clin Oncol 5: 756–767; 1987.
58. Carde P, MacKintosh F, Rosenberg S. A dose and time response analysis of the treatment of Hodgkin's disease with MOPP chemotherapy. J Clin Oncol 1: 1776–1782; 1989.
59. Van Rijswijk R, Haanen C, Dekker A, de Meijer A and Verbeek J. Dose intensity of MOPP chemotherapy and survival in Hodgkin's disease. J Clin Oncol 7: 1776–1782; 1989.
60. Klasa R, Murray N, Coldman A. Dose intensity meta-analysis of chemotherapy regimens in small cell carcinoma of the lung. J Clin Oncol 9: 499–508; 1991.
61. Bishop J, Mathew J, Young G, Szer J, Joshua D, Dodds A, Laidlaw C, Cobcroft R, Herman R, Ma D, Page F. The influence of induction chemotherapy dose and dose intensity on the duration of remission in acute myeloid leukemia. Leukemia and Lymphoma 15: 79–84; 1984.
62. Plunkett W, Iacoboni S, Keating M.J. Cellular pharmacology and optimal therapeutic concentrations of 1-β D-arabinofuranosylcytosine. 5'-triphosphate in leukemic blasts during treatment of refactory leukemia with high dose 1-β D-arabinofuranosylcytosine. Scand J. Haematol 44: 51–59, 1986.
63. Rustum Y.M., Preisler H.D. Correlation between leukemic cell retention of 1-β D-arabinofuranosylcytosine 5-triphosphate and response to therapy. Cancer Res 39: 42–49, 1979.
64. Hines J.D., Oken M.M., Mazza J, Keller A.M, Streeter R.R, Glick J.H et al. High dose cytarabine and M-AMSA is effective therapy in relapsed non-lymphocytic leukemia. J. Clin Oncol 2: 2 supp 1, 545–549, 1984.
65. Champlin R, Ho W, Winston D, Decker R, Greenberg P, Burnison M, Holly F.H., Gale R.P. Treatment of adults with acute myelogenous leukemia: prospective evaluation of high dose cytarabine in consolidation chemotherapy and with bone marrow transplantation. Semin Oncol 14: 1–6, 1987.
66. Mayer R.J., Schiffer C.A., Peterson B.A., Budman D.R., Silver R.T., Rai K.R., Cornwell G.G., Ellison R.R., Maguire M, Berg D.T., Davis R.B., McIntyre O.R., Frei E. Intensive post-remission therapy in adults with acute non-lymphocytic leukemia using various dose schedules of cytarabine: a progress report from CALGB. Semin. Oncol. 14: 2 suppl 1, 25–31, 1987.
67. Brito-Babapulle F, Catovsky D, Newland A.C, Goldman J.M, Galton D.A.G. Treatment of acute myeloid leukemia with intermediate dose cytarabine and mitoxantrone. Semin.Oncol.14: 2 suppl 1, 51–52, 1987.
68. Bishop J, Matthews J, Young G, Szer J, Gillet A, Joshua D, Bradstock K, Enno A, Wolf M, Fox R, Cobcroft R, Herrman R, Van Der Weyden M, Rowenthal R, Page F, Juneja S. A randomised study of high dose cytarabine in induction in acute myeloid leukemia. Blood 87: 1710–17, 1996
69. Weick J, Kopecky J, Appelbaum F et al. A randomised investigation of high dose versus standard dose cytoside arabinoside with daunorubicin in patients with acute myelogenous leukemia (abstract) Proc Amer Soc Clin Oncol 11: 261, 1992.
70. Plunkett W, Liliemark J.O, Estey E, Keating M.J. Saturation of cytarabine TP accumulation during high-dose cytarabine therapy: pharmacologic rationale for intermediate-dose cytarabine. Semin Oncol 14: 2 Suppl 1, 159–166, 1987.
71. Mayer R.J, Davis R.B, Schiffer C.A, Berg D.T, Powell B.L, Schulman P, Omura G.A, Moore J.O, McIntyre O.R, Frei IIIE. Intensive post-remission chemotherapy in adults with acute myeloid leukemia. New Engl J. Med 331: Vol 14, 896–903, 1994.
72. Gorin N.C, Labopin M, Meloni G, Korbling M, Carella A, Herve P, Burnett A, Rizzoli V, Alessandrino E.P, Bjorkstrand B, Ferrant A, Lowenberg B, Coser P, Simonsson B, Helbig W, Brunet Mauri S, Verdonck L.F, Iriondo A, Polli E, Colombat P, Franklin I.M, Souillet G, Willemze R. Autologous bone marrow transplantation for acute myeloblastic leukemia in Europe: further evidence of the role of marrow purging by mafosfamide. Leukemia 5: 896–904, 1991.
73. Clift R.A, Buchkner C.D, Thomas E.D, Kopecky K.J, Appelbaum F.R, Tallman M, Storb R, Sanders J, Sullivan K, Banaji M, et al. The treatment of acute non-lymphoblastic leukemia by allogeneic marrow transplantation. Bone Marrow Transplant. 2: 243–58, 1987.
74. Cassileth PA, Lynch E, Hines JD, Oken MM, Mazza JJ, Bennett JM, McGlave PB, Edelstein M, Harrington DP, O'Connell MJ. Varying intensity of post-remission therapy in acute myeloid leukemia.
75. Bishop J.F. Intensified therapy for acute myeloid leukemia. New Engl J. Med 331: Vol 14, 941–942, 1994.

Acute Leukemias VI
Prognostic Factors
and Treatment Strategies
Büchner et al. (eds)

Results of All-Trans Retinoic Acid Treatment in Acute Promyelocytic Leukemia (European Experience)

L. Degos[1] and P. Fenaux[2]

Introduction

Acute promyelocytic leukemia (APL) is a specific subtype of acute myeloid leukemia (AML) in the French–American–British classification of AML[1], characterized by the morphology of blast cells (M3), the t(15;17) translocation which fuses the PML gene on chromosome 15 to the retinoic acid receptor alpha (RARα) gene on chromosome 17 [2], and by a coagulopathy combining disseminated intravascular coagulation (DIC), fibrinolysis, and proteolysis [3]. Intensive chemotherapy, including anthracycline was the most effective treatment of APL [4] with a high mortality due to the exacerbation of coagulopathy.

Recently, all-trans retinoic acid (ATRA) has been shown as a differentiating agent of APL blasts [5] and could give complete remission (CR) in 95% of patients without worsening of coagulopathy, and without aplasia in de novo [6] or in relapsed patients [7]. However, ATRA has two major side effects: the risk of a rapid rise in leukocytes and of ATRA syndrome, and the risk of rapid relapse unless intensive chemotherapy is administered in CR.

Methods and Results

The French cooperative group started a treatment approach combining ATRA followed by intensive chemotherapy in newly diagnosed APL; We first performed a pilot study between 1990 and 1991 where treatment with ATRA was given until CR and followed by a combination of daunorubicin (DNR) (4 days) and cytosine arabinoside ara-C (7 days), then three "2 + 5" courses, and finally, prolonged continuous maintenance with 6-mercaptopurine and methotrexate. The first DNR-ara-C course was, however, administered as an emergency treatment if leukocytes were above 6000/μl by day 5 or 10 000/μl by day 10, or 15 000/μl by day 15 of ATRA treatment in order to prevent ATRA syndrome.

Twenty-six patients were included. All had leukocytes under 10 000/μl; 96% achieved CR, 14 with ATRA alone, 11 after the addition of chemotherapy (only one early death) as compared to 76% CR in a historical control treated by chemotherapy alone between 1984 and 1989 [8].

With a minimum follow up of 38 months from CR achievement, event-free survival (EFS, including as events: resistance, relapse, and death in CR) disease-free interval (DFI, taking into account relapse in patients who had reached CR, and censoring deaths in CR) and survival were 62%, 70%, and 77% at 4 years, as compared to 28%, 42%, and 42% in the historical control group and these differences were all significant.

The prolonged follow up now available in both cohorts of patients shows that the combination of ATRA and chemotherapy mainly reduces the risk of early relapses, within 18

[1]Institut d'Hématologie, Hôpital Saint Louis, 1, avenue Claude Vellefaux, 75010 Paris, France
[2]Hematology Department, Hôpital Claude Huriez, Place de Verdun, 59037 Lille Cedex, France

months of CR achievement, whereas the risk of later relapses is similar to that of the chemotherapy group. This suggested that combination therapy did not delay relapses but actually reduced their frequency [9].

A European trial comparing ATRA follwed by chemotherapy and chemotherapy alone in newly diagnosed APL was started in April 1991 after the favorable results obtained in the pilot study. In the chemotherapy group, patients received three successive courses of DNR and ara-C. In the ATRA group, patients received ATRA until CR, followed by the same three chemotherapy courses. The first course was, however, rapidly administered if white blood cells (WBC) were greater than 5000/mm^3 at diagnosis, or increased above thresholds defined in the pilot study. The trial was prematurely closed in December 1992, because the EFS was significantly better in the ATRA group [10].

The last analysis, performed at the reference date of September 1, 1994, showed actuarial EFS, relapse rate, and survival at 2 years of 68%, 25%, and 81% in the ATRA group, as compared to 23%, 56%, and 51%, respectively, in the chemotherapy group ($p = 10^{-4}$, $p = 10^{-4}$, and $p = 0.009$, respectively) [11].

Whether this additive effect is better achieved by administering ATRA and chemotherapy together or one after the other is unknown. The current Euopean APL trial (APL 93 trial) is trying to answer this question by randomizing ATRA followed by chemotherapy and ATRA plus chemotherapy (started on day 3 of ATRA) in newly diagnosed APL. Up to now more than 180 patients have been included and 95 % of patients obtained a CR in both arms.

In the European APL 93 trial, after two consolidation courses, patients in CR are randomized between no maintenance, intermittent treatment with ATRA (15 days every 3 months), continuous low-dose chemotherapy (6-mercaptopurine plus methrotrexate) or both. (This part of the APL 93 trial is organized in cooperation with the GIMEMA Italian group).

Discussion

In Vivo Differentiation of APL Blasts by ATRA

Terminal differentiation of bone marrow cells appears progressively during the treatment and Auer rods are sometimes observed in mature cells, thus confirming the differentiation process of the leukemic cells [12].

Nuclear bodies are ultrastructurally defined granules predominantly found in dividing cells. PML protein, in normal cells, gives a speckled pattern of staining using a PML antibody in the cell nucleus and is specifically bound to a nuclear body [13]. PML and several nuclear body-associated proteins found as autoantigens in primary biliary cirrhosis (PBC) are co-localized and co-regulated. In APL cells, the PML-RARα fusion protein is predominantly localized in the cytoplasm, whereas a fraction is nuclear and delocalizes PML protein to multiple micropunctated dots in the cytoplasm and the nucleus without ultrastructural organization [14]. ATRA administration causes the aggregation of PML and PBC proteins into the nuclear bodies with return to a speckled pattern of PML staining in the nucleus. These findings show that PML-RARα fusion appears to disrupt the function of PML-associated nuclear bodies and that this disruption could be important in APL pathogenesis.

Retinoic Acid Syndrome

Incidence and Clinical Symptoms. Frankel et al. [15] gave a precise description of the clinical symptoms of retinoic acid (RA) syndrome. RA syndrome mainly includes fever and respiratory distress, weight gain, edema, pleural or pericardial effusions, hypotension, and sometimes renal failure. They are preceded by an increasing of WBC counts in the majority of cases, but few patients develop symptoms at WBC counts < 10 000/mm^3. The spontaneous incidence of RA syndrome in de novo patients was 35% in our experience and 23% in the New York experience but was very low in the Chinese experience. Hyperleucocytosis is more frequent (70% of de novo patients, 35% of relapse patients) and also not found in China.

Prevention and Treatment. Once RA syndrome has developed, addition of low-dose chemotherapy is ineffective in lowering WBC counts and leucophereses are unable to reverse symptoms, so two different approaches are currently proposed. The first approach, used by the European and Japanese groups, is to prevent RA syndrome by the addition of chemotherapy for patients presenting with WBC counts above 5000/mm^3, or when a WBC increase above the WBC thresholds defined earlier is seen. This approach has proved very effective on a multicenter basis, as RA syndrome was seen in only three of 54 patients treated in the European APL 91 trial, three of 71 first patients included in the currently ongoing European APL 93 trial, and seven of 109 patients treated by the Japanese group. Only one patient died in the three series (totalling 234 patients) treated with the combination of ATRA and chemotherapy. The second approach, used by the United States and Australian groups, is to treat RA syndrome by administering high-dose intravenous corticosteroids (dexamethasone, 10 mg i.v. twice daily for 3 or more days) as soon as the first symptoms occur. Results of the corticosteroids as treatment of RA syndrome are available from one experienced group and its efficacy will have to be confirmed in a large multicenter study. It will therefore be important to know the results of the United States intergroup study which also uses steroids for the treatment of RA syndrome. In fact, it could be dangerous to give high-dose corticosteriods to patients with fever and dyspnea if an infectious disease is suspected [19].

Coagulation Disorders

Coagulopathy of APL and Its Evolution with ATRA. The coagulopathy associated with APL results from at least three distinct mechanisms due to thrombin activation by the release of pro-coagulant activities, plasmin activation by plasminogen activators, and lysosomal neutrophil enzyme free activities (human leukocyte elastase, cathepsin G, proteinase 3) from the leukemic cells. Thrombin activation may lead to DIC, plasmin activation to plasmin-dependent primary fibrinogenolysis, while leukocyte-mediated proteolysis is able to cleave various substrates including von Willebrand factor and fibrinogen itself, both in vitro and in vivo [3]. The rapid normalization of the fibrinogen level found in APL patients treated with ATRA seems to be chronologically related to the disappearance of plasmin-dependent primary fibrinogenolysis. However, the persistence of a moderate thrombin activation not compensated by primary fibrinolysis during the first weeks of ATRA treatment could lead to a transient period of hypercoagulability, and a few well-documented cases of thromboembolic events in APL patients treated with ATRA have been reported [20–20]. This observation justifies the use of prophylactic heparin therapy during the first 2–3 weeks of ATRA treatment.

Resistance to ATRA

Primary resistance is rare (less than 2%) in APL confirmed by the t(15; 17) translocation or the PML-RARα product. Secondary resistance to ATRA is, however, observed in almost all patients on treatment or after withdrawal of ATRA with early relapse (0–6 months).

Prolonged administration of high doses of ATRA results in an increase of proteins that induce ATRA catabolism, leading to the reduced plasma levels observed during ATRA therapy (induction of cytochrome P450 enzymes [16] and of cytoplasmic retinoic acid-binding protein [17].

After ATRA withdrawal, this hypercatabolytic state persists for a period of several months which may vary according to the duration, dose of ATRA therapy, and level of ATRA cell sequestration. Recovery of ATRA sensitivity after sufficient ATRA withdrawal (more than 6 months) is frequently observed.

Minimal Residual Disease in APL

The PML-RARα product persists in almost all APL patients after ATRA-induced CR. Although RT-PCR does not allow to distinguish differentiated from proliferating APL cells, the fact that all patients relapse after ATRA-induced remission, if not consolidated by chemotherapy, suggests that the leukemic clone is not sufficently eradicated by ATRA. On the contrary, RT-PCR is generally found negative after consolidation chemotherapy [18]. However, the sensitivity of RT-PCR for PML-RARα fusion transcript is low compared to the tests performed in other types of leukemia. RT-PCR studies will also define whether any of the PML-RAR transcript (bcr1, bcr2, and bcr3) has an influence in the clinical, cytological, or biological features and prognosis of APL. It has been suggested in some studies that bcr3 transcript was more frequent in children, was correlated to higher leukocyte counts, higher incidence of microgranular APL variant and of CD2 expression, and to poorer prognosis (C. Chominna, personal communication). The higher risk of relapse when bcr3 is present (small transcript) [E23] seems to be a feature of European-American populations and was not found in Japan.

Role of Bone Marrow Transplantation in APL

Patients who have relapsed after ATRA plus chemotherapy are obvious candidates for allogeneic bone marrow transplantation (BMT). Because more than 70% of the patients in CR and treated with ATRA and intensive chemotherapy have long survival, the role of allogeneic BMT in first CR in these patients is questionable even if results of allogeneic BMT seem to be better in APL than in other AML. The relatively prolonged follow up in the APL 91 trial, however, suggests that patients presenting with high WBC counts (who also often have a microgranular variant of APL) are still at relatively high risk of relapse (about 40%) and could be candidates for allogeneic BMT if an HLA-identical sibling is available. Conversions to positive RT-PCR findings for the PML-RAR rearrangement during follow up are inevitably associated with subsequent relapse. Regular monitoring of residual disease by RT-PCR, especially if initial high WBC counts were observed, may allow to plan an allograft in the case of positive findings.

Conclusion

The confirmation that in vitro differentiation of APL blasts by ATRA could be efficiently transposed in vivo has not only modified the therapeutic approach to APL but has also opened new perspectives for differentiation therapy in oncology as well as novel research on retinoic acid receptor function in the hematopoietic tissue.

The reduced number of cases of RA syndrome by appropriate treatments, the control of coagulation disorders, the better understanding of resistance due to hypercatabolism of ATRA, and the surveillance of the minimal residual disease by RT-PCR increase the accuracy of the dual treatment (ATRA plus chemotherapy). Up to now the EFS estimated at 68% at 2 years when ATRA is added to chemotherapy compared to 23% when chemotherapy is given alone is a great improvement in the treatment of APL.

References

1. Bennett JM, Catovsky D, Daniel MT, Flandrin G, Galton D, Gralnick M, Sultan C. Proposals for the classification of the acute leukemias. Br. J. Haematol., 1976, 33: 451.
2. de The H, Chomienne C, Lanotte M, Degos L, Dejean A: The t(15;17) translocation of acute promyelocytic leukemia fuses the retinoic acid receptor alpha gene to a novel transcribed locus. Nature 1990, 347 : 558-561.
3. Dombret H, Scrobohaci ML, Ghorra P., Zini JM, Daniel MT, Castaigne S, Degos L : Coagulation disorders associated with acute promyelocytic leukemia: corrective effect of all-trans retinoic acid treatment. Leukemia 1993, 7: 2
4. Bernard J, Weil B, Boiron M et al.: Acute promyelocytic leukemia. Results of treatment with daunorubicin. Blood 1973, 41 : 489-496
5. Chomienne C., Ballerini P, Balitrand N, Daniel MT, Fenaux P, Castaigne S, Degos L : All trans retinoic acid in promyelocytic leukemias. II. In vitro studies structure function relationship. Blood 1990, 76 : 1710
6. Huang M, Yu-Chen Y, Shu-Rong C, Lu MX, Zhoa L, Gu LJ, Wang ZY : Use of all trans retinoic acid in the treatment of acute promyelocytic leukemia. Blood 1988, 73 : 567
7. Degos L, Chomienne C, Daniel MT, Berger R, Dombret H, Fenaux P, Castaigne S : Treatment of first relapse in acute promyelocytic leukemia with all trans retinoic acid. Lancet 1990, 2 : 1440
8. Fenaux P, Castaigne S, Dombret H, Archimbaud E, Duarte M, Morel P, Lamy T, Tilly H, Guerci A, Maloisel F, Bordessoule D, Sadoun A, Tiberthien P, Fenueux N, Daniel MT, Chomienne C, Degos L : All-trans retinoic acid followed by intensive chemotherapy gives a high complete remission rate and may prolong remissions in newly diagnosed acute promyelocytic leukemia: a pilot study on 26 cases. Blood 1992, 80 : 2176-2181
9. Fenaux P, Wattel E, Archimbaud E, Sanz M, Hecquet B, Guerci A, Link H, Feguex N, Fey M, Castaigne S, Degos L: Prolonged follow up confirms that all trans retinoic acid (ATRA) followed by chemotherapy reduces the risk of relapse in newly diagnosed acute promyelocytic leukemia (APL). Blood 1994, 84: 666-667
10. Fenaux P, Le Deley MC, Castaigne S, et al.: Effect of all trans retinoic acid in newly diagnosed acute promyelocytic leukemia. Results of a multicenter randomized trial. Blood 1993, 82:3241-3249
11. Degos L, Dombret H, Chomienne C, Daniel MT, Miclea JM, Chastang C, Castaigne S, Fenaux P: All-trans retinoic acid as a differentiating agent in the treatment of acute promyelocytic leukemia. Blood 1995 (in press)
12. Castaigne S, Chomienne C, Daniel MT, Berger R, Fenaux P, Degos L : All-trans retinoic acid as a differentiation therapy for acute promyelocytic leukemias. I.Clinical results. Blood 1990, 76:1704
13. Koken MHM, Puvion-Dutilleul F, Guillemin MC, V iron A, Linaret-Cruz G, Sturman W; de Jong L, Szostecki C, Calvo F, Chomienne C, Degos L, Puvion E, de The H: The t(15;17) translocation alters a nuclear body in a retinoic and reversible fashion. EMBO J. 1994, 13: 1073-1083

14. Daniel MT, Koken M, Romagne O, Barbey S, Bazarbachi A, Stadler M, Guillemin MC, Degos L, Chomienne C, de The H: PML protein expression in haematopoietic and APL cells. Blood 1993, 82: 1858–1867
15. Frankel SR, Eardley A, Lauwers G, Weiss M, Warrell R: The "retinoic acid syndrome" in acute promyelocytic leukemia. Ann. Intern. Med. 1992, 117: 292
16. Muindi JRF, Frankel ST, Huseltion C, DeGrazia F, Garland WA, Young CW, Warrell RP: Clinical pharmacology of oral all-trans retinoic acids in patients with acute promyelocytic leukemia. Cancer Res. 1992, 52: 2138–2142
17. Cornic M, Delva L, Guidez F, Balitrand N, Degos L, Chomienne C: Induction of retinoic acid-binding protein in normal and malignant human myeloid cells by retinoic acid in acute promyelocytic leukemia patients. Cancer Res 1992,52: 3329–3334
18. Castaigne S, Balitrand N, de The H, Dejean A, Degos L, Chomienne C: A PML/RARα fusion transcript is constantly detected by RNA-based polymerase chain reaction in acute promyelocytic leukemia. Blood 1992, 79: 3110
19. Frankel SR, Eardley A, Lauwers G, Weiss M, Warrell R. The retinoic acid syndrome in acute promyelocytic leukemia Ann Intern Med 1992, 117: 292
20. Runde V, Aul C, Sudhoff T, Heyll A, Schneider W. Retinoic acid in the treatment of acute promyelocytic leukemia: Inefficacy of the 13-cis isomer and induction of complete remission by the all-trans isomer complicated by thromboembolic events. Ann. *Hematol.* 1993, 64,270
21. Forjaz De Lacerda J, Alves Do Carmo J. Lurdes Guerra M, Geraldes J, Forjaz De Lacerda JM. Multiple thrombosis in acute promyelocytic leukemia after tretinoin. *Lancet* 1993, 342, 114
22. Hashimoto S, Koike T, Tatewaki W, Seki Y, Sato N, Azegami T, Tsukada N, Takahashi H, Kimura H, Ueno M, Arakawa M, Shibata A. Fatal thromboembolism in acute promyelocytic leukemia during all-trans retinoic acid therapy combined with antifibrinolytic therapy for prophylaxis of hemorrhage. *Leukemia* 1994, 8, 1113–1115

Acute Leukemias VI
Prognostic Factors
and Treatment Strategies
Büchner et al. (eds)

Intensified Post-Remission Chemotherapy for Adults with Acute Myeloid Leukemia: An Update of CALGB 8525

R.J. Mayer[1], R.B. Davis[2], C.A. Schiffer[3], D.T. Berg[1], B.L. Powell[4], P. Shulman[5], G.A. Omura[6], G.O. Moore[7], O.R. McIntyre[8], and E[1]. Frei III

Abstract. While complete remission may be achieved in 65% of adults with de novo AML, such remissions lack durability when conventional post-remission therapy is administered. Uncontrolled trials have suggested that intensive post-remission therapy may prolong these responses. To assess this concept, the Cancer and Leukemia Group B administered induction therapy (cytarabine and daunoribucin) to 1088 adults (median age: 52 years). Of these 1088 patients, 693 (64%) achieved complete remission of whom 596 were randomly assigned to receive four courses of single-agent cytarabine in one of three dose schedules: 3 gm/m^2 in a 3-h infusion every 12 h $\times$ 2 on days 1, 3, and 5 (HiDAc; 187 patients); 400 mg/m^2 per day $\times$ 5 days continuous infusion (206 patients); or 100 mg/m^2 per day $\times$ 5 days continuous infusion (203 patients). All patients then received four courses of monthly maintenance treatment. After a median follow-up time of 63.5 months, the three treatment cohorts had significantly different disease-free survivals ($p = 0.001$). The probability of remaining in continuous complete remission after 5 years for patients 60 years of age or younger was 42% for HiDAc, 29% for 400 mg/m^2, and 19% for 100 mg/m^2 ($p = 0.0007$). In contrast, for patients older than age 60 years, the probability of continuous complete remission after 4 years was 14% or less in each of the three cytarabine groups. With further maturation of the data, the outcome of this trial continues to support the concept of a dose-response effect for cytarabine in patients with AML and 60 years of age or younger. The results observed with the HiDAc dose schedule in this age group are similar to those reported in patients with AML who undergo allogeneic or autologous bone marrow transplantation during first remission.

Introduction

Complete remission can be achieved in approximately 65% of previously untreated adults with de novo acute myeloid leukemia (AML) who are treated with cytarabine and an anthracycline with or without 6-thioguanine [1]. These responses, however, are not durable when conventional maintenance or consolidation therapy is utilized; fewer than 25% of such individuals remain in extended remission [1]. The results of recent clinical trials have suggested that the duration of remission of patients with AML may be prolonged through the use of post-remission

[1]Division of Medical Oncology, Dana-Farber Cancer Institute and the Department of Medicine, Harvard Medical School, Boston, MA, USA
[2]Division of General Medicine and Primary Care, Beth Israel Hospital, Harvard Medical School, Boston, MA, USA
[3]University of Maryland Cancer Center, Baltimore, MD, USA
[4]Bowman Gray School of Medicine, Winston-Salem, NC, USA
[5]Northshore University Hospital, Manhasset, NY, USA
[6]University of Alabama, Birmingham, AL, USA
[7]Duke University Medical Center, Durham, NC, USA
[8]Dartmouth Medical School, Norris Cotton Cancer Center, Lebanon, NH, USA

programs utilizing higher drug doses than those given as part of induction regimens [2, 3]. During the past 25 years, cytarabine has become the mainstay of induction regimens for the management of AML. Preclinical studies have revealed the presence of a steep dose-response curve for this antimetabolite [4] and higher doses of the drug have become a fundamental component of recent intensive post-remission programs for patients with AML [5].

To provide an objective assessment of post-remission intensification in patients with AML, the Cancer and Leukemia Group B (CALGB) focused post-induction therapy on cytarabine and designed an investigative program (CALGB protocol 8525) comparing the effects of intermittent high-dose cytarabine (HiDAc) to standard and intermediate doses of the drug administered by continuous infusion on the duration of complete remission. The dose schedules for the HiDAc regimen and the intermediate continuous infusion program were determined during an initial phase of the program which was conducted by the CALGB between 1982 and 1985 [6].

Methods

The eligibility criteria, study design, criteria for response, and method of statistical analysis utilized in this trial have been previously reported [7]. In brief, patients 16 years of age or older with de novo AML who had received no prior anti-leukemia therapy were treated with an induction regimen which included a 7-day continuous intravenous infusion of cytarabine (200 mg/m^2 per day accompanied by daily bolus administrations of daunorubicin (45 mg/m^2 per day given on the first 3 days of cytarabine therapy for patients aged 60 years of age or younger, 30 mg/m^2 per day for patients aged older than 60). If persistent leukemia was present at the time of bone marrow examination 14 days after the start of treatment, a second course of induction therapy including 5 days of cytarabine and 2 days of daunorubicin at identical daily doses was initiated.

Patients entering complete remission were stratified by the number of induction courses required to achieve a remission bone marrow (one or two) and their age (<40 years, 40–60 years, >60 years) and were randomized to receive four courses of single-agent cytarabine in one of three dose schedules: 3 mg/m^2 administered in a 3-h infusion every 12 h twice daily on days 1, 3, and 5 for a total of six doses per course (i.e., HiDAc); 400 mg/m^2 per day for 5 days as a continuous intravenous infusion; or 100 mg/m^2 for 5 days as a continuous intravenous infusion. Hematopoietic growth factors such as granulocyte colony-stimulating factor (G-CSF), granulocyte-macrophage CSF (GM-CSF), or erythropoietin were not utilized. Following four courses of cytarabine therapy, all patients received four identical courses of monthly maintenance treatment consisting of cytarabine (100 mg/m^2 every 12 h, 200 mg/m^2 per day for 5 days by subcutaneous injection) and daunorubicin (45 mg/m^2 by rapid infusion on the first treatment day) after which all treatment was discontinued.

Disease-free survival was measured as the time from randomization in patients who had achieved a complete remission to relapse or death from any cause. Survival comparisons of post-remission therapies were measured from the time of randomization in patients who had achieved a complete remission to death from any cause. Patients who underwent allogeneic or autologous bone marrow transplantation were considered censored for disease-free survival on the date of the procedure but were still followed for survival.

Results

Between October, 1985 and October, 1990, a total of 1088 evaluable patients (median age: 52 years; range 16–86 years) were registered onto this trial. The morphologic distribution of the patients, utilizing the French–American–British (FAB) classification system, was similar to that of previous reports [8]. Complete remission was achieved in 693 (64%) of patients. The likelihood of response was age dependent, occurring in 75% of 340 patients less than age 40, 68% of 402 individuals 40–60 years of age, and 47% of 346 patients older than age 60. Complete response rates were similar among morphologic subsets as defined by FAB criteria, ranging from 60% (M4) to 74% (M3).

Of the 693 patients who achieved complete remission, 596 were randomized to receive four courses of post-remission cytarabine at the HiDAc level (187 patients; median age: 43 years), the 400 mg/m^2 dose level (206 patients;

median age: 49 years), or the 100 mg/m^2 dose level (203 patients; median age: 48 years). The three cohorts were well balanced with regard to leukocyte count at the time of diagnosis and FAB subtype. The median follow-up time from randomization is 63.5 months. The full four courses of post-remission cytarabine therapy were administered to 56% of the HiDAc group, 74% of the 400 mg/m^2 cohort, and 76% of the 100 mg/m^2 cohort. For patients 60 years of age or younger, the likelihood of receiving the full four courses was 62%, 76%, and 78% for the three different dose levels while for patients older than age 60, there was a similar probability of receving four courses of treatment for individuals randomly assigned to receive the 400 mg/m^2 or 100 mg/m^2 but only 29% could tolerate a full four courses of HiDAc. A clear-cut relationship between hematologic toxicity and cytarabine dose schedule was noted; the probability for hospitalization because of fever and neutropenia and for platelet transfusions was 71% and 86% per course in individuals treated with HiDAc, 59% and 80% for patients receiving 400 mg/m^2, and 16% and 28% in patients receiving 100 mg/m^2, respectively. Central nervous system abnormalities were reported only in the group of patients assigned to receive HiDAc. The probability for developing significant neurotoxicity was related to age, being noted in only 5% of 76 patients under age 40 and 10% of 80 patients aged 40–60, but 32% of 31 patients older than age 60. Of the 22 patients who experienced neurologic toxicity, the symptoms totally resolved within several days in about 20% of patients and receded in a more gradual fashion in about 40% of patients; however, persistent disability persisted in about 40% of individuals. Further HiDAc therapy was not administered following recovery from an episode of neurotoxicity. Treatment-related deaths during remission, primarily due to infection, occurred in 5% of patients assigned to the HiDAc regimen, 6% of those assigned to the 400 mg/m^2 level, and 1% of patients assigned to the 100 mg/m^2 level.

The probability of remaining alive and free of recurrence for patients who had achieved complete remission was closely related to age and post-remission cytarabine treatment schedule. An analysis of all 596 patients randomized to receive post-remission cytarabine reveals an estimated probability of being alive and disease-free after 5 years of 31% and 29% for patients younger than age 40 and 40–60 years of age, respectively; this probability falls to 13% in individuals older than age 60. When analyzed by cytarabine treatment schedule, the likelihood of remaining alive and disease free after 5 years is 37% for the HiDAc group, 26% for the 400 mg/m^2 cohort, and 18% for the 100 mg/m^2 subset ($p = 0.0014$). Relapses continued to occur at a steady rate in the 100 mg/m^2 and 400 mg/m^2 groups during the initial 3 years of follow up but became far less frequent after 2 years in patients receiving HiDAc. The probability of remaining disease free in relation to post-remission cytarabine treatment schedule was statistically similar in the 225 patients under age 40 and 242 patients aged 40–60, so these two groups were combined into a single cohort of 467 individuals. The likelihood of remaining disease free after 5 years for this cohort is 42% for the HiDAC group, 29% for the 400 mg/m^2 group, and 19% for the 100 mg/m^2 ($p = 0.0007$) (Fig. 1a.). In contrast, for the 129 patients older than age 60, the probability of remaining disease free after 5 years is 14% or less for each of the three post-remission cytarabine subsets (Fig. 1b). The probability of remaining alive 5 years following randomization for patients 60 years of age or younger is 49% for the HiDAc group, 41% for the 400 mg/m^2 cohort, and 33% for the 100 mg/m2 group ($p = 0.0355$) (Fig. 2). For the entire population of 1088 evaluable patients who entered the study, the likelihood for remaining alive 5 years following the diagnosis of AML is 35% for patients under age 40, 26% for those ages 40–60, and 8% for individuals older than age 60 ($p < 0.001$).

Discussion

The preliminary results of this trial were presented after a median follow-up time of 37.5 months [9]. More mature data appeared after a median follow-up time of 52 months [7]. The present update reflects a median follow-up time of 63.5 months. The results of the study continue to demonstrate a significant dose-response effect when cytarabine is given as post-remission therapy. Patients 60 years of age or younger who were randomly allocated to HiDAc treatment has a statistically superior likelihood of remaining in remission and an improved survival when compared to similar individuals who received lower dose; 42% of this HiDAc cohort remain in remission after 5 years of follow up

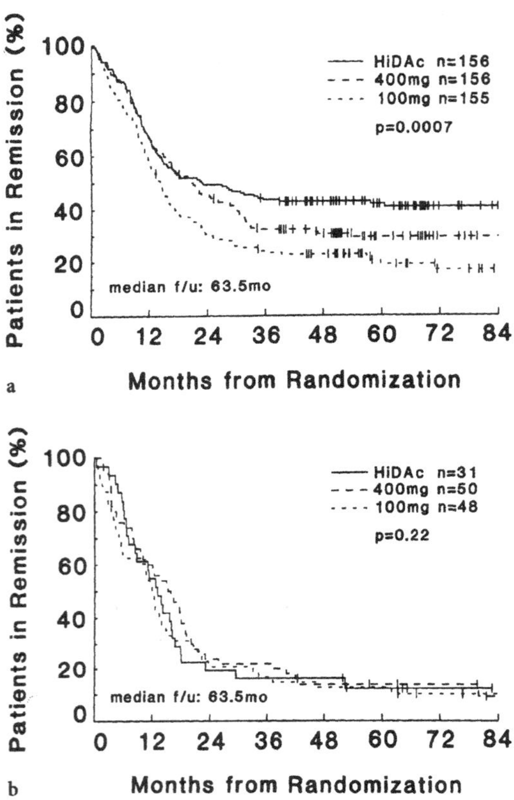

Fig. 1a,b. Probability of disease-free survival for randomized patients by cytarabine dose for: **a** patients 60 years of age or younger; **b** patients older than age 60

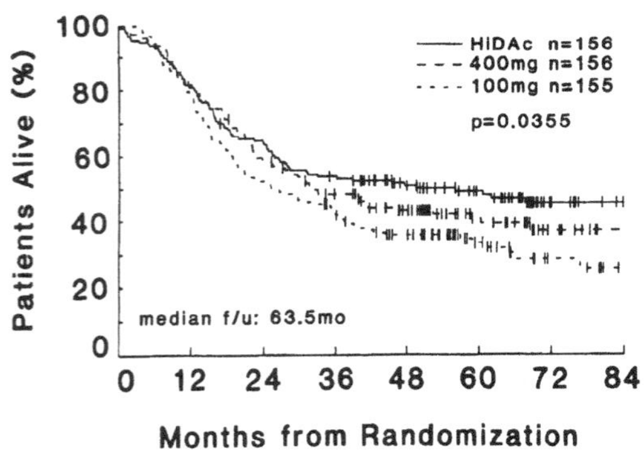

Fig. 2. Probability of survival for randomized patients 60 years of age or younger by cytarabine dose

with few relapses having occurred beyond 20 months of observation.

Unresolved questions regarding the use of HiDAc therapy remain (Table 1).

1. Significant myelosuppression, as characterized by the need for hospitalization due to fever at a time of neutropenia as well as frequent platelet transfusions, represented the major toxicity observed in the HiDAc cohort. Could the use of hematopoietic growth factors reduce the extent of myelosuppression [10], thereby increasing tolerance for this intensive treatment?
2. Is there an optimal dose schedule for HiDAc in terms of drug dosage, duration of infu-

Table 1. Unresolved questions in the use of HiDAc for AML

- Can toxicity from drug-induced myelosuppression be reduced?
- Can an optimal dose schedule be defined?
- What is the role of additional drugs?
- Can the probability of neurotoxicity be reduced?
- If post-remission HiDAc is more active than conventional cytarabine, why is HiDAc not more effective during remission induction?

sion, and number of doses per course? High-dose schedules of cytarabine have ranged from 1 to 3 gm/m^2, administered in an infusion ranging from 1–3 h, every 12 h for 6–12 doses per course [11]. None of these dose schedules has been compared in a prospective, randomized manner. Pharmacologic studies have demonstrated saturation of the kinase enzyme which is required to activate the drug at a dose of 1.5 gm/m^2 [12], suggesting that higher doses of HiDAc, such as the 3 gm/m^2 which we utilized, may not provide further therapeutic benefit but may contribute additional toxicity.

3. What is the role of additional drugs when added to HiDAc? The CALGB, in protocol 9222 (Fig. 3), is presently comparing three doses of post-remission HiDAc to one course of post-remission HiDAc followed by a single course of etoposide and cyclophosphamide and a single course of mitozantrone and AZQ with G-CSF support.
4. Is there a manner to overcome cerebellar toxicity as was experienced by 22 of the 187 patients in our study assigned to HiDAc therapy? A multivariate analysis has revealed that age over 40 years, serum creatinine levels >1.2 mg/dl and a threefold elevation in the serum alkaline phosphatase titer are predictive factors for neurotoxicity in the patients who received HiDAc in our trials [13]; the risk for neurotoxicity was $<1\%$ if none or one of these criteria was present but rose to 37% if two or more criteria were documented. Because of the potential of neurotoxicity, concern has been raised about the use of HiDAc in elderly patients who, ironically, have a higher likelihood of having drug-resistant leukemia and most likely would benefit from more intensive treatment if it were tolerable [14].
5. Why is HiDAc, shown in our study to be highly effective in prolonging the duration of remission compared to standard-dose cytarabine, not equally superior when utilized during remission induction? Comparisons of HiDAc to standard-dose cytarabine in induction programs conducted in Australia [15] and the United States [16], have failed to show any difference in the remission rate in previously untreated adults with AML.

The outcome of our study utilizing HiDAc in patients 60 years of age or younger merits comparison with the results of two alternative strategies of post-remission management—allogeneic and autologous bone marrow transplantation. Eligibility for an allogeneic transplant is generally restricted to patients 45 years of age or younger who have a histocompatible sibling

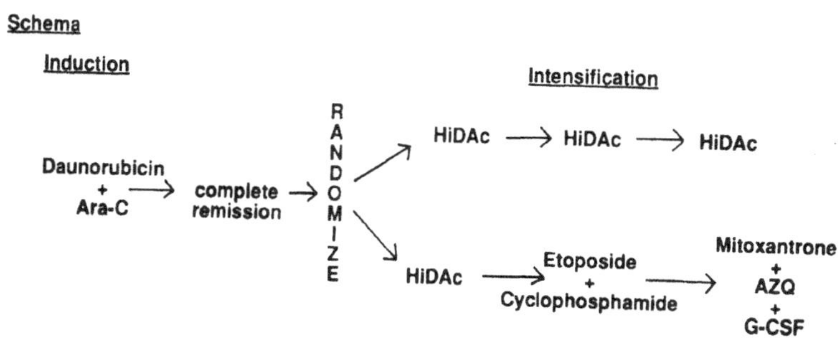

Fig. 3. Design of CALGB protocol 9222: phase III trial of intensification therapy in patients < 60 years of age with AML in first remission

Table 2. Comparison of high-dose cytarabine chemotherapy with allogeneic and autologous bone marrow transplantation as post-remission therapy for patients with AML in first remission

Treatment modality	Source	Patients (*n*)	Median age (years)	Median folllow-up time (months)	Probability of 4 year disease-free survival (%)
High-dose cytarabine	CALGB	156	40	64	43
Autologous transplant	EBMTR[17]	660	30	~48	47
Allogeneic transplant	MSKCC [18]	31	29	72	45
	Fred Hutchinson Cancer Research Center [19]	71	26	40	58
	IBMTR [20]	1343	27	49	52

[a]EBMRT, European Cooperative Group for Bone Marrow Transplantation; MSKCC, Memorial Sloan-Kettering Cancer Center; IBMTR, International Bone Marrow Transplantation Registry.
[b]Includes patients 60 years of age or younger.

while autologous transplantation may be performed on individuals as old as 55 years. A comparison of the data from our study to the results from some of the more recent autologous (registry) [17] and allogeneic (single institution [18, 19] and registry [20] transplant experiences reveals a similarity in the probability of disease-free survival after 4 years (Table 2); this is particularly true in view of the higher median age in our patient population (40 years) than that of most transplantation programs (less than 30 years). Prospective comparisons of HiDAc chemotherapy and allogeneic transplantation in trials conducted by investigators at the Univeristy of California—Los Angeles (UCLA) [21] and the Eastern Cooperative Oncology Group [5] have reached similar conclusions. A recent European study [22] comparing a single course of post-remission HiDAc chemotherapy to autologous bone marrow transplantation (randomized comparison) or allogeneic bone marrow transplantation (assigned comparison) showed there to be a higher probability of relapse in patients who received the HiDAc but a statistically indistinguishable likelihood of overall survival when the three treatment approaches were compared. Conceivably the administration of additional courses of post-remission HiDAc, such as were used in our study, might further reduce the relapse rate and make the three management approaches even more comparable [23].

References

1. Mayer RJ. Current chemotherapeutic treatment approaches to the management of previously untreated adults with de novo acute myelogenous leukemia. Semin Oncol 1987; 14: 384–396.
2. Mayer RJ, Weinstein HJ, Coral FS, Rosenthal DS, Frei E III. The role of intensive postinduction chemotherapy in the management of patients with acute myelogenous leukemia. Cancer Treat Rep 1982; 66: 1455–1462.
3. Wolff SN, Herzig RN, Fay JW, et al.: High-dose cytarabine and daunorubicin as consolidation therapy for acute myeloid leukemia in first remission: long-term follow-up and results. J Clin Oncol 1989; 7; 1260–1267.
4. McCulloch EA, Buick RN, Curtis JE, Messner HA, Senn JS. The heritable nature of clonal characteristics in acute myeloblastic leukemia. Blood 1981; 58: 105–109.
5. Cassileth PA, Lynch E, Hines JD, et al.: Varying intensity of postremission therapy in acute myeloid leukemia. Blood 1992; 79: 1924–1930.
6. Mayer RJ, Schiffer CA, Peterson BA, et al.: Intensive postremission therapy in adults with acute nonlymphocytic leukemia using various dose schedules of ara-C: a progress report from the CALGB. Semin Oncol 1987; 14(suppl 1): 25–31.
7. Mayer RJ, Davis RB, Schiffer CA et al.: Intensive post-remission chemotherapy in adults with acute myeloid leukemia. N Engl J Med 1994; 331: 896–903.
8. Dick FR, Armitage JO, Burns CP. Diagnostic concurrence in the subclassification of adult acute leukemia using French-American-British criteria. Cancer 1982; 49: 916–920.
9. Mayer RJ, Davis RB, Schiffer CA et al.: Comparative evaluation of intensive post-remission therapy with different dose schedules of cytarabine in adults myeloid leukemia (AML): initial results of a CALGB phase III study. Proc Am Soc Clin Oncol 1992; 11: 261 (abstract)

10. Moore JO, Schiffer CA, Amrein PC, et al.: G-CSF reduces the duration of both granulocytopenia and thrombocytopenia after AZQ/mitoxantrone consolidation in acute myelogenous leukemia—CALGB 9022. Blood 1992; 80(suppl 1): 291a. (abstract)
11. Bolwell BJ, Cassileth PA, Gale RP. High dose cytarabine: a review. Leukemia 1988; 2: 253–260.
12. Plunkett W, Liliemark JO, Estey E, Keating MJ, Saturation of ara-CTP accumulation during high-dose ara-C therapy: pharmocologic rationale for intermediate-dose ara-C. Semin Oncol 1987; 14(suppl 1): 159–166.
13. Rubin EH, Andersen JW, Berg DT, et al.: Risk factors for high-dose cytarabine neurotoxicity: an analysis of a Cancer and Leukemia Group B trial in patients with acute myeloid leukemia. J Clin Oncol 1992; 10: 948–953.
14. Stone RM, Mayer RJ. The approach to the elderly patient with acute myeloid leukemia. Hematol Oncol Clinics N America 1993; 7: 65–79.
15. Bishop JF, Young GA, Szer J, et al.: Randomized trial of high dose cytosine arabinoside (ara-C) combination in induction of acute myeloid leukemia (AML). Proc Am Soc Clin Oncol 1992; 11: 260. (abstract)
16. Wieck J, Kopeckk K, Appelbaum F, et al.: A randomized investigation of high-dose (HDAC) versus standard dose (SDAC) cytosine arabinoside with daunorubicin (DNR) in patients with acute myelogenous leukemia.Proc Am Soc Oncol 1992; 11: 261. (abstract)
17. Gorin NC, Labopin M, Meloni G, et al.: Autologous bone marrow tranplantation for acute myeloblastic leukemia in Europe: further evidence of the role of marrow purging by manfosfamide. Leukemia 1991; 5: 896–904.
18. Young JW, Papadopoulous EB, Cunningham I, et al.: T-cell depleted allogeneic bone marrow transplantation in adults with acute non-lymphocytic leukemia in first remission. Blood 1992; 79: 3380–3387.
19. Clift RA, Buckner CD, Appelbaum FR, et al.: Allogeneic marrow transplantation in patients with acute myeloid leukemia in first remission: a randomized trial of two irradiation regimens. Blood 1990; 76: 1867–1871.
20. Bortin MM, Horowitz MM, Rowlings PA, et al.: 1993 progress report from the International Bone Marrow Transplant Registry. Bone Marrow Transplantation 1993; 12: 97–104.
21. Schiller GJ, Nimer SD, Territo MC, et al.: Bone marrow transplantation versus high-dose cytarabine-based consolidation chemotherapy for acute myelogenous leukemia in first remission. J clin Oncol 1992; 10: 41-46.
22. Zittoun RA, Mandelli F, Willemze R et al.: Autologous or allogeneic bone marrow transplantation compared with intensive chemotherapy in acute myelogenous leukemia. N Eng J Med 1995; 332: 217–223.
23. Löwenberg B. Post-remission treatment of acute myelogenous leukemia. N Engl J Med 1995; 332: 260–262.

Acute Leukemias VI
Prognostic Factors
and Treatment Strategies
Büchner et al. (eds)

Postremission Therapy: The Role of Allogeneic Bone Marrow Transplantation in Acute Myelogenous Leukemia: An Analysis of the AML8A EORTC-GIMEMA Protocol

T. De Witte[1], S. Keating[2], S. Suciu[2], F. Mandelli[3], R. Willemze[4], P. Muus[1], M.C. Petti[3], G. Solbu[2], M. Dardenne[2], M.L. Vegna[5], M. Peetermans[2], and R. Zittoun[6]

Abstract. The AML8A protocol of the European Organization for Research on Treatment of Cancer (EORTC) and GIMEMA Cooperative Groups studied the value of allogeneic (allo-BMT) and autologous bone marrow transplantation (autoBMT) in adult acute myelogenous leukemia (AML) when performed during first complete remission (CR). Following one or two courses of remission induction treatment, 66% of patients achieved a CR. Then 168 patients who had an HLA-identical sibling were assigned to alloBMT, while 254 were randomized for an autoBMT or for a second intensive consolidation course. Disease-free survival (DFS) of the intensive chemotherapy arm was 30% at 4 years, the DFS in the alloBMT and autoBMT arms were 55% and 48%, respectively. The two BMT arms gave significantly better results than the intensive chemotherapy arm ($p = 0.03$). The main reason for failure is relapse in both the autoBMT and the chemotherapy arms, while treatment-related mortality is higher in the alloBMT arm.

Several selection biases are operational during selection for alloBMT. A preliminary, retrospective analysis of the role of alloBMT showed that patients in whom no HLA typing was performed had a poor prognosis. Furthermore, only 68% of the patients in CR1 with a donor received an alloBMT. Patients with a donor and who received no alloBMT in CR1 had a poor prognosis. AlloBMT was performed in 170 patients in CR1, including patients who achieved CR1 after salvage treatment. The DFS for this group of patients is 59% at 4 years. Of the 170 patients allografted in CR1 122 patients needed just one course of remission induction treatment to achieve CR. The DFS at 4 years was 66% and this was significantly better compared to the DFS of 41% for the 48 patients who needed more than one course of remission induction treatment to achieve CR ($p = 0.003$). The disease-free interval for early versus late remitters is 84% vs. 57% at 4 years ($p = 0.0003$), which shows that the relapse rate of early remitters is significantly lower than that of late remitters. The treatment-related mortality (TRM) for early remitters is 21% compared to 28% for late remitters at 4 years. Patients transplanted shortly after achieving CR (< 8 weeks) appeared to have a worse prognosis than those patients transplanted further into remission (DFS at 4 years: 33 vs. 67%; $p = 0.01$).

Only 60% of the CR patients without a donor were randomized between chemotherapy and autoBMT. Moreover, only 75% of the patients randomized for autoBMT received an autograft. An intention-to-treat analysis resolved this last selection bias partly. The rate of patients completing the full treatment protocol is still relatively low. In the AML8A study only 33.5% of registered patients completed the full treatment protocol. Results of BMT are difficult to interpret because of these selection biases. Most

[1]St. Radboud Hospital, Nijmegen, The Netherlands
[2]EORTC Data Center, Bruxelles, Belgium
[3]Università La Sapienza, Rome, Italy
[4]University Leiden, The Netherlands
[5]GIMEMA Data Center, Rome, Italy
[6]Hôtel-Dieu, Paris, France

selection biases, such as delay of BMT after achieving CR, are similar for autoBMT and alloBMT. Genetic selection bias is not operational in autoBMT, but exclusion of patients due to an insufficient number of colony forming units—granulocyte macrophage (CFU-GM) in the harvest forms a specific selection bias in autoBMT. Careful analysis of these selection biases is needed. Prospective randomized trials are extremely useful for this approach.

Introduction

Intensification of induction chemotherapy regimens [1, 2] and improvement of supportive care have significantly increased the rate of complete remission (CR) in acute myelogenous leukemia (AML) [1, 3–7]. Thus, 60%–80% of adult patients younger than 60 years of age achieve a CR after one to three courses of induction treatment [3]. With conventional consolidation and maintenance chemotherapy, the duration of CR has remained relatively short, with the median remission duration ranging from 10 to 20 months in most studies. The reported 5-year disease-free survival (DFS) rates were less than 25% [3, 4–6, 8]. Intensive chemoradiotherapy followed by allogeneic bone marrow transplantation (alloBMT) has resulted in long-term DFS in 45%–60% of cases if the alloBMT was performed in first CR [9]. The role of alloBMT is difficult to determine as treatment results are biased. AlloBMT for AML patients in first remission is generally restricted to patients with an HLA-identical sibling donor. Selection of patients for BMT who are in good condition occurs, excluding patients who have persistent infections or other medical complications. Bias also occurs because of the variability of interval between the achievement of CR and the time when BMT is performed [4]. This bias excludes patients who relapse rapidly.

The results obtained by alloBMT, when performed during first CR, are mainly due to the activity of combined high-dose cyclophosphamide and supralethal total body irradiation (TBI) [10]. AlloBMT may also confer an immunologically mediated graft-vs.-leukemia effect [9, 11]. The major reasons for failure following alloBMT are toxicities related to the transplant procedure itself [10], such as graft-vs.-host disease, interstitial pneumonia, and other infections [9]. Approximately 20% of patients die from transplant-related complications within 6 months. Delayed complications such as chronic graft-vs.-host disease may occur. The incidence of transplant-related complications increases with advancing age and most centers do not perform BMTs in patients who are more than 45 years of age [9].

The AML8A protocol of the European Organization for Research on Treatment of Cancer (EORTC) Leukemia Cooperative Group in collaboration with GIMEMA is the first prospective study comparing alloBMT with autologous BMT (autoBMT) and intensive consolidation chemotherapy. The main data have been published recently [12]. In this communication we emphasize some of the core results. In addition, we evaluated the influence of several prognostic factors on the survival of the patient after alloBMT.

Patients and Methods

The study is a prospective registration study conducted from November 1986 to December 1993 in 60 European centres. Patients included those with untreated newly diagnosed AML, providing ⩾30% blast cells in bone marrow smears, aged between 10 and 45 years old, with no blast crisis of chronic myeloid leukemia, and no leukemias supervening after other myeloproliferative diseases or myelodysplastic disorders of more than 6 months' duration. Patients with severe heart, renal, hepatic, or neurological concomitant disease were excluded from registration. All patients were informed of the treatment, the involved risks and gave their formal consent.

Patients were registered at diagnosis and induction treatment was subsequently given. The induction regimen consisted of daunomycin (DNR): 45 mg/m^2 on days 1, 2, and 3, i.v. push injection; cytarabine (aRA-C): 200mg/m^2 per day continuous i.v. infusion from day 1 to day 7. Patients entering a CR after one or two courses of induction regimen received a first intensive consolidation course 4 weeks after the beginning of the (last) induction course. The intensive consolidation (IC1) consisted of: aRA-C 500mg/m^2, every 12 h, by a 2-h i.v. infusion, for 6 days; amsacrine (AMSA): 120mg/m^2 i.v., on days 5, 6, and 7.

Complete remission was confirmed by blood and BM examination 3 weeks after the end of this consolidation course. At that time, in the case of HLA-A and -B identical sibling(s), the mixed leucocyte culture (MLC) was performed, followed eventually by an alloBMT. This can be considered as a randomization by genetic chance. Patients not elected for alloBMT, with confirmed CR were randomized for either a second intensive consolidation (IC2) or for autoBMT.

Duration of survival was calculated from the date of diagnosis until death. The disease-free survival (DFS) was calculated from the date of first CR until the date of first relapse or date of death in first CR. For the disease-free interval (DFI), patients who did not relapse were censored at the time of death in first CR. The duration of survival from CR corresponds to the time from first CR to the date of death. The time from the date of randomization (alloBMT, autoBMT, or IC2) until the date of death in first CR (date of relapse = censored observation) was called treatment-related mortality (TRM). Actuarial curves were calculated according to the Kaplan-Meier technique. The differences between curves were tested for statistical significance using the two-tailed logrank test.

Results

Overall Results of the AML8A Study. Out of 990 patients registered, 49 patients were either ineligible or inevaluable because of inadequate diagnosis or missing data. Following one or two courses, 623 patients (66%) achieved CR; 576 patients received a consolidation course. Then 168 patients who had an HLA-identical sibling were assigned to alloBMT, while 254 were randomized for an autoBMT using an unpurged bone marrow, or for an IC2 course. At a median follow-up of 3 years, DFS of the intensive chemotherapy arm was 30% at 4 years, the DFS in the alloBMT and autoBMT arms was 55% and 48%, respectively. The two BMT arms gave significantly better results than the intensive chemotherapy arm ($p = 0.03$). The overall survival following CR was not significantly different between the three treatment arms. More patients who relapsed after IC2 were salvaged with autoBMT in second remission. The main reason for failure is relapse in both the autoBMT and the chemotherapy (CT) arms while TRM is higher in the alloBMT arm. A significant difference was observed for the relapse rate (alloBMT < autoBMT < IC2, $p < 0.001$). The TRM was higher after alloBMT, 23%, than after autoBMT, 10%, or IC2, 6%. These analyses were performed on an intention-to-treat basis. Only 144 out of 168 patients with a donor completed alloBMT, 95 autoBMT, and 104 IC2. The data have been published recently [12].

Results of Patients Potentially Available for AlloBMT. Some minor discrepancies with regard to the overall analysis are due to the time when this analysis was made (January 1994 v. November 1993 for the overall results). Patients from some centers treated according to the granulocyte–macrophage colony-stimulating factor (GM-CSF) amendment [13] during the last phase of the study were also included in this analysis. In view of the fact that alloBMT is not performed within 8 weeks of diagnosis or in patients more than 45 years of age, all patients who died within 8 weeks registration were excluded from this analysis of the AML8A study. The total number of patients of this analysis was 827. All 827 patients were treated according to the protocol with remission induction therapy. A total of 496 patients achieved a CR after one course (60%); 108 additional patients achieved a CR after a second course of remission-induction therapy (13%); 104 patients achieved a CR after receiving salvage therapy (13%). Salvage therapy was given outside the protocol and consisted mainly of high-dose aRA-C and mAMSA. Altogether, 708 out of 827 patients who survived more than 8 weeks after registration achieved a CR. The remaining patients achieved a partial remission (1%), showed absolute resistance to treatment (11%), or had leukemic regrowth (2%). The overall DFS at 4 years for these 708 patients in CR is 39%.

Donor Availability and HLA Typing. Family HLA typing was reported in 661 patients (80%) of the 827 patients included in this analysis: 274 patients had an HLA-identical sibling donor and 387 did not. Of the patients with a histocompatible sibling 199 eventually underwent transplantation. Reasons for not performing alloBMT are listed in Table 1. Altogether 170 patients were transplanted in first CR, 29 patients at another stage in the disease. The overall survival at 4 years for the 170 patients allografted in first CR was 63%. The DFS at 4 years was 59%. The relapse rate at 4 years was 24% and the TRM 22%.

Table 1. Reasons for not performing allo BMT in patients with histocompatible sibling donors

Reason	Number
No complete remission	12
Refusal	18
Lost to follow up	2
Toxic/early death	7
Early relapse	14
Medical decision	5
Toxicity	17

Number of Courses and Time to Achieve First CR. The patients were divided into early and late remitters. Early remitters are the 122 patients who achieved CR after one course of remission induction treatment. Late remitters are the remaining 48 patients who needed more courses of remission induction treatment to achieve CR. Table 2 shows the survival statistics for patients according to the number of courses to achieve CR (early and late remitters), as well as according to the time taken to achieve CR (<5 weeks, 5–10 weeks, and ≥10 weeks). The number of courses of remission induction treatment corresponded to the actual time taken to achieve a CR. Early remitters had a significantly better survival and DFS and a significantly lower relapse rate compared to late remitters. TRM was essentially the same for both groups of patients (Table 2).

Interval Between CR and AlloBMT. Patients allografted shortly (within 8 weeks) after achieving CR have a significantly worse survival and DFS at 4 years post transplant compared to patients allografted after a longer period of CR. The survival (29%) and DFS (29%) was significantly ($p=0.01$) lower in those patients who were allografted within 8 weeks following achievement of CR compared to the other three groups. This was due to a combination of a higher chance of relapse (53%) and TRM (38%) compared to the other groups of patients who were transplanted later after achieving CR. The relapse rate and TRM were not significantly different when all four groups were compared despite the higher relapse risk and higher TRM in the patients transplanted within 8 weeks after achieving remission (Table 3).

Table 2. Results at 4 years from allo BMT in first CR according to number of courses to achieve CR or the time from diagnosis to CR

	Patients	Survival (%)	DFS (%)	Relapse rate (%)	TRM (%)
Early remitters	122	70	66	16	21
Late remitters	48	46	41	43	28
p		0.02	0.003	0.0003	0.43
Time to CR					
< 5 weeks	101	69	65	17	21
5–10 weeks	48	60	58	27	21
≥ 10 weeks	21	40	34	47	37
p		0.10	0.01	0.002	0.48

Table 3. Results at 4 years from allo BMT in first CR according to time from CR to BMT

	Patients	Survival (%)	DFS (%)	Relapse rate (%)	TRM (%)
Time CR–BMT					
≤ 8 weeks	13	29	29	53	38
9–15 weeks	81	62	60	23	22
16–24 weeks	56	72	64	22	18
≥24 weeks	20	65	60	20	25
p		0.015	0.07	0.11	0.31

Discussion

The AML8 study of the Leukemia Cooperative Groups of the EORTC and GIMEMA was undertaken to assess prospectively the role of intensive post-consolidation chemotherapy, alloBMT and autoBMT following CR in the treatment of AML. The patients registered at diagnosis represented a standard population of patients with AML (with an underrepresentation of M3 features) less than 45 years of age. The proportion of patients who entered first CR was comparable to results of large chemotherapy trials [4, 9]. Studies intended to assess these types of post-remission treatment are controversial. Often the number of patients is limited and selection biases occur. The superior results following alloBMT could be due to selection of patients before alloBMT is performed. To avoid this bias, one should start the follow up of patients at the time of HLA typing. At this time all patients would be considered for alloBMT, providing an HLA-identical sibling donor is available. In this study 73% of patients with an HLA-identical sibling donor actually received alloBMT. The remaining patients who did not receive the alloBMT had a poor prognosis (21%) or refused treatment (6%).

The number of cycles required to reach CR had an influence on the outcome of treatment. For patients transplanted in first CR the DFS was significantly higher for early remitters than for late remitters. The relapse rate was significantly higher for later remitters, but the TRM is virtually identical for both groups of patients. One would expect that patients who had received more chemotherapy to reach CR would respond worse to the intensive conditioning regimen for transplantation, resulting in a higher TRM. This did not appear to be the case. The higher DFS rate in the early remitters must therefore be due to the lower relapse rate. The actual time taken to achieve CR corresponded to the number of courses of remission induction treatment needed to achieve CR. Forman et al. [14] evaluated 69 patients who were allografted in first CR. They concluded that the length of remission induction therapy had no significant influence on the survival of the patient post transplant. In most other analyses, the length of remission induction therapy is not taken into account [15–17].

Patients transplanted shortly after achieving CR(< 8 weeks) had a worse prognosis than those patients transplanted further into remission. This could be due to the fact that these patients might have had a relapse before the transplant if they had had to wait longer for the allograft. On the other hand, patients transplanted after a longer period of time might have already been cured without the alloBMT.

The AML8A study shows major differences between the three treatment options, especially regarding the risk of TRM and of relapse. To minimize selection bias, the follow up of patients should start at the time of HLA typing of the patient. At this time, the proportion of patients who have an HLA-identical sibling donor is comparable to what could be expected in a random sample of patients with at least one sibling available for typing.

The results of this and other studies justify alloBMT in AML patients under the age of 45 years in first CR if an HLA-identical sibling donor is available. If a donor is not available, further chemotherapy with or without autograft should be considered. Only careful analysis of prospectively registered patients can evaluate treatment modalities such as alloBMT.

References

1. Berman E, Heller G, Santorsa J. Results of a randomized trial comparing idarubicin and cytosine arabinoside with daunorubicin and cytosine arabinoside in adult patients with newly diagnosed acute myelogenous leukemia. Blood 1991; 77: 1666–1674.
2. Vogler WR, Velez-Garcia E, Weiner RS, et al. A phase III trial comparing idarubicin and daunorubicin in combination with cytarabine in acute myelogenous leukemia: a Southeastern Cancer Study Group study. J Clin Oncol 1992; 10: 1103–1111.
3. Preisler H, Davis RB, Kirschner J, et al. Comparison of three remission induction regimens and two post induction strategies for the treatment of acute non-lymphocytic leukemia:a Cancer and Leukemia Group B study. Blood 1987;69: 1441–1449.
4. Zittoun R, Jehn U, Fiere C, et al. Alternating repeated postremission treatment in adult acute myelogenous leukemia: a randomized phase III study (AML 6) of the EORTC Leukemia Cooperative Group. Blood 1989; 73: 896–906.
5. Buchner T, Urbanitz D, Hiddeman W, et al. Intensified induction and consolidation with or without maintenance chemotherapy for acute myeloid leukemia (AML): two multicenter studies of the German AML Cooperative Group. J Clin Oncol 1985; 3: 1583–1589.

6. Rees JKH, Gray RG, Swinsky D, et al. Principal results of the Medical Research Council's 8th acute myeloid leukaemia trial. Lancet 1986; 2: 1236–1241.
7. Bishop JF, Lowenthal RM, Joshua D, et al. Etoposide in acute non-lymphocytic leukemia. Blood 1990; 75: 27–32.
8. Cassileth PA, Harrinton DP, Hines JD, et al. Maintenance chemotherapy prolongs remission duration in adult acute nonlymphocytic leukemia. J Clin Oncol 1988; 6: 583–587.
9. Gale RP, Champlin RE. How does bone marrow transplantation cure leukemia? Lancet 1984; 2:28–31.
10. Working Party on Leukemia. European Group for Bone Marrow Transplantation. Allogeneic bone marrow transplantation for leukemia in Europe. Lancet 1988; 2: 1379–1382.
11. Pizzolo G, et al. Natural killer cell function and lymphoid subpopulations in acute non-lymphoblastic leukemia in complete remission. Br J Cancer 1988; 58: 368–372.
12. Zittoun RA, Mandelli F, Willemze R, De Witte T, et al. Autologous or allogeneic bone marrow transplantation compared with intensive chemotherapy in acute myelogenous leukemia. N Engl J Med 1995; 332: 217–223.
13. Zittoun R, Mandelli F, De Witte T, et al. Recombinant human granulocyte-macrophage colony-stimulating factor (GM-CSF) during induction-treatment of acute myelogenous leukemia (AML). A randomized trial from the EORTC-GIMEMA cooperative groups (abstract #909). Blood 1994; 84 (suppl. 1): 231a.
14. Forman SJ, et al. Bone marrow transplantation for acute non-lymphoblastic leukemia during first complete remission: an analysis of prognostic factors. Transplantation 1987; 5: 650–653.
15. Thomas ED, Clift RA, Buckner CD. Marrow transplantation for patients with acute non-lymphoblastic leukemia who achieve a first remission. Canc Treatm Rep 1982; 7: 1463–1466.
16 .Bostrom B, Brunning RD, McGlave P, et al. Bone marrow transplantation for acute nonlymphocytic leukemia in first remission: analysis of prognostic factors. Blood 1985; 65: 1191–1196.
17. Tallman MS, Kopecky KJ, Amos D, et al. Analysis of prognostic factors for the outcome of marrow transplantation or further chemotherapy for patients with acute nonlymphocytic leukemia in first remission. J Clin Oncol 1989; 7: 326–337.

Acute Leukemias VI
Prognostic Factors
and Treatment Strategies
Büchner et al. (eds)

Impact of Marrow Transplantation in Acute Myeloid Leukemia in First Complete Remission: Experience from MRC AML-10 Trial

A.K. Burnett, A.H. Goldstone, I. Hann, R. Stevens, J.H.K. Rees, and K. Wheatley
on behalf of the Adult and Paediatric Leukemia Working Parties of the Medical Research Council, UK

Abstract. A total of 1900 patients under 56 years of age were entered into the Medical Research Council (MRC) AML-10 trial, which aimed to compare the induction schedules, and the additional impact of a bone marrow transplantation (BMT) after all patients had received four courses of intensive chemotherapy. The overall remission rate was 80% and the survival from trial entry was 40%. Of the first 1225 evaluable patients who entered complete remission (CR), 26% had a sibling donor and are expected to have an allogeneic BMT. Of the rest, 40% were randomised to autologous BMT or no further treatment (STOP). No survival benefit has been demonstrated for the addition of autoBMT although there is a significant reduction in relapse risk.

Karyotype and the percentage blasts in the bone marrow after course 1 have a considerable impact on the subsequent prognosis for the patient, irrespective of what treatment is applied. Based on a donor-available versus no-donor-available analysis, which is demonstrated to be a potentially valid way to evaluate allogeneic BMT, no survival benefit has yet been demonstrated for good and poor-risk groups. However, standard-risk patients with a donor have a modest, but significant, survival advantage compared with those who have no donor and receive chemotherapy only.

Introduction

The first studies of autologous bone marrow transplantaion (BMT) in acute myeloid leukaemia (AML) were initiated in the late 1970s, initially as a strategy to enable dose escalation at the time of relapse [1]. Shortly thereafter, studies in first and second remission were initiated. There were two main theoretical reservations about this approach. First, the assumption was that the myeloblative treatment used for allogeneic BMT was the major anti-leukaemic effect in that setting. At that time the statistical association between the relapse and the incidence and severity of graft-versus-host disease (GVHD) was known but had not actually been shown for AML in remission [2, 3]. During the 1980s as further data accumulated and the results of T cell depletion in AML became known, it became clear that a component of the curative effect of allogeneic BMT is immune mediated and that this might not operate in the autologous context. However, in vitro studies which suggest that this may not be the case and that T-cell, autoreactive against the patients own blasts, are demonstrable post autograft that are not seen with chemotherapy alone [4]. The second objection was, since the majority of AML cases would in due course relapse, then it was probable that the autologous harvest would have occult disease present which was beyond the routinely available methods of detection. This led to the development of techniques of in vitro purging, usually with a cyclophosphamide derivative [5]. However, comparative studies have never validated the value of purging, while registry data suggest that the major benefit may be confined to patients who are slow to enter complete remission (CR) or who have the autograft early

Department of Haematology, University of Wales College of Medicine, Heath Park, Cardiff CF4 4XN, UK

in CR [6]. The in vitro approach is not easy to standardise for multicentre use, and its in vitro efficacy is not easily measured. In spite of evidence from gene marking that the autograft can contribute to subsequent relapse [7], the major priority in recent years has been to conduct prospective randomised studies to ascertain the value, if any, of autograft in AML rather than evaluating purging per se.

The single-centre studies and the collected registry data suggested that patients autografted in CR1-could expect durable survival of 45%–50%, whereas when the autograft is deployed in CR2 about 30% will survive. However encouraging these results may be, there has been increasing concern that the patients presented for the procedure have been unconsciously selected [8, 9]. There is a danger that these patients were selected because they were considered to be haematologically, physically and psychologically fit to go forward to the procedure. This issue has been highlighted when the effect of time censoring is taken into account. There has therefore been a compelling need for the proper perspective evaluation of autograft in the clinical trial setting.

MRC AML-10 Trial

In the summer of 1988, the Medical Research Council (MRC) Adult and Paediatric Working Parties opened a prospective trial (AML-10) with the principal aims of comparing two induction schedules for the first two courses comprising daunorubicin, cytosine arabinoside and thioguanine (DAT) versus daunorubicin, cytosine arabinoside and etoposide (ADE) (Fig. 1). All patients who entered CR received a third amsacrine, cytosine arabinoside and etoposide, (MACE) and fourth mitoxantrone and cytosine arabinoside, (MidAc) course of chemotherpy. Those who lacked, an HLA-matched sibling donor had marrow harvested (minimum dose 1.0×10^8 nucleated cells/kg) and were randomised to an early autograft (Auto) or no further treatment (STOP). Those with a sibling donor would undergo allogeneic (allo) BMT after completing the fourth course of chemotherapy.

The intention was to evaluate any additional benefit of transplant (allo or auto) in patients who have already received four intensive courses of chemotherapy. Under these circumstances it was not felt that purging of the harvested marrow was feasible or necessary. patients in the STOP arm are eligible for an autograft if they relapse and achieve a second remission using the marrow already harvested. The myeloblation in CR1 is cyclophosphamide and TBI, and in CR2 busulphan/cyclophosphamide. Individual transplant units can choose whatever methods of GVHD prophylaxis or supportive care considered necessary. Haemopoietic growth factors are not routinely used. Patients from 0–55 years were eligible for entry, while those with a prior antecedent hematological disorders were not excluded.

Patient Entry

The trial was closed in November 1994 when 1900 patients from over 120 institutions in the United Kingdom, Ireland and New Zealand had been recruited. The median age was 36 years; 20% of entrants were children under 15 years. The French-American-British (FAB) distribution was MO = 1.7%, M1 = 17.4%, M2 = 28.2%, M3 = 15.2%, M4 = 20.6%, M5 = 9.3%, M6 = 2.9%, M7 = 2.7%. All-trans retinoic acid (ATRA) was introduced as an add-on randomised study in the FAB M3 group in January 1993. Ninety-two of the total 267 M3 patients were included in this trial which compared 5 days of ATRA only, immediately followed by chemotherapy against ATRA given together with the initial chemotherapy and continued daily until complete remission (blasts < 5% was confirmed.

At present, cytogenetic data are available on the first 1327 patients, where an evaluable result is available in 1170. A favourable karyotype (t8: 21; t15: 17, inv16) was observed in 24% of cases, whereas 12% were designated as being unfavourable (abnormalities of chromosomes 5 or 7 or a complex karyotype). The remainder were designated as standard risk and included 42% of the total with a normal karyotype.

Results

Remission Induction. The overall remission rate was 80%, being higher in the paediatric patients (91%) and lower in those > 45 years (75%); 70% of patients who achieved CR did so after the first course. There was no difference between DAT or ADE with respect to remission rate, reasons for induction failure or subsequent disease free survival.

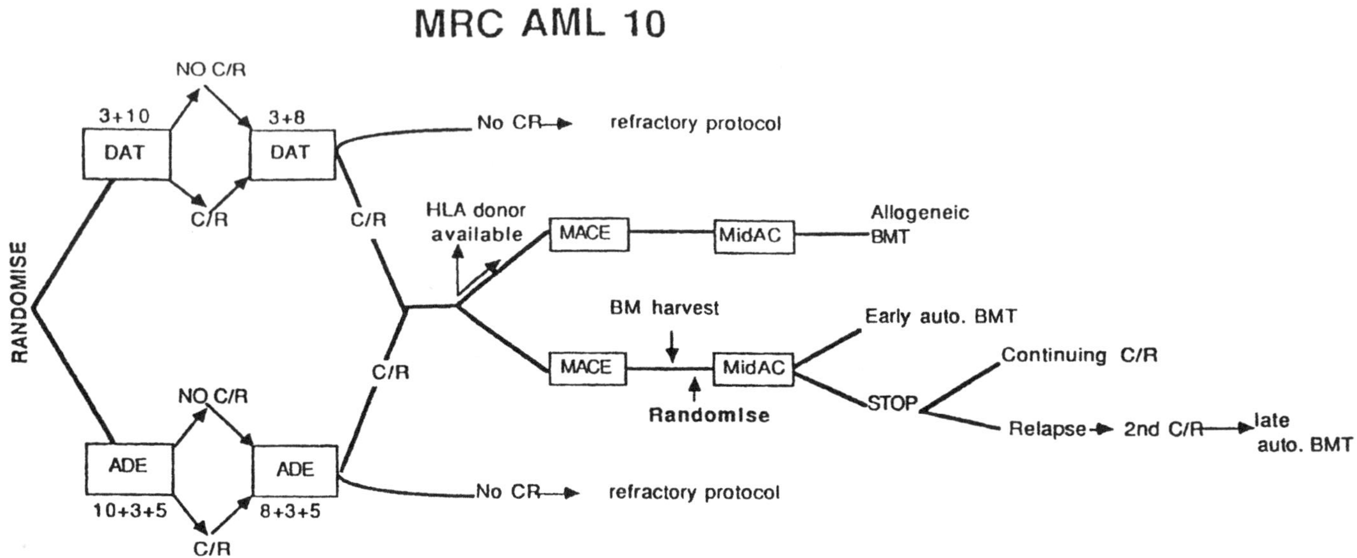

Fig. 1. MRC AML-10 trial. DAT, 10+3+5: daunorubicin 50 mg/m^2 days 1, 3, 5; cytosine arabinoside 100 mg/m^2 every 12 h; thioguanine 100 mg/m^2 days 1–5; ADE 10+3+5: daunorubicin 50 mg/m^2 days 1, 3, 5; cytosine arabinoside 100 mg/m^2 hourly; etoposide 100 mg/m^2 days 1–5; MACE, amsacrine 100 mg/m^2 days 1–5; Cytosine arabinoside 200 mg/m^2 day 1–5 by continuous infusion; by continuous infusion; etoposide 100 mg/m^2 days 1–5; MidAC, Mitozantrone 100 mg/m^2 days 1–5; cytosine arabinoside 1.0 g/m^2 every 12 h days 1–3

Progression Through the Treatment. Each successive course resulted in progressively longer periods of neutropenia and thrombocytopenia. This contributed to some difficulties in eligible patients in CR getting randomised to the AUTO or STOP option. However, only a small number of patients failed to do so because of relapse which only happened in about 3.5% of patients. Of 1225 evaluable patients, 318 (26%) had a matched donor and were expected to undergo allo BMT, data on 213 are available at the data centre. Of the remaining 907 patients, 365 (40%) were randomised to Auto ($n = 183$) or STOP ($n = 182$). The reasons for randomisation failure are illustrated in Fig. 2. This lower than expected ability to randomise has become a feature of multicentre trials of this type.

Auto vs. STOP Randomisation. A preliminary analysis of the 365 randomised patients has been reported on an intention-to-treat basis. The respective overall survivals at 5 years from the point of randomisation for auto and STOP were 55% vs. 48%. Of the 183 patients who were allocated to the auto arm, 140 are currently known to have received the procedure. The remission durations are 52% and 37% ($p = 0.1$). However the risk of relapse is substantially reduced in the auto arm, 39% vs. 61% ($p = 0.008$). The ability of the auto to reduce relapse has not been translated into a survival benefit because 13% of the auto arm died in CR, compared with none of the STOP group ($p = 0.0001$). It is clear that delayed engraftment following the auto is linked with post-auto deaths.

Overall Survival and Key Risk Factors

The overall survival of the 1900 patients entered into the trial is 41%. There is no difference in overall outcome between DAT or ADE allocations, but the prospects of survival are influenced by the patient age group, with the survival at 5 years for patients under 35 years being around 50%, and for the older patients being around 30%. In the first 1200 patients in whom successful cytogenetic analysis was available and who are evaluable, the cytogenetic group was a powerful predictor of remaining in CR.

Favourable cytogenetics comprise t15: 17, t8; 21 and inverted chromosome 16, which together applied to 16% of the patients evaluable. The overall survival of the group is 62% at 5 years. The unfavourable group demonstrated abnormalities of chromosome 5 or 7 or a complex karyotype. This group comprise 5% of the evaluable patients and is characterised by a more rapid rate of relapse and a poor overall

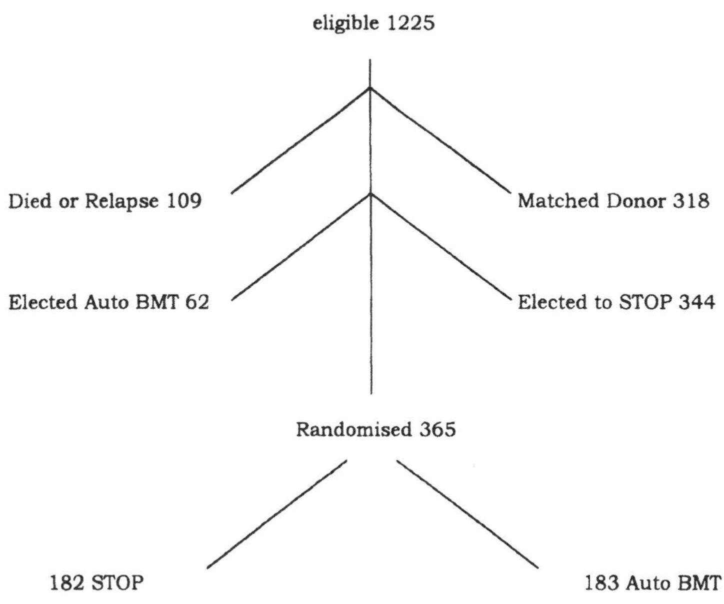

Fig. 2. Randomisation for patients in complete remission

survival at 5 years (27%). All other karyotypes—including normal—were designated as standard risk and had an intermediate overall survival (41%) at 5 years. The reason for the difference in outcome on this trial schedule was entirely attributable to relapse, since the death rate in CR was identical within the groups.

The second powerful predictor of the probability of remaining in CR was the percentage blasts recorded in the marrow on recovery from the first course of chemotherapy. This was normally undertaken on day 28–30 after the start of therapy. Based on these data, it is clear that patients with >20% residual blasts have a bad prognosis—even if they subsequently enter CR (24% at 5 years), whereas those with <5% or between 5% and 20% blasts have a similar long-term outcome (44% and 47% at 5 years) once they enter remission. This parameter is therefore of value in identifying poor-risk patients for whom alternative approaches to treatment might be appropriate.

These two parameters are independently strongly predictive of relapse in multivariate analysis ($p < 0.0001$ in both cases). Using both factors as a risk index provides a robust predictor which could form the basis of different treatment modalities. when cytogenetics or blast percentage after course 1, or the combined risk index, is examined in the context of the subsequent mode of treatment, i.e. chemotherapy alone, allo or auto BMT, it is highly predictive of the outcome in each case. This indicates that the biology of the disease is potentially more influential on the subsequent outcome than the therapeutic intervention—at least in the context of this trial schedule.

Allogeneic BMT

Of the 318 patients who have an HLA-matched sibling donor and are in CR, the data centre is aware of the outcome of 213 patients who have received a BMT. The missing 105 patients will broadly fall into three categories which are not quantifiable at this stage. There will be a proportion of patients who are moving through the treatment protocol and will come to BMT. Some will have had the BMT but the follow-up form is not yet returned, but some who are eligible for allo on the basis of having a donor available will not get a BMT, either because they are medically unfit, refuse or relapse before the transplant can be done.

In order to eliminate bias as far as possible from the alloBMT, our patients have been evaluated on an intention-to-treat basis (i.e. donor availability). In order to reduce the bias resulting from "time censoring" the comparative assessments between the allo group (donor available) and the chemotherapy only group, only patients in remission at the time of the first BMT were included in the analysis.This eliminated those patients with a donor who may have relapsed or died before that point and also the equivalent cohort of chemotherapy patients.

The importance of time censoring has been clearly demonstrated in the auto setting, and may also be operating in those patients who receive an allo BMT. The important of attempting to compare allo BMT outcome in an intention-to-treat-basis is illustrated in this trial. If the survivals at 5 years are compared in three groups, namely patients with a donor available who have received BMT, patients with a donor available who have not received BMT, and the no-donor group who received only the four course of chemotherapy, the survivals are, respectively, 70% 51%, 63%.

The fact that those with a donor and without BMT do worse than the chemotherapy only group implies that those who got the allo were subjected to selection biases which could explain the modestly superior outcome. Based on this form of anlaysis, the comparative outcomes for patients overall in terms of survival are donor 57% vs. no donor 50% ($p = 0.2$) event-free survival; donor 54%, no donor 42% ($p = 0.006$) and probability of relapse: donor 32% vs. nodonor 50% ($p = < 0.0001$).

Impact of Risk Groups

Since the risk index, as defined above, is a key parameter in defining subsequent outcome, patients have been analysed within each risk category. The relative 5-year outcomes are shown in Table 1. In terms of survival, alloBMT confers significant further benefit on standard-risk patients—who comprise 72% of all eligible patients. This is primarily because of a highly significant reduction in relapse risk which more than outweighs the procedural mortality. In good-risk patients, survival benefit cannot be demonstrated. Although the relapse risk is very small, this does not outweigh the procedural related death risk. Poor-risk patients with a donor do not survive better, largely

Table 1. Allogeneic transplant outcomes based on donor vs no donor analysis

Group	Donor (*n*)	No donor (*n*)	Surivival *p*	Remission duration *p*	Relapse *p*
Good	62	123	0.3	0.7	0.007
Standard	235	519	0.03	0.006	0.001
Poor	28	49	0.7	0.9	0.7

because there is no evidence of a reduction in relapse risk.

Discussion

The preliminary results from this large trial demonstrate a high initial remission rate and an encouraging overall survival. In common with all other trials of this design, it has proved problematic to randomise the majority of the patients to the auto option [10]. However, at the moment there is no early survival advantage of adding an auto to the four intensive courses used in this protocol. Already, however, there is a significant reduction in relapse risk, so a later survival benefit may yet emerge with longer follow up. The actuarial risk of death following auto BMT is 13% which is higher than that reported in the original single-centre series, but may be remediable since it is associated with delayed recovery of neutrophils or platelets.

Of particular importance in this trial has been the emergence of a risk index which can identify patients whose outlook is sufficiently favourable that the additional benefit of alloBMT has not yet been demonstrated—despite a highly significant reduction in relapse. The survival of those patients who actually received the allo BMT is 70% overall from the time of transplant which is a very respectable result in a multicentre trial, but is limited by the inevitable procedural-related deaths.

There is a modest, but significant advantage in survival for standard-risk patients in this trial—even when analysed on an intention-to-treat bias, i.e. even though some of the patients did not receive the therapy. The poor-risk cohort are also identified by the risk index, in whom allo BMT made no impact either in terms of survival or reduction in relapse risk. Clearly these patients have biologically unresponsive disease. It should be noted, however, that this group of patients relapse quickly, so the relatively small number who qualified for a BMT were a selected group. It is conceivable that BMT might be effective if applied at an earlier stage of disease. It might be a mistake to generalise from this study to all patients. The characteristics which have defined risk reflect what is being observed in several different trials involving different therapies. However, the failure to demonstrate benefit for auto or allo in good or poor-risk disease must be seen in the context of this protocol where four intensive courses of chemotherapy had already been given. This does not exclude the possibility of benefit for patients treated less aggresively in other schedules. The median follow up in this trial is 3 years, so clearly longer follow up is merited.

References

1. Dicke A, Spitzer G, Peters L et al. (1979) Autologous bone marrow transplantation in relapsed adult acute leukaemia. Lancet, i 514–517.
2. Weiden PL, Flournoy N, Thomas ED et al. (1979) Anti-leukemic effect of graft-versus-host disease in recipients of allogeneic marrow grafts. New England Journal of Medicine, 300. 1068–73.
3. Weiden PL, Sullivan KM, Flournoy N et al. (1981) Anti-leukemic effect of chronic graft-versus-host disease. Contribution to improved survival after allogeneic marrow transplantation. New England Journal of Medicine, 304: 1529–33.
4. Reittie JE, Gottlieb D, Heslop HE et al. (1989) Endogenously generated activated killer cells circulate after autologous and allgeneic marrow transplantation but not after chemotherapy. Blood, 73: 1351–8.
5. Rowley SD, Jones RJ, Piantadosi S, Braine HG, Colvin OM, Davis J, Saral R, Sharkis S, Wingard J, Yeager AM and Santos GW (1989) Efficacy of ex vivo purging for autologous bone marrow transplantation in the treatment of acute nonlymphoblastic leukemia. Blood, 74: 501–506.
6. Gorin NC, Labopin M, Meloni G, Korbling M, Carella A, Herve P, Burnett A, Rizzoli V, Alessandrino EP, Bjorkstrand B, Ferrant A, Loweberg Coser P, Simonsson B, Helbig W, Mauri SB, Verdonck LF, Iriondo A, Polli E, Colombat P,

Franklin IM, Souillet G and Willemze R. (1991) Autologous bone marrow transplantation for acute myeloid leukemia in Europe: further evidence of the role of marrow purging by masfosfamide. Leukemia, 5(10): 896–904.
7. Brenner MK, Rill DR, Moen RC et al (1993) Gene marking to trace origin of relapse after autologous bone marrow transplantation. Lancet 341, 85–6.
8. Burnett AK (1988) Autologous bone marrow transplantation in acute leukaemia. Leukaemia Research, 12: 531–6.
9. Gale RP & Butturini A (1989) Autotransplant in leukaemia. Lancet, ii, 315–17.
10. Zittoun RA, Mandelli F, Willemze R. et al (1995) Autologous or allogeneic bone marrow transplantation compared with intensive chemotherapy in acute myelogenous leukaemia. New England Journal of Medicine, 332: 217–223.

Acute Leukemias VI
Prognostic Factors
and Treatment Strategies
Büchner et al. (eds)

Bone Marrow Transplantation for Acute Myelogenous Leukemia

M.M. Horowitz[1], R.P. Gale[2], T. Büchner[3], A. Keating[4], P.A. Rowlings[1], K.A. Sobocinski[1], M.J. Zhang[1], and P.J. Klein[1]

Abstract. Options for post-remission therapy for acute myelogenous leukemia include consolidation chemotherapy with or without maintenance, allogeneic bone marrow transplantation, and autologous bone marrow transplantation. Rare individuals may receive a transplant from an identical twin. Risks of treatment-related mortality and relapse differ with these approaches. Leukemia-free survival appears higher with allogeneic transplants than with conventional therapy. Leukemia-free survival at 4 years is similar with allogeneic, identical twin and autologous transplants.

Introduction—Increasing Use of Bone Marrow Transplants

Bone marrow transplants are increasingly used to treat diverse diseases. A survey from the International Bone Marrow Transplant Registry (IBMTR) indicated more than 5000 allogeneic transplants in 1990 with about a 15% annual increase over the preceding 5 years [1]. Over 45000 persons received allogeneic transplants between 1970 and 1993. Widespread use of autologous transplants (including bone marrow and peripheral blood) began more recently than the use of allogeneic transplants [2]. The annual number of autologous transplants now exceeds 6000 yearly and is increasing by about 20% a year, with over 35000 recipients since 1980. About 25% of allogeneic and 15% of autologous transplants are for acute myelogenous leukemia (AML). Most of these are done in first remission. Below are summarized results of allogeneic, identical twin, and autologous transplants for AML as reported to the IBMTR and Autologous BMT Registry (ABMTR).

Methods—IBMTR and ABMTR

The IBMTR and ABMTR are voluntary working groups of over 350 transplant teams that contribute detailed data on their consecutive allogeneic and identical twin (IBMTR) or autologous (ABMTR) bone marrow and blood cell transplants to a stastistical center at the Medical College of Wisconsin [3, 4]. The IBMTR collects data on allogeneic and identical twin transplants from over 200 institutions in more than 30 countries. The IBMTR database includes 40%–45% of all allogeneic transplant recipients since 1970. The ABMTR collects data from autologous transplants in over 100 institutions in North America. The ABMTR database includes about 50% of all autologous transplant recipients in North America since 1989. IBMTR and ABMTR participants are required to report all consecutive transplants; compliance is monitored by on-site audits. Patients are followed

[1]International Bone Marrow Transplant Registry/ Autologous Blood and Marrow Transplant Registry, Health Policy Institute, Medical College of Wisconsin, Milwaukee, Wisconsin 53226, USA
[2]Bone Marrow and Stem Cell Transplantation, Salick Health Care Inc., Los Angeles, California, 90048-4520, USA
[3]Department of Internal Medicine, University of Münster, Münster 48149, Germany
[4]University of Toronto Autologous Bone Marrow Transplant Program, The Toronto Hospital, Toronto, Ontario M5G 2C4, Canada

longitudinally. Computerized error checks, physician review of submitted data, and on-site audits of participating centers ensure data quality.

Results

HLA-Identical Sibling Transplants for AML. Results of HLA-identical sibling transplants for AML correlate with the pretransplant remission state. Among recipients of HLA-identical sibling transplants reported to the IBMTR between 1988 and 1993, 5-year actuarial probabilities of relapse are 23% $\pm$ 3% for transplants done in first remission ($n=1124$), 37% $\pm$ 7% in second remission ($n=231$), and 65% $\pm$ 7% in relapse ($n=415$). Five-year probabilities of leukemia-free survival are 56% $\pm$ 3%, 37% $\pm$ 7%, and 19% $\pm$ 4%, respectively. Disease-related factors predicting outcome of conventional chemotherapy also predict outcome of HLA-identical sibling transplants for AML in first remission [5–7]. Patients with high leukocyte counts at diagnosis, French-American-British (FAB) classification M4 or M5, and certain chromosome abnormalities have lower leukemia-free survival. However, a recent IBMTR study comparing outcome of HLA-identical sibling transplants with chemotherapy in a trial of the German AML Cooperative Group suggests that leukemia-free survival is higher with transplants even after adjustment for prognostic factors like age, leukocyte count, and FAB type. A recent IBMTR study suggests that results of HLA-identical sibling transplants are improving [8]. This analysis demonstrated a decrease in transplant-related mortality of about 10% during the 1980s. Possible reasons were altered radiation schedules, use of cytomegalovirus (CMV)-negative blood products, improved antiviral therapy, and better graft-versus-host disease (GVHD) prophylaxis. There was no significant change in the risk of post-transplant relapse during this time.

Identical Twin Transplants for AML. Immune-mediated antileukemia effects (graft-versus-leukemia, GVL) appear to be important in preventing relapse after allogeneic transplants for AML [9–11]. Relapse rates after identical twin transplants (no GVL effect) are about 60%, which is similar to that reported with conventional chemotherapy. Despite higher relapse rates, leukemia-free survival after twin transplants is similar to HLA-identical sibling transplants because of decreased transplant-related mortality with a twin donor [11].

Autologous Transplants for AML. Autologous transplants for AML use cells obtained during remission and, is some cases, treated with drugs or monoclonal antibodies to remove residual leukemia cells [12–15]. Among recipients of autologous transplants for AML between 1989 and 1993, reported to the ABMTR, 3-year leukemia-free survival was 52% $\pm$ 5% for 598 patients transplanted in first remission, 37% $\pm$ 6% for 275 transplanted in second remission, and 15% $\pm$ 9% for 81 patients transplanted in relapse, with corresponding relapse rates of 42% $\pm$ 5%, 56% $\pm$ 7%, and 81% $\pm$ 10%. An IBMTR/ABMTR study comparing leukemia-free survival after HLA-identical sibling and autologous transplants in first remission shows similar leukemia-free survival at 4 years [16].

Summary

High-dose therapy followed by an HLA-identical sibling, identical twin, or autologous transplant is effective therapy for AML in first remission with leukemia-free survival rates of about 50%. Although outcome has improved over the last decade, transplant-related mortality after allogeneic transplants and relapse after identical twin and autologous transplants remain important problems.

Acknowledgments. This work was supported by Public Health Service Grant PO1-CA-40053 from the National Cancer Institute; the National Institute of Allergy and Infectious Diseases; and the National Heart, Lung and Blood Institute; and Contract No. CP-21161 from the National Cancer Insitute of the US Department of Health and Human Services; the US Army Medical Research and Development Command; and grants from Activated Cell Therapy; Alpha Therapeutic Corporation; Amgen, Inc.; Applied Immune Science; Armour Pharmaceutical Company; Astra Pharmaceutical; Baxter Healthcare Corporation; Biogen; Lynde and Harry Bradley Foundation; Bristol-Myers Squibb Company; Frank G. Brotz Family Foundation; Burroughs-Wellcome Company; Caremark, Inc.; Cell Pro, Inc; Center for Advanced Studies in Leukemia; COBE BCT Inc.; Charles E. Culpeper Foundation; Eleanor Naylor Dana Charitable Trust; Deborah J. Dearholt Memorial Fund; Eppley Foundation for Research; Glaxo Pharmaceutical; Hewlett-Packard Company; Immunex Corporation; Kabi Pharmacia; Kettering Family Foundation; Robert J. Kleberg, Jr. and Helen C. Kleberg Foundation; Herbert H. Kohl Charities; Lederle Laboratories; Eli Lilly Company Foundation; Nada and Herbert P. Mahler Charities; Marion Merrell Dow, Inc.; Milstein Family Foundation; Milwaukee Foundation/Elsa Schoeneich Research Fund; Samuel Roberts Noble Foundation; Ortho Biotech Corporation; John Oster Family Foundation; Elsa U. Pardee Foundation; Jane and Lloyd Pettit Foundation; Pharmacia; Quadra Logic Technologies; RGK Foundation; Roche Laboratories; Roerig Division of Pfizer Pharmaceuticals; Sandoz Oncology; Schering-Plough International; Walter Schroeder Foundation; Stackner Family Foundation; Starr Foundation; StemCell Technologies; Joan and Jack Stein Charities; SyStemix, Upjohn Company; and Wyeth-Ayerst Research.

References

1. Bortin MM, Horowitz MM, Rimm AA. Increasing utilization of allogeneic bone marrow transplantation III. Results of the 1988–1990 survey. Ann Intern Med 116: 505–512, 1992.
2. Cheson BD, Lacerna L, Leyland-Jones B, et al. Autologous bone marrow transplantation: current status and future directions. Ann Intern Med 110: 51–65, 1989.
3. Rimm AA, Barr JT, Horowitz MM, Bortin MM. Use of a clinical data registry to evaluate medical technologies. Int J Technol Assess Health Care 7: 182–193, 1991.
4. Horowitz M, Bortin M. The role of registries in evaluating the results of bone marrow transplantation. Treleavan J, Barrett J, eds. In: bone marrow transplantation in practice. New York: Churchill Livingstone; 1992, pp. 367–77.
5. Clift RA, Buckner CD, Thomas ED, et al. The treatment of acute nonlymphoblastic leukemia by allogeneic marrow transplantation. Bone Marrow Transplant 2: 243–258, 1987.
6. Gale RP, Horowitz MM, Biggs JC, et al. Transplant or chemotherapy in acute myelogenous leukaemia. Lancet 1: 1119–1122, 1989.
7. Tallman MS, Kopecky KJ, Amos D, et al. Analysis of prognostic factors for the outcome of marrow transplantation or further chemotherapy for patients with acute nonlymphocytic leukemia in first remission. J Clin Oncol 7: 326–337, 1989.
8. Bortin MM, Horowitz MM, Gale RP, et al. Changing trends in allogeneic bone marrow transplantation for leukemia in the 1980's. JAMA 268: 607–612, 1992.
9. Horowitz MM, Gale RP, Sondel PM, et al. Graft-versus-leukemia reactions after bone marrow transplantation. Blood 75: 555–562, 1990.
10. Weiden PL, Flournoy N, Thomas ED, et al. Antileukemic effect of graft-versus-host disease in human recipients of allogeneic-marrow grafts. N Engl J Med 300: 1068–1073, 1979.
11. Gale RP, Horowitz MM, Ash RC, et al. Identical-twin bone marrow transplants for leukemia. Ann Intern Med 120: 646–652, 1994.
12. Ball ED, Mills LE, Cornwell GG III, et al. Autologous bone marrow transplantation for acute myeloid leukemia using monoclonal antibody-purged bone marrow. Blood 75: 1199–1206, 1990.
13. Gorin NC, Aegerter P, Auvert B, et al. Autologous bone marrow transplantation for acute myeloid leukemia in first remission: a European survey of the role of marrow purging. Blood 75: 1606–1614, 1990.
14. Lowenberg B, Verdonck LJ, Dekker AW, et al. Autologous bone marrow transplantation in first remission: results of a Dutch prospective study. J Clin Oncol 8: 287–294, 1990.
15. McMillan AK, Goldstone AH, Linch DC, et al. High-dose chemotherapy and autologous bone marrow transplantation in acute myeloid leukemia. Blood 76: 480–488, 1990.
16. Keating A, Rowlings PA, Horowitz MM, et al: Comparison of HLA-identical sibling and autologous bone marrow transplants for acute myelogenous leukemia. Blood 84 (Suppl 1): 201a, 1994.

Acute Leukemias VI
Prognostic Factors
and Treatment Strategies
Büchner et al. (eds)

Autologous Bone Marrow Transplantation Versus Chemotherapy in Acute Myeloblastic Leukemia Patients: Argentinean Study Results

S. Pavlovsky, I. Fernandez, F. Lastiri, E. Bullorsky, and B. Koziner

Abstract.

Purpose. The aim of this study was to compare the impact of autologous progenitor cell transplantation (APCT) versus chemotherapy alone (CMT) in acute myeloid leukemia (AML) patients in first complete remission (CR1), in event-free survival (EFS), and overall survival (OS).

Patients and Methods. A total of 56 patients registered at the Argentine Group of Bone Marrow Transplantation (GAMTO) who received an APCT between June 1991 and November 1994 were compared to 55 patients receiving CMT registered at the Argentine Group of Treatment of Acute Leukemia (GALTA) from March 1986 to March 1994. Patients in the CMT group had to be more than 5 months in CR to be eligible. Patients of both groups were matched by age. Median age was 35 years (range 3–65 years) for APCT, and 34 years (range 3–64 years) for CMT. Eleven patients of both groups were under 16 years old. Twenty-six with APCT and 25 with CMT were males. The ablative regimen in 37 patients was the classical busulfan 16 mg/kg for 4 days, plus cyclophosphamide 120 mg/kg for 2 days. In addition, 15 patients received etoposide (VP-16) 2400 mg/m^2 in 36 h continous infusion and four received other regimens.

Results. At present 21 out of 56 patients with APCT have an event (eight treatment-related deaths, TRD and 13 relapses). No relapse were observed after 20 months. Of the 55 patients with CMT, 35 had an event (one TRD and 34 relapses) with relapses until 43 months. At 36 months, EFS and survival are 54% and 56% versus 33% and 39% in APCT and CMT groups, respectively ($p = 0.035$ and $p = 0.217$).

Conclusions. Patients who received an APCT had better EFS and OS than the CMT group. This is mainly due to lack of relapses after 20 months in the group with APCT. The small number of patients and short follow up probably preclude the observation of statistical differences in survival.

Introduction

Around 70%–80% of previously untreated patients with acute myeloid leukemia (AML) achieve complete remission (CR) with an induction therapy including 7 days of continous infusion of cytarabine and 3 days of an anthracycline (mitoxantrone or idarubicine). However, with standard-dose consolidation, with or without maintenance therapy, fewer than 25% of patients remain disease-free at 5 years [1,2]. Recently, the Cancer and Leukemia Group B [2] has confirmed the superiority of high-dose cytarabine as consolidation in terms of disease-free survival. In this randomized study, the probability of remaining in continous CR at 4 years for patients of less than 61 years was 24% in the 100 mg/m^2 cytarabine group, 29% in the 400 mg/m^2 group and 44% in the 3 gr group

The Argentine Group of Treatment of Acute Leukemia (GALTA) and Argentine Group of Bone Marrow Transplantation (GAMTO), Buenos Aires, Argentina

($p = 0.002$). Allogeneic bone marrow transplantation as consolidation in AML patients in first Cr (CR1) has resulted in a disease-free survival of 45%–60% of the patients at 5 years [1, 3]. Autologous progenitor cell transplantation (APCT) has been increasingly used following ablative therapy in AML in CR1 especially in Europe [3–5]. Most of the trials have obtained results similar to those of allogeneic transplantation with fewer transplant-related deaths (TRD), though with a higher relapse rate due to the lack of graft-versus-leukemia effect [6, 7]. Several cooperative groups have organised large randomized studies comparing allogeneic versus autologous transplant versus only consolidation therapy. The results of most of these studies suggest that the transplant groups have better long-term leukemia-free survival than the chemotherapy ones. However, many results are controversial and a statement cannot be obtained. This is mainly because, inspite a large number of initially eligible patients, only a small fraction can undergo transplantation, making the final evaluation of these studies complex [8].

The purpose of this presentation is to compare the outcome of 56 patients with AML in CR1 who received an APCT and were treated by members of GATMO with 55 patients matched by age who received the same induction, but not only chemotherapy (CMT) post CR in terms of disease-free survival and overall survival.

Material and Methods

Patients. Data from 56 patients with AML autografted in CRI were reported to the GATMO registry between June 1991 and November 1994. These patients were compared to 55 patients entered to GATLA protocols from March 1986 to March 1994, who maintained at least a CR1 for 6 months. Patients of both groups were matched by age. Eleven patients in both groups were under 16 years old, and received the same induction and intensification phase according to our current pediatric protocol 4-AML-90 [9]. The intensification phase consisted of cytarabine 3 g/m^2 every 12 h for six doses plus etoposide 125mg/m^2 daily × 4. According to the decision of each institution, after intensification children received maintenance therapy or Granulocyte colony-stimulating factor (G-CSF) was added and primed progenitor cells were collected and the patient autografted. All adult patients received similar induction with continous infusion of cytarabine 100 mg/m^2 per day for 7 days, plus 3 days of an anthracycline (daunomycin or mitoxantrone) [10]. Twenty-two patients on CMT received two courses of intensification with the same dosage of anthracycline for 2 days and cytarabine for 5 days [10], while 23 received high-dose cytarabine, as did the APCT group. No maintanence treatment was given. Patients in the APCT group received one or two intensification with high-dose cytarabine (2g/m^2 every 12 h for six doses) plus an anthracycline (mitoxantrone), followed by cytokines as a mobilzation prior to the progenitor cell collection. In 37 patients, days followed by cyclophosphamide 60mg/kg/per day for 2 days. In 15 patients etoposide 2.4 g/m^2 in 36 h infusion was added to busulfan-cyclophosphamide; four patients received other regimens.

Six patients were rescued with non-mobollised bone marrow, 25 received mobilized peripheral blood and bone marow, and 25 patients only mobilized peripheral blood progenitor cells. The hematological reconstitution according to the source of progenitor cells has been previously reportred by our group [11] and was faster with the use of peripheral blood. After the infusion of the progenitor cells, all the patients received hematopoietic growth factors (G-CSF orgranulocyte-macrophage CSF GM-CSF) until recovery of neutrophils to > 1.0 × 109/l.

Statistical Analysis. All the patients were prospectively registered at the GATLA or GATMO Data Center. Both are located in the same place and the analysis performed by the same statistician (FL).The homogenecity of the treatment groups was tested with the Kruskal-Wallis method for numerical data and the χ^2 test to compare propotions.

Disease-free survival was calculated from date of diagnosis until date of first relapse, date of death in CR1, or last follow up in CR. Overall survival was estimated from date of diagnosis to date of death or last follow up alive.

Survival and EFS survivorship functions were estimated by the Kalpan-Meier product limit method. Comparsion between curves was tested for statistical significance with the two-tailed log rank test. Treatment-related death (TRD) proportions were tested with the two-tailed Fisher exact test. The final analysis was done in Febraury 1995.

Results

Parameters at diagnosis of both groups are summarized in Table 1. Comparison of all the characteristics showed a similar distribution by sex age, French–American–British (FAB) subtypes, and number of white blood cells (WBC) Median follow up was longer in the CMT group (53 months) than the APCT group (24 months), this was due to the difficulties in finding in the GATLA Data Registry.

The TRD was higher in the APCT group with eight out of 56 (14%) deaths in a median of 51 days (range 9–111 days). The causes of death were bleeding in four cases, sepsis in one case, Cytomegalovirus (CMV) infection in two cases, and venous occlusive disease (VOD) in one case. In the CMT group only one patient (2%) had a TRD with a meningitis at 7 months ($P = 0.032$).

Thirteen patients (23%) of the APCT group relapsed, compared to 34 (62%) in the CMT group. The actuarial EFS at 36 months in 54% for the A PCT group and 32% for the CMT group ($P = 0.035$) Fig. 1. No relapses were observed after 20 months in the APCT group,

Table 1. Characteristics of autograft and chemotherapy-treated patients

Characteristics		APCT	CMT
Patients (*n*)		56	55
Male / female (*n*)		25/31	26/29
Median Age — (years)		35	34
Range — (years)		3–65	3–64
	Unclassified(*n*)	5	6
Fab Classification	M1/M2(*n*)	8/16	2/16
a	M3 / M4 (*n*)	5/18	7/21
b	M5 / M6 (*n*)	3/0	2/0
	M7/biphenotypic (*n*)	0/1	1/0
WBC × 10^3 cells/μl—Median		14.1	17.0
	Range	1.0–690	0.5–317
Time to APCT or eligible—Median (months)		7	>5
	Range (months)	4–15	
Follow up Median—(months)		24	53
	Range(months)	5–45	6–68

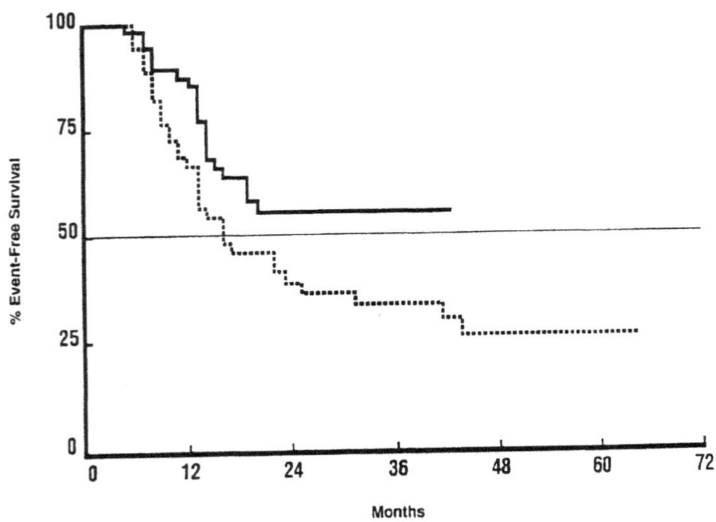

Fig. 1. Event-free survival in AML in first complete remission according to treatment. *Solid line*, APCT, $n = 21/56$, 54%; *dotted line*, CMT, $n = 35/55$, 33%; $p = 0.035$

while the last relapse in the CMT group occured at 44 months.

A total of 21 patients in the APCT group died due to TRD or leukemia-related complications, compared to 35 patients in the CMT group. At 36 months, the actuarial OS is 56% for the APCT and 39% for the CMT group ($P = 0.217$, Fig. 2). The last deaths were reported at 20 and 57 months, respectively.

Discussion

Our non-randomized study comparing chemotherapy alone versus high-dose chemotherapy followed by autologous transplantation in AML patients in CR1 showed a higher EFS in the autograft group despite a higher TRD. The difference in OS did not reach statistical significance. These results confirm several recent non-random and randomized series, using either allogeneic or autologous transplantation versus chemotherapy and reporting the better EFS of the transplant groups, without differences between the two transplant modalities [1, 3, 12]. Usually the allogeneic transplant produces, higher TRD and lower relapse rates, due to the graft-versus-leukemia effect, though with a similar number of events when compared to the autograft [1, 3]. Also most of the studies have not shown statistically significant differences in OS. This is mainly due to the higher probability of achieving a CR2 in the chemotherapy group and the chance being treated at that stage with transplantation. Longer follow up and a larger number of patients will be needed in order to see a difference between transplanting patients in CR1 or waiting until CR2.

Most of the transplant series have shown no relapses after 2 years, while later relapses are frequently seen in all the chemotherapy series, specially with low or intermediate doses of cytarabine as intensification [1–5].

The results of allogeneic or autologous transplantion in children with AML in CR1 compared to intensive courses of chemotherapy alone are much more controversial. Series from the Pediatric Oncology Group (POG) or Childrens Cancer Study Group (CCSG) in the United States as well as others in Europe, have not clearly demonstrated a benefit in EFS or OS. However, most of the studies have a short follow up; longer follow up will be needed to determine if any differences will emerge as regards the durability of the remissions [12–15].

In our study, none of the patients received purged APCT, though the benefit of using purging in CR1 has not been clearly demonstrated. Recently, Laporte et al. [5] reported the results of 64 AML patients transplanted in CR1 with mafosfamide-purged bone marrow with a leukemia-free survival of 58% at 8 years. The

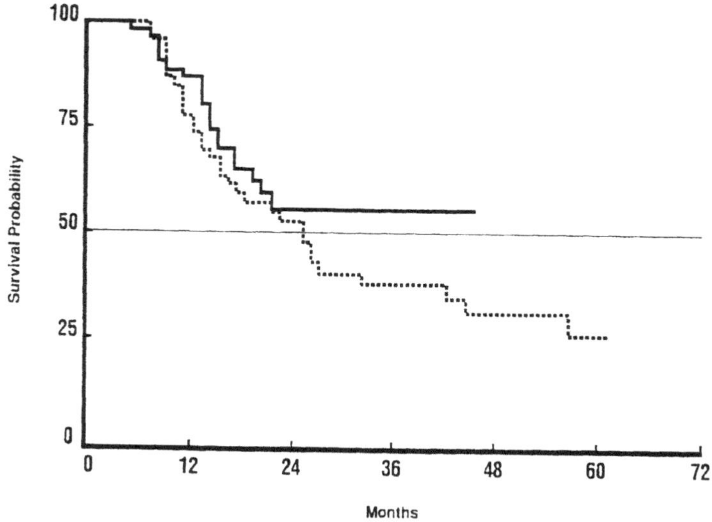

Fig. 2. Overall survival in AML in first complete remission according to treatment. *Solid line*, APCT, $n = 20/56$, 56%; *dotted line*, CMT, $n = 33/55$, 39%; $p = 0.217$

patients had 30 days to engraftment of neutrophils and 90 days for platelets.

The use of perpheral blood progenitor cells has shorted the time to engraftment; however, AML patients usually show a slower engraftment compared to other hematological malignancies and solid tumors [11]. This is probably due to the use of high-dose cytarabine during intensification.

We conclude the unpurged APCT in AML in CR1 resulted in longer EFS when compared to CMT. Up to now, we not have been able to demonstrate a significant difference in survival; however the follow up in the APCT group is still short.

Acknowledgments. The following centers and investigators included patients: FUNDALEU, Buenos Aires (S. Pavlovsky, I. Fernandez, G. Milone, J. Martinez-Rolon, P. Desmery); Instituto de Investigaciones Hematologicas, Buenos Aires (C. Corrado, S. Bruno, M.E. Aris Cancela); Hospital Nacional de Pediatria Garrahnan, Buenos Aires (F. Sackmann-Muriel, M.A. Fernandez-Barbieri); Hospital Ramos Mejia, Buenos Aires (M. Eppinger-Helft, M. Lluesmo-Goñalons); Hospital Britanico, Buenos Aires (E. Bullorsky, G.R. Stemelin, C.M. Shanley); Clinica Independencia, Munro (B. Koziner, R. Bayo, C. Dengra); Institutos Medicos Antartida, Buenos Aires (L. Feldman, V. Milovic, G. Jaimovich); Hospital Privado, Cordoba (E. Palazzo, J.J. Garcia, A. Berreta); Sanatorio Parque, Rosario (I. Cerruti, A. Gabriel); Hospital Britanico, Rosario (J. Saslavsky, J.M. Lein, S. Cheringoy). We thank Mariana Juni for collecting data and preparing and editing the manuscript.

References

1. Tallman MS, Kopecky KJ, Amos D, et al.: Analsis of prognostic factors for the outcome of marrow transplantation or further chemotherapy for patients with acute nonlymphocytic leukemia in first remission . J Clin Oncol 7: 326–337, 1989.
2. Mayer RJ, Davis RB, Schiffer CA, et al.: Intensive postremission chemotherapy in adults with acute myeloid leukemia N Engl J Med 331: 896–903, 1994.
3. Zittoun RA, Mandelli F, Willemze R, et al.: Autologous or allogeneic bone marrow transplantation compared with intensive chemotherapy in acute myelogenous leukemia. N Engl J Med 332: 217–223, 1995.
4. Cahn JY, Labopin M, Mandelli F, et al.: Autologous bone marrow transplantation for first remission acute myeloblastic leukemia in patients older than 50 year: a retrospective analysis of the European Bone Marrow Transplant Group. Blood 85: 575–579, 1995.
5. Laporte JPh, Douay L, Lopez M, et al.: One hundred twenty-five adult patients with primary acute leukemia autografted with marrow purged by mafosfamide: a 10-year single institution experience. Blood 84: 3810–3818, 1994.
6. Carella AM, Frassoni F, van Lint MT, et al.: Autologous and allogeneic bone marrow transplantation in acute myeloid leukemia in first complete remission: an update of the Genoa experience with 159 patients. Ann Hematol 64: 128–131, 1992.
7. Beelen DW, Quabeck K, Mahmoud HK, et al.: Maintenance of remission in acute myeloid leukemia by allogeneic or autologous bone marrow transplantation. Dtsch Med Wochenschr 116: 401–410, 1991.
8. Gamberi B, Bandini G, Visani G, et al.: Acute myeloid leukemia from diagnosis to bone marrow transplantation: experience from a single centre. Bone Marrow Transplant: 14: 69–72, 1994.
9. Sackmann Muriel F, Zubizarreta P, Felice M, et al.: Results of treatment with an intensive induction regimen using idarubicin in combination in children with acute myeloblastic leukemia. Blood 81: suppl 1, 145a, 1994.
10. Pavlovsky S, Gonzalez Llaven J, Garcia Martinez MA, et al.: A randomized study of mitoxantrone plus cytarabine versus daunomycin plus cytarabine in the treatment of previously untreated adult patients with acute nonlymphocytic leukemia. Ann Hematol 69:11–15, 1994.
11. Pavlovsky S, Milone G, Fernandez I, et al.: Comparison of hematological recovery and supportive care requirement according to source of mobilized progenitor cells: bone marrow + peripheral blood (PB) vs. PB alone. Proc ASCO 13: 382, 1994.
12. Nesbit ME, Buckley JD, Feig SA, et al.: Chemotherapy for induction of remission of childhood acute myeloid leukemia followed by marrow transplantation or multiagent chemotherapy: a report from the Childrens Cancer Group. J Clin Oncol 12: 127–135, 1994.
13. Creutzig U, Bender-Gotze C, Klingebiel T, et al.: Comparison of chemotherapy alone with allogeneic bone marrow transplantation in first full remission in children with acute myeloid leukemia in the AML-BFM-83 and AML-BFM-87 studies. Matched pair analysis. Klin Padiatr 204: 246–252, 1992.
14. Woods WG, Kobrinsky N, Buckley J, et al.: Intensively timed induction therapy followed by autologous or allogeneic bone marrow transplantation for children with acute myeloid leukemia or myelodysplastic syndrome: a Childrens Cancer

Group pilot study. J Clin Oncol 11: 1448–1457, 1993.
15. Ravindranath Y, Yeager A, Krischer J, et al.: Intensive consolidation chemotherapy vs purged autologous bone marrow transplantation early in remission for treatment of childhood acute myeloid leukemia: Preliminary results of Pediatric Oncology Group study 8821. Proc ASCO :13: 320, 1994.

Acute Leukemias VI
Prognostic Factors
and Treatment Strategies
Büchner et al. (eds)

Granulocyte–Macrophage Colony-Stimulating Factor in the Therapy of Adults with De Novo Acute Myeloblastic Leukemia: An Update of a Double-Blind Randomized, Placebo-Controlled Trial

G. Heil[1], L. Chadid[1], D. Hoelzer[2], G.Seipelt[2], P. Mitrou[2], C. Huber[3], K. Kolbe[3], R. Mertelsmann[4], A. Lindemann[4], J. Frisch[5], U. Nicolay[5], W. Gaus[6], and H. Heimpel[1]

Abstract. We investigated whether granulocyte-macrophage colony-stimulating factor (GM-CSF) given concomitantly with chemotherapy (CT) improves the outcome of adults with de novo acute myeloblastic leukemia (AML) by increasing the efficacy of CT and reducing infections. CT included cytarabine (ara-C) daunorubicin, and etoposide (DAV) for induction and early consolidation therapy and one cycle with high-dose (patients aged ≤50 years) or intermediate-dose ara-C (patients aged >50 years) /daunorubicin for late consolidation therapy. Eighty patients were randomized after DAV 1 to receive either GM-CSF (*Escherichia coli*, 250 μg/m² per day, s.c.) or placebo starting 48 h prior to DAV II and the subsequent courses and given throughout CT until the absolute neutrophil count had recovered to >500/μl. The CR was 81% in the GM-CSF and 79% in the placebo group (p=0.57; Fisher's exact test). After a median follow up of 35 months the probability of relapse-free survival (RFS) at 41 months was 42% in the GM-CSF and 41% in the placebo group (p=0.89; log-rank test). The probability of RFS for patients aged ≤50 years was 65% in the GM-CSF versus 58% in the placebo group (p=0.31; log-rank test). In patients aged >50 years the probability of RFS under GM-CSF was 20% versus 31% in the placebo group (p=0.28; log-rank test).

Granulocyte macrophage CSF did not shorten the period of neutropenia ≤500/μl, while it prolonged the duration of thrombocytopenia ≤25000/μl, especially in patients aged over 50 years. Taken together, although GM-CSF does not have a significant effect on treatment outcome, an age-dependent effect on treatment outcome cannot be excluded for the present.

Introduction

Recent advances in the treatment of adults with de novo acute myelogenous leukemia (AML) have led to complete remission (CR) rates of 60%–80%, and about 20%–30% of the patients remain free of recurrence and are probably cured (for review see [1,2]. This progress is the result of the identification of effective chemotherapeutic agents, improved supportive care, and finally the intensification of both remission induction and postremission therapy. Further improvement of the prognosis may be achieved by an even more intensified chemotherapy (CT).

In this context, hematopoeitic growth factors such as granulocyte–macrophage colony-stimulating factor (GM-CSF) and granulocyte colony-stimulating factor (G-CSF) are of interest, because of their capability to ameliorate CT-induced myelosuppression and associated complications and thereby reduce the dose-limiting toxicity (for review see [3–9]). In addition, GM-CSF as well as G-CSF have been found to

[1]Department of Internal Medicine III, University of Ulm, Germany
[2]Department of Hematology/Oncology, University of Frankfurt, Germany
[3]Department of Hematology/Oncology, University of Mainz, Germany
[4]Department of Hematology/Oncology, University of Freiburg, Germany
[5]Behringwerke AG, Marburg, Germany
[6]Department of Biometry and Medical Documentation, University of Ulm, Germany

enhance the cytotoxic effect of chemotherapeutic agents on AML blasts in vitro [10,11] and in vivo (for review see [7]). However, a negative impact on treatment outcome cannot be excluded in that they might increase the susceptibility of normal hematopoeitic progenitors to CT and/or stimulate the leukemic re-growth after CT, since its stimulatory effect on normal and malignant progenitors is well documented [8, 9, 12, 13]. For further analysis of the role of GM-CSF in AML therapy, a double-blind, placebo-controlled multicenter trial was conducted. We felt this study necessary since data from clinical trials comparing the effect of GM-CSF in AML therapy to historical controls were contradictory in that both a positive effect of GM-CSF on CR rate and/or on neutrophil recovery after CT [14, 15], as well as a negative effect on CR rate and survival probability (16) had been described. The aim of this study was to test the hypotheses that (a) the efficacy of CT is increased by "priming" of the AML blasts by GM-CSF given prior to and concomitant with the CT; and (b) that the period of CT-induced neutropenia and the incidence of infections is reduced by GM-CSF given after CT. The median follow up of this study is now 35 months.

Patients and Methods

Patients. The entry criteria included: diagnosis of de novo AML French-American-British classification (FAB) M1-M6 [17], age of the patient between 15 and 75 years, women after exclusion of pregnancy, and written informed consent of the patient or legal guardian. According to these criteria 82 patients were eligible for this study between May 1990 and November 1991.

Treatment. The first induction course (DAV I) included cytarabine (ara-C, 100 mg/m^2, on days 1-8 continuous intravenous infusion (civi), daunorubicin (60 mg/m^2, i.v. bolus infusion on days 3-5) and etoposide (100 mg/m^2, on days 4-8, 2-h i.v. infusion). The second induction course (DAV II) was started on day 21 including ara-C (100 mg/m^2, on days 1-7 24-h civi), daunorubicin (45 mg/m^2, bolus i.v. infusion on days 3-4), and etoposide (100 mg/m^2, on days 3-7, 2-h i.v. infusion). Patients in CR after DAV II received an identical third cycle of the DAV regimen (DAV III) as early consolidation after recovery of the neutrophil count above 1500/µl and of the thrombocytes above 100 000/µl. Patients not in CR after DAV II were regarded as treatment failures and excluded from further-protocol therapy. Late consolidation therapy was intitated 4 weeks after recovery from DAV III and included one cycle with high-dose ara-C (3 g/m^2, 2-h i.v. infusion, 12 doses) and daunorubicin (30 mg/m^2, bolus i.v. infusion on days 7-9) (HDA-DNR) for patients aged $\leqslant 50$ years, who were not candidates for an allogeneic bone marrow transplantation. Patients aged >50 years received a reduced dose of ara-C (0.6 g/m^2, 12 doses; IDA-DNR).

Randomization. The patients were randomized after DAV I to receive either recombinant human GM-CSF (*Escherichia coli*, 250 µg/ m^2 per day, s.c.) or placebo. The participating centers received GM-CSF/placebo in numbered, unlabeled vials, which were assigned to the individual patients by the statistical center. GM-CSF/placebo therapy was started 48 h prior to DAV II and the subsequent courses and was continued until the patients had recovered from CT- induced neutropenia with an absolute neutrophil count over 500/µl on at least 3 consecutive days.

The treatment protocol and informed consent form had been approved by the Ethics Committee of the University of Ulm.

Supportive Care. Prophylactic platelet transfusions were given when platelet counts dropped below 20 000/µl. Antimicrobial prophylaxis and interventional antibiotic and/or antifungal therapy were performed as previously described [18].

Evaluation. The remission status was evaluated after the second induction course (DAV II) according to the Cancer and Leukemia Group B (CALGB) criteria. Toxicity was quantitated according to the Eastern Cooperative Oncology Group (ECOG) grading system. Life tables were calculated according to the method of Kaplan and Meier for overall survival (calculated from the 1st day of chemotherapy to death) and for relapse-free survival (calculated from the 1st day of CR to relapse or death in first CR [19]. Patients, who underwent bone marrow transplantation (BMT) were censored at the time of transplantation. The closing data for statistical evaluation was March 30, 1994.

Results

Patient Characteristics

Eighty out of 82 patients could be randomized. The median age of the 80 randomized patients was 50 years (range 17–73 years). Sex, leucocyte count, and FAB subtypes were equally distributed between the GM-CSF and placebo groups.

Results of the Induction Therapy

The results of the induction therapy are detailed on Table 1.

Relapse Free Survival

Sixteen patients of the GM-CSF group (four ⩽50 years old, 12 > 50 years old) and 14 patients of the placebo group (five ⩽50 years old, nine > 50 years old) relapsed. In addition, a 47-year-old patient of the placebo group died in CR during late consolidation therapy.

Five GM-CSF patients aged ⩽50 years underwent BMT in first CR. Another two GM-CSF patients with persistent disease after DAV II underwent BMT after an alternate salvage therapy.

Eleven patients of the placebo group underwent BMT including seven patients in first CR (five ⩽50 years old, two ⩽50 years old). Three patients aged ⩽50 years with persistent disease after DAV II underwent BMT after an alternate salvage therapy and one 51-year old patient underwent BMT in second CR.

After a median follow up of 35 months, the probability of relapse-free survival (RFS) at 41 months was 42% (95% confidence intervals, CI, 22%–61%) for the GM-CSF patients versus 41% (95% CI, 21%–61%) for the placebo group (P=0.89; log-rank test). Median remission duration (MRD) was 24 months for the GM-CSF and and 17 months for the placebo group respectively. The probability of RFS for patients aged ⩽50 years was 65% (95% CI, 36%–95%) under GM-CSF versus 58% (95% CI, 31%–85%) in the placebo group (p=0,31; log-rank test; Fig. 1). In patients aged > 50 years the probability of RFS under GM-CSF was 20% (95% CI, 0%–40%; MRD=9 months) versus 31% (95% CI, 6%–56%) in the placebo group (MRD=17months; p=0, 28; log-rank test; Fig. 2.).

Overall Survival

Nineteen patients of the GM-CSF group (five ⩽50 years old, 14 > 50 years old) died including five patients with progressive disease after the second induction course (DAV II) and another 14 patients who died in relapse. In the placebo group, 16 patients (eight ⩽50 years, eight > 50 years old) died including one patient in CR during late consolidation therapy, five patients with progressive disease after DAV II, and ten patients in relapse.

The probability of survival after 43 months was 45% (95% CI, 28%–62%) in the GM-CSF versus 49% (95% CI, 31%–67%) in the placebo group with a median survival time (MST) of 19 months of the GM-CSF versus 31 months of the placebo group (p=0.66; log-rank test).

Probability of survival was 70% (95% CI, 47%–93%) for the GM-CSF patients aged ⩽50 years versus 50% (95% CI, 24%–76%) in the placebo group (p=0.26; log-rank test; Fig. 3). The probability of survival of the GM-CSF patients aged >50 years was 24% (95% CI, 3%–44%; MST=14 months) versus 50% (95% CI, 26%–75%) in the placebo group (p=0.08; log-rank test; Fig. 4).

Toxicity

The hematological toxicity is detailed on Table 2. The duration of thrombocytopenia ⩽25 000/μl was longer after all treatment courses in the GM-CSF group, with a significant difference after the DAV II, DAV III, and IDA/DNR course. This effect was more pronounced in those patients aged > 50 years.

GM-CSF has neither a significant effect on the incidence of severe documented infections nor on the non-hematological toxicity.

Discussion

The strategy to give GM-CSF prior to, concomitantly, and after chemotherapy aimed at conditioning of priming AML blasts for CT and thereby promoting drug-induced cell kill as well as an accelerating neutrophil recovery after CT. The study design differed from recent trials [14, 16, 20] in that the GM-CSF therapy was only initiated with the second induction course. As a consequence, no dose modification or patient selection on the basis of leukemic blast number

Table 1. Results of induction therapy in the randomized patients

	All patients				Patients aged ≤ 50 years				Patients aged > 50 years			
	GM-CSF (n = 41)		Placebo (n = 39)		GM-CSF (n = 22)		Placebo (n = 21)		GM-CSF (n = 19)		Placebo (n = 18)	
	(*n*)	(%)	(*n*)	(%)	(*n*)	(%)	(*n*)	(%)	(*n*)	(%)	(*n*)	(%)
Complete remission	33	81	31	79	18	82	16	76	15	79	15	83
Partial remission	1	2	1	3	0	0	1	5	1	5	0	0
Failure	6	15	7	18	3	14	4	19	3	16	3	17
Not evaluable	1	2	0	0	1	4	0	0	–		–	

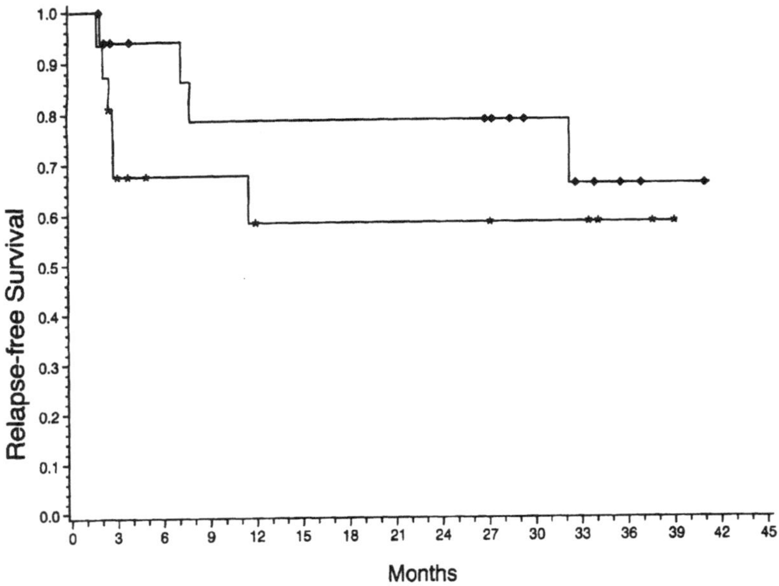

Fig. 1. Relapse-free survival of patients aged ⩽50 years. *Rhombi*, GM-CSF: $n = 18$; *Stars*, placebo: $n = 16$. The probability of relapse-free survival after 41 months is 65% (95% CI, 35%–95%) for the GM-CSF patients and 58% (95% CI, 32%–84%) for the placebo patients. *Marks* indicate patients remaining in remission and alive. $p = 0.31$, log-rank test

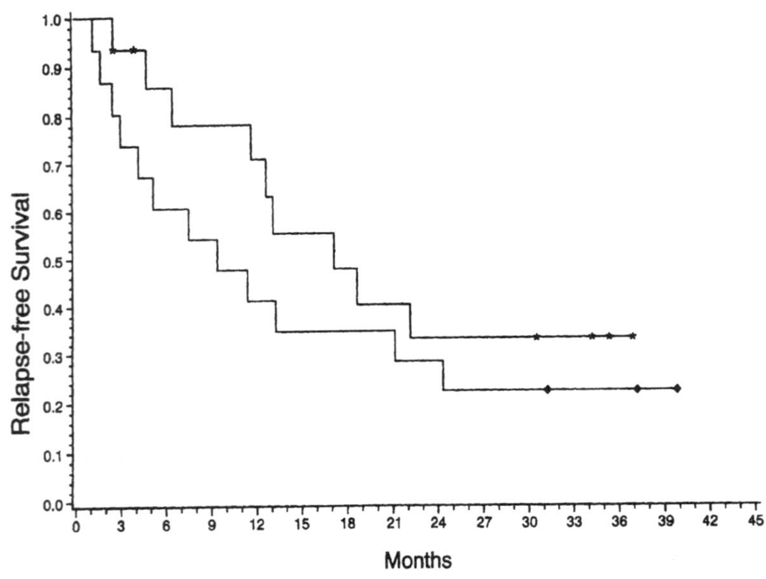

Fig. 2. Relapse-free survival of patients aged >50 years. *Rhombi*, GM-CSF: $n = 15$; *Stars*, placebo: $n = 15$. The probability of relapse-free survival after 41 months is 20% (95% CI, 0%–40%) for the GM-CSF patients and 31% (95% CI, 5%–57%) for the placebo patients. The median duration of the relapse-free survival is 9 months for the GM-CSF and 17 months for the placebo group. *Marks* indicate patients remaining in remission and alive. $p = 0.28$, log-rank test

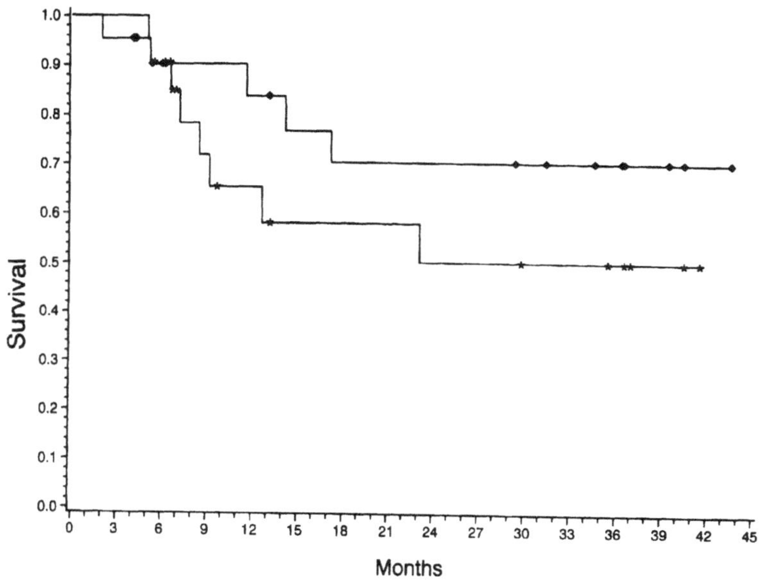

Fig. 3. Overall survival of patients aged ⩽ 50 years. *Rhombi*, GM-CSF: $n = 22$; *Stars* placebo: $n = 21$). The probability for ongoing survival at 42 months is 70% (95% CI, 48%92%) for the GM-CSF and 50% (95% CI, 24%–76%) for the placebo group with a median survival time of 23 months for the placebo group. The *marks* represent surviving patients. $p = 0.26$; log-rank test

Table 2. Hematological toxicity

Chemotherapy cycle	Study drug	Patients (n)	Duration of neutropenia ⩽ 500/µl	Duration of thrombopenia ⩽ 25 000/µl
			Median (days)	Median (days)
DAV I	—	82	19.5	16.5
DAV II	GM-CSF	40	12.5	10.0
	Placebo	39	11.0	7.0*
DAV III	GM-CSF	29	12.0	11.0
	Placebo	30	11.5	5.5*
HDA / DNR	GM-CSF	11	25.0	26.0
	Placebo	8	22.5	21.5
IDA / DNR	GM-CSF	6	17.0	21.0
	Placebo	11	16.0	12.0

*$p < 0.05$ (Wilcoxon test).

was required. The favorable CR rate of 81% in the GM-CSF group argues in favor of an equivalent antileukemic activity of this strategy and largely excludes a negative effect of GM-CSF on treatment outcome, e.g., by a restimulation of the leukemic clone [21] and/or a protective effect on the clonogenic leukemic blasts from the cytotoxic effect of ara-C [22, 23]. On the other hand, GM-CSF has no significant impact on the outcome of the patients. This is in line with previous data of Witz and co-workers [24] in 220 elderly AML patients and suggests that GM-CSF did not exert a priming effect in vivo. Residual blasts may have an altered GM-CSF response shortly after a preceding chemotherapy (DAV I). Supporting evidence for this hypothesis is provided by recent data of te Boekhorst and co-workers [25] who found a reduced growth factor-enhanced cytotoxicity in blasts of relapsed or primary refractory AML

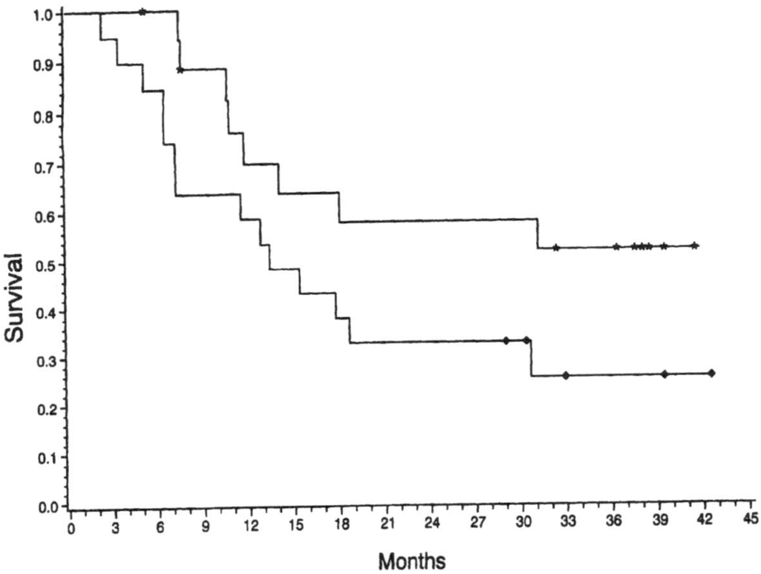

Fig. 4. Overall survival of patients aged < 50 years. *Rhombi*, GM-CSF: *n*-19; *Stars* placebo: $n = 18$). The probability for ongoing survival at 42 months is 24% (95% CI, 4%–44%) for the GM-CSF and 50% (95% CI, 26%–74%) for the placebo group with a median survival time of 14 months for the GM-CSF group. The marks represent surviving patients. $p = 0.008$; long-rank test

blasts compared with the effect on blasts isolated at diagnosis of these patients. Finally, the priming effect of GM-CSF might be age dependent as suggested by a separate analysis of the two age groups which differed in the late consolidation therapy they received. This analysis suggests opposite effects in the two age groups, which may cancel each other out and thus obscure GM-CSF activity in the GM-CSF group as a whole. Büchner and co-workers [26] made similar observations with respect to the RFS with a trend in favor of GM-CSF in patients aged 60 years or less (63% versus 52%; $p = 0.07$).

Further evidence that elderly patients respond in a different way to GM-CSF is provided by the observation that the GM-CSF-induced delay in platelet recovery was more pronounced in that particular age group. In contrast to recent reports (for review see [7]), in our trial GM-CSF did not accelerate neutrophil recovery. One possible explanation for this phenomenon and the delayed platelet recovery is that GM-CSF given concomitantly with chemotherapy primed normal prognitors and thereby in-creased the cytotoxic effect of the chemotherapy on these cells.

As previously reported [27], GM-CSF had no significant effect on the incidence of severe infectious episodes and did not increase the non-hematological toxicity.

In conclusion, GM-CSF as an adjunct to AML chemotherapy seems feasible in the selected strategy. The treatment outcome of the patients aged $\leqslant 50$ years makes this concept worth pursuing, while the outcome of the older patents under GM-CSF calls this strategy for therapy of de novo AML patients aged > 50 years into question.

Acknowledgment. The authors are indebted to M. Steinke for his help in preparing the manuscript.

References

1. Stone R.M. and Mayer RJ. Treatment of the newly diagnosed adult with de novo acute myeloid leukemia. In: Hematology/oncology: Clinics of North America: Management of acute leukemia, edited by Bloomfield, C.D., Herzig, G.P., Chohan, N. and Kaiser, N.Piladelphia, London, Toronto, Montreal, Sydney, Tokyo: W.B. Saunders Company, 1993, p. 47–64.
2. Stone, R.M. and Mayer, R.J. The approach to the elderly patient with acute myeloid leukemia. In: Hematology/Oncology: Clinics of North America: Management of acute leukemia, edited by Bloomfield, C.D., Herzig, G.P., Chohan, N. and

Kaiser, N. Philadelphia, London, Toronto, Montreal, Sydney, Tokyo: W: B. Saunders Company, 1993, p. 65–80.
3. Bernstein SH (1993) Growth factors in the management of adult acute leukemia. Hematol Oncol Clin North Am 7: 255–274
4. Löwenberg B, Touw IP (1992) Haemopoietic growth factors in acute myeloblastic and lymphoblastic leukaemia. Baillieres Clin Haematol 5: 599–618
5. Robinson BE, Quesenberry PJ (1990) Hematopoietic growth factors: overview and clinical applications, Part II. Am J Med Sci 300: 237–244
6. Williams ME, Quesenberry PJ (1992) Hematopoietic growth factors. Hematol Pathol 6: 105–124
7. Hoelzer D, Seipelt G (1995) Granulocyte colony-stimulating factor and granulocyte-macrophage colony-stimulating factor in the treatment of myeloid leukemia. Current Opinion in Hematology 2: 196–203
8. Lieschke GJ, Burgess AW (1992) Granulocyte colony-stimulating factor and granulocyte-macrophage colony-stimulating factor (Second of two parts). N Engl J Med 327: 99–106
9. Lieschke GJ, Burgess AW (1992) Granulocyte colony-stimulating factor and granulocyte-macrophage colony-stimulating factor (First of two parts). N Engl J Med 327: 28–35
10. Andreef M, Welte K (1989) Hematopoietic colony-stimulating factors. Seminars in Oncology 16: 211–229
11. Tafuri, A. and Andreeff, M. Cell kinetic modulation of hematological malignancies by cytokines: recruitment therapy to overcome cytokinetic resistance. In: Hematopietic growth factors in clinical application, edited by Mertelsmann, R. and Herrmann, F. New York, Basel: Marcel Dekker, 1990, p. 381–399.
12. Griffin JD, Young D, Herrmann F, Wiper D, Wagner K, Sabbath KD (1986) Effects of recombinant human GM-CSF on proliferation of clonogenic cells in acute myelobsastic leukemia. Blood 67: 1448–1453
13. Vellenga E, Young DC, Wagner K, Wiper D, Ostapovicz D, Griffin JD (1987) The effects of GM-CSF and G-CSF in promoting growth of clonogenic cells in acute myeloblastic leukemia. Blood 69: 1771–1776
14. Bettelheim P, Valent P, Andreeff M, Tafuri A, Haimi J, Gorischek C, Muhm M, Sillaber C, Haas O, Vieder L, Maurer D, Schulz G, Speiser W, Geissler K, Kier P, Hinterberger W, Lechner K (1991) Recombinant human granulocyte-macrophage colony-stimulating factor in combination with standard induction chemotherapy in de novo acute myeloid leukemia. Blood 77: 700–711
15. Büchner T, Hiddemann W, Koenigsmann M, Zuhlsdorf M, Wormann B, Boeckmann A, Freire EA, Innig G, Maschmeyer G, Ludwig WD, Sauerland M, Heinecke A, Schulz G (1991) Recombinant human granulocyte-macrophage colony-stimulating factor after chemotherapy in patients with acute myeloid leukemia at higher age or after relapse. Blood 78: 1190–1197
16. Estey E, Thall PF, Kantarjian H, O'Brien S, Koller CA, Beran M, Gutterman J, Deisseroth A, Keating M (1992) Treatment of newly diagnosed acute myelogenous leukemia with granulocyte-macrophage colony-stimulating factor (GM-CSF) before and during continuous-infusion high-dose ara-C + daunorubicin: comparison to patients treated without GM-CSF. Blood 79: 2246–2255
17. Bennett JM, Catovsk D, Daniel MT, Flandrin G, Galton DAG, Gralnick HR, Sultan C (1976) Proposals for the classifcation of the acute leukaemias. Br J Haematol 33: 451–458
18. Kurrle E, Ehninger G, Fackler-Schwalbe E, Freund M, Heil G, Hoelzer D, Link H, Löffler B, Lösch A, Mitrou PS, Öhl S, Queisser W, Schlimok G, Wandt H (1990) Consolidation therapy with high-dose cytosine arabinoside. Experiences of a prospective study in acute myleoid leukaemia. Haematology and Blood Transfusion 33: 254–260
19. Kaplan EL, Meier P (1958) Nonparametric estimation from incomplete observations. J Amer Stat Assoc 53: 457–481
20. Visani G, Damiani D, Cenacchi A, Russo D, Revignas G, Gamberi B, Fanin R, Fogli M, Baccarani M, Tura S (1991) Granulocyte-macrophage colony-stimulating factor in acute non-lymphocytic leukemia before and after chemotherapy. A hematol 63: 276–281
21. Königsmann M, Hiddemann W, Büchner T (1991) Reversible leukaemic regrowth under GM-CSF treatment after chemotherapy for AML. Leuk Res 15: 37–41
22. Koistinen P, Wang C, Curtis JE, McCulloch EA (1991) Granulocyte-macrophage colony-stimulating factor and interleukin-3 protect leukemic blast cells from ara-C toxicity. Leukemia 5: 789–795
23. Sachs L, Lotem J (1993) Control of programmed cell death in normal and leukemic cells: new implications for therapy. Blood 82: 15–21
24. Witz F, Harousseau JL, Cahn JY, Abgrall JF, Briere J, Sadoun A, Guyotat D, Hurteloup P, Mercier M, Berthaud Pon behalf of the GOELAM group (1994) GM-CSF during and after remission induction treatment for elderly patients with acute myeloid leukemia (AML). Blood 84, Suppl. 1: 231 (abstract)
25. te Boekhorst PA, Löwenberg B, Sonneveld P (1994) Hematopietic growth factor stimulation and cytarabine cytotoxicity in-vitro: effects in untreated and relapsed or primary refractory acute myeloid leukemia cells. Leukemia 8: 1480–1486
26. Büchner T, Hiddemann W, Wörmann B, Rottmann R, Zühlsdorf M, Maschmeyer G, Ludwig WD, Sauerland MC, Frisch J, Schulz G (1994) GM-CSF multiple course priming and long-term administration in newly diagnosed AML. Hematopietic and therapeutic effects. Blood 84, Suppl. 1 (abstract 95)
27. Heil G, Chadid L, Hoelzer D, Seipelt G, Mitrou P, Huber C, Kolbe K, Mertelsmann R, Lindemann A, Frisch J, Nicolay U, Gaus W, Heimpel H (1995) GM-CSF in a double-blind randomized, placebo controlled trial in therapy of adult patients with de-novo acute myeloid leukemia (AML). Leukemia 5: 3–9

Acute Leukemias VI
Prognostic Factors
and Treatment Strategies
Büchner et al. (eds)

Long-term Follow Up of a Prospective Multicenter Trial with a High-Dose Cytosine Arabinoside and Daunorubicin Postremission Therapy in Adults with De Novo Acute Myeloid Leukemia

G. Heil[1], P.S. Mitrou[2], D. Hoelzer[2], M. Freund[3], H. Link[3], G. Ehninger[4], B. Steinke[4], S. Öhl[5], H. Wandt[5], E. Fackler-Schwalbe[6], G. Schlimok[6], A. Lösch[7], W. Queißer[7], B. Löffler[8], W. Gaus[9], J. Högel[9], H. Heimpel[1], and E. Kurrle[1]

Abstract. A total of 149 consecutive de novo acute myeloid leukemia (AML) patients aged 50 years or less (median age = 37 years) were enrolled in this prospective multicenter trial initiated in May 1985. All patients received the same induction and early consolidation therapy with daunorubicin (DNR), high-dose cytosine arabinoside (HD-ara-C), and etoposide. HD-ara-C/DNR therapy included ara-C at 3 g/m^2, 12 doses (HD-ara-C/DNR 1) and eight doses (HD-ara-C/DNR II), respectively followed by DNR 30 mg/m^2 for 3 days. A complete remission (CR) was achieved in 104 (70%) patients. sixty-one complete responders received at least one cycle with HD-ara-C/DNR. After a median follow up of 95 months, the median relapse-free survival (MRFS) of all 104 patients was 20 months with a probability of relapse-free survival (RFS) at 116 months of 33% (95% confidence interval, Cl, 21%–43%). The MRFS of the HD-ara-C/DNR-consolidated patients was 32 months with a probability of RFS at 116 months of 38% (95% Cl, 26%–50%).

The median survival time (MST) of all 149 patients was 23 months with a probability to be alive at 118 months of 29% (95% Cl, 20%–38%). MST of the HD-ara-C/DNR-consolidated patients was 58 months with a survival probability of 49% (95% Cl, 34%–63%) at 118 months. Prognostic factor analysis did not reveal any significant influence of age, sex, French–American–British (FAB) subtype, white blood cell count, hemoglobin level, thrombocyte count, lactate dehydrogenase (LDH), and response to the first induction course on RFS of the HD-ara-C/DNR-consolidated patients. In summary, HD-ara-C/DNR consolidation can improve the long-term outcome of a subgroup of denovo AML patients. Further improvement of the outcome depends on the identification of patients with an inferior outcome under that strategy who might benefit from alternative treatment strategies.

Introduction

The development of effective chemotherapeutic agents together with a substantial improvement of the supportive care provide a high likelihood of achieving a complete remission (CR) for adults with newly diagnosed denovo acute myeloid leukemia AML; for review see [1, 2]. Although it is acknowledged that achievement of a CR should be followed by additional chemotherapy (CT) to eliminate residual leukemic blasts, which most likely account for the relapse the optimal approach still remains controversial (for review see [2, 3]). Based on laboratory [4] and clinical studies [5], it was reasoned that a

[1]Department of Internal Medicine lll, University of Ulm,Germany
[2]Department Hematology/Oncology, University of Frankfurt,Germany
[3]Department Hematology/Oncology, University of Hannover, Germany
[4]Department Hematology, University of Tübingen, Germany
[5]Department Internal Medicine and Institute for Medical Oncology/Hematology Nürnberg, Germany
[6]Department Internal Medicine, Zentralklinikum Augsburg, Germany
[7]Department Oncology, Klinikum Mannheim, Germany
[8]Department Internal Medicine, Robert-Bosch-Krankenhaus, Stuttgart, Germany
[9]Department Biometry and Medical Documentation, University of Ulm, Germany

significant increase in the dose of such drugs as cytarabine can overcome certain patterns of cellular resistance and thereby may eliminate residual leukemic cells which have survived induction therapy. During the mid-1980s, several investigators reported initial results of uncontrolled trials involving the use of high-dose ara-c (HD-ara-C) after CR had been achieved in patients with AML (for review see [1]). These promising results with a likelihood of remaining in CR 2 years after diagnosis of 30%–62% (reviewed in [3]) have prompted us to 50 years who are not candidates for allogeneic bone marrow transplantation (BMT) according to usual critera. The median follow up of the patients enrolled in this prospective multicenter trial initiated in May 1985 is now 95 months.

Patients and Methods

Patients

The entry criteria were: diagnosis of denovo AML, French-American-British Classification (FAB) M1-M6; age 15–50 years; exclusion of pregnancy; absence of severe organ dysfunction, absence of severe complications of the leukemia such as shock, pneumonia with hypoxia, and/or uncontrolled bleeding unless these complications had been treated successfully; and informed consent of the patient or legal guardian. Between April 1985 and March 1990, 149 patients were consecutively enrolled into this study.

Treatment

The first induction course (DAV I) included daunorubicin (DNR, 60 mg/m^2 per day rapid intravenous (i.v.) infusion on days 3–5), ara-C 100 mg/m^2 per day 24-h continuous i.v. infusion on days 1–8, and etoposide (VP16–213, 100 mg/m^2 per day 2-h i.v. infusion, on days 4–8. The second induction course (DAV II) was given after day 21: DNR (45 mg/m^2 per day rapid i.v. infusion on days 3–4), ara-C (100 mg/m^2 per day 2-h i.v. infusion on days 3–7). Patients not in CR after DAV II were regarded as treatment failures and excluded from further protocol therapy.

Patients in CR after DAV II received a third course of the DAV regimen for early consolidation (DAV III).

Patients in CR who did not fulfil the eligibility criteria for allogeneic BMT (histocompatible family donor, age $\leqslant$ 50 years, good performance status) received one or two courses of HD-ara-C and DNR (HD-ara-C/DNR) for late consolidation.

High-dose ara-C/DNR I, including ara-C (3 g/m^2 2 h i.v. infusion every 12 h) on days 1–6 and DNR (30 mg/m^2 per day rapid i.v. infusion) on days 7–9, was scheduled to start 4 weeks after recovery from early consolidation. Eight weeks after recovery from HD-ara-C/DNR I patients received HD-ara-C/DNR II with ara-C (3 g/m^2, 2-h i.v. infusion every 12 h) on days 1–4 and DNR (30 mg/m^2 per day rapid i.v. infusion) on days 5–7. Patients who experienced severe infectious or pulmonary complications during HD-ara-C/DNR I and those with prolonged bone marrow aplasia were not given the second course of HD-ara-C/DNR. After late consolidation no maintenance therapy was administered.

Supportive Care

The patients were nursed in single-bed or two-bed rooms under conventional ward conditions. Glucocorticoid eye drops were used during the HD-ara-C treatment. Prophylactic platelet transfusions were given to keep the platelet count above 20 000/µl. Selective decontamination was used to prevent bacterial and fungal infections [6].

Evaluation

The remission status was evaluated after the second induction course (DAV II) according to the Cancer and Leukemia Group B (CALGB) criteria [7]. Survival curves were calculated according to the method of Kaplan and Meier [8] for overall survival (calculated from the 1 day of chemotherapy to death) and relapse-free survival (RFS) (calculated from 1 day of CR to relapse or death in first CR). Survival curves (e.g., of the different FAB subtypes) were compared by the log-rank test. The Cox proportional hazards model [9] was used to determine the influence of age, sex, white blood cell count (WBC), hemoglobin level, thrombocyte count, serum lactate dehydrogenase (LDH) and response to DAV I on RFS of the HD-ara-C/DNR-consolidated patients.

Patients who underwent BMT in first CR ($n = 26$) were censored at the date of transplantation. The closing date for statistical evaluation was June 30, 1995.

Toxicity was quantitated according to the World Health Organization (WHO) criteria [10].

Results

Patients Characteristics

The characteristics of the 149 study patients are outlined in Table 1.

Results of Induction Therapy

A total of 104 (70%) out of the 149 study patients achieved a CR, seven patients (5%) a partial remission, 22 patients (15%) were treatment failures, and 14 patients (9%) died during induction therapy. In another two patients (1%), response to therapy was not evaluable. All 104 CR patients received one course of early consolidation.

Table 1. Characteristics of the study patients

Patients (n)	149
Sex	
Male (n)	74
(%)	50
Female (*n*)	75
(%)	50
Age	
Median(years)	37
Range(years)	15–50
FAB	
M1 (*n*)	22
(%)	15
M2 (*n*)	58
(%)	39
M3 (*n*)	11
(%)	7
M4 (*n*)	35
(%)	23
M5 (*n*)	19
(%)	13
M6 (*n*)	4
(%)	3
WBC ($\times 10^9$/l)—median	16.8
Hemoglobin—median(g/dl)	9.1
Platelet count—Median ($\times 10^9$/l)	44
LDH median—*(U/l)*	401

WBC, white blood cell count; *LDH*, lactate dehydrogenase (*normal*: < 240 U/l).

Late Consolidation Therapy

Of the 104 CR patients, 61 (59%) received late consolidation with HD-ara-C/DNR, including 42 patients with one and 19 patients with two HD-ara-C/DNR courses. The median interval in days from CR to HD-ara-C/DNR consolidation was 75 days (range 42–191 days). Forty-three patients did not receive HD-ara-C/DNR therapy. Seventeen patients underwent allogeneic BMT in first CR. Twenty-six patients neither received BMT nor HD-ara-C/DNR due to either refusal ($n = 1$), loss to follow up ($n = 1$), medical reasons against HD-ara-C/DNR consolidation therapy ($n = 16$), death during early consolidation ($n = 1$), or relapse before HD-ara-C/DNR ($n = 7$). Medical reasons against HD-ara-C/DNR I included refractoriness to HLA-matched platelet transfusions ($n = 1$), persistence of toxicity from induction therapy ($n = 8$), prolonged myelosuppression under induction therapy ($n = 1$), severe infections during prior therapy ($n = 4$), and pyschological problems during prior therapy ($n = 2$).

Forty-two patients did not receive HD-ara-C/DNR II due to either refusal ($n = 1$), life-threatening infections and/or prolonged myelosuppression after HD-ara-C/DNR I ($n = 21$), allogeneic BMT before HD-ara-C/DNR II ($n = 8$), death during HD-ara-C/DNR I ($n = 2$), or relapse prior to HD-ara-C/DNR II ($n = 10$).

All patients experienced profound neutrohand thrombocytopenia after HD-ara-C/DNR therapy. Median duration of neutropenia <500/µl was 24 days for HD-ara-C/DNR I and 18 days for HD-ara-C/DNR II. Median duration of thrombocytopenia <25 000/µl was 20 days for HD-ara-C/DNR I and 16 days for HD-ara-C/DNR II, respectively. As a consequence, infections were the most frequent and severe complications (38% of the patients experienced a septicemia during HD-ara-C/DNR I versus 32% during HD-ara-C/DNR II) and two patients (3%) died from infections. Nonmyeloid toxicity consisted mainly of nausea, vomiting, liver dysfunction, diarrhea, dermatitis, and conjunctivitis. These adverse reactions did not usually exceed grade II WHO toxicity. Severe cerebellar or other forms of CNS toxicity were not observed.

Relapse Free Survival

Fifty-one of the 104 CR patients relapsed including 31 patients after HD-ara-C/DNR consolidation therapy. In addition, three patients died in CR (one during early and two during late consolidation therapy.

After a median follow up of 95 months, the median duration of RFS (*MRFS*) for all 104 CR patients was 20 months and the probability of RFS at 116 months was 33% (95% confidence interval, CI, 21%–43%). MRFS of patients who had received at least one HD-ara-C/DNR course was 32 months with a probability of RFS of 38% (95% CI, 26%–50%; Fig. 1) at 116 months.

The probability of RFS and 116 months of those patients who had received one cycle with HD-ara-C/DNR was 35% (95% CI, 18%–51%; MRFS = 15 months) versus 45% (95% CI, 22%-68%; MRFS = 57 months) of those patients who had received two cycles with HD-ara-C/DNR (Fig. 2; $p = 0.1$; log-rank test).

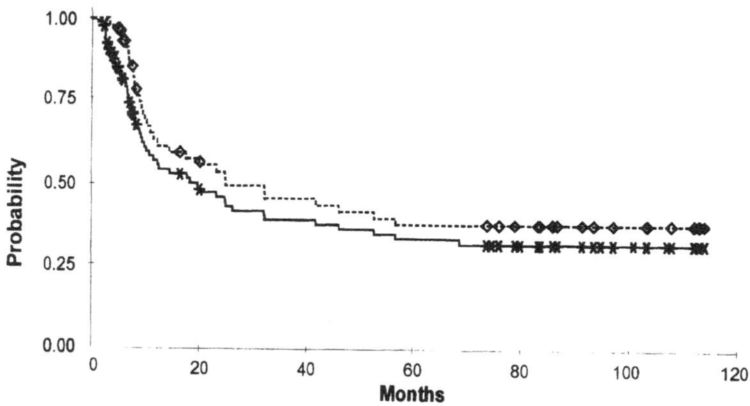

Fig. 1. The median duration of RFS of all patients (*solid line* $n = 104$) is 20 months and the probability of RFS at 116 months is 33% (95% CI, 21%–43%). *Marks* indicate patients remaining in CR and alive ($n = 50$). The median RFS of those patients who had received at least one cycle with HD-ara-C/DNR for late consolidation ($n = 61$) is 32 months and the probability of RFS at 116 months is 38% (95% CI, 26%–50%). *Marks* indicate patients remaining in CR and alive ($n = 28$)

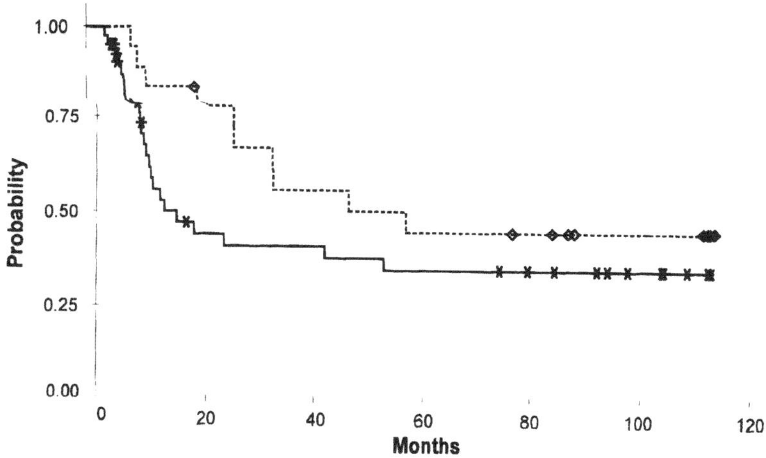

Fig. 2. The median duration of RFS of those patients (*broken line* $n = 42$) who had received one course of HD-ara-C/DNR *solid line* postremission therapy was 15 months and the probability of RFS at 116 months was 35% (95% CI, 20%–50%). *Marks* indicate patients remaining in CR and alive ($n = 19$). The median duration of RFS of those patients ($n = 19$) who had received two courses of HD-ara-C/DNR *broken line* was 57 months and the probability of RFS at 116 months was 45% (95% CI, 23%-67%). *Marks* indicate patients in CR and alive ($n = 9$)

Overall Survival

Of the 149 patients 78 have died: 14 patients during induction therapy, 25 with refractory disease, three in CR and another 36 patients in relapse. The median survival time (*MST*) of all 149 patients was 23 months with a probability to be alive at 118 months of 29% (95% CI, 20%–38%; Fig. 3). The MST of those patients who had received at least one cycle with HD-ara-C/DNR was 58 months with a probability of survival at 118 months of 49% (95% CI, 34%–63%).

Prognostic Factors

The contribution of age, sex, WBC, hemoglobin level, platelet count, LDH, response to the DAV I and FAB subtype on RFS of HD-ara-C/DNR-consolidated patients was evaluated only in those patients who did not undergo BMT in first CR. None of the parameters considered had a significant influence on RFS of these patients.

Discussion

The influence of a HD-ara-C/DNR postremission theapy on unmaintained long-term disease-free survival of de novo AML patients aged $\leqslant 50$ years was analysed after an identical induction and early consolidation therapy. After a median follow up of 95 months with a maximum of 118 months, the probability of RFS at 116 months of the 104 CR patients was 33% (95% CI, 21%–43%) and 38% (95% CI, 26%–50%) for the subgroup of patients who had received at least one cycle of HD-ara-C/DNR consolidation.

In the meantime a series of trials has been published dealing with a HD-ara-C-based consolidation [11–22]. Although these studies differed in the protocol design, the median age of the patients, and the median follow up, they produced comparable results with respect to RFS and overall survival. These data provide evidence that an intensified consolidation therapy may be superior to conventional postremission therapy. This conclusion has been confirmed by two recent randomized trials comparing a HD-ara-C-based postremission therapy with a consolidation program including ara-C at substantially lower doses (100 mg/m^2 or 400 mg/m^2 [16]) or with maintenance therapy (ara-C/6-thioguanine [[12]) in patients 60 years of age or younger.

The results of our trial differ from the studies cited above with respect to one important feature. While a stable plateau for RFS could be obtained in these trials after the first 2–3 years after the achievement of a CR, in our trial 23% of the relapses occurred beyond 2 years with the latest relapse at 57 months in the HD-ara-

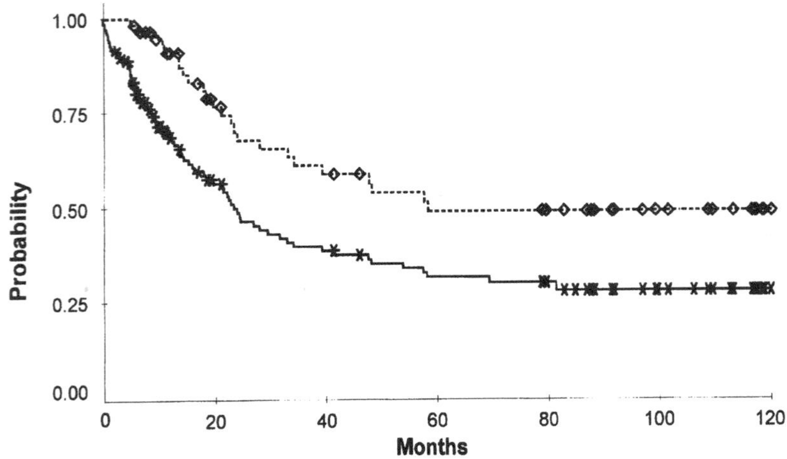

Fig. 3. The median survival time of all patients (*solid line* $n=149$) is 23 months and the probability to be alive at 118 months is 29% (95% CI, 20%–38%). *Marks* represent surviving patients ($n=71$). The median survival time of the HD-ara-C/DNR-consolidated patients ($n=61$) is 58 months with a probability to be alive at 118 months of 49% (95% CI, 34%–63%). *Marks* represent surviving patients ($n=37$)

C/DNR-consolidated patients. The reason for this difference remain unclear. One possible explanation is that they might have missed late relapses due to their substantially shorter follow up.

It cannot be excluded, however, that this phenomenon is due to the delay in the onset of the HD-ara-C/DNR therapy after attaining CR (median interval = 75 days) in our trial. Supporting evidence for this hypothesis is provided by two recent trials. In the study of Zittoun and co-workers [23], postremission chemotherapy including one course of intermediate-dose ara-C (500 mg/m^2) in combination with amsacrine followed by one course of HD-ara-C/amsacrine consolidation (median time between the achievemtn of CR and onest of HD-ara-C/amsacrine: 10 weeks) has produced comparable long-term results with relapses occurring beyond 5 years. Harousseau and co-workers [14] found some evidence that the prognosis was better for patients receiving the intensified consolidation therapy within 60 days after the initial treatment than for those who received the same regimen beyond that time.

Combined data indicate that there is a subgroup of AML patients who benefit from an HD-ara-C-based postremission therapy and may be definitely cured. The overall results, however, remain unsatisfactory in that the majority of patients still relapse and ultimately succumb to their disease.

A further intensification of the HD-ara-C-based regimen is, however, limited by a substantial treatment-related toxicity resulting in a treatment-related mortality of up to 13% in patients aged < 60 years [12]. As a consequence of this well-documented toxicity, only a fraction of patients in recent studies, including our own, have actually completed the scheduled intensive consolidation therapy. In addition, no significant benefit of further therapy following one HD-ara-C cycle could be demonstrated in any of the studies cited above. Thus the identification of those patients with an inferior outcome after intensive consolidation therapy seems necessary since their poor prognosis renders these patients candidates for new treatment strategies. Prognostic factors associated with the RFS and HD-ara-C/DNR consolidation therapy could not be identified in this trial. This might be a statistical problem due to the small numbers of patients enrolled in the intensified therapy. On the other hand, the parameters analysed might not be relevant for the treatment outcome after that therapy.

There is a growing body of evidence that the karyotype is the most important prognostic factor in adult de nove AML patients [24]. In a recent CALGB trial the outcome of the patients with a favourable karyotype, as defined by t(8; 21) or inv. 16, was significantly better than of the "unfavorable group" after an HD-ara-C-based postremission therapy [16, 25]. In the latter group, the dosage of ara-C had no significant influence on the RFS at 4 years.

In summary, this trial with a long follow up provides strong evidence, that an HD-ara-C/ DNR-based postremission therapy can acutally improve the long-term outcome of a subgroup of AML patients. Further improvement of the prognosis of AML patients requires the identification of "poor-risk" patients by karyotype analysis and the development of effective treatment strategies for that particular group.

Acknowledgments. This study was supported by the Deutsche Krebshilfe (contract M37/85 He2). The authors wish to thank B. Hay and D. Österle for excellent assistance in the documentation and M. Steinke for his help in preparing the manuscript.

References

1. Stone RM, Mayer RJ. Treatment of the newly diagnosed adult with de novo acute myeloid leukemia. Hamatol Oncol Clin North Am 1993; 7: 47–64.
2. Büchner T. Acute leukemia. Curr Opin Hematol 1993; 1: 172–182.
3. Mayer RJ. Current chemotherapy treatment approaches in the management of previously untreated adults with de novo acute myelogenous leukemia. Semin Hematol 1987; 14: 384–396.
4. Capizzi RL, Yang J, Rathmell JP, White JC, Cheng E, Cheng Y, Kute T. Dose-related pharmacologic effects of high-dose ara-C and its self-potentiation. Seminars in Oncology 1985; 12, suppl. 3: 65–75.
5. Kantarjian HM, Estey EH, Plunkett W, Keating MJ, Walters RS, Iacoboni S, McCredie KB, Freireich EJ. Phase I-II clinical and pharmacologic studies of high-dose cytosine arabinoside in refractory leukemia. Am J Med 1986; 81: 387–394.
6. Kurrle E, Dekker AW, Gaus W, Haralambie E, Krieger D, Rozenberg-Arska M, de Vries-Hospers G, van der Waaij D, Wendt F. Prevention of infection in acute leukemia: a prospective randomized study on the efficacy of two different regimen for antimicrobial prophylaxis. Infection 1986; 14: 226–232.

7. Rai KR, Holland JF, Glidewell OJ, Weinberg V, Brunner K, Obrecht JP, Preisler HD, Nawabi IW, Prager D, Carey RW, Cooper R, Haurani F, Hutchison JL, Silver RT, Falkson G, Wiernik P, Hoagland HC, Bloomfield CD, James GW, Gottlieb A, Ramanan SV, Blom J, Nissen NI, Bank A, Ellison RR, Kung F, Henry K, Mclntyre OR, Kaan SK. Treatment of acute myelocytic leukemia: a study by Cancer and Leukemia Group B. Blood 1981; 58: 1203–1212.
8. Kaplan EL, Meier P. Nonparametric estimation from incomplete observations. J Amer Stat Assoc 1958; 53: 457–481.
9. Cox DR. Regression models and life tables (with discussion). J R Stat Soc B 1972; 34: 187–202.
10. World Health Organization. WHO handbook for reporting results of cancer treatment. Geneva. WHO Publication 1979; 38:
11. Archimbaud E, Thomas X, Michallet M, Jaubert J, Troncy J, Guyotat D, Fiere D. Prospective genetically randomized comparison between intensive postinduction chemotherapy and bone marrow transplantation in adults with newly diagnosed acute myeloid leukemia. J Clin Oncol 1994; 12: 262–267.
12. Cassileth PA, Lynch E, Hines JD, Oken MM, Mazza JJ, Bennett JM, McGlave PhB, Edelstein M, Harrington DP, O'Connell MJ. Varying intensity of postremission therapy in acute myeloid leukemia. Blood 1992; 79: 1924–1930.
13. Champlin RE, Gajewski J, Nimer S, Vollset S, Landaw E, Winston D, Schiller G, Ho W. Postremission chemotherapy for adults with acute myelogenous leukemia: improved survival with high dose cytarabine and daunorubicin consolidation treatment. J Clin Oncol 1990; 8: 1199–1206.
14. Harousseau JL, Milpied N, Briere J, Desablens B, Leprise PY, Ifrah N, Gandhour B, Cassasus P. Double intensive consolidation chemotherapy in adult acute myeloid leukemia. Semin Hematol 1991; 28: , suppl 4: 80–83.
15. Hines JD, Mazza JJ, Oken MM, Adelstein DJ, Keller A, Bennett JM, O'Connell MJ. Prolonged survival after high-dose cytosine arabinoside and amsacrine induction in patients with previously untreated de novo acute nonlymphocytic leukemia. Semin Oncol 1987; 14 (Suppl. 1): 37–39.
16. Mayer RJ, Davis RB, Schiffer CA, Berg DT, Powell BL, Schulman P, Omura GA, Moore JO, Mclntyre OR, Frei III E for the Cancer and Leukemia Group B. Intensive postremission chemotherapy in adults with acute myeloid leukemia. N Engl J Med 1994; 331: 896–903.
17. Philips GL, Reece DE, Shepherd JD, Barnett MJ, Brown RA, Frei Lahr DA, Klingemann HG, Bolwell BJ, Spinelli JJ, Herzig RH, Herzig GP. High-dose cytarabine and daunorubicin induction and postremission chemotherapy for the treatment of acute myelogenous leukemia in adults. Blood 1991; 77: 1429–1435.
18. Schiller G, Gajewski J, Territo M, Nimer S, Lee M, Belin T, Champlin R. Long-term outcome of high-dose cytarabine-based consolidation chemotherapy for adults with acute myelogenous leukemia. Blood 1992; 80: 2977–2982.
19. Tricot G, Boogaerts MA, Vlietinck R, Emonds MP, Verwilghen RL. The role of intensive remission induction and consolidation therapy in patients with acute myeloid leukemia. Br J Haematol 1987; 66: 37–44.
20. Geller RB, Burke PJ, Karp JE, Humphrey RL, Braine HG, Tucker RW, Fox MG, Zahurak M, Morrell L, Hall KL, Piantadosi S. A two-step timed sequential treatment for acute myelocytic leukemia. Blood 1989; 74: 1499–1506.
21. Preisler HD, Raza A, Early A, Kirshner J, Brecher M, Freeman A, Rustum Y, Azarnia N, Priore R, Sandberg A, Block AM, Browman G, Walker I, Benjer A, Miller K, D Arrigo P, Doeblin T, Stein A, Bloom M, Logue G, Rustagi P, Barcos M, Larson R, Joyce R. Intensive remission consolidation therapy in the treatment of acute nonlymphocytic leukemia. J Clin Oncol 1987; 5: 722–730.
22. Tallman MS, Appelbaum FR, Amos D, Goldberg RS, Livingstone RB, Mortimer J, Weiden PL, Thomas ED. Evaluation of intensive postremission chemotherapy for adults with acute nonlymphocytic leukemia using high-dose cytosine arabinoside with L-asparaginase and amsacrine with etoposide. J Clin Oncol 1987; 5: 918–926.
23. Zittoun R, Mandelli F, Willemze R, de Witte T, Labar B, Resegotti L, Leoni F, Damasio E, Visani G, Papa G, Caronia F, Hayat M, Stryckmans P, Rotoli B, Leoni P, Peetermans M, Dardenne M, Vegna M, Petti MC, Solbu G, Suciu S. Autologous or allogeneic bone marrow transplantation compared with intensive chemotherapy in acute myelogenous leukemia. N Engl J Med 1995; 332: 217–223.
24. Hirsch-Ginsberg CH, Huh YO, Kagan J, Liang JC, Stass SA. Advances in the diagnosis of acute leukemia. Hematol Oncol Clin North Am 1993; 7: 1–46.
25. Bloomfield CD, Lawrence D, Arthur DC, Berg TD, Schiffer CA, Mayer RJ. Curative impact of intensification with high-dose cytarabine (HiDAC) in acute myeloid leukemia (AML) varies by cytogenetic group. Blood 1994; 84, Supplement 1: 111a.

Acute Leukemias VI
Prognostic Factors
and Treatment Strategies
Büchner et al. (eds)

Idarubicin, Cytarabine, Etoposide Versus Risk-Adjusted Daunorubicin Plus Cytosine Arabinoside for Induction Treatment of Acute Myeloid Leukemia: A Randomized Multicenter Trial

J. Holowiecki[1], S. Krzemien[1], Z. Kuratowska[2], A. Hellmann[3], E. Krykowski[4], A. Dmoszyńska[5], A. Skotnicki[6], L. Konopka[7], S. Maj[8], E. Rudzka[1], M. Krawcyzk[1], and B. Holowiecka[1] for the Polish Adult Leukemia Group

Abstract. The aim of study was to evaluate the efficacy and tolerability of the the idarubicin, cytarabine (ara-C), and etoposide (ICE) remission induction protocol in comparison to the modified, risk-adjusted daunorubicin(DNR) and ara-C (DA) schedule. Fifty-six adults with primary acute myeloid leukemia (AML); median age 36 years, range 16–60 years, males 46%) were centrally randomized to receive one of the following two induction treatments: (a) ICE 7/10: idarubicin 10 mg/m^2 per i.v. on days 1, 3, 5 ara-C 100 mg/m^2 per day continuous infusion on days 1–7/10, etoposide 100 mg.m^2 per day on days 1–5; (b) DA 3+7, high dose (HD) ara C: daunorubicin 60 mg/m^2 per day i.v. on days 1, 2, 3 ara-C 100 mg/m^2 per day continuous infusion on days 1–6 and then modified depending upon the day 6 bone marrow biopsy; in responders displaying >30% blast reduction and <20% blasts in the specimen, the initial dose was continued up to day 7–10 (age adjusted). In nonresponders with lower cytoreduction, HD-ara-c 1.5 g/m^2 infusion every 12 h was administered on days 7–10 dependent upon age. In addition, etoposide 65 mg/m^2, i.v. was given in French-American-British classification (FAB) M4/5 patients. Patients reaching Complete remission (CR) received two mitoxantrone+ ara-C consolidation courses and thereafter were submitted to bone marrow transplantation (BMT), autologous BMT (ABMT), or maintanence treatment. Both groups were well balanced with comparable of distribution prognostic factors. The CR rates obtained with ICE and DA 3+7 ±HD-araC were comparable (63% vs 61%). CR was obtained more frequently after one cycle using ICE when compared to DA 3+7±HD-ara-C, and the time to CR was significantly shorter (93% vs 55%, and 31±6 days vs 44±13 days). In the ICE group the following side effects were observed more frequently: diarrhea (31% vs 17%) WHO grade 3/4 infections (60% vs 42%) and hepatotoxicity (24% vs 0%).

The early results obtained with both regimens are comparable. The advantage of the ICE protocol is a quick achievement of CR, mostly with one cycle, but this benefit is paid for by a higher rate of side effects and a more intensive supportive care than with the risk-adjusted DA 3+7 ±HD-ara-C regimen

Introduction

Pharmacokinetic studies suggest that idarubicin is more effective when compared to daunorubicin (DNR) as a result of its longer half-life, faster cellular uptake, and higher activity in

[1]Department of Hematology, Silesian Medical Academy in Katowice, Poland
[2]Department of Hematology, Medical Academy in Warsaw, Poland
[3]Department of Hematology, Medical Academy in Gdansk, Poland
[4]Departmental of Internal Medicine, Medical Academy in Lodz, Poland
[5]Department of Hematology, Medical Academy in Lublin, Poland
[6]Department of Hematology, Medical Academy in Krakow, Poland
[7]Department of Internal Medicine, Institute of Hematology and Blood Transfusion in Warsaw, Poland
[8]Department of Hematology, Institute of Hematology and Blood Transfusion in Warsaw, Poland

inhibiting DNA polymerases and RNA synthesis [1, 2]. The antileukemic activity of idarubicin has been found to be two to five times higher than that of other anthracyclines [3]. Advantages of remission induction programs employing idarubicin have recently been demonstrated in multiple clinical trials [4-10]. The aim of this study was to evaluate the efficacy and tolerability of the idarubicin, cytarabine (ara-C), and etoposide (ICE) remission induction protocol in comparison to the modified risk-adjusted DNR plus ara-C ± high-dose (HD) ara-C schedule in a prospective randomized, cooperative study organised by the Polish Acute Leukemia Group (PALG).

Material and Methods

Starting in 1993, 56 adult patients suffering from acute nonlymphoblastic leukemia (ANLL) were included in a randomized, prospective trial in eight cooperating centers. Newly diagnosed adult patients were registered by telephone and fax to the coordinating center and randomized to receive either ICE or "DA 3+7 ± HD-ara-C remission induction treatment. Both arms were balanced according to the risk factors.

Inclusion criteria were as follows: (a) newly diagnosed ANLL; (b) age 16-60 years; (c) written informed consent; (d) performance status < WHO grade 2 (Karnofsky's index > 50%).

Exclusion criteria included: (a) previous chemotherapy; (b) co-existence of another neoplastic disease; (c) myelodysplastic syndrome in transformation; (d) hepatic or renal failure (serum bilirubin; Serum glutamic oxalo-acetic transaminase, SGOT; serum glutamic Pyruvic transaminase SGPT; and serum creatinin levels twice above the normal levels), pulmonary and myocardial insufficiency, and central nervous system failures; (e) pregnancy.

Twenty eight patients (13 males—46% and 15 females—54%) were included in each arm. The distribution of risk factors in both arms was comparable (Table 1) except for insignificant differences in white blood cell count (WBC) and in FAB subtype distribution

The general design of the study is presented in Fig.1 and the exact chemotherapy schedules were as follows:

ICE. Idarubicin 10 mg/m^2 i.v. on days 1, 3 and 5; ara-C 100 mg/m^2 per day continuous infusion on days 1-7/10, etoposide 100mg/m^2 per day in 60-min infusion on days 1-5.

DA 3+7 ± HD-ara-C. Daunorubicin 60 mg/m^2 per day i.v. on days 1, 2, 3, ara-C 100 mg/m^2 per day continuous infusion on days 1-6 and then modified depending on the day-6 bone marrow biopsy; in responders displaying > 30% blast reduction and < 20% of blasts in the specimen, the initial dose was continued up to day 10 in

Table 1. Characteristics of the randomized groups

	ICE	DA 3+7 ± HD-ara-C
Sex: M/F (*n*)	13/15	13/15
Age (years)	34 ± 13	35 ± 10
Median (years)	33	38
Range (years)	17-59	16-55
WBC (g/I)	51.2 ± 58.3	39.3 ± 48.0
Median	29.0	23.0
Peripheral bold blasts (g/I)	32.1 ± 29.8	28.0 ± 18.4
Bone marrow blasts(%)	77 ± 14	80 ± 14
FAB: M1/2/3/4/5 (*n*)	9/8/1/7/3	5/6/1/11/5
Platelets (g/I)	59.0 ± 39.0	39.0 ± 16
Hb g/dl	8.7 ± 2.1	8.0 ± 2.3
Karnofsky (%)	70 ± 10	70 ± 10
Fever (°C)	37.3 ± 1.0	37.5 ± 0.6
Infections (%)	52	58
Bleeding (%)	46	24
WHO grade	1.6 ± 1.7	2.0 ± 1.0
> Liver (%)	44	54
> Spleen (%)	19	37
> Lymph nodes (%)	50	37

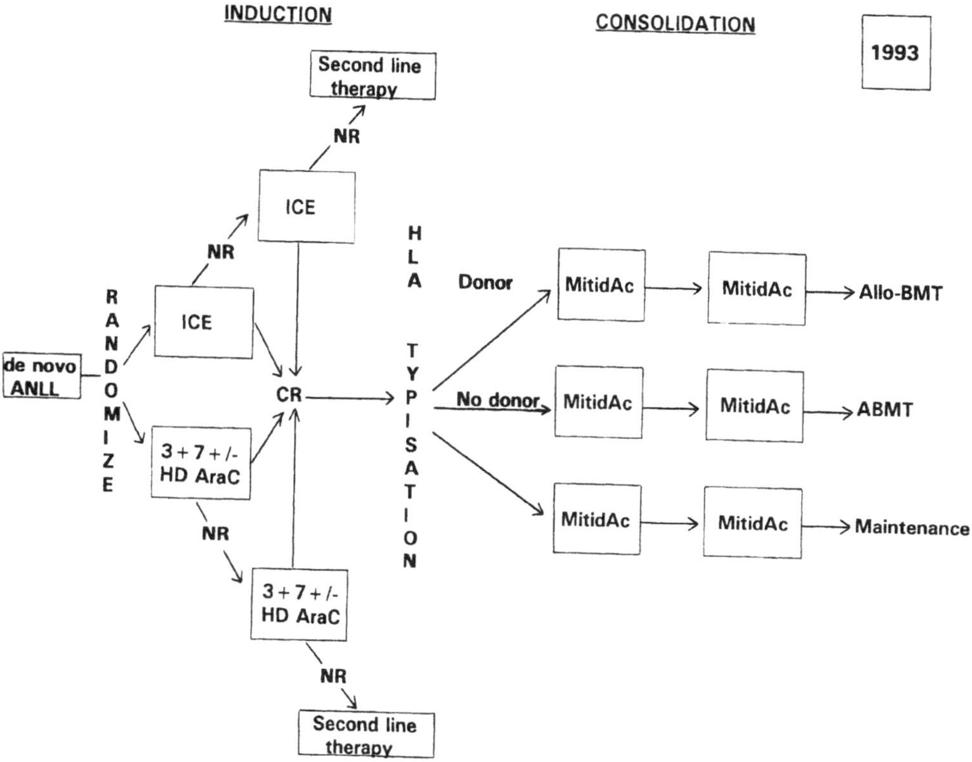

Fig. 1. General Design of the Polish Acute Leukemia Group ANLL Trial, 1993 *MitidAC* mitoxantrone-ara-c

patients aged <30 years, day 9 in patients aged 30–40 years, day 8 in patients aged 40–50 years and day 7–10 in patients aged 50–60 years. In non-responders with lower cytoreduction, HD-ara-C 1.5 g/m^2 infusion every 12 h was administered on days 7–10 in patients aged <30 years, and on days 7 and 8 in patients older than 30 years. In addition, etoposide 65mg/m^2 i.v. per day was given in FAB M4/5 patients. Non-responders received a second cycle before evaluation. Patients reaching CR obtained two mitoxantrone + Ara-C consolidation courses and thereafter were submitted to BMT, ABMT, or maintenance treatment.

Results

The results are presented in Table 2. Fifty-five patients were eligible for final evaluation: 27 in the ICE arm and 28 in the DA 3+7 ± HD-ara-C arm. One female patient was excluded from analysis because she died from pseudomonas sepsis before the induction treatment was initiated. The CR rate was comparable in both arms—63% and 61%, respectively.

In the ICE-treated group, 93% of patients reached CR after one remission induction cycle only, whereas in the DA 3+7 ± HD-ara-C arm only 55% of responders achieved CR with one cycle $\chi^2 = 8.791$, $p < 0.02$), and the remaining 45% needed two induction cycles. In the ICE-treated group, both the average and the median time to achieving CR was about 10 days shorter than in the second arm. Hematopoetic reconstitution as measured by the time of granulocyte recovery to values >0.5 g/l occurred only slightly later in the ICE arm. Young patients appeared to respond better to the treatment and the median age of the CR patients was lower if compared to the non-responder group (30 vs. 40 years).

In the ICE-treated subgroup, 15% of patients (four patients out of ten non-responders) died in the period <30 days from starting of induction therapy. Two patients died from hemorrhage disorders and the other two from sepsis.

Table 2. Results of induction treatment and some factors characterizing induction

	ICE	DA 3+7 ±HD-ara-C
Total (*n*)	28	28
Died before therapy (*n*)	1	0
Evaluable (*n*)	27	28
CR/NR (*n*)	17/10	17/11
CR rate (%)	63	61
Age of CR patients (years)	34.8 ± 13	38.1 ± 10
Median (years)	30.0	40.0
Died < 30 days of induction (*n*)	4	2
(%)	15	8
HD-ara-C treatment (*n*)	-	6
(%)		21
No. of induction cycles	1–78%, 2–22%	1–46%, 2–54%
No. of induction cycles patients	1–93%, 2–7%	1–55%, 2–45%
Time to CR (days)	32.9 ± 8.3	43.8 ± 13.4
Median (days)	30.5	48.0
after one cycle (days)	31.2 ± 5.8	40.0 ± 16.9
Median (days)	29.5	31.5
Nadir of aplasia (days)	13.9 ± 4.5	12.4 ± 1.6
Median (days)	12.0	13.0
Granulocytosis > 0.5	25.6 ± 4.9	22.0 ± 4.5
Median (days)	24.0	22.0

In the DA 3+7 ± HD-ara-C arm, the mortality in the same time period was 8%. The causes of death were sepsis in one case and cerebral bleeding in the other. Out of 28 patients treated with DA 3+7 ± HD-ara-C, in six cases the day-6 bone marrow evaluation revealed resistance to the standard treatment. In all these patients therapy was continued using HD-ara-C, and in three patients it resulted in achieving CR.

The frequency and WHO grading of the side effects are listed in Table 3. In the ICE arm the following side effects were more frequent than in the other group: diarrhea (30% vs. 17%), WHO grade 3/4 infections (60% vs. 42%), and hepatotoxicty (24% vs. 0). No cardiotoxicity was observed in the idarubicin-treated group, whereas in the DNR ara-C arm it was reported in 10% of patients.

Substitution of platelets and erythrocytes was necessary more frequent in the ICE group if compared to the DA 3+7 arm (8.1 ± 5.7 ± 8 units, and 3.2 ± 1.9 vs 2.3 ± 1.6 l, respectively).

Table 3. Side effects

	ICE		DA 3+7 plus	
	WHO 1/2 (*n*)	WHO 3/4 (*n*)	WHO 1/2 (*n*)	WHO 3/4 (*n*)
Nausea/vomiting	90	5	67	17
Diarrhea	21	10	17	0
Infection	15	60	42	42
agranulocytosis	10	75	8	75
Bleeding	20	75	17	83
Cardiotoxicity	0	0	05	5
Alopecia	42	47	25	67
Polyneuropathy	0	0	0	0
Hepatotoxicity	14	10	0	0

Discussion

The CR rate achieved with ICE in this study was comparable to that obtained in the modified DA 3+7 ± HD-ara-C group. The advantage of the ICE protocol was a quick achievement of CR, mostly with one cycle, but this benefit was paid for by a higher rate of side effects and a requirement for more intensive supportive care than with the risk-adjusted DA 3+7 ±HD-ara-C regimen. Some studies do not confirm significant differences between idarubicin and DNR pharmacokinetics [11], but most clinical trials demonstrate essential advantages of the idarubicin-containing regimens [4–10]. However, some of these studies involved a small number of patients and the remission rates obtained in the control arms employing DNR appear to be too low [10, 12].

In the present study we have compared the ICE protocol with a modified risk adjusted DA 3+7 ± HD-ara-C based on earlier results obtained in multi-institutional trails organised by PALG.

The ICE program, employing fixed-dose cytostatic composition, is aggressive and according to the expectations of the European Organization for Research on Treatment of Cancer (EORTC), it should allow CR to be achieved with one single induction course in the maximal number of patients. The DA 3+7 ± HD-ara-C program, based on conventional doses of ara-C and DNR in the first 6 days, is then adjusted to the response (± HD-ara-C) depending upon the response evaluated using a 6-day bone marrow biopsy. The third drug—etoposide—is administered optionally in M4 and M5 FAB subtypes only.

Summarising, in this study the ICE program, applied at its full strength in each case was compared to a risk-adjusted and potentially less hazardous schedule of the DA 3+7 ± HD-ara-C regimen.

In our experience, the overall CR rates were comparable in both chemotherapy groups, but in the ICE arm patients entered CR significantly more frequently after a single cycle. Concurrently, the time to CR was significantly shorter in the ICE group, suggesting a better prognosis. In contrast, in the DA 3+7 ±HD-ara-C group about one half of the patients needed a second induction cycle before CR was reached. These results are in line with some other reports [4–6, 9, 10, 12, 13].

It is noteworthy that CR in the idarubicin-treated group was achieved in patients younger than in the DNR-treated one (median age 30 vs 40 years). This confirms, to some extent, the observations of the GIMEMA group [13]. The results published recently by Ruutu et al. [19] also confirm the advantages of using oral idarubicin for older patients.

Some advantages of the ICE regimen are paid for by more frequent non-hematological adverse events such as diarrhea, hepatotoxicity and infections [4, 5, 7, 9, 10, 13, 14, 16]. In contrast, cardiotoxicity was not observed in the idarubicin-containing regimen, whereas in the DNR treated patients it was present in 10% of cases. This confirms some other reports [1,5]. In the ICE arm only in one case did we notice the first type of resistance according to Preissler and this indirectly confirms the efficacy of idarubicin in patients expressing MDR genes as suggested by some authors [1, 17, 18].

Among non-hematological adverse reactions about one quarter of the idarubicin-treated patients suffered from hepatotoxicity which was also reported by Wiernik et al. [9] and Pagano et al. [15].

Owing to the higher cytotoxic potency of the ICE composition, also resulting in a higher early death rate, the supportive treatment was more intensive in the ICE arm. Red blood cell substitution therapy was used in all patients in both arms. Platelet transfusions were applied in 95% of patients in the ICE arm and in 91% of patients in the DA arm. Both the frequency of platelet substitution and the volume of erythrocyte substitution were significantly higher in the ICE-treated group.

Conclusions

1. The regimens under study produced a comparable CR rate.
2. The advantages of ICE were the following: CR was achieved significantly more frequently after one cycle of induction as compared to DA 3+7 ± HD-ara-C ($p < 0.02$) and the time to CR was significantly shorter.
3. Side effects such as diarrhea, infections and hepatotoxicity were more frequent in the ICE-treated group but cardiotoxicity was noted only in the DA 3+7 arm.
4. A more intensive supportive therapy was required after ICE.

References

1. Berman E, McBride M. Comparative cellular pharmacology of daunorubicin and idarubicin in human multidrug-resistant leukemia cells. Blood 1992; 79: 3267–3273.
2. Robert J, Rigal-Huguet F, Hurterloup P. Comparative pharmacokinetic study of idarubicin and daunorubicn in leukemia patients. Hematol-Oncol. 1992; 10: 111–116.
3. Kuffel MJ, Reid JM, Ames MM. Anthracyclines and their c-13 alcohol metabolites: growth inhibition and DNA damage following incubation with human tumor cells in culture. Cancer Chemother. Pharmacol. 1992; 30: 51–57.
4. Berman E, Heller G, Santorsa J, McKenzie S, Gee T, Kempin S, Gulati S, Andreef M, Kolitz J, Gabrilove J. Results of a randomized trial comparing idarubicin and cytosine arabinoside with newly diagnosed acute myelogenous leukemia. Blood 1991; 77: 1666–1674.
5. Carella AM, Carlier P, Pungolino E, Resegotti L, Liso V, Stasi R, Montillo M, Iacopino P, Mitro S, Pagano L. Idarubicin in combination with intermediate-dose cytarabine and VP-16 in the treatment of refractory or rapidly relapsed patients with acute myeloid leukemia. The GIMEMA Cooperative Group. Leulemia 1993; 7: 196–199.
6. Carella AM, Yaozza E, Piatti G. A new combination of idarubicin, etoposide and cytarabine in untreated acute non-lymphocytic leukemia. Leukemia and lymphoma 1990; 2: 317–322.
7. Ogawa M, Ariyoshi Y. New anthracyclines. Gan. To. Kagaku. Rhyoho. 1993; 20: 27–33.
8. Volger WR, Velez-Garcia E, Weiner RS, Flaum MA, Bertolucci AA, Omura GA, Gerber MC, Banks PL. A phase III trial comparing idarubicin and daunorubicin in combination with cytarabine in acute myelogenous leukemia: a Southeastern Cancer study Group study. J Clin Oncol 1992; 10: 1103–1111.
9. Wiernik PH, Banks PL, Case DC Jr, Arlin ZA, Periman PO, Todd MB, Ritch PS, Enck RE, Weitberg AB. Cytarabine plus idarubicin as induction and consolidation therapy for previously untreated adult patients with acute myeloid leukemia. Blood 1992; 79: 313–319.
10. Wiernik PH, Case DC Jr, Periman PO, Arlin ZA, Weiberg AB, Ritch PS, Todd MB. A multicenter trial of cytarabine plus idarubicin or daunorubicin as induction therapy for adult nonlymphocytic leukemia. Sem. in Oncol. 1989; 17: 25–29.
11. Cersosimo, RJ. Idarubicin: an anthracycline antineoplastic agent. Clim. Pharm. 1992; 11: 152–167.
12. Gale RP. Acute myelogenous leukemia: progress and controversies. Leukemia 1990; 4: 529–531.
13. Mandelli F, Petti MC, Ardia A, Di Pietro N, Di Raimondo F, Ganzina F, Falconi E, Geraci E, Ladogana S, Latagliata R. A randomised clinical trial comparing idarubicin and cytarabine to daunorubicin and cytarabine in the treatment of acute non-lymphoid leukaemia. A multicentric study from the Italian Cooperative Group GIMEMA. Eur. J. Cancer 1991; 27: 750–755.
14. Ogawa M, Masoaka T, Yamada K, Kimura K. Early phase II study of idarubicin, a new anthracycline anticancer drug, in acute leukemia. Idarubicin Study Group. Gan. To. Kagaku. Ryoho 1993; 20 897–906.
15. Pagano L, Sica S, Marra R, Voso MT, Storti S, Di Mario A, Leone G. Oral idarubicin plus cytosine arabinoside in the treatment of acute non-lymphoblastic leukemia in elderly patients. Hematologica 1991; 76: 517–518.
16. Resegotti L. Treatment of acute non-lymphoid leukemia (ANLL) in elderly patients. The GIMEMA experience. Leukemia 1992; 6: 72–75.
17. Michieli M, Michelutti A, Damiani D, Pipan C, Raspadori D, Lauria F, Baccarani M. A comparative analysis of the sensitivity of multidrug resistant (MDR) and non-MDR cells to different anthracycline derivatives. Leukemia and Lymphoma 1993; 9: 255–264.
18. Muller MR, Lennartz K, Bogen C, Nowrousian MR, Rajewsky MF, Seeber S. Cytotoxicity of adrimycin, idarubicin, and vincristine in acute myeloid leukemia: chemosensitization by verapamil in relation to P-glycoprotein expression. Ann. Hematol. 1992; 65: 206–212.
19. Ruutu T, Almqvist A, Hallman H, Honkanen T, Jarvenpaa E, Jarventie G, Koistinen P, Koivunen E, Lantinen R, Lehtinen M, Nousiainen T, Pelliniemi T, Rajmaki A, Remes K, Sarkkinen R, Sinisalo M, Timonen T, Volin L, Elonen E. Oral induction and consolidation of acute myeloid leukemia with etoposide, 6-thioguanine and idarubicin (ETI) in elderly patients: a randomised study with 5-day TAD. Leukemia 1994; 8: 11–15.

Acute Leukemias VI
Prognostic Factors
and Treatment Strategies
Büchner et al. (eds)

"7+3" Versus "7+3+VP-16" as Remission Induction in Acute Myeloid Leukemia Patients Under the Age of Sixty Years: Preliminary Results of a Russian Multicenter Trial

H. Parovitchnikova, V. Savchenko, G. Kliasova, V. Isaev, H. Maslova, and S. Kulikov
for the Russian Leukemia Research Group

Abstract. The goal of the study was to determine the role of etoposide (VP-16) as an additional component to the standard 7+3 regimen applied in two-step induction fashion in de novo acute myeloid leukemia (AML). Treatment for each patient consisted of four cycles 7+3 or 7+3+VP-16 according to the arm of randomization. M3 patients were treated with the 7+3 regimen. The type of maintenance was also defined by randomization: repetition of 7+3 with 6–8 weeks interval or a rotation program (5 days cytarabine, ara-C, with daunorubicin or cyclophosphamide or 6-mercaptopurine) with a 4-week interval for 3 years of complete remission (CR).

From August 1992 until January 1995, 188 patients were enrolled in the study from 18 participating hematological centers. Ninety-three patients were randomized to 7+3 and 96 patients to 7+3+VP-16. Forty-seven patients were excluded from the analysis. Nine M3 patients were analyzed separately. Sixty-two patients (34 males, 28 females; median age 34 years; M1-9, M2-25, M4-20, M5-6, M6-1, M7-1) on 7+3, and 70 patients (30 males, 40 females; median age 33 years; M1-11, M2-27, M4-29, M5-3) on 7+3+VP-16 were finally evaluated. The CR rates were 60% and 66%, drug resistance (DR) 19% and 10%, early death(ED) 21% and 24% respectively. The death rate in consolidation was 11% on 7+3 and 20% on 7+3+VP-16. Among nine M3 patients, four died during induction (cranial hemorrhages), one patient had resistant leukemia, four patients achieved CR. Event-free survival over 2.5 years in the 7+3 arm was 22% (37 patients and in the 7+3+VP-16 arm 36% (46 patients) ($p=0.59$). Event-free survival according to the type of maintenance in the 7+3 group was 32% on the rotation program (13 patients) and 88% on 7+3 maintenance (13 patients) ($p=0.47$); in the 7+3+VP-16 group the rate was 20% on the rotation program (13 patients) and 42% on 7+3 maintenance (11 patients) ($p=0.17$).

These results indicate that VP-16 does not improve CR rate and event-free survival in AML patients in a 2.5 year follow-up period. More intensive maintenance seems to have some, though not statistically significant, benefit over the rotation program. A high death rate in induction and consolidation, especially on 7+3+VP-16, may make the advantages of addition of VP-16 to the standard 7+3 regimen questionable.

Introduction

Though acute myeloid leukemia (AML) treatment seems to have been well defined for more than 15 years, there are still many questions and debates. Conventional chemotherapy with low-dose maintenance provides standard long-term results with almost of 25% event-free survival [1, 2]. For years it has been discussed whether the introduction of new drugs (idarubicin; amsacrine; mitoxantrone; etoposide, VP-16), or high-dose cytarabine (ara-C) in induction/consolidation with or without prolonged maintenance, or usage of time-sequential protocols

National Research Center for Hematology, Moscow, Russia

may improve the outcome in AML patients. The same question is posed regarding new non-cytostatic agents recently introduced in AML therapy, i.e., growth factors and retinoid acid [3]. Allogeneic bone marrow transplantation (BMT) is considered almost unanimously to reduce the risk of relapse thus increasing survival up to 50% in a selected group of patients [4].

Intensified AML therapy is now believed to provide some, though not dramatic, advantages over the gold standard—the 7+3 regimen. This conclusion was reached mostly following the results of single-center studies, and a few large multicenter trials have proved this concept [5].

The goal of our study group was to determine the role of VP-16 as an additional agent to the 7+3 regimen applied in a two-step induction fashion in de novo AML therapy. The results of this multicenter randomized trial comparing 7+3 and 7+3+VP-16 are now discussed in this paper.

Materials and Methods

The study comprised 18 participating centers and was started in August 1992. The criteria for study enrolment were: de novo AML, age 16-60 years, no previous treatment for AML. The study design is shown in Fig. 1.

All patients (except M3) were randomized to 7+3 or 7+3+VP-16. VP-16 was administered for 5 days at a dose of 120 mg/m^2 per day, 30-min infusion started on day 10 after finishing 7+3 (Fig. 2). The treatment for each patient consisted of four induction/consolidation courses. Patients who did not achieve complete remission (CR) after two courses were excluded from the protocol as having resistant leukemia. After finishing the induction/consolidation program, patients were randomized either to 7+3 maintenance with a 6–8 week interval or to a rotation protocol (5 days ara-C 100 mg/m^2 s.c. plus daunorubicin 45/m^2 on days 1,2; or cyclophosphamide 600 mg/m^2 on day 1; or 6-mercaptopurine 60 mg/m^2 on days 1–5) with a 4-week interval between courses. The whole treatment was conducted for 3 years of CR.

Supportive Care. All patients received nistatin and cotrimoxazole p.o. as decontamination and if necessary antibiotic treatment was started according to the protocol of empirical antibiotic therapy (first line—cephalosphorins of the third generation plus aminoglycosides; second—addition on day 3-4 of vancomycin or unasin; third—addition on day 6–7 of antifungal drugs: amphotericin B, or fluconazol, or itraconazol; then according to the positive cultures obtained from blood or catheter, etc.).

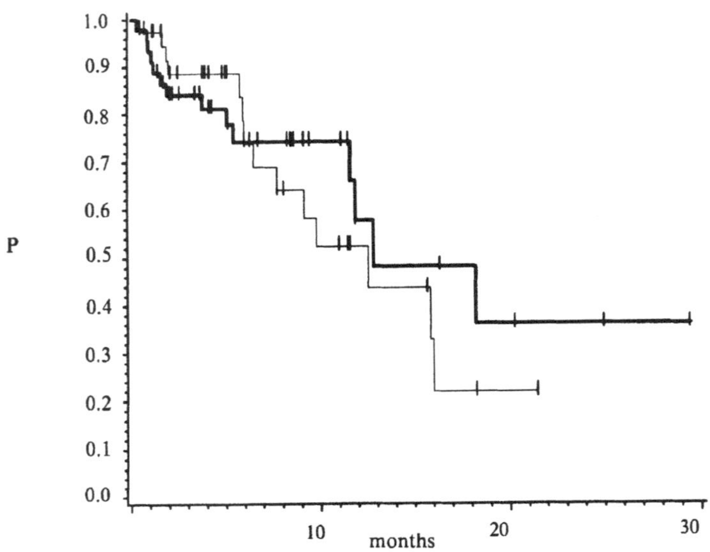

Fig. 1. Design of the study

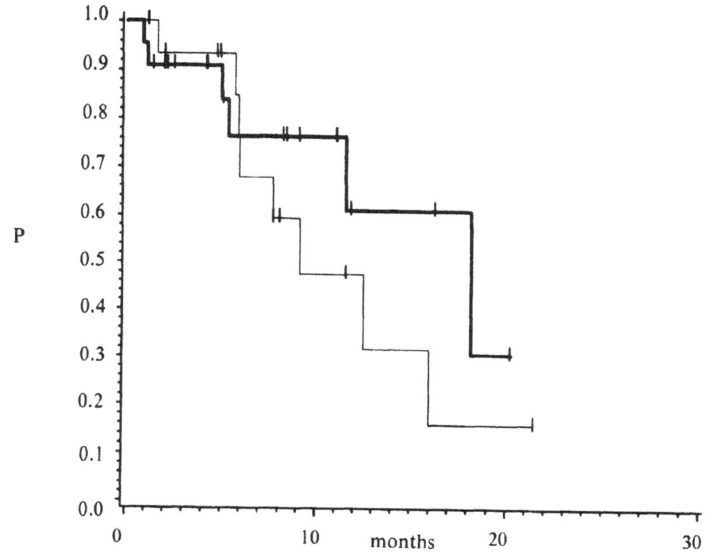

Fig. 2. 7+3+VP-16 schedule

From August 1992 until December 1994, 188 patients less than 60 years old with de novo AML were randomized: 93 to the 7+3 protocol and 95 to the 7+3+VP-16 protocol. The data on excluded and analyzed patients is presented in Fig. 3. As already mentioned, M3 patients were analyzed separately.

Survival analysis was estimated by the Kaplan-Meier method for CR patients according to the type of induction (for M4–5 patients separately) and according to the type of maintenance. Events were deaths or relapses. Four patients underwent transplantation in their first remission, and in the life-table analysis they were censored at the time of BMT.

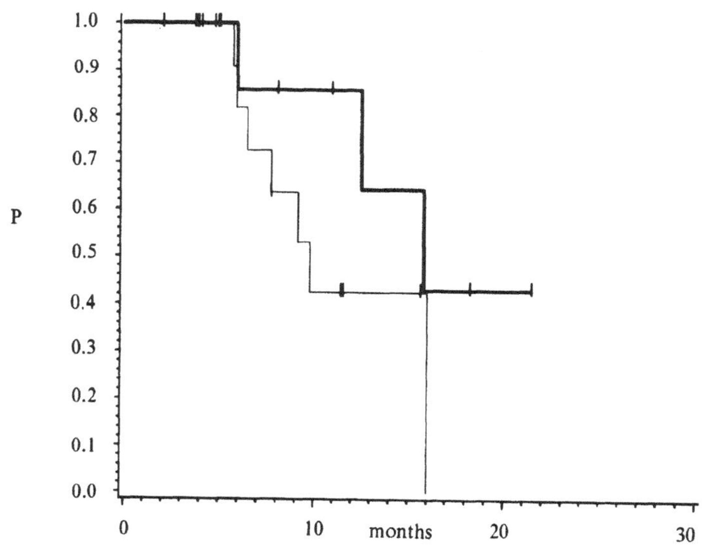

Fig. 3. Data on excluded and analyzed patients

Results

After 2.5 years of on-going trial the data from 132 patients were evaluable. The results of treatment in AML patients according to the type of induction are presented in Table 1. We also compared the results obtained in our center—the National Research Center for Hematology (NRCH)—and in all the other participating centers as this could easily demonstrate the advantages of a single-center trial.

We did not observe any difference between the two protocol arms. The CR rate was almost identical with slightly more patients in the 7+3+VP-16 group achieving CR after the first course of induction (87% vs. 68%). In both treatment groups there was high early death (ED) rate (death within 6 weeks of therapy). The causes of ED are shown in Table 2. As the majority of complications occurred during the neutropenic phase, the comparison of critical neutropenia duration (leukocytes $< 1.0 \times 10^9$/l) and platelet transfusion support was performed (Table 3). One platelet unit presented in this analysis consitutes ~40×10^9 platelets obtained from 500 ml blood. These data again show no differences between the two protocol arms but they do reveal the insufficient transfusion support used in the study.

Among nine M3 patients, only four achieved CR (all after the second course of 7+3), one patients was resistant, and four died in induction due to cranial hemorrhages. Three out of four CR patients relapsed within 1 year of CR.

All patients needed antibiotic treatment during induction. Fever of unknown origin was the reason to start the antibiotic therapy in 90% of cases and pneumonia in 10% of cases. The data for the precise infection analysis were evaluable in 38 patients. The first-line antibiotics (cefoperazon+gentamycin) were effective in 32% (12 patients) of 38 cases; 36% (nine patients) out of 25 patients in whom it was indicated (24% of all patients responded to the second—line therapy with the addition of unasin); an antifungal drug (third line—fluconazol) was applied to 39% (15 patients) of all patients and 53% (8 patients) of them responded. One death occurred during the first-line treatment, one death during the second line, and three deaths during the third line of protocol (in two cases it was fungal sepsis). Of all patients, 10% (4 patients) did not respond to this protocol, so the overall response rate was 76%. There were no differences between induction groups. regarding the antibiotical protocol application.

Among 46 CR patients in the 7+3+VP-16 group, nine (20%) died in consolidation. Until December 1995, 26 had come through four induction/consolidation courses and were randomized to 7+3 maintenance (13 patients) and the rotation protocol (13 patients). Among 37 CR patients in the 7+3 group, four died (11%) in consolidation and 24 were randomized to the maintenance protocol: 11 patients to 7+3 maintenance and 13 patients to the rotation program.

Event-free survival according to the type of induction is presented in Fig. 4. Survival at 2.5 years constitutes 36% in the 7+3+VP-16 group and 22% in the 7+3 group. Event-free survival according to the type of induction for patients with M4 and M5 was evaluated separately and is shown in Fig. 5. M4-M5 patients did slightly better on the 7+3+VP-16 protocol with 30% achieving 2-year survival vs. 18% on 7+3. Figures 6 and 7 show event-free survival according to the type of maintenance in the 7+3 and 7+3+VP-16 groups. Both figures show a slight advantage for the 7+3 maintenance over the rotation program. In no one case of survival analysis was a statistical difference found.

Discussion

Intensification of AML treatment is going in different directions: dose acceleration, incorporation of new cytostatic drugs, and use of time-sequential protocols and priming effects in induction and in postremission therapy. In initiating the study with VP-16 applied as the second step after the 7+3 regimen, we tried to follow two of these principles, i.e., the addition of new drug and time sequence with a priming effect. VP-16 has been reported by some groups to bring some additional effects in AML. Bishop et al. [6] showed statistically better 4-year event-free survival in a younger group of patients treated with 7+3 combined with VP-16 75 mg/m^2 for 7 days in comparison with those treated with 7+3: 36% vs. 15%. In a retrospective analysis, a higher remission rate (72%) was reported by Leoni et al. [7] in 61 patients treated with the daunorubicin, cytarabine, and 6-thioguanine (DAT) regimen where thioguanine was replaced by VP-16 vs 57% in 35 patients who were treated with the original DAT. In the German Berlin-Frankfurt-Münster (BFM) study, the addition of

Table 1. Results of treatment according to the type of induction

Results	7+3						7+3+VP-16					
	NRCH ($n=11$)		Other centers ($n=51$)		Total ($n=62$)		NRCH ($n=12$)		Other centers ($n=58$)		Total ($n=70$)	
	(n)	(%)	(n)	(%)	(n)	(%)	(n)	(%)	(n)	(%)	(n)	(%)
Complete remission	8	73	29	57	37	60	8	67	38	66	46	66
Resistance	2	18	10	20	12	19	3	25	4	7	7	10
Early death	1	9	12	23	13	21	1	8	16	28	17	24
Death in CR	1	13	3	10	4	11	1	13	8	21	9	20

Thirteen patients were excluded.

Table 2. Causes of death during induction

Events	7+3						7+3+VP-16					
	NRCH ($n=11$)		Other centers ($n=51$)		Total ($n=62$)		NRCH ($n=12$)		Other centers ($n=58$)		Total ($n=70$)	
	(n)	(%)	(n)	(%)	(n)	(%)	(n)	(%)	(n)	(%)	(n)	(%)
Early death	1	9	12	23	13	21	1	8	16	28	17	24
Infection	–		5	10	5	38	1	8	11	19	12	71
Hemorrhage	1	9	7	14	8	62	–		5	9	5	29

Thirteen patients were excluded.

Table 3. Neutropenia duration and transfusion support according to induction course

Characteristics	7+3		7+3+VP-16	
	First course	Second course	First course	Second course
Neutropenia (days)	13.5	8.5	15	10
Platelets (units)	16	4	16	14

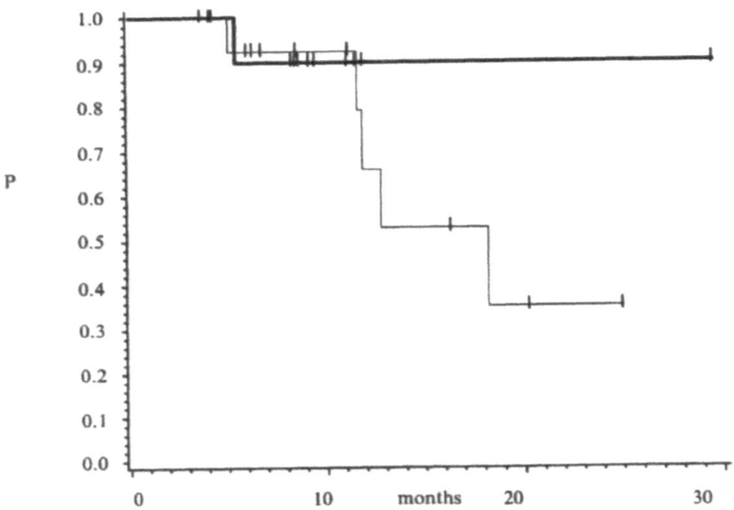

Fig. 4. Event-free survival in AML patients according to the type of induction. *Thick line*, 7+3+VP-16 induction (46 patients); *thin line*, 7+3 induction (37 patients); $p = 0.59$

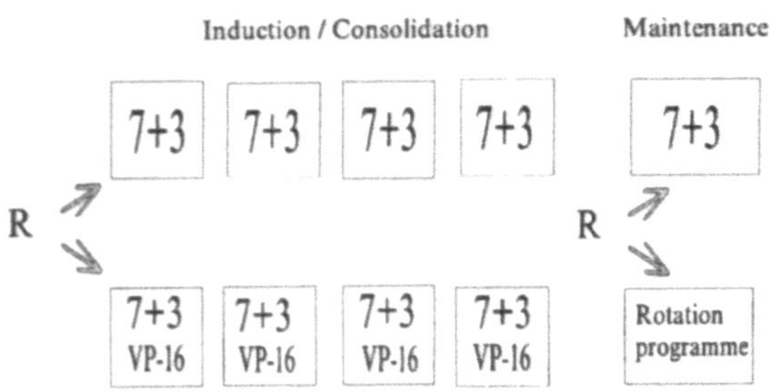

Fig. 5. Event-free survival in patients with M4 and M5 AML according to the type of induction. *Thick line*, 7+3+VP-16 induction (22 patients); *thin line*, 7+3 induction (16 patients); $p = 0.35$

the ara-C+VP-16 course before the main protocol brought substantially better survival results in children in all AML subtypes except M5 [8]. In all these studies VP-16 administered together with ara-C, but some authors reported that the activity of ara-C may be reduced by the concomitant use of VP-16 [9]. Following this data, we decided to infuse VP-16 after finishing the ara-C infusion. Another point that was taken into consideration was the evidence of drug-induced humoral stimulatory activity (HSA) present in serum following initial cytoreduction and associated with endogenous growth factor activity [10]. As a result, there is a predictable peak in in vivo post-drug residual tumor proliferation (day 8) [11]. So the application of the cytostatic drug at days 8–10 after initial chemotherapy (7+3) may increase tumor clearance. These facts

Fig. 6. Event-free survival according to the type of maintenance in patients treated with 7+3 induction protocol. *Thick line*, 7+3 maintenance (11 patients); *thin line*, rotation programme (13 patients); $p = 0.17$

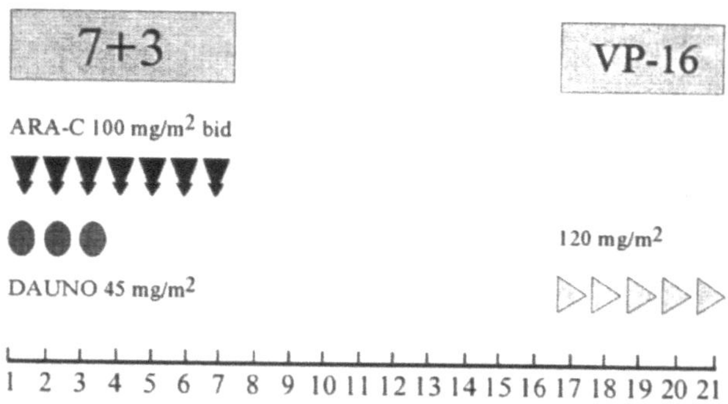

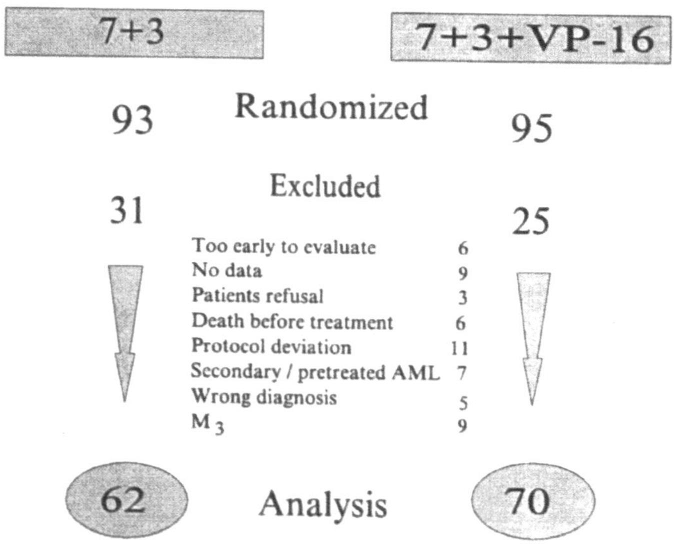

Fig. 7. Event-free survival according to the type of maintenance in patients treated with 7+3+VP-16 induction protocol. *Thick line*, 7+3 maintenance (13 patients); *thin line*, rotation programme (13 patients); $p = 0.47$

became the basis for the two-step induction protocol 7+3+VP-16 that was proposed to be compared with the standard 7+3 in a multicenter randomized study.

In 132 patients were analyzed: 62 patients in the 7+3 induction arm and 70 patients in the 7+3VP-16 arm. Forty-five patients were excluded, mostly (32 patients) due to unprecise fulfillment of the protocol (wrong diagnosis, secondary AML, pretreated AML, dose reductions, no information about the patient, and other protocol deviations). Six patients (3% out of all randomized) died before any treatment was started, this is a common situation in rural regions of Russia where patients are admitted to hospital in the terminal phase of the disease due to a late diagnosis. Both groups were similar in AML subtype distribution and median age. It is worth noting that the median age of patients enrolled in the study is young (33–34 years). There may be two explanations: the caution of participating centers who do not randomize older patients (subjective reason) and a very low median life duration of people in Russia—65 years (objective reason). So the results of the AML chemotherapy discussed here and the conclusions refer, to some extent, to a selected group of patients.

Results of induction treatment do not differ much from those reported elsewhere for multicenter trials: a 60% CR rate on 7+3 and 66% on 7+3+VP-16 [12]. The exception is promyelocytic leukemia as only 44% of patients achieved CR, possibly due to a high incidence of death during induction. There is a real problem with a supportive care as 21%–24% of patients died during induction. We also revealed a very low level of transfusion support during induction (16 units) and this fact can explain the high incidence of hemorrhagic deaths (62% on 7+3 and 29% on 7+3+VP-16). Deaths from infection occurred in 57% (17 patients) of 30 induction patients. Infections were the major cause of death in consolidation too (11% CR patients died in the 7+3 arm and 20% in the 7+3+VP-16 arm). These induction/consolidation deaths affected the event-free survival in CR patients, and the higher death rate in the 7+3+VP-16 group may conceal the antileukemic effect of this protocol.

Event-free survival (36%) during the short period of follow up (2.5 years) in patients treated with the 7+3+VP-16 regimen is almost identical to that reported by Kurrle et al. [13], i.e., 42% at 22 months in patients treated with the DAV regimen (ara-C 100 mg/m^2 continuous infusion on days 1–7, daunorubicin 60-45 mg/m^2 on days 1–3, VP-16 100 mg/m^2 on days 5--7). The remission rate described in this report is also the same as in our study—67%. There was no statistical difference in survival between the 7+3 and 7+3+VP-16 groups in our study.

Results in M4-M5 patients treated with 7+3+VP-16 show some trend in favour of a protocol including VP-16, but only long-term follow up will provide clear conclusions. The event-free survival curve for four CR M3 patients cannot be shown, but three relapses (two of them were early relapses within 6 months of CR) demonstrated the poor efficacy of 7+3 courses.

It is clear that there are few patients in the analysis but perhaps it would be reasonable to increase the dose of daunorubicin for M3 patients up to 60 mg/m^2 in the 7+3 schedule. Retinoids are currently not evaluable in Russia.

The idea of comparing more or less aggressive maintenance treatment within the same period of time (3 years of CR) was tested in our trial. It appeared once again that at this period of follow up no one type of maintenance therapy showed statistically better results; there is only a trend towards better remission duration on 7+3 maintenance than on the rotation protocol. However the groups of patients are small (11–13 patients) and the period of follow up is short. Moreover, almost all the patients on 7+3 maintenance needed hospitalization and supportive measures during their treatment. In approximately 75% of patients on 7+3 maintenance a dose reduction of up to two thirds of the expected dose was needed. There were much fewer problems in the rotation arm.

The conclusions after 2.5 years of this ongoing trial are:

- The addition of VP-16 to the induction protocol did not improve the CR rate but did not worsen the induction death rate in adult AML patients.
- 7+3+VP-16 gives a 36% and 7+3 a 22% 2.5 years event-free survival rate in adult AML patients. -7+3+VP-16 does not improve survival in M4-M5 AML patients at 2.5 years of follow up.
- 7+3 maintenance has no statistically reliable advantages over the rotation program.
- More time and more patients are needed to reach more exact conclusions.

Acknowledgment. The Participating centers in this Russian AML study were: Moscow (five centers), St.Petersburg (two centers), Novosibirsk, Yaroslavl, Ekatherinburg (two centers), Hmelnitsky, Samara, Irkutsk, Ivanovo, Rjasan, Kirov, and Arhangelsk.

References

1. Preisler H., Davis R.B., Kirshner J., Dupre E., Richards F. et al. Comparison of three remission induction regimes and two post induction strategies for the treatment of acute non-lymphocytic leukemia. Blood 1987 v. 69 pp.1441–1449
2. Buchner Th., Urbanitz D., Hiddemann W., Ruhl H., Ludwig W.D., Fisher J. et al. Intensified induction and consolidation with or without maintenance chemotherapy for acute myeloid leukemia (AML): two multicenter studies of German AML Cooperative Group. J.Clin.Oncology 1985 v. 3 pp. 1583–1589
3. Estey E.H., Freireich E. Therapy for acute myelogenous leukemia. Hematology 1991 v.14 pp1–33
4. Formann S.J., Blume K.G., Thomas E.D., (eds) Bone marrow transplantation Blackwell Scientific Publications 1994 pp 607–617
5. Buchner T., Hiddemann W., Wormann B, Loeffler H., Maschmeyer G, Hossfeld D. et al Long term effects of prolonged maintenance and of very early intensification chemotherapy in AML: data from AMLCG. Leukemia 1991 v. 6, suppl 2, pp 68–71

6. Bishop J.F., Lowental R.M., Joshua D. et al Etoposide in acute non-lymphocytic leukemia. Blood 1990 v. 75 pp.27–32
7. Leoni F., Ciolli S., Patriarchi S., Morfini M., Rossi-Ferrini P. Etoposide in remission induction of adult acute myeloid leukemia Acta Haemato. 1990 v. 83 pp.82–85
8. Creuzig U., Ritter J., Schellong G.(eds) Acute myelogenous leukemia in childhood. Berlin 1990
9. Slevin M.L. The clinical pharmacology of etoposide. Cancer (Phil) 1991 v. 67 suppl 1, pp. 319–329
10. Karp J.E., Burke P.J., Donehower R.C. Effects of rhGM-CSF on intracellular ara-C pharmacology in vitro in acute myelocytic leukemia: comparability with drug induced humoral stimulatory activity. Leukemia 1990 v. 4 pp.553–556
11. Karp J.E., Donehower R.C., Enterline J.P., Dole G.B., Burke P.J. In vivo cell growth and pharmacologic determinants of clinical response in acute myelogenous leukemia. Blood 1989 v. 73 pp.24–30
12. Buchner Th., Hiddemann W. Treatment strategies in acute myeloid leukemia (AML). I. First line treatment Blut 1990 v. 60 pp. 60–67
13. Kurrle E., Ehninger G., Freund M., Heil G., Hoelzer D., Link H., Mitrou P.S., Ohl S., Queisser W., Schlimok G., Wandt H. A multicenter study on intensive induction and consolidation therapy in acute myelogenous leukaemia. Blut 1988 v. 56 pp. 233–236

Acute Leukemias VI
Prognostic Factors
and Treatment Strategies
Büchner et al. (eds)

Poor-Risk Acute Myelogenous Leukemia Patients Undergoing the Fludarabine – Cytosine Arabinoside – Filgrastim Regimen: Multidrug Resistance Expression, Granulocyte Colony-Stimulating Factor Priming Activity and Clinical Response

M.C. Petti, M.P. Martelli, S. Tosti, L. De Felice, T. Valentini, A. Tafuri, M.T. Petrucci, and F. Mandelli

Abstract. Eleven poor-risk acute myelogenous leukemia (AML) patients were treated with fludarabine + cytosine arabinoside + granulocyte colony-stimulating factor (FLAG). The median age was 38 (range 31–51 years) and five patients were female. Six patients were resistant to a previous induction chemotherapy (European Organization for Research on Treatment of Cancer, EORTC, AML10 protocol), two patients had AML secondary to myelodysplastic syndrome, one had chronic myelomonocytic leumekia and two patients were in first resistant or subsequent relapse. According to the French-American-British (FAB) classification, patients presented with the following subtypes: four M4/M5, three not classifiable, two M2, one CMML, one M6. Seven patients achieved a complete remission (CR) (63%), of these four patients were MDR positive. The median time to achieve CR was 39.5 days (range 28–49 days). Four patients relapsed after 1, 2, 3, 3 months, respectively, while three patients (all MDR positive) are still in CR after 3, 7, and 12 months. In our experience, no major toxicities were observed during the treatment, except mild mucositis. Our results confirm the feasibility of this schedule and its efficacy in poor-risk AML, suggesting a preferential role in AML patients expressing the MDR phenotype.

Introduction

Treatment of acute myelogenous leukemia (AML) with initial induction chemotherapy induces complete remission (CR) in approximately 70% of patients and cure may be obtained in about 30%–40% [1–4]. Despite these results in the treatment of newly diagnosed AML, refractoriness to multiple chemotherapeutic agents remains a major cause of treatment failure. Although many AML patients can achieve a first CR after a second induction course or a second CR after reinduction chemotherapy, the response duration is usually short and long-term survival is observed in fewer than 5% of patients with a new chemotherapeutic approach Only a bone marrow transplantation (BMT), allogeneic or autologous, may offer a potential curative alternative [5–7]. Two major pathogenetic mechanisms are responsible of refractoriness: (a) failure of initial chemotherapy (primary resistant leukemia); and (b) developement of resistance to chemotherapy in initially responding patients who have then relapsed (early or late). The poor prognosis of these patients has been associated with the presence of leukemic clones resistant to conventional drugs. Thus, patients not achieving CR after one course of intensive induction chemotherapy represent a poor prognosis group.

Multidrug resistance (MDR) is so far a poorly understood phenomenon. Recently it has been proved that an overexpression of MDR1 gene is closely related to clinical drug resistance and is predictive of treatment outcome in several hematologic diseases [8–10]. Therefore, agents not related to MDR are in evaluation with the aim of overcoming MDR. Among these agents, fludarabine phosphate, an adenosine nucleoside

Department of Hematology, University La Sapienza, Roma, Italy

analogue, has been successfully used as single agent in lymphoproliferative disorders. This drug exerts its antileukemic activity by interfering with tumor cell growth by directly or indirectly inhibiting DNA replication. Moreover, recently the association of fludarabine + cytosine arabinoside 'ara-C' was proven to increase the intracellular arabinosylcytosine 5'-triphosphate (Ara-CTP) accumulation beyond that possible with a single dose of ara-C [11].

Cytosine arabinoside is one of the most used and effective agents for the treatment of AML. Its cytotoxic activity depends on the intracellular conversion of ara-C to its active metabolite, the 5'-triphosphate ara-CTP that inhibits DNA synthesis; thus, ara-C is a cell cycle-specific drug that exerts its cytotoxic effects predominantly in S phase [12–13].

The administration of granulocyte colony-stimulating factor (G-CSF), given prior to and during drug administration, has been shown to improve ara-C cytotoxicity in AML [14–15]. Recent clinical trials by Estey et al. [16] have demonstrated that fludarabine infusion prior to ara-C increased ara-CTP accumulation and G-CSF infusion enhanced F-ara-ATP accumulation in AML blasts in vivo. A first study by this group tested this combination in relapsed or refractory AML, producing 59% CR [17]. These results induced these authors to use the association G-CSF and fludarabine/ara-C in poor-prognosis newly diagnosed AML or myelodysplastic syndrome (MDS) patients; 65% of 69 AML patients and 60% of 49 MDS patients achieved CR [18].

Based on these data, we have used the combination of G-CSF and fludarabine/ara-C (FLAG) as a therapeutic synergistic strategy in order to improve the remission rate in patients with poor-prognosis AML.

Patients and Methods

Patients. Since November 1993, 11 poor-risk AML patients have been enrolled. Poor-risk AML was defined as follows: (a) patients with all cytological types of AML according to the French–American–British (FAB) classification, except M3 AML, who are resistant to standard induction chemotherapy (European Organization for Research on Treatment of Cancer, EORTC, AML10 protocol); (b) patients in first relapse resistant to standard reinduction chemotherapy or in second/subsequent relapse; (c) MDS evolved with AML or secondary AML not eligible for standard induction chemotherapy. Inclusion criteria were as follows: (a) performance status of 0–2 according to the World Health Organization (WHO) grading and life expectancy of more than 3 months; (b) bilirubin and creatinine <2 mg/dl; (c) left ventricular ejection $>50\%$ with no cardiac dysfunction; (d) informed consent of the patient. The median age was 38 years (range 31–51 years) and five patients were female. Six patients were resistant to previous induction chemotherapy (EORTC AML10 protocol), two patients had AML secondary to a myelodysplastic syndrome, one had chronic myelomonocytic leukemia (CMML) and two patients are in first resistant or subsequent relapse. According to the FAB classification, patients presented with the following subtypes: four M4/M5, three not classifiable, two M2, one chronic myelomonocytic leukemia (CMML), one M6.

Prophylaxis against *P. carinii* infection was scheduled using cotrimoxazole, and herpetic complications were prevented by acyclovir (5 mg/kg per day). Broad-spectrum antibiotics were given in case of fever during neutropenia. Patients characteristics are listed in Table 1.

Treatment. The patients were treated with 30 mg/m^2 per day fludarabine by 30-min infusion (days 1–5) followed by 4-h infusion of ara-C at 2 g/m^2 per day (days 1–5); G-CSF was administered on days 0–5 in six patients and from day 0 to a polymorphonuclear (PMN) recovery (defined as PMN value greater than 500/mmc) in five patients (FLAG regimen).

Bone marrow (BM) was evaluated on day 26 after the begining of the course. Patients who did not achieve CR received a second identical course after 3–4 days from evaluation of response, with a new BM control 26 days after the initiation of this second cycle.

Patients achieving CR after one or two courses of induction were submitted to a consolidation course starting 4 weeks after the completion of the last induction course. This consolidation course was identical to the induction course with the omission of G-CSF.

The patients in CR after the consolidation course were then planned to a post-remissional program that included allogeneic or autologous BMT or conventional maintenance therapy in patients ineligible for transplantation procedures.

Table 1. Patient characteristics

Patient no.	Sex	Age (years)	FAB	Status	MDR Rhdefflux (mean)	BM Blasts (%)	G-CSF Schedule	Consolidation	Response	Follow up
1	F	31	NC	Resistant	51	80	PMN Recovery	Yes	CR	CCR+12 months
2	M	35	M2	Resistant	7.4	30	PMN Recovery	No	Resistant	Lost to follow up
3	M	50	M5	Resistant	9.3	30	PMN Recovery	Yes	CR	Relapse after 3 months
4	M	38	M4	Resistant	28	54	5 Days	Yes	CR	Relapse after 3 months
5	M	43	M2	Resistant	0	55	5 Days	Yes	CR	Relapse after 2 months
6	F	36	M6	Resistant	6	70	5 Days	Yes	CR	CCR+5 months
7	M	51	M5	Second relapse	4.5	38	PMN Recovery	No*	CR	Relapse after 1 month
8	F	38	NC	Secondary	25.2	32	PMN Recovery	NO	Persistant Hypoplasia	Hypoplasic after 10 months
9	M	48	CMML	Onset	24	14	5 Days	Yes	CR	CCR+8 months
10	M	38	M5	First Relapse Resistant	20	76	5 Days	No	Resistant	Dead after 1 month
11	F	48	NC	Secondary	21.2	55	5 Days	No	Resistant	Alive with Disease after 8 months

Complete remission was defined according to the conventional criteria of the Cancer and Leukemia Group B [19]. Failures to induction therapy were classified according to Preisler et al. [20], whereas toxicity was assessed according to the WHO criteria [21].

Biological Study. All patients included in the study were evaluated for MDR expression and leukemic growth patten. Biological studies were performed before G-CSF administration.

The detection of MDR expression was made using the flow cytometric Rhodamine-123 functional test performed in the presence or absence of cyclosporine A(CSA), used as a MDR-reversing agent [22–23]. Samples were incubated with Rhd-123 (1 μg/l) for 15 s, then washed and exposed to an MDR-reversing agent for 60 min. Evaluation in the presence or absence of CSA was performed at 0, 15 and 60 s comparing within each sample the percentage decrease of mean fluorescence. Flow cytometric measurement was performed using a FACScan (Becton Dickinson) and its software for analysis.

The effect of G-CSF administration on the proliferative potential of clonogenic leukemic cells was assessed by in vitro cultures of BM and peripheral blood samples. Cultures in cytokine-free medium were also established in order to determine the autologous proliferative activity of AML cells. The effect of G-CSF was evaluated by comparing the clonogenic leukemic (CFU-L) growth detected in cultures performed before and 24 h after in vivo G-CSF administration

Results

Clinical Results

Seven out of 11 patients (63%) entered a CR, all of them after one course of FLAG. Among the seven patients who achieved CR, four were MDR positive. The median time to achieve CR was of 39.5 days (range 28–49 days). Five out of six patients with resistant disease achieved CR, while the two patients in first resistant and in second relapse developed resistance and second CR, respectively. The two patients with AML secondary to a myelodysplastic phase did not enter CR because of persistant hypoplasia and resistant disease, respectively.

Reasons for failure were resistance in three patients and persistent hypoplasia in one patient. All but one, of the patients, received a consolidation course; persistent infection was the cause of the one patient not being treated. Four patients relapsed after 1, 2, 3, 3 months respectively with three patients (all MDR positive) are still in CR after 3, 7, and 12 months (see Table 1).

Toxicity

Nine out of 11 patients were evaluable for hematological recovery. The median time to obtain a PMN > 500/mmc was 23 days (range 20–27 days) while a median interval of 28 days (range 20–35 days) was required to achieve a platelets value > 50 000/mmc. No differences were observed among patients receiving G-CSF from day 0 to day 5 or from day 0 until PMN recovery. Generally, the FLAG regimen was well tolerated and only mild mucositis was observed. Eight patients developed fever during the treatment: in patients cases a sepsis by Gramnegative bacteria was detected, in two patients a pulmonary infection by *Aspergillus* had complicated a lung infection observed during the previous induction chemotherapy, one patient developed a Gram-negative sepsis in association with sinusitis caused by *Aspergillus*.

Biological Results

MDR Expression. In ten out of 11 evaluable patients the mean Rhd-efflux value was 19.8% (range 4.5%–51.2%) showing in all cases a high dye efflux, although to a different degree, efficiently blocked by the MDR-reversing agent, indicating a MDR functional expression [18].

Clonogenic Assay. The clonogenic cell growth at time 0 and after 24 h of in vivo G-CSF administration showed only minor changes in standard culture conditions, whereas a rise of the autonomous proliferation of BM clonogenic leukemic cells was detected after G-CSF in all but two cases with a 13-fold mean increase.

Therapy of resistant/relapsed disease remains a major problem in treating AML patients. Several mechanisms of drug resistance, including decreased drug accumulation (antifolate resistance), altered drug metabolism (ara-C and alkylating agents), increased repair (alkylating agents), altered drug targets (topoisomerase II activity), and altered gene expression are most likely involved in the emergency of leukemic clones. In this tissue the role of typical MDR and altered ara-C metabolism seems particularly relevant since standard AML induction regimens are based on ara-C and MDR-related drugs. To circumventing this problem, various strategies have been explored, such as the use of high dose ara-C or of MDR-un related drugs [24]. In this setting, the M.D. Anderson Group [18], among others investigated the efficacy and the safety of the association of fludarabine + ara-C with and without G-CSF in relapsed and refractory AML patients, and obtained promising results. These preliminary data allowed us test the FLAG protocol in a small group of poor-risk AML patients. In our experience, among 11 patients evaluable for clinical response, seven achieved remission, three did not, and one was considered as having persistent hypoplasia; these data confirm the results obtained by other groups using the FLAG protocol [17, 18, 25]. It is worth noting that among seven patients expressing the MDR phenotype, four achieved remission, suggesting that the FLAG regimen may be effective in inducing CR in poor-risk AML patients characterized by high MDR expression. These preliminary data suggest the efficacy of the FLAG protocol in AML patients characterized by high MDR expression and the possibility of an elective use of this association in large series of patients expressing the MDR phenotype at the onset of the disease and/or in relapse.

Furthermore, the FLAG protocol seems to be a tolerable regimen with mild toxicity, as reported by our group and by others. The role of growth factor priming of G-CSF in these patients will be further evaluated in the ongoing study.

References

1. Keating MJ, Kantarjian H, Smith TL et al.: Response to salvage therapy and survival after relapse in acute myelogenous leukemia. J Clin Oncol 7: 1071-1080, 1989
2. Buchner T, Urbanitz D, Hiddeman W et al.: Intensified induction and consolidation with or without maintenance chemotherapy for acute myeloid leukemia (AML): two multicenter studies of the German AML cooperative group. J Clin Oncol 3: 1583-9, 1985
3. Cassileth PA, Lynch E, Hines JD et al.: Varying intensity of postremission therapy in acute myeloid leukemia. Blood 79: 1924-30, 1992
4. Harosseau JL, Milpied N, Briere J et al.: Double intensive consolidation chemotherapy in adult myeloid leukemia. J Clin Oncol 9: 1432-7, 1991
5. Champlin RE, Gale RP. Acute myelogenous leukemia: recent advances in therapy. Blood 69: 1551-1562, 1987
6. Mandelli F, Rees JKH, Gorin NC, Prentice G. Post-remission treatment in acute myeloid leukemia: chemotherapy or autologous or allogeneic bone marrow transplantation. Haematologica 75: 203-211, 1990
7. Hiddemann W, Buchner T. Treatment strategies in acute myeloid leukemia (AML). II Second line treatment. Blut 60: 163-171, 1990
8. Campos L, Guyotata D, Archimbaud E et al.: Clinical significance of multidrug resistance P-glycorprotein expression on acute non-lymphoblastic leukemia cells at diagnosis. Blood, 79: 473-476, 1992
9. Marie JP, Zittoun R, Sikic B. Multidrug resistance (MDR1) gene expression in adult leukemias: correlations with treatment outcome and in vitro drug sensitivity. Blood 78: 586-592, 1991
10. Pirker R, Wallner J, Geissler K et al.: MDR1 gene expression and treatment outcome in acute myeloid leukemia. J Natl CancerInst 83: 708-712, 1992
11. Gandhi V, Estey E, Keating MJ et al.: Fludarabine potentiates metabolism of cytarabine in patients with acute myelogenous leukemia during therapy J Clin Oncol 11: 116-124, 1993Y
12. Kufe DW, Spriggs DR: Biochemical and Cellular pharmacology of cytosine arabinoside. Semin Oncol 12: 34-38, 1985
13. Major PP, Egan EM, Herrick DJ et al.: Effect of ara-C incorporation of deoxyribonucleid acid synthesis in cells. Biochem Pharmacol 31: 2937-2946, 1982
14. Tafuri A, Andreeff M. Kinetic rationale for cytokine-induced recruitment of myeloblastic leukemia followed by cycle—specific chemotherapy in vitro. Leukemia 4: 826-834, 1990
15. Koistinen P, Wang C, Curtis JE, McCulloch EA. Granulocyte—macrophage colony-stimulating factor and interleukin 3 protect leukemic blast cells from ara-C toxicity. Leukemia 5: 704-711, 1991
16. Estey E, Kantarjuan H, Plunkett W et al.: Treatment of refractory acute leukemia with fludarabine+cytosine arabinoside. Proc Am Soc Clin Oncol 11: 268, 1992 (abstr)
17. Estey E, Plunket W, Gandhi V et al.: Fludarabine and arabi-nosylcytosine therapy or refractory and relapsed acute myelogenous leukemia. Leuklymphoma 9: 343-350, 1993
18. Estey E, Thall P. Andreeff M et al.: Use of granulocyte colony stimulating factor before, during and after fludarabine plus cytarabine induction therapy in newly diagnosed acute myelogenous leukemia or myelodysplastic syndromes: comparison with fludarabine plus cytarabine without granulocyte colony stimulating factor. J Clin Oncol 12(4): 671-678, 1994

19. Ellison RR, Holland JF, Weil WM et al.: Arabinosylcytosine: useful agent in the treatment of acute leukemia in adults. Blood 32: 507–513, 1968.
20. Preisler HD. Failure or remission induction in acute myelocytic leukemia. Med Ped Oncol 4: 275–280, 1988
21. Miller AB, Hoogstraten B, Staquet M, Winkler A. Reporting results of cancer treatment. Cancer 47: 207–214, 1981
22. Marie JP, Bastie YN, Colonna F et al. Cyclosporin A as a modifier of agent in the salvage treatment of acute leukemia (AL). leukemia 7: 821–824, 1993
23. Andreeff M, Drzynkiewicz Z, Sharpless TK, Clarkson BD, Melamed MR. Discrimination of human leukemia subtypes by flow cytometric analysis of cellular DNA and RNA. Blood 55: 282–293, 1989
24. Martiat P, Ghilain JM, Ferrat A et al. High dose cytosine arabinoside and amsacrine or mitoxantrone in relapsed and refractory acute myeloid leukemia: A prospective randomized study. Eur J Haem 45: 164–167, 1990
25. Visani G. Tosi P, Zinzani PL et al. FLAG (fludarabine+high-dose cytarabine+G-CSF): An effective and tolerable protocol for the treatment of "poor risk" acute myeloid leukemias. Leukemia 8 (11): 1842–1846, 1994

Acute Leukemias VI
Prognostic Factors
and Treatment Strategies
Büchner et al. (eds)

Granulocyte–Macrophage Colony-Stimulating Factor During and After Remission Induction Treatment for Elderly Patients with Acute Myeloid Leukemia

F. Witz[1], J.L. Harousseau[2], A. Sadoun, D. Guyotat, C. Berthou, J.Y. Cahn, C. Gardin. B. Lioure, B. Witz, B. Desablens, N. Ifrah, B. Pignon, P.Y. Leprise, B. Audhuy, D. Caillot, P. Casassus, B. Christian, P. Linassier, M. Mercier, Z. Tellier, and P. Hurteloup on behalf of the GOELAM Group

Abstract. From May 1992 to November 1994, 240 patients with de novo acute myeloid leukemia (AML) and aged 55–75 years (median 68 years) were enrolled in a multicenter, double-blind randomized study comparing placebo and granulocyte-macrophage colony-stimulating factor (GM-CSF) (*Escherichia coli* derived) (5/μg/kg per day 6-h infusion) during induction chemotherapy (idarubicin 8 mg/m^2 per day i.v. on days 1–5 plus cytarabine, ara-C, 100 mg/m^2 per day continuous infusion on days 1–7) and until recovery of a neutrophil count > 0.5×10^9/l. Post-remission therapy was identical in the two arms. The two groups were comparable regarding the following parameters: age, sex, performance status, fever, organomegaly, initial blood cell counts, French-American-British (FAB) classification, presence of myelodysplastic features, and incidence of karyotypic abnormalities. Of the 209 patients currently evaluable, 130 (62%) achieved complete remission (CR) with no significant difference between patients aged 55–64 (57/90 = 63%) and patients aged 65 to 75 years (73/119 = 61%). There were 17 (8%) early deaths, 18 (9%) deaths in aplasia, and 45 (21%) failures. No significant difference was observed between the GM-CSF group (n = 103) and the placebo group (n = 106) regarding the CR rate (63% vs. 61%), the incidence of early deaths (10% vs. 6%), of deaths in aplasia (8% vs. 9%), and of failures (19% vs. 24%). The duration of neutropenia was shorter in the GM-CSF group (median 22 days vs. 26 days, p = 0.002). However, the incidence of febrile episodes and of bacteriemias and the duration of hospitalization was similar in the two groups. With a median follow up of 19 months, the overall survival of all eligible patients was similar in both groups (39% actuarial survival at 2 years in the GM-CSF group vs. 33% in the placebo group, p = 0.45 log-rank test). Nonetheless, the disease-free survival was longer for patients who achieved CR in the GM-CSF group (44% continuous CR rate at 2 years vs. 19%, p = 0.024). The study medication was prematurely stopped due to toxicity in 17 patients (14 GM-CSF, three placebo; p = 0.003). We conclude that (a) the induction treatment with idarubicin and conventional doses of ara-C obtains a high CR rate in elderly patients (b) the administration of GM-CSF during and after induction chemotherapy results in a faster recovery of neutrophils but does not reduce infectious toxicity and increases neither the efficacy of this chemotherapy nor the overall survival. However, the disease-free survival was significantly longer for patients who received GM-CSF before achieving CR.

Introduction

While it is currently possible to cure an increasing number of younger patients with acute myeloid leukemia (AML), the results in elderly patients have been unsatisfactory. The induction treatment for AML in the elderly remains disappointing for two main reasons. First, a higher incidence of adverse prognostic factors which explain an increased failure rate. Secondly, and most obviously, there is a higher toxicity of

[1]Centre Hospitalier Universitaire, Service de Medicine A, CHu Nancy, France
[2]Centre Hospitalier Regional et Universitaire de Nantes, France

intensive chemotherapy which increases the death rate during aplasia. Therefore the use of hematopoietic growth factors in combination with intensive chemotherapy has appeared as a potentially highly effective approach for improving outcome in fit elderly patients. Two separate mechanisms of granulocyte-macrophage colony-stimulating factor (GM-CSF) have been demonstrated in AML. When given during chemotherapy, GM-CSF can recruit leukemic blast cells into cell cycle thus making them more susceptible to killing by S phase-specific agents [1]; on the other hand, when given after chemotherapy, GM-CSF may reduce the duration of neutropenia and therefore decrease the rate of infection. In early 1992 the French GOELAM group initiated a randomized trial designed to evaluate the effects of GM-CSF given both during and after induction chemotherapy for AML in elderly patients.

Patients and Methods

Design. The trial was designed as a prospective, randomized, double-blind, placebo—controlled study. The objectives were to compare in a GM-CSF group of patients and in a placebo group the complete remission (CR) rate, the duration of neutropenia, the rate of infections, the disease-free survival (DFS), and the overall survival. Patients were eligible for the study if they were aged 55–75 years with a diagnosis of de novo AML and a performance status before diagnosis of less than 2 according to the World Health Organization (WHO) grading system, and no severe organ failure. Patients with previous unexplained cytopenia were included in the study. Conversely, patients with a history of preleukemia syndrome or secondary AML could not enter the study.

Treatment Program. Induction chemotherapy consisted of idarubicin 8 mg/m^2 per day i.v. for 5 days and cytarabine (ara-C) 100 mg/m^2 per day as a continuous infusion for 7 days. Patients were randomized to receive identical study medication, placebo, or GM-CSF. Recombinant human GM-CSF derived from *Esherichia coli* was provided by Pharmacia-Farmitalia Oncology Department and administered at a dose of 5 µg/kg per day. Study medication was started on day 1 and given as a 6-h infusion until neutrophil recovery (with more than 0.5 × 10^9 neutrophils/l for 3 days) or up to day 28. In patients with more than 50 × 10^9 white blood cells (WBC) per liter before treatment, the study medication was delayed by 1–2 days. Randomization was balanced within each center and was stratified according to age with a cut-off at 65 years. Post-remission treatment was identical in the GM-CSF and placebo groups. Two strategies were used according to age. Patients aged 65–75 received maintenance treatment for 1 year with 6-thioguanine and ara-C weekly and every 3 months a reinduction with CCNU, mitoguazone and ara-C. Patients aged 55–64 were randomly assigned to receive consolidation treatment followed by maintenance treatment or maintenance treatment only. Consolidation treatment consisted of intermediate-dose ara-C 1 g/m^2 every 12 h for 4 days and amsacrine 100 mg/m^2 per day for 2 days.

Patients. As of November 15, 1994, 240 patients were registered in the study. Of the 226 patients analysed, 221 were eligible and 209 can be evaluated for efficacy of the induction treatment.

Results

The median age of the overall group was 68 years; 90 patients were aged 55–64 years and 119 patients were 65–75. The initial characteristics of the patients were similar in the GM-CSF group (103 patients) and the placebo group (106 patients). There was no statistical difference between the two groups regarding median age, proportion of older people, sex ratio, history of unexplained cytopenia and incidence of poor clinical condition at presentation, or frequency of fever at diagnosis. The two groups were also comparable considering the initial hematologic characteristics of the patients, especially the French-American-British (FAB) subtype, the blood cell counts, the presence of morphologic features of myelodysplasia and the incidence of cytogenetic abnormalities.

Remission Treatment Outcome. Overall CR rate was 62% (130/209) with no significant difference between patients aged 55–64 years (63%) and patients aged 65–75 (61%). There were 17 (8%) early deaths, 18 (9%) deaths in aplasia, and 45 (21%) failures. No significant difference was observed between the GM-CSF group and the placebo group regarding the CR rate (63% vs.

61%), the incidence of early deaths (10% vs. 6%), deaths in aplasia (8% vs. 9%), and failures (19% vs. 24%). The incidence of early regrowth of blood leukemic blasts was similar in the two groups (9% in the GM-CSF group vs. 7% in the placebo group).

Duration of Neutropenia. Median duration of neutropenia in patients who entered and came out of neutropenia was 22 and 26 days in the GM-CSF and placebo groups, respectively (p = 0.002). However, the incidence of febrile episodes and documented infections like bacteriemias was similar in both groups as was the duration of antibiotic use (median 21 days in the GM-CSF group vs. 23 days in the placebo group; p = 0.28), and the duration of hospitalization (median 30 days vs. 32 days; p = 0.08).

Toxicity. GM-CSF treatment was discontinued in 14% of patients due to intolerance, whereas the rate for placebo discontinuation was only 3% (p = 0.003). The main reasons for discontinuation were fluid overload symptoms (five patients) and side effects like flushing, hypotension, and fever. In four patients with multiorgan failure, the study medication was discontinued only as a precaution. Severe extra-hematologic toxicities (National Cancer Institute NCI, grade ≥3) were comparable in both groups.

Survival. The median follow-up time is 19 months. Despite similar overall outcome after induction treatment in the two groups, the DFS was significantly longer for patients who achieved CR in the GM-CSF group. The probability of continuous CR after 2 years is shown in Fig. 1: 44% in the GM-CSF group vs. 19% in the placebo group (p = 0.024, log-rank test). We have checked that post-CR treatment was actually identical in both groups, especially after the second randomization. Nonetheless, the overall survival of all eligible patients was almost the same in both groups as shown in Fig. 2: the 2-year actuarial survival was 39% in the GM-CSF group vs. 33% in the placebo group (p = 0.45, log-rank test).

Discussion

The results of this last interim analysis of our trial are still preliminary. However, several points are noteworthy. The induction treatment with idarubicin and conventional doses of ara-C achieves a high CR rate in elderly patients.

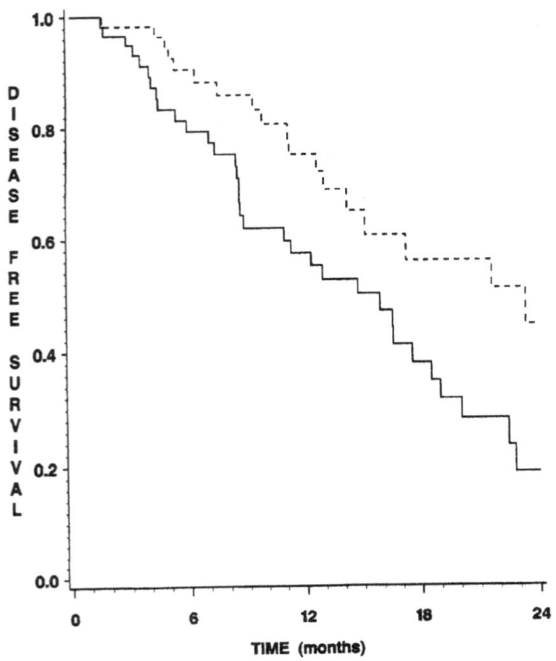

Fig. 1. Disease-free survival in patients in CR, $n = 130$. *Broken line*, GM-CSF, $n = 65$; *Solid line*, placebo, $n = 65$; p = 0.024

Specially in the subgroup of patients aged 65 and older, the 61% CR rate compares favorably with other regimens [2].

The administration of GM-CSF resulted in a faster recovery of neutrophils (22 days vs. 26; $p = 0.002$) but did not reduce either the incidence of severe infections or the duration of anti-infectious treatment and the duration of hospitalization. Several clinical trials of hematopoietic growth factors in conjunction with chemotherapy have been reported in AML since 1989 [3]. Considering comparative trials which have used GM-CSF, the results agree on the reduction of the time to neutrophil recovery [4–8]. However, this accelerated neutrophil recovery did not translate into significant reduction in the rate of severe infections.

In our study, GM-CSF appears ineffective in increasing CR rate and also in reducing early death, toxic death rates and failure rate. Similarly, none of the reported studies in which patients received GM-CSF found an improvement in CR rate whatever the timing for CSF administration had been (either after; or before and during; or before, during, and after chemotherapy) [5, 6, 8–11].

Considering survival, in our study DFS was longer for patients who had received GM-CSF before achieving CR ($p = 0.024$). Nonetheless, overall survival of all patients was almost the same in both groups ($p = 0.45$). The reason for this discrepancy between the DFS and overall survival curves is not yet clear. A somewhat similar result with an equivalent outcome of induction treatment and surprisingly longer DFS in patients having received GM-CSF has already been reported by Buchner et al. [6]. In this study, which included 33% of patients 60 years and over, patients received GM-CSF before, during, and after chemotherapy for induction as well as for consolidation treatment. Only one study, reported by Rowe et al. [8] found chemotherapy associated with GM-CSF to have an improvement in survival rate in elderly patients aged 55–70 years.

Up to now, the clinical use of GM-CSF has not really shown a marked impact on overall survival in elderly patients with AML. The issue remains unsettled and further analysis is required to identify possible subgroups of patients who could benefit the most from GM-CSF treatment.

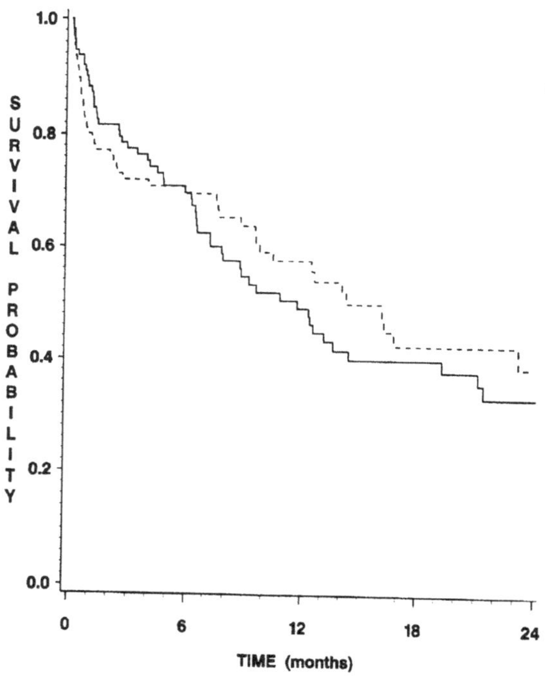

Fig. 2. Overall survival (eligible patients, $n = 221$). *Broken line*, GM-CSF, $n = 107$; *Solid line*, placebo, $n = 114$; $p = 0.45$

References

1. Tafuri A, Andreef M. Kinetic rationale for cytokine-induced recruitment of myeloblastic leukemia followed by cycle-specific chemotherapy in vitro. Leukemia 1990; 4: 826–834.
2. Johnson Pre, Liu Yin JA. Acute myeloid leukemia in the elderly: biology and treatment Br J Haematol 1993; 83: 1–6.
3. Estey EH. Use of colony-stimulating factors in the treatment of acute myeloid leukemia. Blood 1994; 83: 2015–2019.
4. Bettelheim P, Valent P, Andreeff M, et al.: Recombinant human granulocyte-macrophage colony-stimulating factor in combination with standard induction chemotherapy in de novo acute myeloid leukemia. Blood 1991; 77: 700–711.
5. Buchner T, Hiddemann W, Koenigsmann M, et al.: Recombinant human granulocyte-macrophage colony-stimulating factor after chemotherapy in patients with acute myeloid leukemia at higher age or after relapse. Blood 1991; 77: 700–711.
6. Buchner T, Hiddemann W, Rottmann R, et al. Multiple course chemotherapy with or without GM-CSF priming and longterm administration for newly diagnosed AML. Proc Am Soc Clin Oncol 1993; 12: 301 (abstr. 985).
7. Estey E, Thall PF, Kantarjian H, et al. Treatment of newly diagnosed acute myelogenous leukemia with granulocyte-macrophage colony-stimulating factor (GM-CSF) before and during continuous-infusion high dose ara C + daunorubicin: comparison to patients treated without GM-CSF. Blood 1992; 79: 2246–2255.
8. Rowe JM, Andersen J, Mazza JJ, et al. Phase III randomized placebo-controlled study of granulocyte-macrophage colony stimulating factor (GM-CSF) in adult patients (55–70 years) with acute myelogenous leukemia (AML). A study of Eastern Cooperative Oncology Group (ECOG). Blood 1993; 82 (suppl 1): 329a (abstr. 1299).
9. Archimbaud E, Fenaux P, Reiffers J, et al. Granulocyte-macrophage colony-stimulating factor in association to timed-sequential chemotherapy with mitoxantrone, etoposide, and cytarabine for refractory acute myelogenous leukemia. Leukemia 1993; 7: 372–377.
10. Stone R, George S, Berg D, et al. GM-CSF "V" placebo during remission induction for patients $\geqslant 60$ years old with de novo acute myeloid leukemia: CALGB study. Proc Am Soc Clin Oncol 1994; 13: 304 (abstr 992).
11. Zittoun R, Mandelli F, de Witte T, et al. Recombinant human granulocyte-macrophage colony stimulating factor (GM-CSF) during induction treatment of acute myelogenous leukemia (AML). A randomized trial from EORTC-GIMEMA leukemia cooperative groups. Blood 1994; 84 (suppl 1): 231 a (abstr 909).

Acute Leukemias VI
Prognostic Factors
and Treatment Strategies
Büchner et al. (eds)

Prospective Comparison of Allogeneic Bone Marrow Transplantation, Intensive Consolidation Chemotherapy, and Unpurged Autologous Bone Marrow Transplantation as Post-Remission Therapy in Adult Acute Myeloid Leukemia

J.L. Harousseau, B. Pignon, F. Witz, P. Linassier, B. Lioure, P.Y. Le Prise, J.Y. Cahn, B. Desablens, D. Caillot, N. Ifrah, J.F. Abgrall, F. Guilhot, D. Guyotat, A. Mors, P. Casassus, J. Brière, V. Polin, P. Berthaud, Z. Tellier, and P. Hurteloup on behalf of the GOELAM Group

Abstract. From November 1987 to April 1994, 522 adult (15–50 years) patients with de novo acute myeloblastic leukemia (AML) were included in the GOELAM 1 protocol comparing allogeneic bone marrow transplantation (BMT), intensive consolidation chemotherapy (ICC) and autologous BMT (ABMT). For induction treatment, patients were randomized to receive a combination of cytosine-arabinoside (ara-C) (200 mg/m^2 per day continuous infusion on days 1–7) and either idarubicin (IDR) (8 mg/m^2 per day on days 1–5) or rubidazone (RBA) (200 mg/m^2 per day on days 1–4). After achievement, of complete remission (CR) an allogeneic BMT was proposed to patients up to the age of 40 with an HLA-identical sibling. Other patients in CR had to receive a first course of ICC (ICC1) with high-dose ara-C (3 g/m^2 every 12 by 3-h infusion on days 1–4, eight doses) and either IDR (10 mg/m^2 per day on days 5–6) or RBZ (200 mg/m^2 per day on days 5–6). Bone marrow was collected after ICC1 and cryopreserved without any in vitro manipulation. If the hematopoietic quality of the collected marrow was adequate, patients were then randomly assigned to receive a second course of ICC (ICC2) with m amsacrine (AMSA); (150 mg/m^2 per day on days 1–5) and etoposide (VP-16) (100 mg/m^2 per day on days 1–5) or an ABMT after a preparative regimen with busulfan (4 mg/kg per day for 4 days) and cyclophosphamide (50 mg/kg per day for 4 days). As of July 1, 1994 490 patients were evaluable and 361 (74%) achieved CR with no significant difference between IDR and RBZ. An allogeneic BMT was planned in 83 cases and was actually performed in 67. Out of the 278 other patients 227 did receive ICC1. The median duration of neutropenia after ICC1 was 19 days and there were nine toxic deaths (4%). A total of 171 patients were randomized between ICC2 (84) and ABMT (87), and 128 have currently been analyzed (61 ICC2, 67 ABMT). The main reasons for exclusion were toxicity, refusal, poor hematologic reconstituion post ICC1, and relapse. With a median follow up of 44 months, the overall survival of the entire cohort of patients is 37% at 6 years (median 22 months) with no difference between the two induction treatment arms. The 4-year disease-free survival (DFS) of the patients in CR who actually received the assigned treatment was 45% for allogeneic BMT, 53% for ICC2, and 47% for ABMT. When considering intention to treat there was no significant difference in DFS between allogeneic BMT and other forms of post-remission therapy or between ICC2 and ABMT. We conclude that (a) a significant improvement of survival can be obtained for patients with de novo AML up 50 years of age with three different modalities of intensive consolidation; (b) the three approaches give comparable results—after ICC1, ICC2 appears to be as effective as unpurged ABMT and is easier to perform; (c) new strategies are needed to reduce the exclusion rate.

Introduction

The optimal strategy for post-remission therapy in acute myeloid leukemia (AML) remains a controversial issue. Three different approaches are currently being debated: allogeneic bone

Department of Hematology, Hôtel-Dieu, Nantes, France

marrow transplantation (BMT), autologous BMT (ABMT), and chemotherapy. Most reports on allogeneic BMT and ABMT in AML have come from single institutions [1–4] or from international registries [5, 6] and could therefore reflect a selection bias. Several small controlled studies comparing allogeneic BMT, chemotherapy [7–9] or ABMT [10–12] have been published. However, the need for large randomized studies was underlined by the controversy persisting in the literature [13, 14]. Moreover, in these studies the post-remission chemotherapy was used at conventional dosage. The issue of dose intensity in post-remission consolidation chemotherapy has been raised after the publication of several pilot studies showing that disease-free survival (DFS) rates of 30%–50% could be achieved after short-term intensive consolidation chemotherapy (ICC) [15–19]. A first randomized trial addressed the issue of the dose–response effect in AML [20]. The clear demonstration of better results with high-dose schedules has recently been published by the Cancer and Leukemia Group B (CALGB) [21].

We present the results of a prospective multicenter randomized study initiated in 1987 by the GOELAM group with the main goal of comparing allogeneic BMT, ABMT, and ICC as post-remission therapy in adult AML.

Patients and Methods

Patients. Patients aged 15–50 years with de novo AML were eligible for entry into a multicenter trial involving 16 centers of the GOELAM group. Patients with a preexisting myelodysplastic syndrome or with a blastic transformation of a chronic myeloproliferative disorder were ineligible. Patients with preexisting cardiac or renal failure or with liver disease and patients who had previously received chemotherapy and/or radiotherapy were not included.

Remission Induction Therapy. The induction treatment was randomized between cytarabine (ara-C) 200 mg/m^2 per day (continuous infusion) for 7 days plus idarubicin (IDR) 8 mg/m^2 per day for 5 days, and ara-C at the same dosage plus rubidazone (RBZ) 200 mg/m^2 per day for 4 days. A bone marrow aspiration was performed on day 17. In the case of minimal residual leukemia ($\leqslant$50% blasts and reduced cellularity), a second course was administered with 3 days of ara-C plus 2 days of either IDR 10 mg/m^2 per day or ZRB 200 mg/m^2 per day. When the marrow was hypoplastic and non-blastic, no further treatment was given. All other cases were classified as failures and treated with salvage regimens.

Post-remission Therapy. Patients in complete remission (CR) were allografted if they were 40 years and younger and had an HLA-identical sibling. The conditioning regimen and the graft-versus-host disease prophylaxis and treatment varied according to protocols used in the different transplant centers. Patients over 40 years of age or without a suitable donor received a first course of intensive consolidation chemotherapy (ICC1) with ara-C (3 g/m^2 in a 3-h infusion every 12 h for eight doses on days 1–4) and either IDR 10 mg/m^2 on days 5–6 or ZRB 200 mg/m^2 on days 5–6. After hematopoietic recovery, marrow was collected. No in vitro manipulation was done. Patients were then randomized between a second course of ICC (ICC2) with m AMSA 150 mg/m^2 per day on days 1–5 and etoposide (VP-16) 100 mg/m^2 per day on days of 1–5. The preparative regimen to ABMT was the Baltimore combination busulfan 4 mg/kg per day for 4 days and cyclophosphamide 50 mg/kg per day for 4 days.

Statistical Analysis. Comparison of patient characteristics within the two induction treatment arms and of CR rates were evaluated by χ^2 tests. Disease-free survival (DFS) was calculated from the date of the first CR until the date of the first relapse or the date of death in CR. Overall survival was calculated from the date of the 1st day of treatment until the date of death or of last visit. Actuarial curves were drawn according to the Kaplan-Meier technique and differences between curves were based on the log-rank test. The median follow-up time is 44 months. The outcome was analyzed according to the post-remission treatment actually received by the patients. However, a number of patients did not receive their assigned treatments. Therefore the analysis was also performed on an intention-to treat basis.

Results

From November 1987 to April 1994, 522 patients were registered. Eighteen were ruled ineligible (nine inadequate diagnosis, nine other exclusion criteria), 14 could not be evaluated (four deaths before any treatment, seven major violations three missing data). Thus, a total of 490 patients were evaluated (246 in the IDR arm, 244 in the HRBZ arm).

The characteristics of the patients are shown in Table 1. There was no significant difference between the two induction treatment arms regarding the incidence of these initial characteristics.

Remission Induction Therapy. Of the 490 evaluable patients, 361 (74%) achieved CR with no significant difference between IDR (172/246 = 70%) and HRBZ (189/244 = 77.5%) ($p = 0.06$). There were eight early deaths (1.5%), 21 deaths in aplasia (4%), and 100 failures (20.5%). CR was achieved with only one course of induction in 95% of cases.

Feasibility of Post-remission Therapy. Of the 361 patients in CR, 24 were considered as unfit for any intensive therapy. Eighty-three patients aged 15–40 years with an HLA-identical sibling were scheduled for allogeneic BMT. However, at the time of this analysis, only 67 allogeneic BMT have been actually performed. A total of 254 patients were assigned to ICC1. Only 227 ICC1 had been performed by November 1994. Altogether 171 patients were randomized between ABMT (87 patients) and ICC2 (84 patients). In only 128 of these patients was the assigned treatment actually performed. Overall, 195 out of the 361 patients in CR (54%) did receive the planned treatment. Twenty-one patients (6%) are not currently evaluable because of missing data and 145 (40%) were excluded at different steps of the post-remission therapy for the following reasons: major protocol violation or physician's decision (29 patients), poor or slow hematopoietic recovery (27 patients), patient's refusal (22 patients), relapse (22 patients), extrahematological toxicity (20 patients), infection (15 patients), toxic death (nine patients), second cancer (one patient). The median interval between CR achievement and the first intensive treatment was 68 days for allogeneic BMT (range 9–200 days) and 20 days for ICC (range 0–98 days). The median interval between the ICC2 and ABMT was 93 days for ABMT (range 61–137 days), and 76 days between ICC1 and ICC2 (range 33–216 days).

Table 1. Characteristics of the patients

Sex M/F (n)	240/250
Median age (years)	36
Performance status (WHO 0-1/2/3-4)	314/114/62
White blood cell count($10^3/\mu l$)	
—Range	0.4–486
Median	13.7
Platelet count ($10^3/\mu l$)	
—Range	2–999
Median	62
Fever at diagnosis (%)	41
FAB classification (M1, M2, M3, M4, M5,) M6, M7	104/144/36/68/81/7/5[a] (32 unclassified)
Cytogenetic abnormalities	199/350 evaluable karyotypes (57%)

[a]Data missing for 13.

Hematological Toxicity of Post-remission Therapy. The median duration of neutropenia ($< 0.5 \times 10^9/l$) was 19 days after ICC, 24 days after ICC2, and 24.5 days after ABMT. The median duration of hospitalization was 30 days after ICC1, 33 days after ICC2, and 37.5 days after ABMT. There were 15 toxic deaths, 9/227 (4%) patients after ICC1, 1/61 patients (1.5%) after ICC2, and 5/67 patients (7.5%) after ABMT.

Overall Survival. The probability of 6-year survival was 37% for the 490 patients evaluable for induction remission treatment with no significant difference between the two anthracyclines. The overall median survival was 22 months.

DFS of Patients in CR. Out of the 195 patients who actually received the assigned treatment, 72 relapsed (19/67 allogeneic BMT, 26/61 ICC, 27/67 ABMT) and 21 died in first CR (15/67 allogeneic BMT, 1/61 ICC, 5/67 ABMT). The actuarial risk of relapse at 4 years was 38% for the 67 patients undergoing allogeneic BMT, 56% for the 221 patients who received at least ICC1, 43% for the 61 patients who received ICC2, and 44% for the 67 patients undergoing ABMT. The actuarial probability of remaining in first CR after 4 years was 45% after allogeneic BMT, 53% after ICC, and 47% after ABMT (Figs. 1, 2). The intention-to-treat analysis of the 83 patients scheduled for allogeneic BMT and of the 254 patients scheduled for ICC1 showed no difference in the DFS curves (Fig. 3). Similarly, the intention-to-treat analysis of the 84 patients scheduled for ICC2 and of the 87 patients scheduled for ABMT showed no significant difference between the two therapeutic options. The 4-year actuarial DFS was 49% after ICC2 and 42% after ABMT (p not significant)(Fig. 4).

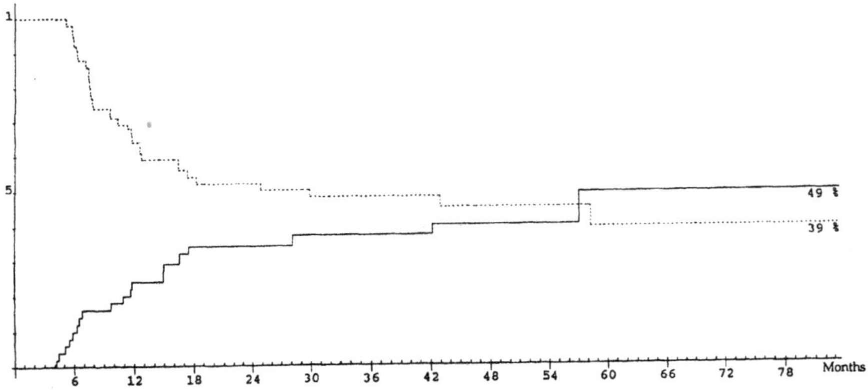

Fig. 1. Disease-free survival (*dotted line*) and probability of relapse (*solid line*) after allogeneic BMT (67 patients)

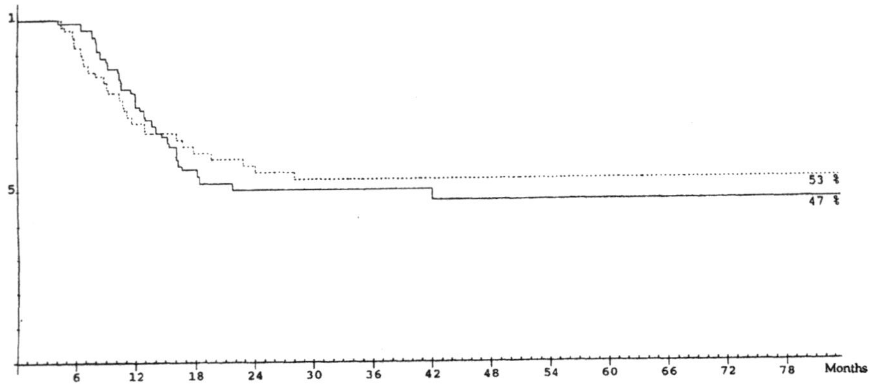

Fig. 2. Disease-free survival after the second course of ICC (*dotted line*; 61 patients) or after unpurged ABMT (*solid line*; 67 patients)

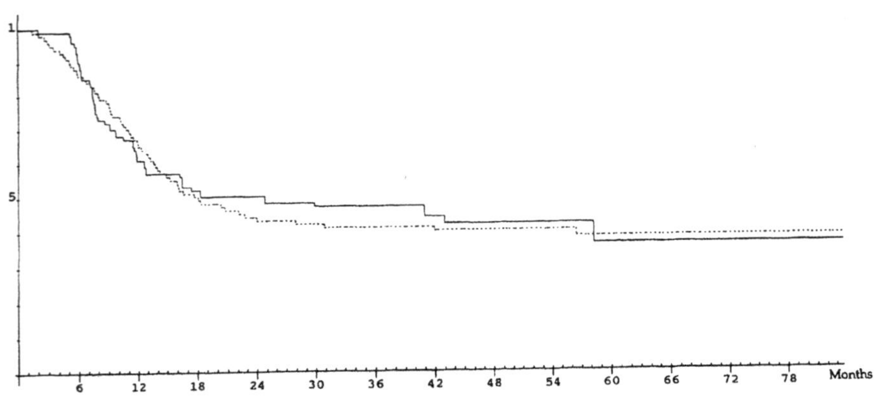

Fig. 3. Disease-free survival. Comparison between allogeneic bone marrow transplantation (*solid line;* 83 patients scheduled for allogeneic BMT) and other intensive therapies (ICC1; *dotted line;* 254 patients scheduled for the first course of ICC) (intention-to-treat analysis)

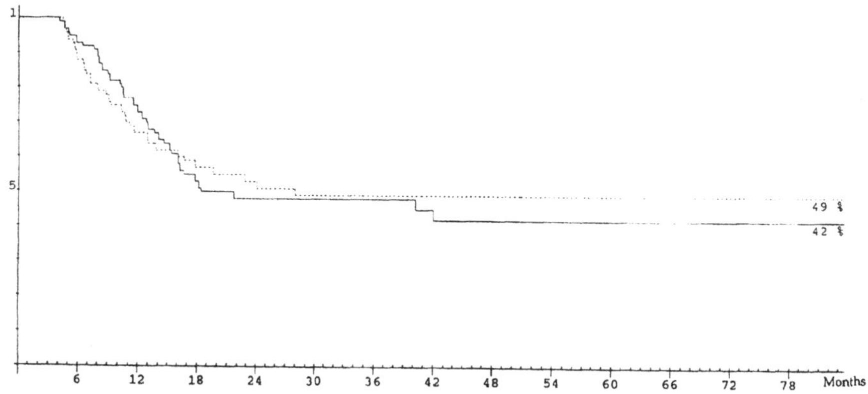

Fig. 4. Disease-free survival. Comparison between the second course of (ICC *dotted line*; 84 patients) and ABMT (*solid line*; 87 patients) (intention-to-treat analysis)

Discussion

The trial was closed for accrual in April 1994 but the final analysis has not yet been done. Therefore the current results must be interpreted with caution. However, they appear to confirm the results of an interim analysis performed previously [22].

The CR rate (74%) is in the range of currently achieved CR rates in the same age population. This result confirms our previous experience with HRBZ [19] together with the good antileukemic activity of IDR shown by other groups [23–25]. However, only 5% of the CR were achieved thanks to the second course of induction and there was a 20.5% failure rate.

The different types of intensive first-remission therapy all raise the issue of feasibility. Only 195 out of the 361 patients in CR (54% of the remitters) could actually receive the intensive treatment assigned by a design of the protocol (allogeneic BMT, ICC, or ABMT). As in other comparable studies [11,26], a large number of patients did not complete the whole program for a variety of reasons including physician's decision, patient's refusal, hematological or extrahematological toxicity of treatment. For instance, in the recently published the European Organization for Research and Treatment of Cancer (EORTC) study [26], only 343 of 623 patients in CR (55%) completed the assigned treatment (allogeneic BMT, ABMT, or intensive chemotherapy). In the CALGB trial comparing three doses of ara-C administered during a four-course post-remission therapy, 62% of patients under the age of 60 years, received the full four courses of the high-dose schedule [21]. New strategies are clearly needed to reduce the toxicity of these intensive regimens. The use of hematopoetic growth factors (granulocyte colony-stimulating factor G-CSF, or granulocyte–macrophage CST GM-CSF) could be of value in this regard, since it appears that after intensive chemotherapy, if any, the risk of leukemic blast stimulation is limited [27]. Another alternative could be the use of peripheral blood stem cell collected during CR.

In our experience, allogeneic BMT does not appear to yield a better outcome than ICC or ABMT, since 4-year DFS was only 45%. These results are in discrepancy with those published by other groups [10, 26]. They are somewhat inferior to those currently achieved for AML in first CR. This was not explained by a higher rate of transplant-related mortality but by a relative high risk of relapse. The actuarial risk of relapse was 38% at 4 years. It should be noticed that in the EORTC trial allogeneic BMT was performed after the first course of ICC and that in this multicenter trial the actuarial risk of relapse after allogeneic BMT was lower (24.4%). Thus new strategies are also being discussed in order to reduce the relapse rate after allogeneic BMT (ICC prior to allogeneic BMT, new conditioning regimens, modulation of graft-versus-host prophylaxis).

Our study does not show any significant difference in terms of DFS between ICC and ABMT. This is true not only when comparing patients who actually received the treatment assigned by randomization but also when comparing the total cohort of randomized patients on an intention-to-treat basis.

These results also differ from those reported by the EORTC-GIMEMA group [26]. With a comparable design, this study showed that ABMT resulted in better DFS than ICC (48% at 4 years versus 30%). Apparently this discrepancy is not explained by differences in the ABMT procedures since in our study DFS after ABMT is quite comparable (47%). The difference between the two studies appears to be a better antileukemic activity of our ICC with a 4-year DFS of 53%. We have no definite explanation for this apparent superiority of our ICC regimen since the design of the two protocols was very similar and since in both studies the interval between each phase of the treatment had to be the shortest possible. We can only underline some differences: the dose of m AMSA is much higher in the GOELAM protocol (600 mg/m^2 total dose versus 360 mg/m^2); VP-16 is used in the GOELAM protocol but not in the EORTC protocol; the EORTC group use daunorubicin for induction and ICC, whereas the GOELAM group use IDR or HRBZ. Our results appear to be comparable to those achieved by the CALGB group with four courses of high-dose ara-C since the 4-year DFS of patients aged 60 years or younger was 44%

Finally, our study confirms that a significant improvement of survival can be obtained in AML for patients up to the age of 50 years thanks to better induction remission treatment and to different modalities of intensive post-remission therapy.

Conclusion

In the GOELAM group experience, after a first course of ICC, a second course of ICC appears to be as effective as an unpurged ABMT and can be offered to a larger number of patients. In our ongoing study, ICC is considered as the reference arm and ABMT is no longer used as consolidation of first CR.

References

1. Clift RA, Buckner CD, Thomas ED et al. The treatment of acute non-lymphoblastic leukemia by allogeneic marrow transplantation. Bone Marrow Transplant 1987, 2: 243–58.
2. Santos GW, Tutschka PJ, Brookmeyer R, et al. Marrow transplantation for acute nonlymphocytic leukemia after treatment with busulfan and cyclophosphamide. N. Engl J Med, 1983, 309: 1347–53.
3. Burnett AK, Tansey P, Watkins R et al. Transplantation of unpurged autologous bone marrow in acute myeloid leukaemia in first remission. Lancet, 1984, 2: 1068–70
4. Körbling M, Hunstein W, Fliedner TM, et al. Disease-free survival after autologous bone marrow transplantation in patients with acute myelogenous leukemia. Blood, 1989, 6:1989–1904.
6. Gorin NC, Aegerter P, Auvert B, et al. Autologous bone marrow transplantation for acute myelocytic leukemia in first remission: a European survey of the role of marrow purging. Blood 1990, 75: 1606–14.
7. Champlin RE, Ho WG, Gale RP et al. Treatment of acute myelogenous leukemia: a prospective controlled trial of bone marrow transplantation versus consolidation chemotherapy. Ann Intern Med 1985, 102: 285–91.
8. Appelbaum FR, Fisher LD, Thomas ED. Chemotherapy versus marrow transplantation for adults with acute non-lymphocytic leukemia: a five-year follow up. Blood 1988, 72: 179–84.
9. Zander AL, Keating M, Dicke K, et al. A comparison of marrow transplantation with chemotherapy for adults with acute leukemia of poor prognosis in first complete remission. J Clin Oncol 1988, 6: 1548–57.
10. Reiffers J, Gaspard MH, Maraninchi D et al. Comparison of allogeneic or autologous bone marrow transplantation and chemotherapy in patients with acute myeloid leukemia in first remission: a prospective controlled trial. Br J. Haematol, 1989, 72: 57–63.
11. Löwenberg B, Verdonck LJ, Dekker AW et al. Autologous bone marrow transplantation in acute myeloid leukemia in first remission: results of a Dutch prospective study. J. Clin. Oncol, 1990, 8: 287-294
12. Ferrant A, Doyen C. Delannoy A et al. Allogeneic or autologous bone marrow transplantation for acute non-lymphocytic leukemia in first remission. Bone Marrow Transplantation, 1991, 7: 303–309
13. Mayer RJ. Allogeneic transplantation versus intensive chemotherapy in first remission acute leukemia: is there a "best choice"? J Clin Oncol, 1988, 6: 1532–6
14. Butturini A, Gale RP. Chemotherapy versus transplantation in acute leukamia. Br J Haematol, 1989, 72: 1–8
15. Cassileth PA, Begg CB, Silber R, et al. Prolonged unmaintained remission after intensive consolidation therapy in adult acute nonlymphocytic leukemia. Cancer Treat Rep, 1987, 71: 137–40.
16. Preisler HD, Raza A, Early A, et al. Intensive remission consolidation therapy in the treatment of acute nonlymphocytic leukemia. J Clin Oncol 1987, 56: 722–30
17. Wolff SN, Herzig RH, Fay JW et al. High-dose cytarabine and daunorubicin as consolidation

therapy for acute myeloid leukemia in first remission: long term follow-up and results. J Clin Oncol 1989, 7: 1260–7.
18. Geller RB, Burke PJ, Karp JE et al. A two-step timed sequential treatment for acute myelocytic leukemia. Blood, 1989, 74: 1499–1506.
19. Harousseau JL, Milpied N, Brière J et al. Double intensive consolidation chemotherapy in adult acute myeloid leukemia. J. Clin Oncol 1991, 9: 1432–7.
20. Cassileth PA, Lyneh E, Hines JD et al. Varying intensity of postremission therapy in acute myeloid leukemia. Blood 1992, 79: 1924–30.
21. Mayer RJ, Davis RB, Schiffer CA et al. Intensive postremission chemotherapy in adults with acute myeloid leukemia. N Engl J Med 1994, 331: 896–903.
22. Harousseau JL, Pignon B, Dufour P et al. Autologous bone marrow transplantation vs intensive chemotherapy in first complete remission: interim results of GOELAM study in AML. Leukemia 1992, 6: suppl 2: 120–3.
23. Berman E, Heller G, Santorsa JA et al. Results of a randomized trial comparing idarubicin with cytosine-idarubicin with daunorubicin and cytosine-arabinoside in adult patients with newly diagnosed acute myelogenous leukemia. Blood 1991, 77: 666–674.
24. Wiernik PH, Banks PLC, Case Jr DC et al. Cytarabine plus idarubicin or daunorubicin as induction and consolidation therapy for previously untreated adult patients with acute myeloid leukemia. Blood 1992, 79: 313–319.
25. Vogler WR, Velez-Garcia E, Weiner RS et al. A phase III trial comparing idarubicin and daunorubicin in combination with cytarabine in acute myelogenous leukemia: a Southeastern Cancer Study Group study. J. Clin. Oncol. 1992, 10: 1103–1111.
26. Zittoun RA, Mandelli F, Willemze R et al. Autologous or allogeneic bone marrow transplantation compared with intensive chemotherapy in acute myelogenous leukemia. N Engl J Med 1995, 332: 217–23.
27. Harousseau JL, Wu D. The use of GM-CSF and G-CSF in the treatment of acute leukemias. Leukemia Lymphoma (in press)

Acute Leukemias VI
Prognostic Factors
and Treatment Strategies
Büchner et al. (eds)

Late Relapses in Adult Acute Myelogenous Leukemia: A Retrospective Study of Characteristics and Outcome in 76 Cases

X. Thomas[1], L. Vila[2], J. Troncy[1], D. Fiere[1], and E. Archimbaud[1]

Abstract. Relapses in acute myelogenous leukemia (AML) are generally considered of poor prognosis. Late relapses are known to represent a special entity with better prognosis. Whether late relapses occur from the original leukemic clone or not is still questioned.

In order to provide clues, the characteristics and outcome of 76 patients with AML who had experienced a first relapse after a first complete remission (CR) duration longer than 18 months (late-relapse AML) were analyzed. Major differences, reflecting exclusively the tumor burden, were noted between presentations at initial diagnosis and after first relapse. Sixteen patients were initially classified as M1, 22 as M2, 12 as M3, 12 as M4, 12 as M5, and two as M6. At the time of first relapse, morphologic changes of blast cells caused assignment to another FAB subgroup in only three patients by comparison with diagnosis. Cytological dyshemopoiesis features, involving at least one lineage, were observed in 29% of patients at diagnosis and 33% at relapse. Metaphase chromosomes were analyzed both at the time of diagnosis and at the time of first relapse only in 15 cases. No differences were noted in karyotypic patterns except in three patients: one patient with normal karyotype at diagnosis presented at relapse with −Y, +8 and +15; one presented at relapse with t(15; 17) not detected at diagnosis; one with del(21) at diagnosis and t(1; 17) at relapse.

Overall, none of the features at time of relapse allow us to suggest a relationship between these late relapses and the development of new leukemias.

Introduction

Complete remission (CR) may be achieved in 50%–80% of adult patients with acute myelogenous leukemia (AML) [1, 2]. However, relapse occurs in 50%–90% of patients with newly diagnosed AML achieving CR when they are treated by chemotherapy only [3]. Relapses are generally considered of poor prognosis [1, 3] and are often diagnosed during the 1st year following CR achievement. However, some relapses arise later and little is still known about these late relapses regarding their pathogenesis and their prognosis. Whether late relapses occur from the original leukemic clone or not is still questioned. Residual leukemic cells could remain uncycling or controlled by the immune system for a long time. Relapse could then occur from the original clone displaying either similar or modified malignant cells, since it is now well established that the cell capacity to mature can be lost to some degree at the time of relapse [4–6]. Another hypothesis in late relapses could be the development of a new leukemia. Late relapses could represent a special entity with better prognosis since several studies have show correlations between the duration of first CR and the ability to achieve a second CR [6–9]. It is now also well established that some patients in first relapse can still achieve long-term second CR when treated with autologous bone marrow transplantation [10, 11] or chemotherapy [12]. We therefore analyzed the characteristics and outcome of patients in our institution who experienced relapse after a first CR duration longer

[1]Service d'Hématologie, Hôpital Edouard Herriot, Lyon, France
[2]Laboratoire Central d'Hématologie, Hôpital Edouard Herriot, Lyon, France

than 18 months (late-relapse AML) with the aim of better evaluating patients with late relapse leading to a better understanding of the pathogenesis of the disease.

Material and Methods

Patient Selection. Among 895 patients with newly diagnosed leukemia treated by chemotherapy in our institution between 1974 and 1991, 76 who experienced their first relapse more than 18 months after CR achievement were included in this study. AML was diagnosed according to the revised French–American–British (FAB) Group criteria [13]. Cytological dyshemopoiesis features were analyzed at the time of diagnosis in 63 cases and at the time of first relapse in 61 cases on May-Grünwald Giemsa-stained bone marrow (BM) smears. The presence of at least one of the following characteristics was taken into account for dyshemopoiesis: nuclear fragmentation, nuclear cytoplasmic maturation asynchrony, large and small erythroblasts for dyserythropoiesis; hypogranulation, monocytoid appearance of neutrophilic granulocytes, Pelger-Huët nuclear abnormality for dysgranulopoiesis; and micromegakaryocytes, hyper- and hyposegmented megakaryocytes for dysmegakaryopoiesis. Metaphase chromosomes were analyzed in 37 patients at diagnosis of whom 22 (59%) displayed a normal karyotype. Twenty-seven patients were analyzed at the time of first relapse, and only 15 both at the time of diagnosis and at the time of first relapse. CR and relapse were defined according to Cancer and Leukemia Group B (CALGB) criteria [14]. All patients presented with medullary relapse except for one with only central nervous system involvement.

Treatment Received by the Patients. At diagnosis, all patients received one or two courses of induction chemotherapy including daunorubicin (67 patients) or mitoxantrone (nine patients) in association with cytosine arabinoside at conventional doses, according to seven successive protocols [15–21]. Once CR was achieved, patients received either maintenance therapy or additional courses of myelosuppressive consolidation according to the protocol design in which they were included. At the time of relapse, eight patients died before any therapeutic attempt or received only palliative therapy, and 68 received reinduction chemotherapy. Among them, 38 patients received a timed-sequential therapy based either on a daunorubicin and cytarabine combination (n = 17) [22], or on mitoxantrone, etoposide, and cytarabine (n = 20) [12]. Seven patients aged over 60 years were treated with daunorubicin from day 1 to day 4 (n = 6) or mitoxantrone from day 1 to day 3 (n = 1) followed by carboplatin from day 4 to day 7 [23]. Fifteen patients received daunorubicin for 3 days in association with cytarabine at conventional doses for 7 days as reinduction at relapse. Two patients with promyelocytic acute leukemia were treated with all-trans retinoic acid associated with daunorubicin and cytarabine [24]. Three patients received amsacrine for 3 days and cytosine arabinoside for 5 days, and four were treated only with low-dose cytarabine. Seven patients underwent allogeneic ($n = 4$) or autologous ($n = 3$) bone marrow transplantation (BMT) while in second CR. For analysis of survival following first relapse, patients in second CR were conventionally censored at the time of transplantation.

Results

Characteristics at Diagonsis and at First Relapse. Forty males and 36 females with a median age of 51 years at presentation (range 17–78 years) and 53 years at first relapse (range 20–81 years) were studied. Pretreatment parameters differed significantly between diagnosis and first relapse particularly for those involving leukemia burden. Twenty-five patients presented with tumoral syndrome at initial diagnosis versus 16 patients at first relapse ($p = 0.1$). Mean percentages ($\pm$ standard deviation, SD) of blast cells in peripheral blood and in bone marrow were respectively 42% $\pm$ 36% and 77% $\pm$ 17% at initial diagnosis, versus, respectively, 26% $\pm$ 34% and 58% $\pm$ 27% at first relapse ($p = 0.0004$ and $p = 0.0001$). Mean value ($\pm$ SD) of lactate dehydrogenase, (LDH) levels was 576 units per liter $\pm$416 units per liter at initial diagnosis versus 431 units per liter $\pm$415 units per liter at first relapse ($p = 0.0001$). Sixteen patients were initially classified as M1, 22 as M2, 12 as M3, 12 as M4, 12 as M5, and two as M6. At the time of first relapse, morphologic changes of blast cells caused assignment to another FAB subgroup in three patients by comparison with diagnosis: one patient classified as M1 was switched to M4, and two patients initially registered as M5 were switched to M4. No differences were noted in karyotypic patterns except in three cases: one patient with normal karyotype at diagnosis presented at relapse with −Y, +8, and +15; one presented at relapse with t(15; 17) not detected at diagnosis; one with del(21) at diagnosis and t(1; 17) at relapse. Cytological dyshemopoiesis features involving at least one lineage were observed in 14 of the 63 studied cases (29%) at diagnosis and in 15 of the 61 studied cases (33%) at relapse. Morphologic changes were noted only in five of the 59 cases studied both at the time of diagnosis and at the time of relapse. Decreases and increases were equally represented since three patients showed acquisition of dyshemopoiesis features at relapse, while two patients lost dyshemopoiesis features initially described.

Overall Outcome. Median time from diagnosis to first relapse was 27 months (range: 18–118 months). After first relapse, eight patients died before any treatment achievement or received only palliative therapy. Among the 68 patients in whom active chemotherapy was attempted, 44 (65%) achieved a second CR and 24 (35%) failed or died during post-relapse induction chemotherapy. Median second CR duration was 8 months (range: 1–64+months). The median overall survival after first relapse was 10 months. Sixteen patients are still in second CR at the time of analysis. Twenty-eight relapsed among whom only five achieved a third CR (18%).

Prognostic Factors for Outcome. Rapid first CR achievement ($p=0.03$), age $\leqslant 50$ at diagnosis ($p=0.004$), low white blood cell (WBC) count at relapse ($p=0.01$), and percentage of circulating blast cells $\leqslant 60\%$ at relapse ($p=0.01$) were associated with a probability of achieving a second CR. Only a low WBC count at relapse appeared to be correlated with the length of second CR duration ($p=0.04$). Rapid first CR achievement was also associated with longer survival after first relapse (median survival: 11 months versus 4 months; $p=0.03$).

Discussion

We studied the clinical and biological characteristics of 76 patients experiencing late relapse, defined as more than 18 months, CR, and their prognostic value for outcome. A decreased cell mass was found between initial diagnosis and first relapse. Careful monitoring of patients in first CR could explain these differences; i.e., there was early diagnosis of relapse before major deterioration of peripheral blood and BM characteristics. Cytological dyshemopoiesis features, involving either erythropoietic, granulocytic, or megakaryocytic lineages, were observed in 29% and 33% of the cases at diagnosis and at relapse, respectively. Similarly to an earlier report [5], acquisition and loss of dyshemopoiesis features were both represented. However, very few patients revealed maturation changes at the time of relapse, confirming that the loss of differentiation at relapse when present was more predictable using immunophenotyping than morphologic examination [6]. A favorable karyotype was shown more frequently in patients whose first CR was > 12 months [8]. This tended to be confirmed in our study since 22 of our patients presented with normal karyotypes. Unfortunately, only 15 of these patients were analyzed at the time of first relapse. Only three showed different karyotypes of whom only one could suggest the involvement of a new leukemia. In our series, the second CR rate was 65%. It is known that a high second remission rate can be achieved using the same chemotherapy for patients whose initial remission ended after 2 years of CR [25]. This suggests the persistance of drug sensitivity and implies that malignant cells belong to a clone initially kinetically quiescent. In our study, some characteristics were found related to prognosis after first relapse, in agreement with previous reports: age [7, 8, 26], high leukocyte count [9], and rapid achievement of the first CR [27]. However, these previous reports selected both early and late relapses.

Overall, none of the features at the time of relapse allows us to suggest a relationship between late relapses and the development of new leukemias. The relapses arising during this period seem to represent the regrowth of leukemic cells which were present at the time of initial diagnosis. A longer first remission duration could involve a leukemic cell population more sensitive to therapy or with a slower doubling time.

References

1. Hiddemann W, Büchner T. Treatment strategies in acute myeloid leukemia (AML). II. Second line treatment (1990) Blut 60: 163–171
2. Büchner T, Hiddemann W. Treatment strategies in acute myeloid leukemia (AML). I. First-line chemotherapy (1990) Blut 60: 61–67
3. Champlin R, Gale RP. Acute myelogenous leukemia: recent advances in therapy (1987) Blood 69: 1551–1562
4. Van Rhenen DJ, Van der Reijden HJ, Van't Veer MB, Engelfriet CP, Von dem Borne AEGK, Langenhuijsen MMAC. Changes in the surface marker pattern related to maturation in adult acute myeloid leukaemia (1983) Leuk Res 7: 357–362
5. Van der Weide M, Van Rhenen DJ, Langenhuijsen MMAC. Maturation changes in relapsing acute myeloid leukaemia (1985) Scand J Haematol 35: 63–65
6. Thomas X, Campos L, Archimbaud E, Shi ZH, Treille-Ritouet D, Anglaret B, Fiere D. Surface marker expression in acute myeloid leukaemia at first relapse (1992) Br J Haematol 81: 40–44
7. Smits P, Schoots L, de Pauw BE, de Witte T, Holdrinet RSG, Janssen JTP, Haanen C. Prognostic factors in adult patients with acute leukemia at first relapse (1987) Cancer 59: 1631–1634
8. Kantarjian H, Keating MJ, Walters RS, McCredie KB, Freireich EJ. The characteristics and outcome of patients with late relapse acute myelogenous leukemia (1988) J Clin Oncol 6: 232–238
9. Uhlman DL, Bloomfield CD, Hurd DD, Peterson BA. Prognostic factors at relapse for adults with acute myeloid leukemia (1990) Am J Hematol 33: 110–116
10. Yeager AM, Kaizer H, Santos GW, Saral R, Colvin OM, Stuart RK, Braine HG, Burke PJ, Ambinder RF, Burns WH, Fuller DJ, Davis JM, Karp JE, Stratford W, Rowley SD, Sensenbrenner LL, Vogelsang GB Wingard JR. Autologous bone marrow transplantation in patients with acute nonlymphocytic leukemia, using ex vivo marrow treatment with 4-hydroperoxycyclophosphamide (1986) N Engl J Med 315: 141–146
11. Ball ED, Mills LE, Cornwell III GG, Davis BH, Coughlin CT, Howell AL, Stukel TA, Dain BJ, McMillan R, Spruce W, Miller WE, Thompson L. Autologous bone marrow transplantation for acute myeloid leukemia using monoclonal antibody-purged bone marrow (1990) Blood 75: 1199–1206
12. Archimbaud E, Leblond V, Michallet M, Cordonnier C, Fenaux P, Travade P, Dreyfus F, Jaubert J, Devaux Y, Fiere D. Sequential therapy with mitoxantrone and continuous infusion etoposide and cytarabine for previously treated acute myelogenous leukemia (1991) Blood 77: 1894–1900
13. Bennett JM, Catovsky D, Daniel MT, Flandrin G, Galton DAG, Gralnick HR, Sultan C. Proposed revised criteria for the classification of acute myeloid leukemia: a report of the French-American-British Cooperative Group (1985) Ann Intern Med 103: 626–629
14. Ellison RR, Holland JF, Weil M, Jacquillat C, Boiron M, Bernard J, Sawitsky A, Rosner F, Gussoff B, Silver RT, Karanas A, Cuttner J, Spurr CL, Hayes DM, Bloom J, Leone LA, Haurani F, Kyle R, Hutchinson JL, Forcier RJ, Moon JH. Arabinosyl cytosine: a useful agent in the treatment of acute leukemia in adults (1968) Blood 32: 507–523
15. Fiere D, Bryon PA, Felman P, Martin C, Peaud PY, Revol L. Treatment of adult acute myeloid leukemia (1977) European Journal of Cancer 13: 403–406
16. Fiere D, Bryon PA, Felman P, Reynaud Y, Coiffier B, Vuvan H. Massive and intermittent chemotherapy induction in 211 patients with acute myeloid leukemia (1979) Symposium on Acute Myeloid Leukemia. International Society of Haematology (Hamburg, Germany)
17. Archimbaud E, Fiere D, Treille-Ritouet D, Adeleine P, Guyotat D, Sebban C, Vuvan H, Viala JJ. Influence of daunorubicin and cytarabine sequencing on the outcome of therapy in acute myelogenous leukemia: a randomized trial (1987) Cancer Treat Rep 71: 571–574
18. Zittoun R, Jehn U, Fiere D, Haanen C, Löwenberg B, Willemze R, Abels J, Bury J, Peetermans M, Hayat M, Suciu S, Solbu G, Stryckmans P. Alternating v repeated postremission treatment in adult acute myelogenous leukemia: a randomized phase III study (AML6) of the EORTC Leukemia Cooperative Group (1989) Blood 73: 896–906
19. Archimbaud E, Thomas X, Michallet M, Jaubert J, Troncy J, Guyotat D, Fiere D. Prospective genetically randomized comparison between intensive postinduction chemotherapy and bone marrow transplantation in adults with newly diagnosed acute myeloid leukemia (1994) J Clin Oncol 12: 262–267
20. Löwenberg B, Fiere D, Zittoun R, Kerkhofs H, Stryckmans P, De Cataldo F, Tura S, Peetermans M, Paulus R, Goudsmit R, Sonnenweld P, Solbu G, Suciu S. Mitoxantrone versus daunorubicin in induction of acute myelogenous leukemia elderly patients and low-dose-ara-C vs control as maintenance. An EORTC phase II trial (AML-9) (1991) Haematologica 76 (suppl.4): 91
21. Castaigne S, Archimbaud E, Fenaux P, Bordessoule D, Tilly H, Simon M, Dupriez B, Auzanneau G, Legros M, Tertian G, Janvier M, Renoux M, Schoenwald M. Place de la double induction dans le traitement des leucémies aiguës myéloblastiques de l'adulte: résultats intermédiaires du protocole LAM90 (1994) Nouv Rev Fr Hematol 36 (suppl.II): 139–140
22. Fiere D, Campos L, Vu Van H, Guyotat D, Archimbaud E, Extra JM, Coiffier B, Viala JJ, Bryon PA, Milan JJ, Ritouet D. Intensive timed chemotherapy protocol for 37 resistant or relapsing acute myeloid leukemias (1986) Cancer Treat Rep 70: 285–286
23. Archimbaud E, Anglaret B, Thomas X, Devaux Y, Ffrench M, Sebban C, Troncy J, Fiere D. Con-

tinuous-infusion daunorubicin and carboplatin of high-risk acute myeloid leukemia in the elderly (1992) Leukemia 6: 776–79
24. Fenaux P, Le Deley MC, Castaigne S, Archimbaud E, Chomienne C, Link H, Guerci A, Duarte M, Daniel MT, Bowen D, Huebner G, Bauters F, Fegueux N, Fey M, Sanz M, Lowenberg B, Maloisel F, Auzanneau G, Sadoun A, Gardin C, Bastion Y, Ganser A, Jacky E, Dombret H, Chastang C, Degos L. Effects of all trans retinoic acid in newly diagnosed acute promyelocytic leukemia. Results of a multicentre randomized trial (1993) Blood 82: 3241–3249
25. Rees JKH, Swirsky D, Gray RG, Hayhoe FGJ. Principal results of the Medical Research Council's 8th Acute Myeloid Leukemia Trial (1986) Lancet i: 1236–1241
26. Keating MJ, Kantarjian H, Smith TL, Estey E, Walters R, Andersson B, Beran M, McCredie KB, Freireich EJ. Response to salvage therapy and survival after relapse in myelogenous leukemia (1989) J Clin Oncol 7: 1071–1080
27. Petersen BA, Bloomfield CD. Re-induction of complete remissions in adults with acute non-lymphocytic leukemia (1981) Leuk Res 5: 81–88

Acute Leukemias VI
Prognostic Factors
and Treatment Strategies
Büchner et al. (eds)

Methods to Detect Prognostic Factors in Acute Myeloid Leukemia

A. Heinecke[1], M.C. Sauerland[1], and T. Büchner[2] for the Acute Myeloid Leukemia Cooperative Group

Abstract. To identify prognostic subgroups, two statistical methods were applied to the data of 1042 adults with acute myeloid leukemia (AML) treated betwen 1986 and 1992 by a protocol of the AML cooperative Group.

Introduction

Risk-adapted treatment in acute myeloid leukemia (AML) requires a clear and practical definition of prognostic subgroups. For this purpose two methods are at hand: the method of classification and regression trees (CART) and Cox regression. Both methods were compared using data of 1042 adults treated between 1986 and 1992 by an intensive and prolonged chemotherapy according to an AML Cooperative Group (AMLCG) protocol [1]. Basic statistics for these 1042 patients are shown in Table 1. A total of 656 patients (63%) had a complete remission (CR). Further analysis is restricted to those 589 (90%) responders with all the covariates shown in Table 1 available.

Method

Prognostic subgroups were defined with respect to disease-free survival (DFS) which is defined as time from CR to relapse or death. The covariates considered for construction of prognostic subgroups were sex, age, platelets, white blood cell count (WBC), serum lactate dehydrogenase (LDH), French-American-British (FAB) subtype, and karyotype. For the purpose of this analysis karyotype was categorized as normal (22% of responders), favorable [t(8, 21), inv16, t(15,17); 7%], unfavorable (-5/5q-, -7/7q-, abnormal 11q23, complex abnormalities; 5%), other karyotype (8%), not evaluable (11%), and not done (47%).

Classification and Regression Trees. This analysis consists of a series of binary splits. At each step the split point is found by maximizing the log-rank statistic over the range of each of the considered covarities [2]. To adjust for different numbers of possible splits, the p value of the log-rank maximum of each covariate is adjusted using the Schumacher-Lausen formula [3]. Only those splits are accepted which are based on an adjusted p value of less than 5%. Splits resulting in subgroups of fewer than 25 patients are rejected. The results of CART are conveniently displayed by means of a binary tree. Besides the splitting condition, each node in the tree contains the group size and the median disease-free survival (DFS) median in months.

For the seven terminal nodes the 5-year DFS rate is included (see Fig. 1).

Cox Regression. Cox regression is based on the well-known proportional hazard model [4]. This model states that DFS prognosis can be calculated from a general baseline prognosis which is modified by a so-called prognostic index (PI). PI is a linear expression of the prognostic covari-

[1]Department of Medical Biostatistics, University of Münster, Germany
[2]Department of Internal Medicine, Hematology/Oncology, University of Münster, Germany

Table 1. Patient Characteristics

	Mean	Median	Range
Observation time (years)	–	5	2–9
Age (years)	50	52	17–83
Platelets (T/cmm)	72	49	0–514
WBC (T/cmm)	42	17	0.1–1038
Serum LDH (U/l)	590	420	86–4362
Sex—			
Male (%)	46.4		
Female (%)	53.6		
FAB subtype			
M1 (%)	18		
M2 (%)	31		
M3 (%)	5		
M4 (%)	29		
M5 (%)	3		
M6 (%)	1		

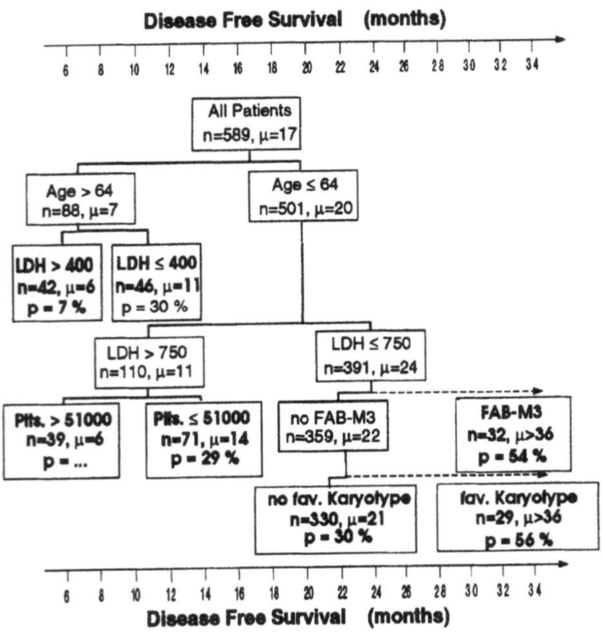

Fig. 1. Prognostic subgroups as identifed by CART, median(months); *p*, 5-year rate

ates. A small PI means good prognosis, a large PI means poor prognosis. A covariate is included into PI on the basis of a stepwise procedure. Considering the same covariates as with CART, the only covariates to be included into PI are LDH, age, FAB M3 (yes = 1, no = 0), and unfavorable karyotype (yes = 1, no = 0). The resulting PI is:

$$PI = .00032 \times LDH + .00947 \times age - .77964 \times (FAB\text{-}M3) + .51794 \times (unfavorable\ karyotype).$$

Discussion

Concentrating the results of CART in to three main groups we get the following: *Good prognosis:* 5-year DFS rate of more than 50%, group size $n = 61$ (10% of evaluable responders). The group is defined by age less than 64 years, LDH less than 750 U/I and FAB M3 or favorable karyotype. *Intermediate Prognosis:* median DFS 21 months, 5-year DFS rate of about 30%, group size $n = 330$ (56%). The group is defined by age less than 64 years, LDH less than 750 U/l and no FAB M3 and no favorable karyotype documented. *Poor prognosis:* median DFS of less than 12 months, group size (n) = 198 (34%). The group is defined by age 64 years, and older or LDH more than 750 U/l. The Kaplan-Meier estimator for these prognostic groups is displayed in Fig. 2.

The result of Cox regression may be described in a similar way by classifying PI into three classes: *Good prognosis:* 5-year DFS rate of

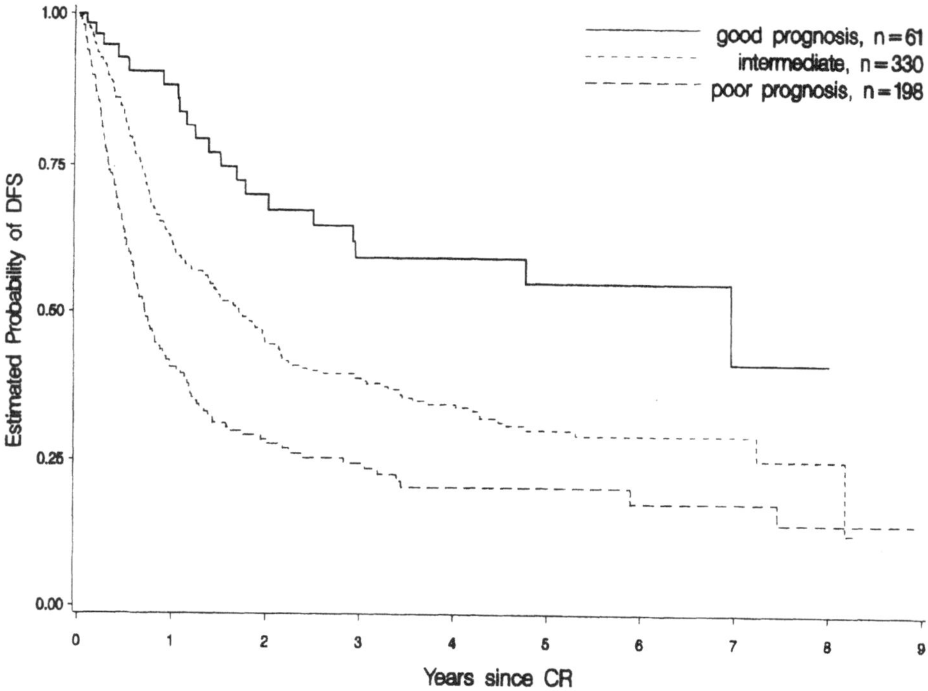

Fig. 2. Kaplan-Meier estimator for prognostic subgroups as identifed by CART

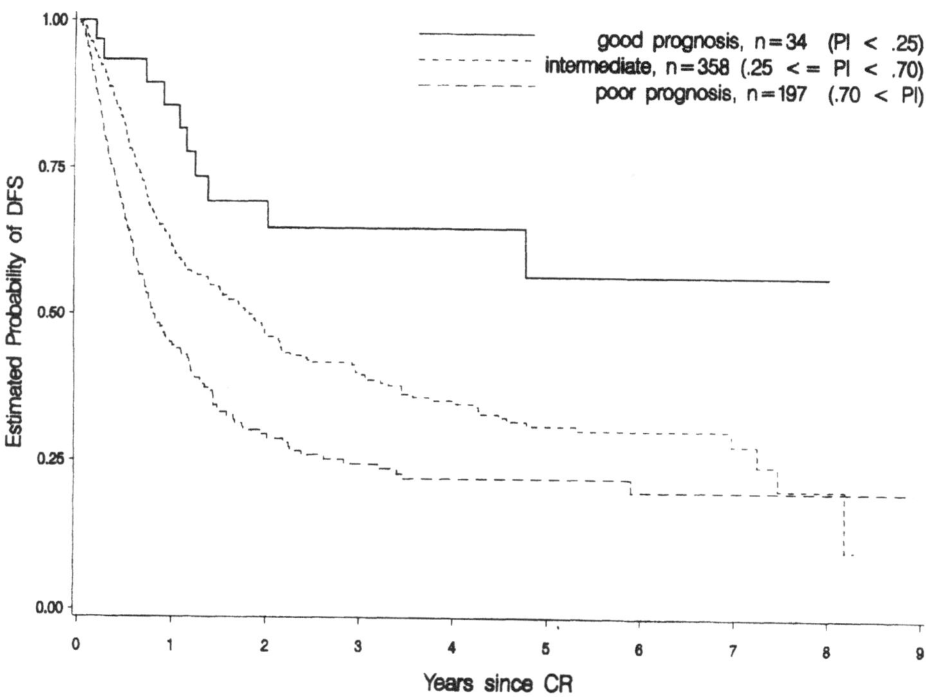

Fig. 3. Kaplan-Meier estimator for prognostic subgroups as identified by Cox regression

more than 50%, group size $n = 34$ (6% of evaluable responders). This group is defined by a PI < .25. *Intermediate prognosis:* median DFS about 15 months, 5-year DFS rate about 30%, group size $n = 358$ (961%). The group is defined by .25 ⩽ PI < .70. *Poor prognosis:* median DFS less than 12 months, 5-year DFS rate less than 20%, group size $n = 197$. This group is defined by a PI ⩾ 0.70. The Kaplan-Meier estimator for these prognostic groups is displayed in Fig. 3.

On the basis of our data, results of CART analysis and Cox regression are in good agreement. Both methods show the same interaction of age and LDH and identify the same group of best DFS prognosis: moderate age and serum LDH together with FAB M3. With CART this group is supplemented by a favorable karyotype. While CART gives a clear-cut definition of prognostic subgroups, Cox regression may give a deeper insight into the dependence of prognosis on the interaction of covariates.

Acknowledgment. The 1986 study of the AMLCG is supported by grant 01 ZP 0123 from the German BMFT.

References

1. Büchner, Th., Hiddemann, W., Löffler, G. et al.: Improved cure rate by very early intensification combined with prolonged maintenance chemotherapy in patients with acute myeloid leukemia: data from the AML Cooperative Group, Seminars In Hematology 28(4), 76–79, 1991.
2. Segal, M.: Regression trees for censored data, Biometrics 44, 35–47, 1988.
3. Lausen, B., Schumacher, M.: Maximally selected rank statistics, Biometrics 48, 73–85, 1992.
4. Cox, D. R.: Regression models and life tables (with discussion), Journal Royal Statistical Society B, 34, 187–220, 1972.

Acute Leukemias VI
Prognostic Factors
and Treatment Strategies
Büchner et al. (eds)

Idarubicin or Mitoxantrone, VP-16, and Cytarabine for Induction/Consolidation Therapy Followed by Autologous Stem Cell Transplantation in Elderly Patients with Acute Myeloid Leukemia: A Feasibility Study

E. Archimbaud[1], U. Jehn[2], F. De Cataldo[3], C. Martin[4], and X. Thomas[1]

Abstract. Seventy-four patients of median age 70 years (range 61–83 years), with acute myeloid leukemia (AML) at diagnosis, 56 of them with de novo AML and 18 with AML secondary to primary myelodysplastic syndrome or toxic exposure (sAML), received inducton therapy with idarubicin, 8 mg/m^2 per day on days 1, 3, and 5, or on a randomized basis, mitoxantrone, 7 mg/m^2 per day on days 1, 3, and 5, both associated with VP-16, 100 mg/m^2 per day on days 1–3 and cytarabine (ara-C), 100 mg/m^2 per day, on days 1–7 Granulocyte colony stimulating factor (G-CSF), 5 µg/kg per day, was administered after chemotherapy in patients aged more than 70 years. Patients in complete remission (CR) received one course of consolidation using the same schedule as for induction except for the shortening of ara-C administration to 5 days. Patients aged less than 70 years were then scheduled to undergo autologous stem cell harvest on days 5–7 of G-CSF, 5 µg/kg per day, initiated after hematopoietic recovery from consolidation. Autologous transplantation was performed after conditioning with carmustine (BCNU), 800 mg/m^2 or busulfan 16 mg/kg. G-CSF was administered when neutrophils were $<0.1 \times 10^9$/l. Among 71 patients evaluable for induction, 39 (55%) achieved CR. The CR rate was 58% in de novo AML and 44% in sAML (p=NS). There was no significant difference in CR rate between the idarubicin (51% CR) and mitoxantrone (58% CR) arms, nor between patients aged <70 years (58% CR) and ≥ 70 years (53% CR). There was no significant difference in aplasia duration between the two arms. Median time to neutrophil recovery was 22 days in patients who received G-CSF and 24 days in patients who did not ($p = 0.1$). Severe toxicities of induction did not differ between the two arms and included sepsis (42%), diarrhea (10%), hyperbilirubinemia (7%), hemorrhage (6%), and vomiting (1%). Overall, four patients (6%), two in each arm, died from toxicity of induction. First consolidation was administered in 31 patients and four (13%) died from toxicity. At this time, eight patients have received transplantation. This procedure was well tolerated, with a median duration of neutrophils $<0.5 \times 10^9$/l of 8 days and of platelets $<50 \times 10^9$/l of 18 days and no lethal toxicity. We conclude that this regimen is well tolerated and has a good efficacy to induce CR. Intensive postinduction is feasible, including transplantation up to the age of 70 years.

Introduction

Results of chemotherapy in elderly patients with newly diagnosed acute myeloid leukemia (AML) have been disappointing, with a complete remission (CR) rate of less than 50% in most series of unselected patients and median CR duration often less than 6 months with very seldom prolonged survival [1]. Some randomized studies in AML suggest the superiority of mitoxantrone

[1]Hôpital Edouard Herriot, Lyon, France
[2]Klinikum Grosshadern, München, Germany
[3]Ospedale Maggiore Ca Grand, Milano, Italy
[4]Centre Hospitalier, Annecy, France

[2, 3] and idarubicin (4, 5, 6) over daunorubicin to induce CR. The addition of etoposide (VP-16) to an anthracycline-cytarabine (ara-C) regimen during induction and consolidation has been shown beneficial for prolongation of CR in young adults with newly diagnosed AML [7].

Postinduction with myeloablative cytotoxic therapy followed by unpurged bone marrow stem cell rescue as postinduction therapy has been shown to be superior to non-myeloablative chemotherapy alone to prevent relapse in patients aged less than 60 years in the large EORTC-GIMEMA AML-8A randomized trial [8]. These results constitute a strong incentive to try to extend the use of postinduction with myeloablative therapy followed by stem cell rescue to older patients.

Nitrosourea compounds exert cytotoxicity against AML cells in vitro [9]. They have been used in AML therapy as part of standard-chemotherapy regimens [10]. They are also part of CBV and BAVC myeloablative regimens which have been used prior to autologous bone marrow rescue in AML, showing good therapeutic efficacy in preventing relapses with decreased toxicity by comparison to total body irradiation (TBI) containing pretransplant regimens [11, 12].

Unlike previously mentioned conditioning regimens, the use of which has been reported in patients aged less than 60 years, the administration of carmustine (BCNU) alone as a single dose of 800 mg/m^2 prior to autologous bone marrow rescue has been shown feasible in more than 125 patients aged up to 66 years, presenting with glioma, with only 12% severe aplasia and 6% toxic death partly attributable to the long-term corticotherapy used in these glioma patients to prevent cerebral edema [13, 14].

Patients and Methods

Patient Selection Criteria

Patients aged more than 60 years, with a newly diagnosed de novo AML or AML secondary to previous primary myelodysplastic syndrome or to toxic exposure (sAML) were eligible for this trial provided they had a good performance status (grade 0, 1 or 2, World Health Organization, WHO, scale) and no severe organ failure. AML was diagnosed according to the French-American-British (FAB) criteria [15].

Therapeutic regimen

Chemotherapy. Induction therapy included idarubicin, 8 mg/m^2 per day on days 1, 3 and 5 or, according to the result of initial randomization, mitoxantrone, 7 mg/m^2 per day on days 1,3, and 5, both associated with VP-16, 100 mg/m^2 per day on days 1–3 and ara-C, 100 mg/m^2 per day as a continuous infusion on days 1–7. Granulocyte colony-stimulating factor (G-CSF), 5 µg/kg per day was administered after chemotherapy in all patients aged more than 70 years. Its use was also allowed in younger patients. CR was defined according to the Cancer and Leukemia Group B (CALGB) criteria [16]. Patients in CR after one or two courses of induction received one course of consolidation administered as early as possible after hematologic recovery from induction using the same schedule as for induction except for the shortening of ara-C administration to 5 days.

Stem Cell Transplantation. Patients treated in Lyon aged less 70 years or, since September 1994, less than 75 years, with a performance status of 0 or 1 (WHO scale) after consolidation chemotherapy were then scheduled to undergo an intensive conditioning regimen followed by autologous stem cell transplantation. peripheral blood stem cell (PBSC) harvest was performed through two to three standard daily aphereses beginning on day 5 of treatment with G-CSF, 5 µg/kg per day, initiated within 2 weeks after hematopoietic recovery from consolidation. PBSC transplantation was performed after conditioning with BCNU, 800 mg/m^2 on day -3, or busulfan, 4 mg/kg per day on days -6 to -3. G-CSF, 5 µg/kg per day was administered after transplantation when the neutrophil count dropped below 0.1 × 10^9/l until recovery.

Results

Patient Characteristics

Seventy-four patients were entered on this trial between April, 1993 and November, 1994. Fifty-six had de novo AML while 18 had sAML. Sixteen patients had AML which could not be classified in the FAB scheme. The main patient characterisitics are listed in Table 1.

Table 1. Initial patient characteristics ($n=74$)

Age—Median (years)	70
Range (years)	61–83
Sex (M/F) (n)	38/36
Etiology of AML	
Primary (*n*)	56
Secondary (*n*)	9
Transformed myelodysplastic syndrome (*n*)	9
Extramedullary involvement (*y*/*n*)	23/51
Hemoglobin—Median (*g*/*l*)	89
Range (g/l)	41–140
Platelet—median ($\times 10^{9/l}$)	63
Range ($\times 10^9$/l)	5–1232
WBC—Median ($\times 10^{9/l}$)	6.9
Range ($\times 10^9$/l)	0.7–295
Blood blasts—Median (%)	28
Range (%)	0–97
Bone marrow blasts—Median (%)	64
Range (%)	10[a]–100
FAB subtype	
M0 (*n*)	1
M1 (*n*)	11
M2 (*n*)	16
M3 (*n*)	0
M4 (*n*)	11
M5 (*n*)	17
M6 (*n*)	2
M7 (*n*)	0
Unclassified (*n*)	16

[a] Two cases with <30% blasts (one FAB M2, one FAB M6).

Results of Induction

Three patients died early, within 7 days of induction therapy, and 71 were evaluable for induction, 35 of them allocated to the idarubicin arm and 36 to the mitoxantrone arm. Thirty-nine patients (55%) achieved CR, including three of six patients in whom a second induction course was attempted after failure of the first induction attempt. A total of 39% of patients had resistant disease while 6% died from toxicity of induction (Table 2). There was no significant difference between the two arms, with 51% and 58% CR, respectively, in patients treated with idarubicin and mitoxantrone. The CR rate was 58% in de novo AML and 44% in sAML ($p=$ NS). There was no significant difference in CR rate between the 33 patients aged <70 years (58% CR) and the 38 patients aged ≥70 years (53% CR), nor between the 44 patients who received G-CSF (55% CR) and the 27 patients who did not (56% CR). Among CR patients, the median time to neutrophil recovery $>0.5\times 10^9$/l and platelets $>50\times 10^9$/l was 23 days (range: 19–40 days) and 23 days (range: 17–34 days), respectively, in patients who received idarubicin, and 24 days (range: 13–32 days) and 25 days (range: 19–79 days) Respectively in patients treated with mitoxantrone. Median time to neutrophil recovery was 22 days (range: 18–40 days) in patients who received G-CSF and 24 days (range: 13–36 days) in those who did not ($p=0.1$). Severe (WHO grade 3 or more) toxicities of induction did not differ between the two arms and included sepsis (42%), diarrhea (10%), hyperbilirubinemia (7%), hemorrhage (6%), and vomiting (1%). Overall, four patients (6%), two in each arm, died from toxicity of induction, three of them from infection and one from hemorrhage.

Results of Post-Induction

First consolidation was performed in 31 patients. Reasons for not undergoing this consolidation included patient refusal (one patient), persisting cytopenia after induction (one patient), persisting infection (three patients) and

Table 2. Efficacy on induction according to treatment arm

Treatment arm	Patients	CR		RD		OF	
	(*n*)	(*n*)	(%)	(*n*)	(%)	(*n*)	(%)
Idarubicin	35	18[a]	(51)	15		2	
Mitoxantrone	36	21[b]	(58)	13		2	
	71	39	(55)	28	(39)	4	(6)

[a] Including two CR after two courses (four second induction courses attempted).
[b] Including one return to previous MDS phase (non-blastic) and one CR after two induction courses (two second induction course attempted).
CR, complete remission; RD, resistant disease; OF, other failure (toxic death).

early relapse (three patients). Median time to neutrophil recovery $>0.5 \times 10^9/l$ and platelets $>50 \times 10^9/l$ was 22 days (range: 16–39 days) and 22 days (range: 13–61 days), respectively, without any difference between the idarubicin and mitoxantrone arms. Four patients (13%), two in each arm, died from toxicity of consolidation, three of them, infection and from hemorrhage.

At this time, eight patients, representing 50% of age-eligible patients who received the first course of consolidation in Lyon, have received autologous stem cell transplantation, one of them from bone marrow and seven from PBSC. Reasons for not undergoing transplantation included death from toxicity of consolidation (one patient), patient refusal (one patient), relapse 2 patients, persisting infection, (two patients), persisting cytopenia (one patient) and inadequate stem cell harvest (one patient). The median age of these patients was 69 years (range: 61–74 years). Pretransplant conditioning used BCNU in six patients and busulfan in two. Patients were grafted with a median 8.05×10^8 MNC/kg (range: 1.5–15.3) containing 23.7×10^4 colony-forming units granulocyte-macrophage (CFU-GM)/kg (range: 5.2–64.1). This procedure was well tolerated, with a median duration of neutrophils $<0.5 \times 10^9/l$ of 8 days (0–12 days) and of platelets $< 50 \times 10^9/l$ of 18 days (3 – 60+ days). Severe (WHO grade 3) or more toxicities included sepsis (three patients), vomiting (one patient) and diarrhea (one patient). No toxic death was observed.

At a median follow-up of 8 months, 22 patients have relapsed after 1–9 months in CR, six of them despite receiving autologous transplantation. Twelve patients are in continuing CR for 1–20 months two of them after receiving autologous transplantation.

Discussion

Our study shows the feasibility and efficacy in elderly patients of a chemotherapy regimen using adapted doses of recent intercalating agents such as idarubicin and mitoxantrone in association with VP-16 and ara-C. Such associations have been found to be highly efficient in inducing CR in young adults with AML and the use of such regimen has already been reported in a short series of 23 patients of median age 65 years in whom association of mitoxantrone, intermediate-dose ara-C, and VP-16 induced a 78% CR rate [17]. The good tolerance of our regimen is reflected by the similar results achieved in patients aged ⩾ 70 years by comparison to younger patients, with a CR rate of more than 50% even in the older group, although these groups are not directly comparable since patient selection for referral to our centers might have occurred in the older age group and G-CSF was more widely used in this group. The use of G-CSF during chemotherapy-induced aplasia has shown to increase CR rate in a recent trial in elderly patients with AML [18]. This potential effect could not be tested in our non-randomized study.

Consolidation chemotherapy using reduced dosages of ara-C could be administered to most patients in CR after one or two courses of induction. However, four toxic deaths were observed and more patients are required to fully evaluate the toxicity of this procedure. Intensive chemotherapy conditioning followed by autologous stem cell rescue could be administered safely to 50% of patients having undergone the first consolidation and potentially eligible according to their age. The use of autologous stem cell transplantation is generally restricted to patients aged less than 60 years and no patient was aged more than 65 years among 919 patients who underwent autologous bone marrow transplantation for AML included in a recent report by the European Bone Marrow Transplantation Group (EBMT) [19]. Extension of this procedure to older age groups might be permitted by using reduced, less intensive, single-agent conditioning regimens, together with PBSC rescue which is known to induce earlier hematopoietic recovery by comparison with bone marrow stem cell rescue [20, 21]. This allowed us to perform transplantation to 50% of potentially eligible patients according to age, representing an exclusion rate similar to that observed in younger patients [8]. In our experience, stem cell transplantation using this less toxic approach appeared better tolerated than consolidation chemotherapy and might even have been carried out in ambulatory patients in some cases. However, early relapses after transplantation were observed in our patients. Therefore, it remains to be seen whether this approach using reduced dosage conditioning will significantly decrease the relapse rate, particularly since the poor tolerance of intensive consolidation in these patients probably precludes adequate disease reduction before stem cell harvest and the graft itself.

References

1. Heineman V, Jehn U. Acute myeloid leukemia in the elderly: biological features and search for adequate treatment. Ann Hematol 179–188, 1991.
2. Arlin Z, Case Jr. DC, Moore J, Wiernik P, Feldman E, Saletan S, Desai P, Sia L, Cartwright K, and the Lederle Cooperative Group. Randomized multicenter trial of cytosine arabinoside with mitoxantrone or daunorubicin in previously untreated adult patients with acute nonlymphocytic leukemia (ANLL). Leukemia 4: 177–183, 1990.
3. Löwenberg B, Fiere D, Zittoun R, Kerkhofs H, Stryckkmans P, De Cataldo F, Tura S, Peetermans M, Paulus R, Goudsmit R, Sonnenweld P, Solbu G, Suciu S. Mitoxantrone versus daunorubicin in aduction of acute myelogenous leukemia elderly patients and low-dose ara-C vs control as maintenance. An EORTC phase II trial (AML-9). Haematologica 76(suppl. 4): 91, 1991.
4. Berman E, Heller G, Santorsa J, McKenzie S, Gee T, Kempin S, Gulati S, Andreeff M, Kolitz J, Gabrilove J, Reich L, Mayer K, Keefe D, Trainor K, Schluger A, Penenberg D, Raymond V, O'Reilly R, Jhanwar S, Young C, Clarkson B. Results of a randomized trial comparing idarubicin and cytosine arabinoside with daunorubicin and cytosine arabinoside in adult patients with newly diagnosed acute myelogenous leukemia. Blood 77: 1666–1674, 1991.
5. Wiernik PH, Banks PLC, Case DC, Arlin ZA, Periman PO, Todd MB, Ritch PS, Enck RE, Weitberg AB, Cytarabine plus idarubicin or daunorubicin as induction and consolidation therapy for previously untreated adult patients with acute myeloid leukemia. Blood 79: 313–319, 1992.
6. Reiffers J, Rigal-Huguet F, Stoppa AM, Michallet M, Marit G, Attal M, Gastaut JA, Corron B, Lepeu G, Routy M, Cony-Makhoul P, Pris J, Hollard D, Maraninchi D, Mercier M, Hurteloup P, for the BGMT Group. Haematologica 76 (suppl 4); 8, 1991.
7. Bishop JF, Lowenthal RM, Joshua D, Matthews JP, Todd D, Cobcroft R, Whiteside MG, Kronenberg H, Ma D, Dodds A, Herrmann R, Szer J, Wolf MM, Young G, for the Australian Leukemia Study Group. Etoposide in acute nonlymphocytic leukemia. Blood 75: 27–32, 1990.
8. Zittoun RA, Mandelli F, Willemze R, de Witte T, Labar B, Resegotti L, Leoni F, Damasio, Visani G, Papa G, Caronia F, Hayat M, Stryckmans P, Rotoli B, Leoni P, Peetermans ME, Dardenne M, Vegna ML, Petti MC, Solbu G, Suciu S, for the European Organization for Research and Treatment of Cancer (EORTC) and the Gruppo Italiano Malattie Ematologiche Maligne dell' Adulto (GIMEMA) Leukemia Cooperative Groups. Autologous or allogeneic bone marrow transplantation compared with intensive chemotherapy in acute myelogenous leukemia. New Engl J Med 332: 217–223, 1995.
9. Gerson SL, Trey JE, Modulation of nitrosourea resistance in myeloid leukemias. Blood 71: 1487–1494, 1988.
10. Oksenhendler E, Landais P, Cordonnier C, Kuentz M, Bagot M, Jais JP, Roujeau JC, Vernant JP: Acral erythema and systemic toxicity related to CHA induction therapy in acute myeloid leukemia. Eur J Cancer Clin Oncol 25: 1181–1185, 1989.
11. Vellekoop L. Jagannath S, Spitzer G, Zander AR, Horwitz LJ, Keating M, McCredie KB, Dicke KA. High-dose cyclophosphamide, BCNU and etoposide followed by autologous bone marrow rescue as treatment for adult acute leukemia in relapse. Am J Clin Oncol 9: 307–310, 1986.
12. Meloni G, De Fabriitis P, Perri MC, Mandelli F. BAVC regimen and autologous bone marrow transplantation in patients with acute myelogenous leukemia in second remission. Blood 75: 2282–2285, 1990.
13. Biron P, Vial C, Chauvin F, Mornex F, Colombat P, Janvier M, Giroux B, Roux N, Philip I. Strategy including surgery, high dose BCNU followed by ABMT and radiotherapy in supratentorial high grade astrocytomas: a report of 98 patients. Proceedings of the Symposium on Autologous Bone Marrow Transplantation. Houston, 1988.
14. Linassier C, Calais G, Velut S, Saudeau D, Jan M, Autret A, Lamagnére JP, Colombat Ph. High dose BCNU with autologous bone marrow transplantation (ABMT) and localised radiotherapy (RT) for patients with high grade astrocytomas. Proceedings of the 18th Annual Meeting of the European Group for Bone Marrow Transplantation, Stockholm, 183, 1992.
15. Bennett JM, Catovsky D, Daniel MT, Flandrin G, Galton DAG, Gralnick HR, Sultan C. Proposed revised criteria for the classification of acute myeloid leukemia: a report of the French-American-British Cooperative Group. Ann Intern Med 103: 626–629, 1985.
16. Ellison RR, Holland JF, Weil M, Jacquillat C, Boiron M, Bernard J, Sawitsky A, Rosner F, Gussoff B, Silver RT, Karanas A, Cuttner J, Spurr CL, Hayes DM, Bloom J, Leone LA, Haurani F, Kyle R, Hutchison JL, Forcier RJ, Moon JH: Arabinosyl cytosine: a useful agent in the treatment of acute leukemia in adults. Blood 32: 507–523, 1968.
17. Shepherd JD, Reece DE, Barnett MJ, Klingemann HG, Nantel SH, Sutherland HJ, Philips GL. Induction therapy for acute myelogenous leukemia in patients over 60 years with intermediate-dose cytosine arabinoside, mitoxantrone and etoposide. Leukemia and Lymphoma 9: 211–215, 1993.
18. Dombret H, Yver A, Chastang C, Degos L. Increased frequency of complete remission by lenograstim recombinant human granulocyte colony-stimulating factor (rhg-CSF) administration after intensive induction chemotherapy in elderly patients with de novo acute myeloid leukemia (AML). Final results of a randomized multicenter double-blind controlled study. Blood 84 (suppl 1.): 231a, 1994.
19. Gorin NC, Labopin M, Meloni G, Korbling M, Carella A, Herve P, Burnett A, Rizzoli V,

Alessandrino EP, Bjorkstrand B, Ferrant A, Lowenberg B, Coser P, Simonsson B, Helbig W, Brunet Mauri S, Verdonck LF, Iriondo A, Polli E, transplantation for acute myeloblastic leukemia in Europe: further evidence of the role of marrow purging by mafosfamide. Leukemia 5: 896–904, 1991.
20. Reiffers J, Stoppa AM, Attal M, Michallet M. Is there a place for blood stem cell transplantation for the younger adult patient with acute myelogenous leukemia? J Clin Oncol 12: 1100, 1994.
21. Reiffers J, Labopin M, Körbling M, Henon Ph, Gorin NC. Autologous blood stem cell transplantation versus autologous bone marrow transplantation for acute myeloid leukemia in first remission: a retrospective analysis of the EBMT registry. Proceedings of the 18th Annual Meeting of the European Group for Bone Marrow Transplantation, Stokholm, 107, 1992.

Acute Leukemias VI
Prognostic Factors
and Treatment Strategies
Büchner et al. (eds)

High-Dose Chemotherapy with Busulfan, Cyclophosphamide, and VP-16 as Conditioning for Allogeneic and Autologous Bone Marrow Transplantation for Patients with Acute Myeloid Leukemia

A.R. Zander[1], C. Berger[1], W. Krüger[1], M. Stockschläder[1], U. v. Eisenhart-Rothe[1], W. Zeller[1], M. Hoffknecht[1], G. Kroschke[2], H. Kabisch[2], P. Schönrock[3], R. Kuse[3], H.J. Weh[4], and D.K. Hossfeld[4]

Introduction

High-dose chemotherapy and total body irradiation (TBI) followed by infusion of bone marrow from a histocompatible sibling have been used extensively in the treatment of acute and chronic leukemias. Long-term disease-free survival has been achieved in 10%–20% of patients with relapsed acute leukemia and in about 50% of selected patients who received this treatment during first remission of their disease. Because of the long-term consequences of TBI, alternative high-dose regimens solely based on chemotherapy have been developed. Tutschka et al. [1] reported on the combination of busulfan (16 mg/kg body weight) and cyclophosphamide (200 mg/kg body weight) without TBI, which allows for full hemopoietic engraftment, hemopoietic chimerism, and control of leukemia in most patients. A variation of this regimen with a lower cyclophosphamide dose (120 mg/kg body weight) was equally effective and less toxic. Other regimens without TBI, such as combinations of cyclophosphamide, BCNU, and VP-16 showed similar activity [2]. VP-16 has been introduced into high-dose therapy in combination with busulfan and busulfan/cyclophosphamide [3–5]. We explored the combination of busulfan, cyclophosphamide, and VP-16 in patients with acute myeloid leukemia in first, second, and third remissions and relapse.

The conditioning arrangements consisted of busulfan (4 mg/kg) on days -8, -7, -6, -5, VP-16 (30–45 mg/kg) on day -4, and cyclophosphamide (60 mg/kg) on days -3 and -2.

Allogeneic bone marrow was given at day -0. Autologous marrow had been purged with mafosfamide (60 μg/ml), frozen, and stored in liquid nitrogen. The marrow was thawed at the bedside and intravenously infused on day 0.

Materials and Methods

Graft-Versus-Host Disease Prophylaxis. Prophylaxis in allogeneic bone marrow transplantation, consisted of cyclosporin A 3 mg/kg and methotrexate 10 mg/kg on days +1, +3, +6, +11, or prednisone instead of methotrexate at a dose of 1 mg/kg.

Infection Prophylaxis. Infection prophylaxis consisted of ciprofloxacin 2 × 500 mg daily p.o. or ofloxacin 2 × 200 mg daily p.o., fluconazole 2 × 100 mg daily, and amphomoronal suspension p.o. Trimethoprim-sulfamethoxazol 2 × 160 mg daily p.o. Friday - Sunday.

Patient Population. A total of 53 patients underwent transplantation. Two out of 53 received busulfan, cyclophosphamide, and VP-16 as a conditioning for the second transplant. Thirty-six patients received an allogeneic transplant: 21 in first complete remission, nine in second complete remission, and three out of six in refractory relapse or primary refractory disease.

[1]Bone Marrow Transplantation Unit, Universitätskrankenhaus Eppendorf, Hamburg, Germany
[2]Department of Pediatric Oncology, Universitätskrankenhaus Eppendorf, Hamburg, Germany
[3]Department of Hematology, AK St. Georg, Hamburg, Germany
[4]Department of Hematology and Oncology, Universitätskrankenhaus Eppendorf, Hamburg, Germany

Seventeen were transplanted autologously, five in first complete remission, 12 in second and third complete remission. The median age was 28 years (range 4–56 years).

Results

Thirty out of 53 patients are alive, 29 in complete remission (Tables 1, 2). Seven of 21 (82%) of allogeneic patients and three of five autologous patients transplanted in first complete remission are alive in continuous complete remission (Fig. 1). Major causes of death for all groups were graft-versus-host disease (two patients) infections (ten patients), relapse (seven patients). All but one patient experienced mucositis grade II, one patient had grade IV.

Discussion

The combination of busulfan, cyclophosphamide, and VP-16 is well tolerated and effective in acute myeloid leukemia in first complete remission [3–5]. The low mortality and low relapse rate in first complete remission justifies allogeneic transplant for all patients in first complete remission who have an HLA-identical donor. The regimen is less effective and more toxic for patients with advanced disease. Patients with refractory leukemia are presently

Table 1. Allogeneic bone marrow transplantation for acute myeloid leukemia

Status pre-bone marrow transplantation	Patients	GVHD grades II–IV	Survival at 12/1994			Cause of death (n)	Survival Median Range (months)	(months)
			Alive	In CCR	Dead			
	(n)	(n)	(n)	(n)	(n)			
First complete remission	21	12	17	17	4	Sepsis 1 Mucositis 1 Pneumonia, GvHD 1 Cerebral bleeding 1	26	0.5–51
Second and third complete remission	9	7	1	1	8	Relapse 3 Cerebral bleeding 1 CMV, GvHD 1 Aspergillus 1 Sepsis 2	2	1–48
Relapse	6[a]	1[a]	1	1	5	Relapse 2 Interstitial pneumonia, GvHD 1 Encephalitis 1 Toxoplasmosis, GvHD 1	3.5	2.5–57

[a]One patient with a hepatic relapse.
GvHD, graft-versus-host disease; cmv, cytomegalovirus.

Table 2. Autologous bone marrow transplantation for acute myeloid leukemia

Status pre-bone marrow transplantation	Patients	Survival at 12/1994			Cause of death (n)	Survival Median Range (months)	(months)
		Alive	In CCR	Dead			
	(n)	(n)	(n)	(n)			
First complete remission	5	4	3	1	Relapse 1	7.5	4–43.5
Second and third complete remission	12	6	6	6	Relapse 4 Aspergillus sepsis 1 Toxic cardiomyopathy + Venous occlusive 1 disease	10	0.5–48

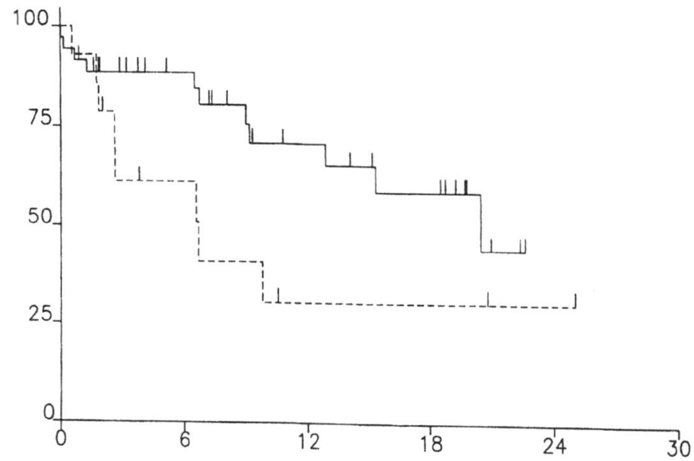

Fig. 1. AML – allogeneic BMT in first CR

conditioned with TBI, VP-16, and cyclophosphamide. For patients with acute myeloid leukemia in first complete remission who have good prognostic factors for long-term survival, i.e., chromosome translocation 8; 21, 15; 17, inversion 16, the option of allogeneic bone marrow transplantation should be offered in view of the fact that they still have a high relapse rate with conventional chemotherapy and in the case of relapse no guarantee of achieving a second remission [6–9]. In view of the uncertainty about the best strategy the patient should be fully informed about the options and offered an allogeneic transplantation.

References

1. Tutschka PJ et al.: BMT for leukemia following a new busulfan and cyslophosphamide regimen. Blood 1987; 70: 1382–1388.
2. Zander AR, Culbert S, Jagannath S et al.: High dose cyclophosphamide, BCNU and VP16 (CBV) as a conditioning regimen for allogeneic bone marrow transplantation for patients with acute leukemia. Cancer 1987; 59: 1083–1086.
3. Linker CA et al.: Autologous BMT for AML using busulfan plus etoposide as a preparative regimen. Blood 1993; 81: 311–318.
4. Chao NJ et al.: Busulfan/etoposide—initial experience with a new preparatory regimen for autologous BMT in patients with ANLL. Blood 1993; 81: 319–323.
5. Spitzer TR et al.: Escalating doses of etoposide with cyclophosphamide and fractionated TBI or busulfan conditioning for BMT. Bone Marrow Transplantation 1989; 4: 559-565.
6. Zander AR, Keating M, Dicke K et al.: A comparison of marrow transplantation with chemotherapy for adults with acute leukemia of poor prognosis in first complete remission. J Clin Oncol 1988; 6: 1548–1557.
7. Keating MJ, Smith TL, Kantarjian H et al.: Cytogenetic pattern in acute myelogenous leukemia: a major reproducible determinant of outcome. Leukemia 1988; 2: 403–412.
8. Bloomfield CD, Lawrence D, Arthur DC, Berg DT, Schiffer CA, Mayer RJ: Curative impact of intensification with high dose cytarabine in acute myeloid leukemia (AML) varies by cytogenetic group. Blood 1994; 84: Suppl. 1: 111a (abstract).
9. Gale RP, Horowitz MM, Weiner RS et al.: Impact of cytogenetic abnormalities on outcome of bone marrow transplants in acute myelogenous leukemia in not remission. Bone Marrow Transplant (in press).

Acute Leukemias VI
Prognostic Factors
and Treatment Strategies
Büchner et al. (eds)

YNK01, an Oral Cytosine Arabinoside Derivative in Acute Myeloid Leukemia and Chronic Myeloid Leukemia

P. Heußner[1], R. Willemze, A. Ganser, A. Hanauske, S. Amadori, G. Heil, E. Schleyer, W. Hiddemann, J. Selbach, M. Schüßler[2], and M. Freund[1] (The European YNK01 Study Group)

Abstract. Twenty-eight patients with acute myeloid leukemia (AML) and chronic myeloid leukemia (CML) were treated in a phase I/II multicenter trial and pilot single-center trial with YNK01 an oral cytosine arabinoside (ara-C) derivative. In contrast to ara-C, YNK01 is resistant to cytidine deaminases. Therefore YNK01 is converted to ara-C in the liver and released slowly into blood. It has been shown in ongoing pharmacokinetic studies that a mean of 16% of YNK01 is secreted as ara-U into the urine. Twenty-two patients with AML (12 patients with relapse, five with secondary AML, five with primary, not qualifying for intensive chemotherapy) were included, median age 67 (range 22–79 years, 13 pretreated /11 with ara-C). In the AML trial the doses of YNK01 were escalated interindividually from a daily 100 mg/kg body weight up to 1200 mg/kg body weight for 14 days. Cycles were repeated every 21–28 days. Major toxicities at the 900- and 1200-mg dose levels were nausea grade 3 (WHO) in one patient; diarrhea grade 3 in five patients, grade 4 in one patient; exanthema grade 3 in one patient; and stomatitis grade 3 in one patient, grade 4 in one patient. At the lower dose levels no grade 3 or 4 organ toxicities were observed. Six patients (median age 53 years, range 26–64 years) were included in the CML pilot trial. Treatment was started with interferon (IFN)-α-2b5 × 10^6 units s.c. daily. After 1 week YNK01 600 mg daily continuously was added. IFN and YNK01 were modified according to toxicity and effectivity. Maximum toxicities were diarrhea grade 3 in one patient bone pain grade 3 in one patient.

In AML patients complete remission (CR) was observed in two of 21 patients, partial remission (PR) in one of 21 patients, and stable disease for up to 70 months in four of 21 patients. In CML six of six patients achieved a complete hematologic response (CHR) after 7 months of continuous treatment and two of six patients had a partial cytogenetic response (PCR), and two of six patients are in minor cytogenetic response (MCR). We conclude that YNK01 has a mild toxicity profile in patients with hematological malignancies. Diarrhea seems to become the dose-limiting toxicity. The maximum tolerable dose of YNK01 seems to be reached at the 1200-mg dose level in AML.

Phase II studies will be performed to further evaluate the efficacy of the drug in AML patients as a maintenance treatment and in CML following the pilot trial.

Introduction

Cytosine arabinoside (ara-C) is one of the most effective drugs in the treatment of hematologic malignancies, especially in the therapy of acute leukemias. Furthermore, the induction of cytogenetic responses has been reported in chronic myeloid leukemia (CML). Ara-C is known to inhibit DNA synthesis by acting as a pyrimidine antagonist. Ara-C is immediately deaminated in the human body and converted to the cytotoxic

[1]Department of Hematology and Oncology, University of Medicine, Rostock, Germany
[2]ASTA Medica Frankfurt, Germany

inactive metabolite ara-U. As a result, ara-C has an extremely short half-life time of about 60 min in blood. Therefore, ara-C derivatives with resistance to cytidine deaminases have been developed. YNK01 (cytarabine ocfosfate, 1-β-D-arabinofuranosylcytosine-5′-stearylphosphate) is an oral prodrug of ara-C. It is metabolized in the liver and is released into blood gradually.

In the ongoing phase I/II study in acute myeloid leukemia (AML) and in the pilot study of YNK01 in combination with interferon α-2b in CML, 28 patients were included from August 1992 until February 1995.

Materials and Methods

The aims of the studies were the determination of the maximal tolerable dose (MTD) of YNK01; the determination of the dose-limiting toxicity (DLT) of YNK01; the collection of information on the efficacy of YNK01; and the determination of the pharmacokinetic parameters of YNK01 and ara-C.

The study design is a multicenter phase I/II study in patients with AML and a monocenter pilot phase I/II trial in patients with CML.

Study I was the administration of YNK01 in AML patients. The treatment plan was as follows. YNK01 100-mg capsules was provided by ASTA Medica AG, Germany. The starting dose and schedule were 100 mg/day absolutely on days 1–14, every 3–7 weeks, depending on hemogram and bone marrow cellularity. Dose escalation was in 100-mg steps with three to six patients per dose level. Treatment duration was for a maximum of six cycles. Specific inclusion criteria included: relapsed AML in second or further relapse; first relapse of AML with complete remission (CR)<6 months; primary refractory AML; AML in elderly or unfit patients; AML secondary to myelodysplastic syndrome (MDS); or AML secondary to previous chemotherapy or radiation. A specific exclusion criterion was any patient qualifying for bone marrow transplantation.

Study IV was the administration of YNK01 and interferon (IFN) α-2b in CML. The treatment plan was as follows. YNK01 was provided by ASTA Medica AG, Germany, and IFN-α-2b was provided by Essex Pharma, Germany. The starting dose and schedule were: days 1–14—3 $\times 10^6$ U/m^2 IFN-α-2b s.c. daily; from day 15 on U/m^2 IFN α-2b s.c. daily; from day 8 on; YNK01 3 × 2 capsules (600 mg) daily; continuous daily application, dose modification according to toxicity and efficacy; dose escalation and de-escalation was directed by white blood cell (WBC) count (goal: 2–3 $\times 10^3$/μl) and tolerability. Treatment duration was until achievement of complete hematologic remission. A specific inclusion criterion was newly diagnosed Ph-positive CML. Specific exclusion criteria included: CML in the accelerated phase; CML in blast crisis; and, pretreatment of the CML.

Twenty-two patients with AML were treated with 48 cycles of YNK01 between August 1992 and December 1992 (Table 1). Six patients with newly diagnosed CML are under continuous treatment with YNK01 in combination with IFN-α–2b in a pilot study since February 1994 (Table 2).

Twenty-two patients with AML were included: 12 relapsed AML patients (one early relapse, six in first relapse) (three in second relapse, two in third relapse); five patients with AML secondary to MDS; and five patients with AML were elderly or unfit, not qualifying for intensive chemotherapy.

Table 1. Number of Patients and cycles per dose level

Dosage (mg)	Patients (*n*)	Cycles (*n*)
100	3	10
300	3	10
400	2	8
600	3	4
600	6[a]	
900	5	10
1200	6	6

[a]Patients with continuous treatment in combination with interferon α-2b; dose modification.

Table 2. Patient characteristics

	AML	CML
Patients (*n*)	22	6
Age—Median (years)	67	53
Range (years)	22–79	24–64
Sex (m/f) (*n*)	10/12	5/1
Pretreated (*n*)	13	0
Pretreated with ara-C	11	0

Results

Clinical Response in AML. Seven of 22 patients with AML responded to YNK01 (Table 3).

Clinical Response in Newly Diagnosed CML. In all six patients with CML, the treatment with YNK01 in combination with IFN-α-2b resulted in hematologic responses. The doses were modified according to the responses and toxicities. All therapies are ongoing (Table 4).

Toxicity. Overall, 59 patients were included for the toxicity analysis. The results of two further clinical phase I/II studies in patients with MDS and low-grade non-Hodgkin lymphoma (NHL) are summarized. The patients were treated with the same schedule as in the AML trial. Neutropenia and thrombocytopenia were dose dependent. Non-hematologic toxicities of WHO grade 3 or 4 were seen only at the 900- and 1200-mg dose levels. In one AML patient at the 1200-mg dose level, therapy had to be stopped because of WHO grade 4 diarrhea. At the 900-mg dose level, one MDS patient had bone marrow aplasia

Table 3. Clinical response in AML

Patient No.	Diagnosis	Dosage (mg/kg body weight)	Cycles (n)	Maximal response/ duration of response
1	Secondary AML	300	8	SD after first cycle for 6 months
2	Secondary AML	400	8	SD after first cycle for 6 months
3	AML in an unfit patient	600	2	CR after second cycle, duration 4 months
4	Second relapse	900	2	CR after second cycle, duration 3 months
5	First relapse	900	1	PR after first cycle, ongoing
6	Secondary AML	1200	4	SD after first cycle for 3 months
7	AML in an elderly patient	1200	1	SD after first cycle

SD, stable disease; CR, complete remission; PR, partial remission.

Table 4. Clinical response in newly diagnosed CML

Patient No.	YNK01 (mg)	IFN (U/m^2 per day)	Treatment duration (months)	Response
1	600 – 0–100 – 200	5×10^6 $- 2.5 \times 10^6$ 3–5 days/week	12	CHR after 7 months MCR after 11 months
2	600 – 200–600 – 400	3×10^6 $- 5\text{–}3 \times 10^6$	9	CHR after 4 months MCR after 6 months
3	600	3×10^6 $- 5\text{–}3 \times 10^6$	9	CHR after 4 months PCR after 6 months
4	600 – 200	3×10^6 $- 1.5 \times 10^6$	9	CHR after 4 months
5	600 – 300	3×10^6 $- 4 \times 10^6$	7	CHR after 1 months PCR after 2 months
6	600 – 300	6×10^6 $- 4 \times 10^6$	3	CHR after 1 month

CHR, complete hematologic response; PHR, partial hematologic response; PCR, partial cytogenetic response; MCR, minor cytogenetic response.

beyond day 50; the patient had hematologic recovery after the treatment was stopped. Another MDS patient at the 900-mg dose level had grade 4 stomatitis. Diarrhea seems to become the DLT. The MTD is defined as organ-toxicity grade 4 in three cases at one dose level. In MDS one of five patients at the 900-mg level had grade 4 diarrhea. In the CML pilot trial YNK01 in combination with IFN-α-2b is well tolerated. Adverse events consisted in depression, fever, chills, and vasculitis which were attributed to IFN-α-2b treatment. These toxicities were not seen in any of the YNK01 monotherapy trials (Table 5).

Pharmacokinetics. The preliminary results of the pharmacokinetic data show the following. There are very long half-life times of YNK01 and its metabolites in the plasma. For ara-C half-life time is about 22 h. After continuous infusion of ara-C, the plasma half-life time is clearly shorter with half-life time for ara-C at 60 min. Up to the 1200 mg/day dose level, absorption and metabolism of YNK01 seem not to be limited. There is a linearity between the excretion of ara-U in the urine and the administered YNK01 dose. Interindividual variability of metabolism is considerable, but intraindividual variability is low. The metabolic bioavailability of YNK01 is about 16%. The maximum plasma concentrations of ara-C after oral application of 900 or 1200 mg YNK01 exceed plasma levels of low-dose ara-C therapy (20 mg/m^2/per day s.c.).

Conclusions

The results of these ongoing studies show a relative mild spectrum of toxicities up to dose levels of 900 mg absolute daily for 14 days. Even continuous administration of 600 mg absolute daily YNK01 in combination with IFN-α-2b is well tolerated. The treatment is feasible in the out-patient setting if monitored regularly for hematologic toxicities. Clinical responses were observed in palliative treatment with a day 1–14 administration in AML. In newly diagnosed CML, YNK01 in combination with IFN-α-2b achieved rapid hematologic and cytogenetic responses in this pilot trial. The pharmacokinetic data show that oral application of YNK01 is able to exceed the ara-C plasma levels reached by conventional low-dose ara-C treatment. Phase II studies will be performed to further evaluate the efficacy of the drug in AML patients as a maintenance treatment and in CML following the pilot trial.

Table 5. Grade 3 and 4 non-hematological toxicities

Toxicity	WHO grade	Dose level (mg)	Patients (*n*)
Stomatitis	3	100	1
	4	900	1
Diarrhea	3	200	1
	3	900	3
	3	1200	1
	4	1200	1
Nausea	3	900	1
Exanthema	3	900	1

References

1. Copplestone J.A., et al. Treatment of acute myeloid leukemia in the elderly: a clinical dilemma. Haemat. Oncol. 7, 53, 1989
2. Hamblin T. The treatment of acute myeloid leukemia preceded by the myelodysplastic syndrome. Leuk Research 16, 89–93, 1992 b
3. Castaigne S, Tilly H, Sigaux F, Daniel MT, Degos L. Treatment of leukemia with low dose ara-C: a study of 159 cases. Haematol Bluttransfus 1985; 29: 56–59
4. Cheson BD, Jaspere DM, Simon R, Friedman NA. Is the use of low dose ara-C (LoA) warranted in acute myelogenous leukemia (AML) and myelodysplastic syndromes (MDS). Proc Am Soc Clin Oncol 1986; 5: 149
5. Arthur CK, et al. Combined interferon alfa-2a and cytosine arabinoside as first-line treatment for chronic myeloid leukemia. Acta Haematol 1993, 89 (Suppl. 1), 15–21
6. Guilhot F, et al. Cytogenetic remissions in chronic myelogenous leukemia using interferon alfa-2a and hydroxyurea with or without low-dose cytosine arabinoside. Leukemia and Lymphoma 1991, Vol. 4, 49–55.
7. Kantarjian HM, et al. Treatment of advanced stages of Ph+CML with interferon alpha and low-dose cytarabine. JCO 1992, 5, 772–778.

Secondary Leukemia, Myelodysplastic Syndrome

Acute Leukemias VI
Prognostic Factors
and Treatment Strategies
Büchner et al. (eds)

Genetic Instability and Evolution of Karyotype in Secondary Acute Myeloid Leukemia

D. Haase [1], C. Fonatsch [2], M. Feuring-Buske [1], H. Gudat [2], C. Schoch [2], B. Wörmann [1], and W. Hiddemann [1]

Abstract. Secondary leukemias occur after a preceding myelodysplastic phase and/or following an exposition to mutagens. On the cytogenetic level, secondary acute myeloid leukemia (S-AML) are well characterized by the extent and special types of karyotypic abnormalities. Furthermore, distinct karyotypic changes can discriminate S-AML from de novo AML and myelodysplastic syndrome (MDS). Patients with S-AML have the highest proportions of clonal abnormalities (72%), of complex abnormalities (37% of abnormal cases), and of karyotype evolution (26% of abnormal cases) as compared to MDS and de novo AML. Both karyotype evolution and complex abnormalities are late manifestations of genetic instability which is already demonstrable in early MDS. They are indicators for a rapid disease progression and therapy refractoriness. Karyotype evolution is the prerequisite for an accumulation of genetic defects which occurs in a nonrandom fashion in S-AML.

Cytogenetic analyses of flow-sorted stem cells revealed that initiating as well as progression-associated cytogenetic changes occur at the level of immature $CD34^+/CD38^-$ progenitor cells in de novo and secondary AML, thus defining the stem cell-like compartment as the target for genetic defects.

Several lines of evidence imply that loss of material from chromosomes 5q and 7q might initiate the multistep process of karyotype evolution in S-AML. To further clarify the molecular basis of genetic instability in myeloid malignancies, genes regulating cell cycle control and DNA repair are promising candidates for future investigations.

Introduction

Secondary leukemias occur after a preceding myelodysplastic prephase and/or following an exposition to mutagens. They evolve via a multistep pathogenetic pathway from a genetically unstable stem cell which expands to a preleukemic cell clone showing primary cytogenetic changes [1, 2]. The occurrence of secondary genetic changes and clonal evolution herald the transformation to secondary leukemia which is characterized by an expansion of genetically unstable cell clones with complex chromosome abnormalities. In secondary acute myeloid leukemia (S-AML), genetic instability is a key mechanism manifesting as karyotype evolution and leading to complex abnormalities. To understand the pathogenetic meaning of genetic instability in myelodysplastic syndrome (MDS) and S-AML, the timepoint of its occurrence, its cellular targets, and the molecular background for this phenomenon have to be delineated.

Material and Methods

Cytogenetic examinations of 179 patients with MDS, of 103 patients with S-AML, and of 498

[1]Zentrum Innere Medizin, Abteilung Hämatologie/Onkologie, Georg-August-Universität, Robert-Koch-Str. 40, 37075 Göttingen, Germany
[2]Arbeitsgruppe Tumorcytogenetik, Institute für Humangenetik, Medizinische Universität zu Lübeck, Ratzeburger Allee 160, 23538 Lübeck, Germany

patients with de novo AML were performed in Lübeck by the tumor cytogenetics working group. Eleven of 13 flow-sorted specimens were analyzed in Göttingen, two in Lübeck. The patients' leukemias and MDS were morphologically classified according to the French–American–British (FAB)-classification [3, 4]. Cell cultivation, chromosome preparation, banding procedures, and staining were performed as described [5]. The documentation of karyotypes was performed according to the ISCN supplement [6]. Immunophenotyping, cell sorting, and the special conditions for the cytogenetic examination of flow-sorted cells are described elsewhere in this issue (Haase et al.).

Results

Cytogenetic analyses of 103 patients with secondary AML and 179 patients with MDS were compared with those of 498 patients with de novo AML. Summarizing our findings, four types of karyotype abnormalities can be distinguished in AML, MDS, and secondary AML (Table 1). Karyotypic changes nearly exclusively associated with de novo AML are inversion 16 together with its variants, and the reciprocal translocations t(8; 21) and t(15; 17). Another group of chromosomal abnormalities is mainly associated with MDS and S-AML. The most important changes in this group are trisomy of 1q, partial or total monosomy 5, monosomy 7, and other chromosome 7 abnormalities as well as trisomy 8. In secondary AML, these abnormalities signal a preceding myelodysplastic prephase. A further group of abnormalities encompassing 12p abnormalities and trisomy 21 can be observed in advanced MDS and secondary AML. They regularly herald or become visible during transformation of MDS to AML. The fourth group of karyotype abnormalities occurs nearly exclusively in secondary AML. Most frequent in our patients were anomalies of 3q, 11q23 and monosomy 18. It is supposed that they are sufficient to cause overt acute leukemia rapidly without any myelodysplastic prephase.

Table 1. Frequency of cytogenetic abnormalities in MDS, S-AML, and de novo AML

Chromosome abnormalities	MDS ($n=179$)	S-AML ($n=107$)	De novo AML ($n=498$)
t(8; 21) t(15; 17) inv(16) and variants	0	4[a]	26
+1q	15	14	4
-5/5q-	32	27	11
-7/7q-	24	10	8
+8	14	16	17
der 3q	3	10	3
der 11q	2	15	4
-18	3	12	3
+21	7	13	4
der 12p	8	15	2

[a]Percentage of abnormal cases der, derivative; n.d., not determined.

Table 2. Cytogenetic findings in MDS, S-AML, and de novo AML

	MDS (%)	S-AML (%)	de novo AML (%)
Abnormal	51	72	59
Complex	10	37	8
Karyotype evolution	9	26	9

Besides these distinct karyotypic changes, one of the most characteristic findings in S-AML is the phenomenon of karyotype evolution which is most frequent in S-AML as compared to MDS and de novo AML. Karyotype evolution is the prerequisite for the accumulation of genetic defects with the endpoint of a complexly rearranged unstable genome. Like karyotype evolution, complex abnormalities are most frequent in secondary AML (Table 2).

There is increasing evidence that in neoplasia the accumulation of genetic defects takes place in a nonrandom sequence as has been demonstrated paradigmatically for colon cancer [7]. To clarify the succession of karyotypic changes in AML, we analyzed patients with complex abnormalities treated in the German AML Cooperative Group trial. It turned out that 5q- or -5 were the initial abnormalities in 64% of cases. Monosomy 7 or 7q- and trisomy 8 were primary in 12% of cases each. The most frequent secondary and tertiary anomalies were +8, −7/7q-, and rearrangements of 11q, 12p, 17p, and trisomy 21.

Myelodysplastic Syndrome and S-AML are considered as stem cell diseases [1, 8]. However, all inferences voting for a stem cell involvement were indirect and not based on the examination of stem cells themselves. Neither had the question been answered whether disease progression was initiated from the stem cell compartment. Thus we performed cytogenetic analysis of highly purified early hematopoetic precursors characterized and flow sorted according to their expression of CD34 and CD38.

We were able to demonstrate clonal chromosomal abnormalities in the $CD34^+$ stem cell-like compartment in two cases of secondary AML, five cases of de novo AML, and in one case of secondary MDS (further details are given in our other paper in this issue). We conclude from our investigations that in de novo AML, S-AML, and MDS clonal chromosome abnormalities occur at the level of immature stem cell-like progenitors independently of the immunophenotype of the bulk leukemic population. This may not be true in promyelocytic leukemia, but we have not examined M3 cases as yet. Furthermore, karyotype evolution and thus the accumulation of genetic defects takes place at a very early level of the hematopoietic hierarchy.

Taken together, our data imply that not only disease initiation but also disease progression are driven from the stem cell compartment in MDS and AML.

An interesting matter concerning genetic instability is the the timepoint of its occurrence. Is it restricted to very advanced disease or is it an early, possibly initiating event, as has been proposed for MDS pathogenesis by Jacobs [2].

Within the scope of a cytogenetic study of patients with MDS we were already able to observe chromosomal breakage in early MDS before the occurrence of clonal chromosome abnormalities [9]. In total, we observed genetic instability without clonal abnormalities in 12% of 179 patients with MDS.

In advanced MDS and S-AML, genetic instability manifests itself not only as chromosomal breakage but also as complex abnormalities, karyotype evolution, single and double minutes, homogenously staining regions, and other bizarre karyotypic changes often occurring as cell-to-cell variations, which was summarized by Sakurai and Sandberg [10] with the term "major karyotypic abnormalities" (MAKA).

The prognostic impact of such complex anomalies is extremely bad even if very recent therapy strategies are applied, which can be inferred from the data of Büchner et al. in this issue.

Discussion

The phenomena of karyotype evolution and complex abnormalities are manifestations of the pronounced genetic instability in S-AML. Our data vote for an immature stem cell-like population as the target for initiating genetic events. Progression likewise seems to be driven from this compartment. Genetic instability is detectable early during the course of MDS before clonal chromosome abnormalities occur. During disease progression, genetic instability is the prerequisite for karyotype evolution and thus for the accumulation of genetic defects for terminating in secondary leukemia with a MAKA karyotype. However, the possible causes for genetic instability in MDS and AML are still obscure.

If we take the very recent findings in hereditary colon cancer as a paradigm for neoplastic transformation [11–13], genetic instability in hematopoietic diseases might result from deficient DNA repair caused by mutations of DNA repair genes. On the other hand, disturbances of cell cycle regulation might likewise, at least indirectly, result in increased genetic instability.

Several lines of evidence imply that the loss of genetic material from 5q and possibly 7q might initiate genetic instability in MDS leading to karyotype evolution and complex abnormalities. The chromosomal localization of DNA repair and cell cycle-regulating genes in the long arm of chromosome 5 [14] and on chromosome 7 [13] is a strong argument for this assumption.

Functional and molecular studies of DNA repair and cell cycle regulation are needed to clarify the molecular basis of genetic instability in MDS and AML.

We have started a research program on DNA repair in MDS. Very recent results show an interesting tendency. Lymphocytes of patients with MDS and healthy controls were irradiated with 0.5 Gray. After 1 h of DNA repair time, a cell cycle analysis was performed. Our hypothesis was that deficient DNA repair in MDS must lead to a higher increase of cells in G2/M phase as compared to normal controls, since damaged cells are not repaired sufficiently to pass the G2 checkpoint [15]. What we observed was the opposite: the G2 increase was significantly lower than in the control group. Thus, we would tentatively like to speculate that in MDS the G2 checkpoint might be defective. However, these results cannot exclude combined defects of cell cycle control and DNA repair.

Molecular and functional studies of DNA repair in MDS have to be performed to elucidate the mechanisms leading to genetic instability in MDS and AML.

References

1. Raskind W.H., Tirumali N., Jacobson R., Singer J., Fialkow P.J. (1984). Evidence for a multistep pathogenesis of a myelodysplastic syndrome. Blood 63: 1318–1323
2. Jacobs A. (1991). Genetic lesions in preleukemia. Leukemia 5: 277–282
3. Bennett J.M., Catovsky D., Daniel M.-T., Flandrin G., Galton D.A.G., Gralnick H.R., Sultan C. (1976). Proposals for the classification of the acute leukaemias. Brit. J. Haematol. 33: 451–458
4. Bennett J.M., Catiovsky D., Daniel M.-T., Flandrin G., Galton D.A.G., Gralnick H.R., Sultan C., The French-American-British (FAB) Cooperative Group (1982). Proposals for the classification of the myelodysplastic syndromes. Br. J. Haematol. 51: 189–199
5. Fonatsch C., Schaadt M., Kirchner H., Diehl V. (1980). A possible correlation between the degree of karyotype aberrations and the rate of sister chromatid exchanges in lymphoma lines. Int. J. Cancer 26: 749–756
6. ISCN (1991): Guidelines for cancer cytogenetics, supplement to an international system for human cytogenetic nomenclature. F. Mitelman (ed). S. Karger, Basel
7. Fearon E.R. and Vogelstein B. (1990): A genetic model for colorectal tumorigenesis. Cell 61: 759–767
8. Janssen J.W.G., Buschle M., Layton M., Drexler H.G., Lyons J., Van Den Berghe H., Heimpel H., Kubanek B., Kleihauer E., Mufti G., Bartram C. (1989). Clonal analysis of myelodysplastic syndromes: evidence of multipotent stem cell origin. Blood 73: 248–254
9. Haase D., Fonatsch C., Freund M. (1992). Karyotype instability in myelodysplastic syndromes—a specific step in pathogenesis preceding clonal chromosome anomalies. Leukemia and Lymphoma 8: 221–228
10. Sakurai M. and Sanberg A.A. (1976). Chromosomes and causation of human cancer and leukemia XIII. An evaluation of karyotypic findings in erythroleukemia. Cancer 37: 790–804
11. Fishel R., Lescoe M.K., Rao M.R.S., Copeland N.G., Jenkins N.A., Garber J., Kane M. and Kolodner R. (1993). The human mutator gene homolog MSH2 and its association with hereditary nonpolyposis colon cancer. Cell 61: 1027–1038
12. Thibodeau S.N., Bren G. and Schaid D. (1993). Microsatellite instability in cancer of the proximal colon. Science, 260: 816–819
13. Nicolaides N.C., Papadopoulos N., Liu B. et al. (1994). Mutations of two PMS homologues in hereditary nonpolyposis colon cancer. Nature 371: 75–80
14. Koken M.H.M., Smit E.M.E, Jaspers-Dekker I., Ooostra B.A., Hagemeijer A., Bootsma D., and Hoeijmakers J.H.J. (1992). Localization of two human homologues, HHR6A and HHR6B, of the yeast DNA repair gene RAD6 to chromosomes Xq24-q25 and 5q23-31. Genomics 12: 447–453
15. Hartwell L.H. and Weinert T.A. (1989). Checkpoints: controls that ensure the order of cell cycle events. Science 246: 629–634

Acute Leukemias VI
Prognostic Factors
and Treatment Strategies
Büchner et al. (eds)

Prognostic Value of Dysmyelopoiesis in 128 Patients with De Novo Acute Myeloid Leukemia

T. Haferlach[1], H. Löffler[1], W. Gassmann[1], C. Fonatsch[2], C. Schoch[2], B. Schlegelberger[3], R. Becher[4], E. Thiel[5], W.-D. Ludwig[6], M.C. Sauerland[7], A. Heinecke[7], and T. Büchner[8] for the AML Cooperative Group

Abstract. In a prospective setting we investigated several cytomorphological features in 128 patients with de novo acute myeloid leukemia (AML) treated in the AML cooperative Group (CG)-92 trial. The most important question to be answered was whether or not dysplasia had a prognostic impact for the remission rate and survival in AML. We could demonstrate a significantly lower remission rate for patients with trilineage dysplasia (TLD) in comparison to those without any dysplastic features. The overall survival was worse for patients with TLD as well but this was not statistically significant at the time of this analysis. Further investigations will help to define new risk factors as a result of this detailed analysis of bone marrow morphology.

Introduction

The prognostic significance of dysplastic features in de novo acute myeloid leukemia (AML) has been investigated by several groups [1–7]. In some studies a poor outcome seemed to be associated with the detection of dysplastic features but the results remain controversial. This may be due to retrospective approaches. Furthermore, the criteria for the presence or absence of dysgranulopoiesis (DysG), dyserythropoiesis (DysE), dysmegakaryopoiesis (DysM), and for trilineage dysplasia (TLD) were different in some studies. This makes it very difficult to compare results or to discuss their prognostic value. In this prospective study, we analysed the incidence and the influence of dysplasia in de novo AML in 128 patients treated in the AML cooperative group (CG)-92 trial.

Material and Methods

Between December 1992 and April 1995 de novo AML was diagnosed in 128 patients treated in the AMLCG-92 study [8, 9]. Treatment results and survival data were available at the time of this interim analysis for all patients. Bone marrow and blood smears were sent for diagnosis and several cytomorphological studies to our reference centre. In all cases a detailed examination of the bone marrow features was performed. All submitted bone marrows were analysed irrespective of whether the patient would be treated or not. This avoided a bias caused by the treatment results.

Bone marrow smears were stained according to standard procedures [10]. For dysplasia

[1]University of Kiel, Second Medical Department, Kiel, Germany
[2]University of Lübeck, Cooperative Group for Tumor Cytogenetics, Institute for Human Genetics, Lübeck, Germany
[3]University of Kiel, Institute for Human Genetics, Kiel, Germany
[4]University of Essen, Department of Internal Medicine, Essen, Germany
[5]University Steglitz, Department of Internal Medicine, Berlin, Germany
[6]Robert-Rössle-Hospital, Department for Medical Oncology and Molecular Biology, Berlin, Germany
[7]University of Münster, Institute for Medical Informatics and Biomathematics, Germany
[8]University of Münster, Department of Internal Medicine, Münster, Germany

Pappenheim and myeloperoxidase staining were examined. Dysplasia was defined according to standard criteria [4]: granulocytic dysplasia (DysG) was defined as >50% of at least ten polymorphonuclear neutrophils (PMN) being agranular or hypogranular, or with hyposegmented nuclei (pseudo Pelger—Huet anomaly). At least 25 cells were observed but usually 100 cells were counted. Myeloperoxidase deficiency in the (PMN) was defined as 50% or more myeloperoxidase-negative cells in at least ten PMN after confirming strong positivity of eosinophils or other PMN.

Erythroid dysplasia (DysE) was defined as 50% or more of dysplastic features in at least 25 erythroid precursors: megaloblastoid aspects, karyorrhexis, nuclear fragments, or multinuclearity. A minimum of 25 cells were counted but usually it was possible to count 100 cells.

Megakaryocytic dysplasia (DysM) was diagnosed when at least three megakaryocytes or >50% in at least six cells showed dysplastic features such as microkaryocytes or multiple separated nuclei.

Trilineage dysplasia was diagnosed when DysG, DysE, and DysM were detectable.

Results

A total of 128 patients with de novo AML were analysed (male, 55; female 73). Median age was 53 years (range 17–74) years. According to the French–American–British (FAB) classification [11] two patients were classified as AML MO, there were 26 M1 (20.3%), 47 M2 (37.1%), five M3 (3.6%), 22 M4 (17.2%), seven M4Eo (5.5%), four M5a (3.1%), 10 M5b (7.8%), five M6 (3.8%), and no M7. Table 1 gives the percentage of dysplastic features according to the FAB criteria as mentioned before in comparison to other studies for all FAB subtyps combined.

The percentage of DysG, DysE, or DysM differed widely in the different studies. Even if the same investigator analysed the bone marrow smears [4, 5], variations of 100% were published. This demonstrates the complexity of detecting dysplasia and one should avoid final conclusions from these retrospective studies.

In contrast, the frequency of patients without any dysplasia or with TLD ranged within small limits. Thus, it seems much easier to achieve reliable results especially for these two groups of patients if one starts to analyse dysplasia in AML. For this reason and because of the number of patients in our prospective study recruited so far, we started to compare our results with others regarding the influence of dysplasia in one cell line only or the detection of TLD with no dysplasia at all. The results for remission rates are controversial so far and are shown in Table 2.

The most important factor to achieve complete remission (CR) in our patients was the absence of dysplastic features (CR 86.7%) in comparison to patients with TLD (CR 57.8%, $p = 0.042$). If patients with TLD achieved a CR, the event-free survival was worse than for patients without any dysplasia but this is not significant so far (Table 3, $p = 0.0632$, Fig. 1).

Only two studies could demonstrate the prognostic value of TLD for event-free survival [3, 7]. In one study, DysM seems to influence this parameter [5].

Table 1. Frequency of dysplastic features in de novo AML

Author	Reference	Study	Year	Patients (n)	No Dys (%)	DysG (%)	DysE (%)	DysM (%)	TLD (%)
Brito-Babapulle et al. [a,b]	[1]	MRC,	1987	160					15
Jinnai et al.	[2]		1987	127				12.6	
Estienne et al.	[3]	Lille,	1990	132	28	23	15	23	11
Goasguen et al.	[4]	ECOG,	1992	336	46	24.7	33.6	24.1	11.6
Goasguen et al.	[5]	AMLCG,	1993	219	38.4	54.8	20.1	20.5	7.8
Ballen et al. [a,b]	[6]		1994	106	7	7	18	17	9
Kuriyama et al.	[7]		1994	230					17
Haferlach et al.		AMLCG,	1995	128	29.7	21.1	14.8	35.8	14.8

[a]The criteria for dysplastic features were different to this analysis. Data were adapted to the FAB criteria as defined by Goasguen [4].
[b]Several therapy regimens were used in this study.

Table 2. Influence of dysplastic features on remission rates in de novo AML

Author	Reference	Study	Year	Patients (n)	DysG	DysE	DysM	TLD
Brito-Babapulle et al.	[1]	MRC,	1987	160	n.d.	n.d.	n.d.	■ $p = 0.001$
Jinnai et al.	[2]		1987	127	n.d.	n.d.	■ $p = 0.025$	n.d
Estienne et al.	[3]	Lille,	1990	132	0	0	0	■ p = 0.003
Goasguen et al.	[4]	ECOG,	1992	336	■ $p = 0.013$	0	0	■ $p = 0.03$
Goasguen et al.	[5]	AMLCG,	1993	219	0	0	■ $p = 0.017$	n.d.
Ballen et al.	[6]		1994	106	0	0	0	0
Kuriyama et al.	[7]		1994	230	n.d.	n.d.	n.d	■ $p = 0.01$
Haferlach et al.		AMLCG,	1995	128	0	0	0	■ $p = 0.042$

n.d., not done; 0, no influence; ■, bad influence.

Table 3. Influence of dysplasia for event-free survival in de novo AML

Author	Reference	Study	Year	Patients (n)	DysG (n)	DysE	DysM	TLD
Brito-Babapulle et al.	[1]	MRC,	1987	160	n.d.	n.d.	n.d.	0
Jinnai et al.	[2]		1987	127	n.d.	n.d.	0	n.d.
Estienne et al.	[3]	Lille,	1990	132	0	0	0	■ $p = 0.0001$
Goasguen et al.	[4]	ECOG,	1992	336	0	0	0	0
Goasguen et al.	[5]	AMLCG,	1993	219	0	0	■ $p = 0.002$	n.d.
Ballen et al.	[6]		1994	106	0	0	0	0
Kuriyama et al.	[7]		1994	230	0	0	0	■ $p = 0.0005$
Haferlach et al.		AMLCG,	1995	128	0	0	0	0 $p = 0.0632$

n.d., not done; 0, no influence; ■, bad influence.

Discussion

The identification of new prognostic factors in AML would be helpful to stratify patients into low-risk and high-risk groups and to modify therapy approaches in the future. Some studies were able to demonstrate the significance of cytogenetic results for the outcome of patients [12–16], others identified age [17] or leucocyte count [18], but these results remain controversial.

We have investigated morphological dysplasia in 128 patients with de novo AML to clarify its clinical significance. All patients were treated in the AMLCG-92 trial. We were able to identify two subgroups of patients with a superior or a worse complete remission (CR) rate. Patients without any dysplasia in the bone marrow had a very high CR rate (86.7%) in comparison to all patients combined (71.8%) and especially in contrast to patients with TLD (CR 57.8%). Even if some other studies were retrospective and criteria for dysplasia differed, it is possible to compare these data. Similar results were reported by some groups [1, 3, 4, 7]. Others failed to demonstrate a significantly lower CR rate for patients with TLD but used unconventional criteria for the definition of dysplasia; this makes it impossible to compare the results with all the other studies [6].

We were not able to clarify the prognostic significance of dysplasia if only one cell line was affected because the number of cases was too small. Further investigations are under way and

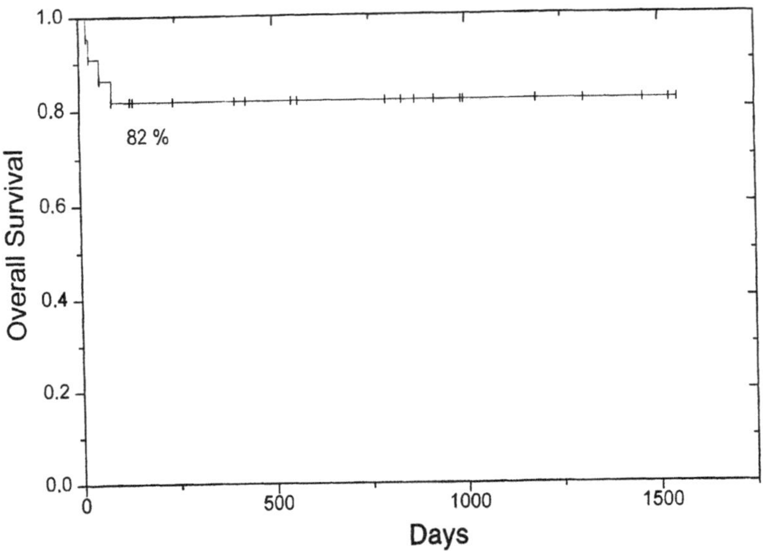

Fig. 1. Trilineage dysplasia (TLD) is a bad prognostic factor in patients with do novo AML. *Solid line*, no dysplasia, $n = 38$ (27 censored); *broken line*, TLD), $n = 19$ (11 censored)

may help to define smaller subgroups of patients with special combinations of dysplastic feature. A multivariant analysis will help to grade the importance of several cytomorphological results.

In conclusion, TLD is correlated with a significantly lower remission rate in de novo AML. This may show that the malignant transformation is near the pluripotent stem cell level which is less sensitive to chemotherapecutic agents. We have not been able to demonstrate the influence of dysplasia for event-free survival yet. The correlation with other prognostic factors such as chromosomal status is necessary as well and will be investigated. It may be that TLD reflects only one of a number of coherent factors with negative influence on the prognosis of AML. Because dysplatic features are detectable at the time of diagnosis in the first bone marrow and seem to give important information about treatment outcome, the search for dysplasia should be inclulded in every bone marrow analysis in AML. Further results could be of interest for different therapeutic strategies such as high-dose chemotherapy or bone marrow transplantation.

References

1. Brito-Babapulle, F., Catovsky, D., Galton, D.A.G.: Clinical and laboratory features of de novo acute myeloid leukaemia with trilineage myelodysplasia. Br J Haematol 66, 445–450 (1987)
2. Jinnai, I., Tomonaga, M., Kuriyama, K., Matsuo, T., Nonaka, H., Amenomori, T., Yoshida, Y., Kusano, M., Tagawa, M, Ichimaru, M.: Dysmegakaryocytopoiesis in acute leukaemias: its predominance in myelomonocytic (M4) leukaemia and implication for poor response to chemotherapy. Br J Haematol 66, 467–472 (1987)
3. Estienne, M.H., Fenaux, P., Preudhomme, C., Lai, J.L., Zandecki, M., Lepelley, P., Cosson, A.: Prognostic value of dysmyelopoietic features in de novo acute myeloid leukaemia: a report on 132 patients. Clin lab Haemat 12, 57–65 (1990)
4. Goasguen, J.E., Matsuo, T., Cox, C., Bennett, J.M.: Evaluation of the dysmyelopoiesis in 336 patients with de novo acute myeloid leukemia: major importance of dysgranulopoiesis for remission and survival. Leukemia 6, 520–525 (1992)
5. Goasguen, J.E., Büchner, T., Hiddemann, W., Wörmann, B., Heinecke, A., Sauerland, M.C., Fonastch, C., Becher, R., Hossfeld, D., Löffler, H., Schaefer, U.W.: Prognostic importance of myeloid dysplastic features in AML. Blood 82 Suppl 1, 124 (1993)
6. Ballen, K.K., Gilliland, D.G., Kalish, L.A., Shulman L.N.: Bone marrow dysplasia in patients with newly diagnosed acute myelogenous leukemia does not correlate with history of myelodysplasia or with remission rate and survival. Cancer 73, 314–321 (1994)
7. Kuriyama, K., Tomonaga, M., Matsuo, T., Kobayashi, T., Miwa, H., Shirakawa, S., Tanimoto, M., Adachi, K., Emi, N., Hiraoko, A., Tominaga, N., Imai, K., Asou, N., Tsubaki, K., Takahashi, I.,

Minami, S., Yoshida, M., Murakami, H., Minato, K., Oshima, T., Furusawa, S., Ohno, R.: Poor response to intensive chemotherapy in de novo acute myeloid leukaemia with trilineage myelodysplasia. Br J Haematol 86, 767–773 (1994)

8. Büchner, T., Hiddemann, W.: Treatment strategies in acute myeloid leukemia (AML). Blut 60, 61–67 (1990)
9. Büchner, T., Hiddemann, W., Schaefer, U.W., Löffler, H., Maschmeyer, G., Ludwig, W.-D., Aul, C., Lathan, B., Heinecke, A.: Combined effect of early intesification and prolonged post-remission chemotherapy in patients with AML. Leukemia 6 Suppl. 4, 68–70 (1992)
10. Löffler, H.: Zytochemische Methoden. In: Huber, H., Löffler, H., Faber, V. (Hrsg.): Methoden der diagnostischen Hämatologie. Berlin u.a.O.: 125–136 (1991)
11. Bennett, J.M., Catovsky, D., Daniel, M.T., Flandrin, G., Galton, D.A.G., Gralnick, H.R., Sultan, C.: Proposed revised criteria for the classification of acute myeloid leukemia: a report of the French-American-British Cooperative Group. Ann Intern Med 103, 626–629 (1985)
12. Fourth International Workshop on Chromosomes in Leukemia: Cancer Genet Cytogenet 11, 259–350 (1984)
13. Haferlach, T., Gassmann, W., Löffler, H., Jürgensen, C., Noak, J., Ludwig, W.-D., Thiel, E., Haase, D., Fonastch, C., Becher, R., Schlegelberger, B., Nowrousian, M.R., Lengfelder, E., Eimermacher, H., Weh, H.J., Braumann, D., Maschmeyer, G., Koch, P., Heinecke, A., Sauerland, M.C., Büchner , Th.: Clinical aspects of acute myeloid leukemias of the FAB types M3 and M4Eo. Ann Hematol 66, 165–170 (1993)
14. Haferlach, T., Bennett, J.M., Löffler, H., Gassmann, W., Andersen, J., Tuzuner, N., Cassileth, P.A., Fonatsch, C., Schlegelberger, B., Thiel, E., Ludwig, W.-D., Sauerland, M.C., Heinecke, A., Büchner, T. for AML Cooperative Group and ECOG: Cytomorphology results and dysplastic features as prognostic factors in 41 cases with acute myeloid leukemia (AML) and translocation (8; 21). Leuk Res 18 Suppl, 45 (1994)
15. Keating, M.J., Cork, A., Broch, Y., Smith, T., Waltes, R.S., McCredie, K.B., Trujillo, J., Freireich, E.J.: Toward a clinically relevant cytogenetic classification of acute myelogenous leukemia. Leukemia Res 11(2), 119–133 (1987)
16. Keating, M.J., Smith, T.L., Kantarjian, H., Cork, A., Walters, R., Trujillo, J.M., McCredie, K.B., Gehan, E.A., Freireich, E.J.: Cytogenetic pattern in acute myelogenous leukemia: a major reproducible determinat of outcome. Leukemia 2, 403–412 (1988)
17. Schiffer, C.A., Lee, E.J., Tomiyasu, T., Wiernik, P.H., Testa, J.R.: Prognostic impact of cytogenetic abnormalities in patients with de novo acute nonlymphocytic leukemia. Blood 73, 263–270 (1989)
18. Keating, M.J., Smith, T.L., Gehan, E.A., McCredie, K.B., Bodey, G.P., Freireich, E.J.: A prognositic factor analysis for the use in development of predictive models for response in adult acute leukemia. Cancer 50, 457–465

Acute Leukemias VI
Prognostic Factors
and Treatment Strategies
Büchner et al. (eds)

Incidence of Secondary Leukemias After Therapy of Childhood Hodgkin's Disease Without Nitrogen-Mustard. Results of the German-Austrian Study Group

G. Schellong[1], M. Riepenhausen[1], U. Creutzig[1], J. Ritter[1], J. Harbott[2], G. Mann[3], and H. Gadner[3]
for the German-Austrian Pediatric Hodgkin's Disease Group

Introduction

For more than 20 years now, secondary leukemias following treatment of Hodgkin's disease (HD) have been reported in the literature [1-7]. Most of these reports refer to adults—corresponding to the higher incidence of HD in adults compared to children but cases following treatment in childhood have also been published. Usually these secondary leukemias present as acute myeloid leukemia (AML), with or without a myelodyplastic prephase, and have a very poor prognosis. As to causative factors, it became increasingly evident that specific elements of the chemotherapy are dicrectly responsible. Retrospective studies were able to identify alkylating cytotoxic agents as the main risk factor, especially nitrogen-mustard (synonyms:mechlorethamine, mustargen) [8-12]. Today it is widely accepted that the mustine vincristine procarbazine and prednisone (MOPP) combination is associated with a considerably higher risk for secondary leukemias than ABVD which includes no alkylating drug [8, 12].

For a long time, precise statements on the incidence and risk factors of secondary leukemias following HD in children could not be given as reports on large series were lacking. In 1989, data from a large pediatric patient group ($n = 979$) were published by Meadows with the international Late Effect Study Group (LESG) [13]. Within 11 years after the diagnosis of HD, 20 events of secondary hematologic malignancies (SHM) were observed: 16 AML, one chronic myelogenous leukemia (CML) and three non-Hodgkin's lymphoma (NHL). The cumulative risk of SHM after 15 and 20 years was 4% for the total group, 6% for the patients who has received chemotherapy (predominantly MOPP) and 8% for those who had been additionally treated with salvage therapy. No SHM were found after radiotherapy alone. Using a specially developed score, the applied cumulative dose of alkylating agents was identified as a clearly significant risk factor. In addition, splenectomized patients showed a higher risk for SHM than those without splenectomy.

We have tried to determine the risk of SHM in those patients treated in four consecutive German-Austrian studies for HD since 1978 [15-18]. Against the background of the high overall survival rate which can be reached with modern treatment strategies in childhood Hodgkin's disease, the risk of secondary malignancies evidently deserves general close attention. An additional aim of our analysis was to compare our data with those of the LESG considering the aspect that in the chemotherapy of the German-Austrian pediatric studies much lower cumulative doses of alkylating agents were used and no nitrogen mustard at all.

Patients and Methods

The total patient group for this analysis comprised all 667 patients of the German-Austrian studies HD-78, -82, and -87 enrolled by 70 par-

[1]University Children's Hospital, Münster, Germany
[2]University Children's Hospital, Gießen, Germany
[3]St. Anna Children's Hospital, Wien, Austria

ticipating centers [15–18]. The median age of patients at the time of primary diagnosis was 12 years 2 months with a range of 1 year 11 months to 16 years 3 months. The sex ratio was 418 boys / 249 girls (1.7/1). As of 31 August, 1994, the Kalpen-meier analysis for all 667 patients (Fig. 1) reveals a probability for survival at 15 years of 95% (SD 1%).

Combined modality treatment was used for patients at all disease stages. The number of chemotherapy blocks in front-line therapy was two in 330 patients (50%), four in 140 (21%), six in 168 (25%) and eight in 29 (4%). Drug combinations in blocks 1 and 2 were OPPA (vincristine, prednisone, procarbazine, adriamycin) or OPA (without procarbazine) and in the subsequent courses COPP (C, cyclophosphamide) or COMP (M, methotreaxate). Thus, alkylating agents in the primary treatment were procarbazine, applied to 65% of the patients, and cyclophosphamide, given to about 50% at a cumulative total dose of 2000, 4000, or 6000 mg/m^2. Nitrogen mustard was never used. The cumulative total dose of adriamycin was 160 mg/m^2 in all patients. Radiotherapy, which followed chemotherapy was applied as extendedfield irradiation with maximum doses of 36–40 Gy in study HD—78 and as involved-field irradiation with 20–35 Gy (depending on treatment group and study) in HD-82, HD-85, and HD-87.

Seventy-five patients (11%) had to undergo salvage therapy due to resistant or recurrent disease. Second-and third-line therapy was less uniform than front-line therapy. Beside ABVD and COPP, combinations containing etoposide and ifosfamide were used [19].

Major efforts on a cooperative basis were made in 1994 to collect information about the current status of the patients. The median follow-up time is 7 years 10 months (range 1–16 years), the median age at the last examination or information 20 years 1months (range 3 years 9 months to 31 years 1 month).

The cumulative probabilities of the incidence of SHM after HD were estimated with the Kalpan-Meier method [20] using the SAS statistical software where the corresponding estimate of the standard error and the confidence limits are computed with Greenwood's formula [21]. Differences between groups were assessed with the log-rank test and Wilcoxon test [22].

Results

A total of five patients developed SHM: four AML and one Myelodyplastic syndrome MDS. Non-Hodgkin's lymphomas were not observed. Some data concerning primary disease and treatment three as well as secondary malignancy are shown in Table 1. The sex ratio was two boys/three girls. Three patients were in first remission of Hodgkin's disease (stage IA, IIIA, IVB), two had developed a relapse and were additionaly treated by salvage therapy. The median time between day 1 of primary therapy and diagnosis of the secondary malignancy was 5 years 3 months (range 2 years 7 months –

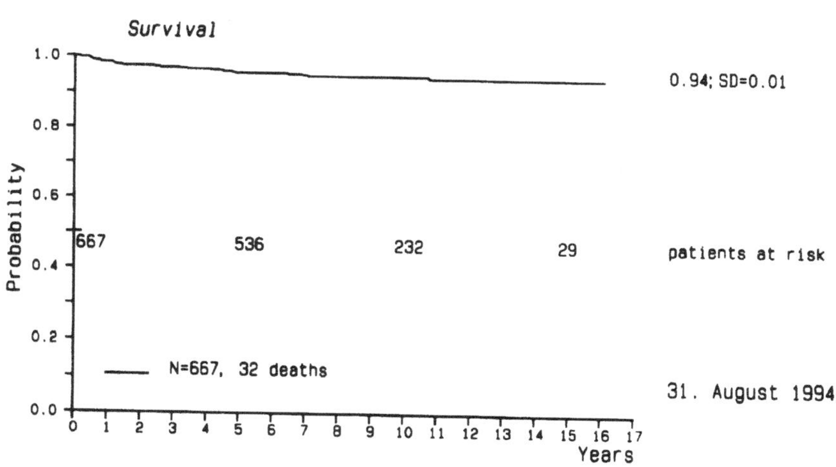

Fig. 1. Kalpan-Meier analysis of survival for the total group of 667 patients in the four German-Austrian trials HD-78, HD-82, HD-85, HD-87

Table 1. Data of five patients with secondary leukemias / MDS regarding HD and secondary malignancy

1 Patient no.	2 Sex	3 Age (years; months)	4 Stage	5 Splen-ectomy	6 Therapy	7 Interval (years; months)	8 SHM	9 Cytoge-netics	10 Therapy	11 Status August 1994
1	f	7;5	III A	+	2 OPPA/6 COPP/TR	10;5	AML	47,XX,+8	Chemotherapy,	Died
2	f	12;2	$IV_{L+}B$	+	2 OPPA/4 COPP/RT	5;3	MDS	Complex, with chromosomes 1,5,7,17 involved	Chemotherapy, ABMT	Died
3	f	10;7	II B	+	2 OPPA/4 COPP/RT + salvage (2x)	2;7	AML	46,XX del(5)(q13q31)	Chemotherapy	Died
4	m	9;7	III A	+	2 OPA/2 COP/RT + salvage	3;6	AML	47,XY,t(1;11) (p32;q23),+8	Chemotherapy	Died
5	m	7;3	I A	–	2 OPA/RT	4;1	AMl	47, XY,t(10;21) (p12;q22),+19?	Chemotherapy	Died

Interval, time between day 1 of therapy for HD until diagnosis of leukemia/MDS; columns 3–6, HD; 7–11, secondary malignancy

10 years 5 months). The median age at diagnosis of AML/MDS was 13 years 2 months (range 11 years 4 months - 1 years 10 months). All five patients died after treatment with chemotherapy and (in two cases) additional autologous bone marrow transplantation (ABMT).

The cumulative risks for AML/MDS at 5, 10 and 15 years in the total group of all patients are 0.5% (SD 0.3%), 0.7% (SD 0.3%), and 1.2% (SD 0.6%), respectively (Table 2). Patients were subdivided in to three groups for further evaluations (Table 2).

Group 1: 296 patients who had received chemotherapy only with two blocks of OPPA or OPA and have remained in first remission. Survival rate at 15 years of this group is 99.6% one case of AML was observed after 4 years 5 months. The cumulative risk for AML/MDS is 0.4% (SD 0.4%) at 5, 10, and 15 years.

Group 2: 296 patients who had received, in addition two blocks of OPPA or OPA, chemotherapy with COPP or COMP and have remained in first remission. One AML after 10 years 5 months and one MDS after 5 years 3 × were observed. The prospective survival rate at 15 years in this group is 94% (SD 2%). The cumulative risks for AML/MDS are 0 at 5 years, 0.4% (SD 0.4%) at 10 years and 1.4% (SD 1.0%) at 15 years.

Group 3: 75 patients who had received salvage therapy in addition to primary treatment. Two casees of AML were observed after 2 years 7 months and 3 years 6 months. The prospective survival rate at 12 years in this group 7% (SD 5%). The cumulative risk for AML/MDS is 3.3% (SD 2.3%) at 5 and 10 years. The value for 15 years cannot yet be given, but the risk at 14 years is identical (3.3%).

The differences between group 3 (salvage therapy) versus group 1 or 2 are statistically significant: group 1 vs group 3: $p = 0.02$ (Wilcoxon), 0.03 (log-rank test); group 2 vs group 3: $p=0.02$ (Wilcoxon), 0.05 (log-rank test). The difference between groups 1 and 2 is not significant (Fig. 2)

Splenectomy was not identified as a risk factor. Four of 329 splenectomized patients developed AML/MDS, compared with one of 338 non-splenectomized patients (cumulative risk at 15 years 1.7% vs. 0.3%). However, the difference is not significant ($p = 0.23$).

Discussion

In our analysis five SHM (four AML, one MDS, no NHL) were observed in 667 children treated for HD in four German-Austrian trials between 1978 and 1990 (follow-up time up to 16 years, median 7years 10 months). Four of the five SHM were diagnosed between the 3 and 6 year after onset of therapy for HD and the last one in the 11 year. It is consistent with other published data that secondary leukemias and MDS after HD in adults and children arise nearly exclusively during the first 10–12 years [10, 12–14]. After this period the risk for further SHM approaches zero.

Compared to most of the recent reports in the literature, the incidence of SHM in our group of HD patients is relatively low: the cumulative risk for SHM in our total group is 0.7% at 10 years and 1.2% at 15 years, wereas risks of 4%–6% were found in several other analyses after HD in adults [10, 12, 14] and children [13]. Of special interest in the comparsion

Table 2. Overall survival, number of secondary hematologic malignancies and cumulative risk (%) at 5, 10 and 15 years for the entire group of patients and the three subgroups with different chemotherapy for HD

	(*n*)	SV	SHM	Cumulative risk					
				5 years		10 years		15 years	
	(%)			(%)	(SD)	(%)	(SD)	(%)	(SD)
Total group	667	95	5	0.5	0.3	0.7	0.3	1.2	0.6
Group 1 2 × OPPA or OPA	296	99	1	0.4	0.4	0.4	0.4	0.4	0.4
Group 2 plus COPP or COMP	296	95	2	0	0.4	0.4	0.4	1.4	1.0
Group 3 salvage therapy	75	77	2	3.3	2.3	3.3	2.3		

The differences between group 1 vs 3 ($p = 0.02$) and group 2 vs. 3 ($p = 0.02$) are significant. sv, overall survival; SHM, secondary hematologic malignancy.

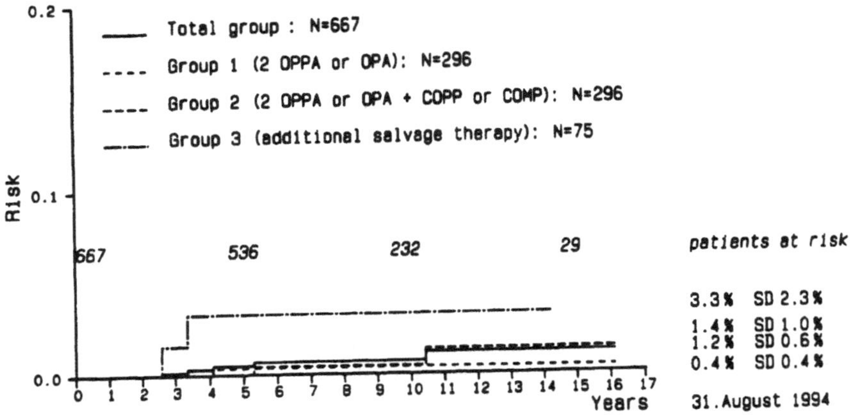

Fig. 2. Cumulative percentage of patients who developed a secondary leukemia / MDS among the entire population of patients ($n = 667$) and those of group 1 ($n = 296$), group 2 ($n = 296$), and group 3 ($n = 75$), respectively

of our results with those of international pediatric LESG [13]. In the total group of 997 LESG patients the risk is 3% at 10 years and 4% at 15 years in the 698 patients who had received chemotherapy (with or without radiotherapy) 5% at 10 years and 6% at 15 years. Using confidence limits we compared these data with our own findings (Table 3). After a follow up of 10 years, there is no overlap of the confidence limits at the 5% level. After 15 years we found no overlap with the group treated with chemotherapy and a marginal overlap between the total groups. Thus, there is strong support for the conclusion that the incidence of SHM in our group is significantly lower than in the LESG patients. A similar difference is found for the patients who underwent salvage therapy as well: 3.3% at 10 years in our 75 patients versus 6% at 10 years and 8% at 15 years in the 365 patients of the LESG. As the standard deviations for this subgroup were not published by the LESG [13] a statistical comparsion is not possible.

Discussing potential causes for these differences in the risk of SHM we recognize that the main features of the two patient groups are quite similar, partly identical. This is true for the size of the groups, patient age at diagnoses of HD, sex ratio, percentage of stage I and II patients and time of follow up [13]. In contrast, major differences exist in important details of the front-line therapy and in the percentage of patients who needed salvage therapy (11% in our group 37% in the LESG). While MOPP was the chemotherapy predominantly used for the LESG patients, front-line chemotherapy in our group included no nitrogen mustard at all, but cyclophosphamide in about 50% of the patients at relatively low cumulative doses. Procarbazine

Table 3. Estimated confidence limits (at 5% level) for the risk of SHM after HD. Comparison of our results with the data of the LESG [13]

	(n)	Own data Risk (%)	(n)	LESG data Risk (%)
After 10 years—				
all patients	667	0.2–0.7–1.2	997	2–3–4
patients with Chemotherapy	Identical group		698	3–5–7
After 15 years—				
all patients	667	0–1.2–2.1	997	2–4–6
Patients with chemotherapy	Identical group		698	4–6–9

All 667 patients in our group had received chemotherapy in contrast to 698/997 patients in the LESG group.

was administered in 65% of our patients, but mostly limited to two to four blocks. It is obivious from the published data that the cumulative total doses of alkylating drugs are considerably lower in our patients. Applying the LESG score for alkylating agents (range in LESG patients 0 - 10), more than 60% of our patients have score of$\leq$ 1.

In general, the differences in the exposition toward alkylating cytotoxic agents explains both the different risk of secondary leukemia in our own study compared to the LESG results and the significantly increased risk after additional salvage therapy. Our comparative evaluation cannot answer the question whether nitrogen—mustard has a specifically high leukemogenic effect, i.e., whether or not omitting this drug was the decisive factor in the lower incidence of leukemia in the German-Austrian studies. Henry-Amar et al. [12] concluded, from a multivariate analysis of 872 adult HD patients that, among the alkylating agents used, only nitrogen—mustard was shown to be significantly associated with an increased risk of secondary leukemias. In view of the fact that nitrogen—mustard is still widely used in the treatment of HD, it is of major importance to clarify this question, especially for children.

Owing to the low absolute count of AML/MSD in our studies, our results cannot contribute to the discussion of whether or not splenectomy increases the risk for SHM after HD [13, 23, 24, 25].

Conclusions. This analysis gives strong evidence that the lower incidence risk of SHM in the patients of the German-Austrian trials compared to those of the LESG is mainly due to the lower cumulative doses of alkylating agents. The question of a specific impact of omitting nitrogen-mustard within this framework needs to be evaluated in further studies. Moreover, the high efficacy of front-line therapy with a relatively small percentage of patients needing salvage therapy is a major factor because relapse treatment considerably increases the cumulative doses of alkylating agents as well as of etoposide and other drugs targeting at DNA topoisomerase II. Hence, differences in the incidence of SHM reflect complex differences between the overall treatment strategies for HD.

References

1. Canellos G.P., V.T. De Vita, J.C. Arseneau, et al.: Second malignancies complicating Hodgkin's disease in remission. Lancet 1 (1975) 94–949
2. Cadman, E.C., R.L. Capizzi, J.R. Bertino: Acute non-lymphocytic leukemia. A delayed complication of Hodgkin's disease therapy: analysis of 109 cases. Cancer 40 (1977) 1280
3. Coleman, C.N., C.J. Williams, A. Flint, E.J. Glatstein, S.A. Rosenberg, H.S. Kaplan: Hematologic neoplasis in patients treated for Hodgkin's disease. N.Engl. J.Med.29 (1977) 1249
4. Valagussa P., A. Santro, R. Kenda, F. Fossati-Bellani, F. Franchi, A. Banfi, F. Rilke, G. Bonadonna: Second malignancies in Hodgkin's disease: a complication of certain forms of treatment. Br.Med.J. 280 (1980) 216
5. Pedersen-Bjergaard J., S.O. Larsen: Incidence of acute non-lymphocytic leukemia, preleukemia, and acute myeloproliferative syndrome up to 10 years after treatment of Hodgkin's disease. N.Engl.Journ.Med. 16 (1982) 966–971
6. Sullivan, M.P., I. Ramirez, H.L.Ried: Second malignancies following Hodgkin's disease in children differ from those of adults: incidence occurring among 228 pediatric HD patients. Proc. Am. Assoc Cancer Res. 24 (1983) 160
7. Tester W.J., T.J. Kinsella, B. Waller, et al.: Second malignant neoplasms complicating Hodgkin's disease: the National Cancer Institute experience. J. Clin. Oncol. (1984) 2: 762–769
8. Valagussa P., A. Santoro, F. Fpssato-Bellani, A. Banti, G. Bonadonna: Second acute leukemia and other malignancies following treatment for Hodgkin's disease. J.Clin.Oncol. 4 (1986) 830–837
9. Tucker M.A., A.T. Meadows, J.D. Boice, M. Stovall, O. Oberlin, B.J. Stone, J. Birch, P.A. Voute, R.N. Hoover, J.F. Fraumeni for the Late Effects Study Group: Leukemia after therapy with alkylating agents for childhood cancer. J.Nat.Cancer Oncol. 4 (1987) 459–464
10. Pedersen-Bjergaard J., S.O. Larsen, J. Struck, H.H. Hansen, L. Specht, J. Ersboll, M.M. Hansen, N.I. Nissen: Risk of therapy-related leukemia and preleukemia after Hodgkin's disease. Lancet 2 (1987) 83–88
11. Van der Velden J.W., W.L.J. van Putten, V.F. Guinee et al.: Subsequent development of acute nonlymphatic leukemia in patients treated for Hodgkin's disease. Int. J. Cancer 42 (1988) 252–255
12. Henry-Amar M., B. Pellae-Cosset, C. Bayle-Weisgerber, M.Hayat, J.M. Cosset, P. Carde, M. Tibina: Risk of secondary acute leukemia and preleukemia after Hodgkin's disease: the institut Gustave Roussy experience. Rec.Results Cancer Res. 11 (1989) 270–283
13. Meadows A.T., A.C. Obringer, O. Marrero, O. Oberlin, L. Robinson, F. Fossati-Bellani, D. Green, P.A. Voute, P. Morris-Jones, M. Greenberg, E. Baum, F. Ruymann: Second malignant neoplasms following childhood Hodgkin's disease: treatment

and splenectomy as risk factors. Med. Ped. Oncology 17 (1989) 477–484
14. Blayney D.W., D.L. Longo, R.C. Young, M.H. Greene, S.M. Hubbard, M.G. Postal, P.L. Duffey, V.T.Jr. DeVita: Decreasing risk of leukemia with prolonged follow-up after chemotherapy and radiotherapy for Hodgkin's disease. N. Engl. J. Med. 316 (1987) 710–714
15. Breu H., G. Schellong, I. Grosch-Wönner, A. Jobke, H. Riehm, J. Ritter, J. Treuner, E.-W. Schwarze, M. Wannenmacher: Chemotherapy of different intensity and reduced radiotherapy of Hodgkin's disease in childhood—a report on 170 patients of the cooperative study HD-78. Klin.Pädiat. 194 (1982) 233–241
16. Schellong G., J. Brämswig, R. Ludwig, V. Gerein, A. Jobke, H. Jürgens, H. Kabisch, B. Stollmann, P. Weinel, H. Gadner, E.-W. Schwarze, M. Wannenmacher: Combined modality treatment in over 200 children with Hodgkin's disease: risk - adapted chemotherapy, low dose involved field irradiation and selective splenectomy. A report of the cooperative therapy study DAL-HD-82. Klin.Pädiat. 198 (1986) 137–146
17. Schellong G., I. Hörnig, J. Brämswig, J.P.M. Bökkering, A. Steinhoff, R. Ludwig, D. Niethammer, A. Reiter, H.J.v. Lengerke, H. Heinecke, E.-W. Schwarze, R. Pötter, R.P. Müller, M. Wannenmacher: The value of procarbazine in the chemotherapy of Hodgkin's disease—a report of the cooperative therapy study DAL-HD-85.Klin.Pädiat.200 (1988) 205–213
18. Schellong G., I. Hörnig-Franz, B. Rath, J. Ritter, M. Riepenhausen, H. Kabisch, B. Goldschmitt-Wuttge, P. Schmidt, D. Niethamer, G. Gaedicke, E.-W. Schwarze, R. Pötter, M. Wannenmacher: Reduction of radiation dosage to 20–30 Gy in the frame work of a combined chemo-/radiotherapy in childhood Hodgkin's disease - a report of the cooperative therapy study DAL-HD-87. Klin. Pädiat. 206 (1994) 253–262
19. Schellong G., I. Hörnig-Franz, for the German Study Group for Hodgkin's disease in children and adolescents: Salvage therapy in childhood Hodgkin's disease. In: Zander A.R., B.Barlogie (Eds) Autologous bone marrow transplantation for Hodgkin's disease, non-Hodgkin's lymphoma and multiple myeloma. Springer Verlag Berlin Heidelberg 1993, 8–10
20. Kalpan E.L., P. Meier: Non-parametric estimation from incomplete observations. J.A. Stat. Assoc53 (1968) 457–481
21. Kalbfleisch J.D., R.L. Prentice: The statistical analysis of failure time data. New York, John Wiley & Sons, 1980
22. Mantel N.: Evaluation of survival data and two new rank order statistics arising in its consideration. Cancer Chemoth. Rep.50 (1966) 163–170
23. van Leeuwen, F.E., R. Somers, A.A.M. Hart: Splenectomy in Hodgkin's disease and second leukemias. Lancet 2 (1987) 210–211
24. Nelson, D.F., S. Cooper, M.G. Weston, P. Rubin: Second malignant neoplasms in patients treated for Hodgkin's disease with radiotherapy or radiotherapy and chemotherapy. Cancer 48 (1981) 2386–2393
25. Henry-Amar, M.: Second cancer after treatment for Hodgkin's disease: a report from the International Database on Hodgkin's Disease. Ann. Oncol. 3, Suppl. 4 (1992)

Acute Leukemias VI
Prognostic Factors
and Treatment Strategies
Büchner et al. (eds)

Intensive Therapy of Myelodysplastic Syndromes and Secondary Leukemias: Preliminary Findings of the French Experience

E. Wattel, E. Solary, D. Caillot, N. Ifrah, A. Brion, N. Milpied, M. Janvier, A. Guerci, H. Rochant, C. Cordonnier, F. Dreyfus, A. Veil, A.M. Stoppa, N. Gratecos, A. Sadoun, H. Tilly, P. Brice, B. Lioure, B. Desablens, B. Pignon, J.P. Abgrall, M. Leporrier, B. Dupriez, D. Guyotat, A. Merlat, and P. Fenaux for the Groupe Français des Myelodysplasies (GFM) and Groupe GOELAMS

Introduction

Low-dose chemotherapy in myelodysplastic syndromes (MDS) gives overall limited results in high-risk MDS [1-3]. Intensive chemotherapy in MDS and secondary leukemias (i.e., acute myeloid leukemia, AML, following de novo or therapy-related MDS) gives lower complete remission (CR) rates and shorter CR duration than in de novo AML [4-11]. This may be due in part to a higher incidence of mdr gene expression in MDS than in de novo AML as mdr gene expression is associated in our experience, with very low CR rates with intensive chemotherapy [12]. These recent results suggested that the use of agents capable of reverting mdr gene expression could improve the CR rate in MDS and secondary leukemias.

Patients and Treatment

We designed a trial of intensive chemotherapy: mitoxantrone 12 mg/m^2 on days 2–5 plus cytosine arabinoside (ara-C) 1 g/m^2 every 12 h on days 1–5, with or without (randomized) quinine 30 mg/kg per day (continuous infusion, maximum 2 g per day), an agent capable of reverting the mdr phenotype [13].

Patients younger than 65 and older than 15 with high-risk MDS were eligible. High-risk MDS was defined as (a) AML following a proven MDS phase; (b) refractory anemia with excess of blasts in transformation (RAEB-T); or (c) RAEB or chronic myelomonocytic leukemia (CMML) with neutrophils $<500/mm^3$ and/or with infectious episodes or with platelet count $<50\ 000/mm^3$ and/or bleeding symptoms or with a transfusion requirement > two red cell units per month or with rapid worsening of cytoipenias. Patients should have given their informed consent.

Patients younger than 55 years achieving CR were scheduled to be autografted (ABMT) after bone marrow (and more recently peripheral blood: three cases) stem cell collection. The conditioning regimen was: cyclophosphamide: 50 mg/kg per day and busulfan 4 mg/kg per day for 4 days.

Complete remission criteria were stringent and included normalization of cytopenias and of karyotype (if initially abnormal), in addition to the presence of $\leqslant 5\%$ blasts and disappearance of MDS features on bone marrow smears. Partial response was defined by (a) presence of $\leqslant 5\%$ bone marrow blasts with an increase of the neutrophil and platelet count of at least 1000 and 50 000/mm^3, respectively, and with an increase of the hemoglobin level of 2g/dl; or (b) normalization of both peripheral blood and bone marrow cell count with persistent myelodysplastic features and/or abnormal karyotype. Patients older than 55 years or who could not be autografted received three courses of consolidation chemotherapy with mitoxantrone 12 mg/m^2 on days and ara-C 100 mg/m^2 every 12 h on days 1–5.

Expression of mdr gene was assessed by flow cytometry on bone marrow or blood mononuclear cells (in patients having progressed to

---

Services des Maladies du Sang, CHU, 1 place de Verdun, 59037 Lille, France

AML) using MRK16 monoclonal antibodies (MAb) or immunocytochemistry on bone marrow slides using JSB1 MAb (in patients treated in MDS phase)

Results

From October 1992 to October 1994, 84 patients were included: median age was 54 (range: 18–68 years, 34 patients older than 55); 49 patients had progressed to AML and 35 were still in the MDS phase (eight RAEB, 26 RAEB-T, one CMML).

Seventy-two patients are currently evaluable for response. Twenty-nine patients (40%) achieved complete remission (CR), eight patients (11%) achieved partial response, 15 (21%) had early death, and 20 (28%) had resistant disease. Analysis of pretreatment prognostic factors of complete remission is currently underway. Of the 16 patients aged $\leqslant$55 years who achieved CR, ten were actually autografted. Reasons for not doing bone marrow transplantation were: early relapse (three patients), poor clinical condition (one patient), allogeneic bone marrow transplantation (one patient), patient refusal (one patient). One patient in whom stem cells were collected was awaiting bone marrow transplantation.

Bone marrow was harvested in 11 patients. Despite several collections, the quality and/or quantity of harvested cells was insufficient in three patients of whom one relapsed. Consequently, peripheral stem cell harvesting was proposed in order to reduce the interval between CR achievement and stem cell collection. This procedure was successfully performed in three patients and allowed transplantation in a patient for whom bone marrow stem cell collection had failed.

Hematological reconstitution occurred in all patients after delays similar to AML. A significantly more prolonged duration of aplasia was observed in patients treated with quinine (29 vs 25 days with ANC $\leqslant 1000/mm^3$; $p<0.03$). Sixteen of the 29 patients who achieved CR had relapsed after 2–18 months and 13 were still in complete remission after 1–19 months. Six of the autografted patients had relapsed, after 4–18 months, one died after the procedure and three were still in CR after 8–9 months.

Median overall survival from the onset of treatment was 8 months. Median CR duration was 10.5 months. The CR rate, CR duration, and survival from treatment were 42% and 38%, 11 months and 10 months, 8 months and 7.5 months, respectively, in patients treated with and without quinine (differences not significant).

The effect of quinine was particularly analysed in patients expressing mdr at the onset of treatment. Results of the mdr gene expression are currently available in 44 patients of whom 14 are positive. The CR rate was 28% in these 14 mdr-positive patients as compared to 40% in the 30 mdr - negative cases. In the 14 mdr-positive cases, four of the nine patients (44%) treated with quinine and none (0%) of the five treated without quinine achieved CR ($p=0.07$). Median survival was 6.4 months in mdr-positive patients treated with quinine and was not reached in mdr - positive patients treated without quinine.

Discussion

Our results confirm the relatively low CR rates previously obtained with intensive chemotherapy in MDS and the short CR duration [4–11]. In our previous report [12], a CR rate of only 14% had been obtained after intensive chemotherapy without quinine in mdr - positive MDS patients. We found an increase of the CR rate to 44% in mdr-positive cases treated with quinine although in a small patient population. These findings are of course preliminary but they suggest a potential benefit of quinine in mdr-positive MDS. Accrual of a larger number of patients in this randomized study should help us answer this issue.

Complete remission duration after intensive chemotherapy appears to be generally very short in MDS [5–11]. Very few previous works have assessed the feasibility of autologous bone marrow in MDS after CR achievement [14]. A prerequisite for bone marrow or peripheral blood stem cell harvest for autologous transplantation is good quality remission. This led us to use stringent CR criteria. In spite of this, our preliminary findings suggest a higher rate of relapse after autologous transplantation in MDS than in AML, as previously described in two reports [14, 15]. Only prolonged follow up will permit an assessment of the benefit of this form of intensive consolidation in MDS and whether, contrary to intensive chemotherapy, it provides prolonged CR. Finally, no previous studies of MDS transplanted with peripheral stem cells are available in the literature, to our knowledge. Our preliminary results suggest that peripheral stem cell collection is of interest in cases of failure of bone marrow harvest and this procedure may now be proposed as soon as CR is obtained in order to reduce the risk of early relapse, a frequent event in MDS treated with intensive chemotherapy.

References

1. Miller K.B., Kyungmann K., Morrison F.S., Winter J.N., Bennett J.M., Neiman R.S., Head D.R., Gassileth P.A., O'Connell M.J. The evaluation of low-dose cytarabine in the treatment of myelodysplastic syndromes: a phase III intergroup study. Ann. Hematol., 1992, 65, 162–168.
2. Hellstrom-Lingberg E., Robert K.H., Gahrton G., Lindberg G. A predictive model for the clinical response to low dose ara-C : a study of 102 patients with myelodysplastic syndromes or acute leukaemia.Brit.J.Haematol., 1992,81,503–511.
3. Cheson B.D., Jasperse D.M., Simon R., Friedman MA. A critical appraisal of low dose Ara C in patients with acute non lymphocytic leukemia and myelodysplastic syndromes. J. Clin. Oncol., 1986, 4, 1857–1864.
4. Mertelsmann R., Thaler H.T., To L. et al. Morphological classification, response to therapy and survival in 263 adult patients with acute nonlymphoblastic leukemia. Blood, 1980, 56, 773–781
5. Hoyle C., De Bastos C., Wheatley K. et al. AML associated with previous chemotherapy. MDS or myeloproliferative disorders: results from the MRC's 9th AML trial. Brit. J. Haematol., 1989, 72, 45–53.
6. Gajewski J., Ho W., Nimer S. et al. Efficacy of intensive chemotherapy for acute myelogenous leukemia associated with a preleukemic syndrome. J. Clin. Oncol., 1989, 7, 1637–1645.
7. De Witte T., Muus P., De Pauw B., Haanen C. Intensive antileukemic treatment of patients younger than 65 years with myelodysplastic syndromes and secondary acute myelogenous leukemia. Cancer, 1990, 66, 831–837.
8. Fenaux P., Morel P., Rose C. et al. Prognostic factors in adult de nove myelodysplastic syndromes treated by intensive chemotherapy. Brit. J.Haematol., 1991, 77, 497–501.
9. Fenaux P., Preudhomme C., Hebbar M. The role of intensive chemotherapy in myelodysplastic synromes. Leukemia and Lymphoma, 1992, 8, 43–49.
10. Michels S.D., Mc Kenna R.W., Arthus D.C., Brunning R.D. Therapy-related acute myeloid leukemia and myelodysplastic syndrome: a clinical and morphologic study of 65 cases. Blood, 1985, 65, 1364–1372.
11. Estey E., Thall P., Andreeff M., Beran M., Kantarjian H., O'Brien S., Escudier S., Robertson L.E., Koller ., Kornblau S., Pierce S., Freireich E., Deisseroth A., Keating M. Use of granulocyte colony-stimulating factor before, during, and after fludarabine plus cytarabine induction therapy of newly diagnosed acute myelogenous leukemia or myelodysplastic syndromes: comparison with fludarabine plus cytarabine without granulocyte colony-stimulating factor. J. Clin. Oncol., 1994, 12, 671–678.
12. Lepelley P., Soenen V., Preudhomme C., Lai J.L., Cosson A., Fenaux P. Expression of the multidrug resistance P glycoprotein and its relationship to hematological characteristics and response to treatment in myelodysplastic syndromes. Leukemia, 1994, 8, 998–1005.
13. Chauffert B., Corda C., Pelletier H., Solary E., Bedenne L., Cailliot D., Martin F. Potential usefulness of quinine for the circumvention of the anthracycline resistance in clinical practice. Br.J.Cancer, 1990, 62, 395–397.
14. Laporte J.P., Isnard F., Lesage S., Fenaux P., Douay L., Lopez M., Schachowiak J., Najman A., Gorin N.C. Autologous bone marrow transplantation with marrow purged by mafosfamide in seven patients with myelodysplastic syndromes in transplantation (AML-MDS): a pilot study. Leukemia, 1993, 7, 2030–2033.
15. Oberg G., Simonsson B., Smedmyr B. Is haematological reconstitution seen after ABMT in MDS patients? Bone Marrow Transpl., 1989, 4, suppl.2, 52, abstr.

Acute Leukemias VI
Prognostic Factors
and Treatment Strategies
Büchner et al. (eds)

Preliminary Results of a Placebo-Controlled, Double-Blind Trial Evaluating Sequential HD-AraC/Mitoxantrone Induction Chemotherapy with or Without Granulocyte–Macrophage Colony-Stimulating Factor in Patients with High-Risk Myelodysplastic Syndromes

W. Verbeek[1], B. Wörmann[1], P. Koch[2], C. Aul[3], H. Hinrichs[4], J. Balleisen[5], J. Bennett[6], T. Büchner[2], and W. Hiddemann[1]

Introduction

Patients with high-risk myelodysplastic syndromes (MDS) face a poor prognosis with a median survival time of less than 12 months. The only curvative treatment known so far is allogeneic bone marrow transplantation which is available for younger patients with an HLA-matched sibling and hence for a minority of cases only. Acute myeloid leukemia (AML)-type combination chemotherapy can achieve complete remissions (CR) in the range of 15%–51%, however, remission duration is short (1, 2). Treatment failures are due to primary drug resistance and a high early death rate. The latter may be related to a longer duration of treatment-induced aplasia as compared to AML.

Sequential high-dose cytosine arabinoside (ara-C) (1.0 g/m^2 on days 1, 2; 8, 9) and mitoxantrone (10 mg/m^2 on days 3, 4; 10, 11) has proven an effective antileukemic therapy in refractory and relapsed AML with a CR rate exceeding 50% even in patients with an age >60 years old [3]. In an earlier study Büchner et al. [4]. showed that 250 μg/m^2 granulocyte- macrophage colony-stimulating factor (GM-CSF) given after sequential HD-AraC/mitoxantrone (S-HAM) chemotherapy for relapsed AML was able to reduce the duration of critical granulocytopenia $<500/\mu l$ by 9 days. This translated into a reduction of the early death rate from 39% to 14% ($p=0.009$). In 1990 Bettelheim et al. [5] first applied GM-CSF prior to AML induction chemotherapy to recruit quiescent leukemic blasts into the cell cycle to overcome a cell kinetic resistence to S phase-specific chemotherapeutic agents like ara-C. We therefore initiated a double-blinded, placebo-controlled trial to assess the role of GM-CSF (250 μg/m^2 once daily s.c.) starting 48 h prior to S-HAM chemotherapy and continuing until the end of aplasia in patients with high-risk MDS. The aim of the GM-CSF application is: (a) to increase the efficacy of S-HAM induction chemotherapy; (b) to reduce early death rate by shortening the time of bone marrow hypoplasia. We report here the overall results of the first 32 patients enrolled into the study. Because the trial is still blind, no data concerning the impact of GM-CSF is available at the present time.

Patients, Protocol, and Methods

Patients. Eligibility criteria included adult patients of all ages with a diagnosis of refractory anemia with excess of blasts (RAEB), RAEB in transformation (RAEB-T), and chronic meylomonocytic leukemia (CMML). Patients with abnormal hepatic, renal, or cardiac function were excluded. A written informed consent was obtained from every patient upon entrance into

[1]Department of Hematology/Oncology, Georg-August-University, Göttingen, Germany
[2]Department of Internal Medicine A, Westf. Wilhelms-University, Münster, Germany
[3]Department of Hematology/Oncology Heinrich-Heine University Düsseldorf, Germany
[4]Department of Internal Medicine, Evangelisches Krankenhaus, Oldenburg, Germany
[5]Department of Internal Medicine, Evangelisches Krankenhaus, Hamm, Germany
[6]Department of Medical Oncology, University of Rochester Medical Center, Rochester, USA

the trial. All investigations were performed after approval by the local ethics committee and are in accordance with the declaration of Helsinki.

Study Design. Therapy according to the S-HAM protocol consisted of ara-C (1 g/m^2) on days 1, 2, 8, and 9 and mitoxantrone (10 mg/m^2) on days 3, 4, 10, 11, respectively. All patients received glucocorticoid eye drops during the ara-C administration for the prophylaxis of photophobia and conjunctivitis. GM-CSF (250 µg/m^2) or placebo given as single subcutaneous injection once daily was started 48 h prior to chemotherapy and continued until neutrophil recovery. GM-CSF or placebo was discontinued if the day 14 bone marrow showed more than 5% blasts. In order to avoid selection of patients with different prognosis, the randomization was balanced for the following *stratification criteria*: (a) age < and >60 years; (b) RAEB, RAEB-T, CMML; (c) Düsseldorf risk score. Antileukemic response was judged according to Cancer and Leukemia Group B (CALGB) criteria and side effects were evaluated following World Health Organization (WHO) definitions. The interval between the onset of therapy and the post-treatment achievment of more than 20 000 platelets/mm^3 and more than 500 granulocytes/mm^3 was defined as time to recovery (TR).

Results

Until February 1995, 32 patients were entered into the study from six participating centers (Göttingen, Münster, Düsseldorf, Hamm, Oldenburg) in Germany and the United States (Rochester). Patient's characteristics are listed in Table 1. From the 32 patients randomized, four patients were not evaluable for response due to protocol violation (two) and false diagnosis (one: aplastic anemia). One patient was still undergoing therapy at the time of writing. Of the 28 evaluable patients, 11 (39%) achieved a complete remission (CR), seven (25%) had persistent MDS, ten patients (36%) died within the first 6 weeks after the start of therapy (early deaths, ED). The percentage of cases with an adequate blast clearance to less than 5% leukemic cells in a day-14 bone marrow was 84%. Median time to CR was 44 days. The median time to hematologic recovery (neutrophils >500/µl and platelets >20 000/µl) and time to neutrophil recovery above 1500/µl was 29 and 35 days, respectively. Median remission duration of patients achieving CR was 190 days (6.35 months) (range: 25–416 days). One patient received allogeneic bone marrow transplantation(BMT) in first CR and is disease-free 100 days+, one patient transplanted in second CR died of venoocclusive disease. Two patients underwent transplantation with persistent MDS: one allogeneic one, autologous transplant. Both are disease free 1558 and 1480 days post BMT. Figure 1 depicts the Kaplan-Meier survival plot censored for patients treated by allogeneic or autologous BMT. A subanalysis according to Düsseldorf risk score indicates a higher CR rate of 48% for patients with risk score C as opposed to 14% for risk score B (Table 2).

Analysis of ED revealed infection as the major cause of death (eight of ten cases). In five of these, fungi could be documented either in blood cultures or bronchoalveolar lavage: *Aspergillus fumigatus* (one), *Candida tropicalis* (one), *Candida* species without further differentiation (three). In two bleeding was considered as cause of death. Nonhematological toxicity consisted mainly of nausea and vomiting, mucositis, and diarrhae, In one patient an increase of bilirubin and liver enzymes of WHO grade IV was associated with a systemic candidiasis. No CNS toxicity due to high-dose ara-C (1g/m^2) was observed. Toxicity data are listed in Table 3.

Table 1. Patient characteristics

Age	— Median(years)	57
	— Range (years)	24–73
FAB type	RAEB (*n*)	6
	RAEB-T (*n*)	20
	CMML (*n*)	3
Risk score	Düsseldorf B (*n*)	8
	C (*n*)	21

Discussion

Complete remission rates of patients with MDS and secondary AML are usually lower than those of patients with de novo AML treated with similar chemotherapeutic regimens. The higher failure rate can be explained partly by the longer duration of hypoplasia after chemotherapy, but also by a higher drug resistence of the leukemic clone. The CR rate of 39% achieved in the first 28 patients treated in the current study is in the

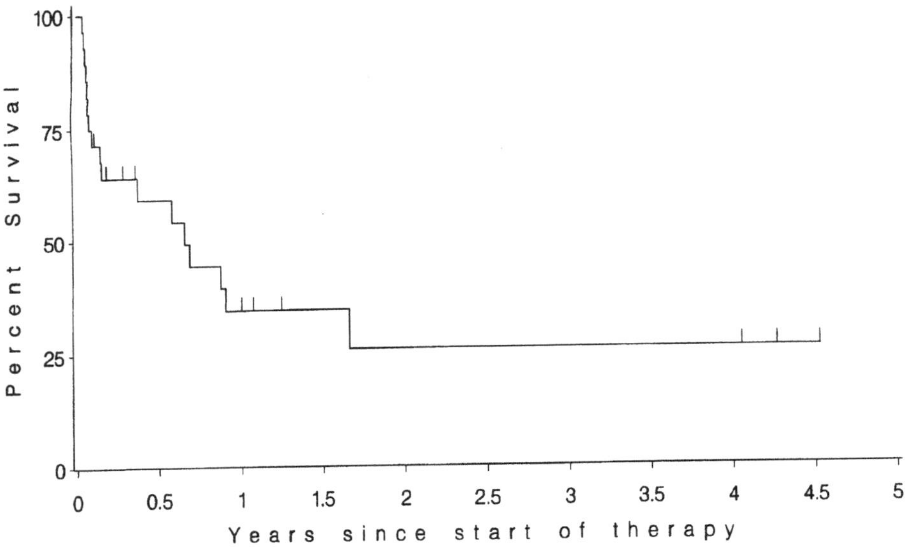

Fig. 1. Treatment of high-risk MDS with intermediate-dose ara-C and mitoxantrone with or without GM-CSF (protocol URCC 4990): all evaluable patients

Table 2. Response to S-HAM chemotherapy ±GM-CSF

Risk score	CR		Persistent-MDS		ED	
	(*n*)	(%)	(*n*)	(%)	(*n*)	(%)
Düsseldorf B	1	14	3	43	3	43
Düsseldorf C	10	48	4	19	7	33
	11	39	7	25	10	36

Table 3. Toxicity according to WHO grade

	Grade I/II (%)	Grade III/IV (%)
Nausea/vomiting	25	30
Renal	5	–
Hepatic	25	15
Infection	26	47
Bleeding	33	19

range of results reported by other groups in high-risk MDS [1, 6–8]. Unfortunately, the ED rate is high (36%). Our preliminary results are similar to those reported by Preisler and coworkers [9] who treated 67 patients with secondary AML with high-dose ara-C. In this study persistent leukemia occurred in only 22%, but a high ED rate of 34% was responsible for the low CR rate of 42%. The median time of neutrophil recovery above 500/µl was 29 days in our study, 5 days longer than compared to a historical control group of relapsed AML patients treated with S-HAM (24 days). These, data confirm the prolonged duration of bone marrow hypoplasia in MDS patients. It is likely that the high incidence of infectious complications, especially of fungal infections with lethal outcome, is due to this fact. However, the acquisition of infectious foci in the period of disease-related immunosuppression before the initiation of treatment may also play a role. The results of Preisler and our data stress the potential benefit of a cytokine given after high-dose ara-C which reduces the time of critical granulocytopenia. This question will hopefully be answered in the future when the number of patients is sufficient to unblind the study. Interestingly, there is a trend toward a higher CR rate in risk group C (48%) than risk group B (14%) as defined by the Düsseldorf score. Because the numbers are still to small, this finding has no significance yet. The median remission duration of 6 months is short, but comparable to results achieved in patients with relapsed AML without consolidation or maintenance treatment. The potentially lower CR rate and the short remission duration of patients with Düsseldorf risk score B contrasts with a longer natural disease history. Thus chemotherapy cannot be recommended for patients in this risk group unless an allogeneic BMT can be performed as consolidation therapy.

Acknowledgments. We would like to thank Mrs. Birgit Teigel for the documentation of patient's data.

References

1. Tricot G, De Bock R, Dekker AW The role of aggressive chemotherapy in the treatment of myelodysplastic syndromes. Br.J. of Haematology (1986)63: 477-483
2. De Witte T New treatment approaches for myelodysplastic syndromes and secondary leukaemias.Annals of Oncology (1994)5: 401-408
3. Hiddemann W, Aul C, Maschmeyer G, Schönrock-Nabulsi, Ludwig WD, Bartholomäus A, Bettelheim P, Becker K, Balleisen L, Lathan B. Köppler H, Grüneisen T, Donhuijsen-Ant, Reichle A, Heinecke A, Sauerland C. Büchner Th High dose versus intermediate dose cytosine arabinoside combined with mitoxantrone for the treatment of relapsed and refractory acute myeloid leukemia: results of an age adjusted randomized comparison. Leukemia and Lymphoma (1993)10: 133-137
4. Büchner Th, Hiddemann W, Koenigsmann M, Zühlsdorf M, Wörmann B, Boeckmann A, Aguion-Freire E, Innig G, Maschmeyer G, Ludwig W.D., Sauerland M, Heinecke A, Schulz G. Recombinant human granulocyte-macrophage colony-stimulating factor after chemotherapy in patients with acute myeloid leukemia at higher age or after relapse. Blood (1991) 78(5): 1190-1197
5. Bettelheim P, Valent P, Andreeff M, Tafuri A, Haimi J, Gorischek C., Muhm M, Sillaber Ch, Haas O, Vieder L, Maurer D, Schulz G, Speiser W, Geissler K, Kier P, Hinterberger W, Lechner K Recombinant human granulocyte-macrophage colony-stimulating factor in combination with standard induction chemotherapy in de novo acute myeloid leukemia. Blood (1991) 77(4): 700-711
6. Hiddemann W Cytosine arabinoside in the treatment of acute myeloid leukemia: the role and place of high-dose regimens. Annals of Hematology (1991) 62: 119-128
7. Preisler HD, Raza A, Barcos M, Azarnia N, Larson R, Walker I, Browmann M, Grunwald H, D`Arrigo P, Doeblin T; High dose cytosine arabinoside as the initial treatment of poor risk patients with acute non-lymphocytic leukemia: a leukemia intergroup study. J. of Clin Oncology (1987) 5(1): 75-82
8. De Witte T, Muus P, De Paw Intensive antileukemic treatment of patients younger than 65 years with meylodysplastic syndromes and secondary acute myelogenous leukemia. Cancer (1990) 66: 831-837
9. Preisler HD, Raza M, Barcos M High dose cytosine arabinoside in the treatment of preleukemic disorders: a leukemia intergroup study. Am. J. of Hematology (1986) 23: 131-134

Acute Leukemias VI
Prognostic Factors
and Treatment Strategies
Büchner et al. (eds)

Childhood Myelodysplastic Syndromes Treated with Acute Myeloid Leukemia Regimens

H. Hasle[1] and G. Kerndrup[2]

Abstract. Myelodysplastic syndromes (MDS) in children are often considered as variants of acute myeloid leukemia (AML) and are frequently treated as such. However, there are very few reported data on the outcome after AML treatment in children with MDS. During the period 1984–1991, 19 children with MDS were treated according to the Nordic AML protocol. All children had de novo MDS. The median age at presentation was 4.2 years. The median interval from first admission to first course of AML treatment was 80 days (range 2–961 days). At presentation the children were classified as: two refractory anemia (RA), five RA with excess of blasts (RAEB), five RAEB in transformation (RAEB-T), seven chronic myelomonocytic leukemia (CMML). When the AML treatment was initiated, five had progressed to AML. Seven attained complete remission, four had refractory disease, and eight died during the cytopenia that followed the induction. Two of the responders were later treated with allogeneic bone marrow transplantation (BMT), both died of procedure-related toxicity. Only two of the 19 children are still alive. One never entered remission on therapy, but showed a spontaneous remission several months after the end of all therapy. The only child entering remission on therapy and still alive presented with RAEB and chloroma. Of eight children with MDS treated with allogeneic BMT without previous chemotherapy, five are still alive. Conventional AML regimens in childhood MDS are associated with a low rate of complete remission, a high risk of death in cytopenia, and a very limited curative potential.

Introduction

Myelodysplastic syndromes (MDS) in children have generally been considered to be very rare. However, our population-based study suggested that MDS constitute 9% of all childhood leukemias thus approximating the incidence of acute myeloid leukemia (AML) [1]. MDS in children have been considered as variants of AML and it has been recommended that they should be treated as such [2]. However, there are very few reported data on the results of AML treatment in children with MDS. A review of the sparse published data on the outcome after intensive chemotherapy not follwed by bone marrow transplantation (BMT) showed a 3-year survival probability of only 14% [3].

We present the results of the Danish experience with AML treatment of 19 cases of childhood MDS.

Material

During the period 1984–1991, 19 children with de novo MDS were treated at the four departments of pediatric hematology in Denmark according to the Nordic Organization of Pediatric Hematology/Oncology (NOPHO) AML protocols; NOPHO-84 (11 patients) and NOPHO-88 (eight patients) (Table 1).

All cases were categorized according to the French–American–British (FAB) classification [4, 5], with the exception that in some of the

[1]Department of Pediatrics, Odense University Hospital, 5000 Odense C, Denmark
[2]Department of Pathology, Odense University Hospital, 5000 Odense C, Denmark

Table 1. NOPHO AML induction regimens

	NOPHO-84	NOPHO-88
Course 1	6-Thioguanine 200mg/m^2 × 2 on days 1–4 Cytarabine 200 mg/m^2 on days 1–4 Doxorubicin 75 mg/m^2	6-Thioguanine 200 mg/m^2 × 2 on days 1–4 Cytarabine 200 mg/m^2 on days 1–4 Doxorubicin 75 mg/m^2 VP-16 100 mg/m^2 on days 1–4
Course 2	As course 1	Mitoxantrone 10 mg/m^2 on days 1–3 Cytarabine 200 mg/m^2 on days 1–4
Course 3	As course 1	As course 1

Chronic myelomonocytic leukemia (CMML) patients more than 5% of myeloblasts in the blood was accepted. According to the FAB classification, these cases should have been classified as refractory anemia with excess of blasts in transformation (RAEB-T), but they all showed typical CMML (juvenile chronic myelogenous leukemia, CML) features; leukocytosis, monocytosis, and hepatosplenomegaly, and all had fewer than 20% of myeloblasts in the bone marrow.

Table 2. Patient characteristics at presentation

De novo MDS(*n*)	19
Boys(*n*)	11
Down syndrome(*n*)	2
Cytogenetics	
Monosomy 7(*n*)	6
Other abnormalities (*n*)	4
Normal (*n*)	8
Not done (*n*)	1
Age—Median (years)	4.2
Range (years)	0.2–15.0

Results

The patient characteristics at presentation are shown in Table 2. The disease stage according to the FAB classification at presentation and at the initiation of therapy is shown in Table 3. Five patients had progressed to AML before the initiation of therapy. The median interval from first admission to treatment was 80 days (range 2–961 days). The outcome following each course of induction therapy is shown in Fig. 1. Only three children attained a complete remission following the first induction course, a further four children attained remission after the second induction. Eight died during the cytopenia that followed the induction therapy (six from infection and two from hemorrhage). The outcome was analyzed in separate subgroups to search for prognostic factors (Table 4). All groups fared poorly and no poor-risk group could be identified. There was a tendency to a higher rate of cytopenia-related deaths in children treated with NOPHO-88. This protocol was characterized by a shorter interval between the first and second induction courses than the NOPHO-84 protocol (median 18 versus 24 days).

Only two of the 19 children are still alive and both showed very unusual features of MDS: A 5-month-old boy with RAEB did not attain remission on therapy but showed a spontaneous remission many months after the end of all therapy. He was 8 years old at the time of writing

Table 3. FAB groups at presentation and at the initiation of treatment

Presentation	Treatment start				
	RAEB (*n*)	RAEB-T (*n*)	CMML (*n*)	AML (*n*)	Total (*n*)
RA	1			1	2
RAEB	2			3	5
RAEB-T		4		1	5
CMML			7		7
	3	4	7	5	19

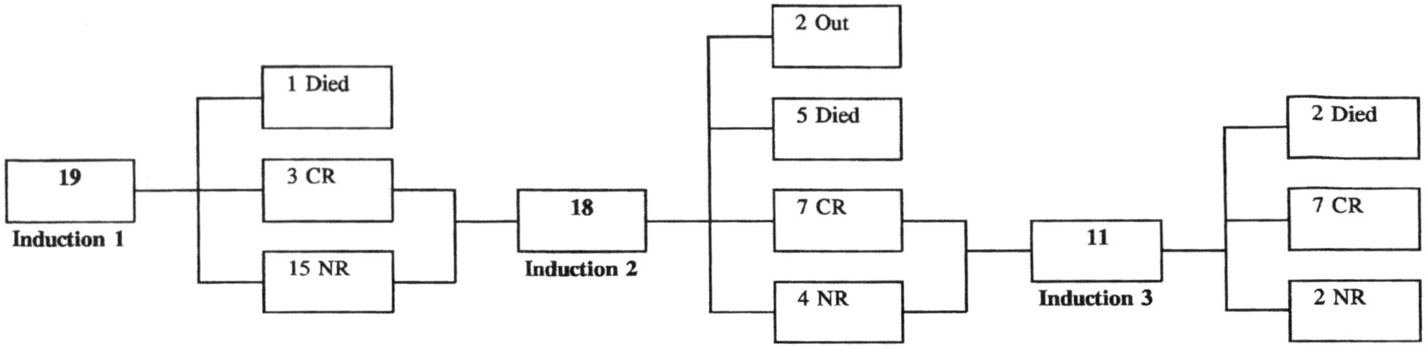

Fig. 1. Treatment outcome following each induction course. *CR*, complete remission; *NR*, no remission; *Out*, withdrawn because of NR

Table 4. Number of children with complete remission, refractory disease, or induction-associated deaths in selected subgroups

	Patients (*n*)	CR (*n*)	RD (*n*)	Deaths (*n*)
All Patients	19	7	4	8
Boys	11	4	3	4
Diagnosis at presentation				
RA	2	1	0	1
RAEB	5	2	2	1
RAEB-T	5	2	0	3
CMML	7	2	2	3
Diagnosis at treatment				
RAEB	3	1	1	1
RAEB-T	4	2	0	2
CMML	7	2	2	3
AML	5	2	1	2
Cytogenetics				
Monosomy 7	6	3	1	2
Other abnormalities	4	1	2	1
Normal	8	2	1	5
Protocol				
NOPHO-84	11	5	3	3
NOPHO-88	8	2	1	5

CR, complete remission; RD, Refractory disease.

without evidence of disease. Only one child entered remission on therapy and is still alive. She presented at the age of 8 years with chloroma. The bone marrow showed slight dysplastic traits with 11% myeloblasts. Cytogenetic studies were not done. At the time of writing, the child is in continued complete remission 10 years from diagnosis.

The 3-year-survival rate of the 19 children was 11% (Fig. 2).

Two of the 19 children were treated with allogeneic BMT following the induction therapy, both died of procedure-related toxicity. During the same period (1984–1991), eight Danish children with MDS were treated with allogeneic BMT without previous induction chemotherapy, five of them are still alive.

Discussion

The poor outcome following intensive chemotherapy in this series is in accordance with the few reported experiences in childhood [3]. The outcome is significantly inferior to the results in children with AML treated with the same protocol [6]. Monosomy 7 was found in a high proportion of the children, none of these survived, but the remission rate was not inferior to chil-

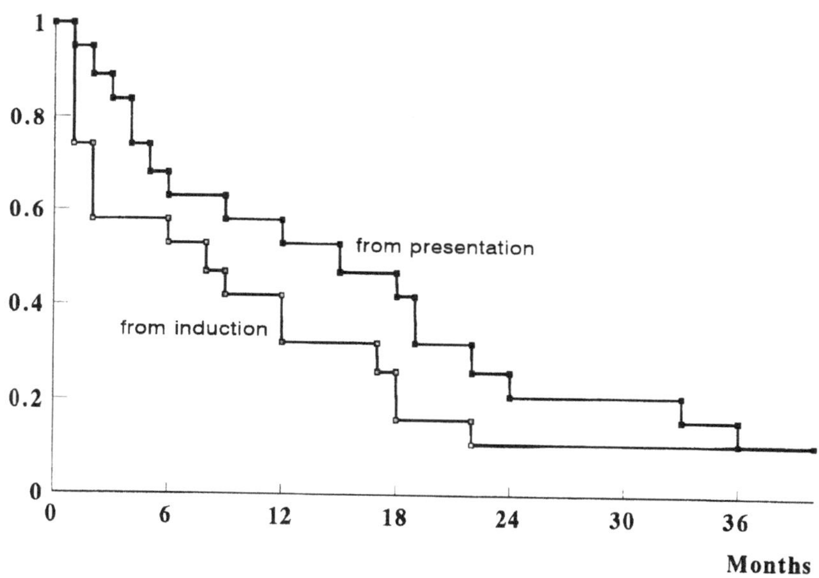

Fig. 2. Survival of 19 children with MDS treated with AML regimens. Survival curves are shown from presentation and from the initiation of induction therapy

dren with other cytogenetic abnormalities or with normal karyotype. The overall survival of childhood MDS is low, and it is uncertain whether monosomy 7 is an independent prognostic factor [3]. Children with CMML may obtain complete remission following intensive chemotherapy, but virtually all relapse [7, 8]. This is in accordance with cell culture studies that showed persistent leukemic cell growth despite clinical remission [9]. The low remission rate in MDS may be related to a low number of nonmalignant progenitor cells and a high expression of the multidrug resistance P-glycoprotein [10].

The poor outcome following intensive therapy is also found in adults. The remission rate in 47 adults was only 47% with 21% hypoplastic deaths and 32% with resistant disease [11]. Patients with RAEB-T and normal karyotype had the longest survival [11]. Higher remission rates have been reported in smaller series of adults [12], a remarkably high remission rate was found in RAEB-T patients treated with idarubicin and high-dose cytarabine [13].

Only two of our patients are still alive, both had very unusual features of MDS. One child with normal cytogenetics experienced what we consider to be a spontaneous remission. The other patient presented with a chloroma. No cytogenetic studies were done. Cases of granulocytic sarcoma are often associated with t(8; 21) and a favorable prognosis and may not represent "true MDS" [14]. If we exclude these two exceptional cases, none of the patients became long-term survivors following these conventional AML induction regimens.

Children with Down syndrome and AML (preceded by MDS or not) show a very favorable response to antileukemic therapy [15, 16]. Of our two patients with Down syndrome, one died during cytopenia and one attained complete remission. The latter relapsed and was not retreated. With our current knowledge he might have been cured following intensive therapy at relapse. Children with Down syndrome may be an exception to the conclusion that standard AML regimens are of little benefit in children with MDS.

Patients with Fanconi anemia are more susceptible to chemotherapy and radiation and not all cases are recognized at the initiation of therapy [17]. Chromosome breakage tests were only performed in three patients (all normal). Cytogenetic studies were performed in all patients except one (one of the survivors). None of the classic cytogenetic studies showed an increased frequency of spontaneous chromosome breakage. We cannot exclude that children with Fanconi anemia were included, but it seems unlikely that they made any significant contribution to the cohort.

Most of the therapy-related deaths occurred following the second induction course which was usually initiated before hematologic recovery. The mortality rate might have been decreased if the treatment had been postponed to hematologic recovery or if the chemotherapy courses were followed by hematopoietic growth factors [18].

The two children who received BMT following intensive chemotherapy died of therapy-related toxicity. In contrast, five of the eight children who received BMT without prior chemotherapy are alive in continued remission. The present study does not allow any firm conclusion concerning the role of chemotherapy prior to BMT but is in accordance with data from the European BMT Group showing a higher risk of transplantaion-related death (41% versus 25%) in patients who received intensive chemotherapy prior to BMT [19], suggesting that prior induction chemotherapy is of no benefit.

Conclusion

Our experience with treatment of childhood MDS with conventional AML regimens can be summarized as follows: (a) a very low rate of complete remission; (b) a high risk of death in cytopenia; (c) a very limited curative potential. The distinction between MDS and AML seems to have major therapeutical implications. Myeloablative therapy supported by allogeneic stem cell infusion may be necessary to cure childhood MDS.

References

1. Hasle H, Jacobsen BB, Pedersen NT (1992): Myelodysplastic syndromes in childhood: a population based study of nine cases. Br J Haematol 81: 495–498.
2. Hann IM (1992): Disorders of the blood and reticuloendothelial system. In: Forfar and Arneil's textbooks of paediatrics, 4th Ed., AGM Campbell, N

McIntosh, eds, Churchill Livingstone, Edinburgh, pp. 919–954.
3. Hasle H (1994): Myelodysplastic syndromes in childhood. Classification, epidemiology, and treatment, Leuk Lymphoma 13: 11–26.
4. Bennett JM, Catovsky D, Daniel MT, Flandrin G, Galton DAG, Gralnick HR, Sultan C (1982): Proposals for the classification of the myelodysplastic syndromes. Br J Haematol 51: 189–199.
5. Bennett JM, Catovsky D, Daniel MT, Flandrin G, Galton DAG, Gralnick HR, Sultan C (1985): Proposed revised criteria for the classification of acute myeloid leukemia. A report of the French-American-British Cooperative Group. Ann Intern Med 103: 620–625.
6. Lie SO, Berglund G, Gustafsson G, Jonmundsson G, Siimes M, Yssing Y (1990): High dose ara-C as a single-agent consolidation therapy in childhood acute myelogenous leukemia. Hamatol Bluttransfus 33: 215–212.
7. Chan HSL, Estrov Z, Weitzman SS, Freedman MH (1987): The value of intensive combination chemotherapy for juvenile chronic myelogenous leukemia. J Clin Oncol 5: 1960–1967.
8. Festa RS, Shende A, Lanzkowsky P (1990): Juvenile chronic myelocytic leukemia: experience with intensive combination chemotherapy. Med Pediatr Oncol 18: 311–316.
9. Estrov Z, Dube ID, Chan HSL, Freedman MH (1987): Residual juvenile chronic myelogenous leukemia cells detected in peripheral blood during clinical remission. Blood 70: 1466–1469.
10. Lepelley P, Soenen V, Preudhomme C, Lai JL, Cosson A, Fenaux P (1994): Expression of the multidrug resistance P-glycoprotein and its relationship to hematological characteristics and response to treatment in myelodysplastic syndromes. Leukemia 8: 998–1004.
11. Fenaux P, Morel P, Rose C, Lai JL, Jouet JP, Bauters F (1991): Prognostic factors in adult de novo myelodysplastic syndromes treated by intensive chemotherapy. Br J Haematol 77: 497–501.
12. de Witte T, Muus P, De Pauw B, Haanen C (1990): Intensive antileukemic treatment of patients younger than 65 years with myelodysplastic syndromes and secondary acute myelogenous leukemia. Cancer 66: 831–837.
13. Estey EH, Kantarjian H, Keating M (1993): Idarubicin plus continuous-infusion high-dose cytarabine as treatment for patients with acute myelogenous leukemia or myelodysplastic syndrome. Semin Oncol 20: 1–5.
14. Xue Y, Yu F, Zhou Z, Guo Y, Xie X, Lin B (1994): Translocation (8; 21) in oligoblastic leukemia: is this a true myelodysplastic syndrome? Leuk Res 18: 761–765.
15. Ravindranath Y, Abella E, Krischer JP, Wiley J, Inoue S, Harris M, Chauvenet A, Alvardo CS, Dubowy R, Ritchey AK, Land V, Steuber CP, Weinstein H (1992): Acute myeloid leukemia (AML) in Down's syndrome is highly responsive to chemotherapy: experience on Pediatric Oncology Group AML Study 8498. Blood 80: 2210–2214.
16. Slødahl SH, Smeland EB, Holte H, Grønn M, Lie SO, Seip M (1993): Leukemic blasts with markers of four cell lineages in Down's syndrome ("megakaryoblastic leukemia"). Med Pediatr Oncol 21: 254–258.
17. Gyger M, Perreault C, Belanger R, Bonny Y, Forest L, Lussier P (1989): Unsuspected Fanconi's anemia and bone marrow transplantation in cases of acute myelomonocytic leukemia. N Engl J Med 321: 120–121.
18. Ganser A, Heil G, Kolbe K, Maschmeyer G, Fischer JT, Bergmann L, Mitrou PS, Heit W, Heimpel H, Huber C, Hoelzer D (1993): Aggressive chemotherapy combined with G-CSF and maintenance therapy with interleukin-2 for patients with advanced myelodysplastic syndrome, subacute or secondary acute myeloid leukemia—initial results. Ann Hematol 66: 123–125.
19. de Witte T, Zwaan F, Hermans J, Vernant J, Kolb H, Vossen J, Lönnqvist B, Beelen D, Ferrant A, Gmür J, Lie Yin J, Troussard X, Cahn J, Van Lint M, Gratwohl A (1990): Allogeneic bone marrow transplantation for secondary leukaemia and myelodysplastic syndrome: a survey by the Leukaemia Working Party of the European Bone Marrow Transplantation Group (EBMTG). Br J Haematol 74: 151–155.

Acute Leukemias VI
Prognostic Factors
and Treatment Strategies
Büchner et al. (eds)

Remission Rates, Survival, and Prognostic Factors in Ninety Patients with Advanced Myelodysplastic Syndromes Treated with Intensive Chemotherapy

C. Aul, V. Runde, U. Germing, M. Burk, A. Heyll, B. Hildebrandt, and R. Willers

Abstract. Previous studies have suggested that intensive chemotherapy in myelodysplastic syndromes (MDS) is associated with low rates of complete remissions and considerable toxicity. These assumptions, however, are based on small patient series. We retrospectively analyzed the outcome of 90 patients (median age 54 years, range 16–74 years) with advanced primary MDS who were treated with intensive antileukemic regimens at our hospital between 1979 and 1994. The median time from diagnosis of MDS to initiation of chemotherapy was 1.5 months. French–American–British (FAB) classification types at treatment begin were refractory anemia with excess of blasts (RAEB) in ten, chronic myelomonocytic leukemia (CMML) in four, and RAEB in transformation (RAEB/T) in 37 cases; 39 patients had already transformed to AML (MDS-AML). The Karnofsky score ranged from 35% to 100% (median, 80%). Chromosome studies were performed in 61 patients of whom 26 (43%) presented with an abnormal karyotype. Sixty-four patients received thioguanine cytosine arabinoside (ara-C) and daunorubicin (TAD), 11 patients idarubicin plus ara-C, ten patients a double-induction regimen, and five patients other protocols for remission induction. Fifty-five patients (61%) entered complete remission (CR), and seven patients (8%) had a partial response. Early death occurred in 14 cases (16%), and 14 patients (16%) had refractory disease. No unusual toxicities of chemotherapy were noted. The median duration of bone marrow aplasia (leukocytes $< 1 \times 10^9/l$ and/or platelets $< 20 \times 10^9/l$) for patients achieving CR after one cycle of induction therapy was 19 days. After entering CR, 47 patients received one to two cycles of consolidation chemotherapy and 18 patients monthly myelosuppressive maintenance chemotherapy over a maximum period of 3 years. Median follow up of the patients is now 21 months. Actuarial overall survival was 33% at 2 years and 21% at 5 years. The projected 2-year and 5-year disease-free survival was 30% and 23%. From these data we conclude that intensive AML-type chemotherapy can be successfully administered to patients with high-risk MDS. In selected patients, this approach offers a chance of long-term remission and potential cure.

Introduction

Myelodysplastic syndromes (MDS) are acquired clonal bone marrow disorders, characterized by progressive peripheral blood cytopenias and an increased risk of transformation into acute myeloid leukemia (AML). The role of aggressive chemotherapy in the treatment of advanced myelodysplastic syndromes is not clearly defined. Early studies suggested that MDS is refractory to intensive chemotherapy. Complete remissions (CR) occurred in fewer than 20% of patients, and a considerable proportion of patients had early deaths due to prolonged chemotherapy-induced bone marrow aplasia [1,2]. More recent trials have questioned these findings by reporting remission rates as high as

Department of Internal Medicine, Hematology and Oncology Division, Heinrich-Heine-University, Düsseldorf, Germany

60% in selected groups of patients [3,4]. However, durable remissions were rarely obtained, suggesting that cure of MDS with standard AML protocols can hardly be achieved. All studies published so far have considerable limitations. Results are difficult to interpret because of low numbers of patients, varied distribution of morphological subgroups, and differences between treatment protocols. In this paper, we describe the clinical course of 90 patients with advanced-stage primary MDS who were treated with standard AML protocols over a time period of 15 years at the University of Düsseldorf.

Patients and Methods

Patients. From February 1979 to December 1994, 90 patients (51 male, 39 female) with an initial diagnosis of primary MDS (refractory anemia RA, three; RA with ring sideroblasts, RARS, one; RA with excess of blasts, RAEB, 22; RAEB in transformation RAEB/T, 51; and chronic myelomonocytic leukemia CMML, five) were treated with intensive antileukemic chemotherapy. Besides hematological parameters, patient selection was guided by performance score, absence of concomitant non-hematological disorders and the patient's wish to be treated. Fifty-seven patients started treatment within 3 months and 33 patients more than 3 months after diagnosis of MDS. Their median age was 54 years (range, 16–74 years). French-American-British (FAB) classification categories at treatment begin were RAEB in ten, CMML in four, and RAEB/T in 37 cases; 39 patients had already progressed to overt AML (MDS-AML). Other clinical and hematological characteristics of the patient population are summarized in Table 1.

Table 1. Clinical and hematological characteristics of 90 patients with advanced primary MDS receiving intensive chemotherapy

Disease duration—Median(months)	1.5
Range (months)	0–41
Age—median (years)	54
Range (years)	16–74
Sex M/F (*n*)	51–39
Karnofsky score—Median(%)	80
Range (%)	25–100
FAB categories	
RAEB(*n*)	10
(%)	11
CMML(*n*)	4
(%)	4
RAEB/T(*n*)	37
(%)	41
MDS-AML(*n*)	39
(%)	43
Neutrophils—Median(10^9/l)	1.4
Range (10^9/L)	0.02–25
Platelets—Median(10^9/l)	50
Range (10^9/L)	1–1300
LDH—MedianU/l	335
Range U/l	129–3485
Bone marrow blasts—Median(%)	27
Range (%)	9–95
Lineage Involvement	
Trilineage dysplasia(*n*)	53
(%)	59
Bilineage dysplasia(*n*)	26
(%)	29
Monolineage dysplasia(*n*)	11
(%)	12
Cytogenetics	
Normal(*n*)	35
(%)	39
Abnormal(*n*)	26
(%)	29
Not obtained(*n*)	29
(%)	32

Treatment Protocols. Chemotherapeutic regimens used for remission induction are summarized in Table 2. In general, treatment followed well-known protocols that were standard therapy for AML in our clinic at the time when individuals MDS patients started chemotherapy. Despite changing protocols, all patients were treated with conventional or high-dose cytosine arabinoside (ara-C) in combination with an anthracycline or an anthrachinone. Sixty-four patients received one or two cycles of ara-C, daunorubicin, and thioguanine (TAD) for remission induction. Eleven patients were treated with ara-C and idarubicin. Ten patients received an intensified induction regimen in which the initial TAD course was shortly followed by chemotherapy with high-dose ara-C and mitoxantrone (HAM). Five patients were treated with other protocols, including HAM, sequential HAM, or polychemotherapy with ara-C and doxorubicin. Supportive care was provided by oral antibiotic and antimycotic prophylaxis as well as transfusion of red blood cells and HLA-matched platelets. After entering CR, 47 patients received one or two cycles of consolidation therapy,

Table 2. Chemotherapeutic protocols used for remission induction of the MDS patients

Patients (n)	Regimen		On days
64	TAD	6-Thioguanine 100mg/m^2 q 12 h orally	3–9
		Ara-C 100 mg/m^2/day continuous infusion	1–2
		100 mg/m^{2}q 12 h i.v.	3–8
		Daunorubicin 60 mg/m^2/day i.v.	3–5
11	IA	Idarubicin 10 mg/m^2/day i.v.	1–3
		Ara-C 100 mg/m^{2}q 12 h i.v.	1–5
10	TAD/HAM	6-Thioguanine 100 mg/m^{2}q 12 h orally	3–9
		Ara-C 100 mg/m^2/day continuous infusion	1–2
		100 mg/m^{2}q 12 h i.v.	3–8
		Daunorubicin 60 mg/m^2/day i.v.	3–5
		Ara-C 3g/m^{2}q 12 h i.v.	21–23
		Mitoxantrone 10 mg/m^2/day i.v.	23–35
5	Other protocols (HAM, sequential HAM, ara-C+doxorubicin		

depending on the type of protocol used. Eighteen patients in remission received monthly maintenance chemotherapy according to the recommendations of the German AML Study Group [5].

Response Criteria. CR and partial remissions (PR) were defined according to Cancer and Leukemia Group B (CALGB) criteria [6]. Early death was defined as death during the first 6 weeks after the start of treatment, and non-response (NR) as failure to achieve CR or PR in patients surviving for at least 6 weeks of therapy.

Results

Fifty-five patients (61%) entered CR, and seven patients (8%) had a PR. Fourteen patients (16%) died of infections, hemorrhages, or anthracycline-induced cardiac failure within 6 weeks following induction chemotherapy. Three patients, all presenting with fever at the start of chemotherapy, died before the induction course was completed. In 14 patients (61%), MDS was refractory to aggressive chemotherapy. CR rates stratified by induction protocol were not different. No unusual toxicities of chemotherapy were noted. The median duration of bone marrow aplasia (leukocytes $< 1 \times 10^9$/l and/or platelets $< 20 \times 10^9$/1) in patients entering CR after one cycle of induction therapy was 19 days (range, 3–46 days). Nearly all induction cycles (98%) were associated with fever, requiring antibiotic or antifungal treatment. Seven patients died from septicemias or proven or suspected fungal pneumonias. Severe bleeding was seen in nine patients, including five fatal hemorrhages. Cardiac toxicity occurred in eight patients. A 32-year-old woman without preexisting heart disease died from intractable congestive heart failure attributed to chemotherapy with daunorubicin and mitoxantrone.

Several patient and disease characteristics at treatment begin were screened by univariate analysis for their association with successful remission induction (Table 3). Using a cut-off level of 50 years, age had no significant influence on remission induction ($p=0.18$). Favorable prognostic factors were good performance status (Karnofsky score > 70%), absence of bleeding symptoms, lactate dehydrogenase (LDH) levels below 500 U/l, low numbers of medullary blast cells, absence of pseudo-Pelger cells and normal karyotype. The CR rate in 54 patients treated while still in MDS phase was 76%, compared to 39% in 36 patients treated after progression to AML ($p=0.0004$). A total of 80% of 35 patients with a normal karyotype entered CR, whereas the respective percentage for 26 patients with an abnormal karyotype was only 42% ($p=0.002$).

Figure 1 shows the overall and disease-free survival for our patient population. After a median follow up of 21 months, 34 to 90 patients remain alive 2–73 months from the start of induction therapy. Twenty patients are alive in continued first CR 1–72 months after remission induction, and six patients are alive with resistant or recurrent MDS 2–42 months from induction treatment. In addition, four of 17 patients

Table 3. CR rates according to various pretreatment characteristics

Variable	Patients (*n*)	CR (%)	*p*
Age			
< 50 years	36	69	0.18
⩾ 50 years	54	56	
Sex			
Male	39	72	0.07
Female	51	53	
Karnofsky score			
> 70%	54	72	0.008
⩽ 70%	36	44	
Disease duration			
⩽ 3 months	61	66	0.20
> 3 months	29	52	
Fever			
Yes	29	52	0.20
No	61	66	
Hemorrhage			
Yes	36	47	0.02
No	54	70	
LDH			
< 500 U/l	67	67	0.02
⩾ 500 U/l	22	41	
Peripheral blood blasts			
< 5%	39	72	0.06
⩾ 5%	48	52	
Bone marrow blasts			
⩽ 30%	54	76	0.0004
> 30%	36	39	
Karyotype			
Normal	35	80	0.002
Abnormal	26	42	

who received reinduction therapy after relapse are alive in second CR for 5–12 months after salvage chemotherapy. Actuarial overall survival for the entire group of patients was 33% at 2 years and 21% at 5 years. Achievement of CR was a significant predictor of survival. Median survival for patients entering CR was 27 months, compared with only 4 months for patients failing to achieve CR. Survival curves for partial remitters and patients not responding to induction chemotherapy were not significantly different. Median actuarial disease-free survival for patients achieving CR was 16 months. The projected 2-year and 5-year disease-free survival was 30% and 23%, respectively. No differences were observed between treatment groups.

Univariate analysis of various pretreatment characteristics showed that only two morphological parameters were significantly correlated with the duration of disease-free survival. These included the presence of hyposegmented granulocytes and an abnormal peroxidase staining of neutrophil precursors. Median disease-free survival for patients with or without pseudo-Pelger cells was 6 and 17 months, respectively ($p = 0.005$). The corresponding values for patients with or without peroxidase-deficient neutrophil precursors were 10 and 16 months, respectively ($p = 0.04$). In addition, the presence of pseudo-Pelger cells was negatively correlated with overall survival. Age, bone marrow blast count, and karyotype were not predictive of disease-free survival, but were significantly related to overall survival.

Discussion

Based on previous reports, it has been assumed that aggressive chemotherapy, as employed for treatment of AML, is not very effective in MDS. This view, however, is challenged by our retrospective study which shows that, with appropriate selection of patients, aggressive chemotherapy produces high rates of CR in advanced-stage primary MDS. According to our results, it is particularly successful in patients with a low tumor burden and normal bone marrow karyotype, whose remission rates approach 80%. Contrary to previous clinical observations and in vitro findings of an increased P-glycoprotein expression in MDS [7, 8], drug resistance was uncommon in our series. In the majority of cases, antileukemic chemotherapy was associated with an acceptable degree of toxicity, as assessed by the percentage of lethal complications and the duration of bone marrow aplasia. Overall, 16% of our patients died during the induction phase of chemotherapy, whereas in other series the early death rate was as high as 33% [9].

It should be emphasized that approximately one fifth of the complete responders entered long-term remission. The decreasing slope of the survival curve suggests to us that at least some patients may be cured with intensive chemotherapy. These findings are not only of academic interest. Considering that in recent years nearly one third of MDS patients in our department received intensive treatment, our data emphasize the feasibility and clinical relevance of aggressive chemotherapy in MDS.

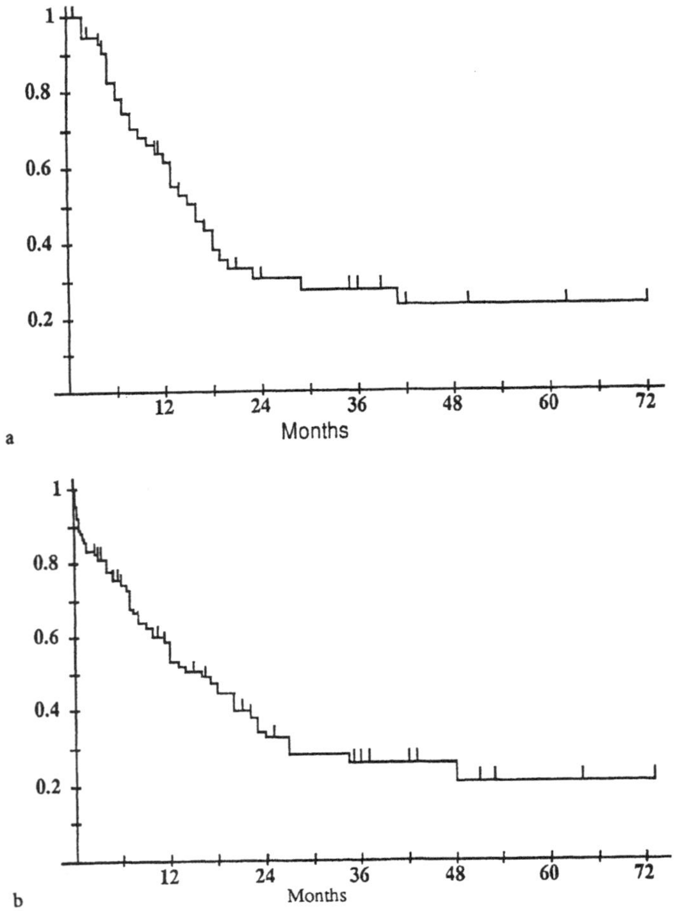

Fig. 1a,b. Actuarial overall (**a**) and disease-free survival (**b**)

References

1. Cohen J, Creger W, Greenberg PL, Schrier SL (1979) Subacute myeloid leukemia. A clinical review. Am J Med 66: 959–966
2. Dreyfus B (1979) Preleukemic states. I. Definition and classification. II. Refractory anemia with an excess of myeloblasts in the bone marrow (smoldering acute leukemia). Blood Cells 2: 33–55
3. De Witte T, Muus P, De Pauw B, Haanen C (1990) Intensive antileukemic treatment of patients younger than 65 years with myelodysplastic syndromes and secondary acute myelogenous leukemia. Cancer 66: 831–837
4. Seymour JF, Estey EH (1993) The prognostic significance of Auer rods in myelodysplasia. Br J Haematol 85: 67–76
5. Büchner T, Hiddemann W (1990) Treatment strategies in acute myeloid leukemia (AML). First-line chemotherapy. Blut 60: 61–67
6. Preisler HD, Rustum Y, Henderson ES (1979) Treatment of acute nonlymphocytic leukemia: use of an anthracycline–cytosine arabinoside induction therapy and comparison of two maintenance regimens. Blood 53: 455–464
7. Holmes J, Jacobs A, Carter G, Janowska-Wieczorek A, Padua RA (1989) Multidrug resistance in haematopoietic cell lines, myelodysplastic syndromes and acute myeloblastic leukaemia. Br J Haematol 72: 40–44
8. List AF, Spier CM, Cline A, Doll DC, Garewal H, Morgan R, Sandberg AA (1991) Expression of the multidrug resistance gene product (P-glycoprotein) in myelodysplasia is associated with a stem cell phenotype. Br J Haematol 78: 28–34
9. Tricot G, Boogaerts MA (1986) The role of aggressive chemotherapy in the treatment of myelodysplastic syndromes. Br J Haematol 63, 477–48

Acute Leukemias VI
Prognostic Factors
and Treatment Strategies
Büchner et al. (eds)

Secondary Myelodysplastic Syndromes: Morphological Findings, Cytogenetics, and Clinical Course in 55 Patients

H. Minning, C. Aul, V. Runde, U. Germing, and W. Schneider

Abstract. Between 1974 and 1994, 55 patients with Myelodysplastic Syndromes (MDS) following previous antineoplastic or immuno-suppressive treatment were identified at the University of Düsseldorf. In a retrospective study, the clinical and hematological features of these patients were examined and compared with those in 918 patients with primary MDS, diagnosed during the same time period.

Morphological subtypes of patients with secondary MDS (sMDS) were refractory anemia (RA) in 21%, RA with ring sideroblasts (RARS) in 21%, RA with excess of blasts (RAEB) in 26% RAEB in transformation (RAEB/T) in 19%, and Chronic myelomonocytic leukemia (CMML) in 13%. On cytogenetic analysis, nine of 11 patients had clonal chromosomal abnormalities including monosomy 7, monosomy 5, and multiple aberrations. The most frequent primary diseases were multiple myeloma in 21%, malignant lymphoma in 20%, and breast cancer in 19% of sMDS patients. Twenty-six patients had been treated with chemotherapy alone, with cylophosphamide, melphalan, or procarbazine being the most frequently administered agents. Twelve patients had been treated with radiotherapy alone and 12 patients with combined radiochemotherapy. Five patients with sMDS had been treated with immunosuppressive therapy because of nonneoplastic diseases such as rheumatoid arthritis, chronic polymyositis, or kidney transplantation. The median latency for development of MDS was 41 months (range, 12–174 months) following combined radiochemotherapy, compared with 60 months (range 17–369 months) after chemotherapy and 132 months (range 71–528 months) after ionizing radiation. Prognosis of patients with sMDS was very poor. Their actuarial median survival was 9 months, as compared with 23 months for patients with primary MDS. Fourteen patients with sMDS died after transformation acute myeloid leukemia (AML), whereas 16% and 21% of patients succumbed to infectious or hemorrhagic complications, respectively, without leukemic tranformation.

Introduction

Myelodysplastic syndromes (MDS) and acute myeloid leukemia (AML) belong to the most feared long-term complications of antineoplastic treatment. According to previous studies, alkylating agents such as cyclophosphamide, melphalan or procarbazine have the strongest leukemogenic potential [1, 2]. Most disturbing is the induction of secondary MDS (sMDS) during the treatment of a nonneoplastic disorder, for example, after immunosuppressive treatment of rheumatoid diseases [3].

Secondary MDS differs from primary MDS (pMDS) in several respects. Patients with sMDS often have a younger age and more profound peripheral blood cytopenia. Former histological studies often found a reduced bone marrow cellularity with varying grades of reticulin fibrosis. The prognosis of patients with sMDS is very poor, with a higher rate of transformation to AML as compared to patients with pMDS [4].

Department of Internal Medicine, Hematology and Oncology, Heinrich-Heine-Universität, Düsseldorf, Germany

Patients with sMDS are also characterized by a higher incidence of clonal karyotype abnormalities, often of a complex nature, which were present in up to 90% of cases in previously published series. Characteristic findings in patients with sMDS include losses of part or all of chromosomes 5 and 7 as well as complex aberrations [5, 6].

Material and Methods

The study population consisted of 55 patients with therapy-related MDS, identified by retrospective analysis of 973 MDS patients diagnosed between 1974 and 1994 at the University of Düsseldorf. The morphological diagnosis of MDS was based on the criteria proposed by the French-American-British (FAB) Cooperative Group [7].

Conventional hematological parameters were determined according to standard methods. In 11 patients, chromosome studies were performed on bone marrow aspirates. Trypsin - Giemsa - banded metaphases obtained from direct preparations and from 24-h or 72-h cultures without added mitogens were examined. In each patient with analyzable mitoses, at least 15 metaphases were karyotyped and classified according to the International System for Human Cytogenetics Nomenclature.

Data analysis was performed using the BMDP statistical package. The Kaplan-Meier product limit method was employed to estimate actuarial survival. Survival was measured from diagnosis of MDS to death or last follow up (December 31, 1994). Survival curves of the different patient groups were compared by the log-rank test.

Results

The number of patients with sMDS diagnosed in our clinic has risen constantly over the last 20 years (three patients in 1974–1978, seven patients in 1979–1983, 21 patients in 1984–1988, and 24 patients in 1989–1994). The relative frequency of sMDS cases, however, remained constant (5.8%–6.3%) since there was a proportional increase in pMDS patients (Fig. 1).

Table 1 summarizes the clinical and hematological features of our 55 patients with sMDS. In addition, it contains the respective findings for our pMDS population ($n = 918$). The median age of sMDS patients was 65 years (range, 27–84 years), as compared to 72 years (range, 13–97 years) in pMDS patients. Morphological subtypes at diagnosis were refractory anemia(RA) in 12 cases, RA with ring sideroblasts (RARS) in 12, RA with excess of blasts (RAEB) in 14, Chronic myelomonocytic leukemia (CMML) in six and RAEB in transformation (RAEB/T) in 11 cases. No subcategory was overrepresented, as compared to the pMDS population. Peripheral blood cytopenia was more profound in patients with sMDS with median hemoglobin levels of 8.1

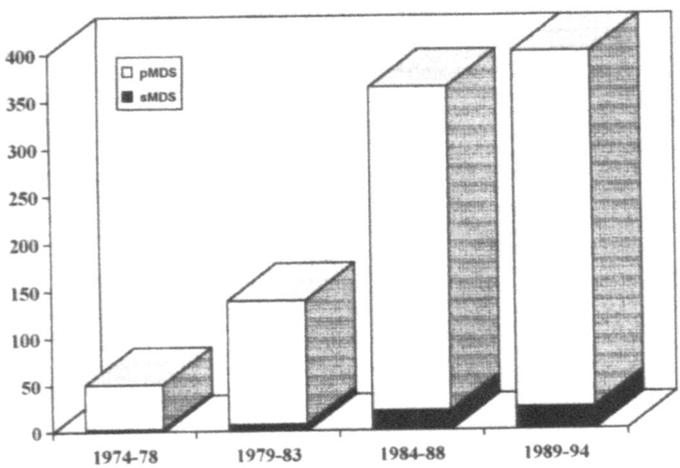

Fig. 1. Incidence of sMDS and pMDS in our clinic between 1974 and 1994

Table 1. Clinical, hematological, and cytogenetic findings at diagnosis of 55 patients with secondary (treatment-related) MDS and 918 patients with primary MDS

	Secondary MDS		Primary MDS	
Patients (n)	55		918	
Age — median (years)	65		72	
Range (years)	27–84		13–97	
Sex M/F (*n*)	20/35		491/427	
Laboratory findings				
Hemoglobin — median (g/dl)	8.1		9.3	
Range (g/dl)	4.0–15.8		3.2–16.6	
WBC — median (10^9/l)	2.8		4.3	
Range (10^9/l)	0.7–143.0		0.2–147.0	
Platelets — median (10^9/l)	78		125	
Range (10^9/l)	3–283		0–999	
Bone marrow cellularity				
Reduced / normal (*n*) (%)	20	36	385	42
Increased (*n*) (%)	35	64	523	58
FAB subtypes				
RA (*n*) (%)	12	21	198	22
RARS (*n*) (%)	12	21	213	23
RAEB (*n*) (%)	14	26	222	24
CMML (*n*) (%)	6	13	138	15
RAEB/T (*n*) (%)	11	19	147	16
Karyotype				
Patients (*n*)	11		163	
Normal (*n*) (%)	2	18	94	58
-5 / 5q- (*n*) (%)	1	10	10	6
-7 / 7q- (*n*) (%)	3	27	2	1
Complex aberrations (*n*) (%)	3	27	20	12
Other aberrations (*n*) (%)	2	18	37	23

g/dl (pMDS: 9.3 g/dl), white blood cell count (WBC) of 2.8×10^9/l (4.3×10^9/l) and platelet count of 78 × 109/l (125×10^9/l). The majority of patients in both diagnostic groups showed an increased bone marrow cellularity (64% versus 58%). On cytogenetic analysis, nine of 11 patients (82%) with sMDS had clonal chromosomal abnormalities, whereas the respective percentage in pMDS patients was only 58%. The most frequent aberrations encountered in sMDS were monosomy 7 and complex aberrations (three patients each).

The most frequent diseases for which antineoplastic treatment was started were malignant lymphoma (21%), multiple myeloma (21%), and breast cancer (19%). The series also included five patients who had been treated with immunosuppressive agents for benign primary diseases, such as rheumatoid arthritis and other collagen vascular diseases, or following kidney transplantation. Twenty-one of 25 MDS patients treated with chemotherapy alone had received alkylating agents: cyclophosphamide (cumulative doses, 1.5–298.5 g), melphalan (1.3–10.2 g), or procarbazine (5.6–33.6 g). Patients treated with ionizing radiation alone had often been exposed to high-dose radiotherapy (40–60 Gy) involving large volumes of the hematopoietic bone marrow. In addition, four patients had received 131-iodine therapy (255–1400 mCi) for metastatic thyroid cancer. Median latency to the development of MDS was strongly influenced by the type of treatment. It was 132 months after radiotherapy, 60 months after chemotherapy, and only 41 months after combined radio chemotherapy.

Our series confirmed the grim outlook of sMDS cases. The actuarial median survival in this patient population was 9 months, whereas the corresponding figure for patients with de novo AML was nearly 2 years (Fig. 2.) Table 2 shows the outcome of sMDS and pMDS patients. Only one patient (2%) in the sMDS group, but 26% of patients in the pMDS group were still alive at the time of last follow up. Transformation to AML was the most frequent cause of

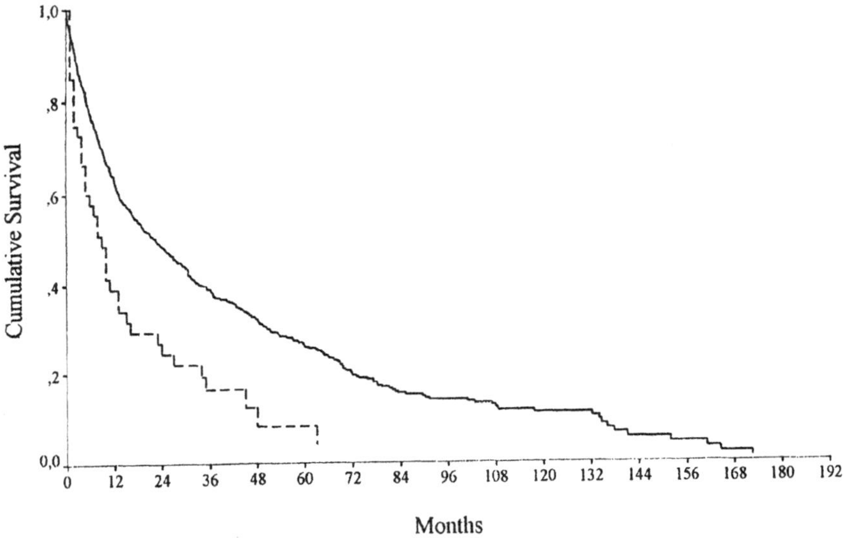

Fig. 2. Kaplan-Meier survival curves of 55 patients with sMDS (*broken line*) and 918 patients with pMDS (*solid line*); $p < 0.00005$

Table 2. Outcome of 55 patients with sMDS and 918 patients with pMDS

	Secondary MDS ($n=55$)		Primary MDS($n=918$)	
	(n)	(%)	(n)	(%)
Causes of death				
Infection	9	16	159	18
Bleeding	12	22	76	9
Transformation to AML	14	26	179	19
Unrelated to MDS	6	11	142	15
Unknown	6	11	91	10
Alive	1	2	236	26
Lost to follow up	7	12	27	3

death in patients with sMDS, followed by hemorrhage (22%) and infections (16%).

Discussion

This study was performed in an attempt to analyze in greater detail the risk, clinical course, and outcome of patients with therapy-related MDS. The absolute number of sMDS cases rose constantly during our study period (1974–1994), emphasizing the increasing importance of this MDS category. Our data confirm previous observations according to which sMDS represents a prognostically unfavorable entity. Although more than 40% of our MDS patients belonged to the RA and RARS categories, their clinical course was characterized by rapid deterioration, high incidence of transformation to AML, and a significantly reduced life expectancy (9 months versus 23 months for pMDS; $p<0.00005$). Considering the poor prognosis of therapy-related MDS patients and their generally poor response to conventional aggressive chemotherapy, new strategies to minimize their incidence are urgently required. These could include the use of non-leukemogenic cytostatic drugs, reduction in dosage and duration of alkylating agents, and avoidance of long-term chemotherapy at low dosages. Chemotherapeutic agents should not be used for treatment of nonneoplastic diseases.

Finally, there is still a lack of systematic investigations into risk factors for therapy-related myeloid malignancies. A more meaningful analysis of antineoplastic treatment and MDS would require prospective studies that could provide detailed information on the multistep development of secondary hematopoietic neoplasms.

References

1. Levine, E.G. and Bloomfield, C.D. (1992) Leukemias and myelodysplastic syndromes secondary to drug, radiation and enviromental exposure. Semin. Oncol., 19,47–84.
2. Deiss, A. (1993) Non-neoplastic diseases, chemical agents and hematologic disorders that may procede hematologic neoplasms. In: Wintrobe's clinical hematology, edited by G.R.Lee, T.C.Bithell, J. Foerster, J.W. Athens and J.N. Lukens, 9th ed., pp. 1946–1968. Philadelphia: Lea & Febiger.
3. Aul, C., Gattermann, N. and Schneider, W. (1992) Age-related incidence and other epidemiological aspects of myelodysplastic syndromes. Br. J. Haematol., 82, 358–367.
4. Kantarjian, H.M. and Keating, M.J.(1987) Therapy-related leukemia and myelodysplastic syndromes. Semin Oncl., 14,435–443.
5. Pedersen-Bjergaard, J., Philip, P., Mortensen, B.T., Ersboll, J., Jensen, G.,Panduro, J. and Thomsen, M. (1981) Acute nonlymphocytic leukemia, preleukemia and acute myeloproliferative syndrome secondary to treatment of other malignant diseases. Clinical and cytogenetic characteristics and results of in vito culture of bone marrow and HLA typing. Blood, 57, 712–723.
6. Heim, S. (1992) Cytogenetic findings in primary and secondary MDS. Leuk.Res., 16, 43–46.
7. Bennett, J.M.,Catovsky, D., Daniel, M.T., Flandrin, G.,Galton, D.A.G., Gralnick, H.R. and Sultan, C. (1982) Proposals for the classification of the myelodysplastic syndromes. Br.J.Haematol., 51, 189–199.

Acute Leukemias VI
Prognostic Factors
and Treatment Strategies
Büchner et al. (eds)

Myelodysplastic Syndromes or Leukemia Following MDS Treated with Allogeneic Bone Marrow Transplantation: A Survey of the Working Party on Chronic Leukemia of the European Cooperative Group for Blood and Marrow Transplantation

V. Runde, T. de Witte, C. Aul, A. Gratwohl, D. Niederwieser, A. van Biezen, J. Hermans, J. Vernant, H. Kolb, J. Vossen, B. Lönqvist, D. Beelen, A. Ferrant, R. Arnold, J. Cahn, M. van Lint, L. Verdonk, and J. Apperley

Abstract. Allogeneic bone marrow transplantation (BMT) offers potential cure for younger patients with myelodysplastic syndromes (MDS) or secondary acute myeloid leukemia (sAML). Until now 450 patients from more than 45 European centers have been reported to the European BMT group (EBMTG). We retrospectively analyzed those patients who received allogeneic BMT without prior remission induction chemotherapy ($n = 107$). Ninenty-one marrow donors were genotypically HLA-identical siblings and 16% received T cell-depleted marrow. The 4-year disease-free and overall survival for the entire group of patients was 31% and 39%, respectively. Forty-three patients (40%) died from transplantation-related complications, most often graft-versus-host disease and/or infections. MDS/AML recurred in 27 patients between 1 and 36 months after transplant, for an actuarial probability of relapse of 34% at 4 years. Disease-free and overall survival was dependent on the pretransplant bone marrow blast count. Patients with refractory anemia (RA)/RA with ring sideroblasts (RARS), RA with excess of blasts (RAEB), RAEB in transformation (RAEB/T), and sAML had a 4-year disease-free survival of 45%, 33%, 24%, and 20%, respectively. The 4-year overall survival for the respective patient groups was 52%, 46%, 23%, and 22%. Younger age was a favorable prognostic factor for overall survival and transplant-related mortality. In addition, a longer interval between MDS/sAML and BMT was associated with a higher incidence of transplant-related mortality. From these data, we conclude that allogeneic BMT without prior remission induction chemotherapy can be recommended for younger patients with early-stage MDS.

Introduction

Myelodysplastic syndromes (MDS) comprise a heterogeneous group of hematopoietic stem cell disorders with varying clinical, laboratory, and morphological features. According to the proposals of the French-American-British Cooperative Group (FAB), five morphological entities can be distinguished, including refractory anemia (RA), RA with ring sideroblasts (RARS), RA with excess of blasts (RAEB), RAEB in transformation (RAEB/T), and chronic myelomobocytic leukemia (CMML) [1]. Treatment of MDS has generally been unsatisfactory. Because of their advanced age, most patients are solely treated with supportive measures. Limited success has been reported with low-dose cytosine arabinoside [2], retinoic acid [3], corticosteroids [4], and hematopoietic growth factors [5]. Young patients with advanced MDS may achieve prolonged, disease-free survival when treated with intensive antileukemic chemotherapy [6]. However, remission duration has generally been short. Nowadays, allogeneic bone marrow transplantation (BMT) is considered the treatment of choice for younger patients with histocompatible siblings. Most MDS patients in North America have been transplanted without prior induction chemotherapy, whereas European BMT centers generaly administer

Heinrich-Heine-University, Moorenstr. 5, 40225 Düsseldorf, Germany

remission induction treatment prior to BMT, at least in advanced cases of MDS [7]. The purpose of this study was to retrospectively analyze the outcome of allogeneic BMT in 107 MDS patients not receiving conventional induction treatment prior to BMT.

Patients and Methods

Study Population. Questionnares were sent to all centers which had reported cases of MDS, sAML, and therapy-related MDS/AML to the Leukemia Working Party of the European Cooperative Group for Blood and Marrow Transplantation (EBMT). Centers were asked to report all patients transplanted for these diseases, to provide additional clinical information, and to send peripheral blood smears, bone marrow smears, and trephine biopsies of patients who received no intensive remission induction chemotherapy before BMT. Data of 107 patients (Table 1) from 31 centers and bone marrow slides of 43 patients treated between 1978 and 1993 were collected. Four patients received one or more courses of low-dose cytosine arabinoside (ara-C) without achieving remission before BMT was performed. In 24 of 38 cases, a central bone marrow cytology review confirmed the FAB diagnosis reported by the local center. In the remaining 14 cases, morphology classification was different (Table 2). In three cases the quality of the bone marrow aspirate was too poor to allow an accurate diagnosis by the reviewer. In two cases the exact FAB type was not specified by the BMT center, and central review led to a diagnosis of RA and RAEB, respectively. The analysis of treatment outcome only referred to the FAB diagnosis made by the centre at the time of transplant.

Treatment. Median time from diagnosis of MDS/AML to BMT was 6 months (range, 1–126 months). Ninety-three donors were HLA-identical siblings, four were identical twins, four were other family donors. Four patients had matched unrelated donors, and two had haploidentical unrelated donors. Detailed information on patients and treatment is given in Table 1.

Statistical Analysis. The Kaplan-Meier product limit method was employed to estimate survival and disease-free survival. Survival was measured from the day of BMT to death or last follow up. Multivariate modeling was performed using the stepwise proportional hazard Cox regression model. The covariates age and disease duration were entered in three different age (≤ 20, 21–40, and >40 years) and disease duration categories (≤ 3, 3–12, and >12 months), respectively.

Results

Cumulative overall survival, disease-free survival (DFS), relapse risk, and transplant-related mortality (TRM) 4 years after BMT for the entire group of patients ($n = 107$) and for patients with HLA-identical sibling donors ($n = 93$) are given in Table 3.

Survival. At the time of analysis 44 patients (41%) were aliive with a median follow up of 39 months (range, 3–179 months). The 4-year overall survival for the entire group of patients was 39%. The 4-year overall survival for patients with RA/RARS ($n = 37$), RAEB ($n = 27$), RAEB T ($n = 24$) and sAML ($n = 17$) was 52%, 46%, 23%, and 22%, respectively (Fig. 1). Chromosomal characteristics at the time of BMT had a strong influence on survival. The 4-year survival for patients with single chromosomal aberrations was 52%, whereas it was 37% for patients with normal karyotypes and 17% for patients with complex aberrations ($p = 0.02$). Other pretreatment factors that were correlated with longer survival of patients were a low medullary blast cell count and younger age.

Transplant-Related Mortality. Forty-three patients (40%) died of transplant-related complications, most often graft-versus-host disease and/or infections. Four years after transplant, patient aged less than 21 years had an actuarial TRM of 20% compared to 44% in patients aged 21–40 years, and 65% in patients older than 40 years. In addition, a longer interval between diagnosis of MDS/AML and BMT was associated with a higher rate of TRM.

Relapse. Recurrence of MDS/AML occurred in 27 patients between 1 and 36 months (median, 6 months) following transplant. The 4-year actuarial probability of relapse in patients with RA/RARS, RAEB, RAEBT, and sAML was 25%, 52%, 44%, and 43%, respectively. Patients with normal karyotypes had a lower relapse risk

Table 1. Clinical and transplantation characteristics of 107 patients with myelodysplasia or postcytotoxic AML

Characteristic		Data
Patients studied (*n*)		107
Age—Median (years)		31
Range (years)		2-58
Males/females (*n*)		63/44
Disease duration	—Median (months)	7
	Range (months)	1-126
Disease etiology	Idiopathic (*n*)	94
	Cytotoxic treatment for	
	Hodgkin's disease (*n*)	10
	ALL (*n*)	1
	Cutaneous sacroma (*n*)	1
	Multiple sclerosis (*n*)	1
FAB subtype at BMT	RA (*n*)	35
	RARS (*n*)	2
	RAEB (*n*)	27
	RAEB/T (*n*)	24
	CMML (*n*)	2
	sAML/tAML (*n*)	17
Cytogenetics	Normal karytope	15
	5q-,-5 (*n*)	2
	8+ (*n*)	1
	7q-,-7 (*n*)	8
	Miscellaneous single aberrations (*n*)	10
	7q-,-7 with other aberrations (*n*)	3
	Miscellaneous complex aberrations (*n*)	3
	No results (*n*)	65
Marrow donar	Identical twin (*n*)	4
	HLA-identical sibling (*n*)	93
	Phenotyp. HLA-matched family member (*n*)	1
	1-3 HLA-AG mismatched family member (*n*)	3
	HLA-identical unrelated donor (*n*)	4
	1-3 HLA-AG mismatched unrelated donor (*n*)	2
Conditioning regimen	Chemotherapy + TBI (*n*)	79
	Chemotherapy alone (*n*)	28
GVHD prevention	None (*n*)	4
	Cylocosporin A (*n*)	26
	Cyclosporine A and MTX (*n*)	53
	MTX (*n*)	7
	T cell depletion (*n*)	3
	T cell depletion and others (*n*)	14

ALL, acute lymphocytic leukemia; RA, refractory anemia; RARS, refractory anemia with ring sideroblasts; RAEB, refractory anemia with excess of blasts; RAEB/T, refractory anemia with excess of blasts in transformation; CMML, chronic myelomonocytic leukemia; AML, acute myeloid leukemia; tMDS/tAML, postcytotoxic MDS/AML; HLA, human leukocyte antigen; TBI, total body irradiation; MTX, methotrexate: GVHD, graft-versus-host disease.

compared to patients with clonal cytogenetic abnormalities, but these differences failed to reach statistical significance.

Disease-Free Survival. At the time of analysis, 37 patients (35%) were alive and disease free. The 4-year disease-free survival for the entire group of patients was 31%. Four years after BMT, patients with RA/RARS, RAEB, RAEBT, and sAML had an actuarial DFS of 45%, 33%, 24%, and 20%, respectively ($p = 0.04$; Fig. 2). Patients with single chromosomal aberrations had a 4-year DFS of 38%, whereas patients with a normal karyotype or complex chromosomal aberrations had a DFS of 24% and 18%, respectively ($p = 0.045$).

Table 2. Results of central bone marrow morphology review in 38 patients

	FAB diagnosis after central review				
	RA/RARS (*n*)	RAEB (*n*)	RAEB T (*n*)	AML (*n*)	CMML (*n*)
FAB diagnosis reported					
RA/RARS	13	2			
RAEB	2	6	1	1	
RAEB/T	1	3	1	2	
AML			2	2	
CMML					2

Consistent diagnosis = 24/38 (63%). Ra, refractory anemia; RARS, refractory anemia with ring sideroblasts; RAEB, refractory anemia with excess of blasts; RAEB/T, refractory anemia with excess of blasts in transformation; CMML, chronic myelomonocytic leukemia; AML, acute myeloid leukemia.

Table 3. Cumulative probability at 4 years for overall survival, disease free survival, relapse risk, and transplant-related mortality. All patients ($n = 107$) and patients with HLA-identical sibling donor ($n = 93$) (results in parentheses)

		Cumulative probability 4 years after BMT								
		Patients	Overall survival		DFS	Risk	Relapse		TRM	
		(*n*)	(%)	(*p*)	(%)	(*p*)	(%)	(*p*)	(%)	(*p*)
All patients		107 (93)	39 (40)		31 (32)		44 (42)		44 (45)	
Ra/RARS		37 (30)	52 (45)	0.02	45 (40)	0.04	25 (27)	0.60	40 (45)	0.07
RAEB		27 (24)	46 (54)	(0.17)	33 (38)	(0.23)	52 (45)	(0.72)	32 (31)	(0.28)
RAEB/T		24(20)	23(28)		24 (29)		44 (40)		57 (51)	
CMML		2 (2)								
AML		17 (17)	22		20		43		65	
Age (years)	≤ 20	26 (21)	57 (54)	0.03	35 (32)	0.09	56 (60)	0.64	20 (20)	0.01
	21–40	54 (47)	41 (44)	(0.05)	33 (36)	0.15	41 (36)	(0.33)	44 (44)	(0.01)
	> 40	27 (25)	20 (22)		21 (23)		(38 (33)		65 (66)	
Interval	≤ 3	37 (34)	54 (56)	0.09	39 (42)	0.25	44 (41)	0.50	31 (29)	0.04
diagnosis–	4-12	43 (39)	32 (32)	(0.04)	28 (28)	(0.08)	47 (45)	(0.74)	47 (50)	(0.03)
BMT (months)	12	25 (18)	26 (23)		23 (17)		45 (52)		59 (64)	
tMDS/	No	94 (81)	40 (41)	0.33	31 (32)	0.41	47 (46)	0.92	41 (42)	0.38
tAML	Yes	13 (12)	29 (31)	(0.41)	29 (31)	(0.60)	22 (14)	(0.42)	63 (63)	(0.30)
T cell	No	90 (82)	42 (41)	0.31	33 (33)	0.33	43 (42)	0.86	42 (43)	0.31
depletion	Yes	17 (11)	23 (27)	(0.34)	19 (18)	(0.24)	53 (45)	(0.35)	59 (67)	0.43

DFS, disease free survival; TRM, transplant-related mortality; RA, refractory anemia; RARS, refractory anemia with ring sideroblasts; RAEB, refractory anemia with excess of blasts; RAEB/T, refractory anemia with excess of blasts in transformation; CMML, chronic myelomonocytic leukemia; AML, acute myeloid leukemia; BMT, bone marrow transplantation, tMDS/tAML, postcytotoxic MDS/AML.

Discussion

In this retrospective study, 107 patients with MDS who underwent allogeneic BMT without prior remission induction chemotherapy were analyzed. At a median follow up of 39 months, 37 patients (35%) were alive and free of disease. Our results are similar to those reported in four other series [8–11]. Only the study from Detroit which included relatively few patients with a

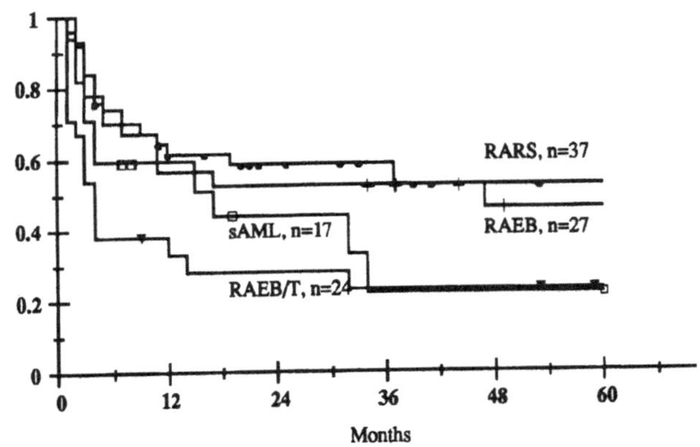

Fig. 1. Overall survival according to FAB classification at the time of BMT ($p = 0.02$; Breslow and Mantel-Cox)

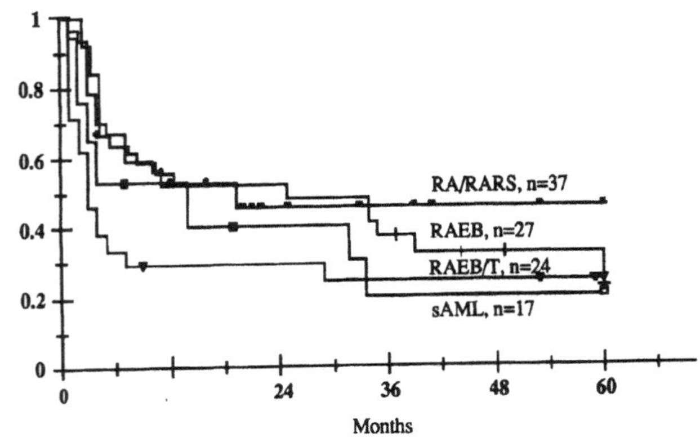

Fig. 2. DFS according to FAB classification at the time of BMT ($p = 0.04$; Breslow and Mantel-Cox)

short follow up (median, 20 months) reported better results with a DFS of 62% [12]. Our analysis, therefore, strongly supports the conclusion that BMT performed as primary treatment in MDS cures approximately one third of patients.

The DFS of our MDS patients was dependent on the pretransplant bone marrow blast count. Results in patients with RA/RARS were comparable to those achieved in CML patients transplanted in first chronic phase. On the other hand, we could demonstrate that BMT in sAML patients without prior remission induction therapy produced an unfavorable long-term outcome comparable to CML patients grafted in accelerated phase. Patients with RAEB or RAEB T had an intermediate outcome with a 4-year DFS of 33% and 24%, respectively. In contrast to the Seattle series in which no relapses occurred after more than 2 years [8], 40% of the RAEB patients in our cohort relapsed during the 3rd year after BMT.

Which patients should receive remission induction treatment prior to BMT? Previous reports have shown that patients with RAEB/T have an excellent response to conventional antileukemic therapy, with remission rates of 69% [6]. These cases and patients with AML following MDS should probably undergo BMT in first CR. The data of our study suggest that allogeneic BMT without prior remission induction chemotherapy should be primarily used for younger patients with early-stage MDS whose cure rates approach 50%. With regard to the results of our central review of bone marrow slides, it should be emphasized that in one third of reviewed cases differences in morphological classification between the central reviewers and local morphologist were found. Therefore, comparison of results from different single centers should be interpreted with caution.

References

1. Bennett J, Catovsky D, Daniel M, Flandrin G, Galton DAG, Gralnick H, Sultan C. Proposals for the classification of myelodysplastic syndromes. British Journal of Haematology. 1982; 51: 189-299
2. Aul C, Schneider W. The role of low-dose cytosine arabinoside and aggressive chemotherapy in advanced myelodysplastic syndromes. Cancer. 1989; 64: 1812-8
3. Aul C, Runde V, Gattermann N. All-trans retinoic acid in patients with myelodysplastics syndromes: results of a pilot study. Blood. 1993; 82: 2967-74
4. Bagby GC, Gabourel JD, Linman JW. Glucocorticoid therapy in the preleukemic syndrome (hemopoietic dysplasia). Annals of Internal Medicine. 1980; 92: 55-8
5. Greenberg PL. Treatment of myelodysplastic syndromes with hemopoietic growth factors. Seminars in Oncology. 1992; 19: 106-14
6. Fenaux P, Preudhomme C, Hebbar M. The role of intensive chemotherapy in myelodysplastic syndromes. Leukemia and Lymphoma. 1992; 8: 43-9
7. De Witte T, Gratwohl A. Bone marrow transplantation for myelodasplastic syndromes and secondary leukemias. British Journal of Haematology. 1993; 84: 361-4
8. Anderson JE, Appelbaum FR, Fisher LD, Schoch G, Shulman H, Anasetti C, Bensinger WI, Bryant I, Buckner D, Doney K, Martin PJ, Sanders JE, Sullivan KM, Thomas ED, Witherspoon RP, Hansen JA, Storb R. Allogeneic bone marrow transplantation for 93 patients with myelodysplastic syndromes. Blood. 1993; 82: 677-81
9. Longmore G, Guinan EC, Weinstein HJ, Gelber RD, Rappeport JM, Antin JH. Bone marrow transplantation for myelodysplatic and secondary acute nonlymphoblastic leukemia. Journal of Clinical Oncology. 1990; 8: 1707-14
10. Nevill TJ, Shepherd JD, Reece DE, Barnett MJ, Nantel SH, Klingemann HG, Phillips GL. Treatment of myelodysplastic syndromes with busulfan-cyclophosphamide conditioning followed by allogeneic BMT. Bone Marrow Transplantation. 1992; 10: 445-50
11. O'Donnell MR, Nademanee AP, Snyder DS, Schmidt GM, Parker PM, Biermann PJ, Fahey JL, Stein AS, Krance RA, Stock AD, Forman SJ, Blume KG. Bone marrow transplantation for myelodysplastic and myeloproliferative syndromes. Journal of Clinical Oncology. 1987; 5: 1822-6
12. Ratanatharathorn V, Karanes C, Uberti J, Lum LG, de Planque MM, Schultz KR, Cronin S, Dan ME, Mohamed A, Hussein M, Sensenbrenner LL. Busulfan-based regimens and allogeneic bone marrow transplantation in patients with myelodysplastic syndromes. Blood. 1993; 81: 2194-9
13. Appelbaum FR, Barrall J, Storb R, Fischer LD, Schoch G, Ramberg RE, Shulman H, Anasetti C, Bearman SI, Beatty P, Bensinger WI, Buckner D, Clift RA, Hansen JA, Martin P, Petersen FB, Sanders JE, Singer J, Stewart P, Sullivan KM, With erspoon RP, Thomas ED. Bpne marrow transplantation for patients with myelodysplasia—pretreatment variables and outcome. Annals of Internal Medicine. 1990; 112: 590-7

Acute Leukemias VI
Prognostic Factors
and Treatment Strategies
Büchner et al. (eds)

Cyclosporin A in the Treatment of Myelodysplastic Syndrome

V.G. Savchenko, E.N. Parovitchnikova, and E.A. Mihailova

Abstract. Cyclosporin A (CsA) was tested in the treatment of five patients with different forms of myelodysplastic syndrome (MDS). Three patients (two with refractory anemia, RA, and one with RA with excess of blasts, RAEB) were pretreated with prednisone and interferon α. In two patients (one with RA, one with RAEB in transformation, RAEB/T) CsA was applied as the first-line treatment. Four out of five patients were transfusion dependent and all had a median of 6 months disease course. CsA was administered orally at an initial dose of 10 mg/kg per day constantly with modifications according to tolerability and creatinine level. The duration of treatment was about 6 months with a final dose of CsA to be 4–5 mg/kg per day. In one case (MDS relapse after autologous bone marrow transplantation, BMT) there was no effect and CsA was stopped after 1 month of treatment. There was a clear response in three cases (RA, RA, RAEB) regarding peripheral blood cytopenia, percentage of bone marrow blasts, and transfusion requirements. In one case we observed freedom from progression. Two patients received one CsA cycle, one–two cycles, and one–three cycles. We conclude that in some MDS patients CsA can improve the clinical course of the disease, but the repeated prolonged applications of the drug seem to be necessary.

Introduction

Myelodysplastic syndrome (MDS) is a clonal disorder of multipotential stem cell comprising a variety of different clinical forms with common morphological features of dysmyelopoiesis and peripheral blood (PB) cytopenia [1–3]. Usually PB cytopenia is in striking contrast to normal or hypercellular bone marrow. However, in some cases severe hypoplasia is noted in bone marrow biopsies and the most important criteria for differentiating MDS from aplastic anemia (AA) is dysmyelopoiesis determined in bone marrow smears [4]. Another commonly recognizable characteristic of MDS is its frequent transformation into acute myeloid leukemia (AML), especially in refractory anemia (RA) with excess of blasts (RAEB) and RAEB in transformation (RAEB/T)[5].

Even if MDS patients do not progress to overt AML they have significantly increased morbidity and mortality rate due to complications of their cytopenias. Though a lot of different therapeutical approaches have been tested in RA, RA with ring sideroblasts (RARS), RAEB, and RAEB/T, no exact well-defined treatment protocols have been established so far. Differential, cytostatic, cytokine therapy provides some, though usually not stable results in a minor proportion of MDS patients. Long-term remissions can be obtained after aggressive chemotherapy followed by bone marrow transplantion (BMT) in younger patients. In most cases the treatment is directed to the improvement of PB cytopenia leading to a decrease in transfusion requirements and incidence of infectious complications.

Recently, some studies have shown that ineffective hematopoiesis in MDS resulting in PB cytopenia is a consequence of a high intrame-

National Reasearch Center for Hematology, Moscow, Russia

dullary cell death rate via apoptosis [6-8]. Thus, the inhibition of programmed cell death (PCD) may become one of the most important mechanisms in the treatment of MDS. Among suppressors of apoptosis are vialability factors (colony-stimulating factors, CSFs). Their efficacy has already been proven in MDS. Inhibition of apoptosis by such immunosuppressive drugs as cyclosporin A (CsA) and FK 506 was also proven in in vitro models: T cell hybridomas, thymocyte cultures, etc. [9,10]. Here we report our experience in the treatment of five MDS patients with CsA.

Material and Methods

Since October 1991 we have treated five patients with different forms of MDS with CsA. Their clinical characteristics before treatment are presented in the Table 1. CsA was administered per os at an initial dose 10 mg/kg per day. After 2-4 weeks of treatment the dose of CsA was modified in all patients according to tolerability and creatinine level. The final CsA dose used in the patients was 4-5 mg/kg per day.

The level of CsA in blood was monitored in the 1st month of treatment by radioimmunoassay done twice a week, and then twice/once a month. The treatment duration in case of response after 1 month of therapy was 6 months. Then it was stopped and started again with the previously adjusted dose if deterioration occurred.

Results

Five patients were treated with CsA at a dose of 10-4 mg/kg per day. Patient N1 received five courses of CsA, patient N4—two courses, patients N2 and N3—one course. In patient N5 the treatment was stopped within 1 month due to non-response. Results of treatment are summarized in Table 2.

In two cases (N3, N5), CsA became the first-line treatment. Patient N5, in whom we started CsA as the first-line therapy, was the most complicated case. He underwent transplantation with autologous bone marrow in April, 1991, in first remission of AML (M4). Duration of complete remission (CR) before BMT was 5 months. Within 1 year, in February, 1992, he relapsed with 60% blasts in bone marrow and was treated with the 7+3 program including mitoxantrone (cytosine arabinoside ara-C, 100 mg/m^2 bid for 7 days, mitoxantrane 10 mg/m^2 once a day on days 1-3). CR was achieved after the first course and afterwards he received five courses. During the last two courses, extremely prolonged and deep cytopenias occurred (leukocytes < 1×10^9/l for 35 days) and PB counts did not restore to normal. Bone marrow was hypoplastic with 2%-5% of blasts and dysmyelopoietic features. The situation was considered to be an MDS relapse. The patient was not treated for 9 months, only regular erythrocyte and platelet transfusions were performed (twice a month). In December, 1993, PB cytopenia was no longer corrected with transfusions, blast cells exceeded 10% in bone marrow, and in January, 1994 we started CsA. However, there was no response for 1 month: bone marrow blasts increased to 25%, PB cytopenia was not improved. The patient died of progressive leukemia 1 month after CsA cessation. In patient N3 CsA stabilized the progressive decrease in PB count. At the moment of diagnosis the Hb level in this patient was 95 g/l, thrombocytes 130×10^9/l, leukocytes 3.5×10^9/l. During the 6 months after MDS diagnosis Hb decreased to 80 g/l, platelets to 70×10^9/l, leukocytes 2.5×10^9/l. At these PB counts the treatment was started and in the following 6 months of treatment there was no further PB count decrease and Hb was slightly elevated to 90 g/l.

In three other patients, CsA was the second or even the third line of treatment. It is of interest that patient N1 suffered his MDS for 18 years before CsA treatment. The disease began in 1974 with leukopenia (2.9×10^9/l) and thrombocytopenia (47×10^9/l). Hb level was normal. Bone marrow biopsy showed partial hypoplasia with a few microforms of megakaryocytes. The diagnosis made in a regional hospital was aplastic anemial (AA). The patient was treated with prednisolone and androgens with some effect. In 1978 he was splenectomized but during the following 10 years thrombocytopenia ($50-70 \times 10^9$/l) and leukopenia ($3-3.5 \times 10^9$/l) persisted without deterioration. In 1989 anemia (Hb 75-80 g/l) developed and levels of thrombocytes and leukocytes decreased. Prednisolone was started again but without any effect. The patient became transfusion dependent. Bone marrow biopsy repeatedly showed hypoplasia. Bone

Table 1. Clinical characteristics of MDS patients before CsA treatment

Patient	Age (years)	Sex	Diag-nosis	Disease duration	Previous treatment	Bone marrow biopsy	Hb (g/l)	Leukocytes ($\times 10^9/l$)	Platelets ($\times 10^9/l$)	Transfusion requirement
N1	42	m	RA	18 years	Prednisone Androgens Splenectomy	Hypo-plasia	75	2.7	18	Weekly RBC and platelets
N2	65	m	RA	1 year	Prednisone Interferon alfa	Hyper-plasia	100	3.1	5	Platelets two times a week
N3	42	m	RA	6 months	None	Hyper-plasia	80	2.5	70	None
N4	18	m	RAEB	1 year 2 months	Prednisone Interferon alfa	Aplasia	51	0.9	2	RBC and platelets three times a week
N5	40	m	RAEB	9 months	None	Hypo-plasia	60	1.2	10	RBC and platelets two times a week

Table 2. Results of CsA treatment in MDS patients

Patient	Follow up on CSA (months)	Hb elevation	Leukocyte elevation	Platelet elevation	Transfusion independence	Freedom from progression
N1	30	+	+	+	+	+
N2	10	+	+	+	+	+
N3	7	+	–	–	+	+
N4	11	+	+	+	+	+
N5	1	–	–	–	–	–

marrow morphology showed the evident features of dysplasia. Since that time (November, 1991) the patient was treated in our clinic. The diagnosis of MDS (RA) was considered to be the most appropriate in this case and CsA treatment was initiated in Spring 1992. He responded within 1 month with an improvement in PB cytopenia followed by a marked decrease in transfusions. Within 3 months of CsA therapy, transfusions could be stopped. After cessation of treatment after 6 months of therapy deterioration occurred quite rapidly (within 1 month). The treatment was restarted. In total there were five CsA courses.

In patient N4 CsA treatment was started after 14 months of disease following unsuccessful prednisolone therapy and severe deterioration of PB cytopenia during the application of mini-dose interferon alpha (1×10^6 U s.c. once every 3 days, five injections). At this moment there was aplastic bone marrow according to biopsy and dysmyelopoiesis in bone marrow smear with 7%–12% of blasts and extremely poor physical status After 1 month of treatment there was sufficient improvement in PB counts and in two months bone marrow contained 0.9% blast cells, Hb level 81 g/1, platelets $32 \times 10^9/1$, leukocytes $2.5 \times 10^9/1$. After 11 months there were 2% bone marrow blasts, Hb was 91 g/1, platelets $43 \times 10^9/1$, leukocytes $2.6 \times 10^9/1$ without any transfusion.

Patient N2 presented with anemia Hb 70 g/1, thrombocytopenia $10 \times 10^9/1$, and leukopenia ($2.5 \times 10^9/1$). Prednisolone was used for 7 months without any effect. After admission to our department prednisolone was stopped and mini-dose interferon-α was started. Interferon α was used for 2 months with substantial improvement in red blood cell (RBC) levels (Hb 100 g/1) with slight but short (1 month) increase in platelet count ($25 \times 10^9/1$). Two months after interferon alpha, CsA was started. Platelet count was $2–5 \times 10^9/1$ with platelet transfusions twice a week. Hb and leukocyte levels were stable. Within 2 months thrombocyte count reached $50–70 \times 10^9/1$. After CsA cessation, platelet count decreased slightly to $35–40 \times 10^9/1$ but remained stable for 2 months. No transfusions were used for 8 months (since CsA initiation).

Toxicity was tolerable with none of these patients showing arterial hypertension, severe gingivitis, renal, hepatic or cerebral side effects. Though during administration of the loading dose of 10 mg/kg per day, CsA levels in blood exceeded normal values of 200–400 ng/ml two to three times, no one showed a creatinine level of more than 1.5 mmol/l. In none of these patients did we notice an increased susceptibility to infections, that means immunosuppression caused by CsA was not so pronounced. Moreover, the PB count improvement correlated with a decrease in the incidence of infectious episodes.

In three cases CsA therapy was conducted on an outpatient basis. Patient N 4 spent 1 month in the department untill CsA treatment brought results, then for 1 year all treatment took place on outpatient basis. Patient N5, who did not respond to treatment stayed in the clinic until his death.

Though the group of patients discussed here is small, we have defined different types of response to CsA treatment. The clinical effects are (a) no response or progression; (b) freedom from progression (stabilization); (c) PB cytopenia improvement; (d) decrease in transfusion requirements or independence from transfusions. The duration of response is (a) stable status for more than 6 months after CsA cessation; (b) stable stauts for more than 2–3 months after CsA cessation with repeated courses of CsA; (c) stable effect on CsA treatment with deterioration after its cessation. In our study we observed each type of response except stable status for more than 6 months after CsA cessation.

Discussion

As already discussed, no totally effective form of therapy has been developed in MDS. In patients in whom the disease does not appear life-threatening at the moment of diagnosis a conservative or "wait and see" approach is warranted.

Corticosteriod, vitamin B12, folic acid, and androgen therapy have generally proven to be ineffective [11,12], though up to 10% responses on corticosteroids have been reported [13]. One of the possible mechanisms of their action, especially in high-dose therapy, is the increase in endogenous granulocyte-macrophage CSF (GM-CSF) levels [14].

Based on the leukemic nature of the disease, various chemotherapeutic options have been tested, ranging from aggressive cytotoxic therapy to low-dose therapy with ara-C or hydroxyurea. However, in the case of chemotherapy, the major point to be taken into consideration is the generally elderly age of these patients (65% are over 65 years old). In addition, a high proportion of these patients have marrow cells with multi-drug resistant phenotype resulting in chemotherapeutic failure [15]. Intensive chemotherapy provides a variable proportion (13%–51%) of CR with a high incidence of toxic deaths, and low-dose ara-C treatment results in a 10%–20% CR rate [11]. The duration of these responses is usually short. For young MDS patients allogeneic BMT may become a treatment of choice as general results in this category of patients are good—40% 7-year disease-free survival [16].

Marrow culture studies have generally demonstrated subnormal clonal growth and defective cellular maturation of myeloid and erythroid precursors [17]. The evidence of cell maturation arrest in MDS became a basis for testing differentiation-inducing agents [18]. These agents can be subdivided into three groups: non-cytotoxic and cytotoxic drugs and hematopoietic growth factors or CSFs. The first group comprises vitamin D3, retinoid acid, interferons, hexamethylene-bisacetamide (HMBA), the second group—5-azacytidine, low-dose ara-C, the third—a variety of CSFs (erythropoietin; G-CSF; GM-CSF; interleukin-3, IL-3; stem cell factor; SCF). All these agents can be used alone or in combination with each other. Neither retinoid acid, vitamin D3, or standard-dose interferons alone nor low-dose ara-C or erythropoietin (EPO) alone has shown consistent or durable responses in a substantial proportion of MDS patients [11,19]. Promising results were reported regarding combined application of retinoid acid, vitamin D3 and interferon α with a 40% CR and partial response (PR) rate, mini-dose interferon α with a 43% CR+PR, 5-azacytidine with a 53% response rate (CR, PR, improvement), and HMBA with a 22% CR+PR rate [19–22].

The vast majority of reports on MDS treatment are now concentrated on CSFs, their combinations and concomitant use with other drugs such as ara-C. The data from in vitro culture techniques provided a biological framework which demonstrated MDS marrow cells to have a proliferative and differentiative response to G-CSF, GM-CSF, IL-3, SCF [23–25]. The clinical use of recombinant human hematopoietic growth factors in patients with MDS shows a distinct but unstable response in white blood cells (G-CSF, GM-CSF, IL-3) plus improvement in platelet and reticulocyte counts (IL-3) [26,27]. However, despite the demonstration of improvements in neutrophil levels and sometimes in platelet count, and of a somewhat better disease course with fewer transfusion requirements, large randomized trials are needed to determine whether the natural history of MDS will be altered by treatment with the CSFs.

Recent studies have demonstrated that MDS is a highly proliferative disorder with a median labeling index in bone marrow biopsies of 26% and cell cycle time (Tc) of 44 h. Moreover, these studies revealed an extensive apoptosis with more than 75% of cells committing suicide in 25 of 40 biopsies examined [6, 7]. The conclusions drawn by the investigators support the hypothesis that increased apoptosis may be the mechanism responsible for the premature intramedullary cell death in MDS [8]. The high birth rate of cells is canceled by the high death rate, resulting in functionally aplastic marrows requiring supportive care for therapy. All CSFs are vialability factors and are proven to suppress the programmed cell death (apoptosis) in normal and leukemic hematopoietic cell cultures [28, 29]. Though there are some exceptions, for example, in murine myeloid leukemia cell line C2M-5A G-CSF induces apoptosis instead of suppression [30]. In human hematopoiesis only IL-3 and GM-SCF were determined as factors maintaining survival in G_0 of the cell progenitors [31]. Thus, beside the proliferative and differentiating action of CSFs in MDS, the inhibition of apoptosis may play one of the most important roles in the improvement of PB cytopenia.

Cyclosporin A is a well-known PCD inhibitor for various thymocyte lines and T cell hybridomas. It is believed that the effect of such immunosuppressive drugs as CsA and FK 506 is based on the regulation of thymocyte sensitivity to clonal deletion via apoptosis. CsA or FK 506 block the TcR-activating signal transduction, in this way protecting cells from activation-induced apoptosis [9].

In our small study the efficacy of CsA is promising. There has only been one report concerning a patient with hypoplastic MDS who responded to CsA treatment by complete normalization of PB count and disappearance of apoptosis in BM biopsy [7]. We had two patients with hypoplastic MDS: RA (patient N1) and RAEB (patient N4). We did not observe complete normalization of PB count, but a dramatic improvement with cessation of transfusion support and a sufficiently better quality of life were attained. Patient N1 had a very prolonged disease course of 18 years before CsA administration. CsA improved PB counts and the patient did not need transfusions during treatment.

Deterioration occurred after CsA cessation. The disease duration on CsA treatment in this case has already exceeded 2.5 years. Patient N4 improved PB and BM counts within 1.5 months of CsA treatment and remained well for 1 year with constant CsA application. This patient is young and we can speculate that, if effective CsA treatment may provide such young MDS patients a chance to undergo transplantation in a stable disease status without constant blood component transfusions, thus decreasing the toxic death rate during the BMT procedure. Two other cases represent a classical MDS picture with hypercellular dysmyelopoietic bone marrow. Patient N2 demonstrated a good response to mini-dose interferon α regarding anemia but continued to require frequent platelet transfusions. CsA treatment for 6 months resulted in a substantial elevation of thrombocytes from $2–5 \times 10^9/l$ to $45–75 \times 10^9/l$. Beside a possible inhibition of increased apoptotic cell death, CsA can also act as a drug converting allosensibilization in the case of heavily transfused patients. Patient N 3 received CsA as first-line treatment and was free from progression of PB cytopenia for 7 months.

We demonstrated good responses to CsA treatment in four cases. It means that CsA is a drug that can be included in the list of remedies possessing some efficacy in MDS. More trials with a good scientific basis are needed to prove these preliminary results.

We have started a study on the CsA treatment of MDS patients together with cytogenetic analysis and apoptotic cell death rate measurements and hope it will contribute new data to our knowledge about this diverse hematological disorder.

Refencences

1. Aul C., Gatterman N., Germing U., Derigs G., Schneider W. Primary myelodysplastic syndromes: analysis of prognostic factors in 235 patients and proposals for an improved scoring system. Leukemia 1992 v.6, pp. 52–59
2. Janssen W.G., Bushle M., Layton M., Drexler H.G., Lyons J., van del Berge H., Heinpel H., Kubanek B., Klerhauer E., Mufti G.J., Bartran R. Clonal analysis of myelodysplastic syndromes: evidence of multipotent stem cell origin. Blood 1989 v.73 pp. 248–254
3. Tefferi A., Thibodeau S.N., Solberg L.A. Clonal studies in the myelodysplastic syndrome using X-linked restriction fragment polimorphisms Blood v.75 pp. 1770–173
4. Fohlmeister I. et al. Aplastic anemia and the hypocellular myelodysplastic syndrome: histomorphological, diagnostic and prognostic features. J.Clin.Pathology 1985 v.38 pp. 1218–1223
5. Jacobs R.H., Cornbleet M.A., Vardiman J.W., Larson R.A., Le Beau M.M., Rowley J.D. Prognostic implications of morphology and karyotype in primary myelodysplastic syndrome. Blood 1986 v.67 pp. 1765–1771
6. Raza A., Mundle S., Ifikhar A., Shetty V., Preisler H. Simultaneous assessment of cell-kinetics and programmed cell death to examine the mechanism of chemo-resistance in myeloid disorders. Ann.-Hematology 1994 v.68 (suppl 1) abstr.22
7. Raza A., Gregory S., Mundle S., Shetty V., Alvi S., Marcus B., Rifkin S., Shoel J., Preisler H. Increased apoptosis as the significant cause of inneffective hematoipoiesis in myelodysplastic syndromes (MDS). Blood 1994 v.84 (suppl 1) abstr.2528
8. Yoshida Y. Hypothesis: apoptosis may be the mechanism responsible for the premature intramedullary cell death in the myelodysplastic syndrome. Leukemia 1993 v. 7 pp.144–146
9. McCarthy S.A., Cachione R.N., Mainwaring M.S., Gairns J.S. The effects of immunosuppressive drugs on the regulation of activation-induced apoptotic cell death in thymocytes. Transplantation 1992 v.53 pp. 543–547
10. Schreier M.H., Zenke G., Borel J.F., Baumann G. The continuing search for new immunomodulators. Transplant.proceedings 1992 v.24 (suppl 2) pp. 19–21

11. Greenberg P.L. Treatment of myelodysplastic syndromes. Blood Reviews 1991 v5 pp. 42–50
12. Najean Y., Pecking A. Refractory anemia with excess of myeloblasts in bone marrow: a clinical trial of androgenes in 90 patients. Br. J. Haematology v.37 pp. 25–33
13. Bagby G.C.Jr., Gabourel J.D., Linmann J.W. Glucocorticoid therapy in preleukemia syndrome (hemopoietis dysplasia): identification of responsive patients using in-vitro techniques. Ann. Int. Medicine 1980 v.92 pp. 55–58
14. Tuncer A.M., Hicsonmez G., Erturk G., Gumruk F., Albayrak D., Oguz H. The effect of high-dose methylprednisolone treatment on GM-CSF level in children with acute leukemia: a pilot study. Leuk.Research 1992 v.16 pp. 615–619
15. Holmes J., Jacobs A., Carter G., Janovska-Wierzorek A., Radua R.A. Multidrug resistance in haemopoietic cell lines, myelodysplastic syndromes and acute myeloblastic leukemia. Br. J. Haematology 1989 v.72 pp. 40–44
16. Bone marrow transplantation; edited by Formann S.J., Blume K.G., Thomas E.D., Blackwell Scientific publications. 1994 pp.629–639
17. Greenberg P.L. The smoldering myeloid leukemic states. Clinical and biologic features. Blood 1983 v.61 pp. 1035–1045
18. Sawyers C.L., Denny C.T., Witte O.N. Leukemia and the disruption of normal hematopoiesis. Cell 1991 v.64 pp.337–350
19. Helistrom E., Robert K-H., Gahrtron G., Mellstedt H., Lindemann C., Einhorm S. Therapeutic effects of low dose cytosine arabinoside, alpha interferon, 1-hydroxyvitamin D3 and retinoid acid in acute leukemia and myelodysplastic syndromes. Eur. J. Haematology 1988 v.40 pp. 449–459
20. Holcombe R.F. Mini-dose interferon alpha-2a in the treatment of myelodysplasia. Leukemia 1993 v. 7 pp.192–195
21. Silverman L.R., Holland K.F., Demakos E.P., Peterson B., Nelson D.A., Clamon G., Powell B.L., Larson R., Bloomfield C.D., McIntyre O.R., Schiffer C. (CALGB). Azacitidine (Aza C) in myelodysplastic syndromes (MDS) Ann.Hematology 1994 v.68 (suppl 1) abstr N 46
22. Andreeff M., Stone R., Michaeli J., Young C.W., Tong W.P., Sogoloff H., Ervin T., Kufe D., Rifkind R.A., Marks P.A. Hexamethylene bisacetamide in myelodysplastic syndrome and acute myelogenous leukemia: a phase II clinical trial with a differentiation-inducing agent. Blood 1992 v.80 pp. 2604–2609
23. Nagler A., Ginzton N., Bangs C., Donlon T., Greenberg P.L. In vitro differentiative and proliferative effects of human recombinant colony stimulating factors on marrow hemopoiesis in myelodysplatis syndromes. Leukemia 1990 v.4 pp. 193–202
24. Nagler A., Mackichan M.L., Negrin R.S., Bangs C., Donlon T., Greenberg P.L. Impact of marrow cytogenetics and morphology on in vitro hemapoiesis in the myelodysplastic syndromes: comparison between human recombinant granulocyte colony stimulating factor and granulocyte-monocyte colony stimulating factor. Blood 1990 v. 766 pp. 1299–1307
25. Maze R., Horie M., Hendrie P., Vadhan-Raj S., Tricot G., Gordon M., Nemunaitis J., Ashman L.K., Broxmeyer H.E. Differential responses of myeloid progenitor cells from patients with myeloid leukemia and myelodysplasia to the costimulating effects of steel factor in vitro. Exp. Hematology 1993 v.21 pp. 545–551
26. Herrmann F., Mertelsmann R., Lindemann A., Ottmann O.G., Seipelt G., Oster W., Hoelzer D., Ganser A. Clinical use of recombinant human hematopoietic growth factors (GM-CSF, IL-3, EPO) in pateints with myelodysplastic syndrome. Biotechnol-Ther.1991 v.2 pp. 299–311
27. Negrin R.S., Nagler A., Kobayashi Y., Sklar J., Donlon T., Souza L., Greenberg P.L. Maintenance treatment of patients with myelodysplastic syndromes using recombinant human granulocyte colony stimulating factor. Blood 1990 v.76 pp. 36–43
28. Sachs L., Lotem J. Control of programmed cell death in normal and leukemic cells: new implications for therapy. Blood 1993 v.82 pp.15–21
29. Bradbury D., Shu Yong-Ming, Russel N. Regulation of Bcl-2 expression and apoptosis in acute myeloblastic leukemia cells by granulocyte-macrophage colony-stimulating factor. Leukemia 1994 v.8 pp. 786–791
30. Bessho M., Yoshida S., Sakate K., Murohashi I., Jinnai I., Hirashima K. Suppression of the development of murine myeloid leukemia with granulocyte colony-stimulating factor by inducing apoptosis of leukemic cells. Leukemia 1994 v.8 pp.1185–1190
31. Ogawa M. Differentiation and proliferation of hematopoietic stem cells. Blood 1993 v.81 pp. 2844–2853

Supportive Care

Acute Leukemias VI
Prognostic Factors
and Treatment Strategies
Büchner et al. (eds)

Mediators in Sepsis and Septic Shock

J. Kienast, H. Ostermann, M. Kiehl, A. Atzeni, J. Bork, D. Wippermann, and T. Büchner

Abstract. Severe sepsis is defined as a systemic inflammatory response to infection associated with organ dysfunction or hypoperfusion abnormalities. The validity of this definition based on readily available clinical and laboratory criteria was prospectively examined in 117 patients with acute myeloid leukemia and chemotherapy-induced leukocytopenia of $<10^9/l$. The results demonstrate that the detection of microorganisms in the blood is of limited value for the identification of patients at high risk of dying from septic complications. The cumulative incidence of severe sepsis and septic shock was found to be linearly related to the duration of leukocytopenia. However, both the rate of progression from severe sepsis to septic shock and sepsis-related mortality disproportionately increased when the duration of leukocytopenia exceeded 20 days. Plasma concentrations of tumor necrosis factor-α, interleukin-6 and -8 were significantly increased at the onset of severe sepsis and septic shock and remained elevated for up to 96 h. Peak cytokine levels were positively associated with the severity of septic complications and fatal outcome, but were unrelated to leukocyte counts and markers of monocyte or granulocyte activation. It is concluded that the cytokine release associated with evolving sepsis or septic shock does not depend on circulating leukocytes. The evaluation of cytokine measurements as an adjunctive tool to assess mortality in septic patients with leukocytopenia is warranted.

Introduction

In recent years sepsis has been conceptually redefined as a systemic inflammatory response to an active infectious process, manifested by fever or hypothermia, tachycardia, tachypnea, and an altered white blood cell count (WBC). The term "severe sepsis" applies to sepsis with organ dysfunction or hypoperfusion disclosed by abnormalities such as lactic acidosis, oliguria, or an altered mental status [1]. According to the revised definition, the presence of demonstrable microorganisms in the blood has limited implications for the diagnosis of sepsis, although the control of the infectious process with appropriage antimicrobial therapy is a fundamental determinant of outcome [2]. The definition of sepsis based on these readily available clinical criteria has been validated in a prospective setting [1, 3], but its applicability to severely leukocytopenic patients has not been examined.

Cytokines, namely interleukins-1, -6, -8 (IL - 1, -6, -8), and tumor necrosis factor alpha (TNF-α), have been identified as key mediators of the systemic host response in patients with severe sepsis and septic shock [4]. In non-leukocytopenic patients with sepsis, the levels of IL-1β, IL-6, TNF-α are directly related to disease severity and outcome [5–7]. However, cytokine levels in leukocytopenic patients with evolving sepsis or septic shock have not been studied. Hence, it is unclear whether the release of cytokines to potentially hazardous levels depends on the presence of at least normal numbers of circulating leukocytes, which are considered a major

Department of Internal Medicine, Hematology/Oncology Section, University of Münster, Germany

endogenous source for proinflammatory cytokines [8].

The present study was initiated to examine the validity of the above clinical criteria for the diagnosis of severe sepsis in leukocytopenic patients and to evaluate the cytokine response during evolving sepsis in this patient group.

Patients and Methods

A total of 117 patients with acute myeloid leukemia (AML) were prospectively recruited to the study before undergoing cytoreductive chemotherapy for remission induction or consolidation. Patients were treated according to standardized protocols with respect to both cytostatic and antimicrobial therapy. All patients provided informed consent to participate. The study protocol was approved by the local ethics committee.

Episodes of severe sepsis of septic shock were documented when occurring during chemotherapy-induced leukocytopenia defined as a total WBC $<10^9/l$. The diagnosis of severe sepsis was made according to the criteria outlined above: (a) evidence of infection; (b) hyperthermia >38°C or hypothermia <36°C; (c) tachycardia >90 beats/min; (d) tachypnea with a respiratory rate >20 breaths/min or $PaCO_2$ <32 torr; (e) signs of inadequate organ perfusion (plasma lactate >1.8 mmol/l, oliguria <30 ml/h for at least 1 h, hypoxemia with PaO_2/FiO_2 <280, or an acute alteration in mental status). Septic shock was diagnosed when the patients met the criteria for severe sepsis as well as those for shock (i.e., systolic blood pressure <90 mm Hg or a fall in systolic blood pressure of more than 40 mm Hg for at least 1 h despite adequate volume replacement). Recurrence of sepsis after defeverescence for at least 5 days was considered a separate event.

Blood samples were taken before chemotherapy was instituted (A) and when the WBC had fallen to $<10^9/l$ (B). During the initial course of the study, additional blood samples were obtained on days 1, 2, 4, and 7 of any febrile episode. Subsequently, blood sampling was restricted to patients who developed severe sepsis or septic shock, with the first sample being obtained within 2 h of onset. Further blood samples were taken after 6, 12, 18, 24, 36, 48, 60, and 96 h.

Cytokine concentrations in plasma samples were determined by enzyme immunoassays according to the instructions provided by the manufacturers. ELISA kits for IL-1β, IL-6, and TNF-α were obtained from Medgenix (Ratingen, Germany). The assay for IL-8 was purchased from Biermann (Bad Nauheim, Germany). Lower limits of detection in plasma were 2 pg/ml for IL-1β, 3 pg/ml for IL-6 and TNF-α, and 18 pg/ml for IL-8. Serum neopterin levels were measured by ELISA (Medgenix) with a lower limit of detection of 0.05 ng/ml and with normal values in healthy individuals ranging below 3 ng/ml. Neutrophil elastase in plasma was determined as elastase-α_1-proteinase inhibitor complex using an immunoactivation method (IMAC-Elastase, Diagnostica Merck, Darmstadt, Germany). The lower limit of detection was 8 ng/ml, with normal values ranging below 40 ng/ml.

For statistical analyses, cytokine concentrations were log-transformed in order to obtain normal distributions. The influence of time and patient group on the evolution of median cytokine levels was examined using analysis of variance. For univariate within or between group comparisons, the non-parametric Mann-Whitney test was employed.

Results

Data on 138 courses of cytoreductive chemotherapy for remission induction or consolidation in 117 patients with AML were evaluable. Forty-one patients experienced a total of 47 independent episodes of severe sepsis ($n=25$) or septic shock (survived $n=10$; fatal $n=12$). Bacteremia was documented by positive blood cultures in 16 out of 47 episodes (34%). Patients with severe sepsis and positive blood cultures were more likely to develop septic shock (50% versus 14%, $p<0.03$). However, neither the total sepsis-related mortality nor the mortality for patients with septic shock differed significantly between patients with and without positive blood cultures (Fig. 1).

The cumulative incidence of severe sepsis or septic shock was a linear function of the duration of leukocytopenia, i.e., the incidence of sepsis remained constant over time (Fig. 2). However, the severity of septic episodes increased during prolonged leukocytopenia. In severe sepsis occurring beyond day 20, the rate of progression to septic shock increased from 17% to 50% ($p<0.05$) and the mortality rose from 14% to 42% ($p<0.03$) when compared to septic episodes arising within the first 20 days of

Fig. 1. Prognosis of patients with severe sepsis or septic shock according to the presence or absence of documented bacteremia

47 episodes			
Bacteremia	(+)		(−)
	34 %		66 %
Shock at onset of sepsis	13 %	p = 0.14	32 %
Progression to shock	50 %	p < 0.03	14 %
Mortality			
- shock	56 %		54 %
- total	31 %		23 %

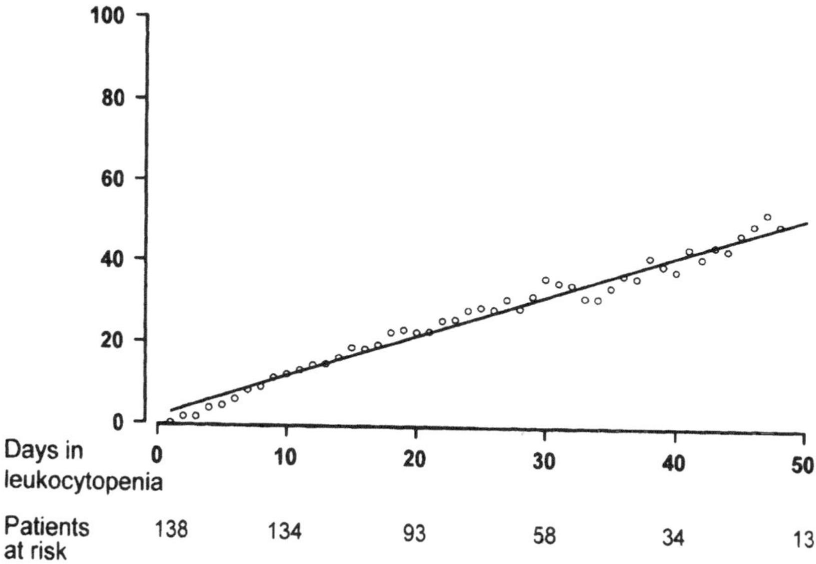

Fig. 2. Cumulative incidence of severe sepsis or septic shock in relation to the duration of leukocytopenia

leukocytopenia. A leukocyte count below 10^8/l at the onset of severe sepsis tended to be associated with a higher rate of progression to septic shock (35% versus 17%) and a higher mortality (31% versus 8%) than observed at leukocyte counts > 10^8/l and < 10^9/l. However, these differences were statistically not significant ($p = 0.26$ and $p = 0.11$, respectively).

Median plasma concentrations of TNF-α, IL-6, and IL-8 peaked within ⩽ 12 h of onset of severe sepsis or septic shock and remained elevated for up to 96 h at levels significantly above those measured in patients with uncomplicated febrile episodes (time course not shown). Maximum cytokine concentrations were significantly higher in patients who developed septic shock than in those who did not (Fig. 3). In contrast, IL-1β was detected in fever than 5% of all plasma samples.

In order to examine the relationship between plasma cytokine release and sepsis-related mortality, a score was established based on the number of cytokines (TNF-α, IL-6, IL-8) that exceeded arbitrarily chosen threshold concentrations within 48 h of onset of severe sepsis or septic shock. Figure 4 demonstrates a significant increase in mortality with the cytokine score.

Markers of monocyte or neutrophil activation (neopterin and elastase, respectively) remained low in patients with severe sepsis or

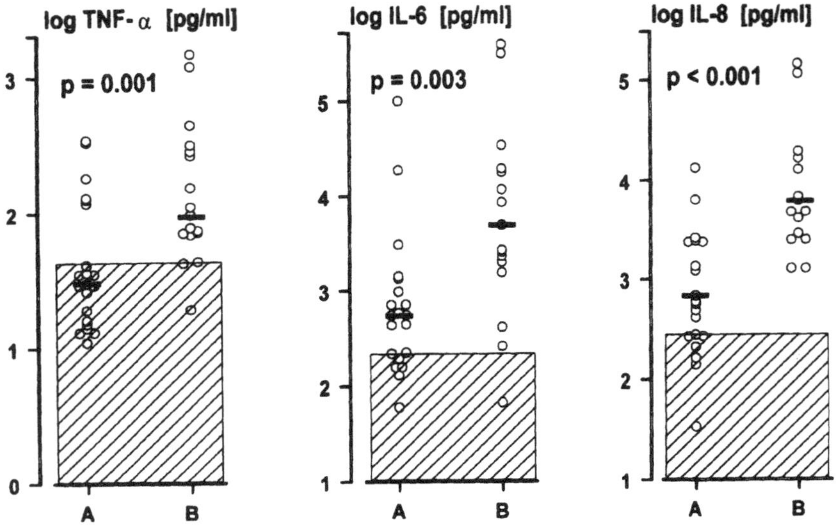

Fig. 3. Peak plasma concentrations of TNF-α, IL-6, and IL-8 in patients with severe sepsis or septic shock. The *p*-values indicate the significance levels between group comparisons. *Hatched areas*, range of cytokine concentrations measured during the course of uncomplicated febrile episodes; *A*, severe sepsis, $n = 21$; *B*, septic shock, $n = 17$

Fig. 4. Relationship between sepsis-related mortality and plasma cytokine score. The score was based on the number of cytokines (TNF-α, IL-6, IL-8) that exceeded arbitrarily chosen threshold levels within 48 h of the onset of severe sepsis or septic shock

septic shock and were unrelated to the increase in plasma cytokine concentrations. In addition, there was no association between TNF-α, IL-6, and IL-8 concentrations and leukocyte counts.

Discussion

The adapted consensus criteria for the definition of severe sepsis and septic shock [1] proved to be valid for the identification of AML patients with chemotherapy-induced leukocytopenia who are at high risk of dying from severe infectious complications. In our study as well as in an earlier report on non-leukocytopenic patients [3], the presence of documented bacteremia was associated with a higher rate of progression to circulatory shock. Nonetheless, the detection of microorganisms in the blood had little impact on sepsis-related mortality and, thus, is not a requirement for the diagnosis of severe sepsis or septic shock. This may be due to the fact that many patients develop septic complications while receiving antibiotics and these may prevent bacterial growth in blood cultures. We conclude that the diagnosis of severe sepsis and septic shock in leukocytopenic patients can be made on the basis of readily available clinical and laboratory criteria and that these criteria allow the identification of candidate patients for clinical trials on new treatment strategies. However, our findings do not obviate the need for a thorough search for causative microorganisms in order to guide adequate antimicrobial therapy for the control of the underlying infection.

The duration of leukocytopenia was linearly related to the cumulative percentage of patients who developed severe sepsis or septic shock. This observation is in line with an early report by Bodey and coworkers [9] who demonstrated a linear association between the duration of granulocytopenia and the frequency of infection. An important novel aspect from our study is that both the progression rate to circulatory shock and the mortality from septic complications disproportionately increased when the duration of leukocytopenia exceeded 20 days. Thus patients with severe sepsis during prolonged leukocytopenia are at high risk for the imminent development of septic shock and organ failure. This observation may have important bearing on the design of clinical trials evaluating the benefit of hematopoietic growth factors and progenitor cell support in patients after cytoreductive chemotherapy.

The peak levels of IL-6, IL-8, and immunoreactive TNF-α measured in our patients with sepsis in leukocytopenia are within the range of plasma concentrations reported for non-leukocytopenic patients with sepsis [7, 10]. Peak concentrations were related to the severity of the septic inflammatory response and to outcome, suggesting that sepsis in leukocytopenic patients with AML can be considered a cytokine release syndrome. On the other hand, cytokine concentrations were unrelatred to leukocyte counts and neither elastase and neopterin increased at the onset or during the course of sepsis in this patient group. This indicates that activation of circulating monocytes or granulocytes is not required for the inflammatory cytokine response to occur. The association of cytokine plasma levels and outcome warrants further evaluation of cytokine measurements as prognostic markers in leukocytopenic patients with sepsis.

References

1. Members of the American College of Chest Physicians/Society of Critical Care Medicine Consensus Conference Committee (1992) American College of Chest Physicians/Society of Critical Care Medicine Consensus Conference: Definitions for sepsis and organ failure and guidelines for the use of innovative therapies in sepsis. Crit Care Med. 20: 864–874
2. An expert report of the European Society of Intensive Care Medicine (1994) The problem of sepsis. Intensive Care Med 20: 300–304
3. Bone RC, Fisher CJ, Clemmer TP, Slotman GJ, Metz CA, Balk RA, the Methylprednisolone Severe Sepsis Study Group (1989) Sepsis syndrome: a valid clinical entity. Crit Care Med 17: 389–393
4. Bone RC, (1991) The pathogenesis of sepsis. Ann Intern Med 115: 457-469
5. Calandra T, Baumgartner JD, Grau GE, Wu MM, Lambert PH, Schellekens, J, Verhoef J, Glauser MP and the Swiss-Dutch J5 Immunoglobulin Study Group (1990) Prognostic values of tumor necrosis factor/cachectin, interleukin-1, interferon alpha and interferon gamma in the serum of patients with septic shock. J Infect Dis 161: 982–987
6. Pinsky MR, Vincent JL, Deviere J, Alegre M, Kahn RJ, Dupont E (1993) Serum cytokine levels in human septic shock: relation to multiple-system organ failure and mortality. Chest 103: 565–575
7. Casey LC, Balk RA, Bone RC (1993) Plasma cytokine and endotoxin levels correlate with survival in patients with the sepsis syndrome. Ann Interm Med 119: 771–778
8. Christman JW, Wheeler AP, Bernard GR (1991) Cytokines and sepsis: what are the therapeutic implications. J Crit Care 6: 172–182
9. Bodey GP, Buckley M, Sathe YS, Freireich EJ (1966) Quantitative relationship between circulating leukocytes and infection in patients with acute leukemia. Ann Intern Med 64: 328–340
10. Endo S, Inada K, Inoue Y, Kuwata Y, Suzuki M, Yamashita H, Hoshi S, Yoshida M (1992) Two types of septic shock classified by the plasma levels of cytokines and endotoxin. Circ Shock 38: 264–274

Acute Leukemias VI
Prognostic Factors
and Treatment Strategies
Büchner et al. (eds)

Interventional Antimicrobial Strategy in Neutropenic Infections

H. Link[1], G. Maschmeyer[2], P. Meyer[3], W. Hiddemann[4], W. Stille[5], M. Helmerking, and D. Adam[6]
for the study group of the Paul Ehrlich Society for Chemotherapy

Abstract. Different treatment strategies for 1573 patients with neutropenia < 1000/µl and fever 38.5 °C after cytotoxic chemotherapy were compared. 79% of patients had acute leukemia, 11.5% high-grade non-Hodgkin's lymphoma, and 9.5% blast crisis of chronic myeloid leukemia or advanced myelodysplastic syndrome. Patients with unexplained fever were randomized to a three-phase sequential study for different established drug regimens. If an infection could be defined microbiologically or clinically, treatment modifications were determined.

In phase I, treatment for all patients consisted of acylaminopenicillin (PEN) plus aminoglycoside (AMG), or third-generation cephalosporin (CEPH) plus AMG, or PEN plus CEPH. In 800 patients with unexplained fever the response rates were: PEN/AMG ($n = 258$): 74.4%, CEPH/AMG ($n = 252$): 73.4%; PEN/CEPH ($n = 290$): 70.0%. Total response rate was 72.5%. In phase II, patients not responding after 3 days received PEN/CEPH/vancomycin ($n = 70$) or PEN/CEPH/AMG ($n = 74$). The respective response rates were 52.9% and 55.4%, total 54.2%. If fever did not resolve,the patients received either PEN/CEPH ($n = 40$) orimipenem/cilastatin ($n = 59$) both in combination with amphotericin-B/5-flucytosin/rifampin. The response rates were 62.5% and 79.7%, respectively ($p = 0.07$), total 72.7%. Overall the differences between the treatment results were not significant. Analyzing all three phases together, 91.3% of patients with unexplained fever were cured. The response rates were also analyzed in patients with documented infections: in Gram-positive bacteremia ($n = 183$) the response rate was 82.5%, with Gram-negative organisms ($n = 145$) it was 78.6%, and in fungemia ($n = 51$) 43.1% ($p < 0.001$). In patients with lung infiltrates ($n = 269$), the response rate was 61.3% ($p < 0.001$), in clinically documented infections ($n = 198$) it was 84.4%, and in clinically and microbiologically documented infections ($n = 84$) 82.1%. If infections were defined after at least 5 febrile days, more lung infiltrates and fungal infections occurred ($p < 0.001$). Leukocytes recovering above 500/µl during the infection predicted better response rates ($p < 0.001$): in unexplained fever 97.8% vs. 86.5% and lower death rates 1.5% vs. 8.5%. In documented infections the response rates were then 89.9% vs. 62.3% and the death rates 7.0% vs. 20.5%. Therapy of neutropenic fever and infections must be adapted according to risk factors and should include early empiric antifungal therapy, especially in patients with lung infiltrates. The duration of neutropenia must be limited by hematopoietic growth factors.

[1]Medizinische Hochschule, Abteilung Hämatologie und Onkologie, 30625 Hannover, Germany
[2]Universitätsklinikum Rudolf Virchow, Robert-Rössle-Klinik, Abteilung Medizinische Onkologie und Angewandte Molekularbiologie, 13122 Berlin, Germany
[3]Medizinische Klinik und Poliklinik der Universität, 97070 Würzburg, Germany
[4]Medizinische Universitätsklinik, Abteilung Hämatologie und Onkologie, 37075 Göttingen, Germany
[5]Zentrum Innere Medizin, Universitätsklinik, 60590 Frankfurt/Main, Germany
[6]Paul Ehrlich Gesellschaft für Chemotherapie (PEG), Studienzentrale, 81701 Munich, Germany

Introduction

Infections due to severe neutropenia are a major cause of death in patients with hematological malignancies who are undergoing intensive cytotoxic chemotherapy [1–3]. Up to 75% of fatal complications in these patients are caused by infections during neutropenia [4–7]. Studies on the efficacy of antimicrobial treatment regimens resulted in response rates of 40%–70% [2, 3, 8–13]. Neutropenic infections demand a rapid initial therapy without knowing the causative organism. Therefore, treatment must cover a broad spectrum of probable harmful bacteria. Beside Gram-negative bacteria, Gram-positive organisms have gained increasing importance. In unresponsive patients, fungi and even opportunistic organisms have to be considered. However, the place for empirical antimicrobials directed against Gram-positive bacteria or fungi is still controversial. The aim of this prospective multicenter trial was the investigation of different treatment strategies in neutropenic patients with unexplained fever and of defined approached for documented infections [14, 15].

Materials and Methods

Patient Eligibility

Patients over 15 years of age with high-grade, malignant hematological disorders, including acute myeloid leukemia ($n=976$), acute lymphoblastic leukemia ($n=267$), blast crisis of chronic myeloid leukemia, advanced myelodysplastic syndrome ($n=149$), or high-grade lymphoma ($n=181$) were treated with this protocol. A granulocyte count $<1000/\mu l$ and fever $\geqslant 38.5$ °C after cytotoxic chemotherapy not related to the administration of drugs or blood products were the entry criteria for the study. Patients who had received parenteral antimicrobial drugs within the 7 preceding days or who had been in the study within the past 4 weeks were not eligible. In total 1573 patients were studied.

Treatment Protocol

Patients with unexplained fever were randomized to a three-phase sequential study for different established drug regimens. If an infection could be defined microbiologically or clinically, treatment modifications were determined.

In phase I, treatment for all patients consisted of acylaminopenicillin (PEN) plus aminoglycoside (AMG) or third-generation cephalosporin (CEPH) plus AMG or PEN plus CEPH (see Fig. 1, 2).

Unexplained Fever. In phase I, all patients were randomized to one of three treatment groups: PEN plus AMG, CEPH plus AMG, or PEN plus CEPH. Initial response was evaluated on days 4–6 of the study (Fig. 1). In responders, the applied regimen was maintained for at least 2 days post defervescence in patients with increasing neutrophil counts $>1000/\mu l$ or for 7 days in patients with persistent neutropenia ($<1000/\mu l$). In phase II, non-responders with persistent unexplained fever were randomized at days 4–6 to one or two new treatment groups: PEN plus CEPH in combination with either vancomycin (VAN) or AMG, and checked for response on days 8–11. Responders to the phase II regimen were maintained on treatment as described above. Patients with persistent unexplained fever or secondary non-responders were randomized in phase III to further two treatment groups: amphotericin B (AM-B) plus 5-flucytosine (5-FC) plus rifampin (RIFA) in combination with either the continued PEN/CEPH regimen or with imipenem/cilastatin (IMI). The maximum duration of the study was 21 days.

Defined Infections. The initial therapy of defined infections was identical to phase I therapy of unexplained fever. Modifications were defined according to the type and the response of the infection (Fig. 2).

Microbiologically Defined Infections. Treatment for infections with proven pathogens could be modified according to the respective susceptibility patterns if necessary. These patients were included in the analysis.

Clinically Defined Infections. In the case of clinically defined infections (CDI), the initial combination was supplemented with RIFA in patients with lung infiltrates, with VAN for skin or venous access inflammation or with metronidazole in the case of abdominal or perianal symptoms. If no clear microbiological definition of infection was possible, non-responders were treated with

Fever ≥38.5°C, granulocytes < 1000/µl

Randomized comparisons

Phase I

Penicillin Aminoglycoside	Cephalosporin Aminoglycoside	Penicillin Cephalosporin

No response: persistence of fever ≥38.5 °C : day 4 - 6

Phase II

Penicillin Cephalosporin Aminoglycoside	Penicillin Cephalosporin Vancomycin

No response: persistence of fever ≥38.5 °C: day 8 -11

Phase III

Penicillin, Cephalosporin Rifampin Amphotericin-B, 5-Flucytosine	Imipenem/Cilastatin Rifampin Amphotericin-B, 5-Flucytosine

Fig. 1. Treatment protocol in unexplained fever

Fever ≥38.5°C, granulocytes < 1000/µl

Randomized comparisons and treatment strategy

Phase I

Penicillin Aminoglycoside	Cephalosporin Aminoglycoside	Penicillin Cephalosporin

Phase II: modification

Pneumonia *+ Rifampin*	*Skin/venous access:* *+ Vancomycin* *Abdomen, perianal :* *+ Metronidazole*	*Microorganism* *Modification ?*

No response: persistence of fever ≥38.5 °C : after 4 - 6 days

Phase III: Modification and addition of antifungal therapy

Imipenem, Cilastatin
Rifampin
Amphotericin-B, 5-Flucytosine

Fig. 2. Treatment protocol in defined infections

IMI, RIFA, AM-B plus 5-FC starting from days 4–6 of the study.

Selection and Dosage of Antimicrobial Drugs

The dosage of all antimicrobial agents used in the study was prescribed according to approved manufacturer guidelines. To allow for the local susceptibility patterns of Gram-negative aerobic bacilli and *Staphylococcus aureus*, the following options were available to the participating centers: azlocillin (5.0 g every 8 h) or piperacillin (4.0 g every 8 h) as the PEN; cefmenoxime, cefotaxime, ceftazidime, or ceftizoxime (2.0 g every 8 h) as the third-generation CEPH; amikacin (7.5 mg/kg of body weight every 12 h), gentamicin, tobramycin (both 1.5 mg/kg every 8 h), or netilmicin (2.0 mg/kg every 8 h) as the AMG; For other trial agents daily dosages were: IMI 1.0 g every 8 h; VAN 0.5 g every 6 h; metronidazole 0.5 g every 8 h; RIFA 0.6 g once daily; 5-FC 37.5 mg/kg every 6 h; and AM-B 0.5 mg/kg every 24 h or 1.0 mg/kg every 48 h. Dosages were adjusted according to renal function if required.

Randomization Procedure and Control

Sequential randomization was performed by attaching three sealed and numbered envelopes to the case record form assigned to each patient selected for the study. The second and third envelope were to be opened only for non-responders in the previous study phase. Case record forms were reviewed for correct handling by the study centers before data analysis.

Response Criteria

In the case of unexplained fever, response was defined as defervescence with no requirement for further antimicrobial treatment for at least 7 days after the termination of treatment. In clinically defined infections, resolution of the respective clinical signs was also required, without a recurrence of the infection for at least 1 week after the initial antibacterial regimen had been stopped. The causative pathogen also had to be eliminated. Patients fulfilling response criteria on days 4–6 of the respective treatment phase, but subsequently relapsing with fever and/or clinical symptoms under continuing antimicrobial therapy or within 2 days after cessation of treatment were regarded as secondary non-responders. The addition of any antibacterial, a change to the initial therapy, or proceeding to a subsequent treatment phase, was recorded as non-response [16]. Patients with initial response and relapse of fever within 7 days were assessed as non-responders. Patients who did not respond during any of the study phases or who died as a result of infection were recorded as failures.

Results

Unexplained Fever

In 800 patients with unexplained fever the response rates were: PEN/AMG ($n=258$): 74.4%, CEPH/AMG ($n=252$): 73.4%; PEN/CEPH ($n=290$): 70.0%. Total response rate was 72.5%. In phase II, patients not responding after 3 days received PEN/CEPH/VAN ($n=70$) or PEN/ CEPH/ AMG ($n=74$). The respective response rates were 52.9% and 55.4%, total 54.2%. If fever did not resolve, the patients received either PEN/ CEPH ($n=40$) or IMI ($n=59$) both in combination with AM-B/5-FC/RIFA. The response rates were 62.5% and 79.7%, respectively ($p=$ 0.07), total 72.7%. No significant differences between the treatment modalities compared were found. Analyzing all three phases together, 91.3% of patients with unexplained fever were cured.

Documented Infections

The response rate was also analyzed by patients with Gram-positive bacteremia ($n=183$), response rate: 82.5%; Gram-negative organisms ($n=145$) 78.6%; fungemia ($n=51$) 43.1% ($p<$ 0.001) (see Table 1); lung infiltrates ($n=269$) 61.3% ($p<0.001$); clinically documented infections (n = 198) 84.4%; and in clinically and microbiologically documented infections ($n=$ 84) 82.1%. Table 2 shows the results bacterial bloodstream infections and clinically defined infections according to the initial treatment modalities.

If the causes of infections were diagnosed after at least 5 febrile days, more lung infiltrates and fungal infections occurred ($p<0.001$; see Table 3).

Table 1. Response in patients with microbiologically defined infections

Pathogen	Total		Complete response		Non-response		Death	
	(*n*)	(%)	(*n*)	(%)	(*n*)	(%)	(*n*)	(%)
Gram-positive	18	40.5	151	82.5[a]	14	7.7	18	9.8
Gram-negative	145	32.1	114	78.6[a]	10	6.9	21	14.5
Fungi	51	11.3	22	43.1[a]	12	23.5	17	33.3
G-pos. + G-neg.	37	8.2	29	78.4	2	5.4	6	16.2
G-pos. + fungi	16	3.5	8		4	4		
G-neg. + fungi	14	3.1	9		1	4		
G-pos.+G-neg.+fungi	2 0.4	1	1					
Others	4	0.9	4	-				
	452	100.0	337	74.6	44	9.7	71	5.7

[a] CR rate bacterial vs. fungal infections: $p<0.001$ (Fisher's exact test).

Table 2. Treatment results in defined infections according to antibiotic therapy

Defined infection	Result	Treatment group							
		PEN AMG		CEPH AMG		PEN CEPH		Modified	
		(*n*)	(%)	(*n*)	(%)	(*n*)	(%)	(*n*)	(%)
Bactermia	Response	21	87.5	17	89.4	25	89.2	24	82.7
Gram-positive	NR	-		1	5.2	1	3.5	3	10.3
	Death	3	12.5	1	5.2	3	10.7	2	6.8
Bacteremia -	Resp	15	93.7	21	87.5	16	76.1	24	82.7
Gram-negative	NR	-		-		1	4.7	1	3.4
	Death	1	6.2	3	12.5	4	19.0	4	13.7
Clinically	Resp	44	91.6	51	86.4	51	86.4	22	68.7
defined	NR	3	6.2	4	7.1	5	8.4	7	21.8
infection	Death	1	2.8	4	7.1	3	5.0	3	9.3

Patients who were initially treated with different or additional drugs are analyzed in the group "modified", there were no significant differences in response rates; NR, no response.

Table 3. Changes of patterns in patients with defined infections under study

			Defined at				
			Days 1–5		Days 6–21		
	(*n*)	(%)	(*n*)	(%)	(*n*)	(%)	p[a]
Site of infection							
Lung infiltrate	269	30.5	171	24.4	98	53.6	< 0.001
Venous access infection	184	20.8	142	20.3	42	23.0	
Abdominal infection	71	8.0	60	8.6	11	6.0	
Bacteremia/fungemia	222	25.1	213	30.4	9	4.9	< 0.001
Other	137	15.5	114	16.3	23	12.6	
Total no. of infections (superadditive)[b]	883	100.0	700	100.0	183	100.0	
Pathogens							
Gram-positive	269	46.2	244	51.5	25	23.1	< 0.001
Gram-negative	213	36.6	188	39.7	25	23.1	0.01
Fungi	95	16.3	39	8.2	56	51.9	< 0.001
Other	5		3		2	n.s.	
Total no. of pathogens	582		474		108		

[a] Fisher's exact test.
[b] In case of multiple sites of infection, each site was counted separately.

In patients with lung infiltrates (LI), response rates among the three initial treatment groups in phase I: PEN/AMG4 ($n = 68$): 55.9%; vs. CEPH/AMG ($n = 69$): 62.2% vs. PEN/CEPH ($n = 72$): 63.9%, were not significantly different ($p = 0.78$). In 60 patients the initial treatment regimen was modified, resulting in a response rate of 60%. In 67 patients, RIFA could not be administered as scheduled, mostly due to elevated liver enzymes. However, they were assessed and evaluated as study patients. Their response rate (58.2%) did not differ from those patients administered RIFA as scheduled (response rate, 62.4%, $p = 0.57$). In 123 patients, LI were only clinically defined and in 79 patients they were also defined microbiologically. In 67 patients, LI were associated with another defined infection.

The response rates among these three subgroups were not significantly different (63.4% vs. 58.2% vs. 60.8%, $p = 0.77$). In patients with microbiologically defined LI, fungi were most common (42.7%), followed by Gram-negative (31.3%), and Gram-positive pathogens (22.3%), while *Pneumocystis carinii* was detected in four cases (3.9%). The response rate in LI with fungal involvement (46.3%) was significantly inferior to that of LI from bacterial origin (76.3%, $p = 0.01$). Among 44 documented fungal pneumonias, there were 19 cases of aspergillosis, seven patients were non-responders and six died during the study.

Leukocyte Counts and Response. Leukocytes rising above 500/µl during the infection predicted better response rates ($p < 0.001$): in unexplained fever 97.8% vs. 86.5% and lower death rates 1.5% vs. 8.5%. In documented infections the response rates were then 89.9% vs. 62.3% and the death rates 7.0% vs. 20.5%.

Discussion

Despite marked differences in their in vitro activity, and in contrast to other clinical studies on agents used in this trial in a comparable patient population, no significant differences with respect to response and death rates could be detected between the different first-line treatment regimens or between the different eligible agents within the treatment groups. In unexplained neutropenic fever, a first-line regimen combining a modern β-lactam and an aminoglycoside antibiotic or two β-lactams with reliable efficacy against Gram-negative aerobic pathogens and *Staphylococcus aureus* results in an initial response rate of 70%–74%. Similar results were reported by others [10, 17, 18]. The treatment modifications in unresponsive fever with added VAN or AMG are equivalent, but have only moderate success. The change at second modification to carbapenem antibiotics and the addition of antifungal therapy was effective and should be considered earlier during the course of the infection. Thus, after stepwise modifications, the overall response in unexplained fever was 91.6%.

In documented bacterial infections, the different treatment schedules were not significantly different, either in Gram-negative or in Gram-positive organisms. However, the response rate in Gram-negative organisms is lower. Thus improvement of therapy is necessary.

Patients with fungal infections had the worst outcome. The rate of these infections was significantly increased when the pathogen was isolated beyond 5 febrile days. Hence antifungal therapy is warranted earlier during the course of the fever. LI are caused by fungi in a high proportion of cases and patients have a poor prognosis. Therefore they should also be treated initially with antifungal drugs. The failure rate declined in all types of infection if leukocytes recovered during the course of infection. Therefore the stimulation of leukocyte recovery with hematopoietic growth factors should be evaluated during neutropenia [19–21]. Finally, this study has shown that risk factors can be identified in neutropenic patients with fever, which should be considered in the treatment strategy.

References

1. Bodey GP, Buckley M, Sathe YS, Freireich EJ. Quantitative relationships between circulating leukocytes and infection in patients with acute leukemia. Ann Intern Med 1966; 64: 328–340.
2. EORTC, International Antimicrobial Therapy Cooperative Group. Ceftazidime combined with a short or long course of amikacin for empirical therapy of Gram-negative bacteremia in cancer patients with granulocytopenia. N Engl J Med 1987; 317: 1692–1698.
3. Klastersky J, Glauser MP, Schimpff SC, Zinner SH, Gaya H, EORTC, International Antimicrobial Therapy Cooperative Group. Prospective randomized comparison of three antibiotic regimens for empirical therapy of suspected bacteremic infection in febrile granulocytopenic patients. Antimicrob. Agents Chemother. 1986; 29: 263–270.
4. Estey EH, Keating MJ, McCredie KB, Bodey GP, Freireich EJ. Causes of initial remission induction failure in acute myelogenous leukemia. Blood 1982; 60: 309–315.
5. O'Hanley P, Easaw J, Rugo H, Easaw S. Infectious disease management of adult leukemic patients undergoing chemotherapy: 1982 to 1986 experience at Stanford University Hospital. Am J Med 1989; 87: 605–613.
6. Brown AE. Neutropenia, fever, and infection. Am.J.Med. 1984; 76: 421–428.
7. Barcos M, Lane W, Gomez GA, Han T, Freeman A, Preisler H, Henderson E. An autopsy study of 1206 acute and chronic leukemias (1958 to 1982). Cancer 1987; 60: 827–837.
8. Freifeld AG, Walsh T, Marshall D, Gress J, Steinberg SM, Hathorn J, Rubin M, Jarosinski P, Gill V, Young RC, Pizzo PA. Monotherapy for fever

and neutropenia in cancer patients: a randomized comparison of ceftazidime versus imipenem. J Clin Oncol 1995; 13: 165–176.
9. Anaissie EJ, Fainstein V, Bodey GP, Rolston K, Elting L, Kantarjian H, Cabanillas F, McCredie KB. Randomized trial of beta-lactam regimens in febrile neutropenic cancer patients. Am J Med 1988; 84: 581–589.
10. Rolston KV, Berkey P, Bodey GP, Anaissie EJ, Khardori NM, Joshi JH, Keating MJ, Holmes FA, Cabanillas FF, Elting L. A comparison of imipenem to ceftazidime with or without amikacin as empiric therapy in febrile neutropenic patients. Arch.Intern.Med. 1992; 152: 283–291.
11. Winston DJ, Barnes RC, Ho WG, Young LS, Champlin RE, Gale RP. Moxalactam plus piperacillin versus moxalactam plus amikacin in febrile granulocytopenic patients. Am.J.Med. 1984; 77: 442–450.
12. Pizzo PA. Management of fever in patients with cancer and treatment-induced neutropenia. N Engl J Med 1993; 328: 1323–1332.
13. de Pauw BE, Deresinski SC, Feld R, Lane Allman EF, Donnelly JP. Ceftazidime compared with piperacillin and tobramycin for the empiric treatment of fever in neutropenic patients with cancer. A multicenter randomized trial. The Intercontinental Antimicrobial Study Group. Ann Intern Med 1994; 120: 834–844.
14. Link H, Maschmeyer G, Meyer P, Hiddemann W, Stille W, Helmerking M, Adam D, for the study group of the Paul Ehrlich Society for Chemotherapy. Interventional antimicrobial therapy in febrile neutropenic patients. Ann Hematol 1994; 69: 231–243.
15. Maschmeyer G, Link H, Hiddemann W, Meyer P, Helmerking M, Eisenmann E, Schmitt J, Adam D. Pulmonary infiltrations in febrile neutropenic patients. Risk factors and outcome under empirical antimicrobial therapy in a randomized multicenter study. Cancer 1994; 73: 2296–2304.
16. European Organization for Research and Treatment of Cancer (EORTC) International Antimicrobial Therapy Cooperative Group and the National Cancer Institute of Canada-Clinical Trials Group. Vancomycin added to empirical combination antibiotic therapy for fever in granulocytopenic patients. J Inf Dis 1991; 163: 951–958.
17. Winston DJ, Ho WG, Bruckner DA, Champlin RE. Beta-lactam antibiotic therapy in febrile granulocytopenic patients. A randomized trial comparing cefoperazone plus piperacillin, ceftazidime plus piperacillin, and imipenem alone [see comments]. Ann Intern Med 1991; 115: 849–859.
18. EORTC. Piperacillin/tazobactam plus amikacin versus ceftazidime plus amikacin as therapy for fever in patients with granulocytopenia: a prospective, randomized, multicenter study. The International Antimicrobial Therapy Cooperative Group of the EORTC. American Society for Microbiology, Proceedings of the 33rd Interscience Conference on Antimicrobial Agents and Chemotherapy, New Orelans 1993; 237
19. Fleischmann R. South-Western Internal Medicine Conference: Clinical use of hematopoietic growth factors. Am.J.Med.Sci. 1994; 30: 248–273.
20. Link H, Herrmann F, Welte K, Aulitzky WE, Ganser A, Kern W, Meyer P, Schrappe M, Schmoll HJ, Werdan K, Kern P. Rationale Therapie mit G-CSF und GM-CSF. Med Klin 1994; 89: 429–441.
21. Maher DW, Lieschke GJ, Green M, Bishop J, Stuart Harris R, Wolf M, Sheridan WP, Kefford RF, Cebon J, Olver I, et al. Filgrastim in patients with chemotherapy-induced febrile neutropenia. A double-blind, placebo-controlled trial [see comments]. Ann Intern Med 1994; 121: 492–501.

Appendix 1

Participating Investigators at 23 Centers

Berlin Rudolf Virchow	W. Siegert
Berlin Benjamin Franklin	G. Hoeffken
Bonn	J. Hartlapp
Dortmund	W. Freund
Düsseldorf	H. Wolf, R. Scharf
Duisburg	J. Selbach
Essen-Werden	G. Maschmeyer, F. Wendt†
Frankfurt	A. Böhme, W. Stille
Frankfurt-Hoechst	K. Burkhardt
Hannover	H. Link
Heidelberg	A. Deboben
Kiel	D. Duncker
Köln	B. Lathan
Krefeld	M. Planker
Lübeck	R. Marre
Mannheim	A. Loesch
Munich-Großhadern	S. Sauer
Munich-Harlaching	N. Brack
Munich-Schwabing	T. Lipp
Münster	W. Hiddemann
Oldenburg-Städt. KH	R. Siegmund
Tübingen	K. Jaschonek
Würzburg	P. Meyer

Acute Leukemias VI
Prognostic Factors
and Treatment Strategies
Büchner et al. (eds)

Acyclovir and Cytomegalovirus Immunoglobulins as Prophylaxis for Cytomegalovirus Infections in Allogeneic Bone Marrow Transplant Recipients

J. Meharchand, A. Dmytrijuk, G. Phillips, A. Smith, L. Huebsch, T. Shore, N. Buscard, and H.A. Messner
for the Canadian Bone Marrow Transplant Group

Abstract. It is now possible to either prevent or successfully treat cytomegalovirus (CMV)-related disease in a significant number of bone marrow transplant recipients using multiple approaches. The clinical study performed by the Canadian Bone Marrow Transplant Group (CMBTG) testing resulted in a decreased rate of severe acute graft-versus-host disease and a more favorable response of patients that developed CMV disease in spite of the prophylaxis was observed for patients in the CMV immunoglobulin (CMV-Ig)-treated group. Acyclovir and CMV-Ig did not result in a significant survival advantage of the group treated with the combined strategy over the group receiving acyclovir alone. Preemptive therapy with ganciclovir holds promise to represent a successful and cost-effective strategy to prevent development of CMV disease in patients at risk.

Introduction

The survival of recipients of bone marrow allografts has significantly improved over the past 15 years. This has been demonstrated in reports by various single institutions and bone marrow transplant (BMT) registries. A review of 97 consecutive patients undergoing transplantation at the Princess Margaret Hospital 1979–1994 for acute myeloid leukemia in first complete remission demonstrated a significant improvement over time. Patients undergoing transplantation between 1979 and 1986 showed a 5-year event-free survival of 42%. At 10 years 32% were alive and free of disease. In comparison, the event-free 5-year survival of patients undergoing transplantation since 1986 amounts to 67%. Since all patients were prepared with the same transplant regimen, it is likely that the improved survival resulted from better support as well as more effective prophylaxis against and therapy for transplant-related complications. The improvement coincided with the routine use of prophylactic cyclosporin and the advent of effective antiviral agents. A retrospective review of 177 consecutive patients undergoing transplantation at the Princess Margaret Hospital between 1979 and 1986 revealed 21 cases of biopsy or autopsy-proven cytomegalovirus (CMV) related interstitial pneumonitis. Twenty of these patients died as a result of their CMV infection (Table 1). The high fatality rate confirmed the universally poor experience of BMT centers with this complication [1]. The availability of acyclovir, ganciclovir, and immunoglobulin preparations with high anti-CMV titers led to the development of various strategies to improve the outcome of patients at risk for life-threatening CMV infections. These strategies have included prophylactic approaches [2–7] and preemptive therapies [8, 9] as well as treatment trials for established CMV infections [10, 11].

The focus of the present report is the description of a study that was designed to test the prophylactic value of acyclovir and CMV immunoglobulins (CMV-Ig) in the prevention of CMV infections. It also includes a preliminary assessment of preemptive therapy with ganci-

University of Toronto, The Princess Margaret Hospital, Toronto, Canada

Table 1. CMV-related disease in three cohorts of consecutive patients undergoing transplantation at Princess Margaret Hospital

Parameters	Group I (1979–1986)	Group II (1989–1992)	Group III (1992–1994)
Patients (n)	177	166	129
Patients at risk for CMV[a] (n)	-**	91	66
Patients at risk (%)	-	54.8	51.1
Mode of detection	Histology	Histology culture, immunofluorescence	Histology culture, immunofluorescence
CMV positive (n)	21	22	17
% of total	11.8	13.0	13.2
% of at risk	-	24.1	25.7
Died from CMV			
Number	20	6	1
% of CMV positive patients	95	27	5.9
% of patients	13.3	3.6	0.8
% of at risk	-	6.6	1.5

[a] CMV-positive recipients and/or donor
[b] Not available

clovir for patients found to be CMV positive on screening bronchoscopy around day 35 after BMT.

Study Background

A number of studies have demonstrated that the development of CMV disease may be influenced by the prophylactic, preemptive, or therapeutic administration of agents with antiviral activities. There is evidence for the beneficial therapeutic effect of ganciclovir combined with immunoglobulines in the treatment of established CMV-related pneumonitis [10, 11]. In addition, it has been shown that prophylaxis with acyclovir may prevent the development of CMV disease in patients at risk [5].

A multicenter, randomized study was conducted under the auspices of the Canadian Bone Marrow Transplant Group (CBMTG) to evaluate whether or not the prophylactic effect of acyclovir could be enhanced by the intravenous administration of an immunoglobulin (CMV-Ig) preparation with high anti-CMV titers (CMV IVEEGAM, Immuno, NY, NY, USA). The study was supported by the Canadian Red Cross and Immuno Clinical Research Corporation.

Study Design

Adult BMT recipients that were either CMV positive or who underwent transplantation with marrow from a CMV-positive donor, or both, were eligible for the study.

All patients received acyclovir at an intravenous dose of 500 mg/m^2 every 8 h for 28 days starting on the day of the transplant. Patients were randomized to receive or not to receive intravenous immunoglobulins at a dose of 500 mg/kg every 14 days × 4 months (nine doses) starting 1 week before the transplant. Patients were stratified according to transplant center, age, disease-related risk group, and availability of a related or unrelated donor. Predetermined endpoints of the study included: (a) development of CMV disease; (b) frequency and severity of acute graft-versus-host disease; (c) overall survival. Patients that developed CMV disease were treated at the discretion of their physicians.

Results

A total of 180 patients were entered into the study and randomized. At the time of this preliminary assessment complete data were available on 151 patients. The data are summarized in Tables 1 and 2. As can be seen, the prophylactic use of CMV-Ig, in addition to acyclovir, did not reduce the incidence of CMV-related disease. Patients receiving CMV-Ig, however, had a lower incidence of severe graft-versus-host disease compared to patients receiving only acyclovir. Similarly, patients in the CMV-Ig group that developed CMV disease seemed to have a more favorable survival compared to the acyclovir group. The study did not demonstrate a significant survival advantage for CMV-Ig treated individuals. Survival at one year was 68% for the CMV-treated group compared to 59% of the controls only treated with acyclovir ($p =$ not significant). The projected 4-year survival amounted to 60% versus 42%. Again, the differences in favor of combined therapy at this time are not statistically significant. The study would have to be expanded to include 328 or 396 patients, respectively, for a one-or two-sided test of sufficient statistical power to determine whether or not the observed difference of 18% reflects a real difference between the two areas of the study. This approach did not seem to be prudent in the light of promising therapeutic benefits of preemptive therapy with ganciclovir for individuals at risk of developing CMV disease as defined by a positive broncho-alveolar lavage performed around 35 days after the transplant.

Preemptive Therapy with Ganciclovir

Subsequent to the previous study, 69 consecutive patients that fulfilled the same eligibility criteria underwent transplantation at the Princess Margaret Hospital and, as patients in the above study, followed with a strategy that included a screening bronchoscopy with bronchoalveolar lavage. Patients demonstrating the presence of CMV either by immunofluorescence or shell vial culture were started on ganciclovir at a dose of 5 mg every kg 12 h for 14 days, followed by maintenance treatment of 5 mg per day × 5 days per week for 8 weeks and 5 mg/kg three times weekly for a further 8 weeks. Seventeen of the 69 patients were found to shed CMV (Table 1). All 17 patients responded to ganciclovir. However, one patient died 6 months later with CMV-related interstitial pneumonitis that was unresponsive to further therapy. As shown in Fig. 1, this highly effective therapy is associated with a significantly reduced cost compared to the tested prophylactic regimen, if one only takes into account the direct costs related to medications and diagnostic procedures.

Table 2. Patient Description and Outcome Measures

Parameters		Acyclovir CMV-Ig	Acyclovir	
Patients	(n)	71	80	
Median age (years)		38	37	
Standard risk	(n)	41	43	
High risk	(n)	30	37	
Related donor	(n)	59	68	
Unrelated donor	(n)	12	12	
Frequency of CMV disease and resolution				
CMV pneumonitis		5/8	7/11	
CMV enteritis		4/7	3/3	
CMV retinitis		2/2	–	
Mortality of patients with CMV infection				
Alive (n)		10	2	
Dead (n)		7	12	$p < 0.005$
Acute GVHD[a]				
Grade 0–1		27	32	
Grade 2		32	20	$p < 0.005$
Grade 3–4		8	26	

[a]GVHD, graft-versus-host disease, six, patients died before they were at risk of developing GVHD.

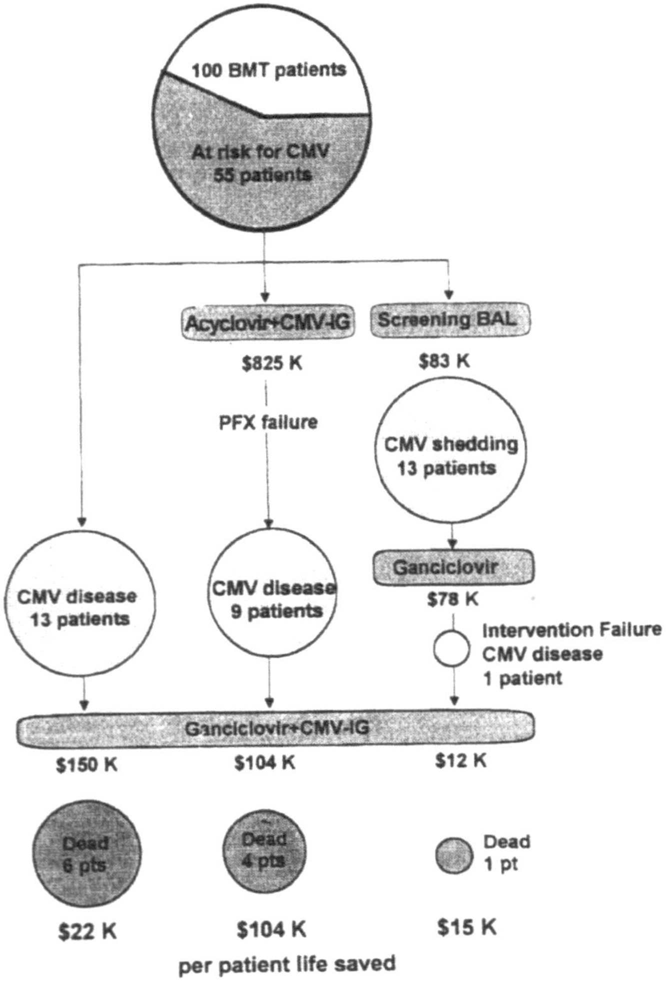

Fig. 1. Cost comparisons of three different strategies to manage CMV disease. They include treatment of established CMV disease using ganciclovir and CMV-Ig. Prophylaxis with acyclovic plus/minus CMV-lg, and preemptive therapy of patients found to shed CMV on a screening bronchoscopy performed around day 35 after BMT. The costs are based on current Canadian figures. They include only the cost for relevant diagnostic procedures and therapies. Secondary costs such as management of complications are not included

References

1. Meyers JD, Fluornoy N, Wade JC et al. Biology of interstitial pneumonia after marrow transplantation. In: Gale RP, ed. Recent advances in bone marrow transplantation. New York: Alan R. Liss, 1983.
2. Meyers JD, Leszczynski J, Zaia JA, et al. Prevention of cytomegalovirus infection by cytomegalovirus immune globulin after marrow transplantation. Ann Intern Med 1983; 98: 442–446.
3. Condie RM, O'Reilly RJ. Prevention of cytomegalovirus infection by prophylaxis with an intravenous, hyperimmune, native, unmodified cytomegalovirus globulin randomised trial in bone marrow transplant recipients. Am J Med 1984; 76 (Suppl 3A): 134–141.
4. Winston DJ, Ho W., Lin C-H, et al. Intravenous immune globulin for prevention of cytomegalovirus infection and interstitial pneumonia after bone marrow transplantation. Ann Intern Med 1987; 106: 12–18.

5. Meyers JD, Reed EC, Shepp DH, et al. Acyclovir for prevention of cytomegalovirus infection and disease after allogeneic marrow transplantation. N Engl J Med. 1988, 318; 70-75.
6. Atkinston K, Downs K, Golenia M, Biggs J, Marshall G. Prophylactic use of ganciclovir in allogeneic bone marrow transplantation: absence of clinical cytomegalovirus infection. Br J Haematol 1991; 79: 57-62.
7. Goodrich JM, Bowden R, Kellar E, et al. Prevention of cytomegalovirus disease after allogeneic marow transplant by ganciclovir prophylaxis. Fifth International Conference on Antiviral Research, 1992 (Vancouver, British Columbia).
8. Schmidt GM, Horak DA, Niland JC, et al. A randomised, controlled trial of prophylactic ganciclovir for cytomegalovirus pulmonary infection in recipients of allogeneic bone marrow transplants. N Engl J Med 1991; 324: 1005-1011.
9. Goodrich J, Mori M, Gleaves C, et al. Early treatment with ganciclovir to prevent cytomegalovirus disease after allogeneic marrow transplant. N Engl J Med 1991; 325: 1601-1607.
10. Reed EC, Bowden RA, Dandliker PS, et al. Treatment of cytomegalovirus pneumonia with ganciclovir and intravenous cytomegalovirus immunoglobulin in patients with bone marrow transplants. Ann Intern Med 1988; 109: 783-788.
11. Schmidt GM, Kovacs A, Zaia JA, et al. Ganciclovir/immunoglobulin combination therapy for the treatment of human cytomegalovirus-associated interstitial pneumonia in bone marrow allograft recipients. Transplantation 1988; 46: 905-907.

Acute Leukemias VI
Prognostic Factors
and Treatment Strategies
Büchner et al. (eds)

Challenge of Alloimmunization and Refractoriness to Platelet Transfusion

C.A. Schiffer

Abstract. Alloimmunization and refractoriness to platelet transfusion remains the major problem following repeated platelet transfusions. Approaches to donor selection for alloimmunized recipients include a variety of strategies for HLA matching and platelet crossmatching of random donor units of platelet concentrates as a means of identifying new compatible apheresis donors. Some patients can be managed with platelets obtained by apheresis during remission and cryopreserved for transfusion during subsequent periods of thrombocytopenia. Trials are under way evaluating the role of leukocyte depletion by platelet filtration and UVB irradiation of platelet preparations as a means of preventing alloimmunization. These approaches remain investigational at this time.

Introduction

Technologic advances permitting efficient collection and longer-term storage of platelets for transfusion represent one of the important success stories of leukemia treatment in the last 2 decades. It is now unusual for patients to succumb to hemorrhage prior to receiving adequate courses of treatment for leukemia and other hematologic malignancies. Nonetheless, platelet transfusion remains expensive and occasionally clinically ineffective, and can be associated with a number of side effects. Alloimmunization to antigens expressed on platelets with refractoriness to platelet transfusion remains the major problem following repeated platelet transfusions. This article will discuss new approaches to the management of this problem as well as techniques to reduce the incidence of alloimmunization.

Alloimmunization should be suspected when patients fail to have adequate platelet count increments following transfusion. In general, at least two ABO-compatible transfusions stored less than 72 h with poor increments should be documented prior to searching for histocompatible transfusions because, for reasons that are sometimes impossible to explain, patients can have poor increments to a single transfusion with subsequent sustained excellent responses to subsequent transfusions. Approximately 90% of patients refractory to platelet transfusion will have antibody detected by either platelet antibody testing or lymphocytotoxic antibody testing, the latter detecting antibody directed against HLA antigens [1]. Inadequate count increments measured 10 min after the completion of transfusion correlate well with the presence of lymphocytotoxic antibody [2, 3].

Matching of donor and recipient for HLA A and B antigens has been the mainstay of support for alloimmunized recipients. Overall, about 50%–60% of HLA-selected transfusions produce satisfactory increments in alloimmunized patients [4]. The ability to identify adequate numbers of donors in part depends on the frequency of the recipient's HLA antigens. For some patients, sometimes depending on the ethnic diversity of the donor pool, few if any available

Division of Hematologic Malignancies, University of Maryland Cancer Center, Division of Hematology/Medical Oncology, University of Maryland School of Medicine, Baltimore, MD 21201, USA

donors can be found [5]. The heterogeneity in the published response to HLA-matched transfusions is a consequence of a number of factors including: the titer and degree of reactivity of the recipient's antibody; the persistence of the antibody (anti-HLA antibodies can disappear in some patients over time and therefore should be monitored periodically) [6]; other complicating clinical conditions and particularly the presence of splenomegaly; the avoidance of donors with HLA types which have not produced successful increments in the past (and conversely, repeated use of donors with HLA types whose platelets have produced good increments in the past); inclusion of some patients in whom refractoriness is a consequence of medication-associated antiplatelet antibodies [7]; differing selection strategies for mismatching certain antigens between donor and recipient. The latter strategy can be quite successful and biologically intriguing. For example, HLA B44 and B45 can have variable expression on the lymphocytes and the platelets from the same individual. This antigen is often strongly expressed on leukocytes but weakly expressed on platelets. Thus, even when adiministered to patients with antibody against these antigens, platelets mismatched for HLA B44 or 45 can produce satisfactory increments approximately 75% of the time. Because this antigen is relatively commonly expressed, it is often possible to substantially increase donor availability for some patients [8]. Conversely, one can rarely successfully mismatch donors and recipients for HLA A2, an antigen found in 40%-50% of the Caucasian population [4].

There is some controversy about whether platelet antibody testing using the platelet as the target cell adds substantially to the results of donor selection by HLA typing [9]. This approach has the advantage of decreasing the requirement for recruitment of large numbers of HLA-typed platelet donors. We have utilized a solid-phase platelet crossmatching assay, which can be performed within 30-60 min, as a means of identifying donors for patients for whom HLA donors cannot be readily identified, either because of unusual HLA type or if HLA typing could not be performed, and as a supplement when only a small number of HLA-matched donors are available [10]. Samples are obtained sterilely from single units of platelet concentrates and units identified as compatible in vitro are transfused in aliquots of one to three units. If the transfusion produces an adequate corrected count increment, then the original red blood cell donor is contacted and asked to serve as an apheresis platelet donor. In a sense, the donor has "passed" both in vitro as well as in vivo crossmatch testing. This approach has worked quite well both as a means providing immediate platelet transfusion support as well as identifying new donors. Interestingly, some of the successful donors identifed in this fashion would not have been selected by HLA-matching criteria. In more heavily alloimmunized patients, it is sometimes necessary to crossmatch more than 100 units to identify even a single potentially compatible donor, and it is in this group of patients that we have found this approach to be of particular value. It is unknown whether this platelet crossmatching technique is more likely to be successful or cost effective than selection by HLA typing in less strongly alloimmunized recipients.

If compatible donors cannot be identified, the management of alloimmunization can be quite difficult. It is generally inadvisable to continue to provide prophylactic transfusions if the patient is not bleeding. Hemorrhage can be managed by the administration of "massive" doses of pooled random donor platelets. An occasional response is seen with this approach, which may sometimes be related to transient decrease in antibody titer, allowing subsequently administered platelets to circulate and exert a hemostatic effect [11]. It is also possible that, if many units of platelets from multiple donors are given, a histocompatible unit may be transfued fortuitously. Therapies that are of value in patients with immune thrombocytopenic purpura, such as intravenous gammaglobulin [12], corticosteroid therapy, splenectomy [13], and aggressive plasma exchange [14] are not of value in such alloimmunized patients. For many years, we have had a program of platelet cryopreservation in which alloimunized patients with leukemia in remission undergo platelet pheresis with cryopreservation of autologous Platelets using dimethylsulfoxide as a cryoprotective agent. These autologous platelets, which can be stored successfully for many years, are utilized during subsequent periods of thrombocytopenia. While the results are variable, on average, these frozen platelets produce increments approximately two thirds of those expected from fresh, histocompatible allogeneic platelets [15].

Prevention of Alloimmunization

There is strong evidence both from in vitro studies and murine platelet transfusion experiments demonstrating that it is the residual leukocytes contaminating platelet transfusions rather than the platelets themselves which provide the primary antigenic stimulus for the development of antibody against HLA antigens on platelets [16]. Because of this, there has been great interest in either reducing the level of contaminating leukocytes or "neutralizing" their antigenicity by UVB irradiation as a means of preventing the development of alloantibody. A number of highly efficient filters have been developed which are capable of relatively reliable, 3–4 log reduction in leukocyte contamination of platelets obtained either by apheresis or prepared as platelet concentrates. A "target level" of fewer than 5×10^6 leukocytes per transfusion has generally been stated, although there are virtually no data about how many leukocytes suffice to serve as an immunologic stimulus [17]. Leukocyte filtration is not without its problems, however. The filters are expensive, associated with appreciable loss of platelets (up to 25%–35% and sometimes greater when fresh apheresis platelets are filtered) and sometimes "fail" and permit excessive numbers of leukocytes to be transfused [18]. All red blood cell transfusions also have to be adequately leukodepleted, further adding to the cost of this treatment.

Although a number of small studies [19–23] suggested reduction of alloimmunization in patients receiving filtered platelets, these studies can be faulted because of: small patient numbers with low statistical power; heterogeneity in the patient population and the type of cytotoxic treatment administered; variability in quality control testing of the platelet product; different criteria for definition of alloimmunization and refractoriness; imbalances in known predisposing factors for alloimmunization such as prior pregnancies or transfusions; differing approaches to leukocyte depletion of red blood cell transfusions. Two recently published small trials failed to show benefit from leukocyte filtration including one in which filtration was done at the bedside, rather than in the blood bank [23, 24]. Similarly, a small trial evaluating UVB irradiation also failed to show a significant decrease in recipient alloimmunization [25]. Two editorials in *Blood*, published 4 years apart, reached similar conclusions, cautioning that leukocyte depletion is not yet proven to be a reliable means of preventing alloimmunization and refractoriness and should not be considered as standard care [26, 27].

A large, randomized, multi-insitutional trial (in the United States) (Trial to Reduce Alloimmunization to Platelets, TRAP) has recently completed registration of approximately 600 patients. This study evaluates both the rate of alloimmunization as assessed by antibody development and associated platelet refractoriness, in four groups of patients with newly diagnosed acute myeloid leukemia (AML) receiving standard induction therapy. The control group receives standard pooled platelet concentrates and is being compared to leukodepletion of platelet concentrates by filtration, UVB irradiation of pooled platelet concentrates, and leukodepleted single—donor platelets prepared by apheresis. The results of this large trial should be available within 1 year and hopefully will resolve many of the remaining issues about the value of different approaches to reduce alloimmunization.

It has also been suggested that leukocyte depletion of red blood cells prior to platelet concentrate preparation and storage might be more efficient and also might have a favourable effect on transmission of cytomegalovirus infections and the incidence of febrile transfusion reactions [28]. There is, however, at least a theoretical concern that this leukocyte depletion could have an adverse effect on the incidence of bacteremias following transfusion of stored platelets because leukocyte removal could allow increased proliferation of organisms inadvertently contaminating the platelets at the time of venipuncture. This is an uncommon, but well-described consequence of platelet transfusion [29] and represents a consideration as more modifications of blood products prior to transfusion are utilized and evaluated. It should also be noted that only a subfraction of patients would benefit from any successful approach to reduce the rate of alloimmunization. Only 30%–40% of patients become alloimmunized using standard, nonleukocyte-depleted platelets and red blood cells [30]. Not all of these 30%–40% of patients achieve complete remission and receive intensive post-remission therapy. It has therefore been estimated that only 10%–15% of patients with newly diagnosed AML might actually benefit clinically from any successful method of reducing alloimmunization [25]. Therefore, even if leukodepletion is proven to be partly effective in reducing the rate of alloimmunization, cost considerations will be of importance in deciding the widespread applicability of this approach.

In summary, although most alloimmunized patients can be managed successfully utilizing donor selection by other HLA typing or platelet crossmatching, it is hoped that ongoing clinical trials will demonstrate that the rate of alloimmunization can be decreased by modification of the transfused platelets. Until this time, it is advisable to monitor patients serologically to anticipate the need for histocompatible platelets and to treat patients in an environment in which such sophisticated transfusion support is readily available.

References

1. Hogge DE, Dutcher JP, Aisner J, Schiffer CA: Lymphocytotoxic antibody is a predictor of response to random donor platelet transfusion. Am J Heme 14: 363–70, 1983.
2. Daly PA, Schiffer CA, Aisner J, Wiernik PA: Platelet transfusion therapy—one hour post-transfusion increments are valuable in predicting the need for HLA-matched preparations. JAMA 243: 435–438, 1980.
3. O'Connell B, Lee EJ, Schiffer CA. The value of 10-minute posttransfusion platelets counts. Transfusion 28: 66–67, 1988.
4. Duquesnoy RJ, Filip DJ, Rodney GE, Rimm AA, Aster RH: Successful transfusion of platelets "mismatched" for HLA antigens to alloimmunized thrombocytopenic patients. Am J Hematol 2: 219–226, 1977.
5. Schiffer CA, Keller C, Dutcher JP, Aisner J, Hogge DE, Wiernik PH: Potential HLA matched platelet donor availability for alloimmunized patients. Transfusion 23: 286–289, 1983.
6. Lee EJ, Schiffter CA. Serial measurement of lymphocytotoxic antibody and response to nonmatched platelet transfusions in alloimmunized patients. Blood 70: 1727–29, 1987.
7. Christie DJ, van Buren N, Lennon SS, Putnam JL: Vancomycin-dependent antibodies associated with thrombocytopenia and refractoriness to platelet transfusion in patients with leukemia. Blood 75: 518–23, 1990.
8. Schiffer CA, O'Connel B, Lee EJ. Platelet transfusion therapy for alloimmunized patients: selective mismatching for HLA B12, an antigen with variable expression on platelets. Blood 74: 1172–76, 1989.
9. Freedman J, Gafni A, Garvey MB, Blanchette V: A cost-effectiveness evaluation of platelet crossmatching and HLA matching in the management of alloimmunized thrombocytopenic patients. Transfusion 29: 201–07, 1989.
10. O'Connell BA, Lee EJ, Rothko K, Hussein MA, Schiffer CA. Selection of histocompatible apheresis platelet donors by crossmatching random donor platelet concentrates. Blood 79: 527–531, 1992.
11. Nagasawa T, Kon BK, Baldini MG: Temporary suppression of circulating antiplatelet alloantibodies by the massive infusion of fresh, stored or lyophilized platelets. Transfusion 18: 429, 1978.
12. Schiffer CA, Hogge DE, Aisner J, Dutcher JP, Lee EJ, Papenberg D: High dose intravenous gammaglobulin in alloimmunized platelet transfusion recipients. Blood 64: 937–40, 1984.
13. Hogge DE, Dutcher JP, Aisner J, Schiffer CA: The ineffectiveness of random donor platelet transfusion in splenectomized, alloimmunized recipients. Blood 62: 253–256, 1984.
14. Bensinger WI, Buckner CD, Clift RA, Slichter SJ, Thomas ED: Plasma exchange for platelet alloimmunization. Transplantation 41: 602, 1986.
15. Schiffer CA, Aisner J, Wiernik PH: Frozen autologous platelet transfusion for patients with leukemia. N Eng J Med 299: 7–12, 1978.
16. Class FHJ, Smeenk RJT, Schmidt R, et al: Alloimmunization against the MHC antigens after platelet transfusions is due to contaminating leukocytes in the platelet suspension. Exp Hematol 9: 84–89, 1981.
17. Meryman HT: Transfusion-induced alloimmunization and immunosuppression and the effects of leukocyte depletion. Transfusion Med Rev 3: 180–93, 1989.
18. Kao KJ, Mickel M, Braine HG, Davis K, Enright H, Gernsheimer T, Gillespie MJ, Kickler TS, Lee EJ, McCullough JJ, McFarland JG, Nemo GJ, Noyes WD, Schiffer CA, Sell K, Slichter SJ, Woodson RD and the TRAP Study Group. White cell reduction in platelet concentrates and packed red cells by filtration: a multicenter clinical trial. Transfusion 35: 13–19, 1995.
19. Oksanen K, Kekomaki R, Ruutu T, Koskimies S, Myllyla G. Prevention of alloimmunization in patients with acute leukemia by use of white cell-reduced blood components—a randomized trial. Transfusion 31: 588–594, 1991.
20. Saarinen UM, Kekomäki R, Siimes MA, Myllylä G: Effective prophylaxis against platelet refractoriness in multitransfused patients by the use of leukocyte-free blood components. Blood 75: 512, 1990.
21. Sniecinski I, O'Donnell MR, Nowicki B, Hill LR: Prevention of refractoriness and HLA-alloimmunization using filtered blood products. Blood 71; 1402, 1988.
22. van Marwijk Kooy M, van Prooijen HC, Moes M, Bosma-Stants I, Akkerman JWN: The use of leukocyte-depleted platelet concentrates for the prevention of refractoriness and primary HLA alloimmunization; a prospective, randomized trial. Blood 77: 201, 1990.
23. Sintnicolaas K, van Marwijk Kooij M, van Prooijen HC, van Dijk BA, van Putten WLJ, Claas FHJ,

Novotny VMJ, Brand A. Leukocyte depletion of random single-donor platelet transfusions does not prevent secondary human leukocyte antigen-alloimmunization and refractoriness: a randomized prospective study. Blood 85: 824–828, 1995.
24. Williamson LM, Wimperis JZ, Williamson P, Copplestone JA, Gooi HC, Morgenstern GR, Norfolk DR, for the Alloimmunization Group: Bedside filtration of blood products in the prevention of HLA alloimmunization—a prospective randomized study. Blood 83: 3028, 1994.
25. Grijzenhout MA, Aarts-Riemens MI, de Gruijl FR, van Weelden H,van Prooijen HC. UVB irradiation of human platelet concentrates does not prevent HLA alloimmunization in recipients. Blood 84: 3524–3531, 1994.
26. Schiffer CA. Preventation of alloimmunization against platelets. Blood 77: 1–4, 1991.
27. Heddle NM, Blajchman MA. The leukodepletion of cellular blood products in the prevention of HLA-alloimmunization and refractoriness to allogeneic platelet transfusions. Blood 85: 603–606, 1995.
28. Stack G, Snyder EL. Cytokine generation in stored platelet concentrates. Transfusion 34: 20–25, 1994.
29. Braine HG, Kickler TS, Charache P, Ness PM, Davis J, Reichart C, Fuller AK: Bacterial sepsis secondary to platelet transfusion: an adverse effect of extended storage at room temperature. Transfusion 26: 391–93, 1986.
30. Dutcher JP, Schiffer CA, Aisner J, Wiernik PH: Long-term follow-up of patients with leukemia receiving platelet transfusions: identification of a large group of patients who do not become alloimmunized. Blood 58: 1007–11, 1981.

Acute Leukemias VI
Prognostic Factors
and Treatment Strategies
Büchner et al. (eds)

Polymerase Chain Reaction for Detection of Various *Aspergillus* Species in Clinical Samples

H. Hebart[1], U. Schumacher[2], G. Roller[1], J. Löffler[1], I. Rothenhöfer[1], G. Ehninger[1], C.A. Müller[1], and H. Einsele[1]

Abstract. To improve the detection of clinically relevant *Aspergillus* species a polymerase chain reaction (PCR) technique was designed to amplify a DNA sequence out of the 18ssu rRNA gene which is highly conserved among a variety of different fungal pathogens. Thus, by computer-assisted alignment of DNA sequences of various infectious agents, primers were chosen allowing specific and sensitive detection (100 fg of genomic fungal DNA) of all clinically relevant *Aspergillus* species. A wide variety of clinical isolates of *Aspergillus* species was reliably amplifiable by this PCR assay. To assess clinical applicability of the assay, blood samples from 15 healthy control persons and blood and plasma samples from 12 patients with proven aspergillosis were tested. All blood samples from the control persons were negative by PCR. Blood samples obtained from nine patients with proven invasive aspergillosis were found PCR positive. Moreover, five out of nine plasma samples of another three patients with proven invasive aspergillosis proved to be PCR positive and hybridized specifically with the *Aspergillus* oligonucleotide probe. Thus, this assay allows sensitive and specific detection of *Aspergillus* DNA in blood and plasma samples of patients with proven aspergillosis.

Introduction

In recent years, *Aspergillus* species have emerged as important nosocomial pathogens [1]. The diagnosis of invasive pulmonary aspergillosis, a life-threatening condition in the immunocompromised host, is often made only at autospy [2] with blood cultures being positive only in rare occassions. Serological kits available for the detection of *Candida* and *Aspergillus* infections often have problems in sensitivity or specificity or both [3–6]. Consequently, in immunosuppressed patients, the potentially highly toxic antifungal therapy is administered more often for presumed than for proven fungal infection.

Thus, more sensitive techniques for detection of fungal pathogens are urgently needed to earlier diagnose fungemia. In recent years, molecular biological techniques, hybridization assays with fungus-specific DNA probes [7, 8] and the polymerase chain reaction (PCR) assays [9–15] have been developed and applied to the detection of pathogenic fungi.

Here we present a PCR assay which allows sensitive detection of all clinically relevant *Aspergillus* species.

Material and Methods

Materials

Various *Aspergillus* species (see Table 1) were collected in the department of Medical Microbiology in Tübingen. Further *Aspergillus* strains were kindly provided by the Fred Hutchinson Cancer Research Center, Seattle, USA.

[1]Medizinische Klinik and Poliklinik, Abt eilung II and Sektion für Transplantationimmunologie and Immunhämatologie, Universität Tübingen, 72076 Tübingen, Germany
[2]Medizinische Klinik and Poliklinik, Institut für Medizinische Mikrobiologie, Universität Tübingen, 72076 Tübingen, Germany

Table 1. Fungal pathogens (species/strains) analyzed in this study

Fungal species (strains detected)	Clinical isolates tested (*n*)
A. fumigatus	8
A. flavus	6
A. terreus	5
A. niger	7
A. nidulans	5
A. versicolor	3

All these isolates and laboratory strains were obtained from the Department of Medical Microbiology, Tübingen, Germany, from the FHCRC in Seattle, USA, and the Department of Medical Microbiology of the University of Innsbruck, Austria.

Fungal Cultures. Blood samples were cultured in culture medium (Bactec Fungal Medium, Becton Dickinson, Heidelberg, Germany) for 7 days at 30°C and tested daily for microbial growth by infrared detection (Bactec 860, Becton Dickinson). When detected positive, samples were subcultured on Sabouraud medium. Other clinical specimens (bronchoalveolar lavage, pleural effusions, cerebrospinal fluid, and biopsy specimens) were cultured for 7 days on Columbia blood, brain heart infusion, and Sabouraud agar.

DNA Extraction. Fungal suspensions were centrifuged at 5000 rpm for 15 min and then the pellet was incubated with 5 ml white cell lysis buffer consisting of proteinase K 200 µg/ml (Boehringer Mannheim, Germany) and 0.2% sodium dodecyl sulfate (SDS).

The pellets were treated with 500 µg zymolyase (300 mg/ml) (ICN, Biomedicals, Coast Mesa, California, USA) to lyse the fungal cell wall. After centrifugation at 3000 rpm, the pellet was resuspended in 0.5 ml Tris/EDTA and then incubated with 50 ml 10% SDS to lyse the spheroblasts. After protein precipitation with 5 M potassium acetate (30 min on ice), DNA was precipitated with ice-cold isopropanol. The precipitate was collected by microcentrifugation and airdried after washing twice with ice-cold 70% ethanol. After resuspension in 30–50 µl double-distilled H_2O, DNA content and purity were determined by spectral photometry at 260, 280, and 320 nm.

Seeded blood culture medium, EDTA-anticoagulated blood, and all other clinical materials (plasma, pleural effusions, cerebrospinal fluid, bronchoalveolar lavage, and homogenized biopsies) were preincubated with white cell lysis buffer (WCLB) and further processed as already described.

Oligonucleotide Design. The design of oligonucleotide primers used in this study was based on comparison of the sequences of 18ssu ribosomal RNA genes (rDNA) in the GenBank database (EMBL, DDBJ databases). The amplification product amplified by these primers is 503 bp in length. Oligonucleotide probes were designed for specific hybridization with *A. fumigatus*, *A. flavus*, and *A. versicolor*, as well as one probe for *A. fumigatus*, *A. flavus*, *A. niger*, *A. terreus*, *A. nidulans*, and *A. versicolor*.

PCR Assay. Amplification reactions were performed on 50-µl volumes consisting of 10 m*M* Tris pH 9.6, 50 m*M* NaCl, 10 m*M* $MgCl_2$, 200 µg/ml bovine serum albumin, 0.5 mmol/l deoxyribonucleotide triphosphates, 100 pmol forward and reverse primer and 1.5 U of Taq polymerase (Amersham, Braunschweig, Germany). Template DNA (100 ng and if negative in a second experiment 500 ng) was added and 35 cycles of repeated denaturation, primer annealing, and enzymatic chain extension performed in a Biomed thermocycler (model 60). The amplification program included 30 s at 94°C, 1 min at 62°C, and 2 min at 72°C. The latter program was preceded by an incubation step of 4 min at 94°C and, after 35 cycles, followed by a 5-min incubation at 72°C. To monitor for false-positive results caused by contamination of clinical specimens during the extraction of DNA, aliquots of saline were prepared concurrently by the same procedure. Each PCR analysis of clinical samples included a positive control as well as negative controls (DNA extracted from human fibroblasts) to ascertain standardized conditions and specific amplification in each experiment.

Detection of the Amplification Products. 10 µl Aliquots of each amplification product were elctrophoretically separated in a 2% agarose gel in 50 × TAE buffer pH 8.0 (2 *M* Tris acetate pH 7.5, 0.1 *M* Na-EDTA). Amplification products were visualized by ethidium bromide staining. Transfer of the amplicon was performed by vacuum filtration onto nylon membranes (Hybond, Amersham, Braunschweig, Germany). Digoxigenin-labeled oligonucleotide probes were used for specific hybridization in the southern blot assay.

Sensitivity Studies. To determine the sensitivity limit of fungal DNA detection by PCR, PCR assays were performed on 100 ng, 10 ng, 1 ng, 100 pg, 10 pg, 1 pg, 100 fg, 50 fg, 10 fg genomic DNA of the *Aspergillus* species.

Patients

To assess clinical applicability of the assay, blood samples from 15 control persons and blood and plasma samples were obtained from 12 immunocompromised patients with proven invasive aspergillosis.

Results

Detection of Various *Aspergillus* Species

All the clinical isolates of the *Aspergillus* species shown in Table 1, either isolated from clinical material or obtained from the FHCRC in Seattle, USA, or the Department of Microbiology in Innsbruck, Austria, could be successfully amplified and detected in the ethidium bromide-stained gel.

Two oligonucleotide probes for specific detection of *Aspergillus* species were designed and synthesized. One of these probes showed specific hybridization with all the *Aspergillus* species, the other one hybridized with *A. fumigatus*, *A. flavus*, and *A. versicolor* only. To be able to detect all the *Aspergillus* species, especially *A. terreus* and *A. versicolor*, the DNA extraction protocol had to be slightly modified by the addition of NaOH because zymolyase and SDS treatment alone only induced insufficient DNA release from these *Aspergillus* species. By this modification, DNA release could be considerably improved to ascertain high sensitivity of detection of all the *Aspergillus* species.

Sensitivity

Different dilutions of purified extracted DNA (10 ng, 1 ng, 100 pg, 10 pg, 1 pg, 500 fg, 100 fg, 50 fg) from each of the *Aspergillus* species listed in Table 2 were amplified according to the PCR protocol shown. After electrophoresis in a 2% agarose gel and ethidium bromide staining, 100 fg of isolated DNA from all the *Aspergillus* species could be detected. By Southern blot hybridization, the sensitivity of fungus detection could be further increased to 50 fg isolated DNA of *A. fumigatus*, *A. flavus*, *A. terreus*, *A. niger*, *A. nidulans*, and *A. versicolor*.

Specificity

A wide range of template DNA extracted from different bacterial and viral pathogens, non-infected cells, tissues and cell lines was analyzed for DNA amplification in the ethidium bromide-stained agarose gel and in the Southern blot assay. None of the bacterial and viral pathogens analyzed nor DNA from human cells and tissues showed amplification products after PCR with the fungus-specific primers in the ethidium bromide-stained agarose gel or after hybridization with the *Aspergillus*-specific oligonucleotides, which hybridized either with *A. fumigatus*, *A. flavus*, *A. versicolor*, *A. niger*, *A. nidulans*, and *A. terreus*, or with *A. fumigatus*, *A. flavus*, and *A. versicolor* only.

Application to Clinical Material

Screening of Healthy Blood Donors. Fifty-three blood samples from 15 healthy control persons were analyzed by PCR assay. None of the 53 blood samples from these patients without evidence of local or systemic fungal infection showed fungus-specific amplicons after amplification with the pair of primers described.

Screening of Patients with Proven Aspergillosis. Twelve patients were diagnosed to suffer from invasive pulmonary aspergillosis. Five of these 12 patients with nodular pulmonary infiltrates were found to be culture-positive for *A. fumigatus* in the broncholaveolar lavage, in seven further patients diagnosis of invasive pulmonary aspergillosis was made post mortem (three of them had additional brain lesions). Blood samples obtained at the time of clinical manifestation from nine patients and five out of nine plasma samples of three patients were found PCR positive for fungus-specific DNA segments in the agarose gel, and all these amplicons showed hybridization only with the *Aspergillus*-specific oligonucleotide probes.

Screening of Clinical Material Apart from Blood Samples for the Presence of Fungal Pathogens. Five bronchoalveolar lavage samples and one pleural effusion specimen were analyzed for the presence of *Aspergillus* DNA. Amplicons of the DNA extracted from these samples hybridized with the *Aspergillus*-specific oligonucleotide probe.

Discussion

The PCR assay presented allows highly sensitive and specific detection of all clinically relevant *Aspergillus* species. A high sensitivity of the PCR assay is essential to detect fungal pathogens in blood samples obtained from patients with invasive aspergillosis as positive blood cultures in these patients are found in only about 1%. For clinical isolates of all *Aspergillus* species (*A. fumigatus, A. niger, A. nidulans, A. flavus, A. versicolor, A. terreus*), as few as 100 fg purified DNA could be detected after amplification and additional hybridization with a labeled internal oligonucleotide corresponding to two fungal genomes.

To achieve this high sensitivity of detection, the method of DNA extraction from molds had to be improved by the addition of NaOH which markedly increased the yield of DNA from these cells, epecially from *A. terreus* and *A. versicolor*.

Invasive pulmonary aspergillosis (IPA), usually caused by *A. fumigatus* or *A. flavus*, is a life-threatening condition of the immunocompromised host. Again, early diagnosis and treatment of this condition results in a more favorable outcome, so it is important that rapid methods for detecting the fungus are developed. Culture of *A. fumigatus* or *A. flavus* from respiratory tract specimens of immunosuppressed patients is usually indicative of IPA, but the diagnosis is not excluded by a negative result for the sensitivity ranges from only 50%-70%. Thus, improving the sensitivity of detection of *Aspergillus* species in broncho-alveolar lavage samples is essential. Using the 18ssu-rRNA-based PCR assay *Aspergillus*-specific DNA fragments could be detected in five broncho-alveolar lavage and in one pleural effusion specimen obtained from five patients with invasive aspergillosis. Three of these specimens, but not the pleural effusion sample, were also found to be culture positive for *A fumigatus*.

The high sensitivity of our assay encouraged us to also screen for *Aspergillus* DNA in blood samples obtained from patients with invasive aspergillosis. In 12 patients with histopathologically and/or broncho-alveolar lavage-proven invasive pulmonary aspergillosis-positive PCR signals were obtained from DNA extracted from blood nine or plasma three samples. In none of these patients were blood samples, drawn three times per week, found culture positive for *Aspergillus* in spite of the use of lysis culture assays. The higher sensitivity of detection of *Aspergillus* species in broncho-alveolar lavage as demonstrated for the PCR assay described compared to culture assays has been confirmed for another PCR assay [12].

Thus, PCR assays obviously provide improved sensitivity for detection of fungal pathogens in clinical material and thus might help to earlier diagnose and treat patients at risk of developing invasive aspergillosis.

References

1. Meyers JD: Fungal infections in bone marrow transplant patients. Sem Oncol 17 (Suppl. 6): 10–13, 1990
2. Aisner J, Schimpff SC, Wiernik PH: Treatment of invasive aspergillosis: relation of early diagnosis to outcome. Ann Intern Med 86: 539–543, 1977
3. Bodey GP: The emergence of fungi as major hospital pathogens. J Hosp Infect 11, Suppl. A: 411–426, 1988
4. Sabetta JR, Miniter P, Andriole VT: The diagnosis of invasive aspergillosis by an enzyme-linked immunosorbent assay for circulating antigen. J Infect Dis 152: 946–953, 1985
5. Kurup VP, Kumar A: Immunodiagnosis of aspergillosis. Clinical Microbiological Reviews 4: 439–456, 1991)
6. Buckley HR, Richardson MD, Evans EGV, Wheat LJ: Immunodiagnosis of invasive fungal infection. J Met Vet Mycol 30 Suppl 1: 249–260, 1992
7. Gabal MA: Development of a chromosomal DNA probe for the laboratory diagnosis of aspergillosis. Mycopathologica 106: 121–129, 1992
8. Holmes AR, Lee YC, Cannon RD, Jenkinson HF, Shepherd MG: Yeast-specific DNA probes and their application for the detection of Candida albicans. J Med Microbiol 37: 346–351, 1992
9. Buchman TG, Rossier M, Merz WG, Charache P: Detection of surgical pathogens by in vitro DNA amplification. I. Rapid identification of Candida albicans by in vitro amplification of a fungus-specific gene. Survery 108: 338–347, 1990
10. Miyakawa Y, Mabuchi T, Kagaya K, Fukazawa Y: Isolation and characterization of a species-specific DNA fragment for detection of Candida albicans by polymerase chain reaction. J Clin Microbiol 30: 894–900, 1992
11. Spreadbury C, Holden D, Aufauvre-Brown A, Bainbridge B, Cohen J: Detection of Aspergillus

fumigatus by polymerase chain reaction. J Clin Microbiol 31: 615–621, 1993
12. Tang CM, Holden DW, Aufauvre-Brown A, Cohen J: The detection of Aspergillus spp. by the polymerase chain reaction and its evaluation in bronchoalveolar lavage fluid. Am Respir Dis 148: 1313–1317, 1993
13. Jordan JA: PCR identification of four medically important Candida species by using a single primer pair. J Clin Microbiol 32: 2962–2967, 1994
14. Anaissie E, Bodey GP, Kantarjian H et al. New spectrum of fungal infections in patients with cancer. Rev Infect Dis 11: 369–378, 1989

Acute Leukemias VI
Prognostic Factors
and Treatment Strategies
Büchner et al. (eds)

Screening with Sensitive Detection Methods Allows a Reduction in the Incidence of Cytomegalovirus Disease After Allogeneic Bone Marrow Transplantation

H. Einsele[1], G. Ehninger[1], H. Hebart[1], G. Jahn[3], P. Mackes[1], M. Herter[2], T. Klingebiel[2], J. Löffler[1], and C.A. Müller[1]

Abstract. To improve the detection of cytomegalovirus (CMV) infection following allogeneic bone marrow transplantation (BMT), three highly sensitive detection methods (Polymerase chain reaction PCR, from whole blood, plasma PCR and antigenemia assay) were applied to weekly screen blood samples in patients receiving an allogeneic marrow transplant. By standardizing the number of blood cells analyzed, similar sensitivity and specificity of CMV detection could be achieved with all three highly sensitive techniques. To prove that highly sensitive screening actually allows earlier detection of CMV infection after BMT, the virus culture technique and PCR from whole blood were compared for the detection of CMV infection in this patient cohort. PCR assays allowed detection of the virus a median of 15 days prior to the culture technique. Following these promising findings, PCR-based preemptive therapy was administered to patients receiving an allogeneic marrow transplant and compared to preemptive therapy based on a positive virus culture assay from blood, urine, and throat washings. In a prospective study, 66 patients either received preemptive therapy based on the much more senstitive PCR technique (34 patients) or on culture assays (32 patients). Therapy was continued in both groups until clinical signs disappeared and PCR negativity was documented. Twenty-two patients in the PCR and 15 patients in the culture group received antiviral therapy. PCR allowed detection of the virus (median day + 32 compared to day + 49) and introduction of antiviral therapy significantly earlier than in the culture group (median day + 44 compared to day + 54). The incidence of CMV disease (2/34 vs. 8/32, $p = 0.02$) and CMV-associated mortality (0/34 vs. 5/32, $p = 0.02$) was significantly lower in the PCR group. Thus, preemptive therapy based on more sensitive detection methods like the PCR assay enables a reduction in the incidence of CMV disease and CMV-related mortality. Additionally, stopping and withholding antiviral therapy in a PCR-negative patient is safe and might help to reduce the duration of antiviral therapy.

Introduction

Cytomegalovirus (CMV) infection is still associated with a substantial proportion of the infectious morbidity and mortality following allogeneic bone marrow transplantation (BMT). Prior to the introduction of new antiviral agents such as ganciclovir and foscarnet, the case fatality rate was 85% among patients diagnosed with CMV pneumonia after allogeneic BMT [1]. Thus, until recently, approximately 15%–20% of the deaths occurring after transplant could be attributed to CMV disease of the lung [2].

In two recent studies [3,4], prophylactic ganciclovir administered to CMV-seropositive allogeneic BMT recipients in a randomized trial was

[1]Medizinische Klinik und Poliklinik, Abteilung II und Sektion für Transplantationsimmunologie und Immunhämatologie, Universität Tübingen, 72076 Tübingen, Germany
[2]Medizinische Klinik und Poliklinik, Kinderlinik, Universität Tübingen, 72076 Tübingen, Germany
[3]Medizinische Klinik und Poliklinik, Institut für Virologie, Universität Tübingen, 72076 Tübingen, Germany

shown to reduce the incidence and severity of CMV infection, but was found to be frequently associated with neutropenia and increasing rates of bacterial and fungal infections. No reduction in early post-transplant mortality could be demonstrated for the patient group receiving prophylactic ganciclovir. Recent studies have demonstrated that preemptive therapy with ganciclovir for culture-proven CMV infection is effective in reducing CMV disease and transplant-related mortality in seropositive allogeneic BMT recipients [5, 6]. However, approximately 12%–13% of patients presented with CMV disease before or coincident with CMV excretion as determined by conventional and shell vial culture assays [5, 6].

Thus, rapid, specific, and sensitive methods are essential for early diagnosis of CMV infection as well as for the monitoring of antiviral therapy. We have described the use of the polymerase chain reaction (PCR) for more rapid and sensitive detection of CMV infection after allogeneic BMT compared with the use of virus culture technique [7]. PCR proved to be a better predictor of the efficacy of antiviral therapy than virus culture or clinical assessment [8] and could be shown to provide a negative predictive value of 100% [9]. In recent publications, the amplification of DNA in plasma samples and the CMV antigenemia assay also proved to be rapid, sensitive, and specific methods for early detection of CMV infection [10–14].

Thus, these techniques were compared for sensitive CMV detection in blood samples obtained from BMT recipients. To evaluate clinical applicability of these new techniques, preemptive therapy with ganciclovir based on the PCR assay was compared with early intervention based on the conventional culture technique.

Patients and Methods

Patients and Clinical Specimens. To compare the three sensitive detection methods, 15 consecutive patients undergoing allogeneic or autologous BMT (median age 36 years, range 18–51 years) were monitored weekly between days +15 to > +100 for CMV infection by CMV DNA PCR, plasma PCR, pp65 antigenemia, and conventional as well as rapid shell vial culture technique.

Preparation of Target DNA. DNA was extracted from plasma or blood cells after proteinase K digestion using phenol/chloroform/isoamylalcohol extraction and precipitation as described before [7,8]. Plasma samples obtained from EDTA blood were maintained at −80°C in a period ranging from 1 week to 6 months; 100 ng extracted cellular DNA or the total amount of DNA extracted from 70 µl plasma (after two cycles of phenol/chloroform/isoamylalcohol extraction and precipitation) were used for PCR.

Polymerase Chain Reaction. Amplification of a 147-bp DNA fragment between positions 1767 and 1913 of the fourth exon of the immediate early gene of the HCMV strain AD169 using primers I and II has been described before [7, 8]. Briefly, 100 ng extracted DNA or the total amount of DNA extracted from 70 µl plasma was denatured at 94°C for 5 min and specifically amplified. Thirty-two cycles, each of which included 3 min for annealing and primer extension at 66°C followed by 1 min of denaturation at 94°C, were administered. To exclude the presence of polymerase inhibitors and to test the quality of the extracted DNA, a fragment of the human HLA class I genes (fourth exon, 129 bp long) was amplified in all samples in parallel. In all plasma samples no HLA class I signals could be detected. Therefore 100 ng DNA extracted from peripheral blood lymphocytes obtained from a CMV-seronegative person were added to each specimen to exclude the presence of polymerase inhibitors. Results were considered valid only if consistent in at least two independent experiments and when none of the negative controls showed amplification in either the agarose gel or after hybridizaion. Detection of the amplification products in a 2% agarose gel or by Southern blot analysis with a gamma ^{32}P-dATP-end-labeled internal oligonucleotide has been described previously [7, 8]. Each PCR analysis of clinical samples from patients before and after BMT included titrated cloned pCM5018 as positive control and several samples of DNA from peripheral blood of sero- and culture-negative normal donors as negative control. A semiquantitative analysis was performed with titrated amounts from 100 to 0.1 fg cloned HCMV DNA fragment pCM5018. After Southern bolt hybridization, the signal of 100 fg HCMV DNA fragment pCM5018 was scored + + +, the signal of 10 to 1 fg pCM5018 + +, and the signal of the lowest amount detectable, almost 0.1 fg, was scored +. The intensity of the signals of the titration curve was compared to the clinical samples and a semiquantative analysis from + to +++ was performed.

Detection of CMV Antigenemia. Polymorphonuclear leukocytes (PMNL) were isolated from 6 ml freshly collected citrate-anticoagulated blood using a dextran sedimentation method [10]. After two washes with phosphate-buffered saline (PBS) 2×10^5 leucocytes were cytocentrifuged on glass slides (Cytospin 3, Shandon Scientific Ltd., Astmoor, UK). Cytospin preparations were fixed with acetone/methanol (1:1) for 90 s at 4°C, air dried and stored at −80°C. After 1 h of incubation with a combination of 25 µl of each of two monoclonal antibodies directed against pp65 (Clonab,C10 and C11, Biotest AG, Dreieich, Germany) in a humid chamber, the slides were washed with Tris-buffered saline (TBS, 0.05 *M*, pH 7.6) and incubated for 30 min with 25 µl rabbit anti-mouse Ig (Dakopatts a/s, Glostrup, Denmark) diluted 1:20 in TBS. After washing three times with TBS, the slides were incubated with the alkaline phosphatase anti-alkaline phosphatase (APAAP) immune complex (Dako APAAP kit, Dakopatts) for 30 min at room temperature and washed thereafter with TBS, followed by incubation with 50 µl substrate (Neufuchsin solution K698, Dako, Carpenteria, USA) for 15 min. Counterstaining was performed with hematoxylin. The number of positive cells per 2×10^5 cells was counted using a Zeiss ZS500 microscope. CMV-infected fibroblasts were used as positive controls. A semiquantitative evaluation of the cytospin preparates was performed with 1–10 positive cells/2×10^5 leukocytes being +, 11–100 positive cells/ 2×10^5 leukocytes ++, and >100 positive cells/2×10^5 leukocytes +++, respectively.

Virus Culture. Blood, urine, and throat washings were conventionally inoculated on human embryonic lung fibroblasts maintained according to standard tissue culture techniques. CMV was identified by production of its characteristic cytopathic effects on human embryonic lung fibroblasts after at least 4 weeks of culture. Monoclonal antibodies directed against the early and immediate early antigen were additionally applied 48 h after inoculation of the fibroblasts for detection of viral antigen expression.

CMV Disease. CMV pneumonia, enteritis, or hepatitis were diagnosed according to the criteria that were defined by the Fourth International Cytomegalovirus Workshop in Paris 1993 [14].

Patients Receiving Preemptive Therapy. To evaluate the clinical utility of the sensitive techniques, 66 patients either received PCR-based or culture-based preemptive antiviral therapy with ganciclovir. These patients had received an allogeneic BMT at the BMT unit in Tübingen (Kinderklinik and Medizinische Universitätsklinik) for a hematological malignancy. The CMV serostatus of patients and bone marrow donors as well as of blood donors was determined by the ELISA technique. CMV-seronegative patients receiving a transplant from a CMV-seronegative donor and blood products from CMV-seronegative blood donors were also included to screen for false-positive results. Criteria for study entry included age > 6 years, no documented CMV infection at the time of BMT, and a serum creatinine of less or equal to 220 µmol/l. For the conditioning regimen, total body irradiation (TBI) was performed on 3 successive days (2 Gy twice a day, lung shielding 10 Gy). Cyclophosphamide 2×60 mg/kg was infused following TBI (Cy/TBI). In patients with accelerated chronic myelogenous leukemia (CML) or acute leukemia not in first remission, etoposide (VP-16/Cy/TBI) was added at a dosage of 40 mg/kg on day 3. Patients treated with busulfan and cyclophosphamide received busulfan at a dosage of 4×4mg/kg per day and cyclophosphamide at a dosage of 2×60 mg/kg.

Antiviral Treatment. Patients were followed by weekly viral cultures and PCR monitoring starting on the day of transplant. Patients were thoroughly screened until day + 100 after BMT. Patients received antiviral therapy either at the time of the second consecutive positive PCR signal (PCR group) or of a positive culture from urine, throat washings, and/or blood samples (culture group). To reduce overtreatment, only patients with two consecutive PCR-positive blood samples received preemptive therapy. Ganciclovir was given at a dose of 5 mg/kg body weight, administered intravenously twice daily for 14 days plus CMV hyperimmunoglobulin at a dosage of 0.2 g/kg body weight administered on days, 1, 3, 5, 7, and 14. Maintenance treatment with ganciclovir 5 mg/kg per day was administered when PCR monitoring still showed a positive result after cessation of antiviral therapy. If two consecutive positive PCR results were obtained in a patient who had been successfully treated (documented clearance of the virus by PCR), ganciclovir was reinstituted at a dosage of 5 mg/kg intravenously twice daily.

Results

CMV Detection: Comparison of PCR, Plasma PCR, CMV Antigenemia, and Conventional Virus Culture. A total amount of 109 blood samples of the 15 patients were tested simultaneously by PCR, plasma PCR, and CMV antigenemia. Overall, 96 to 109 blood samples showed identical results in the three assays ($p < 0.01$). Thirty-nine blood samples were found to be positive and 57 to be negative by all the assays applied. Discordant results between the three assays were only found when a low amount of virus was present. Only nine of the 15 patients developed culture-proven viremia and/or viruria, whereas all the 15 patients were found to be CMV positive by PCR, plasma PCR, and CMV antigenemia. CMV was diagnosed prior to a positive result in the virus culture by all three assays, confirming our previously reported results. All three assays proved to be negative at the end of antiviral therapy.

Preemptive Therapy. Sixty-Six patients who received an allogeneic BMT at the BMT unit in Tübingen were included in the study entry. About one third of the patients in each group received their transplant from a family donor not completely HLA matched or from an unrelated donor representing a population at very-high risk of developing CMV disease. The patients in the two groups were balanced for source of transplant and CMV serostatus of donor and recipient. The patients who received preemptive therapy based on culture technique did not differ from those receiving PCR-based preemptive therapy concerning age, conditioning regimen, graft-versus-host-disease (GVHD) prophylaxis and grade of acute GVHD prior to the development of CMV infection.

CMV Detection: Comparison of PCR and Culture Assay. Twenty-two patients were found to be PCR positive in the PCR group, and culture assays revealed 15 patients to be CMV infected in the culture group. Fifteen of 34 PCR-monitored patients excreted CMV in the PCR group compared to 15 of 32 patients in the culture group. The number of patients who became culture positive for CMV in blood, urine, and/or throat washings was not different. None of the PCR-negative patients; CMV was culture positive. None of the blood samples obtained from CMV-seronegative patients with a CMV-seronegative donor was found to be PCR- or culture-positive. The median day of diagnosis of CMV infection was day +32 in the PCR group and day +49 in the culture group (Fig. 1). PCR positive always preceded a positive culture assay in the patients analyzed simultaneously by both techniques. Among the patients of the PCR group, CMV infection was diagnosed by PCR assay a median of 15 days prior to culture positivity. In ten PCR-monitored patients, therapy had already been started at the time of first detection of the virus by culture technique.

Antiviral Therapy Based on PCR or Culture Assay. Treatment was started a median of 44 days after BMT in the PCR and a median of 54 days after BMT in the culture group. The duration of treatment was shorter for the PCR-monitored patients (see Fig. 1)

CMV Disease. All CMV-infected patients who developed CMV disease presented with disease as first manifestation and did not progress to disease during or following antiviral therapy. In seven of the ten patients who suffered from CMV disease, the marrow donor was CMV seropositive. Whereas only two PCR-monitored patients developed CMV disease (one CMV interstitial pneumonia, one CMV enteritis) a total of eight culture-monitored patients were found to have symptomatic CMV infection (six CMV interestitial pneumonia, two CMV enteritis). Two patients with CMV disease in the PCR group survived, whereas five patients died due to CMV disease in the culture group. Thus, CMV-related mortality was higher among the culture-monitored patients (five of 32 patients) compared to the PCR-monitored ones (0/34)($p = 0.02$). Overall survival until day +100 was better for the PCR group (32/34) compared to the culture group (23/32) ($p < 0.05$).

Discussion

In recent studies we demonstrated the PCR technique as allowing CMV detection in blood

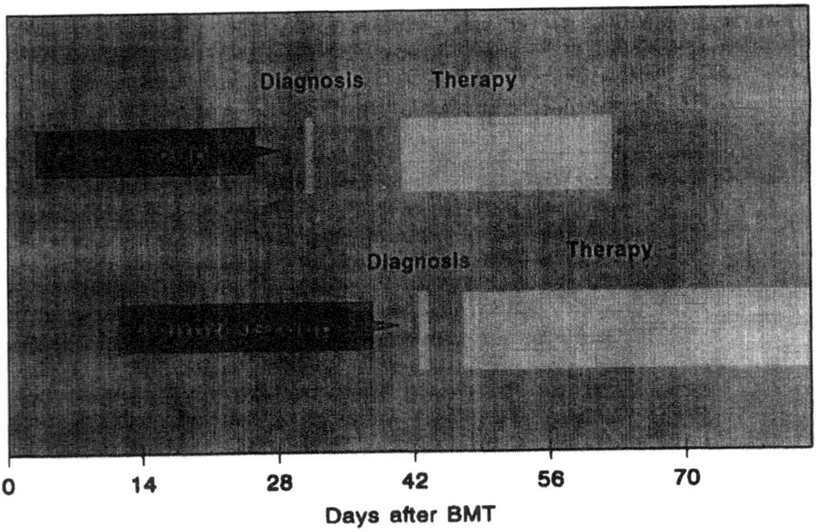

Fig. 1. Time schedule of diagnosis of CMV infection and treatment. Time points of diagnosis of CMV infection and of initiation and of termination of antiviral therapy are given for the two treatment groups. *PCR group*: preemptive therapy was initiated when PCR assays were positive for CMV DNA from two consecutive blood samples. *Culture group*: preemptive therapy was initiated when CMV could be cultivated from urine, throat washing and/or blood samples

and urine samples in BMT recipients earlier than the virus culture technique [7]. Additionally, PCR was successfully used to monitor antiviral therapy for CMV infection after allogeneic BMT [8,9]. The aim of the first part of the study was to compare the CMV antigenemia assay and the plasma PCR with the established PCR from whole blood for early diagnosis of CMV infection and assessment of the efficacy of antiviral treatment. Recently, clinical application of these techniques in the surveillance of patients after BMT at risk of developing CMV infection was reported [7, 8, 10–15, 17]. A total of 109 blood samples of 15 consecutive patients transplanted in the BMT unit in Tübingen for different hematological malignancies were simultaneously analyzed for CMV infection by PCR, CMV antigenemia assay, plasma-PCR and CMV shell vial culture. All 15 patients proved to be CMV positive by PCR, plasma PCR, and CMV antigenemia after BMT, whereas only nine of 15 patients developed culture-proven viremia and/or viruria, confirming our recently published results [8, 9]. In total 96 of 109 blood samples revealed identical results by PCR, plasma-PCR, and pp65 antigenemia. Discordant results in 13 blood samples could be attributed to the different sensitivity of the assays applied and occurred exclusively when a low amount of virus in the blood samples was present as, for example, in the early phase of CMV infection or after cessation of antiviral therapy.

Quantitative evaluation of CMV content of blood samples could be easily performed by the CMV antigenemia assay, but also DNA PCR from whole blood and plasma PCR, provided a semiquantitative analysis of the amplicons. No obvious advantage for either of the assays for the evaluation of the efficacy of antiviral therapy could be demonstrated.

Thus PCR, CMV antigenemia, and plasma PCR all seem to be suitable in monitoring BMT in recipients for CMV infection and controlling the efficacy of antiviral therapy in this patient population.

In two recent studies [3, 4], preemptive therapy with ganciclovir could be shown to reduce the incidence of CMV disease and CMV-related mortality in recipients of an allogeneic BMT. Preemptive therapy was started when a positive culture was obtained either from bronchoalveolar lavage [5] or from blood, urine, and throat washings [6]. Unfortunately, in these studies 12%–13% of patients developed CMV disease before or at the time of a positive surveillance culture. Thus, earlier therapeutic intervention based on more sensitive techniques was suggested [13]. In the second part of the study, the highly sensitive PCR assay was applied for early CMV detection and institution of antiviral therapy. PCR monitoring revealed 65% of patients to be CMV-DNA positive, whereas culture assays only demonstrated 50% of the patients as developing active CMV infection. This corresponds to our previous findings [7] showing 80% of PCR-positive patients to be or to become also culture positive for CMV. As already reported before [7, 8], PCR could be shown to detect the virus earlier after BMT than culture assays—in this study by a median of 15 days.

Thus treatment was started earlier in PCR- than in culture-monitored patients. This resulted in a significant reduction not only in the incidence of CMV disease (2/34 vs. 8/32), but also in a prevention of CMV-related and a reduction in overall mortality, as demonstrated in this study. The high incidence of CMV disease among the culture-monitored patients (24%) is most likely due to the high percentage of patients in both groups receiving a transplant from an unrelated or from a mismatched family donor. This patient cohort had been shown to represent a group at very high risk to develop CMV disease (19).

Polymerase chain reaction-based preemptive therapy appears to allow introduction of antiviral treatment at a time of still low virus load in blood and organs and thus to effectively prevent fatal CMV disease in recipients of an allogeneic BMT, even from an HLA-mismatched family or unrelated marrow donor.

Treatment was stopped in all patients in both groups when blood samples were found to be PCR negative after antiviral therapy. None of the PCR-negative patients in either group developed CMV disease following cessation of therapy. Thus, withholding antiviral therapy in a PCR-negative patient was found to be safe.

Thus, sensitive screening for CMV infection in recipients of an allogeneic BMT and consequent early introduction of antiviral therapy help to reduce CMV-associated mortality following BMT.

References

1. Meyers JD, Flournoy N, Wade JC, et al. Biology of interstitial pneumonia after marrow transplantation. In: Gale RP, ed. Recent advances in bone marrow transplantation. New York; Alan R. Liss. 1983; 405–23.
2. Meyers JD, Flournoy N, Thomas ED: Nonbacterial pneumonia after allogeneic bone marrow transplantation. A review of ten years experience. Rev Infect Dis 4. 1119–32. 1982
3. Goodrich JM, Bowden RA, Fisher L, Keller C, Schoch G, Meyers JD. Ganciclovir prophylaxis to prevent cytomegalovirus disease after allogeneic BMT. Ann Intern Med 118: 173. (1993)
4. Winston DJ, Winston GH, Bartoni K, DuMond C, Ebeling DF, Buhles WC, Champlin RE. Ganciclovir prophylaxis of cytomegalovirus infection and disease in allogeneic bone marrow transplant recipients. Ann Intern Med 118: 179. (1993)
5. Schmidt GM, Horac DA, Niland JC, Duncan SR, Forman SJ, Zaia A. A randomized, controlled trial of prophylactic ganciclovir for cytomegalovirus pulmonary infection in recipients of allogeneic bone marrow transplants. N Engl J Med 324: 1005.(1991)
6. Goodrich JM, Mori M, Gleaves CA, DuMond C, Cays M, Ebeling DF, Buhles WC, DeArmond B, Meyers JD. Early treatment with ganciclovir to prevent cytomegalovirus disease after allogeneic bone marrpw transplantation. N Engl J Med 325: 1601. (1991)
7. Einsele H, Steidle H, Vallbracht A, Saal JG, Ehninger G, Müller CA (1991) Early occurrence of human cytomegalovirus infection after bone marrow transplantation as demonstrated by the polymerase chain reaction technique Blood 77: 1104. 1991
8. Einsele H, Ehninger G, Steidle M, Vallbracht A, Müller M, Schmidt H, Saal JG, Waller HD, Müller CA. Polymerase chain reaction to evaluate antiviral therapy for cytomegalovirus disease. Lancet ii: 1170. (1991)
10. Storch GA, Buller RS, Bailey TC, et al. Comparison of PCR and pp65 antigenemia assay with quantitative shell vial culture for detection of cytomegalovirus in blood leukocytes from solid-organ transplant recipints. J Clin Microbiol 1994; 32: 997–1003.
11. Einsele H, Vallbracht A, Jahn G, Kandolf R, Müller CA. Hybridization techniques provide superior sensitivity for HCMV detection compared to immunhistological analysis and allow quantitation of the virus in clinical samples. J. Virol Methods 4: 91.(1989)
12. Vlieger AM, Boland GJ, Jiwa NM, et al. Cytomegalovirus antigenemia assay or PCR can be used to monitor ganciclovir treatment in bone marrow transplant recipients. Bone Marrow Transplant 1992; 9: 247–53.
13. Wolf DG, Spector SA, Early diagnosis of human cytomegalovirus disease in transplant recipients by DNA amplification in plasma. Transplantation 1993; 56: 330–34.
14. Zweyberg Wirgart B, Claesson K, Erikson BM, Tufveson G, Tötterman T, Grillner L. CMV pp65 antigen detection in leukocytes compared to CMV DNA amplification from plasma for early diagno-

sis of CMV infection in kidney transplanted patients. In: Multidisciplinary approach to understanding cytomegalovirus disease, eds Michelson S, Plotkin SA, Elsevier Science Publishers B.V. (1993) p 195–99.
15. Jiwa NM, Van Gemert GW, Raap AK, et al. Rapid detection of human cytomegalovirus DNA in peripheral blood leukocytes of viremic transplant recipients by the polymerase chain reaction. Transplantation (1989) 48: 72–77.
16. Ljungman P, Griffiths P. Definitions of cytomegalovirus infection and disease. In Multidisciplinary approach to understanding cytomegalovirus disease, eds Michelson S, Plotkin SA, Elsevier Science Publishers B.V. (1993) p 233–37.
17. Einsele H, Ehninger G, Steidle M, et al. Lymphocytopenia as an unfavourable prognostic factor in patients with cytomegalovirus infection after bone marrow transplantation. Blood 1993; 82: 1672–78.
18. Rubin RH. Preemptive therapy in immunocompromised hosts. N Engl J Med 324: 1057. (1991)
19. Lanino E, Anasetti C, Longton G, Etzioni R, Bowden R, Hanson JA. Prevention of cytomegalovirus disease with ganciclovir in recipients of marrow transplants from unrelated donors. Blood 82, Suppl. 1: 1359 (Abstract). (1993)

Acute Leukemias VI
Prognostic Factors
and Treatment Strategies
Büchner et al. (eds)

Therapy of Sepsis Syndrome with Human Polyclonal IgM-Enriched Immunoglobulins: Interim Analysis of a Randomized Trial in Neutropenic Cancer Patients

G. Behre[1], H. Ostermann[2], M. Rothenburger[3], X. Schiel[1], D. Bockelmann[3], S. Geiger[1], M. Dedroogh[1], M. Helmerking[3], B. Wörmann[1], J. Kienast[2], and W. Hiddemann[1]

Abstract. Sepsis is a major cause of death in neutropenic cancer patients. We have shown the prognostic significance of endotoxin plasma levels in neutropenic patients with sepsis syndrome, and other groups have suggested the efficacy of polyclonal IgM-enriched immunoglobulins in the treatment of endotoxin-positive sepsis in non-neutropenic patients. To evaluate the efficacy of polyclonal IgM-enriched immunoglobulins in the treatment of sepsis syndrome in neutropenic patients with hematologic malignancies, a randomized, placebo-controlled trial was initiated at our institutions. The patients were randomly assigned to either the human polyclonal immunoglobulin preparation every 6 h for 3 days (total dose, 1.3 l with 49.4 g IgG, 7.8 g IgM, 7.8 g IgA) or the equivalent dose of 5% human albumin. In the 52 entered patients with sepsis syndrome followed to death or day 28, there were ten deaths among the 22 recipients of albumin (46%) and nine deaths among the 30 recipients of immunoglobulin (30%; $p > 0.05$). In the subgroup of patients with sepsis syndrome but without shock at entry, the mortality was 11% (one of nine) in the albumin and 12% two of seventeen in the immunoglobulin group. However, the immunoglobulin administration reduced mortality from 69% nine of thirteen to 54% (seven of thirteen) in the subgroup of patients with shock at entry and from 89% to 67% in the subgroup of patients with organ failure at entry, (acute lung, renal or hepatic failure or disseminated intravascular coagulation). This interim analysis suggests that human polyclonal IgM-enriched immunoglobulins may reduce the mortality from sepsis syndrome in neutropenic cancer patients. A completion of the ongoing trial is needed to substantiate these findings taking into account that randomization has to be stratified for sepsis syndrome with and without septic shock at entry because of the different risk of death.

Introduction

Sepsis is a major cause of death in neutropenic cancer patients [1], and, on the other hand, cancer is one of the most common underlying diseases in patients with sepsis [2]. Thus, neoplasmas were 37% of the underlying diseases in 200 patients with Gram-negative bacteremia and severe sepsis [2]. In patients with severe neutropenia from hematologic malignancy, the incidence of Gram-negative bacteremia is considered 15% of [3, 4] with an associated mortality of 15% [3, 4] and the incidence of severe sepsis and/or septic shock 25% [5] with a death rate of 35% [5]. However, most of the urgent questions concerning definition, pathophysiology, and therapy of sepsis in neutropenic cancer patients are still open.

Until now, the absence of firm definitions for sepsis has had little practical consequence because the only therapy available has been antibiotics and supportive care. Given the abundance of new agents under active investigations, however, more precice diagnostic guidelines are

[1]Department of Hematology/Oncology, University of Göttingen, Robert-Koch-Str. 40, 37075 Göttingen, Germany
[2]Department of Hematology/Oncology, University of Münster, Albert-Schweitzer-Str. 33, 48161 Münster, Germany
[3]Clinical Research Organisation, Albert-Schweitzer-Str. 62/1, 81735 München, Germany

needed to evaluate efficacy, to determine which patients might benefit from such therapy, and to compare the results of different clinical trials. Therefore, new firm definitions of sepsis and its sequelae have been proposed, such as sepsis syndrome and septic shock by Bone et al. [6] or systemic inflammatory response syndrome (SIRS)/ sepsis, severe sepsis, septic shock, and multiple organ dysfunction syndrome (MODS) by the American College of Chest Physicians/ Society of Critical Care Medicine consensus conference [7]. However, the clinical practicability of the new terminology "sepsis syndrome", defined as the earliest stage during an infectious process at which evidence of altered organ perfusion can be detected [6], has not been evaluated and proven in patients with neutropehia yet.

With respect to the pathophysiology of sepsis, it has become clear that endotoxin, (LPS) triggers humoral mechanisms involving the complement, clotting, fibrinolytic, and kinin pathways [8]. Fever and inflammation are mediated by cytokines, such as tumor necrosis factor (TNF)-α and interleukin-1 (IL-1) [9], which are released from host defense cells such as monocytes and macrophages in response to the lipid A moiety of endotoxin [10]. In this sense, sepsis syndrome may be considered a constellation of signs and symptoms which represents the host's response to infection, whereby the effects of cytokines or substances triggered by cytokines are responsible for most of the clinical manifestations [8].

In spite of this pathogenetic hypothesis, no new anti-endotoxin or anti-cytokine therapy for sepsis has shown clinical efficacy yet [11, 12]. Ten clinical trials using anti-endotoxin core antibodies produced inconsistent results and did not conclusively establish the safety or benefit of this approach [11–14]. Both IL-1 receptor antagonist and a murine monoclonal anti-TNF antibody have been beneficial in some animal models of sepsis, but did not clearly improve survival in human trials [15, 16].

However, one group has suggested the efficacy of human polyclonal IgM-enriched immunoglobulins in the treatment of endotoxin-positive sepsis in non-neutropenic patients [17]. Therefore, after having shown the prognostic significance of endotoxin plasma levels in neutropenic patients with sepsis syndrome in a pilot study [18], we carried out a randomized trial to evaluate the efficancy of therapy with human polyclonal IgM-enriched immunoglobulins in neutropenic patients with hematologic malignancies and sepsis syndrome.

Materials and Methods

Patients. Patients fulfilling all of the following criteria were eligible for the study: (a) acute leukemia or high-grade lymphoma; (b) neutropenia $<1000/\mu l$; (c) sepsis syndrome or septic shock; (d) informed consent. Patients fulfilling one of the following criteria were excluded from the study: (a) age $\leqslant 18$ years; (b) Pregnancy or lactation; (c) prior allergic reaction to study drugs; (d) HIV infection; (e) prior enrollment into the study during the last 4 weeks.

Definitions of Sepsis. Sepsis syndrome or septic shock were defined according to Bone et al. [6] and Glauser et al. [8]. *Sepsis syndrome*: clinical evidence of infection, tachypnea (respirations >20/min; if mechanically ventilated >10 l/min), tachycardia (pulse >90/min), hyperthermia or hypothermia (core or rectal temperature >38.3°C or 35.6°C), and evidence of inadequate organ perfusion, including one or more of the following : hypoxemia ($PaO_2/FiO_2 \leqslant 280$, without other pulmonary or cardiovascular disease as the cause), elevated plasma lactate concentration (exceeding upper limits of normal for the laboratory), or oliguria (documented urine output <0.5 ml/kg of body weight for at least 1 h, in patients with catheters); *septic shock*: sepsis syndrome with hypotension (sustained decrease in systolic blood pressure to <90 mmHg or drop by >40 mmHg for at least 1 h when volume replacement is adequate, the patient is taking no antihypertensive medication, and other causes of shock such as hypovolemia, myocardial infarction, and pulmonary embolism are absent). Organ failures such as acute lung, renal, or hepatic failure, or disseminated intravascular coagulation were defined according to Schuster [19]. *Acute lung failure*: hypoxemia ($PaO_2 < 75$ mmHg or $PaO_2/FiO_2 \leqslant 280$), pathologic chest X-ray, and mechanical ventilation; *acute renal failure*: increase of serum creatinine >3 mg/dl and/or dialysis; acute hepatic failure: increase of serum bilirubin >2mg/dl and increase of aspartate aminotransferase or alanine aminotransferase levels more than twice the normal laboratory value; *disseminated intravascular coagulation*: decrease of platelet count (thrombocytopenia or drop by 150 000/μl), decrease of fibrinogen (hypofibrinogenemia or drop by 150 mg/dl), and at least two abnormal plasmatic coagulation tests (PT, PTT, TT, factor II, factor V, factor X).

Interventions. After enrollment into the study, the patients were randomly assigned to either the human polyclonal immunoglobulin preparation Pentaglobin (Biotest, Dreieich, Germany) or the equivalent dose of 5% human albumin. Pentaglobin is obtained from the Cohn fraction III out of the pooled plasma of at least 1000 normal donors, and treated with ß-propiolactone for inactivation of potentially contaminating viruses. It contains 50 g/l total protein comprising approximately 6 g/l IgG (12%), 6 g/l IgA (12%), and 38 g/l IgG (76%). After an initial loading dose of 0.2 l, patients received 0.1 l of immunoglobulin preparation every 6 h for 72 hours as slow intravenous infusions for a total dose of 1.3 l corresponding to 49.4 g IgG, 7.8 g IgM, and 7.8 g IgA. All patients received a standardized antibiotic therapy according to the interventional antimicrobial strategy of the German multicenter trials I and II of the Paul Ehrlich society [20,21].

Statistics. Patients with sepsis syndrome were followed to death or day 28. The primary endpoint of the randomized trial was the 28-day all-cause mortality. A total of 164 patients are planned to be enrolled into the study to detect a significant ($\alpha < 0.05$) difference between the two treatment groups with an 80% power ($ß = 0.2$) in the χ^2test by Mantel-Haenszel, assuming that the mortality from sepsis syndrome can be reduced from 50% in the albumin group to 30% in the immunoglobulin group. After 50 enrolled patients, an intent-to-treat interim analysis has been scheduled.

Results

Demographic Characteristics. Fifty-two patients from the Departments of Hematology and Oncology of the University of Göttingen and University of Münster entered the randomized trial between August 1992 and September 1994. The median age was 50 years in the immunoglobulin and 55 years in the albumin group. The majority of patients suffered from acute myelogenous leukemia: 74% (22/30) of the immunoglobulin group and 64% (14/22) of the albumin group.Of the immunoglobulin group, 13% (4/30) and 13% (4/30) suffered from acute lymphoblastic leukemia and high-grade lymphoma in comparison to 23% (5/22) and 13% (3/22) of the albumin group (Table 1). Of the patients with sepsis syndrome, 50% (26/52) revealed septic shock at

Table 1. Demographic characteristics by treatment group: age, underlying disease, and severity of sepsis syndrome at study entry

		Albumin	Immunoglobulin
Patients (*n*)	(*n*)	22	30
Age—Median (years)		55	50
Underlying disease			
AML	(*n*)	14	22
	%	64	74
ALL	(*n*)	5	4
	%	23	13
High-grade NHL	(*n*)	3	4
	%	13	13
Severity of sepsis syndrome at entry			
No septic shock at entry	(*n*)	9	17
	%	41	57
Septic shock at entry	(*n*)	13	13
	%	59	43
Organ failure at entry	(*n*)	9	9
	%	41	30
Disseminated intravascular coagulopathy	(*n*)	7	8
Acute lung failure	(*n*)	3	3
Acute renal failure	(*n*)	1	2
Acute hepatic failure	(*n*)	2	2

entry, and 35% (18/52) initial organ failure [acute lung ($n=6$), renal ($n=3$), or hepatic ($n=4$) failure, or disseminated intravascular coagulation ($n=15$)] (Table 1).

Mortality. In the 52 patients with sepsis syndrome, there were ten deaths among the 22 recipients of albumin (46%) and nine deaths among the 30 recipients of immunoglobulins (30%) (Table 2). This reduction of the 28-day mortality by immunoglobulin administration from 46% to 30% was not statistically significant ($p>0.05$, chi-square α test),). In the subgroup of patients with sepsis syndrome but without shock at entry, the 28-day mortality was 11% (one of nine) in the albumin and 12% (two of 17 in the immunoglobulin group. However, the immunoglobulin administration reduced mortality from 69% (nine of 13) to 54% (seven of 13) in the subgroup of patients with shock at entry and from 89% (eight of 9) to 67% (six of 9) in the subgroup of patients with organ failure at entry (Table 2).

Discussion

The current randomized trail tries to elucidate the impact of a thereapeutic intervention with an IgM-enriched human polyclonal immunolgobulin preparation (Pentaglobin) on the clinical out- come of neutropenic patients with hematologic malignancies and sepsis syndrome.

No anti-endotoxin core or anti-cytokine therapy for sepsis has shown clinical efficacy yet [11, 12]. The efficacy of the human or murine monoclonal IgM antibodies against endotoxin core, HA-1A [2, 13] and E5 [14], and of the IL-1 receptor antagonist [15] and a murine monoclonal anti-TNF antibody [16] could not be proven by randomized clinical trials, and a recombinant human dimeric anti-TNF antibody actually produced harm [22]. Perhaps more accurate clinical and laboratory predictors are needed to identify patients who may benefit from a given treatment strategy. On the other hand, the therapeutic premises may be wrong. Targeting a single microbial toxin such as endotoxin may not represent a viable strategy for treating a complex inflammatory response to diverse bacteria. Similarly, the strategy of inhibiting the host inflammatory response may not be beneficial because immune cells and cytokines play both pathogenetic and protective roles. Finally, our scientific knowledge of the complex timing of mediator release and balance during sepsis may be insufficient to develop successful therapeutic interventions for sepsis syndrome.

Because of the failure of anti-endotoxin core and anti-cytokine therapies in the treatment of sepsis, human polyclonal immunoglobulins have become a major interest of sepsis research under the hypothesis that they may provide a broad-spectrum antibacterial [23], antitoxic [24], and antiinflammatory [25] efficacy. In particular, experimental data strongly suggest a greater antitoxic and protective effect of polyclonal IgM rather than IgG preparations [26–28]. The applied IgM-enriched human polyclonal immunoglobulin preparation Pentaglobin was shown to contain antibody titers to a variety of Gram-negative bacteria [23]. In the preceding pilot study of the current randomized trial, anti-endotoxin core antibodies like IgM and IgG antibodies against lipid A and Re LPS increased significantly under immunoglobulin therapy [18]. Because it is prepared from pooled human plasma, the immunoglobulin preparation may also contain a greater amount [29] of several

Table 2. Twenty-eight day mortality for all patients with sepsis syndrome and the subgroups of patients without septic shock at entry, with septic shock at entry, and with organ failure (acute lung, renal, or hepatic failure, or disseminated intravascular coagulation) at entry

Subset		28-day mortality			
		Albumin		Immunoglobulin	
	(n)	(%)	(n)	(%)	(n)
Sepsis syndrome	52	46	10/22	30	9/30
No septic shock at entry	26	11	1/9	12	2/17
Septic shock at entry	26	69	9/13	54	7/13
Organ failure at entry	18	89	8/9	67	6/9

antibodies to the immunodominant, species-specific endotoxin side chains, which may be protective against the homologous endotoxin [26]. Moreover, Pentaglobin was shown to protect non-neutropenic animals from endotoxemic and Gram-negative bacteremic death [23, 24]. In a therapeutic trial, it reduced mortality from, endotoxin-positive sepsis in non-neutropenic patients [17], and it decreased the risk of infectious death (0/29 versus 6/34 deaths) after bone marrow transplantation when applied prophylactically [30].

The interim analysis of the present ongoing randomized trial suggests that the polyclonal immunoglobulins administered every 6 h for 3 days (total dose: 49.4 g IgG, 7.8 g IgM, 7.8 g IgA) may reduce the mortality from sepsis syndrome in comparison to 5% human albumin. Immunoglobulin administration reduced mortality from 46% (ten of 22) to 30% (nine of 30) in patients with sepsis syndrome, from 69% (nine of 13) to (seven of 13) in the subgroup of patients with septic shock at entry, and from 89% to 67% in the subgroup with initial organ failure (Table 2). A completion of the ongoing trial is needed to substantiate these findings, taking into account that randomization has to be stratified for sepsis syndrome with and without septic shock at entry because of the different risk of death.

References

1. Pizzo PA: Management of fever in patients with cancer and treatment-induced neutropenia. N Engl J Med 1993; 328: 1323-32
2. Ziegler EJ, Fisher CJ, Sprung CL, Straube RC, Sadoff JC, Foulke GE, Wortel CH, Fink MP, Dellinger RP, Teng NNH, Allen IE, Berger HJ, Knatterud GL, LoBuglio AF, Smith CR, the HA-1A sepsis study group. Treatment of Gram-negative bacteremia and septic shock with HA-1A human monoclonal antibody against endotoxin.N Engl J Med 1991; 324: 429-36
3. Deresinski S, De Pauw BE, Feld R. Empirical treatment of Gram-negative bacteremia in granulocytopenic patients with leukemia. Program Abstr 30th Intersci Conf Antimicrob Agents Chemother 1990; abstract 251
4. The EORTC International Antimicrobial Therapy Cooperative Group. Ceftazidime combined with a short or long course of amikacin for empirical therapy of Gram-negative bacteremia in cancer patients with granulocytopenia. N Engl J Med 1987; 317: 1692-8
5. Ostermann H, Rothenburger M, Mesters RM, van de Loo J, Kienast J. Cytokine release during sepsis in leukocytopenic patients: results of a prospective study. Blood 1993; 82 (Suppl 1): abstract 997
6. Bone RC, Fisher CJ, Clemmer TP, Slotman GJ, Metz GA, Balk RA. A controlled clinical trial of high-dose methylprednisolone in the treatment of severe sepsis and septic shock. N Engl J Med 1987; 317: 653-8
7. Bone RC, Balk RA, Cerra FB, Dellinger RP, Fein AM, Knaus WA, Schein RMH, Sibbald WJ. ACCP/SCCM consensus conference: definitions for sepsis and organ failure and guidelines for the use of innovative therapies in sepsis. Chest 1992; 101: 1644-55
8. Glauser MP, Heumann D, Baumgartner JD, Cohen J. Pathogenesis and potential strategies for prevention and treatment of septic shock: an update. Clin Infect Dis 1994; 18 Suppl 2: 205-16
9. Dinarello CA, Wolff SM, The role of interleukin-1 in disease. N Engl J Med 1993; 328: 106-12
10. Rietschel ET, Kirikae T, Schade FU, Mamat U, Schmidt G, Loppnow H, Ulmer AJ, Zahringer U, Seydel U, Di Padova F: Bacterial endotoxin: molecular relationships of structure to activity and function. FASEB J 1994; 8: 217-25
11. Natanson C, Hoffman WD, Suffredini AF, Eichacker PQ, Danner RL. Selected treatment strategies for septic shock based on proposed mechanisms of pathogenesis. Ann Intern Med 1994; 120: 771-83
12. Stone R: Search for sepsis drugs goes on despite past failures. Science 1994; 264; 365-7
13. McCloskey RV, Straube RC, Sanders C, Smith SM, Smith CR, and the CHESS Trial Study Group. Treatment of septic shock with human monoclonal antibody HA-1A—a randomized, double-blind, placebo-controlled trial. Ann Intern Med 1994; 121: 1-5
14. Greeman RL, Schein RMH, Martin MA, Wenzel RP, MacIntyre NR, Emmanuel G, Chmel H, Kohler RB, McCarthy M, Plouffe J, Russell JA, the XOMA Sepsis Study Group. A controlled clinical trial of E5 murine monoclonal IgM antibody to endotoxin in the treatment of Gram-negative sepsis. JAMA 1991; 226: 1097-102
15. Fisher CJ, Dhainaut JF, Opal SM, Pribble JP, Balk RA, Slotman GJ, Iberti TJ, Rackow EC, Shapiro MJ, Greeman RL, Reines HD, Shelly MP, Thompson BW, LaBrecque JF, Catalano MA, Knaus WA, Sadoff JC, for the Phase III rhIL-1ra Sepsis Syndrome Study Group. Recombinant human interleukin 1 receptor antagonist in the treatment of patients with sepsis syndrome—results from a randomized, double-blind, placebo-controlled trial. JAMA; 271: 1836-43
16. Wherry J, Wenzel R, Wunderink R, Silverman H, Perl T, Nasraway S. Monoclonal antibody to human tumor necrosis factor (TNF MAb): multicenter efficacy and safety study in patients with the sepsis syndrome. Program Abstr 33th Interci Conf Antimicrob Agents Chemother 1993; abstract 696
17. Schedel I, Dreikhausen U, Nentwig B, Höckenschnieder M, RauthmannD, Balikcioglu S,

Coldewey R, Deicher H. Treatment of Gram-negative septic shock with an immunoglobulin preparation: a prospective, randomized clinical trial. Crit Care Med 1991; 19: 1104–13
18. Behre G, Schedel I, Nentwig B, Wörmann B, Essink M, Hiddemann W. Endotoxin concentration in neutropenic patients with suspected Gram-negative sepsis: correleation with clinical outcome and determination of anti-endotoxin core antibodies during therapy with polyclonal immunoglobulin M-enriched immunoglobulins. Antimicrob Agents Chemother 1992; 36: 2139–46
19. Schuster HP, Definition und Diagnose von Sepsis und Multiorganversagen. In: Schuster HP, editor. Intensivtherapie bei Sepsis und Multiorganversagen. Berlin: Springer, 1993: 3–19
20. Link H, Maschmeyer G, Meyer P, Hiddemann W, Stille W, Helmerking M, Adam D, for the study group of the Paul Ehrlich Society for Chemotherapy (PEG). Interventional antimicrobial therapy in febrile neutropenic patients. Ann Hematol 1994; 69: 231–43
21. Meyer P, Adam D, Hiddemann W, Link H, Maschmeyer G, Helmerking M für die Studiegruppe Infektionen in der Hämatologie/Onkologie der Paul-Ehrlich-Gesellschaft für Chemotherapie e.V.. Interventionstherapie von Infektionen und Fieber unklarer Genese bei neutropenischen Patienten mit malignen hämatologischen Grunderkrankungen-Studien II-Zeitschrift für antimikrobielle antineoplastische Chemotherapie 1992; 10: 1–27
22. Sadoff J. Soluble TNF receptors. Presentation on the Third International Congress of the Immune Consequences of Trauma, Shock and Sepsis: Mechanisms and Therapeutic Approaches, München, March 1994
23. Stephan W, Dichtelmüller H, Schedel I. Properties and efficacy of a human immunoglobulin M preparation for intravenous administration. Drug Res 1985; 35: 933–6
24. Berger D, Beger HG. Adjuvant septic therapy with immunoglobulin—in vivo and in vitro studies. Intensive Care Med 1990; 16 Suppl 1: 20
25. Andersson UG, Björk L, Skansen-Saphir U, Andersson JP. Down-regulation of cytokine production and interleukin-2 receptor expression by pooled human IgG. Immunol 1993; 79; 211–16
26. Baumgartner JD, Heumann D, Gerain J, Weinbreck P, Grau GE, Glauser MP. Association between protective efficacy of anti-lipopolysaccharide (LPS) antibodies and suppression of LPS-induced tumor necrosis factor alpha and interleukin 6. Comparison of O side chain-specific antibodies with core LPS antibodies. J Exp Med 1990; 171: 889–96
27. Garbett ND, Munro CS, Cole PJ. Opsonic activity of a new intravenous immunoglobulin preparation: Pentaglobin compared with Sandoglobulin. Clin Exp Immunol 1989; 76: 8–12
28. McCabe WR, DeMaria A, Berberich H, Johns MA. Immunization with rough mutants of Salmonella minnesota: protective activity of IgM and IgG antibody to the R595 (Re chemotype) mutant. J Infect Dis 1988; 158: 291–300
29. Cross AS, Sidberry H, Sadoff JC. The human antibody response during natural bacteremic infection with Gram-negative bacilli against lipopolysaccharide core determinants. J Infect Dis 1989, 160: 225–36
30. Poynton CH, Jackson S, Fegan C, Barnes RA, Whittaker JA. Use of IgM enriched intravenous immunoglobulin (Pentaglobin) in bone marrow transplantation. Bone Marrow Transplant 1992; 9: 451–7

Acute Leukemias VI
Prognostic Factors
and Treatment Strategies
Büchner et al. (eds)

The 10/NL Trigger for Prophylactic Platelet Transfusion in Acute Myeloid Leukemia: A Prospective Comparative Multicenter Study

H. Wandt[1], M. Frank[1], H. Link[2], C. Schneider[2], N. Brack[3], A. Daoud[4], G. Ehninger[5], E. Fackler-Schwalbe[6], J. Fischer[7], R. Gäckle[8], T. Geer[9], M. Gramatzki[10], P. Harms[11], B. Löffler[12], S. Öhl[13], B. Otremba[14], M. Raab[15], P. Schönrock-Nabulsi[16], and R. Winter[17]

Abstract. This study shows that the 10/nl trigger for prophylactic platelet transfusion according to the inclusion criteria of our transfusion protocol is as safe as the traditional platelet transfusion threshold of 20/nl. The main cause of severe acute bleeding complications in acute myeloid leukemia patients is not the absolute count of thrombocytes but local problems such as gastrointestinal lesions, local infiltrations or hyperleucocytosis and coagulation disorders such as disseminated intravascular coagulopathy during septic shock. A total of 78% of our patients with severe bleeding complications were classified as M4 or M5 (FAB). These myeloid leukemias are often complicated by hyperleucocytosis and local infiltrations. Successful therapeutic management of these problems, beside platelet transfusions, is most important to stop bleeding complications. In no case was the major cause of death fatal bleeding. Our observation confirms the analysis of recent studies in this field.

The 38% reduction of platelet products ($p < 0.05$) in the stringent transfusion group A, despite the longer thrombocytopenia, is clinically relevant:

- lower need of platelet transfusions in the light of limited numbers of donors
- Reduction in cost of about DM-400 000 in our study period or DM-3700 per treatment cycle. This may be important in reducing the complications following multiple transfusions such as transfusion-associated infections and refractoriness.

Introduction

As we know from patients with Myelodysplastic Syndrome (MDS) and (ITP), a thrombocyte count of 20/nl is not a magic threshold for bleeding complications. Patients with thrombocytes of 10/nl or even lower can live for long

[1]Städtisches Klinikum, Nürnberg, Germany
[2]Medizinische Hochschule, Hannover, Germany
[3]Städtisches Krankenhaus, München-Harlaching, Germany
[4]Medizinische Akademie, Magdeburg, Germany
[5]Medizinische Universitäts-Klinik, Tübingen, Germany
[6]Klinikum, Augsburg, Germany
[7]Stätisches Krankenhaus, Karlsruhe, Germany
[8]Bürgerhospital, Stuttgart, Germany
[9]Diakonie-Krankedhaus, Schwäbisch-Hall, Germany
[10]Medizinische Universitäts-Klinik, Erlange, Germany
[11]Städtisches Klinikum, Minden, Germany
[12]Robert-Koch-Krankenhaus, Stuttgart, Germany
[13]Klinik St. Antonius, Wuppertal, Germany
[14]Evangelisches Krankenhaus, Oldenburg, Germany
[15]Diakonissen-Krankenhaus, Stuttgart, Germany
[16]Krankenhaus St. Georg, Hamburg, Germany
[17]Städtisches Krankenhaus, Wolfsburg, Germany

times without bleeding complications. One clinical study and some reviews for platelet transfusion in recent years favorize a lower trigger for prophylactic transfusion (1-3).

Patients and Methods

From April 1992 to July 1993 we studied prospectively the safety and economy of the routine morning 10/nl trigger for prophylactic platelet transfusion in AML patients (FAB M3 excluded) compared to the traditional 20/nl trigger. Exclusion criteria for routine platelet transfusion below this 10/nl trigger were as follows: in the case of fever >38.5°C and rapid decrease of platelet count the morning trigger should be 15/nl; a minimum of 20/nl of platelets should be maintained in any of the following situations: disseminated intravascular coagulopathy (DIC) or other coagulation disorders, major bleeding (WHO grade>2), any kind of biopsy, deterioration of sight by retinal bleeding, use of drugs affecting platelet function.

Eight centers of our AML group accepted this experimental prophylactic transfusion protocol (group A) and nine centers were reluctant and used the traditional 20/nl trigger (group B). From April 1992 to July 1993, 105 consecutive patients of our AML group were included in the study and evaluated regarding bleeding complication according to the WHO criteria. The numbers of platelet transfusions in both groups were compared. The economics of both transfusion protocols were calculated . In both groups random single-donor and multiple-donor platelets, as available, were mainly transfused with leukocyte filters. HLA-compatible transfusions were performed only after refractoriness to unmatched transfusions.

Results

We examined prospectively 2198 days of thrombopenia (<25/nl) during 110 treatment cycles in group A and 1645 days during 106 cycles in group B, respectively. Mean age of all patients was 47 years (range 17-73 years). The groups were comparable for age, sex, and FAB classification. Pretreatment blood cell counts and the Complete Remission (CR) rate were both in favor of group B (See Table 1). The relationship of single-donor vs. multiple-donor platelets used in groups A and B was well balanced, 1: 5.1 vs. 1:5.3, respectively. The median time of thrombopenia per treatment cycle was longer for the stringent transfusion group A as expected: 18 days for group A vs. 13 days for group B. Bleeding WHO grade 0/1 was 82% vs. 83%, grade 2 was 18% vs. 9% and grades 3 and 4 was 0% vs. 8%. There was no statistically significant difference between the two groups for clinically relevant bleeding complications (>grade 2).

The reduction of platelet transfusion in group A compared to group B was 38% ($p<0.05$) despite the longer median time of thrombocytopenia in group A. The nine patients with grade 3 and 4 bleeding were all in group B. Six of these patients had a platelet count >30/nl at the time of seven complication. Seven out of nine had AML M4 or M5. Four patients died the day following bleeding, but none of fatal bleeding. The causes of death were: two irreversible septic shock with acute respiratory distress syndrome, (ARDS), one acute heart arrest during hyperleu-

Table 1. Patient characteristics

	Group A	Group B
Median (years)	45.2	49.1
Range (years)	17-72	25-73
female/male (%)	50/50	49/51
Leucocyte count before treatment >100/nl(%)	6	3.6
Platelet count before each cycle <100 n/l	56.9	36.6
>100/nl	43.1	63.4
AML (M0/M1/M2)(%)	50	46.7
AML (M4/M5)(%)	44.6	46.7
AML (M6/M7) (%)	5.4	6.6
Complete remission rate (%)	53.5	68.1

Table 2. Analysis of major bleeding complications of WHO grades 3 and 4

Patient No.	AML	WHO grade	Bleeding site	Platelets/nl	Major complications	Outcome
1	M4	3	Diffuse	58	Bacterial sepsis	Resolved
2	M5	3	Vaginal, 1 week post partum	53	None	Resolved
3	M4	3	Rectal	17	Sigmoiditis	Resolved
4	M4	3	Unclear decrease of Hb	9	Pneumonia	Resolved
5	M5	4	Diffuse plasmat. coagulation disorder	36	Hepatic-renal syndrome	Death, hepatic failure
6	M4	3	Unclear decrease of HB	36	Hyperleucocytosis	Death, heart arrest
7	M2	4	Gastrointestinal, stress ulcer	36	Septic shock/ARDS	Death, irreversible shock
8	M2	3	Rectal and vaginal	13	None	Resolved
9	M4	3	Hemorrhagic diarrhea	50	Septic shock/ARDS	Death, irreversible shock

cocytosis, one hepato-renal failure in a patient with liver cirrhosis (see Table 2).

The cost analysis per treatment cycle (platelet transfusions and costs for medical personnel) in group A compared to group B were DM-5932 vs DM-9643. This led to an overall reduction of costs for group A of DM-400 000 in the study period.

Acknowledgment. This was a cooperative AML study by the süddeutsche Hämoblastosegruppe and was supported by the Deutsche Krebshilfe.

References

1. J.Gmür, J. Burger, U.Schanz, J. Fehr, A. Schaffner: Safety of stringent prophylactic platelet transfusion policy for patients with acute leukaemia. Lancet 338: 1233–1226,1991.
2. Ernest Beutler: Platelet transfusion: The 20.000/μl trigger Blood 81: 1411–1413,1993.
3. J.Bux, C. Mueller-Eckhardt: Leitlinien für die Substitutionstherapie mit Thrombozyten. Dtschemed Wschr 118: 1367–1370,1993.

Acute Leukemias VI
Prognostic Factors
and Treatment Strategies
Büchner et al. (eds)

Transplantation of Allogeneic Peripheral Blood Progenitor Cells Alone or in Addition to Bone Marrow

H. Link[1], L. Arseniev[1], O. Bähre[1], R.J. Berenson[2], J.G. Kadar[1], K. Battmer[1], R. Jacobs[1], J. Casper[1], H. Diedrich[1], J. Schubert[1], J. Kühl[1], H. Poliwoda[1]

Introduction

The transplantation of allogeneic peripheral blood progenitor cells (PBPC) could provide durable hematopoietic engraftment. In healthy bone marrow (BM) donors, large amounts of PBPC can be mobilized with hematopoietic growth factors (1–7). However, the high content of immunocompetent T cells in apheresis products may expose recipients of allogeneic PBPC to an elevated risk of acute graft-versus-host disease (aGVHD) [2, 8, 9]. Thus, the use of an appropriate T cell reduction, but not depletion technique might reduce this risk [9, 10]. The hazards of rejection and of a higher relapse rate should be avoided by maintaining a portion of the T cells in the graft [10, 11]. The positive selection of $CD34^+$ cells from peripheral blood preparations simultaneously provides an approximately 1000-fold reduction of T cells [8, 12]. Purified $CD34^+$ cells containing committed and pluripotent stem cells [13–16] may be sufficient for allogeneic transplantation [17]. The aim of the study was the development of a protocol for allogeneic transplantation of PBPC instead of BM cells.

Materials and Methods

Three patient groups were studied: group I received unmanipulated (BM), 4.5×10^6 $CD34^+$ and 172.3×10^5 $CD3^+$ cells/kg and stored immunoselected (IS) PBPC, 3.3×10^6 $CD34^+$ and 3.7×10^5 $CD3^+$ cells/kg; group II was transplanted with both IS BM, 1.6×10^6 $CD34^+$ and 0.6×10^5 $CD3^+$ cells/kg and stored IS PBPC 2.3×10^6 $CD34^+$ and 2.7×10^5 $CD3^+$ cells/kg; group III received only fresh IS PBPC, 6.2×10^6 $CD34^+$ and 9.4×10^5 $CD3^+$ cell/kg. Granulocyte colony-stimulating factor (G-CSF) primed (2×5 μg/kg) PBPC were collected on days 4 and 5 (groups I and II) or on days 4–7 (group III) of mobilization. BM harvest was performed on day 0. $CD34^+$ cells were selected from the pooled PBPC concentrates or BM harvests by immunoadsorption onto avidin with the biotinylated anti-CD34 monoclonal antibody 12.8 (Ceprate SC^R, Cellpro, Seattle, USA). A historical control group transplanted with a mean of 5.2×10^6 $CD34^+$ cells/kg and 156×10^5 $CD3^+$ cells/kg from BM alone was assembled for comparison. Patients were conditioned with either busulfan (16 mg/kg) or 12 Gy total body irradiation (TBI) followed by 120 mg/kg cyclophosphamide. Cyclosporin A (CsA) and short methotrexate were used for GVHD prophylaxis. Group III patients only received CsA. After transplantation all study and control patients received G-CSF (5 μg/kg per day iv.) and erythropoietin (150 U/kg per day, continuous i.v. infusion).

Results

Median recovery times of neutrophils, platelets, and reticulocytes (Ret) are shown in Table 1. The rates of acute GVHD in groups I–III were similar to control patients. So far no graft rejection or leukemic relapse has occurred.

[1]BMT Unit, Medical School Hannover, Germany
[2]CellPro Inc., Bothell, WA, USA

Table 1. Median recovery time

	Group I($n=5$) (days)	Group II ($n=5$) (days)	Group III ($n=3$) (days)	Controls ($n=12$) (days)
Neu > 100/μl	12	14	9	17
Neu > 500/μl	15	15	10	18
Neu > 1000/μl	17	18	11	20
Plt > 50000/μl	24	35	15	41
Ret > 10000/μl	14	16	13	20

Neu, neutrophils; plt, platelets; Ret, reticulocytes.

Discussion

The addition of allogeneic PBPC to bone marrow cells accelerated the hematopoietic recovery as compared to historical control patients. Also, in comparison with published data, this effect was evident in neutrophil and erythrocyte regeneration. The platelet recovery of our control group was longer than the usual 12–24 days [18]. However, patients who received PBPC alone had a short interval of 15 days to platelet recovery. Similar data have been published with unselected PBPC by other groups [19–21].

With this protocol of combined transplantation we were able to switch the allogeneic transplantation program in adult patients from bone marrow to blood stem cells. We are now investigating whether immunoselected PBPC along with low numbers of T cells (1×10^5/kg) are suitable for stem cell grafting. However, there are several open questions, if PBPC are transplanted:

1. What number and quality of blood stem cells are required for durable engraftment?
2. Is the incidence of acute and chronic GVHD increased if large amounts of T cells from peripheral blood are transplanted without prior T cell depletion?
3. Will the graft-versus-leukemia effect be more potent, if more T cells are transplanted?
4. If T cells are depleted, will the known problems of this method, such as rejection, graft failure or leukemic relapse recur?
5. Are there late sequelae of using G-CSF for a healthy donor?

Several prospective studies have now begun, in order to find answers to these questions.

References

1. Baumann I, Testa NG, Lange C, de Wynter E, Luft T, Dexter TM, van Hoef MEHM, Howell A. Haemopoietic cells mobilised into the circulation by lenograstim as alternative to bone marrow for allogeneic transplants. Lancet 1993; 34: 369
2. Weaver CH, Buckner CD, Longin K, Appelbaum FR, Rowley S, Lilleby K, Miser J, Storb R, Hansen JA, Bensinger W. Syngeneic transplantation with peripheral blood mononuclear cells collected after the administration of recombinant human granulocyte colony-stimulating factor. Blood 1993; 82: 1981–1984.
3. Matsunaga T, Sakamaki S, Kohgo Y. Ohi S, Hirayama Y, Niitsu Y. Recombinant human granulocyte colony-stimulating factor can mobilize sufficient amounts of peripheral blood stem cells in healthy volunteers for allogeneic transplantation. Bone Marrow Transplant. 1994; 11: 103–108.
4. Tjonnfjord GE, Steen R, Evensen SA, Thorsby E, Egeland T.Characterization of CD 34+ peripheral blood cells from healthy adults mobilized by recombinant human granulocyte colony-stimulating factor. Blood 1994; 84: 2795–2801.
5. Suzue T, Kawano Y, Takaue Y, Kuroda Y. Cell processing protocol for allogeneic peripheral blood stem cells mobilized by granulocyte colony-stimulating factor. Exp Hematol 1994; 22: 888–892.
6. Lane TA, Law P, Maruyama M, Young D, Burgess D, Mullen M, Mealiffe M, Terstappen LWMM, Hardwick A, Moubayaed M, Oldham F, Corringham RET, Ho AD. Harvesting and enrichment of hematopoietic progenitor cells mobilized into the peripheral blood of normal donors by granulocyte-macrophage colony stimulating factor (GM-CSF) or G-CSF: potential role in allogeneic marrow transplantation. Blood 1995; 85: 275–282.
7. Arseniev L, Tischler H-J, Battmer K, Südmeyer I, Casper J, Link H. Treatment of poor marrow graft function with enriched allogeneic CD34+ cells immunoselected from G-CSF mobilized peripheral blood progenitor cells of the marrow donor. Bone Marrow Transplant. 1994; 14: 791–797
8. Link H, Arseniev L, Löhmann D, Andres J, Battmer K, Südmeier I, Schmoll HJ, Freund M, Bokemeyer C. Mobilization kinetics of CD34+ cell subsets in

blood and bone marrow after G-CSF alone following repetitive dose-intensive chemotherapy or BMT. Bone marrow Transplant. 1994; 14, Suppl. 1: S17

9. Kernan NA, Collins NH, Juliano L, Cartagena T, Dupont B, O'Reilly RJ. Clonable T lymphocytes in T cell-depleted bone marrow transplants correlate with development of graft-v-host disease. Blood 1986; 68: 770–773.
10. Verdonck LF, de Gast GC, van Heugten HG, Dekker AW. A fixed low number of T cells in HLA-identical allogeneic bone marrow transplantation. Blood 1990; 75: 776–780.
11. Verdonck LF, Dekker AW, de Gast GC, van Kempen ML, Lokhorst HM, Nieuwenhuis HK. Allogeneic bone marrow transplantation with a fixed low number of T cells in the marrow graft. Blood 1994; 83: 3090–3096.
12. Brugger W, Henschler R, Heimfeld S, Berenson RJ, Mertelsmann R, Kanz L. Positively selected autologous blood $CD34^+$ cells and unseparated peripheral blood progenitor cells mediate identical hematopoietic engraftment after high-dose VP16, ifosfamide, carboplatin, and epirubicin. Blood 1994; 84: 1421–1426.
13. Berenson RJ, Andrews RG, Bensinger WI, Kalamasz D, Knitter G, Buckner CD, Bernstein D. Antigen $CD34^+$ marrow cells engraft lethally irradiated baboons. J Clin Invest 1988; 81: 951–955.
14. Berenson RJ, Bensinger WI, Hill RS, Andrews RG, Garcia-Lopez J, Kalamasz DF, Still BJ, Spitzer G, Buckner CD, Bernstein ID, Thomas ED. Engraftment after infusion of $CD34^+$ marrow cells in patients with breast cancer or neuroblastoma. Blood 1991; 77: 1717–1722.
15. Terstappen LW, Huang S, Safford M, Lansdorp PM, Loken MR. Sequential generations of hematopoietic colonies derived from single non-lineage-committed $CD34^+CD38$-progenitor cells. Blood 1991; 77: 1218–1277.
16. Huang S,Terstappen LW,Formation of haematopoietic microenvironment and heamatopoietic stem cells from single human bone marrow stem cells. Nature 1992; 360: 745–749.
17. Andrews RG, Bryant EM, Bartelmez SH, Muirhead DY, Knitter GH, Bensinger W, Strong DM, Bernstein ID. $CD34^+$ marrow cells, devoid of T and B lymphocytes, reconstitute stable lymphopoiesis and myelopoiesis in lethally irradiated allogeneic baboons. Blood 1992; 80: 1693–1701.
18. Link H, Boogaerts M, Fauser AA, Slavin S, Reiffers J, Gorin NC, Carella AM, Mandelli F, Burdach S, Ferrant A, Linkesch W, Tura S, Bacigalupo A, Schindel F, Heinrichs H. A controlled trial of recombinant human erythropoietin after bone marrow transplantation. Blood 1994; 84: 3327–3335.
19. Bensinger WI, Weaver CH, Appelbaum FR, Rowley S, Demirer T, Sanders J, Storb R, Buckner CD. Transplantation of allogeneic peripheral blood stem cells mobilized by recombinant human granulocyte colony stimulating factor. Blood 1995; 85: 1655–1658.
20. Körbling M, Przepiorka D, Van Besien K, Giralt S, Andersson B, Huh YO, Kleine HD, Seong D, Deisseroth AB, Andreeff M, Champlin R. Allogeneic blood stem cell transplantation for refractory leukemia and lymphoma: potential advantage of blood over marrow allografts. Blood 1995; 85: 1659–1665.
21. Schmitz N, Dreger P, Suttorp M, Rohwedder EB, Haferlach T, Löffler H, Hunter A, Russell NH, Primary transplantation of allogeneic peripheral blood progenitor cells mobilized by filgrastim (granulocyte colony stimulating factor). Blood 1995; 85: 1666–1672.

Acute Leukemias VI
Prognostic Factors
and Treatment Strategies
Büchner et al. (eds)

Quality of Life in Patients with Acute Myeloid Leukemia – A Longitudinal Study

A. Schumacher, T. Kessler, T. Büchner, and J. van de Loo

Abstract. In oncology, quality of life (QL) has become an essential criterion for evaluating the effects of therapy in clinical trials. So far, in adult patients suffering from acute leukemia assessment of QL has not been considered possible due to poor prognosis and the acute course of the disease. Advances in chemotheraphy significantly prolong survival of patients with acute myeloid leukemia (AML) and may cure a significant percentage (25%–30%) of patients. Therefore, the assessment of QL of patients undergoing chemotherapy is of growing interest. This study was designed to evaluate QL in patients with AML treated according to the protocol of the German AML Cooperative Group (Münster).

The dynamic concept of QL can change as an adaptational process interacting with life circumstances. The assessment of QL is usually achieved by an evaluation of specific components contributing to the QL construct. Based on conceptual, methodological, and practical criteria, the European Organization for Research on Treatment of Cancer (EORTC)-QLQ c30 questionnaire was used. Patients' individual perception of their disease and therapy was evaluated by a semi-structured interview. QL will be analysed during induction therapy and maintenance therapy over 3 years, evaluating defined specific parameters at 12 different time points. The questionnaire is administered in the first four courses of chemotherapy (double induction, consolidation, first cycle of maintenance therapy) during in-patient treatment, before and after drug-induced myeloid aplasia. Every 6 months during out-patient treatment, patients assess a set of mailed questionnaires up to the end of their treatment.

Currently, 74 patients are enrolled in the protocol. Those patients having completed the course of in-patient treatment are evaluated for changes in the conceptually distinct QL domains: physical functioning ($p=.000$) and emotional functioning ($p=.001$) improve significantly from beginning of chemotherapy to the end of in-patient treatment. Individual assessment of global health status and subjective QL ($p=.000$) improve significantly over the same time. Patients suffer significantly less from fatigue, nausea/emesis, and loss of appetite ($p=.000$). The content analysis of the interviews shows to what extent aspects of the in patient setting influence patients' QL. As clarified by the qualitative data, a substantial number of patients experience a secondary benefit from their disease. Although only a minority of patients with AML remain in continuous complete remission, the evaluation of QL in patients undergoing treatment shows that subjective benefit outweighs the adverse effects of anti-leukemic therapy.

Introduction

In hematology, quality of life (QL) has become an essential criterion for evaluating the effects of therapy in clinical trials. So far, in adult patients suffering from acute leukemia, assessment of QL has not been considered possible due to poor

University of Münster, Department of Internal Medicine A, 48129 Münster, Germany

prognosis and the acute course of the disease [1]. Advances in chemotherapy significantly prolong survival of patients with acute myeloid leukemia (AML) and may even cure a significant percentage (25%–30%) of patients [2]. Therefore, the assessment of QL of patients undergoing chemotherapy is of growing interest. This study was designed to evaluate QL in patients with AML treated according to the protocol of the German AML Cooperative Group in Münster

Table 1. EORTC-QLQ C30 subscales

Functional scales	Symptom scales
Physical functioning	Fatigue
Role functioning	Nausea and vomiting
Emotional functioning	Pain
Cognitive functioning	Dyspnea
Social functioning	Sleep disturbance
Global health status/ quality of life	Appetite loss
	Constipation
	Diarrhea
	Financial impact

Material and Methods

According to current standards [3,4] at least three domains should be included in order to evaluate QL: physical, psychological, and functional status. The dynamic concept of QL can change as an adaptational process interacting with life circumstances. The assessment of QL is usually achieved by an evaluation of specific components contributing to the QL construct. Based on conceptual, methodological, and practical criteria, we used the QL questionnaire developed by the European Organization for Research on Treatment of Cancer (EORTC): EORTC-QLQ C30 [5]. The EORTC QLQ-C30 is a 30-item questionnaire composed of multi-item scales and single items that reflect the multidimensionality of the QL construct (Table 1).

Quality of life will be analysed during induction therapy and maintenance therapy over 3 years, evaluating defined specific parameters at 12 different time points. The questionnaires are administered in the first four courses of chemotherapy (double induction, consolidation, first cycle of maintenance therapy) during in patient treatment, before and after drug-induced myeloid aplasia. Every 6 months during outpatient treatment, patients assess a set of mailed questionnaires up to the end of their treatment. Patients' individual perception of their disease and therapy is evaluated by a semi-structured interview during the first cycle of maintenance therapy (Fig. 1).

Results

Currently, 74 patients are enrolled in the protocol. Those patients having completed the course of in-patient treatment are evaluated for changes in the conceptually distinct QL domains: physical functioning (from 62.92 to 92.36, $p = .000$) and emotional functioning

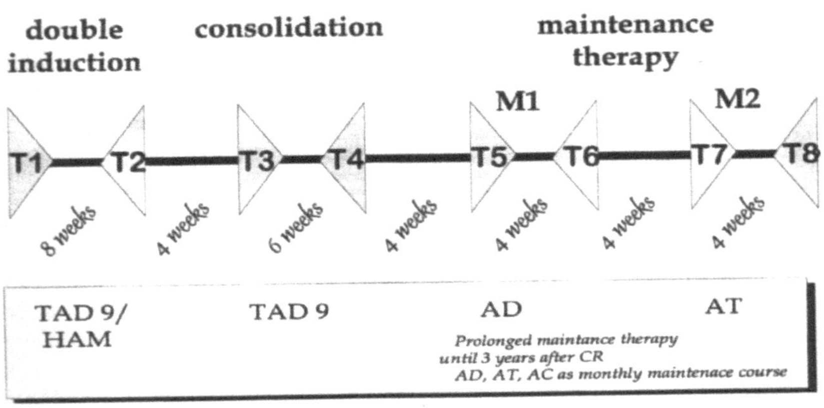

Fig. 1. Design of the study

(59.38 to 74.27, $p = .001$) significantly improve from the beginning of chemotherapy to the end of in-patient treatment (Fig. 2). This means that at the end of in-patient treatment, patients' physical fitness has improved and patients do not worry that much anymore. Individual assessment of global health status and subjective QL (Fig. 3) significantly improve over the same time (42.71 to 69.94, $p = .000$). The symptoms fatigue, nausea/emesis, and loss of appetite vary during the course of treatment (Fig. 4). Accordingly, patients suffer significantly less from fatigue (61.81 to 28.18, $p = .000$), nausea/ emesis (22.22 to 14.58, $p = .000$), and loss of appetite (45.14 to 18.75, $p = .000$) at the end of in-patient treatment.

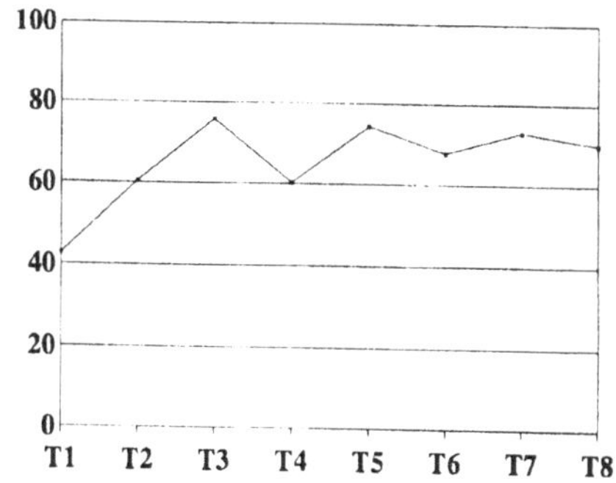

Fig. 3. EORTC-QLQ C30 subscale "Global health status/quality of life" ($n = 24$; $p = .000$) (a higher scale score representing a higher level of QL).

Discussion and Outlook

Although only a minority of patients with AML remain in continuous complete remission, the evaluation of QL in patients undergoing treat-

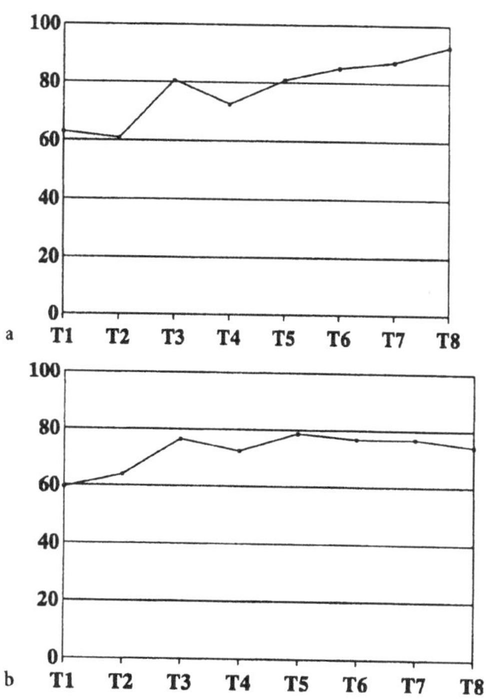

Fig. 2a,b. EORTC-QLQ-C30 subscales "physical functioning," "(**a**,$n = 24$; $p = .000$)" emotional functioning ("**b**, $n = 24$',$p = .001$) (a higher scale score representing a higher level of functioning)

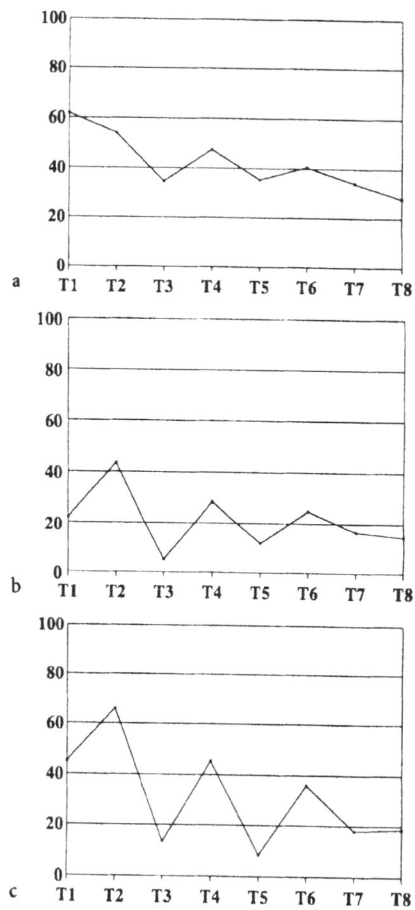

Fig. 4a–c. EORTC-QLQ C30 subscales "fatigue" (**a**, $n = 24$; $p = .000$) Nausea and vomiting "**b**)$n = 24$; $p = .001$)" Appetite loss (**c**, $n = 24$; $p = .000$) (a higher scale score representing a higher level of symptomatology)

ment shows that subjective benefit outweighs the adverse effects of antileukemic therapy. This seems to be somewhat unexpected since one would assume that treatment toxicity and poor prognosis would be associated with poor QL. However, for example, a number of studies with breast cancer patients [6–8] highlight the fact that patients set different priorities in defining their individual QL to what doctors and nurses would consider, e.g., they may trade more toxicity for a brief extension of life [9].

The interviews in our study underline these results and highlight the different aspects of patients' QL. The content analysis of data (spontaneous statements) shows to what extent patients rely on the emotional support they get, not only from their family but from nurses, medical staff, and psychologists as well. This is a very important factor contributing to patients QL during in-patient treatment (Fig. 5). Other aspects of the in-patient setting diminish patients' QL. Patients complain about the lack of entertainment facilities when staying in hospital for such a long time. Lack of privacy bothers quite a number of patients. The quality of hospital food is obviously one of the most important aspects of QL. At first glance, this may seem to be a minor fact. However, if one takes into account the fact that patients usually have only very reduced ways of experiencing the outside world, the sensual enjoyment of food intake plays a dominant role in their subjective well-being.

The analysis of the interviews reveals certain major factors influencing patients' psychosocial well-being. Undergoing treatment for such a long time makes it difficult for patients to cope with their disease. Of 23 patients, 78% find it hard to set up a daily routine at home as they frequently have to go back to hospital for several courses of in-patient therapy. During outpatient treatment, the monthly course of therapy means an interruption in their everyday routine like work, family and household tasks.

- Emotional support (51%) (+)
- Quality of hospital food (35%) (−)
- Boredom (13%) (−)
- Lack of privacy (18%) (−)

Fig. 5. Aspects of in-patient treatment setting contributing to patients' QL ($n = 23$)

"Leading a plain, ordinary life, back in my daily routine" is a highly desired aim for most patients. Uncertainty about long term remission is another threat to patients' psychosocial well-being (23%). Recurrent offers to talk about whatever seems vital to them can help patients adjust to their situation and can even encourage them to see positive changes in their life. We find some patients experience a kind of secondary benefit from their disease: many of them (65%) claim they get a different perspective on life, being ill makes them readjust their priorities, life has become more valuable to them and therefore they are able to enjoy it in a very intensive way.

Acute myeloid leukemia patients have to undergo treatment for a long period of time without ever being sure about long-term remission. To support these patients and help them cope with the uncertainity is a major challenge for all medical personnel.

References

1. Zittoun, R.: Quality of life in adults with acute leukemia. In: Aaronson, N.K. Beckmann, J. (eds.): The quality of life of cancer patients. Raven, New York 1987, 183–192.
2. Büchner, Th.: Acute leukemia. In: Adamson, J.W. (ed.) Current opinion in hematology. Current Science, Philadelphia 1993, 172–182.
3. Aaronson, N.K. Beckmann, J. (eds.): The quality of life of cancer patients. Raven, New York 1987.
4. Osaba, D.: Effect of Cancer on quality of life. CRC Press, Boca Raton 1991.
5. Aaronson, N.K. Ahmedzai, S. Bergman, B. et al.: The EORTC-QLQ-C30: A quality-of-life instrument for use in international clinical trials in oncology. J. natl. Cancer Inst. 1993, 85, 365–376.
6. Tannock, I.F., Boyd, N.F. De Boer, G. et al.: A randomised trial of two dose levels of cyclophosphamide, methotrexate and fluorouracil chemotherapy for patients with metastatic breast cancer. J. Clin. Oncol. 1988, 6, 1377–87.
7. Coates, A. Gebski, M. Bishop, J., et al.: Improving the quality of life during chemotherapy for advanced breast cancer. A comparison of intermittent and continous treatment strategies. N. Engl. J. Med. 1987, 317, 1480–95.
8. Richards, M.A., Hopwood, P. Ramirez A.J. Twelves C.J. et al.: Doxorubicin in advanced breast cancer: influence of schedule on response, survival and quality of life. Eur. J. Cancer 1992, 28A (12), 1731–40.
9. Slevin, M.L. Stubbs, L. Plant, H.J. et al.: Attitudes to chemotherapy: comparing views of patients with cancer with those of doctors, nurses and general public. B.M.J. 1990, 300, 1458–60.

Subject Index

Kolibri 360 GmbH
Ferdinand-Jühlke-Straße 7
99095 Erfurt, Deutschland
produktsicherheit@kolibri360.de